The AARP Guide to Pills

The AARP Guide to Pills

Essential Information on More Than 1,200 Prescription and Nonprescription Medications, Including Generics

EDITOR IN CHIEF

MaryAnne Hochadel, PharmD, BCPS

Gold Standard Publishers
Tampa, Florida, USA

GOLD
STANDARD
A Gold Standard Product
www.goldstandard.com

Produced by
StayWell®
A MediMedia USA Company
www.medimedia.com

Sterling Publishing Co., Inc.
New York

Patient education drug information is provided by Clinical Pharmacology, a product of Gold Standard, leading developers of drug information databases, software, and clinical information solutions. www.goldstandard.com

AARP Books publishes a wide range of titles on health, personal finance, lifestyle, and other subjects to enrich the lives of older Americans. For more information, go to www.aarp.org/books. AARP, established in 1958, is a nonprofit organization with more than 35 million members age 50 or older. The AARP name and logo are registered trademarks of AARP, used under license to Sterling Publishing Co., Inc.

The AARP Guide to Pills is designed to provide you with information about commonly prescribed drugs—and a few common over-the-counter medications—for your personal information and to help you become a better-informed, more active health care consumer. The book is not intended to be exhaustive, nor does it substitute for the advice of your prescriber or pharmacist. The science of pharmacology is continually advancing and expanding. Therefore, it is recommended that the reader always check product information inserts for changes in dosage or administration before taking any medication. This is particularly important with new or rarely used drugs. Whereas every attempt has been made to check the content for accuracy, all information is presented without guarantees by the publishers and consultants, who disclaim all liability in connection with its use.

Library of Congress Cataloging-in-Publication Data

The AARP guide to pills : essential information on more than 1,200 prescription and
    nonprescription medicines, including generics / edited by Maryanne Hochadel ; foreword
  by Jerry Avorn ; introduction by Bill Thomas.
      p. cm.
    ISBN 1-4027-4446-3
      1. Drugs—Handbooks, manuals, etc. 2. Drugs—Popular works. I. Hochadel, Maryanne.
  II. AARP (Organization)

  RM301.12.A22 2005
  615'.1—dc22

  10 9 8 7 6 5 4 3 2 1   2005054444

Published by Sterling Publishing Co., Inc.
387 Park Avenue South, New York, NY 10016
Distributed in Canada by Sterling Publishing
c/o Canadian Manda Group, 165 Dufferin Street
Toronto, Ontario, Canada M6K 3H6
Distributed in Great Britain by Chrysalis Books Group PLC
The Chrysalis Building, Bramley Road, London W10 6SP, England
Distributed in Australia by Capricorn Link (Australia) Pty. Ltd.
P.O. Box 704, Windsor, NSW 2756, Australia

Printed in China

Sterling ISBN 1-4027-4446-3

For information about custom editions, special sales, premium and corporate purchases, please contact Sterling Special Sales Department at 800-805-5489 or specialsales@sterlingpub.com.

Contents

Contents

Editorial Board—Gold Standard

Editorial Review Board—*The AARP Guide to Pills*

AARP Reviewers

Preface

Medications and Older Americans

Jerry Avorn, MD

Prescription drugs can be a medical paradox for older Americans. They are one of the most effective ways we have to restore health and prevent disability, but they are also a major cause of unintended illness. Prescribed and used well, they can be one of the best bargains in medical care. Yet prescription drugs also represent the fastest-rising component of health care costs—and they impose a heavy financial burden on many patients.

Each year, on all these fronts, the ante grows higher. New drugs are introduced that are more effective than anything our parents could have dreamed of. At the same time, they are far more costly—and they carry the risk of side effects unknown even a decade ago.

These trends will only intensify in the coming years, making it increasingly important that patients become active participants with their doctors and other health care professionals in making these crucial medical choices. That kind of teamwork is necessary to craft a regimen of prescription drugs that can bring the greatest benefit at the lowest possible risk—and cost.

MAXIMIZING THE BENEFITS

Debate over the Medicare drug-benefit legislation passed in 2003 prompted many people to ask this question: Why didn't the original Medicare plan cover prescriptions filled outside hospitals when it was designed in the mid-1960s?

The answer reveals how dramatically our use of medications has changed in the last 40 years. Controversy reigned in 1965 over whether it was helpful (or even safe) to lower blood pressure in people with mild to moderate elevations. Medical experts of the time argued whether it was worth measuring cholesterol levels, much less trying to control them with drugs. Depression, a stigmatized condition, was either ignored, or treated with a handful of inexpensive drugs. Lacking any real means to deal with the bone thinning caused by osteoporosis, physi-

cians rarely made that diagnosis—and even more infrequently attempted to manage it.

Most of the prescriptions doctors wrote in those days were designed to treat specific diseases. They prescribed antibiotics for infections, morphine-derived analgesics for pain, insulin for diabetes. The concept of medicines intended to "manage risk factors" was largely unknown.

All that has changed, of course, in the four decades since the enactment of original Medicare. Large clinical trials proved that controlling even modest elevations of blood pressure could prevent strokes and heart ailments or kidney disease; that lowering cholesterol could reduce the risk of heart attack; and that taking an anticoagulant could sharply lower the likelihood of a devastating stroke in patients with the heart-rhythm abnormality known as atrial fibrillation.

Oddly enough, older people were omitted from the studies that led to many of these important discoveries. People age 65 and older make up only 14 percent of the U.S. population, but they consume over a third of all prescriptions. Despite this population's disproportionate role, older Americans have often been underrepresented in crucial clinical trials of drugs. Because of this, debate raged for years about the wisdom of treating many chronic conditions in patients in their 70s and beyond. Several more years passed before studies focusing on such patients made it clear that they too could benefit from preventive treatments.

Once that was done, the contents of Americans' medicine cabinets changed forever. Today it no longer suffices to treat acute medical problems. Many patients now take a host of pills to control ongoing "risk factors" such as blood pressure, cholesterol, or thin bones. These problems may not cause symptoms in their own right, but they do increase the chances that a major problem—stroke, heart disease, fracture—will occur in the future. True, each new pill may confer some protection. Yet each also adds its own expense—often substantial—as well as the potential for side effects. The risk/benefit/cost equation has become much more complex, and that complexity deepens as we age.

CONTROLLING THE RISKS

As we get older, we become more vulnerable to the side effects of medication. With each passing decade, even if we remain in good health, our bodies grow slightly less able to process drugs. For example, the kidneys are a major way we clear drugs from our system. But even in the absence of any medical problems, we lose about one-third of kidney function between age 20 and age 90. The liver, our primary organ for breaking down and inactivating drugs, also becomes somewhat less robust with the passage of time. And our tissues—brain, heart, lungs, and other organs—don't always react to drugs the same way they did when we were in our 20s.

Does this mean that drugs are inherently dangerous in older patients? Far from it. It simply means that they must be used with greater care by doctor and patient alike. The "correct" dose determined in studies of young and middle-aged people may not be the right one for older consumers. Yet the clinical trials on which drug approvals are based often do not include large enough numbers of truly old subjects—and that can cause problems once those drugs are marketed and used heavily by precisely that type of patient.

Most medication side effects do not appear overnight. Instead, they are often preceded by certain warning signals, which patients and doctors can use to detect and defuse a problem before it looms out of control. One rule of thumb I teach medical students is this: "Any new symptom in an older patient should be evaluated to see if it's a drug side effect." The reason is simple: Of all the clinical problems that physicians encounter in this age group, drug-induced illness is one of the "best" to treat; once the correct diagnosis is made and the offending medicine is stopped or reduced in dose, the difficulties it has been causing may disappear completely within days. If only all conditions were that easy to fix!

In 2004 Vioxx, one of the most commonly prescribed painkillers, was abruptly with-drawn from the market after it was established that it doubles the risk of heart attack and stroke. By then, the drug had been widely used for more than five years by tens of millions of patients. The incident triggered concern that the drug industry and the U.S. Food and Drug Administration (FDA) appeared unable to detect important side effects even for drugs that had been in widespread use for years.

Since then, a number of methods have been proposed for improving the FDA's capacity to uncover side effects sooner, and much work is still needed in this area. In the end, however, the safest course for any patient is to inform his or her doctor if a new problem arises while taking any drug. It may or may not be related to the medicine—but only a conversation with a health care professional can begin to sort that out.

One major obstacle to identifying drug-related problems is known as "ageism." In health care, ageism sometimes rears its head as the mistaken belief that symptoms that develop in people over age 60 must be the result of "just getting old." That kind of sloppy thinking can derail the thoughtful evaluation of a new problem—an evaluation that might have found the problem to be a treatment side effect, or perhaps a new disease requiring a new prescription.

Many doctors have heard a colleague describe a patient this way: "She has low energy, some confusion, and shortness of breath. But what do you expect? She's 79." In teaching medical students to avoid this kind of bias, I suggest that they substitute their own age in such a description: "The patient is forgetful, incontinent, and has aches in all his joints. But what do you expect? He's 23." If that sentence makes no sense, I tell them, neither should the other. At any age, the search for the origin of each symptom must be a careful one. If the problem is caused by a drug side effect, we may have a chance to relieve it entirely. If a new diagnosis is made, we may be able to treat that as well.

Doctors aren't the only ones guilty of age-related stereotyping. Sometimes it's the patient who thinks, "I won't bother the doctor with that new symptom; it's probably just my age." That's never a safe assumption; let the doctor know about it so he or she can evaluate the problem and decide. Most important, make sure your doctor knows about all the medicines you're taking—including those bought over the counter, as well as nontraditional treatments such as dietary supplements and herbal remedies. (Unfortunately, the latter are so poorly regulated that consumers have no way of knowing whether these products are effective, or even safe. Many nonprescription remedies may even interfere with the prescription medicines a doctor has prescribed.)

MANAGING YOUR MEDICINES

Even with Medicare drug coverage starting in 2006, deductibles and co-payments can turn a drugstore bill into a humbling experience. Some of the burden may be lifted at the doctor's office, where you should not hesitate to ask whether a generic drug is available that will work as well as a costlier brand-name product.

Generics must pass the same FDA standards of manufacturing excellence that brand-name drugs do, and they can provide the same clinical benefit, often at a fraction of the cost. Generic drugs are available to manage most (but not all) of the conditions for which costlier brand-name products are commonly prescribed. Here, too, a knowledgeable patient is the best catalyst for starting the conversation with the doctor. Many physicians may not be in the habit of prescribing a generic initially, but most will do so if asked. It's far better to have a conversation about costs before a prescription is written than to suffer sticker shock at the drugstore when asked to pay $100 or more for a 30-day supply of pills.

Even the most conscientious doctor has a hard time trying to compare drugs that are chemically different from one another. This is partly because the sole hurdle related to effectiveness that the FDA often requires a drug to clear on its way to market is for its manufacturer to document that its product is better—sometimes only a little bit better—than a placebo or sugar pill. But since the day I started practice more than 30 years ago, I've never once had a patient come into my office and say, "Dr. Avorn, I'd like you to write me a prescription for a pill that's a little bit better than nothing." What patients want—and what we doctors want to prescribe—are medications that are clearly improvements over the alternatives we could have used.

Unfortunately, that testing is usually not required. Drug companies are generally reluctant to perform such head-to-head comparisons, perhaps because many newly introduced products do not confer clinically significant improvements over what's already out there. So by all means ask your doctor which of several competing products is stronger, or safer, or more cost-effective than the others in its class. Just don't be surprised if the answer is, "It's hard to tell." Get the best answer you can, then ask your Congressperson why we don't have a more consumer-friendly system of drug evaluation. A growing number of consumer-friendly websites have been developed to help patients search out such information on their own (see page xxi).

In talking to your doctor, also make sure you understand the purpose of every single drug you're using, as well as how you should take it and which potential side effects you should watch out for. Don't hesitate to bring a list of written questions into the exam room, or to write down the answers you get. An informed patient is one of the best ways to ensure that prescription drugs will be used safely and appropriately.

DRUGS VS. LIFESTYLE

The success of modern pharmacology, combined with the drug companies' seemingly infinite marketing resources, has engendered an unhealthy side effect of its own: the notion that "there's a pill for every ill." At a time when critics caution us not to "medicalize" everything from normal grief reactions to our high-calorie, low-activity lifestyles, it's tempting to believe that pharmaceutical manufacturers can provide a chemical solution to every one of life's problems.

The truth is far different.

Especially for drugs meant to make people more relaxed (or more happy, docile, sleepy, peppy, or the like), it's useful to ask some hard questions first: Are we treating an actual underlying disease? Or are we simply resorting to a chemical shortcut in order to gloss over a meaningful and potentially addressable life problem?

In a book about medications, it's all too easy to overlook the many important nondrug ways we can take control of our medical conditions. Yes, modern science has devised a panoply of effective medications, and these are described in detail in the pages that follow. At the same time, however, it's essential to bear in mind that our everyday choices have crucial effects on many aspects of our health. By cutting down the salt in our diet and losing weight, we can lower our blood pressure. By upping our exercise and limiting our intake of saturated fats, we can reduce our cholesterol count. Consuming less caffeine and embracing a more active lifestyle may avert insomnia. And it's crucial to remember that the side effects that sicken and kill the greatest number of older Americans arise from two drugs that doctors don't prescribe: tobacco and (in excessive amounts) alcohol.

For medications to work optimally, we must learn to use them wisely. Yet we also need to prescribe ourselves all those commonsense, healthy-lifestyle practices our grandparents urged upon us. That approach to life, melded with a drug regimen that is well-conceived and carefully managed by clinician and patient working together, can give us the chance to lead lives that are longer and healthier than any previous generation could have hoped for.

The Wise Use of Prescription Drugs
William H. Thomas, MD

A few years ago, I was delighted to have a bright, eager medical student join my practice for a month-long clerkship. As a first step, I arranged for him to interview one of my favorite patients—lively, opinionated Mrs. M. She was 102 years old at the time.

To my surprise, the med student returned from his visit with Mrs. M looking dejected. After some prodding, he confessed that he thought I was not providing quality care for my patient.

Before speaking to Mrs. M, he had reviewed her medical chart. Not surprisingly, he found a lengthy list of diagnoses there. The "Doctor's Orders" section, however, appalled him. It listed but a single medication: "Tylenol, 325 milligrams—two tablets by mouth as needed for pain and fever."

As we talked, he pointed out, rightly, that medical studies supported the use of many different medications in Mrs. M's case. He let me know he thought I should have prescribed all of these drugs in her case.

I heard him out, then asked him to itemize the medications he thought Mrs. M should be taking. The next day, he handed me a laundry list of 17 different medicines. Although the med student had backed up every suggestion with published research articles, his recommended course of treatment would have constituted a death sentence for Mrs. M.

The medical student was confusing care with treatment. We all want—indeed, we all deserve—the maximum amount of care we can get. Medical treatment, on the other hand, is fraught with risk, cost, and uncertainty. That often makes the pursuit of maximum treat-ment a peril. When it comes to prescription drugs, in particular, rarely is the maximum the optimum.

This is especially true for older patients. Geriatricians (doctors who specialize in the care of older people) have long understood that the aging process has a profound effect on how medications are metabolized—that is, how they are absorbed and broken down in the human body. Recognizing this, the best doctors "start low and go slow" when prescribing for older patients. Frequently that means beginning with a dose lower than the one they would prescribe to a younger patient. Changes are then made cautiously, with the dosage increased only if necessary—and only in consultation with the patient.

As a physician caring for residents of nursing homes, I regularly see patients who are among the oldest and frailest in America. These men and women have taught me that prescription drugs can harm just as easily as they can heal. Used foolishly or thoughtlessly, medications can even kill.

Now that prescription drugs have become a linchpin of quality health care in the United States, how can we derive the biggest benefits from them while incurring the fewest risks? One way is to embrace the "wise use" of prescription drugs. Those who adopt the wise use philosophy are eager to ask questions, especially of their doctors. They are willing to search in books such as this one and on the internet for the information they need to make good decisions. They are prepared to view direct-to-consumer advertisements (such as those on television urging you to "ask your doctor about" a certain drug) with a healthy dose of skepticism.

Does all that sound complicated? It needn't be. In fact, the tenets of wise use can be boiled down to three big ideas, detailed below, that should be kept in mind by every savvy consumer of prescription drugs.

PAY CHEVROLET PRICES FOR CADILLAC DRUGS

To reward risk-taking and innovation, the U.S. Patent and Trademark Office grants the makers of new medications a patent that lasts 20 years from the date of first filing. Because a patent is typically obtained early in a drug's development, however, the actual market exclusivity after the drug receives approval can be much shorter. The drug manufacturer may then apply to the US Food and Drug Administration

(FDA) for a patent term extension. Total market exclusivity time cannot exceed 14 years, a period established by the Hatch-Waxman Act, a public law enacted in 1984. As long as the patent term extension remains in force, no other company may manufacture or market that medication. This makes the market exclusivity phase of a drug's development highly profitable for the manufacturer.

Once that exclusivity expires, however, other companies gain the right to make and sell generic versions of the once-exclusive brand-name product—so long as their products meet federal standards. The FDA guarantees that every substitutable generic medication is as safe and effective as its brand-name equivalent. "The standards for quality are the same for brand-name and generic products," says Gary Buehler, director of the FDA's Office of Generic Drugs. (To read a copy of the FDA report "Generic Drugs: What Everyone Should Know," visit www.fda.gov/cder/consumerinfo/ generic-what_everyone_should_know.htm.)

With generic drugs equal in quality to their brand-name cousins, switching to generics can be a very wise—and thrifty—thing to do. In 2004, generic drug costs averaged less than 30 percent of brand-name drug costs.

Because medicines sold under patent are legally protected from price competition, their makers can charge whatever price for them the market will bear. A June 2004 AARP study of 197 brand-name drugs commonly used by those over 50 found that from 2000 to 2003 the manufacturer had raised the price of all but four of the drugs at an average annual rate exceeding inflation. By contrast, an October 2004 AARP study of 75 generic drugs also popular among older adults found that more than half of the drugs had remained constant or dropped in price from 2001 to 2003.

Price disparities show up in nonprescription medications as well. At my local pharmacy, the 325-milligram strength of Bayer aspirin sells for 12 cents a pill. Next to the Bayer sits a bottle of no-name aspirin. The unbranded version is just as effective, yet it costs barely a penny a pill, making it 10 times cheaper.

Generics differ in size, shape, and color from brand-name medications because federal law bars makers of the former from copying the physical attributes of the latter. Do these cosmetic divergences matter once you swallow the pill? Not in the least. Consumers committed to the wise use of prescription drugs resist equating appearance with efficacy.

As many patients taking a maintenance (long-term) dose of a generic drug have observed, the appearance of their pills may change from one prescription renewal to the next. This is not necessarily cause for concern. On the contrary, it may be an encouraging sign of resourcefulness on the part of your pharmacist: It means that she or he is constantly shopping around for the lowest-cost generic version available.

Regrettably—and, one hopes, exceedingly seldom—a change in pill appearance may mean you've been given the wrong medicine. If you suspect this is the case, before you leave the pharmacy counter, ask to check a reference book that shows both a color photograph and the imprint code of the medicine that was supposed to have been dispensed to you.

By understanding the value, economy, and safety of generics, you will have taken the first step on the road to the wise use of prescription drugs. Switching to available generics can also confer that uniquely American thrill: buying Cadillac drugs at Chevrolet prices.

RELY ON OLD RELIABLE

We live in a world where "new" frequently connotes "better." New cars are expected to perform better than older ones. New computer models are invariably cheaper and faster. In an environment that celebrates novelty, it is natural to assume that the latest medications are superior to those already on the market.

When it comes to prescription drugs, however, it's best to question the embrace of the new. A proven medicine can be a surprisingly smart choice. First, established drugs are tried and true. Doctors and patients may have years (as opposed to months) of experience with a medication that has been on the market for some time. When they open their morning papers, they are unlikely to learn that a long-established medication has been recalled. Second, an "old reliable" drug frequently costs much less than a competing newcomer; the patent on the original medicine has often run out, permitting it to be marketed as a generic. Third, certain older medications have been shown to work just as well as their late-model cousins. In the case of drugs designed to treat high blood pressure, to cite just one example, a study published in the *British Medical Journal* in 1997 found "no evidence of superiority for the 'new' classes of antihypertensive drugs (calcium-channel blockers and ACE inhibitors) over beta-blockers and diuretics."

Older people have plenty of reason to cast a skeptical eye on new and relatively untested medications. When a drug company wishes to get a new product approved, it tests the drug primarily on younger people. Thus a good deal of time is required *after* a drug is first brought to market to determine how the medicine will react inside the bodies of older people. Uncertainties about long-term side effects likewise take a considerable length of time to resolve.

It is the FDA's responsibility to make sure that no new medicine is approved for use until it has been proved safe and effective. Given the demands placed on the agency, the system is far from flawless. Certain drugs have been found to be of such high risk that they were abruptly withdrawn from the market, even after several years of use by the general public.

Attempting to gauge the scope of the problem, the *Journal of the American Medical Association* reported that 10 percent of all drugs approved from 1975 to 1999 had later been relabeled with a warning about a serious side effect—or had been removed from sale altogether for safety reasons.

In 2004, this dynamic precipitated the widely publicized withdrawal of the pain reliever Vioxx. During the seven years in which Vioxx was available to doctors and their patients, it was heralded for easing the anguish of millions of arthritis sufferers. Far less known was a persistent concern of researchers: that Vioxx increased the risk of heart attack and stroke among people who used it regularly.

A study conducted by the Vioxx manufacturer itself—part of an effort to have the drug approved as a treatment for colon polyps—confirmed that patients taking Vioxx suffered nearly twice as many heart attacks and strokes as those receiving a placebo. In the fall of 2004, the company therefore voluntarily withdrew Vioxx from the market. Most members of the public had no inkling of the drug's dangers until it was suddenly withdrawn.

The reason new drugs garner so much attention is because, at least in the United States, millions of dollars are often spent to promote them, not because they have bested their older rivals in clinical trials. Can you think of a bigger fool than the patient who consistently transfers his medical records to the youngest, least experienced surgeon he can find? In health care, experience counts. In prescription medicines, new is not always better.

SIMPLE IS SUPERIOR

Common sense tells us that too much of a good thing can readily become a bad thing. Older people in particular run risks when they take more than a handful of daily medications. Wayne Anderson, dean of the State University of New York's School of Pharmacy, has shown that patients who take six different drugs have an 80 percent chance of at least one drug-drug interaction. These complications can range from merely vexatious to downright lethal.

People with multiple medical conditions often must resort to a complex medical regimen that elevates their risk of experiencing drug interactions. According to the Institute of Medicine, medication errors caused an estimated 7,000 deaths in the United States in 1993. That's about 16 percent more deaths than result each year from on-the-job injuries nationwide. In 1997, the *Journal of the American Medical Association* reported that more than 770,000 hospital patients in the United States experience an "adverse drug effect" each year.

For these reasons, a third central precept of the wise-use strategy is to shun complexity. Although complicated drug combinations are necessary sometimes, they are almost always freighted with risk. The vast majority of older patients would be best served by some streamlining of their medical regimens.

This message warrants exploration here because you are unlikely to encounter it in the media. Newspapers, magazines, radio and television stations, and websites are more apt to tout the benefits of drugs designed to treat a "condition" you might not even know you have.

Pandemic advertising of this kind has contributed to "poly-pharmacy"—the regular use of multiple medicines at the same time—which can increase the health risk of millions of Americans. Not only can polypharmacy be dangerous, it is massively expensive. The unwise use of prescription drugs adds billions of dollars of unnecessary costs to our health care system each year.

As we age, polypharmacy is likely to become more common. Fortunately, health care professionals can help manage polypharmacy in a way that minimizes potential drug-related problems. Your own treatment plan may begin the day you start to follow the three big ideas outlined above. Next, consider making a few of the six smart moves detailed below. Finally and throughout, be prepared to work closely with both your doctor and your pharmacist to craft an approach to your health and medicine that makes the wisest possible use of prescription drugs.

Six Smart Moves

What can you do *right now* to raise your "Rx IQ"? Here are six simple but powerful suggestions.

Ask the Right Questions

Anyone who has coached an elementary school student through a homework assignment knows the drill: Confronted with an unfamiliar word, the young scholar asks you to define it. You can both predict your response: "Look it up!"

That was good advice then, and it is good advice now. In fact, you hold in your hands the means to enact it. To get started, read this book's entry for each medication you are currently taking. Mark the relevant passages; even doctors have to work hard to stay informed about the details of prescription drugs.

The AARP Guide to Pills will probably serve you best if it is close at hand whenever a question occurs to you. In fact, the entries that make up the bulk of the book are presented in the form of answers to eight commonsense questions about the wise use of each medication described. All eight questions appear in every drug entry; each is explained in detail below.

"What is this medicine?"

Below this question you will find both the generic name and the brand-name(s) of the drug being profiled, as well as an explanation of the purpose for which the drug is normally prescribed. This section of the book typically discusses why a drug may be preferred in certain instances. It may also include information about other generic forms of the drug.

"What should my health care professional know before I take this medicine?"

The answer to this question usually takes the form of a list of certain diseases and medical conditions, allergies, and personal behaviors (such as alcohol consumption or tobacco use) that, to ensure safe use, should be revealed to your physician before you take the prescribed medication.

"How should I take this medicine?"

A chasm often separates the way patients are *supposed* to take their pills and the way they *actually* take them. The dosage advice on a medication label—notably the medicine's recommended schedule and amount—is meant to help you get the most out of every pill you take. It is also intended to minimize the risk of side effects.

"What if I miss a dose?"

Everyone misses the occasional medication dose. If that happens to you, it's best to know beforehand how to remedy the lapse in the case of each medicine you take.

Basically, you have three options:

1. Take the missed medication immediately upon discovering the   oversight;

2. Wait for your next scheduled dose; or

3. Double your next scheduled dose.

The correct choice hinges on the individual medicine itself, so the old counsel prevails: "Look it up!"

"What may interact with this medicine?"

Modern medicine is constantly striving to learn more about the ways in which medications interact with substances—including other drugs—inside the human body. The odds are high that you could eventually take something that interferes with the proper functioning of one of your own medicines. But you can reduce that likelihood. Use the book's answers to this question to inform yourself how each of the drugs you take might react to special foods, beverages, over-the-counter (OTC) medicines, nutritional supplements, herbal products, or another, recently prescribed medication. Also, for detailed information on interactions, see page xli.

Pay special attention to any advice the label or its accompanying leaflet offers about foods or beverages to avoid when taking the medication. People who take calcium-channel blockers, for example, should avoid drinking more than one glass of grapefruit juice per day. Why? Because certain compounds found in grapefruit juice can triple the level of calcium-channel blockers circulating in the bloodstream. The net effect, equivalent to taking three pills rather than one, can result in headaches, flushing, and light-headedness. Although that's just one instance, it's fair to extrapolate from its particulars to a general truth: All prescription drugs are powerful—so it pays to know how they interact with the food and beverages you enjoy.

"What should I watch for while taking this medicine?"

Right after "Physician, heal thyself!", most practitioners' favorite adage seems to be this old saw: "The doctor who treats himself has a fool for a patient." Even so, many drug consumers opt to treat themselves—and in so doing they too take on a fool for a patient. An experienced, knowledgeable physician or pharmacist can help you understand how certain medications may mask symptoms or interfere with diagnostic test results.

In the final analysis, however, no one knows your body as well as you do. One of the best ways to protect your health is therefore to remain alert to changes in how you feel. If you notice any difference, don't hesitate to seek advice from the people who know these drugs best.

"What side effects may I notice from taking this medicine?"

The primary reason consumers cite for buying and using a pill guide is that it helps them track the potentially dangerous side effects of the medications they are taking. It's no surprise that they would look to other sources. Some of the tiniest lettering ever set in type appears on the "package inserts" that may accompany prescription or OTC medications, as well as in the printed medication-information handout the pharmacy generates for consumers. Neither one of these materials consistently meets its stated purpose—to educate consumers.

If you do nothing more with this book than study and learn the side-effect profile of the drugs you and the people you care about are taking, its purchase will have been well worth the price. What are the most common and significant side effects of the pills on your shelf? If you can't answer that question off the top of your head, look up the information in these pages.

You should also keep nearby any pharmacy-printed handouts that come with your medicines. For certain medications, such as non-steroidal anti-inflammatory prescription drugs, the FDA requires that you be given an FDA-approved "Medication Guide" leaflet as well (see page xxxvii).

"Where can I keep my medicine?"

The improper storage of prescription drugs can undermine their effectiveness. Whereas medications are customarily best stored in a place that is cool and dry, most consumers keep them in a place almost guaranteed to be warm and moist—the bathroom medicine cabinet. Consider storing them in a kitchen cabinet instead. *The AARP Guide to Pills* will also help you take steps to keep your medications off-limits to at-risk populations, such as children, thus avoiding accidental overdose.

Outdated medications are now considered a form of medical waste, so devote some care to disposing of them properly. In the past, people were often advised to flush expired medicines down the toilet. That counsel might have been acceptable in the days before researchers began finding traces of prescription drugs in community water supplies, but no more. So far the amounts have been tiny, but the consequences of higher concentrations could be huge. So don't flush those old drugs. Instead, take them to a pharmacy that accepts returns of outdated drugs (most do).

Make a List—and Check It Twice

When we were young, most of us dreaded the prospect that some adolescent prank would become engraved in our "permanent record." The notion that official records were up to date and accurate was, and often still is, accepted without question. I wish I could assure you that your medical records are always precise and always current. The truth is that they may contain errors—some of which could have serious consequences if not caught and corrected in time.

When my daughter was hospitalized as a child, for example, the attending physician accidentally moved a decimal point when ordering Klonopin, one of her antiseizure medications (she has Otahara's syndrome). Unfortunately, no one caught the error before the drug was administered. As a result, she received 10 times the recommended dose and wound up sleeping continuously for nearly 24 hours. The moral of the story: Even talented doctors working in prestigious hospitals can make mistakes. It pays to be vigilant.

Patients, too, are complicit in the chaos. They have a hard time recalling the details of their treatment precisely, completely, and consistently. No surprise there: Many older people take multiple medications, have multiple chronic conditions, and see multiple specialists.

If you too struggle to keep track of all your medications, important lab results, and medical procedures, start writing things down. Keeping good records is no longer exclusively the doctor's responsibility.

This exercise need not be tedious or time-consuming. A personal health record will serve you best, however, if you update it regularly. Make a habit of writing in your health log and you'll never again have to rummage through records stashed in shoeboxes.

There is no single correct way to record your health information. Some people keep their own personal health record with a notebook and a pen. (I'm partial to those speckled composition notebooks myself.) Others use one of the growing number of software programs that simplify record-keeping. The website www.myphr.com offers a range of options for people interested in maintaining a personal health record. Bookstores stock journals specially designed for this kind of record-keeping; you may want to browse their offerings before making a decision. Increasingly aware of the value of personal health records, doctors' offices sometimes provide free booklets that can be used for this purpose.

The essential details to record fall into three categories:

CONTACT INFORMATION

- Your address and phone number(s), plus those of a close friend or relative.
- Names, addresses, and contact information for all the doctors and pharmacies (including the online variety) that you visit on a regular basis.
- The name of the hospital you prefer.
- Key health-insurance information.
- Information about your living will or health-care proxy.

MEDICATION LIST

List all your prescribed medications, the reason they were prescribed, and the doctors who prescribed them. Include the start and stop dates of each prescription and its dosage. Any regularly consumed vitamins, herbal remedies, dietary supplements, or OTC medicines should also be itemized here. Readers interested in exploring this in greater detail may be interested in the AARP online course "Medicines and You," which can be found at www.aarp.org.

HEALTH CONDITIONS

This section should list any major medical concerns you have at present—arthritis, osteoporosis, high blood pressure, and the like. Also include any hospitalizations, noting their cause and duration. Pertinent facts from your family medical history deserve mention here as well.

People who have not kept careful health records are sometimes overwhelmed by the idea of gathering scattered information from the past. Don't worry—it's never too late to start. Because this is *your* record, you can begin it with an assessment of your current condition. Record the date and reason for your next doctor visit. Put your health record in an easy-to-reach place and add to it whenever you revisit the doctor, have a test done, or get a prescription filled. As you gradually fill in the details you need, your journal will take shape. This is a "permanent record" you can be proud of and rely on. It will prove its worth every time you come in contact with the health care system.

Follow the "Seven-Year Rule"

According to Dr. Sidney Wolfe, who directs the health-watchdog organization Public Citizen Health Research Group in Washington, DC, "Most troublesome drugs do not represent any advance in treatment and are at best no better than older, safer drugs already on the market." In 2002, Wolfe's group published guidelines urging older patients to adopt what it calls the "Seven-Year Rule" (see www.citizen.org/hrg). Many specialists in the field of geriatrics agree that older consumers should wait at least seven years from the release date of a new prescription drug before they use it—unless, of course, it is one of those rare "breakthrough" drugs such as Amevive (used to treat psoriasis) or Epogen (a treatment for certain kinds of anemia) that offer a clear therapeutic advantage over older, proven drugs.

Fill a Pill Caddy

I like the sporty sound of the phrase "pill caddy," the term most often used to describe that little plastic box with seven separate medication compartments, one for each day of the week. This handy device is also referred to as a pill organizer, pill holder, pill box, pill dispenser, or pill carrier. Most pill caddies are simple models that can be purchased from your local drugstore for less than five dollars. Others are more elaborate and expensive affairs.

A pill caddy caters to those committed to the wise use of prescription drugs. The individual receptacles provide convenient visual reminders of whether you have taken your medication dose for the day. Used properly, these devices can help prevent inadvertent double dosing. If you are among the many people who benefit from a little prompting to take your medicine on time, certain pill caddies feature built-in timers and buzzers. These devices are evolving rapidly; ask your pharmacist about new products of this type.

Buy Two for the Price of One

Strange to say, you can sometimes buy twice as much medicine without paying a penny more.

According to my local pharmacist, for example, 50 milligrams of Zoloft sells for an average price of $2.87 per pill. Yet double that dose of Zoloft—100 milligrams—costs the identical price, $2.87 per pill. People whose doctors have prescribed them 50 milligrams of Zoloft a day can therefore buy the 100-milligram tablets and break them in half with a pill splitter, cutting their monthly cost for the medication by $43.05.

In another hypothetical but fact-based case, imagine that you are taking 10 milligrams of Lipitor a day. A perfectly acceptable strategy would be to buy the 20-milligram strength of Lipitor and split each pill in half, saving $1.87 a dose. That's a discount of 28 percent—and a monthly savings of $56.10.

Before you explore the money-saving potential of pill splitting, however, ask your doctor or pharmacist if the practice is safe for the medication you have in mind. Some medicines are unsuited to the tactic; they may have special coatings, for example, designed to make the medicine they contain easy on the stomach or extra long-acting.

For an in-depth discussion of additional price-paring tactics, including the benefits and pitfalls of pill splitting, see "Managing Your Prescription Drug Costs" on page xix.

Brown Bag It

Taking a comprehensive look at an individual's medication use is often nicknamed a "brown bag evaluation." That's because participants are asked to prepare for the session by filling a lunch or grocery bag with all the prescription bottles, OTC medicines, creams, ointments, herbal remedies, and vitamins that they use. Then, during a sit-down meeting with their doctor or pharmacist, the bag is emptied and every item is carefully examined for its appropriateness to current medical conditions, its potential drug-drug interactions, and its side effects. Outdated medications are identified and properly disposed of.

When such a session is combined with a complete review of your medical history, potentially beneficial changes to your drug regimen can be suggested (and relayed to your physician, if a pharmacist conducts the review). The outcome is a new confidence that you are taking the right medications—and at the right doses—for the right reasons. (Better still, such confabs often yield ideas for how you can save money on drugs.)

If the notion of brown bagging your medications appeals to you, how should you proceed? The quickest route may lead to your corner drugstore. Some community pharmacists perform a limited number of brown-bag evaluations for their customers free of charge. Others have developed these medication management sessions into a thriving side business, charging $50 to $100 per session. Before you schedule a brown-bag session with your pharmacist, ask if he or she has special training in this area. The American Society of Consultant Pharmacists maintains a website (www.seniorcarepharmacist. com) that helps people find qualified pharmacists in their area.

If you prefer a brown-bag meeting with your doctor, arrange the session in advance to allow enough time for a thorough job. A complete evaluation can take up to an hour, but—as with most initiatives you undertake to educate yourself about prescription drug use—it is time wisely spent.

Managing Your Prescription Drug Costs
Katharine Greider

Prescription drugs, once a minor act in American medicine, have taken center stage. Many of us now expect to take medication every day for the rest of our lives to manage serious conditions that would already have disabled or killed our ancestors. We're grateful those medicines are available. The problem, for many of us, is how to afford them.

As drugs become more important in medicine and commerce, they also consume a heftier slice of our economic pie. Americans' spending on prescription drugs exceeded $221 billion in 2004—nearly double what we spent in 1999. We are taking more pills. (For every 100 patient visits in 1985, doctors wrote prescriptions for 109 medicines; by 1999 that number had jumped to 146 prescriptions.) We are using more new drugs, which tend to be the priciest products. And increases in the drug prices we pay are outpacing inflation every year.

It is sometimes assumed that only the poor and the uninsured cannot afford prescription drugs. It would be bad enough if that were true—imagine having to choose between a life-saving medicine and food or rent. But in fact the cost of drugs increasingly presses on everyone, even those who have drug coverage. Insurance premiums and co-payments are on the rise, and many people's health plans do not cover all the drugs they need.

Someday, perhaps, these conditions will change for the better. Until they do, this section of *The AARP Guide to Pills* suggests a number of useful ways to cut down your drug costs.

"TALK TO YOUR DOCTOR"

The phrase is a familiar one. It comes at the end of many of the drug advertisements we see on television. It's there in part for commercial reasons—to persuade you to ask your doctor about a particular drug rather than its competitors. Yet the ads never mention price. And price is the one topic that many consumers likewise neglect when we discuss drugs with our doctors.

"I can't afford it": Somehow these words hardly ever pass our lips. In a 2003 study by University of Chicago researchers, nearly 3 in 4 people who skipped medications for cost reasons reported failing to discuss financial pressures with their doctors. As for doctors broaching the subject, one physician described the situation in a 2004 issue of the *Archives of Internal Medicine* as "Don't ask, don't tell."

Instead, when money is tight, we often quietly take matters into our own hands: We accept a prescription written by a doctor—and then don't fill it. Or we stretch a supply of pills to make them last longer: Rather than hewing to the dosage the doctor prescribed, we may take one pill a day instead of two, or skip every other day. In a third common dodge, we may take a prescribed medicine for a while and then simply stop. Twenty-six percent of seniors admitted resorting to one or more of these self-defeating behaviors in 2003.

All three money-saving expedients are understandable, but they carry a great risk. Here's why:

- If a drug is taken below its prescribed dosage, there's a good chance it will not work. Consider the case of statin drugs to lower cholesterol, such as Lipitor and Zocor: Missing doses regularly means that your cholesterol may not be sufficiently reduced, potentially increasing your risk of stroke or heart attack.
- If the doctor, not knowing that you are skipping doses, sees that your condition is not improving, he or she may write a new prescription for a stronger dosage or a stronger drug. This could be medically inappropriate—possibly even perilous.
- Not filling prescriptions means that your condition is not being controlled—and may get worse. Failing to take the drugs that control potentially serious conditions such as high cholesterol, high blood pressure, and diabetes increases the likelihood of premature disability (or even death), with its accompanying expense of surgery, hospitalization, rehabilitation, and long-term care.

So there is every reason to talk frankly to your doctor about what you can afford. Most people who do this get a positive response. Your doctor might be able to help immediately—by giving you free samples of the drug you need, by switching you to a less expensive medicine, or by advising you on programs that help people buy prescription drugs at lower cost.

Having a brass-tacks talk with your physician is the single most important step you can take to lower drug costs while tending to your health. Tell him or her how much you can afford to spend on drugs. Take with you a list of your current medications and the amount each one costs. Above all, go armed with information so that you can talk knowledgeably and make the best use of your time with the doctor.

You can prepare for these conversations by gathering cost-saving ideas beforehand. The good news is that many consumer and other groups have responded to the increasing burden of drug costs by developing tools to help you figure it all out. Many of these are cited below, and most of them are available on the internet. (If you don't have home access to the internet, spend an afternoon at the public library; staffers there can show you how to get online and find the information you need.)

The information below explores ways of achieving cost savings in three critical areas: the drugs you take, where you buy them, and who pays for them.

THE DRUGS YOU TAKE

The obvious first question in any cost-trimming plan is one for your doctor: Do you need all the medications you are currently taking? It may be that you do, and your doctor will explain why. Equally likely, you and your doctor may discover that a drug you started taking years ago is no longer required. Economy is important here, not only for the purse but for the body, because each drug you add to your daily regimen interacts with the others, increasing the chance of side effects and possibly dangerous drug-drug inter-actions. That's one reason why it's so worth-while to take a current list of all your drugs to show your doctor: It guarantees that the doctor will know the whole picture when prescribing.

Next question: Are you taking the best and most cost-effective drug available for your con-dition? This sounds elementary, but many peo-ple use the priciest drug in a category for years (often because the doctor who prescribed it was oblivious to price), overlooking a cheaper alter-native that's just as good. So if you have been prescribed an expensive, brand-name drug, explore with your doctor whether you can try:

- **A cheaper brand.** The slogan "new and improved" often comes with a price hike. "Improved" may mean only added conven-ience—a pill that can be taken once a day instead of twice, for example, or one that works by controlled release. Such newer dosage forms almost always cost more than the original drug. So one question is this: Does the novelty or minor improvement truly justify the higher price? Another point to ponder: Is there an older, less expensive product in the same class of drugs—that is, those that work in similar ways to treat the same condition—that would serve the purpose just as well? In some cases, several drugs in the same class are equally effective, yet they vary widely in price. Information for comparing drugs

within a class is outlined on page xi and on page xxii.

- **A generic drug.** A generic is a copy of a brand-name drug that is allowed onto the market when the brand has lost the patent protection that grants it exclusive market-ing rights (see page xiii). Generic drugs deliver the same active ingredients as their brand-name counterparts—usually at a fraction of the cost. In 2004, for example, the average price of a brand-name drug was $96.01, compared with just $28.74 for a generic drug. This price differential explains why, if you have drug coverage, your insurer probably charges lower co-pays for generics than for brands. To gain the greatest advantage from this system, explore not just whether a generic equiva-lent exists for the brand-name drug you're taking, but also whether any generic is available in that entire class of drugs. If you're taking a new antidepressant, for example, a generic version will not yet be available. But, with your doctor's consent, you could instead try fluoxetine—a generic form of the older antidepressant Prozac.

- **An over-the-counter (OTC) drug.** When drugs are considered safe enough to be sold over the counter (meaning they no longer require a prescription), their prices plum-met. If you're paying 100 percent out of pocket—that is, if your prescription drug costs are not covered by a health plan—an OTC could be less expensive. If you have insurance, by contrast, you may find that your co-pay for the equivalent prescribed drug is still lower than the OTC price.

- **Splitting pills.** For complicated commer-cial reasons, a supply of 40-mg. tablets often costs exactly the same as (or only a little bit more than) the same number of 20-mg. tablets. Some people therefore buy the higher-dosage pills, then cut them—and their drug bill—in half. Drugstores sell inexpensive pill-splitting gadgets that can cut them accurately. Because of the chemi-cal makeup of pills and the way they are designed to work in your body, however, some pills cannot be split safely. It is there-fore crucial to ask your doctor or pharma-cist first before adopting this strategy.

- **Buying a 90-day supply.** Higher-count bottles often get a volume discount—a clear plus for those paying out-of-pocket.

Insurance plans, too, sometimes charge lower co-pays for 90-day (as opposed to three 30-day) supplies. If you have a health condition that is controlled by a "maintenance" drug—one you must take over an extended period of time—it's worth asking your doctor to write you a 90-day prescription.

- **Changing your lifestyle.** There's no question that certain conditions—high blood pressure and heartburn, for example—can be improved by adopting a healthier diet, quitting smoking, and getting more exercise. These measures may not eradicate the health problem, but they could enable you to control it with fewer drugs or lower dosages.

Once you get comfortable with the strategies outlined above, you can vary and combine them to suit your own preferences and requirements. Let's say, for example, that you're one of the countless Americans who helped make Nexium, a treatment for gastric problems, the country's fourth-bestselling drug. Nexium is virtually identical to another drug, Prilosec, made by the same manufacturer. When Prilosec's patent was about to expire in 2001, opening the market to cheaper generic versions, the company used an aggressive marketing campaign to persuade patients to switch to Nexium—for which there would be no generic equivalent for years to come. Canny customers who know this story therefore have a real choice. In April 2005, a large national discount mail-order pharmacy (Costco) was selling a month's supply of Nexium for $126. At the same time, a 30-day supply of the generic version of Prilosec could be purchased from the same source for only $38. And an even cheaper form of Prilosec—its OTC version—can be bought for less than $20 at most pharmacies. Be aware, however, that the dosage strength of the OTC product can differ from that of the prescription product.

So how can you tell which drug gives you good treatment at the best price? One reliable source is the Drug Effectiveness Review Project at Oregon's Health and Science University, which is using the best available research to compare the safety and effectiveness of all medicines within the most commonly used classes of drugs. This "evidence-based" information forms the basis of two handy websites that permit consumers to compare various drugs for clinical effectiveness and cost: For AARP's guide, visit www.aarp.org/health/comparedrugs. For Consumer Reports Best Buy Drugs, go to http://crbestbuydrugs.org.

WHERE YOU BUY YOUR DRUGS

You have a prescription from your doctor and now you want to fill it as economically as possible. As a consumer, you are well aware that the identical brand of shampoo typically costs more at a supermarket than it does at a discount drugstore. To an even greater extent, the price of medicines depends on where you buy them. Here are some options to consider:

- **Comparison shopping locally.** Drug prices can vary dramatically—even among pharmacies in the same neighborhood. In a 2005 survey of drug prices, for example, the New York State Attorney General's office found 30 tablets of cholesterol-lowering Zocor selling for $190.09 at one pharmacy; at another store just four miles away, they were offered for $96.59—about half the price. Some pharmacies offer discounts, most often for seniors. So if you want to buy locally, it's worth comparison-shopping the old-fashioned way: Make a list of your drugs and their dosages, then contact pharmacies within a reasonable distance and ask them what they charge. The following states have created websites that help residents quickly find out the same information:

  Maryland: www.oag.state.md.us/drugprices

  New Hampshire: www.egov.nh.gov/medicine-cabinet

  New York: www.NYAGRx.org

- **Discount programs.** As mentioned above, pharmacies frequently offer discounts, usually for seniors. A number of states also offer pharmaceutical discounts to eligible residents—in most cases, low-income seniors. Or you may be eligible for a limited supply of free or reduced-cost medicines from assistance programs run by pharmaceutical manufacturers. Eligibility requirements vary, and applying can be a complex process. A comprehensive list of programs is available at www.pparx.org; click on "View a list of participating programs." This website is sponsored by the Partnership for Prescription Assistance, a coalition of pharmaceutical companies and health-care practitioners. (You can also call them at 1-888-477-2669.) Also worth looking into is Rx Outreach at www.rxoutreach.com (or 1-800-769-3880), a program run by pharmacy benefits manager Express Scripts. Rx Outreach helps people buy commonly prescribed generic drugs at discounted prices.

- **American mail order.** Unless your local pharmacy can offer a lower price, buying drugs by mail can be both convenient (they're delivered to your door) and money-saving. Many major U.S. pharmacy chains (Costco, Walgreen's, and CVS are among the largest) offer discount mail-order services through their websites. They also list the drugs they sell and what they charge, making it easy to compare prices. (Don't forget to include shipping costs in your calculations, and remember to order refills far enough in advance that the shipping time does not leave you "stranded" without a necessary medicine.) Many drug insurance plans also charge lower co-pays for purchases from their mail-order pharmacy.

- **Mail order from abroad.** Millions of Americans have drastically cut their drug bills by ordering their medicines from other countries, especially Canada, where brand-name drugs are a great deal cheaper—sometimes as much as 70 percent less expensive. (Generics, by contrast, usually cost more abroad than they do in the United States.) This practice is against the law, but as debate about drug importation continues, U.S. authorities generally have not prosecuted Americans who purchase medications from abroad for their own personal use. Increasingly, however, filled orders have been intercepted, delayed, and confiscated. (AARP supports Congressional action to legalize drug importation but recommends that any such imports initially be limited to drugs from licensed pharmacies and wholesalers in Canada.)

Besides illegality, there are other weighty factors to consider in ordering prescription drugs from abroad. One factor is financial: Drugs purchased this way do not qualify for reimbursement under most health insurance programs. Another factor has to do with safety: Canada and the leading nations of Europe regulate drug safety and pharmacy practices as rigorously as

does the United States. If your drugs come from a licensed pharmacy in one of these countries, you can be confident that they are bona fide. However, shady operations abound on the internet, and they may sell counterfeit or otherwise substandard medications. To steer clear of charlatans, choose a pharmacy that observes the following "best practices" of safety and customer service:

- Displays on its website its license number and the name of the regulatory agency that granted it so that its authenticity can be verified. (See discussion of IMPAC and CIPA seals below.)

- Provides its full street address and a toll-free telephone number you can call to speak to a pharmacist or a customer service representative.

- Requires you to send the prescription written by your doctor. (Avoid sites that do not require prescriptions, sell controlled substances or narcotics such as OxyContin, hawk "lifestyle" drugs, or send promotional e-mails.)

- Requires you to submit details of your medical history and clearly states the pharmacy's policies for ensuring medical, personal, and financial privacy.

- Explains the difference between American and its own country's drug names and labeling, and sends drugs with labels that include strength, dosing instructions, expiration date, appropriate warnings of side effects, and a drug identification number.

- Provides on its website full information about shipping fees, payment policies, and refunds.

For those with limited time or enthusiasm for internet sleuthing, a handful of trade groups and other organizations can serve as gateways to pharmacies that meet their standards:

- An independent American research group at www.pharmacychecker.com rates 50 U.S. and international pharmacies, and allows shoppers to compare their services (including prices) free of charge.

- The Internet and Mail Order Pharmacy Accreditation Commission (IMPAC), a U.S.-based group of doctors and pharmacists, lists on its website (www.impac survey.org) American and foreign pharmacies that it has accredited after rigorous evaluation.

- The Canadian International Pharmacy Association (CIPA) website (www .ciparx.ca) lists license numbers and includes links to the websites of its member pharmacies—which, in turn, are authorized to display the CIPA seal of approval.
- The National Association of Boards of Pharmacy (NABP), which regulates the practice of pharmacy in all 50 states, lists on its website (www.nabp .net/vipps) US internet pharmacies that have qualified for its seal of approval, known as VIPPS (Verified Internet Pharmacy Practice Sites).

- **State government.** Finally, look to your state government for savings opportunities. Several states have flouted the federal ban on prescription drug importation by setting up websites that link residents to state-vetted foreign pharmacies where they can save money. For example, people living in Illinois, Wisconsin, Kansas, Missouri, and Vermont can all order drugs through the I-SaveRx program (www.i saverx.net or 1-866-472-8333), whose Canadian and British pharmacies have been inspected by state officials. Minnesota (www.state .mn.us) and the District of Columbia (www.dc.gov) share a similar program.

One caveat about using multiple pharmacies to fill your prescriptions: You must be vigilant to inform each pharmacy what other prescription and nonprescription medicines you are taking, as well as any dietary or herbal supplements. These essential data will allow the pharmacist to check for possible drug interactions. Alternatively, if you rely on just one pharmacy, by all means ask the pharmacist to keep your patient profile (medication list) on her or his computer.

WHO PAYS FOR YOUR DRUGS

If you lack prescription drug insurance, buying the most cost-effective medicines at the lowest available price is one strategy for managing your drug costs. Another is to try to get insurance or some other type of assistance. Some possibilities are described below.

- **State-based programs.** If your income is limited, you may qualify for Medicaid—a state-administered program, jointly funded by the federal and state governments, that covers the cost of both medical care and prescription drugs. Alternatively, you may qualify for a state-sponsored pharmacy assistance program. These programs run the gamut from price discounts to the state's paying much of the cost of prescription medicines. Some are far more generous than others, but all are intended to help people who do not qualify for Medicaid.

There's a shortcut to finding out what's available to you: Once you've assembled details about your income and a list of your medications, you can plug them into a web-based tool that will quickly tell you which public and private assistance programs you qualify for—and how to apply. To do this, go to www.benefitscheckup.org, which is run by the National Council on the Aging and is designed for people 55 and older.

Another excellent source of help, available in every state, is dubbed SHIP, for State Health Insurance Assistance Program. It offers free personal counseling, referrals, and information on a wide range of national and in-state health services, including prescription drug assistance and discount programs. To find your nearest SHIP office, call the Eldercare Locator at 1-800-677-1116 or visit www.shiptalk.org.

- **Free samples.** Americans who have difficulty paying for medicine often rely on free samples they get from their doctors. Pharmaceutical companies hand out $10 billion worth of such samples each year, says Dr. Jerry Avorn, the author of *Powerful Medicines*. In fact, a 2004 survey revealed that 91 percent of patients who talked to their doctors about drug costs received these samples. Free is free, but be aware that pharmaceutical companies furnish free samples to promote their drugs, not as an exercise in charity. The drugs they publicize this way are their newest and costliest—and eventually that free supply will run dry, leaving you to cover the drug's costs. There are safety considerations as well: By accepting samples, you bypass the pharmacist, failing to create any record of your ever having taken those samples when you fill future prescriptions. You may also miss receiving written information, including precautions about potential side effects, that is normally furnished to you at the pharmacy.

CAN MEDICARE HELP?

Prescription-drug insurance is available to everyone who has Medicare—either Part A or Part B—under the optional "Part D" benefit that began in 2006. This has saved money for millions of Medicare beneficiaries who formerly received no help in paying for the drugs they need.

To get Part D drug coverage, you must join a private plan approved by Medicare. There are many such plans, but they all fall into two broad types: "stand-alone" plans, which offer drug coverage only and are intended for people who prefer traditional Medicare for their medical benefits; and Medicare Advantage plans (mainly managed care), which offer comprehensive medical and drug coverage.

Each plan has its own mix of benefits and charges, but all must offer at least (or more than) the level of coverage specified by Congress. Here's a brief overview of how the system works:

Premiums: "Stand-alone" drug plans have monthly premiums that vary a great deal and must be paid in addition to Medicare Part B premiums. These premiums are projected to average roughly $24 per month in 2007. Medicare Advantage (MA) plans usually have one premium that covers both medical care and drugs, but some MA plans charge no premiums for either. (Zero premiums usually occur in areas of heavy plan competition, such as parts of Florida and California.) In most cases, the Part B premium is in addition to any premium required by an MA plan.

Deductibles: Medicare allows plans to charge an annual deductible—the amount you pay at the beginning of each year before your drug coverage begins—of up to $265 (in 2007). Many plans have no deductibles.

Copayments: Depending on the plan you choose, you will pay either copayments (a flat fee for each prescription) or coinsurance (a percentage of the drug's cost). Most plans divide their covered drugs into "tiers." Each tier has a different copay, ranging from generic drugs (the lowest copay) through "preferred" brand-name drugs and "nonpreferred" brands to the highest copay for rare and very expensive drugs.

Coverage: Most drug plans follow the formula originally designed by Congress. This divided drug coverage in each calendar year into three parts: initial coverage, catastrophic coverage and, in between the two, a coverage gap often called the "doughnut hole." In the **initial coverage** phase, once you've paid your deductible (if any), you pay roughly 25 percent of your drug costs and your plan pays about 75 percent until total drug costs (what you have paid plus what your plan has paid) reach $2,400. Beyond that, you fall into the **coverage gap**, where you must pay 100 percent of your drug costs until you have spent $3,850 out of pocket since the beginning of the year (this equals $5,452 in total drug costs). If your costs are high enough to reach this point, you then pass into the third phase, **catastrophic coverage**, in which you pay only 5 percent of your costs for the remainder of the year. (Note: These dollar amounts are for 2007. They change every year.)

Because this cost-sharing can stress your wallet—particularly in the coverage gap—the money-saving strategies described earlier will be key to lowering your expenses. The further you can stretch your drug-purchasing dollars—by choosing a less expensive drug with a lower copay, for example—the longer it will take you to hit the coverage gap.

Some drug plans, however, offer continuous coverage throughout the year, usually for a higher premium than the average. Most of these plans offer coverage only for generic drugs during the gap, meaning you will have to pay full price for any brand-name drugs you may take. A few plans offer continuous coverage for both generic and brand-name drugs.

Extra Help: But what if, like millions of Americans, you simply can't afford these costs? One special part of the Medicare drug benefit is known as "Extra Help." This offers substantial assistance to people with limited incomes and resources who qualify: zero (or greatly reduced) premiums and deductibles, small copayments for prescriptions, and continuous coverage throughout the year. People who get their drugs through Medicaid automatically receive full Extra Help when they become eligible for Medicare. Others can apply for Extra Help by calling 1-800-772-1213 or by visiting www.socialsecurity.gov.

Do you need Medicare drug coverage? You may not need it if you already have drug coverage (such as from a current or former employer or union) that is at least as good as Medicare's. (Seek the advice of the benefits administrator of your current plan before making any decision.) Otherwise, you should seriously consider signing up. For those who currently spend not much money (or nothing at all) on drugs, Medicare coverage may not seem worthwhile; after all, you still have to pay premiums even if you receive no benefit. But it's important to view the program as insurance. And, like all insurance, Medicare drug coverage affords protection from unexpected events—and their attendant costs—in the future. You may be perfectly healthy now, but consider what might happen if you develop a chronic health condition or need treatment for a serious illness in years to come. Drugs for certain conditions could set you back several thousand dollars each month.

Do you have to sign up? No. The Part D benefit is voluntary, so you need not sign up for it if you don't want to. If you ignore it, you will have effectively chosen not to enroll. Note, however, that if you don't have comparable drug coverage already and you opt not to sign up for a Medicare drug plan when you are initially eligible to do so, you will face a late-enrollment penalty if someday you do enroll. The penalty boosts your monthly premium by at least one percent for every month you delay in signing up. Delay enrolling for two years, for example, and your monthly premiums will be 24 percent higher for as long as you are in the program.

Choosing a plan: Plans vary a great deal, not only in how much they charge but also in the drugs they cover and in the "preferred" pharmacies they use. It is therefore essential to compare plans to find the one that is best for you. You can do this by visiting the "plan finder" on Medicare's website at www.medicare.gov or by calling its helpline at 1-800-633-4227. In estimating your total out-of-pocket expenses for the year under any plan, the amount of your copays for the drugs you take is more important than merely looking at premiums and deductibles. So make a list of all your drugs, their dosages, and how often you take them before you compare plans.

Enrolling in a plan: You must normally sign up for a plan (or switch to another plan) during the annual enrollment period, which runs from November 15 to December 31 each year. You can sign up (or switch) at other times only under special circumstances—when you first become eligible for Medicare, for example, or if you qualify for Extra Help, lose employer drug coverage, move out of your plan's service area, or move into or out of a nursing home.

All of these factors are worth mulling as you decide whether or not to enroll in the Medicare drug program. You will also need to find out how any coverage you currently rely on—from employer-sponsored drug benefits to state pharmacy-assistance programs—will mesh with Medicare coverage. For additional help and information, go to:

- The official Medicare website at www.medicare.gov or the Medicare helpline at 1-800-633-4227 (TTY 1-877-486-2048)
- Your State Health Insurance Assistance Program (SHIP), where you can get expert personal help free of charge (call the Eldercare Locator at 1-800-677-1116 or visit www.shiptalk.org)
- AARP information at www.aarp.org/health/medicare or www.aarp.org/bulletin/medicare
- The Medicare Rights Center, a consumer help and advocacy group, at www.medicarerights.org

PERSEVERANCE PAYS

When it comes to medicine, it's a complex new world out there. Drugs have become vital but expensive, and the market in which they are sold has grown devilishly complex. Our situation today recalls that of our grandparents and great-grandparents, who had to decode a brand-new consumer economy in which food came in cans—and in which a bigger can did not necessarily contain more food.

Yet there is reason for optimism. Modern medicines may not constitute a panacea, but they offer doctors and patients more powerful and effective treatment options than have ever existed before. Meanwhile, consumers and their advocates will continue to devise new strategies for managing and minimizing the high price of prescription drugs.

Think of it this way: The tedium of trawling for savings in the marketplace for prescription drugs will prepare you to improve or protect your long-term health. The exercise may return short-term benefits as well—dollars left in your pocket.

Contributors

Dr. Jerry Avorn is Professor of Medicine at Harvard Medical School and director of the Division of Pharmaco-epidemiology and Pharmaco-economics at the Brigham and Women's Hospital, Boston, a major Harvard teaching hospital. Dr. Avorn is the author of *Powerful Medicines: The Benefits, Risks, and Costs of Prescription Drugs* (Knopf, 2004). An internist and geriatrician, he has been studying medications and their effects in older patients for more than 20 years.

Dr. William Thomas is a physician and an internationally recognized authority on the relationship among aging, health, and medicine. Named an AARP visiting scholar in 2004, Dr. Thomas is the author of numerous books and articles. His most recent book is *What Are Old People For?: How Elders Will Save the World* (VanderWyk and Burnham, 2004). Dr. Thomas frequently addresses professional and lay audiences on the importance of making wise use of prescription drugs.

Katharine Greider is a freelance writer based in New York City. Her investigative articles and commentary have appeared in many national magazines and newspapers, including *The New York Times, The Los Angeles Times, Mother Jones,* and the *AARP Bulletin*. Greider is the author of *The Big Fix: How the Pharmaceutical Industry Rips Off American Consumers* (PublicAffairs, 2003).

How to Use This Book

To help you quickly find information about the drugs you are taking, the content of *The AARP Guide to Pills* is succinctly presented. The description below and the examples on the following pages explain the book's organization, helping you gain maximum benefit from using it.

Drugs are presented alphabetically by their generic name. This is done because although drugs may have several brand-names, they have only one generic name. Special design features have been incorporated throughout to enhance access to the book's medication information.

Colored thumb tabs on the edges of the pages designate letters of the alphabet, so you can quickly page through the book to find a particular alphabetic section of drugs and target the one you are searching for.

Two comprehensive, color-keyed indexes are provided to help you locate these sections in the book and the specific medication you are looking for within these sections.

- The Disorder and Disease Index organizes drugs by medical problems, such as allergies, cholesterol levels, infections, or high blood pressure. This index is particularly helpful if you want to look up medications available to treat a specific medical problem. The edges of the pages in the Disorder and Disease Index are tinted blue.
- The Index of Generic and Brand-Name Drugs alphabetically lists all drug names included in the book along with the page number where they can be found—whether they are generic or brand-name, prescription or nonprescription. Generic drugs are shown in italic type, while brand-name drugs are shown in regular type. The pages of the Index of Generic and Brand-Name Drugs are tinted beige along the entire edge of the page to help you find this essential section of the book.

Each drug is presented in monograph format. Essentially, this means all of the information provided on a specific drug can be found in one place. Each drug monograph opens with the name of the generic drug and its particular dosage form(s) in large red type for ease of identification.

Wherever available, a color photo—oftentimes two—is provided to illustrate examples of the particular drug discussed in the monograph. The brand-name, dosage (5 mg, 40 mg, 250 mg, etc.), dosage form (tablet, capsule, injection, patch, etc.), and manufacturer of the illustrated drugs are also provided for each image. These images are designed to aid in the identification of some dosage forms and dosages available. *The AARP Guide to Pills* provides many more images than any other book of its kind. Nevertheless, space limitations do not allow for the inclusion of images of every available dosage form and dosage for each drug presented. Whenever possible, compare the dosage form and dosage in these images to the drug you are taking. Follow up with your health care provider or pharmacist if you have any questions.

The monographs pose a series of eight questions, and provide the answers to each, as described below and illustrated in the examples on the following pages.

What is...(this medication)?

Opens with the generic drug name in capital letters and bold type. Examples of available brand-names are listed in parentheses immediately following the generic name. This section describes the pharmacologic class of each drug: "anticoagulant," "antihypertensive," "decongestant," and so on. It discusses the symptoms and/or medical conditions for which the drug is prescribed and for which the FDA has approved the drug's use; describes how the drug works in your body; and indicates whether generic forms are available.

What should my health care professional know before I take...(this drug)?

Provides a comprehensive, bulleted list of diseases, medical conditions, allergies, and personal behaviors (such as alcohol consumption and tobacco use) you should discuss with your doctor before taking this drug to ensure your safety and maximize the effectiveness of your drug therapy. The bulleted list makes it easy to scan this important information to determine whether any of these factors are relevant to you, so you will know what to discuss with your physician or prescriber.

How should I take...(this medicine)?

Details specific instructions on how to take the drug. It discusses special dietary restrictions that may relate to the drug, to ensure you gain maximum benefit from your prescription. Additionally, this section encourages you to follow the recommended dosage and labeling instructions, and cautions against taking more than the prescribed dosage or administering the drug to special populations, such as children, pregnant or breast-feeding women, or older adults.

What if I miss a dose?

Explains exactly what to do if you accidentally miss a dose—whether you should take it as soon as you remember, or wait until the next scheduled dose—and provides cautions about double dosing.

What drugs may interact with...(this drug)?

Presents a comprehensive, bulleted list of those prescription, nonprescription, and illicit drugs that may have significant side effects when combined with your prescribed drug. Whenever certain dietary supplements, herbal products, foods, or beverages have the potential for serious interactions with the drug you are taking, they will also be included in the bulleted list to highlight the importance of discussing their use in conjunction with your prescribed medication with your prescriber. (See page xli for a general discussion of dietary supplements, herbal substances, foods, and beverages that may interact with prescription drugs.) Otherwise, information about the possible interactions of combining your prescribed medication with certain foods, beverages, nutritional supplements, and herbal products is discussed in the text that follows the bulleted list in this section.

What should I watch for while taking...(this drug)?

Details special considerations specifically related to your prescribed medication. In easy-to-understand terms, this section discusses such important considerations as the need for regular checkups and discussing with your prescriber whether your dosage may need to be changed, foods and/or beverages to avoid, signs of serious complications that should be reported to your prescriber, and information specific to special populations—children, pregnant or breast-feeding women, and older adults.

What side effects may I notice from taking...(this drug)?

Provides critical information about possible side effects in color-keyed bulleted lists to allow you to see at a glance those side effects that may require immediate medical attention and those that do not. Possible side effects requiring immediate medical attention are designated with red bullets; those side effects that you should report if they continue or become troublesome are noted with yellow bullets.

Where can I keep my medicine?

Includes vital information about where and how to store your medications to enable you to maintain the effectiveness of your prescription while you are taking it, as well as information regarding expiration dates of drugs and how to safely dispose of unused drugs.

Red lozenge indicates drug requires an FDA-approved Medication Guide.

Dosage form

Atorvastatin
Atorvastatin tablets

LIPITOR®; 20 mg; Tablet Parke Davis Division of Pfizer Co.

LIPITOR®; 40 mg; Tablet Parke Davis Division of Pfizer Co.

Color thumb tabs indicate where each alphabetic section is located.

Photos with captions that include the brand (or generic) name, dosage, dosage form, and manufacturer of the medication depicted in the photo.

A

Brand-name

What are atorvastatin tablets?

ATORVASTATIN (Lipitor®) blocks the body's ability to make cholesterol. Atorvastatin can help lower blood cholesterol for patients who are at risk for heart disease or stroke. It is only for patients whose cholesterol level is not controlled by diet. It is not a cure. Generic atorvastatin tablets are not yet available.

Generic drug name

Tells you how the drug works in your body, what conditions the drug is used to treat, and whether generic forms are available.

What should my health care professional know before I take atorvastatin?

They need to know if you have any of these conditions:

- an alcohol problem
- any hormone disorder (such as diabetes, underactive thyroid)
- blood salt imbalance
- infection
- kidney disease
- liver disease
- low blood pressure
- muscle disorder or condition
- recent surgery
- seizures (convulsions)
- severe injury
- an unusual or allergic reaction to atorvastatin, other medicines, foods, dyes, or preservatives
- pregnant or trying to get pregnant
- breast-feeding

Comprehensive, bulleted list of diseases, disorders, and personal behaviors you should discuss with your prescriber before taking this drug.

Specifies how this drug should be taken and, if applicable, the best time of day to take it.

How should I take this medicine?

Take atorvastatin tablets by mouth. Follow the directions on the prescription label. Swallow the atorvastatin with a drink of water. Atorvastatin can be taken at any time of the day with or without food. Take your doses at regular intervals. Do not take your medicine more often than directed. Contact your pediatrician or health care professional regarding the use of this medicine in children. Special care may be needed.

Provides cautions about taking more often than directed or administering to special populations.

What if I miss a dose?

If you miss a dose, take it as soon as you can. If it is almost time for your next dose, take only that dose. Do not take double or extra doses.

Explains exactly what to do if you accidentally miss a dose.

Bulleted, alphabetical list of other prescription, non-prescription, and illicit drugs that may cause interactions with your prescribed medication.

Dietary supplements, herbal products, and certain foods and beverages that may interact with the drug you are taking are also listed. See page xli for additional information.

What may interact with atorvastatin?

- alcohol-containing beverages
- amiodarone
- barbiturates (examples: phenobarbital, butalbital, primidone)
- antacids
- birth control pills
- bosentan
- carbamazepine
- certain antibiotics, such as clarithromycin, erythromycin, or troleandomycin
- danazol
- digoxin
- diltiazem
- grapefruit juice
- herbal medicines such as went yeast (Cholestin®) or St. John's wort
- medicines for fungal infections (examples: fluconazole, itraconazole, ketoconazole, voriconazole)
- medicines for treating HIV infections
- medicines that suppress your immune response (cyclosporine)
- medicines to lower cholesterol or triglycerides (examples: colestipol, fenofibrate, gemfibrozil, niacin)
- medicine used to stop early pregnancy (mifepristone, RU-486, or Mifeprex®)
- nefazodone
- nicardipine
- oxcarbazepine
- phenytoin
- pioglitazone
- rifampin, rifabutin, or rifapentine
- verapamil

Tell your prescriber or health care professional about all other medicines you are taking, including non-prescription medicines, nutritional supplements, or herbal products. Also tell your prescriber or health care professional if you are a frequent user of drinks with caffeine or alcohol, if you smoke, or if you use illegal drugs. These may affect the way your medicine works. Check with your health care professional before stopping or starting any of your medicines.

What should I watch for while taking atorvastatin?

Visit your prescriber or health care professional for regular checks on your progress. You will need to have regular tests to make sure your liver is working properly. Tell your prescriber or health care professional as soon as you can if you get any unexplained muscle pain, tenderness, or weakness, especially if you also have a fever and tiredness. Atorvastatin is only part of a total cholesterol-lowering program. Your physician or dietician can suggest a low-cholesterol and low-fat diet that will reduce your risk of getting heart and blood vessel disease. Avoid alcohol and smoking, and keep a proper exercise schedule. If you are going to have surgery, tell your prescriber or health care professional that you are taking atorvastatin.

> Details special considerations related to your condition and prescribed medication in easy-to-understand terms.

What side effects may I notice from taking atorvastatin?

Side effects that you should report to your prescriber or health care professional as soon as possible:

Rare or uncommon:
- dark yellow or brown urine
- decreased urination, difficulty passing urine
- fever
- muscle pain, tenderness, cramps, or weakness
- redness, blistering, or peeling or loosening of the skin, including inside the mouth
- skin rash, itching
- unusual tiredness or weakness
- yellowing of the skin or eyes

Side effects that usually do not require medical attention (report to your prescriber or health care professional if they continue or are bothersome):
- diarrhea
- gas
- headache
- joint pain
- nausea, vomiting
- stomach upset or pain
- tiredness

> Side effects you should report to your health care professional immediately are bulleted in red.

> Side effects that usually do not require immediate medical attention are bulleted in yellow.

Where can I keep my medicine?

Keep out of the reach of children in a container that small children cannot open. Store at controlled room temperature between 20 to 25 degrees C (68 to 77 degrees F). Keep container tightly closed. Throw away any unused medicine after the expiration date.

> Guidelines for proper storage of your medication to ensure that its efficacy is not compromised.

Interactions with Dietary Supplements and Food

Medicines you take may interact with dietary supplements or foods in addition to interacting with other drugs. Discuss with your physician all other medicines you are taking, including nonprescription medicines, nutritional supplements, or herbal products. Dietary supplements include amino acids, vitamins, minerals, herbs, botanicals, and other plant-derived substances, and extracts of these substances. These products are not regulated by the FDA as drugs and must state "Dietary Supplement" on the product label. You should note that rigid quality control standards are not required for dietary supplements, so big differences can occur in the potency and purity of the products. Different brands of herbal products might contain different amounts of the active ingredients, so be careful to use the same brand. It is recommended that you use a brand from a reputable manufacturer, because a standardized product is more likely to contain the same amount of herb from dose to dose. Your health care professional or pharmacist can assist you in finding a reliable product.

It is important to note that many herbal and dietary supplements are combinations of herbal products, vitamins, and other ingredients. Make sure to read labels carefully. In most cases, herbs or dietary supplements that are consumed in normal dietary amounts as a spice or flavoring in foods, such as garlic or ginger, will not interact with medications. However, be careful when *taking* any dietary supplements with your medicines; discuss any dietary supplements or herbs that you are taking with your health care provider.

This information is not intended to cover all possible uses, precautions, interactions, or adverse effects for these drugs. If you have questions about the drug(s) you are taking, check with your health care professional. Contact your physician if you notice a new or different effect from your medications, especially if you have started taking a nonprescription medicine or dietary supplement.

For some dietary supplements, important drug interactions may occur with prescription or non-prescription medicines; for others, the potential for interaction is not known. Important drug interactions are known to be possible with the following dietary supplements:

St. John's Wort

St. John's wort may interact with many prescription and non-prescription medications. Some of these interactions may be very important, including some that could reduce the effectiveness of your prescribed medications. You should check with your health care professional before taking St. John's wort if you are taking other medications. St. John's wort should not be used concurrently with MAOI drugs (e.g., Marplan®, Nardil®, Parnate®, and others) or SSRIs (Celexa®, Prozac®, Lexapro®, Zoloft®, and others) because of the possibility of severe reactions. At least two weeks should elapse between discontinuation of one agent and the initiation of therapy with the other. Do not use St. John's wort if you are currently being treated for a mental or emotional problem such as depression or anxiety, except on the advice of your health care professional, because St. John's wort may interfere with your treatments. Also, do not stop your prescribed treatments without talking to your physician or health care professional. If you are treating yourself with St. John's wort, seek medical advice if your mood does not improve in six to eight weeks or if you have suicidal thoughts. You should check your blood pressure closely while taking St. John's wort if you have high blood pressure. Until more is known about the actions of this herb, it may be advisable to limit intake of certain foods and beverages that contain tyramine (see next page).

Ginger

Important interactions may occur between ginger and anti-inflammatory medications such as aspirin; ibuprofen (Motrin®, Advil®, or others); naprosyn (Aleve®, Naproxen®, and others); and other medications such as Persantine®, blood thinners (such as Coumadin®, Lovenox®, Plavix®, Pletal®, Ticlid®, and others), and medicines for treating diabetes or high blood sugar.

Ginkgo Biloba

While taking ginkgo biloba, be aware of any signs of bleeding, especially if you have a history of bleeding disorders; are taking blood thinners such as Coumadin®, Lovenox®, Plavix®, Pletal®, Ticlid®, or others; or are taking aspirin or any other anti-inflammatory medicines (Motrin®, Advil®, Aleve®, Naproxen®, and others).

Kava Kava

Do not use kava kava if you are currently being treated for a mental or emotional problem such as depression or anxiety. Kava kava may interfere with your treatments. Do not stop your prescribed treatments without talking to your physician or health care professional. Do not drink alcohol while taking kava kava, as alcohol can increase its side effects. Other prescription medicines that may interact with kava kava include medications for depression, anxiety, or other emotional or psychiatric problems; medications for pain; medications to treat Parkinson's disease or other neurologic illness; medications for sleep; and muscle relaxants.

Green Tea

Green tea usually contains caffeine, but some green tea products are decaffeinated. Seek the advice of your health care professional before taking green tea regularly for health purposes. Caffeine-containing products may interact with cold products containing decongestants, Ritalin® and related drugs, theophylline, beta-agonists (such as Proventil®, Alupent®, and others), Ditropan®, and other medicines. In addition, green tea may also interact with MAOI drugs (e.g., Marplan®, Nardil®, Parnate®, and others) or Comtan®. If you are taking any of these medicines, talk to your physician or pharmacist before taking green tea.

SAM-e

Interactions with SAM-e and other medications are unknown, which is why you should always be careful when mixing supplements with traditional medications. If you take any other medications, consult with your health care professional before taking SAM-e. Medicines that may interact with SAM-e include alcohol or alcohol-containing beverages; antacids; lithium; medications for Parkinson's disease such as levodopa; and some medications for the treatment of depression, anxiety, or other mood disorders.

Went Yeast

While taking went yeast (Cholestin™), visit your prescriber or health care professional for your regular evaluation. Cholestin™ is intended as a dietary supplement for healthy adults only and is not recommended to treat a disease. Cholestin™ may interact with the following medicines: alcohol; amiodarone; certain antibiotics such as Biaxin® or erythromycin; diltiazem (Cardizem® and others); grapefruit juice; medicines for fungal infections (examples include Diflucan®, Sporonax®, and Nizoral®); medications used to lower cholesterol or triglycerides such as niacin, Lofibra®, and others; Lopid® and the "Statin" drugs; nefazodone; Dilantin®; verapamil (Calan® and others); St. John's wort; and Coumadin®.

Vitamins and minerals can also interact with certain medicines. Calcium, iron, or zinc supplements and multi-vitamin supplements should not be taken at the same time with certain antibiotics such as tetracycline, Cipro®, or Floxin®. Separate the administration of these products by several hours. Nutritional supplements containing excessive vitamin K should be avoided if you are taking Coumadin®, a type of blood thinner. Carefully read the "Supplement Facts" panel on all vitamin/mineral supplements to check the ingredients before taking the supplement with prescription medicines.

While taking certain medicines, it may be important to play close attention to your diet, as some foods may interact. Certain foods and beverages may contain vitamins or minerals, such as calcium or vitamin K, or other ingredients such as caffeine, alcohol, grapefruit components or tyramine. In most cases, it is important to maintain a consistent diet during your therapy; however, there are some foods that you should avoid altogether depending on the medicine you are taking. Discuss any special dietary needs during your therapy with your physician, pharmacist, or nutritionist.

Vitamin K

Brussels sprouts, kale, green tea, asparagus, avocado, broccoli, cabbage, cauliflower, collard greens, liver, soybean oil, soybeans, certain beans, mustard greens, peas (black-eyed peas, split peas, and chick peas), turnip greens, parsley, green onions, spinach, and lettuce contain moderate to high amounts of vitamin K. Some meal replacement products also contain vitamin K, so read labels carefully.

Although you can still eat these products while taking this medication, it is best to maintain a consistent intake. Discuss your dietary needs with your physician, pharmacist, or nutritionist.

Tyramine

Aged cheeses, yeast extract, protein extract, soy sauce, fava beans or broad bean pods, smoked meats, pickled meats, smoked poultry, pickled poultry, smoked fish (such as lox or smoked salmon), pickled fish (such as pickled herring), fermented sausage (bologna, pepperoni, salami, or summer sausage), bananas, avocados, any overripe fruit, yogurt, and sour cream contain significant amounts of tyramine.

These foods must be avoided when taking selected medications and for a period of time after stopping them, especially MAOI drugs (for example, Marplan®, Nardil®, Parnate®, and others).

Caffeine

Some teas, coffee, chocolate, guarana, cola, "stay awake" products, and certain "energy" drinks contain caffeine.

Caffeine-containing products may interact with cold products containing decongestants, Ritalin® and related drugs, theophylline, beta-agonists (such as Proventil®, Alupent®, and others), Ditropan®, and other medicines.

Grapefruit Juice or Grapefruit-Containing Products

Grapefruit juice and grapefruit-containing foods may increase or decrease the effects of certain medicines. If you think you may be experiencing increased or new adverse effects, or if the medicine does not seem to be working as well, contact your physician.

The following medicines may interact with grapefruit juice or grapefruit products (*Note*: This is not a complete list. Please contact your physician or pharmacist for more information):

- Amiodarone (Pacerone®)
- Calcium-channel blockers (e.g. Calan®, Cardene, Norvasc®, Nimotop®, Plendil®, Procardia®, Sular®, and others)
- Carbamazepine (Tegretol® and others)
- Cyclosporine (Neoral® and Sandimune®)
- Dextromethorphan-containing products (Robitussin® DM and other over-the-counter cough suppressants)
- Erythromycin (E-Mycin®, EryTab®, E.E.S. ®, and other oral products)
- Estrogen-containing products
- Fexofenodine (Allegra®)
- Itraconazole (Sporonox®)
- Sildenafil (Revatio and Viagra®)
- "Statin" Medicines (Lipitor®, Mevacor®, and others)

FDA-Approved Medication Guides

The FDA may require distribution of Medication Guides, which are FDA-approved patient information documents, for selected prescription drugs that pose a serious and significant public health concern.

Medication Guides will be required if the FDA determines that one or more of the following circumstances exist:

- patient labeling could help prevent serious adverse effects;
- the drug product has serious risk(s) (relative to benefits) of which patients should be made aware because information concerning the risk(s) could affect patients' decision to use, or to continue to use, the product;
- the drug product is important to health, and patient adherence to directions for use is crucial to the drug's effectiveness.

Medication Guides are required for these products:*

abacavir; lamivudine (Epzicom)
abacavir (Ziagen)
abacavir sulfate; lamivudine; zidovudine (Trizivir)
acitretin (Soriatane)
alosetron (Lotronex)
amiodarone (Cordarone)
atomoxetine (Strattera)
bosentan (Tracleer)
fluticasone; salmeterol (Advair HFA, Advair Diskus)
formoterol (Foradil Aerolizer)
hydromorphone (Palladone) (no longer on the market)
human insulin, inhaled (Exubera)
interferon alpha-2a, recombinant (Roferon-A)
interferon beta-1a (Rebif)
interferon alfacon-1 (Infergen)
interferon beta-1a (Avonex)
isotretinoin (Accutane, Amnesteem, Claravis, Sotret)
lenolidamide (Revlimid)
lindane shampoo or lotion (Kwell)
mefloquine (Lariam)
mifepristone (Mifeprex)
natalizumab (Tysabri)
nevirapine (Viramune)
peginterferon alfa-2a (Pegasys)
peginterferon alfa 2b (PEG-Intron)
pimecrolimus (Elidel Cream)

pramlintide acetate (Symlin)
ribavirin (Rebetol, Ribasphere, Copegus)
ribavirin; interferon alfa-2b combination (Rebetron)
salmeterol (Servent Diskus)
selegiline transdermal system (Emsam)
sodium oxybate (Xyrem)
tacrolimus (Protopic Ointment)
tamoxifen (Nolvadex, Soltamox)
teriparatide (Forteo)

Antidepressant Class Drugs (Medication Guides required for children and teens only)
- Amitriptyline (Elavil)
- Amoxapine (Asendin)
- Bupropion (Welbutrin)
- Citalopram (Celexa)
- Clomipramine (Anafranil)
- Desipramine (Norpramin)
- Doxepin (Sinequan)
- Duloxetine (Cymbalta)
- Escitalopram (Lexapro)
- Fluoxetine (Prozac)
- Imipramine (Tofranil)
- Isocarboxazid (Marplan)
- Maprotiline (Ludiomil)
- Mirtazapine (Remeron)
- Nefazodone (Serzone)
- Nortriptyline (Pamelor)
- Paroxetine (Paxil)
- Phenelzine (Nardil)
- Protriptyline (Vivactil)
- Sertraline (Zoloft)
- Tranylcypromine (Parnate)
- Trazodone (Desyrel)
- Trimipramine (Surmontil)
- Venlafaxine (Effexor)

Non-Steroidal Anti-Inflammatory Class Drugs (NSAIDs)
- Celecoxib (Celebrex)
- Diclofenac (Cataflam, Voltaren)
- Diclofenac; Misoprostol (Arthrotec)
- Etodolac (Lodine)
- Fenoprofen (Nalfon)
- Flurbiprofen (Ansaid)
- Ibuprofen (Advil, Motrin, Nuprin)
- Indomethacin (Indocin)
- Ketoprofen (Orudis)
- Ketorolac (Toradol)
- Meclofenamate, Mefenamic Acid (Ponstel)

- Meloxicam (Mobic)
- Nabumetone (Relafen)
- Naproxen (Anaprox, Naprelan, Naprosyn)
- Oxaprozin (DayPro)
- Piroxicam (Feldene)

- Sulindac (Clinoril)
- Tolmetin (Tolectin)

*Not all drugs listed below appear as entries in the book. The FDA updates this list periodically; ask your pharmacist if your prescription medication requires a Medication Guide.

Abacavir tablets

ZIAGEN™;
300 mg; Tablet
Glaxo Wellcome

A

This drug requires an FDA medication guide. See page xxxvii.

What are abacavir tablets?

ABACAVIR (Ziagen®) is an antiviral drug called a nucleoside reverse transcriptase inhibitor or NRTI. Abacavir is used to treat human immunodeficiency virus (HIV) infection. Abacavir may reduce the amount of HIV in the blood and increase the number of CD4 cells (T-cells) in the blood. Abacavir is used in combination with other drugs to treat the HIV virus. Abacavir will not cure or prevent HIV infection or AIDS. You may still develop other infections or conditions associated with HIV. Generic abacavir tablets are not yet available.

What should my health care professional know before I take abacavir?

They need to know if you have any of these conditions:
- liver disease
- an unusual or allergic reaction to abacavir, other medicines, foods, dyes, or preservatives
- pregnant or trying to get pregnant
- breast-feeding

How should I take this medicine?

Take abacavir tablets by mouth. Follow the directions on the prescription label. Swallow tablets with a drink of water. Abacavir can be taken with or without food. Take your doses at regular intervals. Do not take your medicine more often than directed. To help to make sure that your anti-HIV therapy works as well as possible, be very careful to take all of your medicine exactly as prescribed. Do not stop taking except on your prescriber's advice. Contact your pediatrician or health care professional regarding the use of this medicine in children. Special care may be needed.

What if I miss a dose?

If you miss a dose, take it as soon as you can. If it is almost time for your next dose, take only that dose. Do not take double or extra doses.

What may interact with abacavir?

- alcohol
- methadone
- ribavirin

Tell your prescriber or health care professional about all other medicines you are taking, including nonprescription medicines, nutritional supplements, or herbal products. Also tell your prescriber or health care professional if you are a frequent user of drinks with caffeine or alcohol, if you smoke, or if you use illegal drugs. These may affect the way your medicine works. Check with your health care professional before stopping or starting any of your medicines.

What should I watch for while taking abacavir?

Visit your prescriber or health care professional for regular checks on your progress. Discuss any new symptoms with your prescriber or health care professional. A small number of people might have a severe allergic reaction to abacavir. If you have a skin rash or two or more of the following symptoms you may be having this type of reaction: fever, nausea, vomiting, stomach pain, severe tiredness, aches, or generally feeling sick. A list of these symptoms is on the Warning Card given to you by your pharmacist. You should carry this Warning Card with you. If you notice these symptoms while taking abacavir, stop taking abacavir and call your prescriber or health care professional immediately. If you have this serious reaction, you must never take abacavir (Ziagen®), abacavir; lamivudine; zidovudine (Trizivir™), or abacavir; lamivudine (Epzicom™) again. If you stop taking abacavir for another medical reason and restart therapy, you may develop an allergic reaction, even if you have taken abacavir before without any problems. If you develop a skin rash or any other symptoms of an allergic reaction, stop taking abacavir and call your prescriber or health care professional immediately. This reaction may occur days to weeks after you restart abacavir therapy. Abacavir will not cure HIV and you can still get other illnesses or complications associated with your disease. Taking abacavir does not reduce the risk of passing HIV infection to others through sexual or blood contact. It is best to avoid sexual contact so that you do not spread the disease to others. For any sexual contact, use a condom. Be careful about cuts, abrasions and other possible sources of blood contact. Never share a needle or syringe with anyone.

What side effects might I notice from taking abacavir?

Some patients may develop a severe allergic reaction to abacavir. You may be having this reaction if you have 2 or more of the following:
- skin rash
- fever
- nausea, vomiting, diarrhea, stomach pain
- sore throat, shortness of breath, wheezing, cough
- fatigue, achiness, general discomfort such as flu-like symptoms

If you think you are having a reaction, STOP taking abacavir and call your prescriber or health care professional right away. Some of these side effects may occur and not lead to an allergic reaction. Check with your prescriber or health care professional if you have any questions. Other side effects that you should report to your prescriber or health care professional as soon as possible:

- bone pain
- changes in body appearance (such as weight gain or loss around the waist and/or face)
- numbness or tingling

Side effects that usually do not require medical attention (report to your prescriber or health care professional if they continue):

- headache
- loss of appetite
- trouble sleeping

Where can I keep my medicine?

Keep out of the reach of children in a container that small children cannot open. Store at room temperature between 20 and 25 degrees C (68 and 77 degrees F). Do not freeze. Throw away any unused medicine after the expiration date.

Abacavir; Lamivudine, 3TC tablets

This drug requires an FDA medication guide. See page xxxvii.

EPZICOM®; 600 mg/300 mg; Tablet GlaxoSmithKline

What are abacavir; lamivudine, 3TC tablets?

ABACAVIR; LAMIVUDINE (3TC) (Epzicom®) is used to treat human immunodeficiency virus (HIV) infection. Abacavir and lamivudine are all antiviral drugs called nucleoside reverse transcriptase inhibitors or NRTIs. This combination may reduce the amount of HIV in the blood and increase the number of CD4 cells (T-cells) in the blood. This product is used in combination with other drugs to treat the HIV virus. This drug will not cure or prevent HIV infection or AIDS. You may still develop other infections or conditions associated with HIV. Generic abacavir; lamivudine tablets are not available.

What should my health care professional know before I receive abacavir; lamivudine, 3TC?

They need to know if you have any of these conditions:

- kidney disease
- liver disease
- pancreatitis
- tingling or numbness in the hands or feet
- an unusual reaction to abacavir, lamivudine, 3TC, other medicines, foods, dyes, or preservatives
- pregnant or trying to get pregnant
- breast-feeding

How should this medicine be used?

Take abacavir; lamivudine tablets by mouth. Follow the directions on the prescription label. Swallow tablets with a drink of water. This drug can be taken with or without food. Take your doses at regular intervals. Do not take your medicine more often than directed. To help to make sure that your anti-HIV therapy works as well as possible, be very careful to take all of your medicine exactly as prescribed. Do not stop taking except on your prescriber's advice. Contact your pediatrician or health care professional regarding the use of this medicine in children. Special care may be needed.

What if I miss a dose?

If you miss a dose, take it as soon as you can. If it is almost time for your next dose, take only that dose. Do not take double or extra doses.

What may interact with abacavir; lamivudine, 3TC?

- alcohol
- indinavir
- methadone
- ribavirin
- sulfamethoxazole; trimethoprim, SMX-TMP (Bactrim®, Septra®)
- zalcitabine, ddC

Tell your prescriber or health care professional about all other medicines you are taking, including non-prescription medicines, nutritional supplements, or herbal products. Also tell your prescriber or health care professional if you are a frequent user of drinks with caffeine or alcohol, if you smoke, or if you use illegal drugs. These may affect the way your medicine works. Check with your health care professional before stopping or starting any of your medicines.

What should I watch for while taking abacavir; lamivudine, 3TC?

Visit your prescriber or health care professional for regular checks on your progress. Discuss any new symptoms with your prescriber or health care professional. A small number of people might have a severe allergic reaction to abacavir. If you have a skin rash or two or more of the following symptoms you may be having this type of reaction: fever, nausea, vomiting, stomach pain, severe tiredness, aches, or generally feeling sick. A list of these symptoms is on the Warning Card given to you by your pharmacist. You should carry this Warning Card with you. If you notice these symptoms while taking abacavir; lamivudine, stop taking this drug and call your prescriber or health care professional immediately. If you have this serious reaction, you must never take abacavir (Ziagen®), abacavir; lamivudine (Epzicom®), or abacavir; lamivudine; zidovudine (Trizivir®) again. If you stop then restart abacavir or abacavir; lamivudine therapy, you may develop an allergic reaction, even if you have taken one of these drugs before without any problems. If you develop a skin rash or any other symptoms of an allergic reaction, stop taking this drug and call your prescriber or health

This drug requires an FDA medication guide. See page xxxvii.

care professional immediately. This reaction may occur days to weeks after you restart abacavir; lamivudine therapy. Tell your prescriber or health care professional if you get tingling, pain or numbness in your hands or feet. Abacavir; lamivudine will not cure HIV and you can still get other illnesses or complications associated with your disease. Taking abacavir; lamivudine does not reduce the risk of passing HIV infection to others through sexual or blood contact. It is best to avoid sexual contact so that you do not spread the disease to others. For any sexual contact, use a condom. Be careful about cuts, abrasions and other possible sources of blood contact. Never share a needle or syringe with anyone.

What side effects may I notice from receiving Abacavir; Lamivudine, 3TC?

Some patients may develop a severe allergic reaction to abacavir. You may be having this reaction if you have 2 or more of the following:
- skin rash
- fever
- nausea, vomiting, diarrhea, stomach pain
- sore throat, shortness of breath, wheezing, cough
- fatigue, achiness, general discomfort such as flu-like symptoms

If you think you are having a reaction, STOP taking abacavir; lamivudine (Epzicom™) and call your prescriber or health care professional right away. Some of these side effects may occur and not lead to an allergic reaction. Check with your prescriber or health care professional if you have any questions. Other side effects that you should report to your prescriber or health care professional as soon as possible:
- bone pain
- changes in body appearance (such as weight gain or loss around the waist and/or face)
- numbness or tingling
- unusual weakness

Side effects that usually do not require medical attention (report to your prescriber or health care professional if they continue):
- dizziness
- headache
- loss of appetite
- trouble sleeping

Where can I keep my medicine?

Keep out of the reach of children in a container that small children cannot open. Store at room temperature between 20 and 25 degrees C (68 and 77 degrees F). Do not freeze. Throw away any unused medicine after the expiration date.

Abacavir; Lamivudine, 3TC; Zidovudine, ZDV tablets

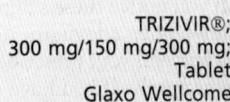

TRIZIVIR®;
300 mg/150 mg/300 mg;
Tablet
Glaxo Wellcome

What are abacavir; lamivudine; zidovudine tablets?

ABACAVIR; LAMIVUDINE (3TC); ZIDOVUDINE (ZDV) (Trizivir™) is used to treat human immunodeficiency virus (HIV) infection. Abacavir, lamivudine, and zidovudine are all antiviral drugs called nucleoside reverse transcriptase inhibitors or NRTIs. This combination may reduce the amount of HIV in the blood and increase the number of CD4 cells (T-cells) in the blood. This product is used in combination with other drugs to treat the HIV virus. This drug will not cure or prevent HIV infection or AIDS. You may still develop other infections or conditions associated with HIV. Generic abacavir; lamivudine; zidovudine (Trizivir™) tablets are not available.

What should my health care professional know before I take abacavir; lamivudine; zidovudine?

They need to know if you have any of these conditions:
- kidney disease
- liver disease
- tingling or numbness in the hands or feet
- an unusual or allergic reaction to abacavir, lamivudine, zidovudine, other medicines, foods, dyes, or preservatives

- pregnant or trying to get pregnant
- breast-feeding

How should I take this medicine?

Take abacavir; lamivudine; zidovudine (Trizivir™) tablets by mouth. Follow the directions on the prescription label. Swallow tablets with a drink of water. This drug can be taken with or without food. Take your doses at regular intervals. Do not take your medicine more often than directed. To help to make sure that your anti-HIV therapy works as well as possible, be very careful to take all of your medicine exactly as prescribed. Do not stop taking except on your prescriber's advice. This medicine is not recommended for use in patients weighing less than 88 pounds (40 kilograms) or children.

What if I miss a dose?

If you miss a dose, take it as soon as you can. If it is almost time for your next dose, take only that dose. Do not take double or extra doses.

What may interact with abacavir; lamivudine; zidovudine?

- alcohol
- atovaquone

- fluconazole
- methadone
- probenecid
- ribavirin
- valproic acid
- zalcitabine, ddC

Tell your prescriber or health care professional about all other medicines you are taking, including nonprescription medicines, nutritional supplements, or herbal products. Also tell your prescriber or health care professional if you are a frequent user of drinks with caffeine or alcohol, if you smoke, or if you use illegal drugs. These may affect the way your medicine works. Check with your health care professional before stopping or starting any of your medicines.

What should I watch for while taking abacavir; lamivudine; zidovudine?

Visit your prescriber or health care professional for regular checks on your progress. Discuss any new symptoms with your prescriber or health care professional. A small number of people might have a severe allergic reaction to abacavir. If you have a skin rash or two or more of the following symptoms you may be having this type of reaction: fever, nausea, vomiting, stomach pain, severe tiredness, aches, or generally feeling sick. A list of these symptoms is on the Warning Card given to you by your pharmacist. You should carry this Warning Card with you. If you notice these symptoms while taking abacavir; lamivudine; zidovudine (Trizivir®), stop taking this drug and call your prescriber or health care professional immediately. If you have this serious reaction, you must never take abacavir (Ziagen®) or abacavir; lamivudine; zidovudine (Trizivir®) again. If you stop then restart abacavir; lamivudine; zidovudine (Trizivir®) therapy, you may develop an allergic reaction, even if you have taken this drug before without any problems. If you develop a skin rash or any other symptoms of an allergic reaction, stop taking this drug and call your prescriber or health care professional immediately. This reaction may occur days to weeks after you restart abacavir; lamivudine; zidovudine (Trizivir®) therapy. Tell your prescriber or health care professional if you get tingling, pain or numbness in your hands or feet. Abacavir; lamivudine; zidovudine (Trizivir®) will not cure HIV and you can still get other illnesses or complications associated with your disease. Taking abacavir does not reduce the risk of passing HIV infection to others through sexual or blood contact. It is best to avoid sexual contact so that you do not spread the disease to others. For any sexual contact, use a condom. Be careful about cuts, abrasions and other possible sources of blood contact. Never share a needle or syringe with anyone.

What side effects might I notice from taking abacavir; lamivudine; zidovudine?

Some patients may develop a severe allergic reaction to abacavir. You may be having this reaction if you have 2 or more of the following:
- skin rash
- fever
- nausea, vomiting, diarrhea, stomach pain
- sore throat, shortness of breath, wheezing, cough
- fatigue, achiness, general discomfort such as flu-like symptoms

If you think you are having a reaction, STOP taking abacavir; lamivudine; zidovudine (Trizivir®) and call your prescriber or health care professional right away. Some of these side effects may occur and not lead to an allergic reaction. Check with your prescriber or health care professional if you have any questions. Other side effects that you should report to your prescriber or health care professional as soon as possible:
- bone pain
- changes in body appearance (such as weight gain or loss around the waist and/or face)
- numbness or tingling
- unusual weakness
- unusual bleeding or bruising

Side effects that usually do not require medical attention (report to your prescriber or health care professional if they continue):
- dizziness
- headache
- loss of appetite
- trouble sleeping

Where can I keep my medicine?

Keep out of the reach of children in a container that small children cannot open. Store at room temperature between 20 and 25 degrees C (68 and 77 degrees F). Do not freeze. Throw away any unused medicine after the expiration date.

Acarbose tablets

PRECOSE®;
50 mg; Tablet
Bayer Corp
Pharmaceutical Div

PRECOSE®;
25 mg; Tablet
Bayer Corp
Pharmaceutical Div

A

What are acarbose tablets?

ACARBOSE (Precose®) lowers blood sugar in patients with diabetes. It slows the entry of certain sugars from food in the intestine into the body. Because it acts to reduce the absorption of sugars or starches in food, it must be taken with meals. Treatment is combined with a balanced diet and exercise. Acarbose may be used with some other diabetic medications. Generic acarbose tablets are not yet available.

What should my health care professional know before I take acarbose?

They need to know if you have any of these conditions:
- hiatal hernia
- kidney disease
- liver disease
- stomach or bowel disease, or obstruction
- an unusual or allergic reaction to acarbose, other medicines, foods, dyes, or preservatives
- pregnant or trying to get pregnant
- breast-feeding

How should I take this medicine?

Take acarbose tablets by mouth. Follow the directions on the prescription label. Swallow the tablets at the start of a main meal, with a drink of water if necessary. Take your doses at regular intervals. Do not take your medicine more often than directed. If you develop severe vomiting or severe diarrhea that prevents you from eating meals, call your health care prescriber for advice. Contact your pediatrician or health care professional regarding the use of this medicine in children. Special care may be needed.

What if I miss a dose?

If you forgot your dose at the start of your meal and you are still eating that meal, take your dose while you are still eating. Otherwise, skip the missed dose. Acarbose is not effective if not taken during a meal. Wait for your next dose at your next main meal, and take only that dose. Do not take double or extra doses.

What may interact with acarbose?

- acetaminophen
- charcoal
- cholestyramine
- colestipol
- digoxin
- neomycin
- other medicines for diabetes
- pancrelipase, pancreatin, amylase, or other digestive enzyme supplements
- warfarin

Many medications may cause changes (increase or decrease) in blood sugar, these include:
- alcohol containing beverages
- beta-blockers, often used for high blood pressure or heart problems (examples include atenolol, metoprolol, propranolol)
- chromium
- female hormones, such as estrogens, progestins, or contraceptive pills
- isoniazid
- male hormones or anabolic steroids
- medications to suppress appetite or for weight loss
- medicines for allergies, asthma, cold, or cough
- niacin
- pentamidine
- phenytoin
- some herbal dietary supplements
- steroid medicines such as prednisone or cortisone
- thyroid hormones
- water pills (diuretics)

Tell your prescriber or health care professional about all other medicines that you are taking, including non-prescription medicines, nutritional supplements, or herbal products. Also tell your prescriber or health care professional if you are a frequent user of drinks with caffeine or alcohol, if you smoke, or if you use illegal drugs. These may affect the way your medicine works. Check with your health care professional before stopping or starting any of your medicines.

What should I watch for while taking acarbose?

Visit your prescriber or health care professional for regular checks on your progress. Learn how to monitor your blood sugar. Acarbose does not cause symptoms of hypoglycemia (too low blood sugar) by itself, but if given with another antidiabetic medicine, it may increase their potential to lower blood sugar. If you do take acarbose in combination with other medications, you and family members must learn to recognize and how to treat symptoms of low blood sugar. *If you are taking acarbose with other diabetic medications:* Because acarbose prevents the breakdown of table sugar you must always keep a supply of glucose or dextrose tablets or solution readily available to treat low blood sugar events if they occur. Ask your pharmacist to help you find these products at the store. Wear a medical identification bracelet or chain to say you have diabetes, and carry a card that lists all your medications.

What side effects may I notice from taking acarbose?

Side effects that you should report to your prescriber or health care professional as soon as possible:

Rare:
- skin rash or itching
- unusual tiredness
- weight loss
- yellowing of the eyes or skin, dark or brown color to the urine, or loss of appetite

In combination with other diabetic medications, (like glyburide, glipizide, metformin or insulin), acarbose may cause hypoglycemia (low blood glucose). Contact your health care professional if you experience symptoms of low blood sugar, which may include:
- anxiety or nervousness
- confusion
- difficulty concentrating
- hunger
- pale skin
- nausea
- fatigue
- sweating
- headache
- palpitations
- numbness of the mouth
- tingling in the fingers
- tremors

- muscle weakness
- blurred vision
- cold sensations
- uncontrolled yawning
- irritability
- rapid heartbeat
- shallow breathing
- loss of consciousness

Side effects that usually do not require medical attention (report to your prescriber or health care professional if they continue or are bothersome):
These side effects with acarbose are usually minor but very common. They include:
- bloated feeling
- diarrhea
- stomach or intestinal gas or rumbling stomach
- stomach pain or discomfort

Where can I keep my medicine?

Keep out of the reach of children in a container that small children cannot open. Store at room temperature between 15 and 30 degrees C (59 and 86 degrees F). Keep away from wet or moist areas, like the bathroom. Throw away any unused medicine after the expiration date.

Acebutolol capsules

SECTRAL®;
400 mg; Capsule
ESP Pharma Inc

ACEBUTOLOL
HYDROCHLORIDE;
200 mg; Capsule
Mylan
Pharmaceuticals Inc

What are acebutolol capsules?

ACEBUTOLOL (Sectral®) belongs to a group of medicines called beta-blockers. Beta-blockers reduce the workload on the heart and help it to beat more regularly. Acebutolol is used to control high blood pressure (hypertension), and to treat or prevent certain heart rhythm problems (ventricular arrhythmias). Acebutolol does not cure high blood pressure. Generic acebutolol capsules are available.

What should my health care professional know before I take acebutolol?

They need to know if you have any of these conditions:
- asthma or bronchitis
- blood vessel disease (such as Raynaud's disease)
- depression
- diabetes
- emphysema
- history of heart attack, or heart disease
- kidney disease
- liver disease
- muscle weakness or disease
- psoriasis
- thyroid disease
- an unusual or allergic reaction to acebutolol, other beta-blockers, medicines, foods, dyes, or preservatives
- pregnant or trying to get pregnant
- breast-feeding

How should I take this medicine?

Take acebutolol capsules by mouth. Follow the directions on the prescription label. Swallow the capsules whole with a drink of water. Take your doses at regular intervals. Do not take your medicine more often than directed. Do not stop taking except on your prescriber's advice. Contact your pediatrician or health care professional regarding the use of this medicine in children. Special care may be needed.

What if I miss a dose?

If you miss a dose, take it as soon as you can. If it is almost time for your next dose, take only that dose. Do not take double or extra doses. There should be at least 4 hours between doses.

What may interact with acebutolol?

- cimetidine
- cocaine
- hawthorn
- medicines for colds and breathing difficulties
- medicines for diabetes
- medicines for high blood pressure
- medicines to control heart rhythm
- water pills

Tell your prescriber or health care professional about all other medicines you are taking, including nonprescription medicines, nutritional supplements, or herbal

products. Also tell your prescriber or health care professional if you are a frequent user of drinks with caffeine or alcohol, if you smoke, or if you use illegal drugs. These may affect the way your medicine works. Check with your health care professional before stopping or starting any of your medicines.

What should I watch for while taking acebutolol?

Check your heart rate and blood pressure regularly while you are taking acebutolol. Ask your prescriber or health care professional what your heart rate and blood pressure should be, and when you should contact him or her. Do not stop taking this medicine suddenly. This could lead to serious heart-related effects. You may get drowsy or dizzy. Do not drive, use machinery, or do anything that requires mental alertness until you know how acebutolol affects you. To reduce the risk of dizzy or fainting spells, do not sit or stand up quickly. Alcohol can make you more drowsy, increase flushing, and cause rapid heartbeats. Therefore, it is best to avoid alcoholic drinks. Acebutolol can affect blood sugar levels. If you are diabetic, check with your prescriber or health care professional before you change your diet or the dose of your diabetic medicine. If you are going to have surgery, tell your prescriber or health care professional that you are taking acebutolol.

What side effects may I notice from taking acebutolol?

Side effects that you should report to your prescriber or health care professional as soon as possible:

- changes in vision
- chest pain
- cold, tingling, or numb hands or feet
- confusion
- difficulty breathing, wheezing
- dizziness or fainting spells
- irregular heartbeat
- muscle aches and pains
- skin rash
- slow heart rate (less than recommended by your prescriber or health care professional)
- sweating
- swollen legs or ankles
- tremor, shakes
- vomiting

Side effects that usually do not require medical attention (report to your prescriber or health care professional if they continue or are bothersome):

- anxiety
- depression, nightmares
- diarrhea
- difficulty sleeping
- dry itching skin
- dry or burning eyes
- headache
- nausea
- unusual tiredness

Where can I keep my medicine?

Keep out of the reach of children in a container that small children cannot open. Store at room temperature between 15 and 30 degrees C (59 and 86 degrees F). Throw away any unused medicine after the expiration date.

Acetaminophen tablets, caplets, or chewable tablets

EQUATE® PAIN RELIEVER;
500 mg; Tablet
Perrigo Company

What are acetaminophen tablets, caplets, or chewable tablets?

ACETAMINOPHEN (Tylenol®, Panadol®, Feverall®, Equate®, and many others) is used to relieve mild to moderate pain and reduce fever. It is the preferred treatment for patients with aspirin allergy, ulcers, or clotting (bleeding) disorders. Patients who are taking medicines to treat gout can safely take acetaminophen. There are many generic variations available for adults and children. Tablets can be plain, extended-release, or chewable. Gelcaps or geltabs are also available.

What should my health care professional know before I take acetaminophen?

They need to know if you have any of these conditions:
- anemia
- drink more than 3 alcohol-containing drinks per day

- infection
- kidney disease
- liver disease
- hepatitis
- phenylketonuria
- an unusual or allergic reaction to acetaminophen, aspirin, other medicines, foods, dyes or preservatives

How should I take this medicine?

Acetaminophen can be taken as needed for the relief of pain or fever, or may be prescribed by the prescriber or health care professional on a more regular basis. Do not take more often than directed, or more than the recommended dose. Acetaminophen tablets come in several strengths for children and adults. Make sure you are taking or giving the correct dose. Take acetaminophen tablets, caplets or gelcaps by mouth. Follow the directions on the label. Chewable tablets can be chewed before swallowing, crushed and taken with tablets whole, do not crush or chew. Drink a full glass of water either with or after taking your medicine. Contact your pediatrician or health care professional regarding the use of this medicine in children. Special care may be needed. Do not administer adult acetaminophen preparations to children.

What if I miss a dose?

If your prescriber or health care professional has prescribed a regular schedule and you miss a dose, take it as soon as you can. If it is almost time for your next dose, take only that dose. Do not take double or extra doses.

What may interact with acetaminophen?

- alcohol
- medicines for seizures
- antacids
- cimetidine
- medicines for mental problems and psychotic disturbances
- warfarin

Tell your prescriber or health care professional about all other medicines you are taking, including non-prescription medicines, nutritional supplements, or herbal products. Also tell your prescriber or health care professional if you are a frequent user of drinks with caffeine or alcohol, if you smoke, or if you use illegal drugs. These may affect the way your medicine works. Check with your health care professional before stopping or starting any of your medicines.

What should I watch for while taking acetaminophen?

Do not treat yourself for pain for more than 10 days (5 days for children) without checking with your prescriber or health care professional. If you are treating a fever, check with your prescriber or health care professional if the fever lasts for more than 3 days. Report any possible overdose promptly to your prescriber or health care professional as soon as possible. The effects of excessive doses may not be obvious for several days. Avoid alcoholic drinks if you are taking acetaminophen on a regular basis. Alcohol can increase possible damage to your liver. Many non-prescription medicines contain acetaminophen as an ingredient. Always read the labels carefully to avoid taking an accidental overdose, which can be dangerous. Certain acetaminophen products containing the artificial sweetener aspartame (Nutrasweet®). Acetaminophen can affect the results from some blood-sugar tests used by diabetic patients. Check with your prescriber or health care professional before you change your diet or the dose of your diabetic medicine. If you are receiving cancer chemotherapy or other immunosuppression medicine, do not take acetaminophen without checking with your prescriber or health care professional. Acetaminophen may hide the signs of an infection such as fever or pain.

What side effects may I notice from taking acetaminophen?

If you take acetaminophen as recommended, serious side effects are uncommon.

Side effects that you should report to your prescriber or health care professional as soon as possible:
- skin rash or hives
- unusual bleeding or bruising, pinpoint red spots on the skin
- difficulty breathing, wheezing
- bloody or black, tarry stools
- decrease in amount of urine passed
- not willing to eat
- fever or sore throat
- nausea, vomiting
- stomach cramps and pain
- unusual tiredness or weakness
- yellowing of the skin or eyes

Where can I keep my medicine?

Keep out of reach of children in a container that small children cannot open. Acetaminophen can be dangerous to children. Avoid accidental overdose of acetaminophen as this may result in severe effects and possibly death. Store at room temperature between 15 and 30 degrees C (59 and 86 degrees F). Protect from moisture and light. Throw away any unused medicine after the expiration date.

Acetaminophen; Aspirin, ASA; Caffeine tablets, caplets, or geltabs

EXCEDRIN®;
250 mg/250 mg/65 mg; Tablet
Bristol Myers Squibb Co

What are acetaminophen; aspirin, ASA; caffeine tablets, caplets, or geltabs?

ACETAMINOPHEN; ASPIRIN, ASA; CAFFEINE (Excedrin® Extra Strength, Excedrin® Migraine) is a combination product used to relieve mild to moderate pain caused by arthritis, colds, headache (including migraine), muscle aches, menstrual discomfort, sinusitis, and toothache. Generic acetaminophen; aspirin, ASA; caffeine tablets, caplets, or geltabs are available.

What should my health care professional know before I take acetaminophen; aspirin, ASA; caffeine?

They need to know if you have any of these conditions:
- anemia

- anxiety
- asthma
- bleeding or clotting problems
- diabetes
- drink more than 3 alcohol-containing drinks per day
- heart disease
- high blood pressure
- infection
- kidney disease
- liver disease
- nasal polyps
- panic disorder
- peptic ulcer disease
- skin problems
- sleeplessness
- stomach ulcers
- thyroid disease
- viral illness, such as the flu or chickenpox
- vitamin K deficiency
- an unusual or allergic reaction to acetaminophen, aspirin, caffeine, other medicines, foods, dyes or preservatives
- pregnant or trying to get pregnant
- breast-feeding

How should I take this medicine?

Take acetaminophen; aspirin, ASA; caffeine tablets, caplets, or geltabs by mouth. Follow the directions on the prescription label. Swallow tablets or capsules whole with a full glass of water; take tablets or capsules in an upright or sitting position. Taking a sip of water first, before taking the tablets or capsules, may help you swallow them. If possible take bedtime doses at least 10 minutes before lying down. If the medication upsets your stomach, you can take it with food or milk. Do not take more than 8 tablets, caplets, or geltabs a day. If taking for migraine headache, stop using if migraine headache worsens or continues for more than 48 hours. Contact your pediatrician or health care professional regarding the use of this medicine in children. Special care may be needed.

What if I miss a dose?

If you miss a dose, take it as soon as you can. If it is almost time for your next dose, take only that dose. Do not take double or extra doses.

What may interact with acetaminophen; aspirin, ASA; caffeine?

- alcohol
- antacids
- anti-inflammatory drugs (NSAIDs such as ibuprofen)
- blood thinners or other drugs which may affect bleeding
- cimetidine
- Ginkgo biloba
- grapefruit juice
- hormones such as prednisone or cortisone
- medicines for colds and breathing difficulties
- medicines for diabetes that are taken by mouth
- medicines for seizures
- methotrexate
- medicines for mental problems and psychotic disturbances
- medicines that stimulate or keep you awake
- probenecid
- warfarin

Tell your prescriber or health care professional about all other medicines that you are taking, including non-prescription medicines, nutritional supplements, or herbal products. Also tell your prescriber or health care professional if you are a frequent user of drinks with caffeine or alcohol, if you smoke, or if you use illegal drugs. These may affect the way your medicine works. Check with your health care professional before stopping or starting any of your medicines.

What should I watch for while taking acetaminophen; aspirin, ASA; caffeine?

Check with your prescriber or health care professional if you are treating yourself for a pain that does not go away after 10 days; and for a fever that does not go away after 3 days or keeps coming back. Stop using if you experience new or unexpected symptoms, ringing in the ears, or loss of hearing. Many non-prescription medicines contain acetaminophen and aspirin as an ingredient. To prevent accidental acetaminophen or aspirin overdose, read labels carefully and do not take more than one product that contains acetaminophen and/or aspirin. Report any possible overdose promptly to your prescriber or health care professional as soon as possible. The effects of excessive doses may not be obvious for several days. If you have had surgery do not take acetaminophen; aspirin, ASA; caffeine for 5 days, unless your prescriber or health care professional tells you to. The aspirin can interfere with your body's ability to stop bleeding. If you are diabetic, acetaminophen; aspirin, ASA; caffeine may alter your blood sugar levels. Check with your prescriber or health care professional before you change your diet or the dose of your diabetic medicine. Acetaminophen; aspirin, ASA; caffeine can irritate your stomach. Drinking alcohol and smoking cigarettes can make this irritation worse and may cause ulcers or bleeding problems. Ask your prescriber or health care professional for help to stop smoking or drinking. Do not lie down for 30 minutes after taking acetaminophen; aspirin, ASA; caffeine to prevent irritation to your throat. Alcohol can also increase possible damage to your liver. If you are receiving cancer chemotherapy or other immunosuppression medicine, do not take acetaminophen; aspirin, ASA; caffeine without checking with your prescriber or health care professional. Acetaminophen; aspirin, ASA; caffeine may hide the signs of an infection such as fever or pain and increase your risk of bleeding. Do not take acetaminophen; aspirin, ASA; caffeine close to bedtime. It may prevent you from sleeping. When you are taking acetaminophen; aspirin, ASA; caffeine, avoid food and drinks that contain additional caffeine. Do not take acetaminophen; aspirin, ASA; caffeine with other non-prescription medicines, especially cold and allergy medicines, without asking your prescriber or health care professional for advice. Do not take acetaminophen; aspirin, ASA; caffeine with grapefruit juice, this can increase the effects of caffeine.

What side effects may I notice from taking acetaminophen; aspirin, ASA; caffeine?

Side effects that you should report to your prescriber or health care professional as soon as possible:
- anxiety or panic reactions
- black, tarry stools
- confusion
- decrease in amount of urine passed
- difficulty breathing, wheezing
- dizziness, drowsiness
- fast or irregular breathing or heartbeat (palpitations)
- fever or sore throat
- lightheadedness or fainting spells
- muscle twitching
- nausea, vomiting
- not willing to eat
- pain on swallowing
- ringing in the ears
- seizures (convulsions)

- skin rash or hives
- stomach cramps and pain
- trembling
- unusual bleeding or bruising, red or purple spots on the skin
- unusual tiredness or weakness
- vomiting up blood, or what looks like coffee grounds
- yellowing of the skin or eyes

Side effects that usually do not require medical attention (report to your prescriber or health care professional if they continue or are bothersome):
- diarrhea
- frequent passing of urine
- headache
- nausea, vomiting
- nervousness, restlessness
- stomach gas, heartburn, or mild upset stomach

Where can I keep my medicine?

Keep out of the reach of children in a container that small children cannot open. Do not share or give this medicine to anyone else. Store at room temperature between 15 and 30 degrees C (59 and 86 degrees F). Keep container tightly closed. Throw away any unused medicine after the expiration date.

Acetaminophen; Butalbital tablets or capsules

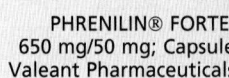
PHRENILIN® FORTE;
650 mg/50 mg; Capsule
Valeant Pharmaceuticals

What are Acetaminophen; Butalbital tablets or capsules?

ACETAMINOPHEN; BUTALBITAL (Sedapap®, Phrenilin® Forte, and others) is a combination product used to treat certain types of headaches. Federal law prohibits the transfer of acetaminophen; butalbital to any person other than the patient for whom it was prescribed. Do not share this medicine with any one else. Generic acetaminophen; butalbital tablets and capsules are available.

What should my health care professional know before I receive acetaminophen; butalbital?

They need to know if you have any of these conditions:
- anorexia or bulimia
- attempted suicide
- drink more than 3-alcohol containing drinks per day
- drug abuse or use of illicit drugs
- heart disease
- high or low blood pressure
- infection
- kidney disease
- liver disease
- lung disease or breathing problems
- mental depression or mental problems
- porphyria
- an unusual or allergic reaction to acetaminophen, butalbital or other barbiturates, other medicines, foods, dyes, or preservatives

- pregnant or trying to get pregnant
- breast-feeding

How should this medicine be used?

Take acetaminophen; butalbital tablets or capsules by mouth. Follow the directions on the prescription label. Swallow the tablets or capsules with a drink of water. If acetaminophen; butalbital upsets your stomach, take it with food or milk. Do not take your medicine more often than directed. If you take acetaminophen; butalbital on a regular basis, do not stop taking the drug suddenly. You may have very bad side effects if you stop taking the drug all at once. Talk with your doctor about how to stop taking acetaminophen; butalbital. Contact your pediatrician or health care professional regarding the use of this medicine in children. Special care may be needed. Do not share this medicine with anyone.

What if I miss a dose?

If it is almost time for your next dose, take only that dose. Do not take double or extra doses.

What may interact with acetaminophen; butalbital?

- alcohol
- female hormones, including contraceptive or birth control pills
- isoniazid

- medicines for depression or other mental health problems
- medicines for pain
- medicines to control heart rhythm
- rifampin
- seizure medicine
- theophylline
- valerian
- warfarin
- zidovudine

Because acetaminophen; butalbital can cause drowsiness, other medicines that also cause drowsiness may increase this effect of acetaminophen; butalbital. Some other medicines that cause drowsiness are:

- alcohol-containing medicines
- certain antidepressants or tranquilizers
- muscle relaxants
- certain antihistamines used in cold medicines

Tell your prescriber or health care professional about all other medicines you are taking, including non-prescription medicines, nutritional supplements, or herbal products. Also tell your prescriber or health care professional if you are a frequent user of drinks with caffeine or alcohol, if you smoke, or if you use illegal drugs. These may affect the way your medicine works. Check with your health care professional before stopping or starting any of your medicines.

What should I watch for while taking acetaminophen; butalbital?

Visit your prescriber or health care professional for regular checks on your progress. After taking acetaminophen; butalbital you may get a residual hangover effect that leaves you drowsy or dizzy. Do not drive, use machinery, or do anything that needs mental alertness until you know how acetaminophen; butalbital affects you. To reduce dizzy or fainting spells, do not sit or stand up quickly, especially if you are an older patient. Avoid alcoholic drinks while you are taking acetaminophen; butalbital. Alcohol can increase possible damage to your liver and can increase possible unpleasant effects. Acetaminophen; butalbital can stop birth control pills (oral contraceptives) from working properly. Use another method of birth control while you are taking acetaminophen; butalbital. Do not take acetaminophen; butalbital more often than you are instructed. If you have been taking butalbital on a regular basis, you can get withdrawal symptoms if you stop taking the product suddenly. Symptoms may include tiredness, dizziness, headache, anxiety, or nervousness. If you need to stop taking acetaminophen; butalbital, talk with your doctor about how to stop gradually. Do not take acetaminophen; butalbital with other non-prescription medicines, especially cold and allergy medicines without asking your prescriber or health care professional for advice. Many non-prescription medicines contain acetaminophen as an ingredient. Always read the labels carefully to avoid taking too much acetaminophen, which can be dangerous. If acetaminophen; butalbital upsets your stomach, you may take it with food. If you are receiving cancer chemotherapy or other immunosuppression medicine, do not take acetaminophen; butalbital without checking with your prescriber or health care professional. Acetaminophen; butalbital may hide the signs of an infection, such as fever or pain. If you think you may have an infection, immediately call your doctor. If you are going to have surgery, tell your prescriber or health care professional that you are taking acetaminophen; butalbital.

What side effects may I notice from taking acetaminophen; butalbital?

Side effects that you should report to your prescriber or health care professional as soon as possible:

- changes in behavior, mood, or mental ability
- seizures
- severe stomach pain
- difficulty breathing or shortness of breath
- fever, sore throat
- hallucinations
- lightheadedness or fainting spells
- redness, blistering, peeling or loosening of the skin, including inside the mouth
- skin rash, itching, hives
- slow or fast heartbeat
- swelling of the face or lips
- unusual bleeding or bruising, pinpoint red spots on the skin
- unusual tiredness or weakness
- yellowing of skin or eyes

Side effects that usually do not require medical attention (report to your prescriber or health care professional if they continue or are bothersome):

- confusion, agitation
- constipation
- clumsiness, unsteadiness, or a "hang-over" effect
- difficulty sleeping or nightmares
- drowsiness, dizziness
- headache
- irritability, nervousness
- nausea or vomiting

Where can I keep my medicine?

Keep out of the reach of children in a container that small children cannot open. Store at room temperature between 15 and 30 degrees C (59 and 86 degrees F). Keep your medicine in the original container and keep the container tightly closed. Throw away any unused medicine after the expiration date.

A

Acetaminophen; Butalbital; Caffeine tablets or capsules

ESGIC®;
325 mg/50 mg/40
mg; Tablet
Gilbert Laboratories

ZEBUTAL™;
500 mg/50 mg/40
mg; Capsule
First Horizon
Pharmaceutical Corp

What are acetaminophen-butalbital-caffeine tablets or capsules?

ACETAMINOPHEN-BUTALBITAL-CAFFEINE (Fioricet®, Esgic®, Endolor®, Zebutal™, and others) is a combination product used to treat certain types of headaches and migraines as well as mild to moderate pain. Federal law prohibits the transfer of acetaminophen-butalbital-caffeine to any person other than the patient for whom it was prescribed. Do not share this medicine with any one else. Generic acetaminophen-butalbital-caffeine tablets and capsules are available.

What should my health care professional know before I take acetaminophen; butalbital; caffeine?

They need to know if you have any of these conditions:
- anemia
- attempted suicide
- diabetes mellitus
- drink more than 3-alcohol containing drinks per day
- drug abuse or use of illicit drugs
- heart disease
- high or low blood pressure
- infection
- kidney disease
- liver disease
- lung disease or breathing difficulties
- mental depression or mental problems
- peptic ulcer disease
- porphyria
- thyroid disease
- an unusual or allergic reaction to acetaminophen, butalbital or other barbiturates, caffeine, other medicines, foods, dyes, or preservatives
- pregnant or trying to get pregnant
- breast-feeding

How should I take this medicine?

Take acetaminophen-butalbital-caffeine tablets or capsules by mouth. Follow the directions on the prescription label. Swallow the tablets or capsules with a drink of water. If acetaminophen-butalbital-caffeine upsets your stomach, take it with food or milk. Do not take your medicine more often than directed. Contact your pediatrician or health care professional regarding the use of this medicine in children. Special care may be needed. Do not share this medicine with anyone.

What if I miss a dose?

If it is almost time for your next dose, take only that dose. Do not take double or extra doses.

What may interact with acetaminophen-butalbital-caffeine?

- alcohol
- cyclosporine
- corticosteroids
- female hormones, including contraceptive or birth control pills
- grapefruit juice
- medicines for high blood pressure or other heart problems
- medicines for depression or other mental health problems
- medicines for pain
- medicines to control heart rhythm
- quinine
- seizure medicine
- theophylline
- warfarin

Because acetaminophen-butalbital-caffeine can cause drowsiness, other medicines that also cause drowsiness may increase this effect of acetaminophen-butalbital-caffeine. Some other medicines that cause drowsiness are:

- alcohol-containing medicines
- certain antidepressants or tranquilizers
- muscle relaxants
- certain antihistamines used in cold medicines

Tell your prescriber or health care professional about all other medicines that you are taking, including non-prescription medicines, nutritional supplements, or herbal products. Also, tell your prescriber or health care professional if you are a frequent user of drinks with caffeine or alcohol, if you smoke, or if you use illegal drugs. These may affect the way your medicine works. Check with your health care professional before stopping or starting any of your medicines.

What should I watch for while taking acetaminophen-butalbital-caffeine?

Visit your prescriber or health care professional for regular checks on your progress. After taking acetaminophen-butalbital-caffeine you may get a residual hangover effect that leaves you drowsy or dizzy. Do not drive, use machinery, or do anything that needs mental alertness until you know how acetaminophen-butalbital-caffeine affects you. To reduce dizzy or fainting spells, do not sit or stand up quickly, especially if you are an older patient. Avoid alcoholic drinks while you are taking acetaminophen-butalbital-caffeine. Alcohol can increase possible damage to your liver and can increase possible unpleasant effects. Acetaminophen-butalbital-caffeine can stop birth control pills (oral contraceptives) from working properly. Use another method of birth control while you are taking acetaminophen-butalbital-caffeine. If you have been taking caffeine or butalbital on a regular basis, you can get withdrawal symptoms if you stop taking them. Symptoms include tiredness, dizziness, headache, anxiety, or nervousness. Try to avoid foods and drinks that contain caffeine while taking acetaminophen-butalbital-caffeine. Do not take acetaminophen-butalbital-caffeine with other non-prescription medicines, especially cold and allergy medicines without asking your prescriber or health care professional for advice. Grapefruit juice may increase the effects of acetaminophen-butalbital-caffeine. Many non-prescription medicines contain acetaminophen as an ingredient. Always read the labels carefully to avoid taking an accidental overdose, which can be dangerous. If you are receiving cancer chemotherapy or other immunosuppression medicine, do not take acetaminophen-butalbital-caffeine without checking with your prescriber or health care professional. Acetaminophen-butalbital-caffeine may hide the signs of an infection such as fever or pain. If you are going to have surgery, tell your prescriber or health care professional that you are taking acetaminophen-butalbital-caffeine.

What side effects may I notice from taking acetaminophen-butalbital-caffeine?

Side effects that you should report to your prescriber or health care professional as soon as possible:
- bone tenderness
- changes in behavior, mood, or mental ability
- seizures
- difficulty breathing or shortness of breath
- eye problems, very small or enlarged centers to the eyes
- fever, sore throat
- hallucinations
- lightheadedness or fainting spells
- redness, blistering, peeling or loosening of the skin, including inside the mouth
- skin rash, itching, hives
- slow or fast heartbeat
- swelling of the face or lips
- unusual bleeding or bruising, pinpoint red spots on the skin
- unusual tiredness or weakness
- yellowing of skin or eyes

Side effects that usually do not require medical attention (report to your prescriber or health care professional if they continue or are bothersome):
- confusion, agitation
- trembling
- increased frequency passing urine
- constipation
- clumsiness, unsteadiness, or a "hang-over" effect
- difficulty sleeping or nightmares
- drowsiness, dizziness
- headache
- irritability, nervousness
- nausea or vomiting

Where can I keep my medicine?

Keep out of the reach of children in a container that small children cannot open. Store at room temperature between 15 and 30 degrees C (59 and 86 degrees F). Keep container tightly closed. Throw away any unused medicine after the expiration date.

Acetaminophen; Butalbital; Caffeine; Codeine capsules

| FIORICET® WITH CODEINE; 325 mg/50 mg/40 mg/30 mg; Capsule Novartis Pharmaceuticals | | ACETAMINOPHEN; BUTALBITAL; CAFFEINE; CODEINE; 325 mg/50 mg/40 mg/30 mg; Capsule Qualitest Pharmaceuticals Inc | |

What are acetaminophen-butalbital-caffeine-codeine capsules?

ACETAMINOPHEN-BUTALBITAL-CAFFEINE-CODEINE (Fioricet® with Codeine) is a combination product used to treat certain types of headaches and migraines as well as mild to moderate pain. Federal law prohibits the transfer of acetaminophen-butalbital-caffeine-codeine to any person other than the patient for whom it was prescribed. Do not share this medicine with any one else. Generic acetaminophen-butalbital-caffeine-codeine capsules are available.

What should my health care professional know before I take acetaminophen-butalbital-caffeine-codeine?

They need to know if you have any of these conditions:
- anemia
- depression
- diabetes mellitus
- drink more than 3-alcohol containing drinks per day
- heart disease
- high or low blood pressure
- infection
- kidney disease

- liver disease
- lung disease or breathing difficulties
- peptic ulcer disease
- porphyria
- thyroid disease
- ulcerative colitis or other intestinal diseases
- an unusual or allergic reaction to acetaminophen, butalbital or other barbiturates, caffeine, codeine, other medicines, foods, dyes, or preservatives
- pregnant or trying to get pregnant
- breast-feeding

How should I take this medicine?

Take acetaminophen-butalbital-caffeine-codeine capsules by mouth. Follow the directions on the prescription label. Swallow the tablets or capsules with a drink of water. If this medicine upsets your stomach, take it with food or milk. Do not take your medicine more often than directed. Contact your pediatrician or health care professional regarding the use of this medicine in children. Special care may be needed. Do not share this medicine with anyone.

What if I miss a dose?

If it is almost time for your next dose (within 2 hours), take only that dose. Do not take double or extra doses.

What may interact with acetaminophen-butalbital-caffeine-codeine?

- alcohol
- carbamazepine
- corticosteroids
- cyclosporine
- divalproex
- female hormones, including contraceptive or birth control medications
- grapefruit juice
- medicines for high blood pressure or other heart problems
- medicines for depression or other mental health problems
- medicines for pain
- medicines to control heart rhythm
- phenobarbital
- phenytoin
- quinine
- theophylline
- valproic acid
- warfarin

Because this medicine can cause drowsiness, other medicines that also cause drowsiness may increase this effect of acetaminophen-butalbital-caffeine-codeine.
Some other medicines that cause drowsiness are:

- alcohol-containing medicines
- certain antidepressants or tranquilizers
- muscle relaxants
- certain antihistamines used in cold medicines

Tell your prescriber or health care professional about all other medicines that you are taking, including non-prescription medicines, nutritional supplements, or herbal products. Also, tell your prescriber or health care professional if you are a frequent user of drinks with caffeine or alcohol, if you smoke, or if you use illegal drugs. These may affect the way your medicine works. Check with your health care professional before stopping or starting any of your medicines.

What should I watch for while taking acetaminophen-butalbital-caffeine-codeine?

Visit your prescriber or health care professional for regular checks on your progress. If you have been taking this medication regularly for a long time, do not suddenly stop taking it without your prescribers advice. Your prescriber may want you to decrease your dose gradually. Acetaminophen-butalbital-caffeine-codeine you may cause drowsiness or dizziness. Do not drive, use machinery, or do anything that needs mental alertness until you know how this medicine affects you. To reduce dizzy spells, do not sit or stand up quickly, especially if you are an older patient. Avoid alcoholic drinks while you are taking acetaminophen-butalbital-caffeine-codeine. Alcohol can increase possible damage to your liver and can increase possible unpleasant effects. Acetaminophen-butalbital-caffeine-codeine can stop birth control pills (oral contraceptives) from working properly. Use another method of birth control while you are taking this medicine. Try to avoid foods and drinks that contain caffeine while taking this medicine. Do not take acetaminophen-butalbital-caffeine-codeine with other non-prescription medicines, especially cold and allergy medicines without asking your prescriber or health care professional for advice. Many non-prescription medicines contain acetaminophen as an ingredient. Always read the labels carefully to avoid taking an accidental overdose, which can be dangerous. If you are receiving cancer chemotherapy or other immunosuppression medicine, do not take acetaminophen-butalbital-caffeine-codeine without checking with your prescriber or health care professional. Acetaminophen-butalbital-caffeine-codeine may hide the signs of an infection such as fever or pain. If you are going to have surgery, tell your prescriber or health care professional that you are taking acetaminophen-butalbital-caffeine-codeine.

What side effects may I notice from taking acetaminophen-butalbital-caffeine-codeine?

Side effects that you should report to your prescriber or health care professional as soon as possible:
- changes in behavior, mood, or mental ability
- difficulty breathing or shortness of breath
- eye problems, very small or enlarged centers to the eyes
- lightheadedness or fainting spells
- redness, blistering, peeling or loosening of the skin, including inside the mouth
- skin rash, itching, hives
- slow or fast heartbeat
- swelling of the face or lips
- yellowing of skin or eyes

Side effects that usually do not require medical attention (report to your prescriber or health care professional if they continue or are bothersome):

- confusion, agitation
- trembling
- increased frequency passing urine
- constipation
- clumsiness, unsteadiness, or a "hang-over" effect
- difficulty sleeping or nightmares

- drowsiness, dizziness
- irritability, nervousness
- nausea or vomiting

Where can I keep my medicine?

Keep out of the reach of children in a container that small children cannot open. Store at room temperature between 15 and 30 degrees C (59 and 86 degrees F). Keep container tightly closed. Throw away any unused medicine after the expiration date.

Acetaminophen; Caffeine; Dihydrocodeine capsules or tablets

PANLOR® SS;
712.8 mg/
60 mg/32 mg; Tablet
PamLab, LLC

What are acetaminophen; caffeine; dihydrocodeine capsules or tablets?

ACETAMINOPHEN; CAFFEINE; DIHYDROCODEINE (Panlor® DC capsules, Panlor® SS tablets) are used to treat moderate to severe pain. Federal law prohibits the transfer of acetaminophen; caffeine; dihydrocodeine to any person other than the patient for whom it was prescribed. Do not share this medicine with anyone. Generic acetaminophen; caffeine; dihydrocodeine capsules or tablets are not available.

What should my health care professional know before I take acetaminophen; caffeine; dihydrocodeine?

They need to know if you have any of these conditions:

- depression
- diabetes mellitus
- drink more than 3-alcohol containing drinks per day
- G6PD deficiency
- heart disease
- high or low blood pressure
- infection
- kidney disease
- liver disease
- lung disease or breathing difficulties
- peptic ulcer disease
- seizures
- thyroid disease
- ulcerative colitis or other intestinal diseases
- an unusual reaction to acetaminophen, caffeine, dihydrocodeine, codeine, other medicines, foods, dyes, or preservatives
- pregnant or trying to get pregnant
- breast-feeding

How should this medicine be taken?

Take acetaminophen; caffeine; dihydrocodeine capsules or tablets by mouth. Follow the directions on the prescription label. Swallow the tablets or capsules with a drink of water. If the medicine upsets your stomach, take it with food or milk. Do not take your medicine more often than directed. Contact your pediatrician or health care professional regarding the use of this medicine in children. Special care may be needed. Do not share this medicine with anyone.

What if I miss a dose?

If it is almost time for your next dose (within 2 hours), take only the next scheduled dose. Do not take double or extra doses.

What may interact with acetaminophen; caffeine; dihydrocodeine?

- alcohol
- antacids
- carbamazepine
- ciprofloxacin
- corticosteroids
- cyclosporine
- grapefruit juice
- lithium
- medicines for high blood pressure or other heart problems
- medicines for depression or other mental health problems, especially MAO inhibitors
- medicines for pain
- medicines to control heart rhythm
- medicines for sleep or anxiety
- medicines to prevent or treat tuberculosis
- phenobarbital
- quinidine
- theophylline
- tramadol
- warfarin

Because this medicine can cause drowsiness, other medicines that also cause drowsiness may increase this effect of acetaminophen; caffeine; dihydrocodeine.
Some other medicines that cause drowsiness are:

- alcohol-containing medicines
- certain antidepressants or tranquilizers
- muscle relaxants
- certain antihistamines used in cold medicines

Tell your prescriber or health care professional about all other medicines you are taking, including nonprescription medicines, nutritional supplements, or herbal products. Also tell your prescriber or health care professional if you are a frequent user of drinks with caffeine or alcohol, if you smoke, or if you use illegal drugs. These may affect the way your medicine works. Check with your health care professional before stopping or starting any of your medicines.

What should I watch for while taking acetaminophen; caffeine; dihydrocodeine?

Visit your prescriber or health care professional for regular checks on your progress. If you have been taking this medication regularly for a long time, do not suddenly stop taking it without your prescribers advice. Your prescriber may want you to decrease your dose gradually. Acetaminophen; caffeine; dihydrocodeine may cause drowsiness or dizziness. Do not drive, use machinery, or do anything that needs mental alertness until you know how this medicine affects you. To reduce dizzy spells, do not sit or stand up quickly, especially if you are an older patient. Avoid alcoholic drinks while you are taking acetaminophen; caffeine; dihydrocodeine. Alcohol can increase possible damage to your liver and can increase possible unpleasant effects. Acetaminophen; caffeine; dihydrocodeine may cause constipation. If your bowel habits (frequency and amount) change, tell your health care professional immediately. Try to avoid foods and drinks that contain caffeine while taking this medicine. Do not take acetaminophen; caffeine; dihydrocodeine with other non-prescription medicines, especially cold and allergy medicines without asking your prescriber or health care professional for advice. Many non-prescription medicines contain acetaminophen as an ingredient. Always read the labels carefully to avoid taking an accidental overdose, which can be dangerous. If you are receiving cancer chemotherapy or other immunosuppression medicine, do not take acetaminophen; caffeine; dihydrocodeine without checking with your prescriber or health care professional. Acetaminophen; caffeine; dihydrocodeine may hide the signs of an infection, such as fever or pain. If you are going to have surgery, tell your prescriber or health care professional that you are taking acetaminophen; caffeine; dihydrocodeine.

What side effects may I notice from taking acetaminophen; caffeine; dihydrocodeine?

Side effects that you should report to your prescriber or health care professional as soon as possible:
- agitation or other changes in behavior or mood
- confusion
- difficulty breathing or shortness of breath
- fainting spells
- redness, blistering, peeling or loosening of the skin, including inside the mouth
- skin rash, itching, hives
- slow or fast heartbeat
- swelling of the face or lips
- yellowing of skin or eyes
- tremors
- vision changes

Side effects that usually do not require medical attention (report to your prescriber or health care professional if they continue or are bothersome):
- constipation
- drowsiness or dizziness
- nausea or upset stomach

Where can I keep my medicine?

Keep out of the reach of children in a container that small children cannot open. Store at room temperature between 15 and 30 degrees C (59 and 86 degrees F). Keep container tightly closed. Throw away any unused medicine after the expiration date.

Acetaminophen; Codeine tablets or capsules

ACETAMINOPHEN; Codeine; 300 mg/15 mg; Tablet Mallinckrodt Inc Pharmaceuticals Group

TYLENOL® WITH CODEINE; 300 mg/30 mg; Tablet OMP Div, Ortho-McNeil Pharmaceuticals

What are acetaminophen-codeine tablets or capsules?

ACETAMINOPHEN-CODEINE (Tylenol® #3, Pyregesic-C™ and others) is a combination of two different types of pain medicine and is used to treat mild to moderate pain. Federal law prohibits the transfer of acetaminophen-codeine to any person other than the patient for whom it was prescribed. Generic acetaminophen-codeine tablets and capsules are available.

What should my health care professional know before I take acetaminophen-codeine?

They need to know if you have any of these conditions:

- drink more than 3 alcohol-containing drinks per day
- anemia
- infection
- heart or circulation problems
- lung disease or breathing difficulties
- kidney disease
- liver disease
- problems urinating
- seizures or other neurologic disorders
- hepatitis
- constipation
- an unusual or allergic reaction to acetaminophen, codeine, other opiate analgesics, foods, dyes or preservatives
- pregnant or trying to get pregnant
- breast-feeding

How should I take this medicine?

Take acetaminophen-codeine tablets or capsules by mouth. Follow the directions on the prescription label. Swallow the tablets whole with a full glass of water. You can take acetaminophen-codeine with food to prevent stomach upset. Do not take your medicine more often than directed. Contact your pediatrician or health care professional regarding the use of this medicine in children. Special care may be needed. Do not share this medicine with anyone.

What if I miss a dose?

If you miss a dose, take it as soon as you can. If it is almost time for your next dose, take only that dose. Do not take double or extra doses.

What may interact with acetaminophen-codeine?

- medicines for seizures
- medicines for high blood pressure
- alcohol
- warfarin
- cimetidine
- antacids

Because acetaminophen-codeine can cause drowsiness, other medicines that also cause drowsiness may increase this effect of acetaminophen-codeine. Some other medicines that cause drowsiness are:

- alcohol-containing medicines
- barbiturates such as phenobarbital
- certain antidepressants or tranquilizers
- muscle relaxants
- certain antihistamines used in cold medicines

Tell your prescriber or health care professional about all other medicines you are taking, including non-prescription medicines, nutritional supplements, or herbal products. Also tell your prescriber or health care professional if you are a frequent user of drinks with caffeine or alcohol, if you smoke, or if you use illegal drugs. These may affect the way your medicine works. Check with your health care professional before stopping or starting any of your medicines.

What should I watch for while taking acetaminophen-codeine?

Tell your prescriber or health care professional if your pain does not go away, if it gets worse, or if you have new or different type of pain. Do not take other pain medicines with acetaminophen-codeine without advice. Use exactly as directed by your prescriber or health care professional. Do not take more than the recommended dose due to the possibility of liver damage or effects on your breathing. If you get flu-like symptoms (fever, chills, muscle aches and pains), call your prescriber or health care professional; do not treat yourself. If you are receiving cancer chemotherapy or other immunosuppression medicine, do not take acetaminophen-containing products without checking with your prescriber or health care professional. Acetaminophen may hide the signs of an infection such as fever or pain. To reduce unpleasant effects on your throat and stomach, take acetaminophen-codeine with a full glass of water and never just before lying down. You may also take it with food or milk. Acetaminophen-codeine may make you drowsy when you first start taking it or change doses. Do not drive, use machinery, or do anything that needs mental alertness until you know how acetaminophen-codeine affects you. Do not sit or stand up quickly. This reduces the risk of dizzy or fainting spells. These effects may be worse if you are an older patient. The drowsiness should decrease after taking acetaminophen-codeine for a couple of days. If you have not slept because of your pain, you may sleep more the first few days your pain is controlled to catch-up on missed sleep. Be careful taking other medicines that may also make you tired. This effect may be worse when taking these medicines with acetaminophen-codeine. Alcohol can increase possible drowsiness, dizziness, confusion and affect your breathing. Alcohol can increase possible damage to your liver. Avoid alcohol while taking acetaminophen-codeine. Acetaminophen-codeine can cause constipation. Make sure to take a laxative and/or a stool softener. Try to have a bowel movement at least every 2 to 3 days. If you do not have a bowel movement for 3 days or more call your prescriber or health care professional. They may recommend using an enema or suppository to help you move your bowels. Many non-prescription medicines contain acetaminophen as an ingredient. Always read the labels carefully to avoid taking an accidental overdose, which can be dangerous. Acetaminophen can affect the results from some blood sugar tests used by diabetic patients. Check with your prescriber or health care professional before you change your diet or the dose of your diabetic medicine. If you are going to have surgery tell your prescriber or health care professional that you are taking acetaminophen-codeine.

What side effects may I notice from taking acetaminophen-codeine?

Elderly patients are more likely to get side effects. Side effects that you should report to your prescriber or health care professional as soon as possible:

- chest pain or irregular heartbeat
- difficulty breathing, wheezing
- severe rash
- cold, clammy skin
- unusual weakness
- fever, chills, muscle aches and pains

Side effects that usually do not require medical attention (report to your prescriber or health care professional if they continue or are bothersome):

- constipation
- dizziness, drowsiness
- confusion
- gas or heartburn

- nausea, vomiting
- dry mouth
- itching
- pinpoint pupils

Where can I keep my medicine?

Keep out of the reach of children in a container that small children cannot open. Do not share or give this medicine to anyone else. Avoid accidental swallowing of acetaminophen-codeine by someone (especially children) other than for whom it was prescribed as this may result in severe side effects and possibly death. Store at room temperature between 15 and 30 degrees C (59 and 86 degrees F). Protect from light. Keep container tightly closed. Throw away any unused medicine after the expiration date.

Acetaminophen; Dichloralphenazone; Isometheptene capsules

MIDRIN®;
325 mg/100 mg/65 mg;
Capsule
Women First Healthcare Inc

What are acetaminophen; dichloralphenazone; isometheptene capsules?

ACETAMINOPHEN; DICHLORALPHENA-ZONE; ISOMETHEPTENE (Amidrine®, Dura-drin™, Midchlor®, Midrin®, Migquin™, Migratine®, Migrazone™, Migrex™, Mitride™) is a combination product used to treat migraine or tension-type headaches. Federal law prohibits the transfer of this drug to any person other than the patient for whom it was prescribed. Do not share this medicine with anyone else. Generic acetaminophen; dichloralphenazone; isometheptene capsules are available.

What should my health care professional know before I take acetaminophen; dichloralphenazone; isometheptene?

They need to know if you have any of these conditions:
- bleeding or clotting problems
- diabetes mellitus
- drink more than 3 alcohol-containing drinks per day
- glaucoma
- head injury
- heart disease
- high blood pressure
- infection
- kidney disease
- liver disease
- lung problems
- porphyria
- skin problems
- stomach ulcer
- suppressed immune function
- thyroid disease
- an unusual or allergic reaction to acetaminophen, dichloralphenazone, isometheptene, other medicines, foods, dyes or preservatives
- pregnant or trying to get pregnant
- breast-feeding

How should I take this medicine?

Take acetaminophen; dichloralphenazone; isometheptene capsules by mouth at the first sign of a migraine headache. Follow the directions on the prescription label. Swallow the capsules with a drink of water, and follow with plenty of liquid. If taking for migraine headache, do not take more than 5 capsules in any 12-hour period. If taking for tension headache, do not take more than 8 capsules a day. Ask your prescriber how many capsules you should take per day. Stop using if headache worsens or continues for more than 48 hours. This medicine is not for use in children.

What if I miss a dose?

If you miss a dose, take it as soon as you can. If it is almost time for your next dose, take only that dose. Do not take double or extra doses.

What may interact with acetaminophen; dichloralphenazone; isometheptene?

- alcohol
- antacids
- antihistamines
- bromocriptine
- certain antibiotics
- cimetidine
- disulfiram
- entacapone
- medicines for anxiety or sleep problem
- medicines for mental problems and psychotic disturbances
- monoamine oxidase inhibitors (MAOIs) such as isocarboxazid and phenelzine—do not take acetaminophen; dichloralphenazone; isometheptene within 2 weeks of stopping MAOI therapy
- omeprazole
- ritonavir
- tramadol
- warfarin

Tell your prescriber or health care professional about all other medicines that you are taking, including nonprescription medicines, nutritional supplements, or herbal products. Also tell your prescriber or health care professional if you are a frequent user of drinks with caffeine or alcohol, if you smoke, or if you use illegal drugs. These may affect the way your medicine works. Check with your health care professional before stopping or starting any of your medicines.

What should I watch for while taking acetaminophen; dichloralphenazone; isometheptene?

Many non-prescription medicines contain acetaminophen as an ingredient. To prevent accidental acetamin-

A

ophen overdose, read labels carefully and do not take more than one product that contains acetaminophen. Report any possible overdose promptly to your prescriber or health care professional as soon as possible. The effects of excessive doses may not be obvious for several days. Avoid drinking alcohol. Alcohol can make your headaches worse and increase the side effects of this medicine. Acetaminophen; dichloralphenazone; isometheptene products can cause dizziness or drowsiness. Driving or operating machinery, or performing other tasks that require mental alertness requires caution when taking this medicine. You should not participate in these activities until you determine how this medicine affects you. If you are receiving cancer chemotherapy or other immunosuppression medicine, do not take acetaminophen; dichloralphenazone; isometheptene without checking with your prescriber or health care professional. Acetaminophen; dichloralphenazone; isometheptene may hide the signs of an infection such as fever or pain. Do not take acetaminophen; dichloralphenazone; isometheptene with other non-prescription medicines, especially cold and allergy medicines, without asking your prescriber or health care professional for advice.

What side effects may I notice from taking acetaminophen; dichloralphenazone; isometheptene?

Side effects that you should report to your prescriber or health care professional as soon as possible:
- difficulty breathing, wheezing
- fast or irregular breathing or heartbeat (palpitations)
- fever or sore throat
- redness, blistering, peeling or loosening of the skin, including inside the mouth
- skin rash or hives
- unusual bleeding or bruising
- unusual tiredness or weakness
- yellowing of the skin or eyes

Side effects that usually do not require medical attention (report to your prescriber or health care professional if they continue or are bothersome):
- dizziness
- drowsiness
- nausea
- mild upset stomach

Where can I keep my medicine?

Keep out of the reach of children in a container that small children cannot open. Do not share or give this medicine to anyone else. Store at room temperature between 15 and 30 degrees C (59 and 86 degrees F). Keep container tightly closed. Throw away any unused medicine after the expiration date.

Acetaminophen; Hydrocodone tablets or capsules

LORCET®-HD; 500 mg/5 mg; Capsule Forest Laboratories Inc

VICODIN®; 500 mg/5 mg; Tablet Abbott Pharmaceutical Product Division

What are acetaminophen-hydrocodone tablets or capsules?

ACETAMINOPHEN-HYDROCODONE (Lortab®, Lorcet®, Vicodin®, and others) is a combination of two different types of pain medicine and is used to treat moderate to severe pain. Federal law prohibits the transfer of acetaminophen-hydrocodone to any person other than the patient for whom it was prescribed. Generic acetaminophen-hydrocodone tablets and capsules are available. Acetaminophen-hydrocodone is also available as caplets.

What should my health care professional know before I take acetaminophen-hydrocodone?

They need to know if you have any of these conditions:
- drink more than 3 alcohol-containing drinks per day
- anemia
- infection
- heart or circulation problems
- lung disease or breathing difficulties
- kidney disease
- liver disease
- problems urinating
- seizures or other neurologic disorders
- hepatitis
- constipation
- an unusual or allergic reaction to acetaminophen, hydrocodone, other opioid analgesics, foods, dyes or preservatives
- pregnant or trying to get pregnant
- breast-feeding

How should I take this medicine?

Take acetaminophen-hydrocodone tablets or capsules by mouth. Follow the directions on the prescription label. Swallow the tablets whole with a full glass of water. You can take acetaminophen-hydrocodone with food to prevent stomach upset. Do not take your medicine more often than directed. Contact your pediatrician or health care professional regarding the use of this medicine in children. Special care may be needed. Do not share this medicine with anyone.

What if I miss a dose?

If you miss a dose, take it as soon as you can. If it is almost time for your next dose, take only that dose. Do not take double or extra doses.

A

What may interact with acetaminophen-hydrocodone?

- medicines for seizures
- medicines for high blood pressure
- alcohol
- warfarin
- cimetidine
- antacids

Because acetaminophen-hydrocodone can cause drowsiness, other medicines that also cause drowsiness may increase this effect of acetaminophen-hydrocodone. Some other medicines that cause drowsiness are:

- alcohol-containing medicines
- barbiturates such as phenobarbital
- certain antidepressants or tranquilizers
- muscle relaxants
- certain antihistamines used in cold medicines

Tell your prescriber or health care professional about all other medicines you are taking, including non-prescription medicines, nutritional supplements, or herbal products. Also tell your prescriber or health care professional if you are a frequent user of drinks with caffeine or alcohol, if you smoke, or if you use illegal drugs. These may affect the way your medicine works. Check with your health care professional before stopping or starting any of your medicines.

What should I watch for while taking acetaminophen-hydrocodone?

Tell your prescriber or health care professional if your pain does not go away, if it gets worse, or if you have new or different type of pain. Do not take other pain medicines with acetaminophen-hydrocodone without advice. Use exactly as directed by your prescriber or health care professional. Do not take more than the recommended dose due to the possibility of liver damage or effects on your breathing. If you get flu-like symptoms (fever, chills, muscle aches and pains), call your prescriber or health care professional; do not treat yourself. If you are receiving cancer chemotherapy or other immunosuppression medicine, do not take acetaminophen without checking with your prescriber or health care professional. Acetaminophen may hide the signs of an infection such as fever or pain. To reduce unpleasant effects on your throat and stomach, take acetaminophen-hydrocodone with a full glass of water and never just before lying down. You may also take it with food or milk. Acetaminophen-hydrocodone may make you drowsy when you first start taking it or change doses. Do not drive, use machinery, or do anything that needs mental alertness until you know how acetaminophen-hydrocodone affects you. Do not sit or stand up quickly. This reduces the risk of dizzy or fainting spells. These effects may be worse if you are an older patient. The drowsiness should decrease after taking acetaminophen-hydrocodone for a couple of days. If you have not slept because of your pain, you may sleep more the first few days your pain is controlled to catch up on missed sleep. Be careful taking other medicines that may also make you tired. This effect may be worse when taking these medicines with acetaminophen-hydrocodone. Alcohol can increase possible drowsiness, dizziness, confusion and affect your breathing. Alcohol can increase possible damage to your liver. Avoid alcohol while taking acetaminophen-hydrocodone. Acetaminophen-hydrocodone can cause constipation. Make sure to take a laxative and/or a stool softener. Try to have a bowel movement at least every 2 to 3 days. If you do not have a bowel movement for 3 days or more call your prescriber or health care professional. They may recommend using an enema or suppository to help you move your bowels. Many non-prescription medicines contain acetaminophen as an ingredient. Always read the labels carefully to avoid taking an accidental overdose, which can be dangerous. Acetaminophen can affect the results from some blood sugar tests used by diabetic patients. Check with your prescriber or health care professional before you change your diet or the dose of your diabetic medicine. If you are going to have surgery tell your prescriber or health care professional that you are taking acetaminophen-hydrocodone.

What side effects may I notice from taking acetaminophen-hydrocodone?

Elderly patients are more likely to get side effects. Side effects that you should report to your prescriber or health care professional as soon as possible:

- chest pain or irregular heartbeat
- difficulty breathing, wheezing
- severe rash
- cold, clammy skin
- unusual weakness
- fever, chills, muscle aches and pains

Side effects that usually do not require medical attention (report to your prescriber or health care professional if they continue or are bothersome):

- constipation
- dizziness, drowsiness
- confusion
- gas or heartburn
- nausea, vomiting
- dry mouth
- itching
- flushing
- pinpoint pupils

Where can I keep my medicine?

Keep out of the reach of children in a container that small children cannot open. Do not share or give this medicine to anyone else. Avoid accidental swallowing of acetaminophen-hydrocodone by someone (especially children) other than for whom it was prescribed as this may result in severe side effects and possibly death. Store at room temperature between 15 and 30 degrees C (59 and 86 degrees F). Protect from light. Keep container tightly closed. Throw away any unused medicine after the expiration date.

Acetaminophen; Oxycodone tablets or capsules

PERCOCET®;
325 mg/5 mg; Tablet
Endo
Pharmaceuticals Inc

TYLOX®;
500 mg/5 mg;
Capsule
Janssen Ortho, LLC

What are acetaminophen-oxycodone tablets or capsules?

ACETAMINOPHEN-OXYCODONE (Percocet®, Roxicet®, Tylox®, Roxilox®) is a combination of two different types of pain medicine and is used to treat moderate to severe pain. Federal law prohibits the transfer of acetaminophen-oxycodone to any person other than the patient for whom it was prescribed. Generic acetaminophen-oxycodone tablets and capsules are available. Acetaminophen-oxycodone is also available as caplets.

What should my health care professional know before I take acetaminophen-oxycodone?

They need to know if you have any of these conditions:
- drink more than 3 alcohol-containing drinks per day
- anemia
- infection
- heart or circulation problems
- lung disease or breathing difficulties
- kidney disease
- liver disease
- problems urinating
- seizures or other neurologic disorders
- hepatitis
- constipation
- an unusual or allergic reaction to acetaminophen, oxycodone, other opioid analgesics, foods, dyes or preservatives
- pregnant or trying to get pregnant
- breast-feeding

How should I take this medicine?

Take acetaminophen-oxycodone tablets or capsules by mouth. Follow the directions on the prescription label. Swallow the tablets whole with a full glass of water. You can take acetaminophen-oxycodone with food to prevent stomach upset. Do not take your medicine more often than directed. Contact your pediatrician or health care professional regarding the use of this medicine in children. Special care may be needed. Do not share this medicine with anyone.

What if I miss a dose?

If you miss a dose, take it as soon as you can. If it is almost time for your next dose, take only that dose. Do not take double or extra doses.

What may interact with acetaminophen-oxycodone?

- medicines for seizures
- medicines for high blood pressure
- alcohol
- warfarin
- cimetidine
- antacids

Because acetaminophen-oxycodone can cause drowsiness, other medicines that also cause drowsiness may increase this effect of acetaminophen-oxycodone. Some other medicines that cause drowsiness are:

- alcohol-containing medicines
- barbiturates such as phenobarbital
- certain antidepressants or tranquilizers
- muscle relaxants
- certain antihistamines used in cold medicines

Tell your prescriber or health care professional about all other medicines you are taking, including non-prescription medicines, nutritional supplements, or herbal products. Also tell your prescriber or health care professional if you are a frequent user of drinks with caffeine or alcohol, if you smoke, or if you use illegal drugs. These may affect the way your medicine works. Check with your health care professional before stopping or starting any of your medicines.

What should I watch for while taking acetaminophen-oxycodone?

Tell your prescriber or health care professional if your pain does not go away, if it gets worse, or if you have new or different type of pain. Do not take other pain medicines with acetaminophen-oxycodone without advice. Use exactly as directed by your prescriber or health care professional. Do not take more than the recommended dose due to the possibility of liver damage or effects on your breathing. If you get flu-like symptoms (fever, chills, muscle aches and pains), call your prescriber or health care professional; do not treat yourself. If you are receiving cancer chemotherapy or other immunosuppression medicine, do not take acetaminophen without checking with your prescriber or health care professional. Acetaminophen may hide the signs of an infection such as fever or pain. To reduce unpleasant effects on your throat and stomach, take acetaminophen-oxycodone with a full glass of water and never just before lying down. You may also take it with food or milk. Acetaminophen-oxycodone may make you drowsy when you first start taking it or change doses. Do not drive, use machinery, or do anything that needs mental alertness until you know how acetaminophen-oxycodone affects you. Do not sit or stand up quickly. This reduces the risk of dizzy or fainting spells. These effects may be worse if you are an older patient. The drowsiness should decrease after taking acetaminophen-oxycodone for a couple of days. If you have not slept because of your pain, you may sleep more the first few days your pain is controlled to catch-up

A

on missed sleep. Be careful taking other medicines that may also make you tired. This effect may be worse when taking these medicines with acetaminophen-oxycodone. Alcohol can increase possible drowsiness, dizziness, confusion and affect your breathing. Alcohol can increase possible damage to your liver. Avoid alcohol while taking acetaminophen-oxycodone. Acetaminophen-oxycodone can cause constipation. Make sure to take a laxative and/or a stool softener. Try to have a bowel movement at least every 2 to 3 days. If you do not have a bowel movement for 3 days or more call your prescriber or health care professional. They may recommend using an enema or suppository to help you move your bowels. Many non-prescription medicines contain acetaminophen as an ingredient. Always read the labels carefully to avoid taking an accidental overdose, which can be dangerous. Acetaminophen can affect the results from some blood sugar tests used by diabetic patients. Check with your prescriber or health care professional before you change your diet or the dose of your diabetic medicine. If you are going to have surgery tell your prescriber or health care professional that you are taking acetaminophen-oxycodone.

What side effects may I notice from taking acetaminophen-oxycodone?

Elderly patients are more likely to get side effects. Side effects that you should report to your prescriber or health care professional as soon as possible:

- chest pain or irregular heartbeat
- difficulty breathing, wheezing
- severe rash
- cold, clammy skin
- seizures
- unusual weakness
- fever, chills, muscle aches and pains

Side effects that usually do not require medical attention (report to your prescriber or health care professional if they continue or are bothersome):

- constipation
- dizziness, drowsiness
- confusion
- gas or heartburn
- nausea, vomiting
- dry mouth
- itching
- flushing
- pinpoint pupils

Where can I keep my medicine?

Keep out of the reach of children in a container that small children cannot open. Do not share or give this medicine to anyone else. Avoid accidental swallowing of acetaminophen-oxycodone by someone (especially children) other than for whom it was prescribed as this may result in severe side effects and possibly death. Store at room temperature between 15 and 30 degrees C (59 and 86 degrees F). Protect from light. Keep container tightly closed. Throw away any unused medicine after the expiration date.

Acetaminophen; Propoxyphene tablets

DARVOCET-N®;
650 mg/100 mg; Tablet
Eli Lilly and Co

What are acetaminophen-propoxyphene tablets?

ACETAMINOPHEN-PROPOXYPHENE (Darvocet-N® 50, Darvocet-N® 100, Darvocet A500™, Wygesic®) is a combination of two different types of pain medicine and is used to treat mild to moderate pain. Federal law prohibits the transfer of acetaminophen-propoxyphene to any person other than the patient for whom it was prescribed. Generic acetaminophen; propoxyphene tablets are available for Darvcocet-N® 100, Darvcocet-N® 50, and Wygesic®.

What should my health care professional know before I take acetaminophen-propoxyphene?

They need to know if you have any of these conditions:
- drink more than 3 alcohol-containing drinks per day
- anemia
- infection
- heart or circulation problems
- lung disease or breathing difficulties
- kidney disease
- liver disease
- problems urinating

- seizures or other neurologic disorders
- hepatitis
- constipation
- an unusual or allergic reaction to acetaminophen, propoxyphene, other opiate analgesics, foods, dyes or preservatives
- pregnant or trying to get pregnant
- breast-feeding

How should I take this medicine?

Take acetaminophen-propoxyphene tablets by mouth. Follow the directions on the prescription label. You can take acetaminophen-propoxyphene with food to prevent stomach upset. Do not take your medicine more often than directed. Contact your pediatrician or health care professional regarding the use of this medicine in children. Special care may be needed. Do not share this medicine with anyone.

What if I miss a dose?

If you miss a dose, take it as soon as you can. If it is almost time for your next dose, take only that dose. Do not take double or extra doses.

What may interact with acetaminophen-propoxyphene?

- medicines for seizures
- medicines for high blood pressure
- alcohol
- warfarin
- cimetidine
- antacids

Because acetaminophen-propoxyphene can cause drowsiness, other medicines that also cause drowsiness may increase this effect of acetaminophen-propoxyphene. Some other medicines that cause drowsiness are:

- alcohol-containing medicines
- barbiturates such as phenobarbital
- certain antidepressants or tranquilizers
- muscle relaxants
- certain antihistamines used in cold medicines

Tell your prescriber or health care professional about all other medicines that you are taking, including non-prescription medicines, nutritional supplements, or herbal products. Also tell your prescriber or health care professional if you are a frequent user of drinks with caffeine or alcohol, if you smoke, or if you use illegal drugs. These may affect the way your medicine works. Check with your health care professional before stopping or starting any of your medicines.

What should I watch for while taking acetaminophen-propoxyphene?

Tell your prescriber or health care professional if your pain does not go away, if it gets worse, or if you have new or different type of pain. Do not take other painkillers with acetaminophen-propoxyphene without advice. Use exactly as directed by your prescriber or health care professional. Do not take more than the recommended dose due to the possibility of liver or kidney damage. If you get flu-like symptoms (fever, chills, muscle aches and pains), call your prescriber or health care professional; do not treat yourself. To reduce unpleasant effects on your throat and stomach, take acetaminophen-propoxyphene with food or milk and never just before lying down. Acetaminophen-propoxyphene may make you drowsy when you first start taking it or change doses. Do not drive, use machinery, or do anything that needs mental alertness until you know how acetaminophen-propoxyphene affects you. Do not sit or stand up quickly. This reduces the risk of dizzy or fainting spells. These effects may be worse if you are an older patient. The drowsiness should decrease after taking acetaminophen-propoxyphene for a couple of days. Be careful taking other medicines that may also make you tired. This effect may be worse when taking these medicines with acetaminophen-propoxyphene. Alcohol can increase possible drowsiness, dizziness, confusion and affect your breathing. Alcohol can increase possible damage to your liver. Avoid alcohol while taking acetaminophen-propoxyphene. Acet-aminophen-propoxyphene can cause constipation. Try to have a bowel movement at least every 2 to 3 days. If you do not have a bowel movement for 3 days or more call your prescriber or health care professional. Many non-prescription medicines contain acetaminophen as an ingredient. Always read the labels carefully to avoid taking an accidental overdose, which can be dangerous. Acetaminophen can affect the results from some blood sugar tests used by diabetic patients. Check with your prescriber or health care professional before you change your diet or the dose of your diabetic medicine. If you are going to have surgery tell your prescriber or health care professional that you are taking acetaminophen-propoxyphene.

What side effects may I notice from taking acetaminophen-propoxyphene?

Elderly patients are more likely to get side effects.
Side effects that you should report to your prescriber or health care professional as soon as possible:
Rare or uncommon:
- breathing difficulties, wheezing
- cold, clammy skin
- seizures
- slow or fast heartbeat
- severe rash
- unusual weakness

More common:
- confusion
- lightheadedness or fainting spells
- nervousness or restlessness

Side effects that usually do not require medical attention (report to your prescriber or health care professional if they continue or are bothersome):
- itching
- clumsiness, unsteadiness
- constipation
- decrease or difficulty passing urine
- dizziness, drowsiness
- dry mouth
- flushing
- headache
- nausea, vomiting
- pinpoint pupils
- sweating

Where can I keep my medicine?

Keep out of the reach of children in a container that small children cannot open. Do not share or give this medicine to anyone else. Avoid accidental swallowing of acetaminophen-propoxyphene by someone (especially children) other than for whom it was prescribed as this may result in severe side effects and possibly death. Store at room temperature between 15 and 30 degrees C (59 and 86 degrees F) or between 20 and 25 degrees C (68 and 77 degrees F) for Darvocet A500™. Protect from light. Keep container tightly closed. Throw away any unused medicine after the expiration date.

Acetaminophen; Pseudoephedrine oral dosage forms

TYLENOL® SINUS NON-DROWSY DAYTIME;
500 mg/30 mg; Tablet
McNeil Consumer Healthcare
Div Mcneil Ppc Inc

What are acetaminophen; pseudoephedrine products?

ACETAMINOPHEN; PSEUDOEPHEDRINE (Actifed® Sinus Daytime, Alka-Seltzer Plus® Cold & Sinus Medicine Liqui-Gels®, Allerest® No-Drowsiness, Aspirin-Free Bayer® Select Sinus Pain Relief, Bayer® Select Head Cold, Children's Tylenol® Sinus, Coldrine®, Contac® Allergy/Sinus Day, Contac® Maximum Strength Sinus, Contac® Non-Drowsy Formula Sinus, Dristan® Cold, Dynafed® Maximum Strength, Infants' Tylenol® Cold Decongestant & Fever Reducer, Maximum Strength Tylenol® Sinus, Naldegesic®, Ornex® Maximum Strength, Ornex® No Drowsiness, PhenAPAP® Without Drowsiness, Sinarest® No-Drowsiness Maximum Strength, Sine-Aid® Maximum Strength, Sine-Off® Maximum Strength No Drowsiness Formula, Sinus Excedrin® Extra Strength, Sinus-Relief®, Sinutab® Sinus Maximum Strength Without Drowsiness, Sinutrol® 500, Sudafed® Cold & Sinus, Sudafed® Sinus Maximum Strength Without Drowsiness, TheraFlu® Sinus Maximum Strength, Tylenol® Sinus Maximum Strength, Vicks DayQuil® Sinus Pressure & Pain Relief and many others) is used to relieve symptoms of nasal congestion, sinus congestion, and/or headache pain caused by allergies, common cold, hay fever, and sinusitis. Generic acetaminophen; pseudoephedrine products are available.

What should my health care professional know before I take acetaminophen; pseudoephedrine?

They need to know if you have any of these conditions:
- anemia
- drink more than 3 alcohol-containing drinks per day
- blood vessel disease
- diabetes
- difficulty urinating (urinary retention)
- glaucoma
- heart disease or heart rhythm problems
- high blood pressure
- infection
- kidney or liver disease
- over active thyroid
- prostate trouble
- an unusual or allergic reaction to acetaminophen, aspirin, pseudoephedrine, other medicines, foods, dyes, or preservatives
- pregnant or trying to get pregnant
- breast-feeding

How should I take this medicine?

Take acetaminophen; pseudoephedrine products by mouth. Follow the directions on the product label. Swallow capsules, caplets, gelcaps, and tablets with plenty of water. Use a specially marked spoon, or container to measure liquids. Ask your pharmacist if you do not have one; household spoons are not always accurate. Do not take medicine more often than directed. Contact your pediatrician or health care professional regarding the use of this medicine in children. Special care may be needed. Do not administer adult preparations to children. Elderly patients over 60 years old may have a stronger reaction to this medicine and may need smaller doses.

What if I miss a dose?

If your prescriber or health care professional has prescribed a regular schedule and you miss a dose, take it as soon as you can. If it is almost time for your next dose, take only that dose. Do not take double or extra doses.

What may interact with acetaminophen; pseudoephedrine?

- alcohol
- ammonium chloride
- amphetamine or other stimulant drugs
- antacids
- bicarbonate, citrate, or acetate products (such as sodium bicarbonate, sodium acetate, sodium citrate, sodium lactate, and potassium citrate)
- bromocriptine
- caffeine
- cimetidine
- cocaine
- furazolidone
- linezolid
- medicines for colds and breathing difficulties
- medicines for diabetes
- medicines known as MAO inhibitors, such as phenelzine (Nardil®), tranylcypromine (Parnate®), isocarboxazid (Marplan®), and selegiline (Carbex®, Eldepryl®)
- medicines for mental problems and psychotic disturbances
- medicines for migraine
- medicines for seizures
- procarbazine
- some medicines for chest pain, heart disease, high blood pressure or heart rhythm problems
- some medicines for weight loss (including some herbal products, ephedrine, dextroamphetamine)
- St. John's wort
- theophylline
- thyroid hormones
- warfarin

Tell your prescriber or health care professional about all other medicines you are taking, including non-pre-

scription medicines, nutritional supplements, or herbal products. Also tell your prescriber or health care professional if you are a frequent user of drinks with caffeine or alcohol, if you smoke, or if you use illegal drugs. These may affect the way your medicine works. Check with your health care professional before stopping or starting any of your medicines.

What should I watch for while taking acetaminophen; pseudoephedrine?

Check with your prescriber or health care professional if your congestion has not improved within 7 days, or if you have a high fever. If the product makes it difficult for you to sleep at night; take your last dose a few hours before bedtime. If nervousness, dizziness, or sleeplessness occur, stop using and consult a health care professional. If you are going to have surgery, tell your prescriber you are taking acetaminophen; pseudoephedrine. Report any possible overdose promptly to your prescriber or health care professional as soon as possible. The effects of excessive doses may not be obvious for several days. Many non-prescription medicines contain acetaminophen as an ingredient. Always read the labels carefully to avoid taking an accidental overdose. Avoid alcoholic drinks if you are taking acetaminophen; pseudoephedrine on a regular basis. Alcohol can increase possible damage to your liver. Acetaminophen can affect the results from some blood-sugar tests used by diabetic patients. Check with your prescriber or health care professional before you change your diet or the dose of your diabetic medicine. If you are receiving cancer chemotherapy or other immuno-suppression medicine, do not take this medicine; check with your prescriber or health care professional first. Acetaminophen may hide the signs of an infection such as fever or pain.

What side effects may I notice from taking acetaminophen; pseudoephedrine?

If you take acetaminophen; pseudoephedrine as recommended, serious side effects are uncommon.

Side effects that you should report to your prescriber or health care professional as soon as possible:
- anxiety or nervousness
- bloody or black, tarry stools
- chest pain
- confusion
- dizziness, or fainting spells
- excessive sweating
- fast or irregular heartbeat, palpitations
- fever or sore throat
- high blood pressure
- numbness or tingling in the hands or feet
- rapid or troubled breathing, or wheezing
- pain or difficulty passing urine
- severe, persistent, or worsening headache
- sleeplessness (insomnia)
- skin rash or hives
- stomach cramps and pain
- tremor
- unusual bleeding or bruising, pinpoint red spots on the skin
- unusual tiredness or weakness
- vomiting
- yellowing of the skin or eyes

Side effects that usually do not require medical attention (report to your prescriber or health care professional if they continue or are bothersome):
- headache (mild)
- loss of appetite
- nausea
- restlessness

Where can I keep my medicine?

Keep out of reach of children in a container that small children cannot open. Acetaminophen can be dangerous to children. Avoid accidental overdose of acetaminophen as this may result in severe effects and possibly death. Store at room temperature between 15 and 30 degrees C (59 and 86 degrees F). Protect from moisture and light. Throw away any unused medicine after the expiration date.

Acetaminophen; Tramadol tablets

ULTRACET®;
325 mg/37.5 mg; Tablet
Janssen Ortho, LLC

What are acetaminophen; tramadol tablets?

ACETAMINOPHEN; TRAMADOL (Ultracet®) is a combination analgesic that is used to relieve moderate, acute pain such as pain following surgical procedures, including dental surgery. Acetaminophen; tramadol may be used for other types of pain as determined by your health care provider. Generic acetaminophen; tramadol tablets are available.

What should my health care professional know before I take acetaminophen; tramadol?

They need to know if you have any of these conditions:
- an alcohol or drug abuse problem

- blood disease, such as anemia
- breathing difficulty or asthma
- drink more than 3 alcohol-containing drinks per day
- drive or operate machinery or perform hazardous activities
- head injury or brain tumor
- kidney disease
- liver disease
- receiving drugs that lower your ability to fight infection
- seizures (convulsions) or seizure disorder (epilepsy)
- stomach or intestinal problems
- an unusual or allergic reaction to acetaminophen,

A

tramadol, codeine, other pain medicines, foods, dyes, or preservatives
- pregnant or trying to get pregnant
- breast-feeding

How should I take this medicine?

Take acetaminophen; tramadol tablets by mouth. Follow the directions on the prescription label. Swallow the tablets with a drink of water. If acetaminophen; tramadol upsets your stomach, take it with food or milk. Do not take more than 2 tablets at a time or more than 8 tablets per day. Higher doses may cause severe side effects, do not take more medication than your prescriber has instructed. Contact your pediatrician or health care professional regarding the use of this medicine in children. Special care may be needed. Older patients (> 60 years of age) may have a stronger reaction to this medicine, especially if they have kidney or liver disease.

What if I miss a dose?

If it is almost time for your next dose, take only that dose. Do not take double or extra doses.

What may interact with acetaminophen; tramadol?

- alcohol
- antacids
- antihistamines (commonly found in allergy or cold products)
- busulfan
- bupropion
- cocaine
- diflunisal
- digoxin
- droperidol
- drugs to regulate heart rhythm such as amiodarone, propafenone, quinidine
- furazolidone
- imatinib
- isoniazid, INH
- linezolid
- medicines called MAO inhibitors-phenelzine (Nardil®), tranylcypromine (Parnate®), isocarboxazid (Marplan®), selegiline (Eldepryl®)
- medicines for anxiety, depression, or sleeping problems
- medicines for nausea or vomiting
- medicines for Parkinson's disease such as entacapone, pramipexole, ropinirole or tolcapone
- medicines for mental problems like schizophrenia
- muscle relaxants
- naloxone
- other medicines for pain such as codeine, morphine, nalbuphine, pentazocine, or propoxyphene
- procarbazine
- rifampin
- ritonavir
- seizure medicines
- stimulants such as amphetamine or dextroamphetamine

- St. John's wort
- sulfinpyrazone
- warfarin

Tell your prescriber or health care professional about all other medicines you are taking, including non-prescription medicines. Also tell your prescriber or health care professional if you are a frequent user of drinks with caffeine or alcohol, if you smoke, or if you use illegal drugs. These may affect the way your medicine works. Check with your health care professional before stopping or starting any of your medicines.

What should I watch for while taking acetaminophen; tramadol?

Tell your prescriber or health care professional if your pain does not go away. Do not drive, use machinery, or do anything that needs mental alertness until you know how acetaminophen; tramadol affects you. Be careful taking other medicines which may also make you tired. This effect may be worse when taking these medicines with acetaminophen; tramadol. Alcohol can increase possible drowsiness, dizziness, confusion and affect your breathing. Do not drink alcoholic beverages while taking tramadol. Your mouth may get dry. Chewing sugarless gum, sucking hard candy and drinking plenty of water will help. If you are going to have surgery, tell your prescriber or health care professional that you are taking Ultracet®. Many non-prescription medicines contain acetaminophen as an ingredient. Additional acetaminophen taken with Ultracet® can be dangerous. Always read the labels carefully to avoid taking an accidental overdose of acetaminophen. Report any possible overdose of acetaminophen; tramadol promptly to your health care provider. Acetaminophen can affect the results from some blood-sugar tests used by diabetic patients. Check with your prescriber or health care professional before you change your diet or the dose of your diabetic medicine.

What side effects may I notice from taking acetaminophen; tramadol?

Side effects that you should report to your prescriber or health care professional as soon as possible:
Rare or uncommon:
- changes in vision
- difficulty breathing, shortness of breath
- fast or irregular heartbeat
- hallucinations (seeing and hearing things that are not really there)
- not passing urine as often as usual
- redness, blistering, peeling or loosening of the skin, including inside the mouth
- skin rash, itching
- seizures (convulsions)
- yellow tint to your skin or whites of your eyes

More common:
- anxiety, agitation
- vomiting

Side effects that usually do not require medical attention (report to your prescriber or health care professional if they continue or are bothersome):

- constipation or diarrhea
- difficulty sleeping
- dizziness, drowsiness
- dry mouth
- false sense of well being, feeling of unreality, mood changes
- headache
- indigestion
- itching
- nausea
- sweating or flushing

Where can I keep my medicine?

Keep out of reach of children in a container that small children cannot open. Store at room temperature between 15 and 30 degrees C (59 and 86 degrees F). Throw away any unused medicine after the expiration date.

Acetazolamide tablets and sustained-release capsules

DIAMOX®;
250 mg; Tablet
Storz Ophthalmics
Inc Sub American
Cyanamid Co

DIAMOX®;
500 mg; Capsule,
Extended Release
Storz Ophthalmics
Inc Sub American
Cyanamid Co

What are acetazolamide tablets and sustained-release capsules?

ACETAZOLAMIDE (Diamox®, Diamox® Sequels®) helps to treat glaucoma, certain types of epilepsy or seizure disorders. It can also help mountain climbers who get altitude or mountain sickness. Generic acetazolamide tablets are available. Generic acetazolamide sustained-release capsules are not yet available.

What should my health care professional know before I take acetazolamide?

They need to know if you have any of these conditions:

- Addison's disease (underactive adrenal gland)
- blood disorders or disease
- kidney disease
- liver disease
- low levels of sodium or potassium in the blood
- lung disease
- an unusual or allergic reaction to acetazolamide, sulfonamides, thiazide diuretics (water pills) other medicines, foods, dyes, or preservatives
- pregnant or trying to get pregnant
- breast-feeding

How should I take this medicine?

Take acetazolamide tablets or capsules by mouth. Follow the directions on the prescription label. Swallow the tablets with a drink of water. Do not crush or chew capsules. Take acetazolamide with food if it upsets your stomach. Take your doses at regular intervals. Do not take your medicine more often than directed. If you are taking acetazolamide for mountain sickness, take the first dose 24 to 48 hours before you start the climb. Continue to take it while at high altitude. If you are unable to swallow the tablets, a liquid can be made by softening (or crushing) a tablet in 2 teaspoonfuls of water and adding 2 teaspoonfuls of honey or syrup. This liquid should be made just before the dose is taken. Contact your pediatrician or health care professional regarding the use of this medicine in children. Special care may be needed.

What if I miss a dose?

If you miss a dose, take it as soon as you can. If it is almost time for your next dose, take only that dose. Do not take double or extra doses.

What may interact with acetazolamide?

- amphotericin B
- aspirin and aspirin-like medicines
- barbiturate medicines for inducing sleep or treating seizures (convulsions)
- carbamazepine
- ciprofloxacin
- dextroamphetamine
- ephedrine
- mecamylamine
- medicines for movement abnormalities as in Parkinson's disease, or for gastrointestinal problems
- methenamine
- mexiletine
- phenytoin
- quinidine
- steroid medicines such as prednisone or cortisone
- water pills

Tell your prescriber or health care professional about all other medicines you are taking, including non-prescription medicines, nutritional supplements, or herbal products. Also tell your prescriber or health care professional if you are a frequent user of drinks with caffeine or alcohol, if you smoke, or if you use illegal drugs. These may affect the way your medicine works. Check with your health care professional before stopping or starting any of your medicines.

What should I watch for while taking acetazolamide?

Ask your prescriber or health care professional about your potassium level. It is important not to have too little or too much potassium. You may need to take a

A

potassium supplement or eat foods that are high in potassium if acetazolamide is making your body lose too much potassium. Do not stop taking acetazolamide suddenly if you are taking it to prevent seizures. Your prescriber or health care professional may want you to reduce your dose gradually. You may get drowsy; until you know how acetazolamide affects you, do not drive, use machinery, or do anything that needs mental alertness. Drink several glasses of water a day. This will help to reduce possible kidney problems. If you are diabetic, monitor blood and urine sugar and ketones regularly. Acetazolamide can increase sugar levels. Check with your prescriber or health care professional if you notice any changes.

What side effects may I notice from taking acetazolamide?

Side effects that you should report to your prescriber or health care professional as soon as possible:
- blood in urine, pain or difficulty passing urine
- black tarry stools
- confusion or mental depression
- dark yellow or brown urine, pale stools, yellowing of the eyes or skin
- difficulty breathing, shortness of breath
- dry mouth or increased thirst
- fever, sore throat
- lower back pain

- muscle weakness
- ringing in the ears
- seizures (convulsions)
- skin rash, itching
- unusual bleeding or bruising
- unusual tiredness

Side effects that usually do not require medical attention (report to your prescriber or health care professional if they continue or are bothersome):
- changes in taste or smell (metallic taste in mouth, loss of taste and smell)
- diarrhea
- drowsiness
- headache
- increased sensitivity of eyes to light
- loss of appetite
- nausea, vomiting
- numbness, tingling, or burning in the hands, fingers, feet, toes, mouth, lips, tongue, or anus
- passing urine more often
- weight loss

Where can I keep my medicine?

Keep out of the reach of children in a container that small children cannot open. Store at room temperature between 15 and 30 degrees C (50 and 86 degrees F). Throw away any unused medicine after the expiration date.

Acetohexamide tablets

ACETOHEXAMIDE;
250 mg; Tablet
Barr Laboratories
Inc

ACETOHEXAMIDE;
500 mg; Tablet
Barr Laboratories
Inc

What are acetohexamide tablets?

ACETOHEXAMIDE helps to treat type 2 diabetes mellitus. Treatment is combined with a suitable diet and balanced exercise. Acetohexamide increases the amount of insulin released from the pancreas and helps your body to use insulin more efficiently. Generic acetohexamide tablets are available.

What should my health care professional know before I take acetohexamide?

They need to know if you have any of these conditions:
- kidney disease
- liver disease
- major surgery
- porphyria
- severe infection or injury
- thyroid disease
- an unusual or allergic reaction to acetohexamide, sulfonamides, other medicines, foods, dyes, or preservatives
- pregnant or trying to get pregnant
- breast-feeding

How should I take this medicine?

Take acetohexamide tablets by mouth. Follow the directions on the prescription label. Swallow the tablets with a drink of water. If you take acetohexamide once a day, take it 30 minutes before breakfast. If you take it twice a day, it is best to take it before breakfast and the evening meal. If acetohexamide upsets your stomach take it with food or milk. Take your doses at the same time each day; do not take more often than directed. Contact your pediatrician or health care professional regarding the use of this medicine in children. Special care may be needed. Elderly patients over 65 years old may have a stronger reaction and need a smaller dose.

What if I miss a dose?

If you miss a dose, take it as soon as you can. If it is almost time for your next dose, take only that dose. Do not take double or extra doses.

What may interact with acetohexamide?

- alcohol
- beta-blockers (used for high blood pressure or heart conditions)
- cisapride
- clofibrate
- diazoxide

- medicines for fungal or yeast infections (examples: itraconazole, ketonazole, voriconazole)
- metoclopramide
- rifampin
- warfarin (a blood thinner)

Many medications may cause changes (increase or decrease) in blood sugar, these include:

- alcohol containing beverages
- aspirin and aspirin-like drugs
- beta-blockers, often used for high blood pressure or heart problems (examples include atenolol, metoprolol, propranolol)
- chromium
- female hormones, such as estrogens or progestins, birth control pills
- isoniazid
- male hormones or anabolic steroids
- medications for weight loss
- medicines for allergies, asthma, cold, or cough
- niacin
- pentamidine
- phenytoin
- quinolone antibiotics (examples: ciprofloxacin, levofloxacin, ofloxacin)
- some herbal dietary supplements
- steroid medicines such as prednisone or cortisone
- thyroid hormones
- water pills (diuretics)

Tell your prescriber or health care professional about all other medicines you are taking, including non-prescription medicines, nutritional supplements, or herbal products. Also tell your prescriber or health care professional if you are a frequent user of drinks with caffeine or alcohol, if you smoke, or if you use illegal drugs. These may affect the way your medicine works. Check with your health care professional before stopping or starting any of your medicines.

What should I watch for while taking acetohexamide?

Visit your prescriber or health care professional for regular checks on your progress. Learn how to monitor blood or urine sugar and urine ketones regularly. Check with your prescriber or health care professional if your blood sugar is high, you may need a change of dose of acetohexamide. Do not skip meals. If you are exercising much more than usual you may need extra snacks to avoid side effects caused by low blood sugar. Alcohol can increase possible side effects of acetohexamide. Ask your prescriber or health care professional if you should avoid alcohol. If you have mild symptoms of low blood sugar, eat or drink something containing sugar at once

and contact your prescriber or health care professional. It is wise to check your blood sugar to confirm that it is low. It is important to recognize your own symptoms of low blood sugar so that you can treat them quickly. Make sure family members know that you can choke if you eat or drink when you have serious symptoms of low blood sugar, such as seizures or unconsciousness. They must get medical help at once. Acetohexamide can increase the sensitivity of your skin to the sun. Keep out of the sun, or wear protective clothing outdoors and use a sunscreen. Do not use sun lamps or sun tanning beds or booths. If you are going to have surgery, tell your prescriber or health care professional that you are taking acetohexamide. Wear a medical identification bracelet or chain to say you have diabetes, and carry a card that lists all your medications.

What side effects may I notice from taking acetohexamide?

Side effects that you should report to your prescriber or health care professional as soon as possible:

- hypoglycemia (low blood glucose) which can cause symptoms such as anxiety or nervousness, confusion, difficulty concentrating, hunger, pale skin, nausea, fatigue, perspiration, headache, palpitations, numbness of the mouth, tingling in the fingers, tremors, muscle weakness, blurred vision, cold sensations, uncontrolled yawning, irritability, rapid heartbeat, shallow breathing, and loss of consciousness
- breathing difficulties, severe skin reactions or excessive phlegm, which may indicate that you are having an allergic reaction to the drug
- dark yellow or brown urine, or yellowing of the eyes or skin, indicating that the drug is affecting your liver
- fever, chills, sore throat; which means the drug may be affecting your immune system
- unusual bleeding or bruising; which occurs when the drug is affecting your blood clotting system

Side effects that usually do not require medical attention (report to your prescriber or health care professional if they continue or are bothersome):

- diarrhea
- headache
- heartburn
- increased sensitivity to the sun
- nausea, vomiting
- stomach discomfort
- skin rash, redness, swelling or itching

Where can I keep my medicine?

Keep out of the reach of children in a container that small children cannot open. Store at room temperature between 15 and 30 degrees C (59 and 86 degrees F). Keep container tightly closed. Throw away any unused medicine after the expiration date.

A

Acitretin capsules

SORIATANE®;
25 mg; Capsule
Connetics Corp

SORIATANE®;
10 mg; Capsule
Connetics Corp

This drug
requires an
FDA
medication
guide. See
page
xxxvii.

What are acitretin capsules?

ACITRETIN (Soriatane®) is used to treat severe forms of psoriasis. Acitretin is not a cure, but it helps reduce the redness, thickness, and scaling that occur with psoriasis. Acitretin can cause serious side effects, including birth defects if given to someone who is pregnant. Do not share this medicine with anyone else. Before you receive your acitretin prescription you should discuss and sign a Patient Information/Consent form with your prescriber. This is to help make sure you understand the risk of birth defects and how to avoid getting pregnant. If you did not talk to your prescriber about this and sign the form, contact your health care provider. Generic acitretin capsules are not yet available.

What should my health care professional know before I use acitretin?

They need to know if you have any of these conditions:
- if you have ever taken Tegison® or Tigason® (etretinate) in the past
- alcoholism
- depression
- diabetes mellitus or high blood sugar
- elevated cholesterol or triglycerides
- heart disease
- kidney or liver disease
- visual problems
- an unusual or allergic reaction to acitretin, etretinate, vitamin A, isotretinoin, tretinoin, other medicines, foods, dyes, or preservatives
- pregnant or trying to get pregnant
- breast-feeding

How should I use this medicine?

Take acitretin capsules by mouth with food. Follow the directions on the prescription label. Swallow the capsules with a drink of water. Do not take your medicine more often than directed. Contact your pediatrician or health care professional regarding the use of this medicine in children. Special care may be needed.

What if I miss a dose?

If you miss a dose, skip the missed dose and resume your normal schedule. Do not take double or extra doses.

What may interact with acitretin?

The following medicines should not be used while you are taking acitretin:
- alcohol, including alcohol that may be in drinks, food, or medicines including over-the-counter medicines
- methotrexate
- other vitamin A analogs ("retinoids") such as isotretinoin, tretinoin

- tetracycline-type antibiotics including tetracycline, doxycycline or minocycline
- vitamin A

Other medicines that may interact with acitretin:
- orlistat
- phenytoin

Tell your prescriber or health care professional about all other medicines you are taking, including non-prescription medicines. Also tell your prescriber or health care professional if you are a frequent user of drinks with caffeine or alcohol, if you smoke, or if you use illegal drugs. These may affect the way your medicine works. Check with your health care professional before stopping or starting any of your medicines.

What should I watch for while taking acitretin?

You may experience worsening of your psoriasis when your first start taking acitretin. You may have to take acitretin for 2 to 3 months before you will see the full benefit of acitretin treatment; although, some patients may have significant improvements in their disease within the first 8 weeks of therapy. Acitretin can cause severe birth defects. Acitretin must not be used by females who are pregnant or who may become pregnant while receiving acitretin or at any time for at least 3 years after treatment is stopped. If pregnancy does occur while receiving acitretin or at any time for at least 3 years after you stop taking acitretin, you should discuss with your physician the possible effects on the pregnancy. You should receive a Medication Guide from your pharmacy every time you receive a new prescription of acitretin, which will explain in greater detail the steps that should be taken to prevent pregnancy while receiving acitretin. If you do not receive a Medication Guide, contact your pharmacist.
- *Female patients who are able to have children*: You must have 2 negative pregnancy tests before you can begin treatment with acitretin. While receiving acitretin, female patients will need to have regular pregnancy tests to make sure they are not pregnant. Discuss effective birth control methods (contraception) with your health care provider. You must use 2 effective forms of birth control at the same time for at least 1 month before beginning acitretin, during treatment, and for at least 3 years after stopping acitretin therapy. If you miss your period or think you may be pregnant, stop taking acitretin right away and contact your health care provider. Do not take acitretin while you are breast-feeding. Acitretin may be passed on to your baby in the milk and may cause side effects. You will need to choose either to breast feed or take acitretin, but not both.

■ *Male Patients:* Small amounts of acitretin may be present in the semen of men taking acitretin. It appears that these small amounts pose little, if any, risk to an unborn child.

During acitretin therapy and for 2 months after stopping treatment, you must avoid drinks, foods, and all medicines that contain alcohol. This includes over-the-counter products that contain alcohol. Avoiding alcohol is important because alcohol changes acitretin into a drug that may take longer than 3 years to leave your body. The chance of birth defects may last longer than 3 years if you take any form of alcohol while taking acitretin or for 2 months after stopping treatment. Do not share your acitretin prescription with anyone else due to the risk of birth defects and other serious adverse effects. Acitretin can increase cholesterol and triglyceride levels and decrease HDL (the 'good' cholesterol) levels. Your health care provider will monitor these levels and recommend appropriate therapy, including dietary changes or prescription drugs, if necessary. You must not donate blood during your treatment with acitretin and for 3 years after you stop taking acitretin. Acitretin in your blood can harm an unborn baby if the blood is given to a pregnant woman. Acitretin does not affect your ability to receive blood transfusions. If you wear contact lenses, they may feel uncomfortable. If your eyes get dry, check with your eye doctor. Use caution when driving or operating machinery, especially at night. Acitretin therapy may cause sudden changes in your vision. If you develop any vision changes, stop taking acitretin and contact your health care provider right away. Acitretin can make your skin more sensitive to sunlight (UV light). Do not use sunlamps, and avoid sunlight as much as possible or wear protective clothing outdoors and use a sunscreen (SPF 15 or higher). If you are receiving light treatment (phototherapy), your prescriber may need to change your light dosages to avoid burns. Your mouth may get dry. Chewing sugarless gum or sucking hard candy, and drinking plenty of water will help. Avoid multivitamins or nutritional supplements that contain vitamin A. Acitretin may affect your blood sugar levels. If you are diabetic check with your prescriber or health care professional if you notice any change in your blood sugar tests. Depression and/or other symptoms such as aggressive feelings or thoughts of self-harm have been reported in patients receiving acitretin. These events have occurred in other drugs similar to acitretin as well.

Since other factors may have contributed to these events, it is not known if they are related to acitretin treatment. If you experience depression or thoughts of suicide, you should stop taking acitretin and contact your health care provider.

What side effects may I notice from using acitretin?

Side effects that you should report to your prescriber or health care professional as soon as possible:
■ dark colored urine
■ decreased vision in the dark
■ depression
■ frequent urination, increased thirst or hunger
■ severe headaches, nausea, vomiting, blurred vision
■ severe or persistent nausea and vomiting and decreased appetite
■ shortness of breath, chest pain, swelling in a leg
■ yellowing of your skin or the whites of your eyes

Side effects that usually do not require medical attention (report to your prescriber or health care professional if they continue or are bothersome):
■ altered taste
■ chapped lips
■ difficulty sleeping
■ dry nose, mouth, and eyes
■ earache
■ easy bruising
■ fatigue
■ fragile (weak) skin
■ hair loss
■ headache
■ increased salivation
■ increased sensitivity to the sun
■ increased sweating
■ itching
■ joint and bone pain
■ peeling of your fingers, palms, or soles of the feet
■ ringing in the ears
■ scaly skin all over
■ weak nails

Where can I keep my medicine?

Keep out of the reach of children. Store at room temperature between 15 and 25 degrees C (59 and 77 degrees F). Protect from light. Avoid exposure to high temperatures and humidity after the bottle is opened. Throw away any unused medicine after the expiration date.

A

Acrivastine; Pseudoephedrine capsules

SEMPREX-D®;
8 mg/60 mg; Capsule
Celltech Pharmaceuticals, Inc

What are acrivastine; pseudoephedrine capsules?

ACRIVASTINE; PSEUDOEPHEDRINE (Semprex-D®) is a combination of an antihistamine and decongestant. It relieves the symptoms of allergies like hay fever (seasonal rhinitis) including nasal and sinus congestion. A generic capsule is not yet available.

What should my health care professional know before I take acrivastine; pseudoephedrine?

They need to know if you have any of these conditions:

- blood vessel disease
- diabetes
- difficulty swallowing
- glaucoma
- heart disease
- high blood pressure
- kidney disease
- liver disease
- overactive thyroid
- stomach ulcer
- urinary tract or prostate trouble
- an unusual or allergic reaction to acrivastine; pseudoephedrine, other medicines, foods, dyes, or preservatives
- pregnant or trying to get pregnant
- breast-feeding

How should I take this medicine?

Take acrivastine; pseudoephedrine capsules by mouth. Follow the directions on the prescription label. Swallow the acrivastine; pseudoephedrine capsules whole with water. Do not break or chew the capsules. Take your doses at regular intervals. Do not take your medicine more often than directed. Contact your pediatrician or health care professional regarding the use of this medicine in children. Special care may be needed. Older patients (> 60 years of age) may have a stronger reaction to this medicine, especially if they have kidney disease.

What if I miss a dose?

If it is almost time for your next dose, take only that dose. Do not take double doses.

What may interact with acrivastine; pseudoephedrine?

- alcohol or illicit drugs such as cocaine
- barbiturate medicines for inducing sleep or treating seizures (convulsions), like phenobarbital
- bromocriptine
- caffeine
- furazolidone
- linezolid

- MAO inhibitors (examples: Eldepryl®, Marplan®, Nardil® and Parnate®)
- mecamylamine
- medicines for anxiety or sleeping problems, such as alprazolam, diazepam or temazepam
- medicines for colds, breathing difficulties or weight loss, such as ephedra
- medicines for hay fever and other allergies such as antihistamines
- medicines for heart disease such as digoxin or beta-blockers
- medicines for mental problems, including anxiety, depression and psychotic disturbances
- medicines for migraine headaches such as dihydroergotamine or ergotamine
- medicines for nasal congestion, such as more pseudoephedrine
- medicines for pain such as codeine or morphine
- procarbazine
- reserpine
- sodium bicarbonate

Tell your prescriber or health care professional about all other medicines you are taking, including non-prescription medicines, nutritional supplements, or herbal products. Also tell your prescriber or health care professional if you are a frequent user of drinks with caffeine or alcohol, if you smoke, or if you use illegal drugs. These may affect the way your medicine works. Check with your health care professional before stopping or starting any of your medicines.

What should I watch for while taking acrivastine; pseudoephedrine?

Do not drive, use machinery, or do anything that needs mental alertness until you know how acrivastine; pseudoephedrine affects you. To reduce the risk of dizzy or fainting spells, do not stand or sit up quickly, especially if you are an older patient. Alcohol may increase dizziness and drowsiness. Avoid alcoholic drinks. Your mouth may get dry. Chewing sugarless gum or sucking hard candy, and drinking plenty of water will help.

What side effects may I notice from taking acrivastine; pseudoephedrine?

Side effects that you should report to your prescriber or health care professional as soon as possible:

- abdominal pain or rectal bleeding
- chest pain
- confusion
- convulsions (seizures)
- difficulty breathing or wheezing
- difficulty swallowing or enlarged tongue
- difficulty urinating
- dizziness or fainting spells
- fast or irregular heartbeat, palpitations

- high blood pressure
- numbness or tingling in the hands or feet
- rash
- severe, persistent, or worsening headache
- tremor, muscle contractions
- visual changes
- vomiting

Side effects that usually do not require medical attention (report to your prescriber or health care professional if they continue or are bothersome):

- dry mouth

- headache (mild)
- loss of appetite or nausea
- nervousness or difficulty sleeping
- tiredness

Where can I keep my medicine?

Keep out of the reach of children in a container that small children cannot open. Store at room temperature or between 15 to 25 degrees C (59 to 77 degrees F). Protect from moisture. Throw away any unused medicine after the expiration date.

Acyclovir tablets or capsules

ZOVIRAX®;
200 mg; Capsule
Glaxo Wellcome Inc

ZOVIRAX®;
800 mg; Tablet
Glaxo Wellcome Inc

What are acyclovir tablets or capsules?

ACYCLOVIR (Zovirax®) treats certain types of viral infections, specifically herpes infections. Acyclovir will not cure herpes infections; it will help the sores heal faster and help to relieve the pain or discomfort. Sometimes acyclovir is given to help prevent the infection from coming back. Acyclovir also treats shingles and chickenpox infections. Generic acyclovir tablets and capsules are available.

What should my health care professional know before I take acyclovir?

They need to know if you have any of these conditions:
- dehydration
- neurological disease
- kidney disease
- seizures (convulsions)
- an unusual or allergic reaction to acyclovir, ganciclovir, valacyclovir, valganciclovir, other medicines, foods, dyes, or preservatives
- pregnant or trying to get pregnant
- breast-feeding

How should I take this medicine?

Take acyclovir tablets or capsules by mouth. Follow the directions on the prescription label. Swallow whole with a full glass of water. You can take acyclovir with or without food. Take your doses at regular intervals. Do not take your medicine more often than directed. Finish the full course prescribed by your prescriber or health care professional even if you think your condition is better. Do not stop taking except on your prescriber's advice. Contact your pediatrician or health care professional regarding the use of this medicine in children. Special care may be needed.

What if I miss a dose?

If you miss a dose, take it as soon as you can. If it is almost time for your next dose, take only that dose. Do not take double or extra doses.

What may interact with acyclovir?

- fosphenytoin
- phenytoin
- probenecid
- zidovudine, AZT

Tell your prescriber or health care professional about all other medicines you are taking, including non-prescription medicines, nutritional supplements, or herbal products. Also tell your prescriber or health care professional if you are a frequent user of drinks with caffeine or alcohol, if you smoke, or if you use illegal drugs. These may affect the way your medicine works. Check with your health care professional before stopping or starting any of your medicines.

What should I watch for while taking acyclovir?

Tell your prescriber or health care professional if your symptoms do not improve after 1 week. Make sure to drink plenty of water or fluids while taking acyclovir to help prevent side effects. Even though you are taking acyclovir, you can still pass herpes or chickenpox to another person. Acyclovir works best when taken very early in the course of an infection. Begin treatment at the first signs of infection (such as tingling, itching, or pain in the affected area). Genital herpes is a sexually transmitted disease. Taking acyclovir will not stop your sexual partner from getting the infection. Do not have sex if you have an active herpes infection; you can use a condom during sex, but this is not foolproof.

What side effects may I notice from taking acyclovir?

The side effects you may notice from acyclovir depend upon the dose you are taking and the infection being treated; not all side effects occur in every patient.

Side effects that you should report to your prescriber or health care professional as soon as possible:

- confusion or hallucinations (i.e., seeing things that are not there)
- increased thirst

- redness, blistering, peeling or loosening of the skin, including inside the mouth
- reduced amount of urine passed
- seizures
- skin rash or hives
- stomach pain
- tremor
- unusual weakness or tiredness

Side effects that usually do not require medical attention (report to your prescriber or health care professional if they continue or are bothersome):

- diarrhea
- dizziness
- headache
- increased sensitivity to the sun
- loss of appetite
- nausea, vomiting

Where can I keep my medicine?

Keep out of the reach of children in a container that small children cannot open. Store at room temperature between 15° and 25°C (59° and 77°F). Protect from light and moisture. Throw away any unused medicine after the expiration date.

Adefovir tablets

HEPSERA®;
10 mg; Tablet
Gilead Sciences Inc

What are adefovir tablets?

ADEFOVIR (Hepsera™) is used to treat infections due to the hepatitis B virus. Adefovir can slow the liver damage caused by hepatitis B. It will not cure or prevent hepatitis B infection. Generic adefovir tablets are not available.

What should my health care professional know before I take adefovir?

They need to know if you have any of these conditions:

- human immunodeficiency virus (HIV) infection or AIDS
- kidney disease
- other liver disease
- an unusual reaction to adefovir, other medicines, foods, dyes, or preservatives
- pregnant or trying to get pregnant
- breast-feeding

How should this medicine be taken?

Take adefovir tablets by mouth. Follow the directions on the prescription label. Swallow tablets with a drink of water. If adefovir upsets your stomach, you can take it with food. Try to take your dose at the same time each day. Do not take your medicine more often than directed. Do not stop taking this medicine except on your prescriber's advice. Contact your pediatrician or health care professional regarding the use of this medicine in children. Special care may be needed.

What if I miss a dose?

If you miss a dose, but then remember it during that same day, take it as soon as you can. Then take your next dose at the regularly scheduled time the following day. Do not take 2 doses at once to make up for a missing dose. If it is almost time for your next dose, take only that dose. Do not take double or extra doses. If you are still unsure about what to do if you miss a dose, check with your prescriber.

What may interact with adefovir?

- certain antibiotics given by injection
- cyclosporine
- ibuprofen or other anti-inflammatory drugs (NSAIDs)
- medicines for HIV infection or AIDS
- metformin
- tacrolimus

Tell your prescriber or health care professional about all other medicines you are taking, including non-prescription medicines, nutritional supplements, or herbal products. Also tell your prescriber or health care professional if you are a frequent user of drinks with caffeine or alcohol, if you smoke, or if you use illegal drugs. These may affect the way your medicine works. Check with your health care professional before stopping or starting any of your medicines.

What should I watch for while taking adefovir?

You must visit your prescriber or health care professional for regular checks on your progress during and after treatment with adefovir. Discuss any new symptoms with your prescriber or health care professional. Tell your prescriber or health care professional at once if you have nausea and vomiting accompanied by severe stomach pain. Some people have worsening of hepatitis after stopping adefovir therapy. Do not stop taking adefovir unless your prescriber instructs you to. Adefovir will not cure hepatitis B infection and you can still get other illnesses or complications associated with your disease. Taking adefovir does not reduce the risk of passing hepatitis B infection to others through sexual or blood contact. Do not have sexual contact without protection; talk to your health care professional about practicing "safe sex," such as using condoms. Be careful about cuts, abrasions and other possible sources of blood contact. Do not share razors, toothbrushes or other personal items that might have contact with blood. Never share a needle or syringe with anyone. Your prescriber may talk to you about being tested for the HIV virus prior to starting or during treatment with adefovir for hepatitis B. The use of adefovir can cause resistance to certain HIV medicines.

What side effects may I notice from taking adefovir?

Side effects that you should report to your prescriber or health care professional as soon as possible:
- breathing difficulties or shortness of breath
- dark yellow or brown urine
- dizziness
- fever, chills, or frequent sore throat
- not passing urine as often as usual
- passing out or fainting
- severe diarrhea
- skin rash
- slow or irregular heart beat
- unusual muscle pain

- unusual weakness, fatigue, or discomfort
- unusual stomach pain or discomfort
- vomiting
- yellowing of the eyes or skin

Side effects that usually do not require medical attention (report to your prescriber or health care professional if they continue or are bothersome):
- headache
- heartburn or indigestion
- itching
- loss of appetite
- nausea
- stomach gas or fullness

Where can I keep my medicine?

Keep out of the reach of children in a container that small children cannot open. Store between 15 and 30 degrees C (59 and 86 degrees F). Keep the container tightly closed. Throw away any unused medicine after the expiration date.

Albendazole tablets

ALBENZA®;
200 mg; Tablet
Smithkline Beecham
Pharmaceuticals Div
Smithkline Beecham Co

What are albendazole tablets?

ALBENDAZOLE (Albenza®) is an anthelmintic. This medicine treats parasitic (worm) infections from roundworms, hookworms, pinworms, whipworms, threadworms and tapeworms. Generic albendazole tablets are not yet available.

What should my health care professional know before I take albendazole?

They need to know if you have any of these conditions:
- anemia
- biliary tract disease
- liver disease
- low white blood cell count
- recent chemotherapy
- an unusual reaction to albendazole, other medicines, foods, dyes, or preservatives
- pregnant or trying to get pregnant
- breast-feeding

How should this medicine be used?

Take albendazole tablets by mouth. Follow the directions on the prescription label. Swallow the tablets whole with a small amount of water. You should take albendazole with a high fat meal to increase how much of the drug gets into the body. Albendazole tablets may be crushed and mixed with applesauce or pudding, which is an easy way to give it to children. Do not take your medicine more often than directed. Finish the full course of medicine prescribed by your prescriber or health care professional even if you feel better. Take at regular intervals. Parasite (worm) death can be slow. To remove all parasites (worms) from the intestines can take several days. Contact your pediatrician or

health care professional regarding the use of this medicine in children. Special care may be needed.

What if I miss a dose?

If you miss a dose, take it as soon as you can. If it is almost time for your next dose, take only that dose. Do not take double or extra doses. If you have to take a missed dose, make sure there are at least 10 to 12 hours between doses.

What may interact with albendazole?

- aminophylline
- caffeine
- carbamazepine
- cimetidine
- clozapine
- dexamethasone
- grapefruit juice
- mexiletine
- olanzapine
- phenobarbital
- phenytoin
- ropinirole
- tacrine
- theophylline
- warfarin

Tell your prescriber or health care professional about all other medicines you are taking, including non-prescription medicines, nutritional supplements, or herbal products. Also tell your prescriber or health care professional if you are a frequent user of drinks with caffeine or alcohol, if you smoke, or if you use illegal drugs. These may affect the way your medicine works. Check

with your health care professional before stopping or starting any of your medicines.

What should I watch for while taking albendazole?

Visit your prescriber or health care professional to check that your infection has gone. Your doctor will request that you have blood drawn every 2 weeks to monitor liver function and blood cell counts while you are receiving treatment. If you have a severe infection you may need a second course of treatment. You may get dizzy. Until you know how albendazole affects you, do not drive, use machinery, or do anything that needs mental alertness. Practice good hygiene to prevent infection of others. Wash your hands, scrub your fingernails and shower often. Every day change and launder linens and undergarments. Scrub toilets often and keep floors clean. Other people in your house may need treatment. Check with your prescriber or health care professional. To prevent worm infections, treat pets regularly for worms. Keep children out of contact with animal feces (wastes). Never eat undercooked (pink) pork meat. You can kill pork worm larvae (trichinosis) by cooking pork meat until it is well done. In females, this drug may cause harm to a developing baby if this drug is taken during pregnancy. Use an effective form of birth control while taking this drug and for 1 month after stopping albendazole; talk to your health care provider regarding birth control options. Tell your health care provider if you think you may be pregnant.

What side effects may I notice from taking albendazole?

Side effects that you should report to your prescriber or health care professional as soon as possible:
- blurred vision
- diarrhea (severe)
- difficulty breathing
- fever or chills, sore throat
- joint aches and pains
- lower back pain
- muscle aches and pains
- redness, blistering, peeling or loosening of the skin, including the inside the mouth
- seizures (convulsions)
- skin rash, hives, or itching
- unusual weakness or tiredness
- yellowing of eyes or skin

Side effects that usually do not require medical attention (report to your prescriber or health care professional if they continue or are bothersome):
- thinning of hair
- dizziness
- loss of appetite
- nausea, vomiting
- stomach pain, which can occur when large numbers of parasites (worms) are present

Where can I keep my medicine?

Keep out of the reach of children in a container that small children cannot open. Store at controlled room temperature between 20 and 25 degrees C (68 and 77 degrees F). Keep container tightly closed. Protect from sunlight. Throw away any unused medicine after the expiration date.

Albuterol tablets or extended-release tablets

ALBUTEROL;
2 mg; Tablet
Mylan
Pharmaceuticals Inc

VOSPIRE ER®;
8 mg; Tablet,
Extended Release
Odyssey
Pharmaceuticals Inc

What are albuterol tablets or extended-release tablets?

ALBUTEROL (Proventil®, Ventolin®, Vospire ER®) is a bronchodilator, a medicine that opens up your air passages and makes you breathe easier. It is a medicine for patients with various lung problems such as asthma or chronic bronchitis. Generic albuterol tablets and extended-release tablets are available.

What should my health care professional know before I take albuterol?

They need to know if you have any of the following conditions:
- diabetes
- heart disease, or irregular heartbeat
- high blood pressure
- low blood levels of potassium
- lung disease
- pheochromocytoma
- seizures (convulsions)
- thyroid disease
- an unusual or allergic reaction to albuterol, levalbuterol, sulfites, other medicines, foods, dyes, or preservatives
- pregnant or trying to get pregnant
- breast-feeding

How should I take this medicine?

Take albuterol tablets or extended-release tablets by mouth. Follow the directions on the prescription label. Swallow the tablets with a drink of water. If albuterol upsets your stomach, take it with food or milk. Swallow extended-release tablets whole; do not crush or chew. Do not take more often than directed. Contact your pediatrician or health care professional regarding the use of this medicine in children. Special care may be needed.

A

What if I miss a dose?

If you miss a dose, take it as soon as you can. If it is almost time for your next dose, take only that dose. Do not take double or extra doses.

What may interact with albuterol?

- arsenic trioxide
- astemizole
- bepridil
- beta-blockers, often used for high blood pressure or heart problems
- caffeine
- certain antibiotics (such as clarithromycin, erythromycin, gatifloxacin, gemifloxacin, grepafloxacin, levofloxacin, linezolid, moxifloxacin, sparfloxacin)
- chloroquine
- cisapride
- droperidol
- halofantrine
- levomethadyl
- medicines for colds and breathing difficulties
- medicines for heart disease or high blood pressure
- medicines known as MAO inhibitors, such as phenelzine (Nardil®), tranylcypromine (Parnate®), isocarboxazid (Marplan®), and selegiline (Carbex®, Eldepryl®)
- medicines to control heart rhythm (examples: amiodarone, disopyramide, dofetilide, flecainide, procainamide, quinidine, sotalol)
- medicines for treating depression or mental illness (amoxapine, haloperidol, maprotiline, pimozide, phenothiazines, risperidone, sertindole, tricyclic antidepressants, ziprasidone)
- methadone
- pentamidine
- probucol
- some medicines for weight loss (including some herbal products, ephedra, ephedrine, dextroamphetamine)
- steroid hormones such as dexamethasone, cortisone, hydrocortisone
- terfenadine
- theophylline
- thyroid hormones
- water pills or diuretics

Tell your prescriber or health care professional about all other medicines you are taking, including non-prescription medicines, nutritional supplements, or herbal products. Also tell your prescriber or health care professional if you are a frequent user of drinks with caffeine or alcohol, if you smoke, or if you use illegal drugs.

These may affect the way your medicine works. Check before starting or stopping any of your medicines.

What should I watch for while taking albuterol?

Tell your prescriber or health care professional if your symptoms do not improve in 1 or 2 days. If your asthma or bronchitis gets worse while you are using albuterol, call your prescriber or health care professional as soon as you can for advice. Your mouth may get dry. Chewing sugarless gum or sucking hard candy, and drinking plenty of water, will help.

What side effects may I notice from taking albuterol?

Side effects that you should report to your prescriber or health care professional as soon as possible:
Rare:
- skin rash or hives
- swelling of the tongue, face, or lips with difficulty breathing, difficulty swallowing, hoarseness, or tightening of the throat (angioedema)

Infrequent:
- difficulty breathing or wheezing which increases or does not go away
- dizziness or fainting spell
- chest pain or palpitations (fast, pounding heartbeat)
- fast or irregular heartbeat
- fever
- headache (severe)
- increased blood pressure
- muscle cramps or weakness
- numbness in fingers or toes
- vomiting

Side effects that usually do not require medical attention (report to your prescriber or health care professional if they continue or are bothersome):
- anxiety, nervousness, trembling
- cough
- diarrhea
- difficulty sleeping
- dry mouth
- mild headache
- nasal congestion, runny nose
- nausea, upset stomach

Where can I keep my medicine?

Keep out of the reach of children in a container that small children cannot open. Store most tablets at controlled room temperature between 2 and 25 degrees C (36 and 77 degrees F). Vospire® extended-release tablets should be stored under refrigeration 2 and 8 degrees C (36 and 46 degrees F). Keep container tightly closed. Throw away any unused medicine after the expiration date.

Albuterol; Ipratropium inhalation aerosol and solution

**COMBIVENT®;
120 mcg/actuation/21 mcg/
actuation; Aerosol, Metered
Boehringer Ingelheim
Pharmaceuticals Inc**

What are albuterol; ipratropium inhalation aerosol and solution?

ALBUTEROL; IPRATROPIUM (Combivent®, DuoNeb™) is a combination of bronchodilators, which are medicines that open up your air passages and make breathing easier. The combination is used for patients with lung problems such as chronic bronchitis and emphysema. This medicine controls acute episodes or prevents recurring bouts of bronchospasm due to these conditions. Generic albuterol; ipratropium inhalation aerosols and nebulizer solutions are not yet available.

What should my health care professional know before I use albuterol; ipratropium inhalation?

They need to know if you have any of the following conditions:
- bladder problems or difficulty passing urine
- diabetes
- glaucoma
- heart disease, angina, or irregular heartbeat
- high blood pressure
- liver or kidney disease
- prostate trouble
- overactive thyroid gland
- pheochromocytoma
- seizures (convulsions)
- an unusual or allergic reaction to albuterol, ipratropium, atropine, bromides, soya protein, soybeans or peanuts, other medicines, foods, dyes, or preservatives
- pregnant or trying to get pregnant
- breast-feeding

How should I use this medicine?

Albuterol; ipratropium inhalation aerosol or inhalation solutions are for inhalation only, do not swallow. Follow the instructions on your prescription. Do not use more often than directed. *If you are using an aerosol inhaler:* Shake the canister well. It is recommended that you "test-spray" the inhaler three times into the air before using your inhaler for the first time. You should also "test spray" the inhaler in cases where you have not used it for more than 24 hours. Tilt your head back slightly. Breathe out fully, emptying as much air as possible from your lungs. Keep the canister upright. Keep the inhaler about 1 inch from your open mouth (or place the mouthpiece loosely between your open lips). Press down on the inhaler (one puff) while breathing in deeply and slowly. If you can, hold your breath to the count of 10 (or as long as you can) and then breathe out (exhale). Wait at least 1 to 2 minutes between puffs. Your inhaler will come with some instructions. Read the instructions carefully; ask your prescriber or pharmacist about instructions you do not understand. Contact your pediatrician or health care professional regarding the use of this medicine in children. Special care may be needed. *If you are using a nebulizer:* Follow your prescriber's instructions for use of the inhalation solution in your nebulizer machine. The albuterol; ipratropium nebulizer solution does not need dilution prior to use in the jet nebulizer.

What if I miss a dose?

If you miss a dose, use it as soon as you can. If it is almost time for your next dose, use only that dose. Do not use double or extra doses.

What may interact with albuterol; ipratropium inhalation?

- arsenic trioxide
- astemizole
- atropine, hyoscyamine, or related medications
- bepridil
- beta-blockers, often used for high blood pressure or heart problems
- caffeine
- certain antibiotics (such as clarithromycin, erythromycin, gatifloxacin, gemifloxacin, grepafloxacin, levofloxacin, linezolid, moxifloxacin, sparfloxacin)
- chloroquine
- cisapride
- droperidol
- halofantrine
- levomethadyl
- medicines for colds and breathing difficulties
- medicines for heart disease or high blood pressure
- medicines known as MAO inhibitors, such as phenelzine (Nardil®), tranylcypromine (Parnate®), isocarboxazid (Marplan®), and selegiline (Carbex®, Eldepryl®)
- medicines to control heart rhythm (examples: amiodarone, disopyramide, dofetilide, flecainide, procainamide, quinidine, sotalol)
- medicines for treating depression or mental illness (amoxapine, haloperidol, maprotiline, pimozide, phenothiazines, risperidone, sertindole, tricyclic antidepressants, ziprasidone)
- methadone
- pentamidine
- probucol
- some medicines for weight loss (including some herbal products, ephedra, ephedrine, dextroamphetamine)
- steroid hormones such as dexamethasone, cortisone, hydrocortisone
- terfenadine
- theophylline
- thyroid hormones
- water pills or diuretics

Tell your prescriber or health care professional about all other medicines you are taking, including non-prescription medicines, nutritional supplements, or herbal products. Also tell your prescriber or health care professional if you are a frequent user of drinks with caffeine or alcohol, if you smoke, or if you use illegal drugs. These may affect the way your medicine works. Check before starting or stopping any of your medicines.

What should I watch for while taking albuterol; ipratropium inhalation?

Check with your prescriber or health care professional as soon as possible if your breathing symptoms do not improve or if they get worse. If you find that your inhalers become less effective in treating your symptoms, you should contact your health care professional as soon as possible. You may be having an increase in your bronchitis symptoms. Do not stop using albuterol; ipratropium except on your prescriber's advice. Do not get the albuterol; ipratropium aerosol spray in your eyes. It can cause irritation, pain, or blurred vision. If you do get any in your eyes, rinse out with plenty of cool tap water. Let your prescriber know if you develop vision problems or eye pain. If you are using other inhaled medicines such as an inhaled steroid, use albuterol; ipratropium first. Wait at least 5 minutes before using the other inhaler. Make sure you are using your inhaler properly. Do not use extra or more frequent inhalations. They will not improve your condition. Once a day, remove the metal canister and rinse the plastic case in warm running water. Replace canister gently without using a twisting motion. Your mouth may get dry. Chewing sugarless gum or sucking hard candy, and drinking plenty of water, will help.

What side effects may I notice from using albuterol; ipratropium inhalation?

Side effects that you should report to your prescriber or health care professional as soon as possible:

- difficulty breathing, wheezing
- dizziness
- chest pain, fast heartbeat (pounding), or irregular heartbeat
- headache (severe)
- muscle cramps
- numbness in fingers or toes
- skin rash or hives
- swelling of the lips, tongue or face
- vomiting
- unusual weakness or tiredness

Side effects that usually do not require medical attention (report to your prescriber or health care professional if they continue or are bothersome):

- anxiety, nervousness, trembling
- blurred vision
- cough
- difficulty passing urine
- difficulty sleeping
- dry mouth
- mouth sores
- nausea
- stuffy nose
- unusual taste or metallic taste in your mouth

Where can I keep my medicine?

Keep out of the reach of children. Store at a room temperature between 15 and 30 degrees C (36 and 86 degrees F); do not freeze. Cold temperature decreases the effectiveness of this medicine. Avoid excessive humidity. The albuterol; ipratropium inhaler contains flammable ingredients under pressure; keep away from heat or flames; do not puncture. Keep nebulizer solution in the foil package until time of use; protect from light. Throw away any unused medicine after the expiration date.

Alendronate tablets

FOSAMAX®;
70 mg; Tablet
Merck and Co Inc

FOSAMAX®;
40 mg; Tablet
Merck and Co Inc

What are alendronate tablets?

ALENDRONATE (Fosamax®) reduces calcium loss from bones. It helps prevent bone loss and increases production of normal healthy bone in patients with Paget's disease, osteoporosis, and other conditions that place someone at risk for bone loss, including after menopause in females or from the long-term use of corticosteroids (like prednisone) in men or women. Generic alendronate tablets are not yet available.

What should my health care professional know before I take alendronate?

They need to know if you have any of these conditions:

- dental disease
- kidney disease
- low level of blood calcium
- stomach, intestinal, or esophageal problems, like acid-reflux or GERD
- problems swallowing
- vitamin D deficiency
- an unusual or allergic reaction to alendronate, other medicines, foods, dyes, or preservatives
- pregnant or trying to get pregnant
- breast-feeding

How should I take this medicine?

Follow the directions on the prescription label. Some patients take alendronate every day. Other patients may only take a dose of alendronate once a week. If you take alendronate only once a week, take the medicine on the same day every week. Take alendronate

A

tablets by mouth in the morning, after you have risen for the day. Swallow the tablets with a full glass (6 to 8 fluid ounces) of plain water first thing in the morning. Do not take the tablets with any other type of liquid except plain water. Do not take with orange juice, coffee or other fluids as these may decrease the absorption of alendronate. Do not chew or suck on the tablets; this may cause mouth ulcers (sores). Do not eat or drink anything before you take your tablets and do not eat breakfast, drink, or take any other medicines for at least 30 minutes after taking alendronate. If you can wait for 2 hours before eating, your body will absorb even more of the medicine. After taking this medicine, remain sitting or standing upright (do not lie down) for at least 30 minutes to avoid irritation of your throat and esophagus (tube connecting mouth to stomach). Do not take this medicine at the same time as antacids, calcium, magnesium or iron supplements, or vitamins with minerals; if you take these medications, take them later in the day. Do not take your medicine more often than directed. Contact your pediatrician or health care professional regarding the use of this medicine in children. Special care may be needed.

What if I miss a dose?

If you take a daily dose of alendronate: If you miss a dose, do not take it later in the day. Continue your normal schedule starting the next morning, before you have eaten. Do not take double or extra doses. If you take a once-weekly dose of alendronate: If you miss a dose of alendronate 35-mg or 70-mg once a week, take the dose on the morning after you remember. Then return to taking your dose just once a week, as originally scheduled on your regular chosen day of the week. Never take 2 tablets on the same day. Do not take double or extra doses.

What may interact with alendronate?

- aluminum hydroxide
- antacids
- anti-inflammatory drugs like ibuprofen, naproxen, and others
- aspirin
- calcium supplements
- iron supplements
- magnesium supplements
- parathyroid hormone
- teriparatide
- vitamins with minerals

Tell your prescriber or health care professional about all other medicines you are taking including non-prescription medicines. Also tell your prescriber or health care professional if you are a frequent user of drinks with caffeine or alcohol, if you smoke, or if you use illegal drugs. These can affect the way your medicine works. Check with your health care professional before stopping or starting any of your medicines.

What should I watch for while taking alendronate?

Visit your prescriber or health care professional for regular checks on your progress. If you have Paget's disease it may be some time before you see the benefit from alendronate. Do not stop taking alendronate except on your prescriber's advice. Low blood levels of phosphorus and calcium can occur but usually do not cause serious problems. Your prescriber or health care professional may order regular blood tests to check for these problems. It is very important to take alendronate with a full glass of water (6 to 8 ounces). Do not take with orange juice, coffee or other fluids as these may decrease the absorption of alendronate. Do not take alendronate with food. Wait at least 30 minutes or longer after taking alendronate before you eat, drink or take other medicines. Because alendronate may irritate your throat, remain sitting or standing upright for at least 30 minutes after taking alendronate; do not lie down. If you begin to have pain when swallowing, difficulty swallowing, heartburn or stomach pain, call your prescriber or health care professional right away. You should make sure you get enough calcium and vitamin D in your diet while you are taking alendronate, unless directed otherwise by your health care provider. Discuss your dietary needs with your health care professional or nutritionist. If you get bone pain, or a worsening of bone pain, check with your doctor. However, many patients have improvement in their bone pain during and after treatment with alendronate. If you are taking an antacid, a mineral supplement like calcium or iron, or a vitamin with minerals, make sure that you wait at least 30 minutes, and preferably 2 hours before or after taking alendronate. Do not take them at same time. Limit your time in sunlight or other UV exposure, such as tanning beds, while taking alendronate. Alendronate may cause a rash that is worsened by exposure to the sun.

What side effects might I notice from taking alendronate?

Side effects that you should report to your prescriber or health care professional as soon as possible:
More common
- stomach pain
- heartburn
- pain or difficulty swallowing

Rare or uncommon:
- allergic reactions such as skin rash or itching, hives, swelling of the face, lips, throat or tongue
- black or tarry stools
- constant jaw pain, especially burning or cramping
- eye inflammation, pain or change in vision
- muscle twitching
- redness, blistering, peeling or loosening of the skin, including inside the mouth
- vomiting

Side effects that usually do not require medical attention (report to your prescriber or health care professional if they continue or are bothersome):

- diarrhea or constipation
- headache
- stomach gas or fullness
- nausea
- changes in taste
- bone, muscle or joint pain
- rash, which may be made worse by prolonged exposure to sunlight

Alfuzosin extended-release tablets

UROXATRAL®;
10 mg; Tablet, Extended Release
Sanofi-Synthelabo Inc

What are alfuzosin extended-release tablets?

ALFUZOSIN (UroXatral®) is used to treat enlargement of the prostate gland in men (benign prostatic hyperplasia or BPH). It is not for use in females. Alfuzosin works by relaxing muscles in the prostate and bladder neck at the site of the obstruction. This improves urine flow and reduces BPH symptoms. Generic alfuzosin sustained-release tablets are not yet available.

What should my health care professional know before I take alfuzosin?

They need to know if you have any of the following conditions:

- chest pain (angina)
- heart disease
- kidney disease
- liver disease
- low blood pressure
- prostate cancer
- an unusual or allergic reaction to alfuzosin, other medicines, foods, dyes, or preservatives

How should I take this medicine?

Take alfuzosin tablets by mouth with food and with the same meal each day. Follow the directions on the prescription label. Swallow the tablets whole with a drink of water; do not crush, cut or chew the tablets. Do not take your medicine more often than directed. Do not stop taking except on your prescriber's advice. Contact your pediatrician or health care professional regarding the use of this medicine in children. Special care may be needed.

What if I miss a dose?

If you miss a dose, take it as soon as you can. If it is almost time for your next dose, take only that dose. Do not take double or extra doses.

What may interact with alfuzosin?

- cimetidine
- drugs used to treat fungal or yeast infections (examples: fluconazole, itraconazole, ketoconazole, voriconazole)
- drugs used to treat HIV infection (examples: ritonavir, saquinavir)
- fluoxetine

Where can I keep my medicine?

Keep out of the reach of children in a container that small children cannot open. Store at room temperature between 15 and 30 degrees C (59 and 86 degrees F). Throw away any unused medicine after the expiration date.

- fluvoxamine
- grapefruit juice
- hawthorn
- imatinib
- medicines for chest pain or high blood pressure
- nefazodone
- sildenafil (doses of sildenafil higher than 25 mg should be taken at least 4 hours apart from taking alfuzosin)
- tadalafil
- vardenafil

Tell your prescriber or health care professional about all other medicines you are taking, including non-prescription medicines, nutritional supplements, or herbal products. Also tell your prescriber or health care professional if you are a frequent user of drinks with caffeine or alcohol, if you smoke, or if you use illegal drugs. These may affect the way your medicine works. Check with your prescriber or health care professional before stopping or starting any of your medicines.

What should I watch for while taking alfuzosin?

You must see your physician regularly for checkups while taking alfuzosin. Follow your physician's advice about when to have these checkups. You may feel drowsy or dizzy. Do not drive, use machinery, or do anything that requires mental alertness until you know how alfuzosin affects you. To reduce the risk of dizzy or fainting spells, do not sit or stand up quickly. If you begin to feel dizzy, sit down until you feel better. Avoid alcoholic drinks; they can make you more drowsy, increase flushing, and cause rapid heartbeats. Take alfuzosin at bedtime to lessen the effects of drowsiness and dizziness, but be careful if you have to get up during the night. Drowsiness and dizziness are more likely to occur after the first dose, after an increase in dose, or during hot weather or exercise. These effects can decrease once your body adjusts to this medicine. Although extremely rare in men taking alfuzosin, contact your health care provider immediately if you experience persistent painful penile erection unrelated to sexual activity (priapism). If not brought to immediate medical attention, priapism can lead to permanent erectile dysfunction (impotence). If you are going to have surgery, tell your prescriber or health care professional that you are taking alfuzosin.

What side effects may I notice from taking alfuzosin?

Side effects that you should report to your prescriber or health care professional as soon as possible:
Rare:
- difficulty breathing, shortness of breath
- painful erections or other sexual problems
- skin rash
- swelling of ankles or legs
- yellowing of skin or eyes

More common:
- fainting spells
- visual problems
- weakness

Side effects that usually do not require medical attention (report to your prescriber or health care professional if they continue or are bothersome):
- constipation or diarrhea
- dizziness
- drowsiness
- fatigue
- headache
- insomnia
- itching
- nausea or upset stomach

Where can I keep my medicine?

Keep out of the reach of children in a container that small children cannot open. Store at room temperature between 15 and 30 degrees C (59 and 86 degrees F). Protect from light and moisture. Throw away any unused medicine after the expiration date.

Allopurinol tablets

ZYLOPRIM®;
300 mg; Tablet
Prometheus
Laboratories Inc

ZYLOPRIM®;
100 mg; Tablet
Prometheus
Laboratories Inc

What are allopurinol tablets?

ALLOPURINOL (Lopurin®, Zyloprim®) reduces the amount of uric acid the body makes. Too much uric acid in the blood can cause damage and produce kidney stones and gout. Allopurinol will help to prevent gout, but will not ease an acute attack. It is also used to help prevent to decrease uric acid levels that occur as a result of some sorts of chemotherapy for certain types of leukemia, lymphoma or solid tumors. Generic allopurinol tablets are available.

What should my health care professional know before I take allopurinol?

They need to know if you have any of these conditions:
- kidney disease
- liver disease
- an unusual or allergic reaction to allopurinol, other medicines, foods, dyes, or preservatives
- pregnant or trying to get pregnant
- breast-feeding

How should I take this medicine?

Take allopurinol tablets by mouth. Follow the directions on the prescription label. Swallow the tablets with a drink of water. If allopurinol upsets your stomach, take it with food or milk. Take your doses at regular intervals. Do not take your medicine more often than directed.

What if I miss a dose?

If you miss a dose, take it as soon as you can. If it is almost time for your next dose, take only that dose. Do not take double or extra doses.

What may interact with allopurinol?

- aluminum hydroxide
- amoxicillin or ampicillin
- azathioprine
- certain medicines used to treat gout
- certain types of water pills (diuretics)
- chlorpropamide
- cyclosporine
- mercaptopurine
- theophylline
- warfarin

Tell your prescriber or health care professional about all other medicines you are taking, including non-prescription medicines, nutritional supplements, or herbal products. Also tell your prescriber or health care professional if you are a frequent user of drinks with caffeine or alcohol, if you smoke, or if you use illegal drugs. These may affect the way your medicine works. Check with your health care professional before stopping or starting any of your medicines.

What should I watch for while taking allopurinol?

Visit your prescriber or health care professional for regular checks on your progress. If you are taking allopurinol to treat gout, you may not have less frequent attacks at first. Keep taking your medicine regularly and the attacks should get better within 2 to 6 weeks. Drink plenty of water (10 to 12 full glasses a day) while you are taking allopurinol. This will help to reduce stomach upset and reduce the risk of getting gout or kidney stones. Call your prescriber or health care professional at once if you get a skin rash together with chills, fever, sore throat, or nausea and vomiting; if you have blood in your urine, or difficulty passing urine; irritation of the eyes; or swelling of the lips and mouth. Alcohol can increase the chance of stomach problems and increase the amount of uric acid in your blood. Avoid alcohol. Do not take vitamin C without asking your prescriber or health care professional. Too much vitamin C can increase the chance of getting kidney stones. You may get drowsy. Do not drive, use machinery, or do anything that needs mental alertness until you know how allopurinol affects you.

What side effects may I notice from taking allopurinol?

Side effects to allopurinol are rare but some can be serious. Side effects that you should report to your prescriber or health care professional as soon as possible:
- any type of skin rash or itching
- any signs of an allergic reaction such as difficulty breathing, wheezing, swelling or irritation of the eyes, or swelling of the lips and mouth
- blood in urine
- muscle aches or pains
- pain or difficulty passing urine, reduced amount of urine
- redness, blistering, peeling or loosening of the skin, including inside the mouth
- sore throat, fever, or chills

Side effects that usually do not require medical attention (report to your prescriber or health care professional if they continue or are bothersome):
- diarrhea
- headache
- indigestion
- loss of appetite
- nausea, vomiting
- nose bleeds
- stomach pain or cramps

Where can I keep my medicine?

Keep out of the reach of children in a container that small children cannot open. Store at room temperature between 15 and 25 degrees C (59 and 77 degrees F). Protect from moisture. Throw away any unused medicine after the expiration date.

Almotriptan tablets

AXERT®;
12.5 mg; Tablet
Ortho McNeil Pharmaceutical Inc

What are almotriptan tablets?

ALMOTRIPTAN (Axert®) helps to relieve a migraine attack that starts with or without aura (a peculiar feeling or visual disturbance that warns you of an attack). Generic almotriptan tablets are not yet available.

What should my health care professional know before I take almotriptan?

They need to know if you have any of these conditions:
- bowel disease or colitis
- diabetes
- family history of heart disease
- fast or irregular heart beat
- headaches that are different from your usual migraine
- heart or blood vessel disease, angina (chest pain), or previous heart attack
- high blood pressure
- high cholesterol
- history of stroke, transient ischemic attacks (TIAs or "mini-strokes"), or intracranial bleeding
- kidney disease
- liver disease
- overweight
- poor circulation
- postmenopausal or surgical removal of uterus and ovaries
- Raynaud's disease
- seizure disorder
- tobacco smoker
- an unusual or allergic reaction to almotriptan, other medicines, foods, dyes, or preservatives
- pregnant or trying to get pregnant
- breast-feeding

How should I take this medicine?

Take almotriptan tablets by mouth. Follow the directions on the prescription label. Almotriptan is taken at the first symptoms of a migraine attack. This medicine is not for everyday use. Swallow the tablets with a drink of water. If your migraine headache returns after one dose, you can take another dose as directed. You must allow at least 2 hours between doses. Do not take more than 25 mg total in any 24 hour period. If there is no improvement at all after the first dose, do not take a second dose without talking to your prescriber or health care professional. Do not take your medicine more often than directed. Contact your pediatrician or health care professional regarding the use of this medicine in children. Special care may be needed.

What if I miss a dose?

This does not apply, almotriptan is not for regular use.

What may interact with almotriptan?

Do not take almotriptan with any of the following medicines:

- amphetamine or cocaine
- dihydroergotamine, ergotamine, ergoloid mesylates, methysergide, or ergot-type medication—do not take within 24 hours of taking almotriptan

- eletriptan, naratriptan, rizatriptan, sumatriptan, zolmitriptan—do not take within 24 hours of taking almotriptan
- medicines for weight loss such as dexfenfluramine, dextroamphetamine, fenfluramine, or sibutramine
- monoamine oxidase inhibitors (MAOIs) such as phenelzine (Nardil®), tranylcypromine (Parnate®), isocarboxazid (Marplan®), and selegiline (Carbex®, Eldepryl®)—do not take almotriptan within 2 weeks of stopping MAOI therapy.

Check with your doctor or pharmacist if you take any of these medications:

- cough syrup or other products containing dextromethorphan
- erythromycin
- feverfew
- itraconazole or ketoconazole
- lithium
- medicines for mental depression, anxiety or mood problems such as buspirone, citalopram, fluoxetine, fluvoxamine, mirtazapine, nefazodone, paroxetine, sertraline, trazodone, tricyclic antidepressants, or venlafaxine
- meperidine
- ritonavir
- St. John's wort
- tryptophan
- verapamil

Tell your physician or health care provider: about all other medicines you are taking, including non-prescription medicines; if you are a frequent user of drinks with caffeine or alcohol; if you smoke; or if you use illegal drugs. These may affect the way your medicine works. Check with your health care professional before stopping or starting any of your medicines.

What should I watch for while taking almotriptan?

Only take almotriptan tablets for a migraine headache. Take it if you get warning symptoms or at the start of a migraine attack. Almotriptan is not for regular use to prevent migraine attacks. Do not take migraine

products that contain ergotamine while you are taking almotriptan; this combination can affect your heart. You may get drowsy or dizzy. Do not drive, use machinery, or do anything that needs mental alertness until you know how almotriptan affects you. To reduce dizzy or fainting spells, do not sit or stand up quickly, especially if you are an older patient. Alcohol can increase drowsiness, dizziness and flushing. Avoid alcoholic drinks. Smoking cigarettes may increase the risk of heart-related side effects from using almotriptan.

What side effects may I notice from taking almotriptan?

Side effects that you should report to your prescriber as soon as possible:
- chest, neck, or throat pain or tightness
- dizziness or faintness
- fast or irregular heart beat, palpitations
- feeling of chest heaviness or pressure
- increased or decreased blood pressure
- persistent severe headache
- severe stomach pain and cramping, bloody diarrhea
- shortness of breath, wheezing, or difficulty breathing
- tingling, pain, or numbness in the face, hands or feet
- unusual reaction or swelling of the skin, eyelids, face, or lips

Stop using almotriptan and call your prescriber as soon as you can if you get any of these side effects.

Side effects that usually do not require medical attention (report to your prescriber or health care professional if they continue or are bothersome):
- drowsiness
- dry mouth
- feeling warm, flushing, or redness of the face
- nausea, vomiting, or stomach upset

Where can I keep my medicine?

Keep out of the reach of children in a container that small children cannot open. Store at room temperature between 15 and 30 degrees C (59 and 86 degrees F). Protect from light and moisture. Throw away any unused medicine after the expiration date.

This drug requires an FDA medication guide. See page xxxvii.

Alosetron tablets

LOTRONEX®;
1 mg; Tablet
Glaxo Wellcome

What are alosetron tablets?

ALOSETRON (Lotronex®) is used to treat irritable bowel syndrome (IBS) in women who have severe diarrhea as the primary symptom and who have not had success with other IBS treatments. Do not use alosetron if you are constipated. Irritable bowel syndrome is also called irritable colon or spastic colon. Alosetron helps to reduce the cramping, abdominal pain, discomfort, urgency (sudden need to move the bowels), and diarrhea caused by IBS. Alosetron has not been shown to work

in men with IBS. Alosetron is available only from health care providers who participate in a special Prescribing Program because this drug may cause serious side effects. Your health care provider will discuss your condition and these side effects with you prior to prescribing this drug. Generic alosetron tablets are not available.

What should my health care professional know before I take alosetron?

They need to know if you have any of these conditions:

- if you are currently constipated or constipated most of the time, have a history of chronic or severe constipation, or if you have had adverse reactions or hospitalizations due to severe constipation
- Crohn's disease
- diverticulitis
- history of ischemic colitis, impaired intestinal circulation, bleeding, or blood clots
- history of a serious stomach or bowel blockage, like stomach or intestinal obstruction, stricture, or adhesions
- history of stomach or intestinal perforation
- kidney disease
- liver disease
- toxic megacolon
- ulcerative colitis
- an unusual or allergic reaction to alosetron, other medicines, foods, dyes, or preservatives
- pregnant or trying to get pregnant
- breast-feeding

How should I take this medicine?

Your health care professional will review a Medication Guide and a Patient-Physician Agreement with you prior to prescribing alosetron. It is important that you read and understand these materials. Let your provider know if you have any questions. If you are unable or unwilling to understand and comply with the Agreement and Medication Guide, you should not take alosetron. Read the Medication Guide before you first take alosetron and each time you refill your prescription. Take alosetron tablets by mouth with or without food. Follow the directions on the prescription label and in the Medication Guide. Swallow the tablets with a glass of water. Take your doses at regular intervals. Do not take your medicine more often than directed. Contact your pediatrician or health care professional regarding the use of this medicine in children. Special care may be needed. Alosetron is not for use in children.

What if I miss a dose?

It is best to skip the missed dose. If it is almost time for your next dose, take only that dose. Do not take double or extra doses.

What may interact with alosetron?

- amantadine
- amiodarone
- amoxapine
- antidiarrheal medications, such as Imodium®, KaoPectate®, Lomotil®
- antimuscarinic medications, such as Donnatal®, hyoscyamine, Librax®
- bethanechol
- bupropion
- cimetidine
- cisapride
- clarithromycin, erythromycin or troleandomycin
- clozapine
- cyclobenzaprine
- diltiazem

- disopyramide
- fluoxetine
- fluvoxamine
- isoniazid, INH
- maprotiline
- metoclopramide
- mibefradil
- nefazodone
- nicardipine
- olanzapine
- opiate pain medications, such as codeine, hydrocodone or morphine
- orphenadrine
- procainamide
- quinine
- St. John's Wort
- tricyclic antidepressants, such as amitriptyline or imipramine
- verapamil
- zileuton

Tell your prescriber or health care professional about all other medicines you are taking, including non-prescription medicines, nutritional supplements, or herbal products. Also tell your prescriber or health care professional if you are a frequent user of drinks with caffeine or alcohol, if you smoke, or if you use illegal drugs. These may affect the way your medicine works. Check with your health care professional before stopping or starting any of your medicines.

What should I watch for while taking alosetron?

Constipation is a common and serious side effect of alosetron. Stop taking alosetron and call your health care provider immediately if you become constipated while taking alosetron. If your constipation does not resolve, contact your prescriber again. Resume alosetron only if your constipation has resolved and you and your prescriber have agreed to restart treatment. You should not start taking alosetron if you are already constipated or constipated most of the time. Ischemic colitis is a serious and potentially life-threatening condition that has been rarely reported with alosetron. If you experience new or worsening abdominal pain, bloody diarrhea or blood in the stool, immediately stop taking alosetron and contact your prescriber. Alosetron may not work for all women who take it. For women who are helped by alosetron, relief may occur within the first week or within four weeks of starting the drug. If alosetron is stopped, it is likely that your symptoms will return within one week. You may get drowsy or dizzy. Do not drive, use machinery, or do anything that needs mental alertness until you know how alosetron affects you. Alcohol can increase drowsiness or dizziness; avoid alcoholic drinks. If you are going to have surgery, tell your prescriber or health care professional that you are taking alosetron.

What side effects may I notice from taking alosetron?

Side effects that you should report to your prescriber or health care professional immediately:

- blood in stool, bloody diarrhea or rectal bleeding
- constipation
- darkened urine
- hemorrhoids
- fever
- irregular heart beat (unusually fast or slow)
- worsening of abdominal pain
- yellowing of the eyes or the skin
- unusual fatigue or weakness

Side effects that usually do not require medical attention (report to your prescriber or health care professional if they continue or are bothersome):
- anxiety
- difficulty sleeping

- drowsiness
- dry mouth
- frequent urination
- gas
- headache
- nausea
- restlessness

Where can I keep my medicine?

Keep out of the reach of children in a container that small children cannot open. Store at room temperature between 15 and 30 degrees C (59 and 86 degrees F). Throw away any unused medicine after the expiration date.

Alprazolam tablets and extended-release tablets

XANAX®;
0.5 mg; Tablet
Pharmacia and
Upjohn Div Pfizer

XANAX XR®;
2 mg; Tablet,
Extended Release
Pharmacia and
Upjohn Div Pfizer

What are alprazolam tablets and extended-release tablets?

ALPRAZOLAM (Xanax®, Xanax® XR) is a benzodiazepine. Benzodiazepines belong to a group of medicines that slow down the central nervous system. Alprazolam relieves anxiety and nervousness and helps to treat panic attacks. Federal law prohibits the transfer of alprazolam to any person other than the patient for whom it was prescribed. Do not share this medicine with anyone else. Generic alprazolam tablets are available. Generic alprazolam extended-release tablets are available.

What should my health care professional know before I take alprazolam?

They need to know if you have any of these conditions:
- alcohol or drug abuse problems
- bipolar disorder, depression, psychosis or other mental health conditions
- glaucoma
- kidney disease
- liver disease
- lung disease, such as chronic obstructive pulmonary disease (COPD), sleep apnea or other breathing difficulties
- myasthenia gravis
- Parkinson's disease
- porphyria
- seizures or a history of seizures
- shortness of breath
- snoring
- suicidal thoughts
- an unusual or allergic reaction to alprazolam, other benzodiazepines, foods, dyes, or preservatives
- pregnant or trying to get pregnant
- breast-feeding

How should I take this medicine?

Take alprazolam tablets by mouth. Follow the directions on the prescription label. Swallow the tablets with a drink of water. If alprazolam upsets your stomach, take it with food or milk. Take your doses at regular intervals. Do not take your medicine more often than directed. Contact your pediatrician or health care professional regarding the use of this medicine in children. Special care may be needed.

What if I miss a dose?

If you miss a dose, take it as soon as you can. If it is almost time for your next dose, take only that dose. Do not take double or extra doses.

What may interact with alprazolam?

Do not take Alprazolam with any of the following:
- alcohol
- grapefruit juice
- ketoconazole
- itraconazole
- some medicines for HIV infection or AIDS

Alprazolam may also interact with the following medications:
- bosentan
- caffeine
- cimetidine
- cyclosporine
- disulfiram
- ergotamine
- female hormones, including contraceptive or birth control pills
- herbal or dietary supplements such as kava kava, melatonin, dehydroepiandrosterone, DHEA, St. John's Wort or valerian
- imatinib, STI-571
- isoniazid
- levodopa
- medicines for anxiety or sleeping problems, such as diazepam, lorazepam or triazolam

- medicines for depression, mental problems or psychiatric disturbances
- medicines for fungal infections (fluconazole, voriconazole)
- mifepristone, RU-486
- prescription pain medicines
- probenecid
- rifampin, rifapentine, or rifabutin
- some antibiotics (clarithromycin, erythromycin, troleandomycin)
- some medicines for colds, hay fever or other allergies
- some medicines for high blood pressure or heart problems (amiodarone, digoxin, diltiazem, nicardipine, verapamil)
- some medicines for seizures (carbamazepine, oxcarbazepine, phenobarbital, phenytoin, primidone)
- theophylline
- troglitazone
- zafirlukast
- zileuton

Tell your prescriber or health care professional about all other medicines you are taking, including non-prescription medicines, nutritional supplements, or herbal products. Also tell your prescriber or health care professional if you are a frequent user of drinks with caffeine or alcohol, if you smoke, or if you use illegal drugs. These may affect the way your medicine works. Check with your health care professional before stopping or starting any of your medicines.

What should I watch for while taking alprazolam?

Visit your prescriber or health care professional for regular checks on your progress. Your body can become dependent on alprazolam, ask your prescriber or health care professional if you still need to take it. However, if you have been taking alprazolam regularly for some time, do not suddenly stop taking it. You must gradually reduce the dose or you may get severe side effects. Ask your prescriber or health care professional for advice. Even after you stop taking alprazolam it can still affect your body for several days. You may get drowsy or dizzy.

Do not drive, use machinery, or do anything that needs mental alertness until you know how alprazolam affects you. To reduce the risk of dizzy and fainting spells, do not stand or sit up quickly, especially if you are an older patient. Alcohol may increase dizziness and drowsiness. Avoid alcoholic drinks. Do not treat yourself for coughs, colds or allergies without asking your prescriber or health care professional for advice. Some ingredients can increase possible side effects. If you are going to have surgery, tell your prescriber or health care professional that you are taking alprazolam.

What side effects may I notice from taking alprazolam?

Side effects that you should report to your prescriber or health care professional as soon as possible:
- confusion, forgetfulness
- depression
- difficulty passing urine
- difficulty sleeping
- difficulty speaking
- lightheadedness or fainting spells
- mood changes, excitability or aggressive behavior
- muscle cramps
- staggering or jerky movements, tremors
- weakness or tiredness

Side effects that usually do not require medical attention (report to your prescriber or health care professional if they continue or are bothersome):
- constipation or diarrhea
- drowsiness, dizziness
- dry mouth, decrease or increase in amount of saliva
- increase or decrease in appetite
- menstrual changes
- sexual dysfunction
- weight changes

Where can I keep my medicine?

Keep out of the reach of children in a container that small children cannot open. Store at room temperature between 15 and 30 degrees C (59 and 86 degrees F). Throw away any unused medicine after the expiration date.

Altretamine capsules

HEXALEN®;
50 mg; Capsule
MGI Pharma Inc

What are altretamine capsules?

ALTRETAMINE (Hexalen®) is a type of chemotherapy for treating cancer of the ovaries. Altretamine interferes with the way cancer cells grow. Generic altretamine capsules are not yet available.

What should my health care professional know before I take altretamine?

They need to know if you have any of these conditions:
- blood disorders
- dental disease

- loss of feeling, pain or numbness in the hands or feet
- recent radiation therapy
- infection (especially virus infection such as chickenpox or herpes)
- an unusual or allergic reaction to altretamine, other chemotherapy, other medicines, foods, dyes, or preservatives
- pregnant or trying to get pregnant
- breast-feeding

How should I take this medicine?

Take altretamine capsules by mouth. Follow the directions on the prescription label. Swallow the capsules

A

with a drink of water. If altretamine upsets your stomach, take it after meals. Take your doses at regular intervals. Do not take your medicine more often than directed. Finish the full course prescribed by your doctor or health care professional, even if the capsules make you feel unwell. Do not stop taking except on your prescriber's advice. Contact your pediatrician or health care professional regarding the use of this medicine in children. Special care may be needed.

What if I miss a dose?

If you miss a dose, take it as soon as you can. If it is almost time for your next dose, take only that dose. Do not take double or extra doses. If you vomit after taking a dose, call your prescriber or health care professional for advice.

What may interact with altretamine?

- cimetidine
- live virus vaccines
- phenobarbital

Tell your prescriber or health care professional about all other medicines you are taking, including non-prescription medicines, nutritional supplements, or herbal products. Also tell your prescriber or health care professional if you are a frequent user of drinks with caffeine or alcohol, if you smoke, or if you use illegal drugs. These may affect the way your medicine works. Check with your health care professional before stopping or starting any of your medicines.

What should I watch for while taking altretamine?

Visit your prescriber or health care professional for regular checks on your progress. Altretamine may make you feel generally unwell. This is not uncommon because altretamine affects good cells as well as cancer cells. Report any side effects as above, but continue your course of medicine even though you feel ill, unless your prescriber or health care professional tells you to stop. While you are taking altretamine, you will be more susceptible to infection. Try to avoid people with

colds, flu, and bronchitis. Do not have any vaccinations without your prescriber's approval and avoid anyone who has recently had oral polio vaccine. Call your prescriber or health care professional for advice if you get a fever, chills or sore throat. Do not treat yourself. Altretamine can cause blood problems. This can mean slow healing and a risk of infection. Try to avoid cutting or injuring yourself. Problems can arise if you need dental work, and in the day to day care of your teeth. Try to avoid damage to your teeth and gums when you brush or floss your teeth.

What side effects may I notice from taking altretamine?

Side effects that you should report to your prescriber or health care professional as soon as possible:
- black tarry stools
- blood in urine
- confusion, agitation, clumsiness
- depression
- fever or chills, sore throat
- lower back pain
- pain or difficulty passing urine
- red spots on the skin
- seizures (convulsions)
- tingling, pain or numbness in the hands or feet
- unusual bleeding or bruising
- unusual tiredness or weakness
- vomiting

Side effects that usually do not require medical attention (report to your prescriber or health care professional if they continue or are bothersome):
- diarrhea
- loss of appetite
- nausea
- stomach pains or cramps

Where can I keep my medicine?

Keep out of the reach of children in a container that small children cannot open. Store at room temperature between 15 and 30 degrees C (59 and 86 degrees F). Throw away any unused medicine after the expiration date.

Aluminum Hydroxide; Magnesium Carbonate chewable tablets

GAVISCON®;
160 mg/105 mg; Tablet
GlaxoSmithKline Consumer
Health

What are aluminum hydroxide; magnesium carbonate chewable tablets?

ALUMINUM HYDROXIDE; MAGNESIUM CARBONATE (Gaviscon® Extra Strength tablets) is an antacid that neutralizes or reduces stomach acid. It helps relieve symptoms of excessive stomach acidity in patients with indigestion, heartburn, or gastroesoph-

ageal reflux disorder (GERD). Aluminum hydroxide; magnesium carbonate also contains the ingredient alginic acid. Alginic acid forms a protective foam that sits on top of the stomach contents. This foam helps to prevent acid irritation to the esophagus (the tube connecting your mouth to your stomach). Generic aluminum hydroxide; magnesium carbonate tablets are available.

What should my health care professional know before I take aluminum hydroxide; magnesium carbonate?

They need to know if you have any of these conditions:

- colostomy
- constipation
- dehydration
- diarrhea
- edema or swelling of the legs and feet
- intestinal problems like colitis or diverticulitis
- kidney disease
- liver disease
- on a sodium (salt) restricted diet
- stomach bleeding or obstruction
- an unusual or allergic reaction to aluminum, magnesium or other antacids, foods, dyes, or preservatives
- pregnant or trying to get pregnant
- breast-feeding

How should I take this medicine?

Take aluminum hydroxide; magnesium carbonate tablets by mouth. Follow the directions on the label. Chew the tablets well so that foam forms in your mouth before swallowing. Do not suck on or crush the tablets; the protective foam will not form if you do this. After taking the medication, drink a full glass of water. Antacids are usually taken after meals and at bedtime, or as directed by your prescriber. Take your doses at regular intervals. Do not take your medicine more often than directed. You should remain in an upright position (do not lie down for 1 to 2 hours) after taking this medicine. Remaining in an upright position will help the protective foam to float on the top of your stomach contents. Contact your pediatrician or health care professional regarding the use of this medicine in children. Special care may be needed.

What if I miss a dose?

Aluminum hydroxide; magnesium carbonate is usually only taken when needed for stomach upset. It is usually not recommended for continued use. Missing a dose is usually not harmful. Do not take double or extra doses.

What may interact with aluminum hydroxide; magnesium carbonate?

- acetaminophen
- alendronate
- antibiotics
- aspirin and aspirin-like medicines
- captopril
- delavirdine
- etidronate
- gabapentin
- heart medicines, such as digoxin or digitoxin
- iron salts
- isoniazid
- itraconazole
- ketoconazole
- medicines for mental problems and psychotic disturbances
- medicines for movement abnormalities as in Parkinson's disease, or for gastrointestinal problems
- medicines for stomach ulcers and stomach problems
- methenamine
- misoprostol
- mycophenolate
- other magnesium-containing antacids, laxatives or supplements
- pancrelipase
- penicillamine
- phenytoin
- quinidine
- risedronate
- rosuvastatin
- sodium fluoride
- sodium polystyrene sulfonate
- sotalol
- sucralfate
- thyroid hormones (example: levothyroxine)
- tiludronate
- valproic acid
- vitamin D

Tell your prescriber or health care professional about all other medicines you are taking, including non-prescription medicines, nutritional supplements, or herbal products. Also tell your prescriber or health care professional if you are a frequent user of drinks with caffeine or alcohol, if you smoke, or if you use illegal drugs. These may affect the way your medicine works. Check with your health care professional before stopping or starting any of your medicines.

What should I watch for while taking aluminum hydroxide; magnesium carbonate?

Check with your prescriber or health care professional if aluminum hydroxide; magnesium carbonate does not relieve your stomach pains; if you get black tarry stools; notice any rectal bleeding; or feel unusually tired. Do not change to another antacid product without advice. Do not treat yourself for stomach problems with aluminum hydroxide; magnesium carbonate for more than 2 weeks without consulting your prescriber or health care professional. If you are taking other medications, leave an interval of at least 2 hours before or after dosing with this aluminum hydroxide; magnesium carbonate. If you are taking prescription medications check with a healthcare professional before taking aluminum hydroxide; magnesium carbonate. Drink several glasses of water a day. This will help to reduce possible constipation and prevent dehydration.

What side effects may I notice from taking aluminum hydroxide; magnesium carbonate?

Side effects that you should report to your prescriber or health care professional as soon as possible:

- confusion, decreased alertness
- drowsiness or dizziness
- headache
- loss of appetite

- nausea, vomiting
- weakness

Side effects that usually do not require medical attention (report to your prescriber or health care professional if they continue or are bothersome):

- chalky taste
- diarrhea
- constipation

Aluminum Hydroxide; Magnesium Hydroxide tablets

What are aluminum hydroxide; magnesium hydroxide tablets?

ALUMINUM HYDROXIDE; MAGNESIUM HYDROXIDE (Maalox®) is an antacid that neutralizes or reduces stomach acid. It helps relieve symptoms of excessive stomach acidity in patients with indigestion, heartburn, gastroesophageal reflux disorder (GERD), or stomach or duodenal ulcers. In large doses, it can act as a laxative. Generic antacid tablets are available.

What should my health care professional know before I take aluminum hydroxide; magnesium hydroxide?

They need to know if you have any of these conditions:

- colostomy
- constipation
- dehydration
- diarrhea
- edema or swelling of the legs and feet
- intestinal problems like colitis or diverticulitis
- kidney disease
- liver disease
- on a sodium (salt) restricted diet
- stomach bleeding or obstruction
- an unusual or allergic reaction to aluminum, magnesium or other antacids, foods, dyes, or preservatives
- pregnant or trying to get pregnant
- breast-feeding

How should I take this medicine?

Take magnesium hydroxide; aluminum hydroxide tablets by mouth. Follow the directions on the prescription label. Chew well, or crush the tablets before swallowing; follow with a glass of water. Antacids are usually taken after meals and at bedtime, or as directed by your prescriber. Take your doses at regular intervals. Do not take your medicine more often than directed. Contact your pediatrician or health care professional regarding the use of this medicine in children. Special care may be needed.

What if I miss a dose?

Aluminum hydroxide; magnesium hydroxide is usually only taken when needed for stomach upset. It is usually not recommended for continued use. Missing a dose is usually not harmful. Do not take double or extra doses.

Where can I keep my medicine?

Keep out of the reach of children in a container that small children cannot open. Store at room temperature between 15 and 30 degrees C (59 and 86 degrees F), do not freeze. Protect from light and moisture. Throw away any unused medicine after the expiration date.

ANTACID EXTRA STRENGTH
CHEWABLE TABLETS;
160 mg/105 mg; Tablet
Leader Brands

What may interact with aluminum hydroxide; magnesium hydroxide?

- acetaminophen
- alendronate
- antibiotics
- aspirin and aspirin-like medicines
- captopril
- delavirdine
- etidronate
- gabapentin
- heart medicines, such as digoxin or digitoxin
- iron salts
- isoniazid
- itraconazole
- ketoconazole
- medicines for mental problems and psychotic disturbances
- medicines for movement abnormalities as in Parkinson's disease, or for gastrointestinal problems
- medicines for stomach ulcers and stomach problems
- methenamine
- misoprostol
- mycophenolate
- pancrelipase
- penicillamine
- phenytoin
- quinidine
- risedronate
- rosuvastatin
- sodium fluoride
- sodium polystyrene sulfonate
- sotalol
- sucralfate
- thyroid hormones (example: levothyroxine)
- tiludronate
- valproic acid
- vitamin D

Tell your prescriber or health care professional about all other medicines you are taking, including non-prescription medicines, nutritional supplements, or herbal products. Also tell your prescriber or health care professional if you are a frequent user of drinks with caffeine or alcohol, if you smoke, or if you use illegal drugs. These may affect the way your medicine works. Check with your health care professional before stopping or starting any of your medicines.

What should I watch for [...]
hydroxide; magnesium h [...]

Check with your prescriber [...]
if aluminum hydroxide; mag [...]
relieve your stomach pains; if [...]
notice any rectal bleeding; [...]
Do not change to another antac [...]
vice. Do not treat yourself for stoma [...]
aluminum hydroxide; magnesium hydrox [...]
than 2 weeks without consulting your presc [...]
health care professional. If you are taking other medi [...]
tions, leave an interval of at least 2 hours before or [...]
after dosing with aluminum hydroxide; magnesium hydroxide. If you are taking prescription medications
check with a healthcare professional before taking aluminum hydroxide; magnesium hydroxide. Drink several glasses of water a day. This will help to reduce
possible constipation.

**What side effects may I notice from taking
aluminum hydroxide; magnesium hydroxide?**

Side effects that you should report to your prescriber
or health care professional as soon as possible:

[...] alcohol [...]
[...] hese [...]

[...] decreased alertness
[...] ion, [...] or dizziness

[...] ly do not require medical atten-
Where c[...]scriber or health care profes-
[...] are bothersome):

Keep out of the [...]
small children canno[...]
between 15 and 30 degree[...]
do not freeze. Protect from ligh[...] container that
away any unused medicine after the [...] temperature
[...] egrees F),
[...] Throw
[...] ate.

Aluminum Hydroxide;
Magnesium Trisilicate
chewable tablets

GAVISCON®;
80 mg/20 mg; Tablet
SmithKline Beecham
Consumer Healthcare LP

**What are aluminum hydroxide; magnesium
trisilicate chewable tablets?**

**ALUMINUM HYDROXIDE; MAGNESIUM
TRISILICATE** (Gaviscon® Regular Strength tablets) is an antacid that neutralizes or reduces stomach
acid. It helps relieve symptoms of excessive stomach
acidity in patients with indigestion, heartburn, or gastroesophageal reflux disorder (GERD). Aluminum hydroxide; magnesium trisilicate also contains the ingredient alginic acid. Alginic acid forms a protective foam
that sits on top of the stomach contents. This foam
helps to prevent acid irritation to the esophagus (tube
that connects your mouth to your stomach). Generic
aluminum hydroxide; magnesium trisilicate tablets are
not available.

**What should my health care professional know
before I take aluminum hydroxide; magnesium
trisilicate?**

They need to know if you have any of these conditions:
- colostomy
- constipation
- dehydration
- diarrhea
- edema or swelling of the legs and feet
- intestinal problems like colitis or diverticulitis
- kidney disease
- liver disease

- on a sodium (salt) restricted diet
- stomach bleeding or obstruction
- an unusual or allergic reaction to aluminum, magnesium or other antacids, foods, dyes, or preservatives
- pregnant or trying to get pregnant
- breast-feeding

How should I take this medicine?

Take aluminum hydroxide; magnesium trisilicate tablets by mouth. Follow the directions on the label. Chew
the tablets well so that foam forms in your mouth before
swallowing. Do not suck on or crush the tablets; the
protective foam will not form if you do this. After taking the medication, drink a full glass of water. Antacids
are usually taken after meals and at bedtime, or as directed by your physician. Take your doses at regular
intervals. Do not take your medicine more often than
directed. You should remain in an upright position (do
not lie down for 1 to 2 hours) after taking this medicine.
Remaining in an upright position will help the protective foam to float on the top of your stomach contents.
Contact your pediatrician or health care professional
regarding the use of this medicine in children. Special
care may be needed.

What if I miss a dose?

Aluminum hydroxide; magnesium trisilicate is usually
only taken when needed for stomach upset. It is not
usually recommended for continued use. Missing a dose

is usually not harmful. [...]
doses.

What may interact [...] magnesium trisilic[...]

- acetaminophen
- alendronate
- antibiotics
- aspirin and [...]
- captopril
- delavirdi[...] digoxin or digitoxin
- etidrona[...]
- gabape[...]
- heart[...]
- iron[...]
- iso[...]
- [...]tes for mental problems and psychotic distur-
- [...]es
- [...]edicines for movement abnormalities as in Parkinson's disease, or for gastrointestinal problems
- medicines for stomach ulcers and stomach problems
- methenamine
- misoprostol
- [...]ycophenolate
- other magnesium-containing antacids, laxatives or supplements
- pancrelipase
- penicillamine
- phenytoin
- quinidine
- risedronate
- rosuvastatin
- sodium fluoride
- sodium polystyrene sulfonate
- sotalol
- sucralfate
- thyroid hormones (example: levothyroxine)
- tiludronate
- valproic acid
- vitamin D

Tell your prescriber or health care professional about all other medicines you are taking, including non-prescription medicines, nutritional supplements, or herbal products. Also tell your prescriber or health care professional if you are a frequent user of drinks with caffeine

[...], if you smoke, or if you use illegal drugs. [...]ay affect the way your medicine works. Check [...] your health care professional before stopping or [...]arting any of your medicines.

What should I watch for while taking aluminum hydroxide; magnesium trisilicate?

Check with your prescriber or health care professional if aluminum hydroxide; magnesium trisilicate does not relieve your stomach pains; if you get black tarry stools; notice any rectal bleeding; or feel unusually tired. Do not change to another antacid product without advice. Do not treat yourself for stomach problems with aluminum hydroxide; magnesium trisilicate for more than 2 weeks without consulting your prescriber or health care professional. If you are taking other medications, leave an interval of at least 2 hours before or after dosing with this aluminum hydroxide; magnesium trisilicate. If you are taking prescription medications check with a healthcare professional before taking aluminum hydroxide; magnesium trisilicate. Drink several glasses of water a day. This will help to reduce possible constipation and prevent dehydration.

What side effects may I notice from taking aluminum hydroxide; magnesium trisilicate?

Side effects that you should report to your prescriber or health care professional as soon as possible:
- confusion, decreased alertness
- drowsiness or dizziness
- headache
- loss of appetite
- nausea, vomiting
- weakness

Side effects that usually do not require medical attention (report to your prescriber or health care professional if they continue or are bothersome):
- chalky taste
- diarrhea
- constipation

Where can I keep my medicine?

Keep out of the reach of children in a container that small children cannot open. Store at room temperature between 15 and 30 degrees C (59 and 86 degrees F), do not freeze. Protect from light and moisture. Throw away any unused medicine after the expiration date.

Amantadine
capsules or tablets

AMANTADINE;
100 mg; Capsule
Upsher-Smith
Laboratories Inc

SYMMETREL®;
Tablet; 100 mg
Endo
Pharmaceuticals Inc

What are amantadine capsules or tablets?

AMANTADINE (Symmetrel®) prevents or treats certain influenza (flu) infections. It is not an effective treatment for colds or other viruses. Amantadine can also improve muscle control and reduce muscle stiffness in patients with Parkinson's disease or similar movement disorders. Generic amantadine capsules are available.

What should my health care professional know before I take amantadine?

They need to know if you have any of these conditions:

- closed-angle glaucoma
- depression or other mental illness
- eczema
- heart or circulation problems
- kidney disease
- liver disease
- low blood pressure
- seizures (convulsions)
- an unusual or allergic reaction to amantadine, rimantadine, other medicines, foods, dyes, or preservatives
- pregnant or trying to get pregnant
- breast-feeding

How should I take this medicine?

Take amantadine capsules or tablets by mouth. Follow the directions on the prescription label. Swallow whole with a full glass of water. If it upsets your stomach you can take amantadine with food. Take your doses at regular intervals. Do not take your medicine more often than directed. Finish the full course prescribed by your prescriber or health care professional even if you think your condition is better. Do not stop taking except on your prescriber's advice. Contact your pediatrician or health care professional regarding the use of this medicine in children. Special care may be needed.

What if I miss a dose?

If you miss a dose, take it as soon as you can. If it is almost time for your next dose, take only that dose. Do not take double or extra doses.

What may interact with amantadine?

- alcohol
- bupropion
- caffeine
- haloperidol
- hydrochlorothiazide, HCTZ; triamterene
- medicines for hay fever and other allergies
- medicines for depression or other mental illness
- metoclopramide
- quinidine
- quinine
- sulfamethoxazole; trimethoprim, SMX-TMP

Tell your prescriber or health care professional about all other medicines you are taking, including non-prescription medicines, nutritional supplements, or herbal products. Also tell your prescriber or health care professional if you are a frequent user of drinks with caffeine or alcohol, if you smoke, or if you use illegal drugs. These may affect the way your medicine works. Check with your health care professional before stopping or starting any of your medicines.

What should I watch for while taking amantadine?

Let your prescriber or health care professional know if your symptoms do not improve in a few days. You may get drowsy or dizzy. Do not drive, use machinery, or do anything that needs mental alertness until you know how amantadine affects you. To reduce the risk of dizzy or fainting spells, do not sit or stand up quickly, especially if you are an older patient. Alcohol can make you more drowsy and dizzy, increase confusion and lightheadedness. Avoid alcoholic drinks. If you are taking amantadine for a movement disorder, do not suddenly stop taking it. You may get muscle stiffness, paralysis, confusion, or find it difficult to pass urine. If you are taking amantadine for Parkinson's disease, be careful not to overdo physical activity as your condition improves. Gradually increase activity so that your body has time to adjust. Your mouth may get dry. Chewing sugarless gum or sucking hard candy, and drinking plenty of water will help. Brush and floss teeth regularly and carefully to avoid problems with the mouth and gums.

What side effects may I notice from taking amantadine?

Side effects that you should report to your prescriber or health care professional as soon as possible:

- changes in vision
- depression or thoughts of suicide
- difficulty passing urine
- fainting spells or lightheadedness
- hallucinations (seeing things that are not really there)
- movement difficulties
- purplish spots or network on the skin
- seizures (convulsions)
- swelling of the feet or legs

Side effects that usually do not require medical attention (report to your prescriber or health care professional if they continue or are bothersome):

- anxiety, irritability, nervousness
- diarrhea or constipation
- difficulty sleeping, or nightmares
- drowsiness
- dry mouth
- headache
- loss of appetite
- nausea or vomiting
- unusual tiredness

Where can I keep my medicine?

Keep out of the reach of children in a container that small children cannot open. Store at room temperature between 15 and 30 degrees C (59 and 86 degrees F). Keep container tightly closed. Throw away any unused medicine after the expiration date.

Amiloride tablets

MIDAMOR®;
5 mg; Tablet
Merck and Co Inc

AMILORIDE;
Tablet; 5 mg;
Par Pharmaceutical
Inc

What are amiloride tablets?

AMILORIDE (Midamor®) is a diuretic (water or fluid pill). Diuretics increase the amount of urine passed, which causes the body to lose water and salt. Amiloride is known as a potassium-sparing diuretic. It does not increase potassium loss, as many other diuretics do, and is useful for treating patients with low levels of potassium. Increased water loss helps to treat high blood pressure and swelling caused by heart disease. Amiloride can be used in combination with other medicines to treat hypertension (high blood pressure). Generic amiloride tablets are available.

What should my health care professional know before I take amiloride?

They need to know if you have any of these conditions:
- diabetes
- elderly patient over 65 years old
- high levels of potassium in the blood
- kidney disease, passing very little urine
- liver disease
- low levels of sodium in the blood
- an unusual or allergic reaction to amiloride, other medications, foods, dyes, or preservatives
- pregnant or trying to get pregnant
- breast-feeding

How should I take this medicine?

Take amiloride tablets by mouth. Follow the directions on the prescription label. Swallow the tablets with a drink of water. Take amiloride with food. Take your doses at regular intervals. Do not take your medicine more often than directed. Remember that you will need to pass urine frequently after taking amiloride. Do not take your doses at a time of day that will cause you problems. Do not take at bedtime. Contact your pediatrician or health care professional regarding the use of this medicine in children. Special care may be needed.

What if I miss a dose?

If you miss a dose, take it as soon as you can. If it is almost time for your next dose, take only that dose. Do not take double or extra doses.

What may interact with amiloride?

- anti-inflammatory drugs (NSAIDs, such as ibuprofen)
- cyclosporine
- digoxin
- dofetilide
- heparin
- lithium
- medicines for high blood pressure or heart failure (ACE inhibitors such as enalapril or ramipril; angiotensin II blockers such as losartan or valsartan; and others)
- potassium salts
- water pills

Tell your prescriber or health care professional about all other medicines you are taking, including non-prescription medicines, nutritional supplements, or herbal products. Also tell your prescriber or health care professional if you are a frequent user of drinks with caffeine or alcohol, if you smoke, or if you use illegal drugs. These may affect the way your medicine works. Check with your health care professional before stopping or starting any of your medicines.

What should I watch for while taking amiloride?

Visit your prescriber or health care professional for regular checks on your progress. Check your blood pressure regularly. Ask your prescriber or health care professional what your blood pressure should be, and when you should contact him or her. Amiloride taken for high blood pressure or fluid retention is not a cure. Amiloride will only control your blood pressure for as long as you continue to take it; do not stop taking amiloride except on your prescriber's advice. Watch your diet while you are taking amiloride. Ask your prescriber or health care professional about both potassium and sodium intake. Avoid salt-substitutes and nutritional supplements that contain potassium, unless your prescriber or health care professional tells you otherwise. Too much potassium can be very harmful. You may need to avoid foods that are high in potassium such as bananas, coconuts, dates, figs, prunes, apricots, peaches, grapefruit juice, tomato juice, and orange juice. Alcohol can make you lightheaded, dizzy and increase confusion. Avoid or limit intake of alcohol while you are taking amiloride.

What side effects may I notice from taking amiloride?

Side effects that you should report to your prescriber or health care professional as soon as possible:
- confusion
- dark yellow or brown urine
- decreased or increased amount of urine passed
- difficult breathing
- fast or irregular heartbeat, palpitations, chest pain
- nervousness
- numbness or tingling in hands, feet, or lips
- pain or difficulty passing urine
- unusual tiredness or weakness
- weakness or heaviness of legs
- yellowing of the eyes or skin

Side effects that usually do not require medical attention (report to your prescriber or health care professional if they continue or are bothersome):

- blurred vision
- dizziness or lig
- headache
- loss of appetite
- muscle cramps
- nausea, vomiting
- sexual difficulty (impoten
- skin rash, itching

- stomach cramps
- constipation, or diarrhea

Where can I keep my medicine?

eep out of the reach of children in a container that
il children cannot open. Store at room temperature
30 degrees C (86 degrees F). Protect from mois-
ow away any unused medicine after the expi-

Amiloride; Hydrochlorothiazide, HCTZ tablets

What are amiloride; hydrochlorothiazide tablets?

AMILORIDE; HYDROCHLOROTHIAZIDE
(Moduretic®) is a diuretic combination which is also known as a 'water pill'. Diuretics increase the amount of urine passed, which causes the body to lose water and salt. This drug is used to treat high blood pressure or water retention and swelling caused by conditions such as heart, kidney, and liver disease. Amiloride does not cause your body to lose potassium the way that many diuretics do. Generic amiloride-hydrochlorothiazide tablets are available.

What should my health care professional know before I take amiloride; hydrochlorothiazide?

They need to know if you have any of these conditions:
- diabetes mellitus
- difficulty breathing or chronic lung disease
- gout or high blood levels of uric acid
- high blood levels of potassium
- kidney disease
- liver disease or jaundice
- low blood levels of sodium
- pancreatitis
- small amount of urine, or difficulty passing urine
- systemic lupus erythematosus (SLE)
- unusual or allergic reaction to, amiloride, hydrochlorothiazide, other diuretics, sulfonamide drugs, other medicines, foods, dyes, or preservatives
- breast-feeding
- pregnant or trying to get pregnant

How should I take this medicine?

Take amiloride-hydrochlorothiazide tablets by mouth. Follow the directions on the prescription label. Swallow the capsules or tablets with a drink of water. Take this medication with food. Take your doses at regular intervals. Do not take your medicine more often than directed. Remember that you will need to pass urine frequently after taking amiloride-hydrochlorothiazide. Do not take your doses at a time of day that will cause you problems. Do not take at bedtime. Contact your pediatrician or health care professional regarding the

use of this med
needed.

MODURETIC®;
mg; Tablet
nd Co Inc

n. Special care may be

What if I miss a dose?

If you miss a dose, take it as soon
almost time for your next dose, take
Do not take double or extra doses.

If it is
that dose

What may interact with amiloride; hydrochlorothiazide?

- alcohol
- allopurinol
- amantadine
- amoxicillin
- amphotericin B
- anti-inflammatory drugs including NSAIDs (such as ibuprofen), aspirin, or salicylates
- arsenic trioxide
- barbiturate medicines for inducing sleep or treating seizures (convulsions)
- bepridil
- cisplatin
- cyclosporine
- dofetilide
- drospirenone; ethinyl estradiol
- griseofulvin
- hawthorn
- heparin
- hormones such as cortisone, hydrocortisone, prednisone
- horse chestnut
- levomethadyl
- lithium
- medicines for asthma such as bronchodilators (such as albuterol)
- medicines for diabetes
- medicines for high blood pressure or heart failure (ACE inhibitors such as enalapril or ramipril, digoxin, angiotensin II antagonists such as losartan or valsartan, and others)
- methazolamide
- neuromuscular blockers used during anesthesia
- some antibiotics which increase sensitivity to sunlight (sulfas, tetracyclines)
- some medicines for mental disorders (phenothiazines)

- vitamin A (retinol) creams or pills (such as ... and others)
- some cholesterol-lowering medications (cholestyramine or colestipol)
- some prescription pain medicines for p... deine, morphine or oxycodone)
- potassium salts
- quinidine
- sotalol
- tacrolimus
- water pills or diuretics

Tell your prescriber or h... ...ional about all other medicines you ... ...uding non-pre-scription medicines, ...lements, or herbal products. Also tell y... or health care profes-sional if you are a... ...er of drinks with caffeine or alcohol, if y... , or if you use illegal drugs. These may aff... ...way your medicine works. Check with your b... are professional before stopping or starting ... your medicines.

What should I watch for while taking amiloride; hydrochlorothiazide?

Visit your prescriber or health care professional for reg-ular checks on your progress. Check your blood pressure regularly. Ask your prescriber or health care profes-sional what your blood pressure should be, and when you should contact him or her. You must not get dehy-drated; ask your prescriber or health care professional how much fluid you need to drink a day. Older patients may be more sensitive to the dehydrating effects of diuretics. This drug will increase the amount of urine you pass. Do not stop taking this medication except on your prescriber's advice. Check with your prescriber or health care professional if you get severe nausea, vomiting or diarrhea. Watch your diet while you are taking this medication. Ask your prescriber or health care professional about diet and your potassium and sodium intake. Too much potassium can be harmful in some patients. Elderly patients, the severely ill, dia-betics, or patients with kidney problems are more likely to suffer from the effects of too much potassium. Avoid salt-substitutes and nutritional supplements that con-tain potassium, unless your prescriber or health care professional tells you otherwise. Too much potassium can be very harmful. You may need to avoid foods that are high in potassium such as bananas, coconuts, dates, figs, prunes, apricots, peaches, grapefruit juice, tomato juice, and orange juice. You may get dizzy or light-headed. Do not drive, use machinery, or do anything that needs mental alertness until you know how this drug affects you. To reduce the risk of dizzy or fainting spells, do not sit or stand up quickly, especially if you are an older patient. Alcohol can make you light-headed, dizzy and increase confusion. Avoid or limit intake of alcoholic drinks. Amiloride; hydrochlorothi-

...lood sugar levels. If you are ...check on blood and urine sugar. ...rescriber or health care professional ...ge the dose of your diabetic medicine. ...hydrochlorothiazide may make your skin ...sitive to sun or ultraviolet light. Keep out of ...un, or wear protective clothing and use a sun-screen. Do not use sun lamps or sun tanning beds or booths. If you are going to have surgery, tell your pre-scriber or health care professional that you are taking amiloride; hydrochlorothiazide.

What side effects may I notice from taking amiloride; hydrochlorothiazide?

Side effects that you should report to your prescriber or health care professional as soon as possible:

- abdominal pain
- confusion
- difficulty breathing
- fast or irregular heartbeat, palpitations, chest pain
- fever, chills
- faintness or moderate dizziness
- hair loss (rare)
- muscle pain or cramps
- numbness or tingling in hands, feet, or lips
- pain or difficulty passing urine, reduced amount of urine passed
- palpitations or chest pain
- redness, blistering, peeling or loosening of the skin, including inside the mouth
- skin rash, itching
- unusual bleeding or bruising, pinpoint red spots on the skin
- unusual tiredness or weakness
- yellowing of the eyes or skin
- blurred vision, change in vision
- worsened gout pain
- decreased sexual function

Side effects that usually do not require medical atten-tion (report to your prescriber or health care profes-sional if they continue or are bothersome):

- constipation
- diarrhea
- mild dizziness
- dry mouth
- fatigue or weakness
- decreased appetite
- headache
- increased sensitivity to the sun
- increased frequency of urination
- nausea, vomiting
- stomach gas or belching

Where can I keep my medicine?

Keep out of the reach of children in a container that small children cannot open. Store at room temperature between 15 and 30 degrees C (59 and 86 degrees F). Protect from light. Throw away any unused medicine after the expiration date.

Amiodarone tablets

CORDARONE®;
200 mg; Tablet
Wyeth Div Wyeth
Pharmaceuticals Inc

PACERONE®;
200 mg; Tablet
Upsher-Smith
Laboratories Inc

This drug requires an FDA medication guide. See page xxxvii.

What are amiodarone tablets?

AMIODARONE (Cordarone®, Pacerone®) is an antiarrhythmic agent and is used to help your heart to beat regularly. Because this drug can have significant side-effects, this is a medicine that is used when irregular heartbeats have not responded to other medicines. It is usually reserved for treating potentially life-threatening heartbeat problems. Generic amiodarone tablets are available

What should my health care professional know before I take amiodarone?

They need to know if you have any of these conditions:
- other heart problems
- liver disease
- thyroid disease
- lung disease
- an unusual or allergic reaction to amiodarone, iodine, other medicines, foods, dyes, or preservatives
- pregnant or trying to get pregnant
- breast-feeding

How should I take this medicine?

Take amiodarone tablets by mouth. Follow the directions on the prescription label. Swallow the tablets with a drink of water. Amiodarone may be taken with or without food, but you should take it the same way each time. Do not take amiodarone with grapefruit juice, as this affects how amiodarone is absorbed and may increase the risk of side effects. Take your doses at regular intervals. Do not take your medicine more often than directed. Keep taking your medicine even if you feel better; do not stop taking except on your prescriber's advice.
- For all uses of this medicine:

Before starting this medication, read the paper (Med-Guide) on your prescription provided by your pharmacist or health care professional. This paper will tell you about the specific product you are taking. Make certain you understand the instructions. Ask your pharmacist or health care provider if you have questions.
Contact your pediatrician or health care professional regarding the use of this medicine in children. Special care may be needed.

What if I miss a dose?

If you miss a dose, take it as soon as you can. If it is almost time for your next dose, take only the next scheduled dose. Do not take double or extra doses.

What drug(s) may interact with amiodarone?

- arsenic trioxide
- astemizole
- beta-blockers or calcium-channel blockers, often used for high blood pressure or heart problems
- bosentan
- certain antibiotics (such as clarithromycin, erythromycin, gatifloxacin, gemifloxacin, grepafloxacin, levofloxacin, moxifloxacin, sparfloxacin, troleandomycin)
- cevimeline
- cholestyramine
- cimetidine
- cisapride
- cyclosporine
- dextromethorphan
- dolasetron
- doxercalciferol
- fentanyl
- grapefruit juice
- ginger
- halofantrine
- hawthorn
- medicines for angina, high blood pressure, or heart failure
- medicines for colds or breathing difficulties (including asthma)
- medicines for HIV infection
- medicines for mental depression such as tricyclic antidepressants
- medicines for mental problems or psychotic disturbances
- medicines for seizures (convulsions) such as phenytoin
- medicines for thyroid problems
- medicines to control heart rhythm (examples: digoxin, disopyramide, dofetilide, sotalol, procainamide, quinidine)
- medicines to lower cholesterol such as atorvastatin, cerivastatin, lovastatin, or simvastatin
- radiopaque contrast agents
- rifampin, rifabutin, or rifapentine
- pimozide
- probucol
- pyridoxine or vitamin B6
- ramelteon
- red yeast rice
- sevelamer
- sirolimus or tacrolimus
- St. John's Wort
- terfenadine
- tramadol
- voriconazole
- warfarin
- water pills (diuretics)

Tell your prescriber or health care professional about all other medicines you are taking, including non-prescription medicines, nutritional supplements, or herbal products. Also tell your prescriber or health care professional if you are a frequent user of drinks with caffeine or alcohol, if you smoke, or if you use illegal drugs. These may affect the way your medicine works. Check with your health care professional before stopping or starting any of your medicines.

...ould I watch for while taking ...arone?

...r condition will be monitored closely when you first ...gin amiodarone therapy. Often, this drug is first start-ed in a hospital or other monitored health care setting. Amiodarone can cause serious side effects including sig-nificant lung damage, liver damage, vision changes, thy-roid dysfunction, skin problems, and potentially heart-beat problems. It is very important to have regular checks with your health care professional. Notify your prescriber immediately if you notice symptoms that are listed in the side effects section, or any other persistent problems or unusual reactions. Amiodarone can be pres-ent in the body for a long time (months); some side ef-fects may persist for a time after treatment is stopped.

Once you are on maintenance therapy, visit your pre-scriber or health care professional for regular checks on your progress. Check with your prescriber or health care professional if you develop a cough or have any difficulty breathing. Because your condition and use of this medicine carry some risk, it is a good idea to carry an identification card, necklace or bracelet with details of your condition, medications, and prescriber or health care professional.

You may get dizzy; to avoid a sudden drop in blood pressure and fainting spells, do not stand or sit up quickly, especially if you are an older person, until you know how amiodarone affects you.

Amiodarone can make your skin more sensitive to the sun. Keep out of the sun, or wear protective clothing outdoors and use a sunscreen. Do not use sun lamps or sun tanning beds or booths.

You should have regular eye exams before and during treatment with amiodarone. Call your doctor if you have blurred vision, see halos, or your eyes become sensitive to light, or experience other changes in vi-sion. Your eyes may get dry while you are using amio-darone. It may be helpful to use a lubricating eye solu-tion or artificial tears solution.

If you are going to have surgery tell your prescriber or health care professional that you are taking amiodarone.

What side effects may I notice from taking amiodarone?

Side effects that you should report to your prescriber or health care professional as soon as possible:
- appetite increase or decrease
- blue-gray coloring of the skin
- blurred vision, seeing blue-green halos, increased sen-sitivity of the eyes to light, loss of vision
- chest pain
- cough, or difficulty breathing
- difficulty walking
- dry or puffy skin or eyes
- feeling faint or light-headed
- heart pounding or skipping a beat
- heart beating very fast or very slow
- intolerance to heat or cold
- nervousness
- numbness or tingling in hands or feet
- pain and swelling of the scrotum
- passing brown or dark-colored urine
- skin rash
- sleep difficulties
- spitting up blood
- sweating
- trembling or shaking hands
- unusual or uncontrolled movements of body
- unusual tiredness or weakness
- vomiting
- weight gain or loss
- yellowing of the eyes or skin

Side effects that usually do not require medical atten-tion (report to your prescriber or health care profes-sional if they continue or are bothersome):
- bitter or metallic taste in the mouth
- constipation
- decreased sexual ability or desire in men
- dizziness
- flushing of the face
- headache
- nausea

Where can I keep my medicine?

Keep out of the reach of children in a container that small children cannot open. Store at room tempera-ture, approximately 25 degrees C (77 degrees F). Pro-tect from light. Keep container tightly closed. Throw away any unused medicine after the expiration date.

This drug requires an FDA medication guide. See page xxxvii.

Amitriptyline tablets

ELAVIL;
100 mg; Tablet
Mutual/United
Research
Laboratories

ENDEP;
10 mg; Tablet
Sandoz
Pharmaceuticals

What are amitriptyline tablets?

AMITRIPTYLINE (Elavil®, Endep®) is an antide-pressant. Amitriptyline can lift your spirits by treating your depression, especially if it is associated with sleep disturbance. Improvement of sleep patterns can be the first benefit of treatment. Your prescriber or health care professional may prescribe amitriptyline for other con-ditions, such as relief from nerve pain. Generic amitrip-tyline tablets are available.

What should my health care professional know before I take amitriptyline?

They need to know if you have any of these conditions:
- an alcohol problem
- asthma, difficulty breathing
- blood disorders or disease
- diabetes
- difficulty passing urine, prostate trouble
- glaucoma
- having intramuscular injections

- heart disease or previous heart attack
- liver disease
- overactive thyroid
- Parkinson's disease
- schizophrenia
- seizures (convulsions)
- stomach disease
- an unusual or allergic reaction to amitriptyline, other medicines, foods, dyes, or preservatives
- pregnant or trying to get pregnant
- breast-feeding

How should I take this medicine?

Take amitriptyline tablets by mouth. Follow the directions on the prescription label. Swallow the tablets with a drink of water. You can take the tablets with or without food. Take your doses at regular intervals. Do not take your medicine more often than directed. Do not stop taking except on your prescriber's advice. Contact your pediatrician or health care professional regarding the use of this medicine in children. Special care may be needed. Adolescents, 12 to 18 years old, and elderly patients over 65 years old may have a stronger reaction to this medicine and need smaller doses.

What if I miss a dose?

If you miss a dose normally taken at bedtime to avoid daytime drowsiness, it may be better to miss that dose. If you take more than one dose a day and miss a dose, take it as soon as you can. If it is almost time for your next dose, take only that dose. Follow your prescriber's advice on missed doses. Do not take double or extra doses.

What may interact with amitriptyline?

Amitriptyline can interact with many other medicines. Some interactions can be very important. Make sure your prescriber or health care professional knows about all other medicines you are taking. Many important interactions are listed below:

Do not take amitriptyline with any of the following medications:

- astemizole (Hismanal®)
- cisapride (Propulsid®)
- probucol
- terfenadine (Seldane®)
- thioridazine (Mellaril®)
- medicines called MAO inhibitors-phenelzine (Nardil®), tranylcypromine (Parnate®), isocarboxazid (Marplan®), selegiline (Eldepryl®)
- other medicines for mental depression (may be duplicate therapies or cause additive side effects)

Amitriptyline may also interact with any of the following medications:

- alcohol
- antacids
- atropine and related drugs like hyoscyamine, scopolamine, tolterodine and others
- barbiturate medicines for inducing sleep or treating seizures (convulsions), such as phenobarbital
- blood thinners, such as warfarin

- bromocriptine
- bupropion
- cimetidine
- clonidine
- cocaine
- delavirdine
- diphenoxylate
- disulfiram
- donepezil
- drugs for treating HIV infection
- female hormones, including contraceptive or birth control pills and estrogen
- galantamine
- herbs and dietary supplements like ephedra (Ma huang), kava kava, SAM-e, St. John's wort, valerian, or others
- imatinib, STI-571
- kaolin; pectin
- labetalol
- levodopa and other medicines for movement problems like Parkinson's disease
- lithium
- medicines for anxiety or sleeping problems
- medicines for colds, flu and breathing difficulties, like pseudoephedrine
- medicines for hay fever or allergies (antihistamines)
- medicines for weight loss or appetite control
- medicines used to regulate abnormal heartbeat or to treat other heart conditions (examples: amiodarone, bepridil, disopyramide, dofetilide, encainide, flecainide, ibutilide, mibefradil, procainamide, propafenone, quinidine, and others)
- metoclopramide
- muscle relaxants, like cyclobenzaprine
- other medicines for mental or mood problems and psychotic disturbances
- prescription pain medications like morphine, codeine, tramadol and others
- procarbazine
- seizure (convulsion) or epilepsy medicine such as carbamazepine or phenytoin
- stimulants like dexmethylphenidate or methylphenidate
- some antibiotics (examples: erythromycin, gatifloxacin, levofloxacin, linezolid, moxifloxacin, sotalol, sparfloxacin)
- tacrine
- thyroid hormones such as levothyroxine

Tell your prescriber or health care professional about all other medicines you are taking, including non-prescription medicines, nutritional supplements, or herbal products. Also tell your prescriber or health care professional if you are a frequent user of drinks with caffeine or alcohol, if you smoke, or if you use illegal drugs. These may affect the way your medicine works. Check with your health care professional before stopping or starting any of your medicines.

What should I watch for while taking amitriptyline?

Visit your prescriber or health care professional for regular checks on your progress. It can take several days before you feel the full effect of amitriptyline. If you have been taking amitriptyline regularly for some time, do not suddenly stop taking it. You must gradually reduce the dose or you may get severe side effects. Ask your prescriber or health care professional for advice. Even after you stop taking amitriptyline it can still affect your body for several days. You may get drowsy or dizzy. Do not drive, use machinery, or do anything that needs mental alertness until you know how amitriptyline affects you. Do not stand or sit up quickly, especially if you are an older patient. This reduces the risk of dizzy or fainting spells. Alcohol may increase dizziness and drowsiness. Avoid alcoholic drinks. Do not treat yourself for coughs, colds or allergies without asking your prescriber or health care professional for advice. Some ingredients can increase possible side effects. Your mouth may get dry. Chewing sugarless gum or sucking hard candy, and drinking plenty of water will help. Amitriptyline may cause dry eyes and blurred vision. If you wear contact lenses you may feel some discomfort. Lubricating drops may help. See your ophthalmologist if the problem does not go away or is severe. Amitriptyline may make your skin more sensitive to the sun. Keep out of the sun, or wear protective clothing outdoors and use a sunscreen. Do not use sun lamps or sun tanning beds or booths. If you are diabetic, check your blood sugar more often than usual, especially during the first few weeks of treatment with amitriptyline. Amitriptyline can affect blood glucose (sugar) levels. Call your prescriber or health care professional for advice if you notice a change in the results of blood or urine glucose tests. If you are going to have surgery or will need an x-ray procedure that uses contrast agents, tell your prescriber or health care professional that you are taking this medicine.

What side effects may I notice from taking amitriptyline?

Side effects that you should report to your prescriber or health care professional as soon as possible:

- abnormal production of milk in females
- blurred vision or eye pain
- breast enlargement in both males and females
- confusion, hallucinations (seeing or hearing things that are not really there)
- difficulty breathing
- fainting spells
- fever with increased sweating
- irregular or fast, pounding heartbeat, palpitations
- muscle stiffness, or spasms
- pain or difficulty passing urine, loss of bladder control
- seizures (convulsions)
- sexual difficulties (decreased sexual ability or desire, difficulty ejaculating)
- stomach pain
- swelling of the testicles
- tingling, pain, or numbness in the feet or hands
- unusual weakness or tiredness
- yellowing of the eyes or skin

Side effects that usually do not require medical attention (report to your prescriber or health care professional if they continue or are bothersome):

- anxiety
- constipation, or diarrhea
- drowsiness or dizziness
- dry mouth
- increased sensitivity of the skin to sun or ultraviolet light
- loss of appetite
- nausea, vomiting
- skin rash or itching
- weight gain or loss

Where can I keep my medicine?

Keep out of the reach of children in a container that small children cannot open. Store at room temperature between 15 and 30 degrees C (59 and 86 degrees F). Throw away any unused medicine after the expiration date.

Amlodipine tablets

NORVASC®;
5 mg; Tablet
Pfizer Laboratories
Div Pfizer Inc

NORVASC®;
10 mg; Tablet
Pfizer Laboratories
Div Pfizer Inc

What are amlodipine tablets?

AMLODIPINE (Norvasc®) is a calcium-channel blocker. It affects the amount of calcium found in your heart and muscle cells. This results in relaxation of blood vessels, which can reduce the amount of work the heart has to do. Amlodipine lowers high blood pressure (hypertension). It also relieves different types of chest pain (angina). It is not a cure. Generic amlodipine tablets are not yet available.

What should my health care professional know before I take amlodipine?

They need to know if you have any of these conditions:
- heart problems, including heart failure or aortic stenosis
- liver disease
- low blood pressure

- an unusual or allergic reaction to amlodipine, other medicines, foods, dyes, or preservatives
- pregnant or trying to get pregnant
- breast-feeding

How should I take this medicine?

Take amlodipine tablets by mouth. Follow the directions on the prescription label. Swallow the tablets with a drink of water. You can take the tablets with or without food. Do not significantly increase grapefruit juice intake while taking this drug, or avoid grapefruit juice if possible. Take your doses at regular intervals. Do not take your medicine more often then directed. Do not stop taking except on your prescriber's advice. Contact your pediatrician or health care professional regarding the use of this medicine in children. Special care may be needed. Elderly patients over 65 years old may have a stronger reaction to this medicine and need smaller doses.

What if I miss a dose?

If you miss a dose, take it as soon as you can. If it is almost time for your next dose, take only that dose. Do not take double or extra doses.

What may interact with amlodipine?

- anti-inflammatory drugs (NSAIDs, such as ibuprofen)
- barbiturates such as phenobarbital
- bosentan
- grapefruit juice
- herbal or dietary supplements such as ginger, gingko biloba, ginseng, hawthorn, ma huang (ephedra), melatonin, St. John's wort, went yeast
- imatinib, STI-571
- local anesthetics or general anesthetics
- medicines for fungal infections (fluconazole, itraconazole, ketoconazole, voriconazole)
- medicines for high blood pressure
- medicines for HIV infection or AIDS
- medicines for prostate problems
- medicines for seizures (carbamazepine, phenobarbital, phenytoin, primidone, zonisamide)
- rifampin, rifapentine, or rifabutin
- some antibiotics (clarithromycin, erythromycin, telithromycin, troleandomycin)
- some medicines for heart-rhythm problems (amiodarone, diltiazem, verapamil)
- some medicines for depression or mental problems (fluoxetine, fluvoxamine, nefazodone)
- water pills (diuretics)
- yohimbine
- zafirlukast
- zileuton

Tell your prescriber or health care professional about all other medicines you are taking, including non-prescription medicines, nutritional supplements, or herbal products. Also tell your prescriber or health care professional if you are a frequent user of drinks with caffeine or alcohol, if you smoke, or if you use illegal drugs. These may affect the way your medicine works. Check with your health care professional before stopping or starting any of your medicines.

What should I watch for while taking amlodipine?

Check your blood pressure and pulse rate regularly; this is important while you are taking amlodipine. Ask your prescriber or health care professional what your blood pressure and pulse rate should be and when you should contact him or her. You may feel dizzy or lightheaded. Do not drive, use machinery, or do anything that needs mental alertness until you know how amlodipine affects you. To reduce the risk of dizzy or fainting spells, do not sit or stand up quickly, especially if you are an older patient. Avoid alcoholic drinks; they can make you more dizzy, increase flushing and rapid heartbeats. Do not suddenly stop taking amlodipine. Ask your prescriber or health care professional how you can gradually reduce the dose. If you are going to have surgery, tell your prescriber or health care professional that you are taking amlodipine.

What side effects may I notice from taking amlodipine?

Side effects that you should report to your prescriber or health care professional as soon as possible:
- fainting spells, dizziness, or lightheadedness
- irregular heartbeat, chest pain, palpitations
- swelling of legs or ankles

Side effects that usually do not require medical attention (report to your prescriber or health care professional if they continue or are bothersome):
- drowsiness
- facial flushing
- headache
- nausea, vomiting
- stomach pain or gas
- weakness or fatigue

Where can I keep my medicine?

Keep out of the reach of children in a container that small children cannot open. Store at room temperature between 15 and 30 degrees C (59 and 86 degrees F). Protect from light. Keep container tightly closed. Throw away any unused medicine after the expiration date.

Amlodipine; Atorvastatin oral tablets	CADUET®; 10 mg/10 mg; Tablet Pfizer Laboratories Div Pfizer Inc		CADUET®; 5 mg/10 mg; Tablet Pfizer Laboratories Div Pfizer Inc	

What are amlodipine; atorvastatin tablets?

AMLODIPINE; ATORVASTATIN (Caduet®) is a combination of 2 drugs. Amlodipine is a calcium-channel blocker used to lower high blood pressure (hypertension). It also relieves different types of chest pain (angina). Atorvastatin blocks the body's ability to make cholesterol. Atorvastatin can help lower blood cholesterol for patients who are at risk of getting heart disease or a stroke. It is only for patients whose cholesterol level is not controlled by diet. This medicine is not a cure. Generic amlodipine; atorvastatin tablets are not yet available.

What should my health care professional know before I take amlodipine; atorvastatin?

They need to know if you have any of these conditions:
- heart problems, including heart failure or aortic stenosis
- liver disease

- kidney disease
- an alcohol problem
- any hormone disorder (such as diabetes, under-active thyroid)
- blood salt imbalance
- infection
- low blood pressure
- muscle disorder or condition
- recent surgery
- seizures (convulsions)
- severe injury
- an unusual reaction to amlodipine; atorvastatin, medicines, foods, dyes, or preservatives
- pregnant or trying to get pregnant
- breast-feeding

How should this medicine be used?

Take amlodipine; atorvastatin tablets by mouth. Follow the directions on the prescription label. Swallow the tablets with a drink of water. You can take the tablets with or without food. Do not significantly increase grapefruit juice intake while taking this drug, or avoid grapefruit juice if possible. Take your doses at regular intervals. Do not take your medicine more often then directed. Do not stop taking except on your prescriber's advice. Contact your pediatrician or health care professional regarding the use of this medicine in children. Special care may be needed. Elderly patients over 65 years old may have a stronger reaction to this medicine and need smaller doses.

What if I miss a dose?

If you miss a dose, take it as soon as you can. If it is almost time for your next dose, take only that dose. Do not take double or extra doses.

What may interact with amlodipine; atorvastatin?

Do not take amlodipine; atorvastatin with any of the following:

- alcohol-containing beverages
- anti-inflammatory drugs (NSAIDs, such as ibuprofen)
- barbiturates (examples: phenobarbital, butalbital, primidone)
- antacids
- birth control pills
- bosentan
- carbamazepine
- danazol
- digoxin
- grapefruit juice
- herbal or dietary supplements such as ginger, gingko biloba, ginseng, hawthorn, ma huang (ephedra), melatonin, St. John's wort, went yeast
- imatinib, STI-571
- local anesthetics or general anesthetics
- medicines for fungal infections (examples: fluconazole, itraconazole, ketoconazole, voriconazole)
- medicines for high blood pressure
- medicines for treating HIV infections
- medicines that suppress your immune response (cyclosporine)
- medicines to lower cholesterol or triglycerides (examples: colestipol, fenofibrate, gemfibrozil, niacin)
- medicine used to stop early pregnancy (mifepristone, RU-486 or Mifeprex™)
- medicines for prostate problems
- medicines for seizures (carbamazepine, oxcarbazepine, phenobarbital, phenytoin, primidone, zonisamide)
- nefazodone
- nicardipine
- rifampin, rifabutin, or rifapentine
- pioglitazone
- some antibiotics (clarithromycin, erythromycin, telithromycin, troleandomycin)
- some medicines for heart-rhythm problems (amiodarone, diltiazem, verapamil)
- some medicines for depression or mental problems (fluoxetine, fluvoxamine, nefazodone)
- water pills (diuretics)
- yohimbine
- zafirlukast
- zileuton

Tell your prescriber or health care professional about all other medicines you are taking, including non-prescription medicines, nutritional supplements, or herbal products. Also tell your prescriber or health care professional if you are a frequent user of drinks with caffeine or alcohol, if you smoke, or if you use illegal drugs. These may affect the way your medicine works. Check with your health care professional before stopping or starting any of your medicines.

What should I watch for while taking amlodipine; atorvastatin?

Visit your prescriber or health care professional for regular checks on your progress. You will need to have regular tests to make sure your liver is working properly. Tell your prescriber or health care professional as soon as you can if you get any unexplained muscle pain, tenderness, or weakness, especially if you also have a fever and tiredness. Amlodipine; atorvastatin contains a cholesterol lowering agent (atorvastatin), but is only part of a total cholesterol-lowering program. Your physician or dietitian can suggest a low-cholesterol and low-fat diet that will reduce your risk of getting heart and blood vessel disease. Avoid alcohol and smoking, and keep a proper exercise schedule. Check your blood pressure and pulse rate regularly; this is important while you are taking amlodipine; atorvastatin. Ask your prescriber or health care professional what your blood pressure and pulse rate should be and when you should contact him or her. You may feel dizzy or lightheaded. Do not drive, use machinery, or do anything that needs mental alertness until you know how amlodipine; atorvastatin affects you. To reduce the risk of dizzy or fainting spells, do not sit or stand up quickly, especially if you are an older patient. Avoid alcoholic drinks; they can make you more dizzy, increase flushing and rapid heartbeats. Do not suddenly stop taking amlodipine; atorvastatin. Ask your prescriber or health care professional how you can gradually reduce the dose. If you are going to have surgery, tell your prescriber or health care professional that you are taking amlodipine; atorvastatin.

What side effects may I notice from taking amlodipine; atorvastatin?

Side effects that you should report to your prescriber or health care professional as soon as possible:
Rare or uncommon:
- dark yellow or brown urine
- decreased urination, difficulty passing urine
- fainting spells, dizziness, or lightheadedness
- fever
- irregular heartbeat, chest pain, palpitations
- muscle pain, tenderness, cramps, or weakness
- redness, blistering, peeling or loosening of the skin, including inside the mouth
- skin rash, itching

- swelling of legs or ankles
- unusual tiredness or weakness
- yellowing of the skin or eyes

Side effects that usually do not require medical attention (report to your prescriber or health care professional if they continue or are bothersome):
- diarrhea
- drowsiness
- facial flushing
- gas
- headache
- joint pain
- nausea, vomiting
- stomach upset or pain
- tiredness, weakness or fatigue

Where can I keep my medicine?

Keep out of the reach of children in a container that small children cannot open. store at controlled room temperature at 25 degrees C (77 degrees F). Short periods of storage at 15 to 30 degrees C (59 to 86 degrees F) are permitted.

Amlodipine; Benazepril capsules

LOTREL®;
5 mg/10 mg;
Capsule
Novartis
Pharmaceuticals

LOTREL®;
2.5 mg/10 mg;
Capsule
Novartis
Pharmaceuticals

What are amlodipine-benazepril capsules?

AMLODIPINE-BENAZEPRIL (Lotrel®) is a combination of two drugs used to lower blood pressure. Amlodipine and benazepril lower, but do not cure high blood pressure (hypertension). Generic amlodipine-benazepril capsules are not yet available.

What should my health care professional know before I take amlodipine-benazepril?

They need to know if you have any of these conditions:
- autoimmune disease (such as lupus), or suppressed immune function
- previous swelling of the tongue, face, or lips with difficulty breathing, difficulty swallowing, hoarseness, or tightening of the throat (angioedema)
- bone marrow disease
- heart or blood vessel disease
- liver disease
- low blood pressure
- kidney disease
- if you are on a special diet, such as a low-salt diet
- an unusual or allergic reaction to amlodipine, benazepril, other medicines, foods, dyes, or preservatives
- pregnant or trying to get pregnant
- breast-feeding

How should I take this medicine?

Take amlodipine-benazepril tablets by mouth. Follow the directions on the prescription label. Swallow the capsules with a drink of water. You can take the capsules with or without food. Do not significantly in-crease grapefruit juice intake while taking this drug, or avoid grapefruit juice if possible. Take your doses at regular intervals. Do not take your medicine more often then directed. Do not stop taking except on your prescriber's advice. Contact your pediatrician or health care professional regarding the use of this medicine in children. Special care may be needed. Elderly patients over 65 years old may have a stronger reaction to this medicine and need smaller doses.

What if I miss a dose?

If you miss a dose, take it as soon as you can. If it is almost time for your next dose, take only that dose. Do not take double or extra doses.

What may interact with amlodipine; benazepril?

Do not take Amlodipine; Benazepril with any of the following:

- alfuzosin
- substitute salts which contain potassium

Amlodipine; Benazepril may also interact with the following medications:

- anti-inflammatory drugs (NSAIDs, such as ibuprofen)
- aspirin
- azathioprine
- barbiturates such as phenobarbital
- bosentan

- cyclosporine
- drospirenone; ethinyl estradiol
- grapefruit juice

- heparin
- herbal or dietary supplements such as gingko biloba, ginseng, hawthorn, ma huang (ephedra), melatonin, St. John's wort, went yeast
- hymenoptera venom
- imatinib, STI-571
- lithium
- local anesthetics or general anesthetics
- medicines for diabetes
- medicines for fungal infections (fluconazole, itraconazole, ketoconazole, voriconazole)
- medicines for high blood pressure
- medicines for HIV infection or AIDS
- medicines for prostate problems
- medicines for seizures (carbamazepine, phenobarbital, phenytoin, primidone, zonisamide)
- potassium salts (examples: potassium chloride, potassium gluconate)
- rifampin, rifapentine, or rifabutin
- some antibiotics (clarithromycin, erythromycin, telithromycin, trimethoprim, troleandomycin)
- some medicines for heart-rhythm problems (amiodarone, diltiazem, verapamil)
- some medicines for depression or mental problems (fluoxetine, fluvoxamine, nefazodone)
- water pills or diuretics (especially amiloride, triamterene, or spironolactone)
- yohimbine
- zafirlukast
- zileuton

Tell your prescriber or health care professional about all other medicines you are taking, including non-prescription medicines, nutritional supplements, or herbal products. Also tell your prescriber or health care professional if you are a frequent user of drinks with caffeine or alcohol, if you smoke, or if you use illegal drugs. These may affect the way your medicine works. Check with your health care professional before stopping or starting any of your medicines.

What should I watch for while taking amlodipine-benazepril?

Check your blood pressure and pulse rate regularly; this is important while you are taking amlodipine-benazepril. Ask your prescriber or health care professional what your blood pressure and pulse rate should be and when you should contact him or her. You may feel dizzy or lightheaded. Do not drive, use machinery, or do anything that needs mental alertness until you know

how amlodipine-benazepril affects you. To reduce the risk of dizzy or fainting spells, do not sit or stand up quickly, especially if you are an older patient. Avoid alcoholic drinks; they can make you more dizzy, increase flushing and rapid heartbeats. Do not suddenly stop taking amlodipine-benazepril. Ask your prescriber or health care professional how you can gradually reduce the dose. If you are going to have surgery, tell your prescriber or health care professional that you are taking amlodipine-benazepril. Check with your prescriber or health care professional if you get an attack of severe diarrhea, nausea and vomiting, or if you sweat a lot. The loss of body fluid can make it dangerous to take amlodipine-benazepril. Avoid salt substitutes or other foods or substances high in potassium salts. Do not treat yourself for coughs, colds, or pain while you are taking amlodipine-benazepril without asking your prescriber or health care professional for advice.

What side effects may I notice from taking amlodipine-benazepril?

Side effects that you should report to your prescriber or health care professional as soon as possible:
- swelling of your face, lips, or tongue
- dizziness, lightheadedness, or fainting spells
- redness, blistering, peeling, or loosening of the skin, including inside the mouth
- uneven or fast heartbeat, chest pain, palpitations
- swelling of your legs and ankles
- decreased amount of urine passed
- difficulty breathing, or swallowing
- skin rash, itching
- persistent dry cough

Side effects that usually do not require medical attention (report to your prescriber or health care professional if they continue or are bothersome):
- occasional cough
- drowsiness or dizziness
- facial flushing
- headache
- nausea, vomiting
- stomach pain or gas
- weakness or tiredness

Where can I keep my medicine?

Keep out of the reach of children in a container that small children cannot open. Store at room temperature below 30 degrees C (86 degrees F). Protect from light. Keep container tightly closed. Throw away any unused medicine after the expiration date.

Amoxapine tablets

ASENDIN;
100 mg; Tablet
Watson Pharmaceuticals Inc

This drug requires an FDA medication guide. See page xxxvii.

What are amoxapine tablets?

AMOXAPINE (Asendin®) is an antidepressant, a medicine that helps to lift mental depression. General amoxapine tablets are available.

What should my health care professional know before I take amoxapine?

They need to know if you have any of these conditions:
- an alcohol abuse problem
- asthma
- bipolar disorder
- blood disorders or disease
- breathing difficulties
- diabetes
- difficulty passing urine
- glaucoma
- having intramuscular injections
- heart disease
- liver disease
- overactive thyroid
- Parkinson's disease
- previous heart attack
- prostate trouble
- schizophrenia
- seizures (convulsions)
- stomach or intestinal disease
- an unusual or allergic reaction to amoxapine, other medicines, foods, dyes, or preservatives
- pregnant or trying to get pregnant
- breast-feeding

How should I take this medicine?

Take amoxapine tablets by mouth. Follow the directions on the prescription label. Swallow the tablets with a drink of water. Take your doses at regular intervals. Do not take your medicine more often than directed. Do not stop taking the tablets except on your prescriber's advice. Contact your pediatrician or health care professional regarding the use of this medicine in children. Special care may be needed. Elderly patients over 65 years old may have a stronger reaction to this medicine and need smaller doses.

What if I miss a dose?

If you miss a dose, take it as soon as you can. If it is less than four hours to your next dose, take only that dose and skip the missed dose. If you only take a single dose at bedtime and forget, do not take it the next morning without checking with your prescriber or health care professional. Do not take double or extra doses.

What may interact with amoxapine?

Amoxapine can interact with many other medicines. An interaction can be very important or fairly insignifi-

cant. Make sure your prescriber or health care professional knows about all other medicines you are taking; the most important are listed below:

- alcohol
- barbiturate medicines for inducing sleep or treating seizures (convulsions)
- blood thinners
- cimetidine or ranitidine
- clonidine
- disulfiram
- erythromycin
- female hormones, including contraceptive or birth control pills
- labetalol
- linezolid
- medicines for anxiety or sleeping problems, such as diazepam or temazepam
- medicines for colds and breathing difficulties
- medicines for hay fever and other allergies
- medicines for high blood pressure
- medicines for mental depression
- medicines for mental problems and psychotic disturbances
- medicines for movement abnormalities as in Parkinson's disease, or for gastrointestinal problems
- medicines for over- or under-active thyroid
- seizure (convulsion) or epilepsy medicine

Tell your prescriber or health care professional about all other medicines you are taking, including non-prescription medicines, nutritional supplements, or herbal products. Also tell your prescriber or health care professional if you are a frequent user of drinks with caffeine or alcohol, if you smoke, or if you use illegal drugs. These may affect the way your medicine works. Check with your health care professional before stopping or starting any of your medicines.

What should I watch for while taking amoxapine?

Visit your prescriber or health care professional for regular checks on your progress. You may have to take amoxapine for several weeks before you feel better. If you have been taking amoxapine for some time, do not suddenly stop taking it. Your prescriber or health care professional may want you to gradually reduce the dose; ask for advice. You may get drowsy, dizzy or have blurred vision. Do not drive, use machinery, or do anything that needs mental alertness until you know how amoxapine affects you. Do not stand or sit up quickly, especially if you are an older patient. This reduces the risk of dizzy or fainting spells. Alcohol may increase dizziness or drowsiness; avoid alcoholic drinks. Amoxapine can make your mouth dry. Chewing sugarless gum, sucking hard candy and drinking plenty of water will help. Amoxapine may make your skin more sensitive to sun or ultraviolet light. Keep out of the sun, or wear protective clothing outdoors and use a sunscreen (at least SPF15). Do not use sun lamps or sun tanning beds or booths. Do not treat yourself for coughs, colds, or allergies without asking your prescriber or health care professional for advice. Some ingredients may increase possible side effects. If you are going to have surgery or will need an x-ray procedure that uses contrast agents, tell your prescriber or health care professional that you are taking this medicine.

What side effects may I notice from taking amoxapine?

Side effects that you should report to your prescriber or health care professional as soon as possible:
- difficulty breathing
- eye pain
- fainting spells
- fast or irregular heartbeat (palpitations)
- fever with increased sweating
- loss of bladder control, or problems passing urine
- muscle stiffness or problems with movement
- pale skin
- seizures (convulsions)
- skin rash or itching (hives)
- swelling or tenderness of breasts or testicles

- unusual and uncontrollable tongue and chewing movements, smacking lips or puffing cheeks
- uncontrollable muscle spasms in the face, hands, arms, or legs
- yellowing of the eyes or skin

Side effects that usually do not require medical attention (report to your prescriber or health care professional if they continue or are bothersome):
- blurred vision
- confusion or nervousness
- constipation or diarrhea
- drowsiness, dizziness or lightheadedness
- dry mouth
- headache
- increased appetite and weight gain
- increased sensitivity to sunlight
- nausea, vomiting
- sexual difficulties (decreased sexual ability or desire)
- trouble sleeping (insomnia)
- unusual tiredness or weakness

Where can I keep my medicine?

Keep out of the reach of children in a container that small children cannot open. Store at room temperature between 15 and 30 degrees C (59 and 86 degrees F). Throw away any unused medicine after the expiration date.

Amoxicillin capsules or chewable tablets

TRIMOX®; 500 mg; Capsule Sandoz Pharmaceuticals

AMOXIL®; 400 mg; Tablet, Chewable Beecham Div Smithkline Beecham Corp

What are amoxicillin capsules or chewable tablets?

AMOXICILLIN (Amoxil®, Trimox®, Wymox®) is a penicillin antibiotic. Amoxicillin kills or stops the growth of bacteria that cause infection. It treats many different kinds of infections of the skin, respiratory tract, sinuses, ear, and kidney. Amoxicillin also treats some sexually transmitted disease. Generic amoxicillin capsules are available, but not generic chewable tablets.

What should my health care professional know before I take amoxicillin?

They need to know if you have any of these conditions:
- asthma
- eczema
- kidney disease
- leukemia
- mononucleosis
- intestinal problems (especially colitis)
- other chronic illness
- phenylketonuria
- viral infection
- an unusual or allergic reaction to amoxicillin, other penicillins, cephalosporin antibiotics, other medicines, foods, dyes, or preservatives
- breast-feeding

How should I take this medicine?

Take amoxicillin capsules or chewable tablets by mouth. Chew or crush the tablets, do not swallow whole. Swallow the capsules or tablets whole with a glass of water; take while in an upright or sitting position. You may take amoxicillin with or without food. Follow the directions on the prescription label. Take your doses at regular intervals. Do not take your medicine more often than directed. Finish the full course prescribed by your prescriber or health care professional even if you think your condition is better. Do not stop taking except on your prescriber's advice.

What if I miss a dose?

If you miss a dose, take it as soon as you can. If it is almost time for your next dose, take only that dose. Do not take double or extra doses. There should be an interval of at least 6 to 8 hours between doses.

What may interact with amoxicillin?

- allopurinol
- birth control pills
- methotrexate
- neomycin
- probenecid

Tell your prescriber or health care professional about all other medicines you are taking, including non-prescription medicines, nutritional supplements, or herbal products. Also tell your prescriber or health care professional if you are a frequent user of drinks with caffeine or alcohol, if you smoke, or if you use illegal drugs. These may affect the way your medicine works. Check with your health care professional before stopping or starting any of your medicines.

What should I watch for while taking amoxicillin?

Tell your prescriber or health care professional if your symptoms do not improve in 2 or 3 days. If you are diabetic and taking large doses of amoxicillin, you may get a false-positive result for sugar in your urine with certain brands of urine tests. Check with your prescriber or health care professional before you change your diet or the dose of your diabetic medicine. If you get severe or watery diarrhea, do not treat yourself. Call your prescriber or health care professional for advice. If you get a skin rash, do not treat yourself. Call your prescriber or health care professional for advice.

What side effects may I notice from taking amoxicillin?

Side effects that you should report to your prescriber or health care professional as soon as possible:
- difficulty breathing, wheezing
- dark yellow or brown urine
- dizziness
- fever or chills, sore throat
- increased thirst
- pain or difficulty passing urine
- pain on swallowing
- redness, blistering, peeling or loosening of the skin, including inside the mouth
- seizures (convulsions)
- skin rash, itching
- stomach pain or cramps
- swollen joints
- severe or watery diarrhea
- unusual bleeding or bruising
- unusual weakness or tiredness
- vomiting
- yellowing of the eyes or skin

Side effects that usually do not require medical attention (report to your prescriber or health care professional if they continue or are bothersome):
- diarrhea
- headache
- loss of appetite
- nausea
- stomach gas or heartburn

Where can I keep my medicine?

Keep out of the reach of children in a container that small children cannot open. Store at room temperature between 15 and 30 degrees C (59 and 86 degrees F). Keep container tightly closed. Throw away any unused medicine after the expiration date.

Amoxicillin; Clarithromycin; Lansoprazole tablets and capsules

 PREVPAC®;
500 mg/500 mg/30 mg;
Capsule
Tap Pharmaceuticals Inc

What is amoxicillin, clarithromycin, lansoprazole administration pack?

AMOXICILLIN; CLARITHROMYCIN; LANSO-PRAZOLE (Prevpac®) is a combination of medications used to treat intestinal ulcers associated with *Helicobacter pylori*, a bacterial infection. The Prevpac® 'kit' contains Trimox® (amoxicillin capsules), Biaxin® (clarithromycin tablets), and Prevacid® (lansoprazole capsules) packaged together. Generic Prevpac® therapy kits are not available.

What should my health care professional know before I take amoxicillin; clarithromycin; lansoprazole?

They need to know if you have any of these conditions:
- asthma
- eczema
- kidney or liver disease
- leukemia
- mononucleosis
- stomach problems (especially colitis)
- virus infection
- other chronic illness
- an unusual or allergic reaction to amoxicillin, clarithromycin, lansoprazole, other antibiotics, other medicines, foods, dyes, or preservatives
- pregnant or trying to get pregnant
- breast-feeding

How should I take this medicine?

Each "dose" of amoxicillin; clarithromycin; lansoprazole contains four pills: one pink and black capsule (Prevacid®), two maroon and light-pink capsules (Trimox®) and one yellow tablet (Biaxin®). Each dose should be taken twice per day before eating. Follow the directions on the prescription label. Swallow capsules and tablets whole with a drink of water; do not crush or chew. Take your doses at regular intervals. Do not take your medicine more often than directed. Contact your pediatrician or health care professional regarding the use of this medicine in children. Special care may be needed.

What if I miss a dose?

If you miss a dose, take it as soon as you can. If it is almost time for your next dose, take only that dose. Do not take double or extra doses.

What may interact with amoxicillin; clarithromycin; lansoprazole?

- arsenic trioxide
- astemizole
- carbamazepine
- cilostazol
- cisapride
- cyclosporine
- digoxin
- diltiazem
- dolasetron
- estazolam
- fentanyl
- grepafloxacin
- imatinib, STI-571
- iron salts
- itraconazole
- ketoconazole
- levomethadyl
- medicines for HIV-infection or AIDS
- medicines for treating heart rhythm problems
- methotrexate
- modafinil
- phenytoin
- sildenafil
- some medicines for migraine (example: dihydroergotamine or ergotamine)
- some medicines for psychosis, depression, anxiety or other mental problems
- soy isoflavones
- sparfloxacin
- some "statin"-type medicines for treating high cholesterol (examples: atorvastatin, lovastatin, simvastatin)
- sucralfate
- tacrolimus
- terfenadine
- theophylline
- verapamil
- voriconazole
- warfarin
- went yeast
- zonisamide

Tell your prescriber or health care professional about all other medicines you are taking, including non-prescription medicines, nutritional supplements, or herbal products. Also tell your prescriber or health care professional if you are a frequent user of drinks with caffeine or alcohol, if you smoke, or if you use illegal drugs. These may affect the way your medicine works. Check with your health care professional before stopping or starting any of your medicines.

What should I watch for while taking amoxicillin; clarithromycin; lansoprazole?

It can take several days of therapy with amoxicillin; clarithromycin; lansoprazole before your stomach pains improve. Check with your prescriber or health care professional if your condition does not improve, or if it gets worse. Call your prescriber or health care professional as soon as you can if you get a fever, watery diarrhea, stomach pain, or vomiting. These could be symptoms of a more serious illness. Do not treat yourself. Call your prescriber for advice. If you get a skin rash, do not treat yourself. Call your prescriber or health care professional for advice. Birth control pills (contraceptive pills) may not work properly while you are taking this medicine. Use an extra method of birth control for at least one month. Do not smoke cigarettes or drink alcohol; these increase irritation of your stomach. If you are going to have surgery, tell your prescriber or health care professional that you are taking amoxicillin; clarithromycin; lansoprazole.

What side effects may I notice from taking amoxicillin; clarithromycin; lansoprazole?

Side effects that you should report to your prescriber or health care professional as soon as possible:
- difficulty breathing, wheezing
- dark yellow or brown urine
- dizziness
- fever or chills, sore throat
- increased thirst
- pain or difficulty passing urine
- redness, blistering, peeling or loosening of the skin, including inside the mouth
- seizures (convulsions)
- skin rash, itching
- stomach pain or cramps
- swollen joints
- severe or watery diarrhea
- unusual bleeding or bruising
- unusual weakness or tiredness
- vomiting
- yellowing of the eyes or skin

Side effects that usually do not require medical attention (report to your prescriber or health care professional if they continue or are bothersome):
- changes in taste
- diarrhea
- headache
- loss of appetite
- nausea
- stomach gas or heartburn

Where can I keep my medicine?

Keep out of the reach of children in a container that small children cannot open. Store at room temperature between 15 and 30 degrees C (59 and 86 degrees F). Protect from light and moisture. Throw away any unused medicine after the expiration date.

Amoxicillin; Clavulanic Acid tablets, chewable tablets and extended-release tablets

AUGMENTIN®;
500 mg; Tablet
Beecham Div
Smithkline Beecham
Corp

AUGMENTIN XR®;
400 mg; Tablet,
Chewable
Beecham Div
Smithkline Beecham
Corp

What are amoxicillin/clavulanic acid tablets, chewable tablets and extended-release tablets?

AMOXICILLIN/CLAVULANIC ACID (Augmentin®, Augmentin XR™) is a penicillin antibiotic. Amoxicillin kills or stops the growth of bacteria that cause infection. Clavulanic acid is added to help the amoxicillin to work better. This medicine treats many different kinds of infections, including those of the ears, kidney, respiratory tract, sinuses, and skin. Generic amoxicillin/clavulanic acid tablets and chewable tablets are available. Generic extended-release tablets are not yet available.

What should my health care professional know before I take amoxicillin/clavulanic acid?

They need to know if you have any of these conditions:
- asthma
- eczema
- kidney disease
- leukemia
- liver disease
- mononucleosis
- intestinal problems (especially colitis)
- other chronic illness
- phenylketonuria
- viral infection
- an unusual or allergic reaction to amoxicillin, other penicillins, imipenem, cephalosporin antibiotics, foods, dyes, or preservatives
- breast-feeding

How should I take this medicine?

Take amoxicillin/clavulanic regular tablets, chewable tablets, or extended-release tablets by mouth. Swallow the regular tablets and the extended-release tablets whole, do not crush or chew. If you are prescribed chewable tablets, crush or chew them before swallowing; do not swallow them whole. Take amoxicillin/clavulanic acid at the start of a meal. Follow the directions on the prescription label. Take your doses at regular intervals. Do not take your medicine more often than directed. Finish the full course prescribed by your prescriber or health care professional even if you think your condition is better. Do not stop taking except on your prescriber's advice.

What if I miss a dose?

If you miss a dose, take it as soon as you can. If it is almost time for your next dose, take only that dose. Do not take double or extra doses. There should be an interval of at least 6 to 8 hours between doses.

What may interact with amoxicillin/clavulanic acid?

- allopurinol
- birth control pills
- methotrexate
- neomycin
- probenecid

Tell your prescriber or health care professional about all other medicines you are taking, including non-prescription medicines, nutritional supplements, or herbal products. Also tell your prescriber or health care professional if you are a frequent user of drinks with caffeine or alcohol, if you smoke, or if you use illegal drugs. These may affect the way your medicine works. Check with your health care professional before stopping or starting any of your medicines.

What should I watch for while taking amoxicillin/clavulanic acid?

Tell your prescriber or health care professional if your symptoms do not improve in 2 or 3 days. If you are diabetic and taking large doses of amoxicillin, you may get a false-positive result for sugar in your urine. Check with your prescriber or health care professional before you change your diet or the dose of your diabetic medicine. If you get severe or watery diarrhea, do not treat yourself. Call your prescriber or health care professional for advice. If you get a skin rash, do not treat yourself. Call your prescriber or health care professional for advice.

What side effects may I notice from taking amoxicillin/clavulanic acid?

Side effects that you should report to your prescriber or health care professional as soon as possible:
- difficulty breathing, wheezing
- dark yellow or brown urine
- dizziness
- fever or chills, sore throat
- headache
- increased thirst
- pain or difficulty passing urine
- redness, blistering, peeling or loosening of the skin, including inside the mouth
- seizures (convulsions)
- skin rash, itching

- stomach pain or cramps
- swollen joints
- severe or watery diarrhea
- unusual bleeding or bruising
- unusual weakness or tiredness
- yellowing of the eyes or skin

Side effects that usually do not require medical attention (report to your prescriber or health care professional if they continue or are bothersome):

- diarrhea
- loss of appetite
- nausea, vomiting
- stomach gas or heartburn

Where can I keep my medicine?

Keep out of the reach of children in a container that small children cannot open. Store at room temperature between 15 and 30 degrees C (59 and 86 degrees F). Keep container tightly closed. Throw away any unused medicine after the expiration date.

Ampicillin capsules

PRINCIPEN®;
500 mg; Capsule
Sandoz
Pharmaceuticals

AMPICILLIN;
250 mg; Capsule
Teva
Pharmaceuticals
USA Inc

What are ampicillin capsules?

AMPICILLIN (Omnipen®, Principen®, Totacillin®) is a penicillin antibiotic. Ampicillin kills bacteria that cause infection, or stops the growth of bacteria. It treats many kinds of infections of the skin, central nervous system, heart, respiratory tract, sinuses, ear, and kidney. Ampicillin also treats some sexually transmitted disease. Generic ampicillin capsules are available.

What should my health care professional know before I take ampicillin?

They need to know if you have any of these conditions:

- asthma
- eczema
- kidney disease
- leukemia
- mononucleosis
- stomach problems (especially colitis)
- virus infection
- other chronic illness
- an unusual or allergic reaction to ampicillin, other penicillins, imipenem, cephalosporin antibiotics, foods, dyes, or preservatives
- breast-feeding

How should I take this medicine?

Take ampicillin capsules by mouth. Follow the directions on the prescription label. Take ampicillin 1 to 2 hours before or at least 2 hours after eating; taking it with food can make it less effective. Swallow the capsules whole with a glass of water; take capsules while in an upright or sitting position. Take your doses at regular intervals. Do not take your medicine more often than directed. Finish the full course prescribed by your prescriber or health care professional even if you think your condition is better. Do not stop taking except on your prescriber's advice.

What if I miss a dose?

If you miss a dose, take it as soon as you can. If it is almost time for your next dose, take only that dose.

Do not take double or extra doses. There should be an interval of at least 6 to 8 hours between doses.

What may interact with ampicillin?

- allopurinol
- certain antibiotics given by injection
- clavulanic acid
- entacapone
- female hormones, including contraceptive or birth control pills
- methotrexate
- probenecid

Tell your prescriber or health care professional about all other medicines you are taking, including non-prescription medicines, nutritional supplements, or herbal products. Also tell your prescriber or health care professional if you are a frequent user of drinks with caffeine or alcohol, if you smoke, or if you use illegal drugs. These may affect the way your medicine works. Check with your health care professional before stopping or starting any of your medicines.

What should I watch for while taking ampicillin?

Tell your prescriber or health care professional if your symptoms do not improve in 2 or 3 days. If you are diabetic and taking large doses of ampicillin, you may get a false-positive result for sugar in your urine. Check with your prescriber or health care professional before you change your diet or the dose of your diabetic medicine. If you get severe or watery diarrhea, do not treat yourself. Call your prescriber or health care professional for advice. If you get a skin rash, do not treat yourself. Call your prescriber or health care professional for advice. Birth control pills (contraceptive pills) may not work properly while you are taking this medicine. Use another method of birth control for at least one month.

What side effects may I notice from taking ampicillin?

Side effects that you should report to your prescriber or health care professional as soon as possible:

- difficulty breathing, wheezing
- dark yellow or brown urine
- dizziness
- fever or chills, sore throat
- headache
- less frequent passing of urine
- redness, blistering, peeling or loosening of the skin, including inside the mouth
- seizures (convulsions)
- skin rash, itching
- stomach pain or cramps
- swollen joints
- severe or watery diarrhea
- unusual bleeding or bruising
- unusual weakness or tiredness

Side effects that usually do not require medical attention (report to your prescriber or health care professional if they continue or are bothersome):

- diarrhea
- loss of appetite
- nausea, vomiting
- sore mouth
- stomach gas or heartburn

Where can I keep my medicine?

Keep out of the reach of children in a container that small children cannot open. Store at room temperature between 15 and 30 degrees C (59 and 86 degrees F). Keep container tightly closed. Throw away any unused medicine after the expiration date.

Amprenavir capsules

AGENERASE℠; 150 mg; Capsule Glaxo Wellcome

GX CC2

What are amprenavir capsules?

AMPRENAVIR (Agenerase℠) is an antiviral drug called a protease inhibitor. Amprenavir is used for the treatment of human immunodeficiency virus (HIV) infection. Amprenavir may reduce the amount of HIV in the blood and increase the number of CD4 cells (T-cells) in the blood. Amprenavir is used in combination with other drugs to treat the HIV virus. Amprenavir will not cure or prevent HIV infection or AIDS. You may still develop other infections or conditions associated with HIV. Generic amprenavir capsules are not yet available.

What should my health care professional know before I take amprenavir?

They need to know if you have any of these conditions:

- diabetes or high blood sugar
- hemophilia A or B
- high cholesterol or triglycerides
- liver disease
- vitamin K deficiency
- an unusual or allergic reaction to amprenavir, sulfa drugs, other medicines, foods, dyes, or preservatives
- pregnant or trying to get pregnant
- breast-feeding

How should I take this medicine?

Take amprenavir capsules by mouth. Follow the directions on the prescription label. You may take amprenavir with or without food but try to avoid taking it with high fat meals. Do not take with antacids. Take your doses at regular intervals. Do not take your medicine more often than directed. To help to make sure that your anti-HIV therapy works as well as possible, be very careful to take all of your medicine exactly as prescribed. Do not stop taking except on your prescriber's advice. Contact your pediatrician or health care professional regarding the use of this medicine in chil-

dren. Special care may be needed. Amprenavir is not recommended for use in children less than 3 years of age.

What if I miss a dose?

If you miss a dose by more than 4 hours, wait and take the next dose at your normal time. However, if you missed the dose by less than 4 hours, take the dose immediately. Then, take your next dose at your normal time. Do not take more or less than your prescribed dose of amprenavir at one time.

What may interact with amprenavir?

Many medicines may interact with amprenavir. If you have a question concerning other medicines you may be taking, talk with your pharmacist, prescriber or other health care professional.
Do not take amprenavir with any of these medicines:

- astemizole
- bepridil
- birth control pills or other hormonal birth control medicines (like the patch, ring, or injections)
- cisapride
- dihydroergotamine
- ergotamine
- lovastatin
- methadone
- methylergonovine
- methysergide
- midazolam
- rifampin
- sildenafil
- simvastatin
- St. John's wort
- triazolam
- vitamin E supplements
- warfarin
- went yeast (Cholestin℠)

Other medicines that may interact with amprenavir:

- amiodarone
- antacids
- bosentan
- certain medicines for anxiety or difficulty sleeping
- certain medicines for depression (e.g., amitriptyline, desipramine)
- certain medicines for high cholesterol (atorvastatin)
- didanosine, ddI
- dofetilide
- lidocaine
- medicines for diabetes
- medicines for seizures
- medicines to lower your cholesterol (e.g., atorvastatin or cerivastatin)
- other medicines for HIV
- quinidine
- rifabutin

Tell your prescriber or health care professional about all other medicines you are taking, including nonprescription medicines, nutritional supplements, or herbal products. Also tell your prescriber or health care professional if you are a frequent user of drinks with caffeine or alcohol, if you smoke, or if you use illegal drugs. These may affect the way your medicine works. Check with your health care professional before stopping or starting any of your medicines.

What should I watch for while taking amprenavir?

Visit your prescriber or health care professional for regular checks on your progress. Discuss any new symptoms with your prescriber or health care professional. Amprenavir will not cure HIV and you can still get other illnesses or complications associated with your disease. Taking amprenavir does not reduce the risk of passing HIV infection to others through sexual or blood contact. It is best to avoid sexual contact so that you do not spread the disease to others. For any sexual contact, use a con-

dom. Be careful about cuts, abrasions and other possible sources of blood contact. Never share a needle or syringe with anyone. If you are a woman of childbearing age and are using hormone contraceptives, then you should use another form of birth control while taking amprenavir. Amprenavir may decrease the effectiveness of hormone birth control agents, including birth control pills and injections. Do not take vitamin supplements containing vitamin E while you are taking amprenavir. Amprenavir contains large amounts of vitamin E. Do not take antacids or didanosine, ddI, within 1 hour of taking amprenavir. Antacids may decrease the amount of amprenavir you may absorb.

What side effects might I notice from taking amprenavir?

Side effects that you should report to your prescriber or health care professional as soon as possible:

- changes in body appearance (such as weight gain or loss around the waist and/or face)
- skin rash or itchy skin
- increased hunger or thirst
- increased urination
- redness, blistering, peeling or loosening of the skin, including inside the mouth
- unusual tiredness or weakness

Side effects that usually do not require medical attention (report to your prescriber or health care professional if they continue or are bothersome):

- changes in taste
- diarrhea
- headache
- nausea and vomiting
- stomach pain
- tingling around the mouth

Where can I keep my medicine?

Keep out of the reach of children in a container that small children cannot open. Store at room temperature. Keep container tightly closed. Throw away any unused medicine after the expiration date.

Anagrelide capsules

AGRYLIN®;
0.5 mg; Capsule
Shire US Inc

AGRYLIN®;
1 mg; Capsule
Shire US Inc

What are anagrelide capsules?

ANAGRELIDE (Agrylin®) is used to treat essential thrombocytosis (too many blood clotting cells [platelets] in the body). Anagrelide lowers the number of platelets and reduces the risk of problems such as intestinal bleeding, stroke, and heart attack caused by having too many platelets. Generic anagrelide capsules are not yet available.

What should my health care professional know before I take anagrelide?

They need to know if you have any of these conditions:

- heart, kidney, or liver disease
- an unusual or allergic reaction to anagrelide, other medicines, foods, dyes, or preservatives
- pregnant or trying to get pregnant
- breast-feeding

How should I take this medicine?

Take anagrelide capsules by mouth. Follow the directions on the prescription label. Swallow the capsules with a drink of water. Contact your pediatrician or health care professional regarding the use of this medicine in children. Special care may be needed.

What if I miss a dose?

If you miss a dose, take it as soon as you can. If it is almost time for your next dose, take only that dose. Do not take double or extra doses.

What may interact with anagrelide?

- supplements that contain garlic, gingko, or ginger
- other medicines that may affect bleeding such as warfarin (Coumadin®)

Tell your prescriber or health care professional about all other medicines you are taking, including non-prescription medicines, nutritional supplements, or herbal products. Also tell your prescriber or health care professional if you are a frequent user of drinks with caffeine or alcohol, if you smoke, or if you use illegal drugs. These may affect the way your medicine works. Check with your health care professional before stopping or starting any of your medicines.

What should I watch for while taking anagrelide?

Visit your prescriber or health care professional for regular checks on your progress. Do not stop taking anagrelide except on your prescriber's advice. If you are going to have surgery, tell your prescriber or health care professional that you are taking anagrelide.

What side effects may I notice from taking anagrelide?

Side effects that you should report to your prescriber or health care professional as soon as possible:
- difficulty breathing
- blood in urine
- fast, slow, or irregular heartbeat
- palpitations, chest pain, or tightness
- seizures
- severe headache
- unusual bleeding
- unusual swelling, not passing urine, or difficulty passing urine
- unusual tiredness or weakness

Side effects that usually do not require medical attention (report to your prescriber or health care professional if they continue or are bothersome):
- abdominal pain
- back pain
- diarrhea
- dizziness
- gas
- headache
- loss of appetite
- nausea, vomiting
- numbness or tingling in hands or feet
- skin itching or rash

Where can I keep my medicine?

Keep out of the reach of children in a child-proof container. Store at room temperature between 15 and 25°C (59 and 77°F) in a light-resistant container. Keep container tightly closed. Throw away any unused medicine after the expiration date.

Anastrozole tablets

ARIMIDEX®;
1 mg; Tablet
AstraZeneca Pharmaceuticals
LP

What are anastrozole tablets?

ANASTROZOLE (Arimidex®) blocks the production of the hormone estrogen. Some types of breast cancer depend on estrogen to grow, and anastrozole can stop tumor growth by blocking estrogen production. Anastrozole is for the treatment of breast cancer in postmenopausal women only. Generic anastrozole tablets are not yet available.

What should my health care professional know before I take anastrozole?

They need to know if you have any of these conditions:
- liver disease
- an unusual or allergic reaction to anastrozole, other medicines, foods, dyes, or preservatives
- pregnant or trying to get pregnant
- breast-feeding

How should I take this medicine?

Take anastrozole tablets by mouth at the same time each day with or without food. Follow the directions on the prescription label. Swallow the tablets with a drink of water. Do not take your medicine more often than directed. Do not stop taking except on your prescriber's advice. Contact your pediatrician or health care professional regarding the use of this medicine in children. Special care may be needed.

What if I miss a dose?

If you miss a dose, take it as soon as you can. If it is almost time for your next dose, take only that dose. Do not take double or extra doses. If you vomit after taking a dose, call your prescriber or health care professional for advice.

What may interact with anastrozole?

- androstenedione
- any medicine containing estrogens (this may include some herbal products and some birth control pills)
- DHEA

Tell your prescriber or health care professional about all other medicines you are taking, including nonprescription medicines, nutritional supplements, or herbal products. Also tell your prescriber or health care professional if you are a frequent user of drinks with caffeine or alcohol, if you smoke, or if you use illegal drugs. These may affect the way your medicine works. Check with your health care professional before stopping or starting any of your medicines.

What should I watch for while taking anastrozole?

Visit your prescriber or health care professional for regular checks on your progress. Let your prescriber or health care professional know about any unusual vaginal bleeding. Do not treat yourself for diarrhea, nausea, vomiting or other side effects. Ask your prescriber or health care professional for advice.

What side effects may I notice from taking anastrozole?

Side effects that you should report to your prescriber or health care professional as soon as possible:

- any new or unusual symptoms
- difficulty breathing
- chest pain
- leg pain or swelling
- vaginal bleeding
- vomiting

Side effects that usually do not require medical attention (report to your prescriber or health care professional if they continue or are bothersome):

- back or bone pain
- cough, or throat infection
- diarrhea or constipation
- dizziness
- headache
- hot flashes
- loss of appetite
- nausea
- stomach pain
- sweating
- weakness and tiredness
- weight gain

Where can I keep my medicine?

Keep out of the reach of children in a container that small children cannot open. Store between 20 and 25 degrees C (68 and 77 degrees F). Throw away any unused medicine after the expiration date.

Aprepitant capsules

EMEND®;
80 mg/125 mg; Capsule
Merck and Co Inc

What are aprepitant capsules?

APREPITANT (Emend®) is used to prevent nausea and vomiting, especially when associated with the treatment of cancer (chemotherapy). This drug may also be used to prevent or treat nausea and vomiting that occurs due to other conditions. Generic aprepitant capsules are not yet available.

What should my health care professional know before I take aprepitant?

They need to know if you have any of these conditions:
- liver disease
- an unusual reaction to aprepitant, other medicines, foods, dyes, or preservatives
- pregnant or trying to get pregnant
- breast-feeding

How should I take this medicine?

Take aprepitant capsules by mouth. Follow the directions on the prescription label. Take aprepitant exactly as prescribed. Usually, you will take your first dose of aprepitant one hour before your chemotherapy begins, and then once daily in the morning for the next 2 days after your chemotherapy treatment. Swallow the capsules whole with a drink of water. This medicine

may be taken with or without food. Do not take more often than directed. Contact your pediatrician or health care professional regarding the use of this medicine in children. Special care may be needed.

What if I miss a dose?

If you miss a dose, take it as soon as you can. If it is almost time for your next dose, take only that dose. Do not take double or extra doses.

What may interact with aprepitant?

Do not take aprepitant with any of these medicines:

- pimozide (Orap®)
- terfenadine (Seldane®)
- astemizole (Hismanal®)
- cisapride (Propulsid®)

Other medicines that may interact with aprepitant include the following:

- alprazolam, diazepam or midazolam which medicines often used for sleep or anxiety disorders
- birth control pills or hormones, including injections or implants
- cilostazol
- cyclosporine

- dexamethasone or methylprednisolone, also known as corticosteroids
- medicines for heart disease, high blood pressure, or to control the heart rhythm
- medicines used for depression or mental disorders (fluoxetine, fluvoxamine, paroxetine)
- medicines for AIDS or HIV infection (amprenavir, delavirdine, efavirenz, indinavir, nelfinavir, ritonavir, saquinavir)
- medicines for seizures or to control epilepsy (carbamazepine, phenytoin, phenobarbital, primidone)
- some chemotherapy medications (etoposide, ifosfamide, vinblastine, vincristine)
- some antifungal medications (fluconazole, griseofulvin, ketoconazole, itraconazole, voriconazole)
- some macrolide antibiotics (clarithromycin, erythromycin, troleandomycin)
- warfarin (Coumadin®), a "blood-thinner" used to help prevent blood clots
- zafirlukast
- ziprasidone

Many other medicines may interact with Aprepitant, if you have a question concerning the medicines you are taking, talk with your pharmacist, prescriber or other health care professional.

Tell your prescriber or health care professional about all other medicines you are taking, including non-prescription medicines, nutritional supplements, or herbal products. Also tell your prescriber or health care professional if you are a frequent user of drinks with caffeine or alcohol, if you smoke, or if you use illegal drugs. These may affect the way your medicine works. Check with your health care professional before stopping or starting any of your medicines.

What should I watch for while taking aprepitant?

Do not take aprepitant if you already have nausea and vomiting. Ask your health care provider what to do if you already have nausea. Women who use birth control pills or other types of birth control that contain hormones while taking aprepitant should also use a non-hormonal back-up method for birth control (for example, a condom) during aprepitant therapy and also for

28-days after stopping aprepitant therapy to avoid pregnancy. Aprepitant may reduce the effectiveness of hormonal birth control. Discuss options for effective contraception and other measures to prevent pregnancy with your health care provider. If you take warfarin (Coumadin®), you may need to have your blood checked within the 2 weeks following each treatment with aprepitant to check to make sure that warfarin is working properly. Aprepitant may decrease the effectiveness of warfarin to thin the blood (the blood may become 'thicker').

What side effects may I notice from taking aprepitant?

Side effects that you should report to your prescriber or health care professional as soon as possible:
- breathing difficulties or shortness of breath
- changes in heart rhythm (fast, slow or irregular heartbeat)
- high or low blood pressure
- rectal bleeding
- serious dizziness or disorientation, confusion
- sharp or severe stomach pain
- sharp pain in your leg
- skin rash

Side effects that usually do not require medical attention (report to your prescriber or health care professional if they continue or are bothersome):
- constipation
- diarrhea
- excessive thirst
- fatigue, drowsiness, or tiredness
- headache
- hiccups
- loss of appetite
- muscle weakness or pain
- nausea or vomiting
- ringing in your ears
- sleep disturbances
- stomach ache or mild pain

Where can I keep my medicine?

Keep out of the reach of children in a container that small children cannot open. Store between 20 and 25 degrees C (68 and 77 degrees F). Throw away any unused medicine after the expiration date.

Aripiprazole tablets

ABILIFY®;
10 mg; Tablet
Otsuka America
Pharmaceuticals Inc

ABILIFY®;
20 mg; Tablet
Otsuka America
Pharmaceuticals Inc

What are aripiprazole tablets?

ARIPIPRAZOLE (Abilify™) helps to treat schizophrenia. Aripiprazole can help you to keep in touch with reality and reduce your other symptoms. It is for patients that have not been helped by other medicines. Occasionally aripiprazole is used to treat other mood disturbances. Generic aripiprazole tablets are not yet available.

What should my health care professional know before I receive aripiprazole?

They need to know if you have any of these conditions:
- frequently drink alcohol or alcohol-containing beverages
- dementia
- diabetes
- difficulty swallowing

- heart disease
- history of brain tumor or head injury
- irregular heartbeat
- low blood pressure
- Parkinson's disease
- previous heart attack
- seizures (convulsions)
- an unusual reaction to aripiprazole, other medicines, foods, dyes, or preservatives
- pregnant or trying to get pregnant
- breast-feeding

How should this medicine be used?

Take aripiprazole tablets by mouth. Follow the directions on the prescription label. Swallow the tablets with a drink of water. If aripiprazole upsets your stomach you can take it with food. Take your doses at regular intervals. Do not take your medicine more often than directed. Do not stop taking except on your prescriber's advice. Contact your pediatrician or health care professional regarding the use of this medicine in children. Special care may be needed.

What if I miss a dose?

If you miss a dose, take it as soon as you can. If it is almost time for your next dose, take only that dose. Do not take double or extra doses.

What may interact with aripiprazole?

Aripiprazole can interact with many other drugs. Some of the possible interactions are listed:

- alcohol
- amiodarone
- carbamazepine
- charcoal
- cimetidine
- citalopram
- clarithromycin
- erythromycin
- fluconazole
- fluoxetine
- fluvoxamine
- grapefruit juice
- imatinib, STI-571
- itraconazole
- ketoconazole
- medicines for diabetes
- medicines for high blood pressure
- medicines for HIV infection
- medicines for sleep
- nefazodone
- paroxetine
- phenobarbital
- phenytoin
- prescription pain medications
- primidone
- quinidine
- rifabutin
- rifampin
- sertraline

- St. John's wort
- voriconazole

Tell your prescriber or health care professional about all other medicines you are taking, including non-prescription medicines, nutritional supplements, or herbal products. Also tell your prescriber or health care professional if you are a frequent user of drinks with caffeine or alcohol, if you smoke, or if you use illegal drugs. These may affect the way your medicine works. Check with your health care professional before stopping or starting any of your medicines.

What should I watch for while taking aripiprazole?

Visit your prescriber or health care professional for regular checks on your progress. It may be several weeks before you see the full effects of aripiprazole. Do not suddenly stop taking aripiprazole. You may need to gradually reduce the dose. Only stop taking aripiprazole on your prescriber's advice. You may get dizzy or drowsy. Do not drive, use machinery, or do anything that needs mental alertness until you know how aripiprazole affects you. Do not stand or sit up quickly, especially if you are an older patient. This reduces the risk of dizzy or fainting spells. Alcohol can increase dizziness and drowsiness. Avoid alcoholic drinks. Aripiprazole can reduce the response of your body to heat or cold. Try not to get overheated or dehydrated from exercise. Avoid temperature extremes, such as saunas, hot tubs, or very hot or cold baths or showers. Dress warmly in cold weather. If you are going to have surgery tell your prescriber or health care professional that you are taking aripiprazole.

What side effects may I notice from taking aripiprazole?

Side effects that you should report to your prescriber or health care professional as soon as possible:

- changes in vision
- confusion
- difficulty swallowing
- fainting spells
- inability to control muscle movements in the face, hands, arms, or legs
- loss of balance or difficulty walking
- muscles or joint pain
- restlessness or need to keep moving
- seizures
- weakness

Side effects that usually do not require medical attention (report to your prescriber or health care professional if they continue or are bothersome):

- constipation
- difficulty sleeping
- drowsiness
- dizziness
- headache
- nausea, vomiting
- weight gain

Where can I keep my medicine?

Keep out of the reach of children in a container that small children cannot open. Store at room temperature between 15 and 25 degrees C (59 and 77 degrees F). Protect the tablets from exposure to bright light. Throw away any unused medicine after the expiration date.

Aspirin, ASA tablets	EXTRA STRENGTH BAYER®; 500 mg; Tablet Bayer Corp Consumer Care Div		ST. JOSEPH® ASPIRIN ADULT EC; 81 mg; Tablet Johnson and Johnson/Merck	

What are aspirin, ASA, tablets?

ASPIRIN, ASA (Ascriptin®, Bayer®, Ecotrin®, Empirin®, ZORprin®, and many others) treats fever, pain, and inflammation (swelling and redness) and reduces the ability of the blood to clot. Aspirin relieves the mild to moderate discomfort caused by a variety of conditions including arthritis, headaches, infections, menstrual cramps or pain, minor injuries, and other conditions. It can also be part of therapy to reduce the risk of a heart attack or stroke. Generic aspirin is available as tablets or caplets. Aspirin tablets can be enteric-coated, extended-release, or chewable.

What should my health care professional know before I take aspirin, ASA?

They need to know if you have any of these conditions:
- anemia
- asthma
- bleeding or clotting problems
- drink more than 3 alcohol-containing beverages a day
- heart failure
- high blood pressure
- gout
- kidney disease
- liver disease
- nasal polyps
- smoke tobacco
- stomach ulcers, or other stomach problems
- systemic lupus erythematosus (SLE)
- thrombotic thrombocytopenic purpura (TTP)
- vitamin K deficiency
- an unusual or allergic reaction to aspirin, tartrazine dye, other medicines, dyes, or preservatives
- pregnant or trying to get pregnant
- breast-feeding

How should I take this medicine?

Take aspirin tablets or capsules by mouth. Follow the directions on the label. Swallow tablets or caplets whole with a full glass of water; take tablets or capsules in an upright or sitting position. Taking a sip of water first, before taking the tablets or caplets, may help you swallow them. If possible take bedtime doses at least 10 minutes before lying down. Extended-release tablets or caplets must be swallowed whole; do not crush or chew. Chewable tablets can be chewed, crushed, mixed in a drink, or swallowed whole. Always follow the dose with a drink of water or other beverage. If aspirin upsets your stomach, take the tablets with food or milk. Take your doses at regular intervals. Do not take your medicine more often than directed. Contact your pediatrician or health care professional regarding the use of this medicine in children. Special care may be needed. Do not give adult preparations to children. Avoid aspirin in children with chickenpox, the flu, or other viral infections.

What if I miss a dose?

If you are taking aspirin on a regular schedule and miss a dose, take it as soon as you can. If it is almost time for your next dose, take only that dose. Do not take double or extra doses.

What may interact with aspirin, ASA?

- alcohol
- alendronate
- antacids (in large doses)
- anti-inflammatory drugs (NSAIDs, such as ibuprofen)
- herbal supplements that contain feverfew, garlic, ginger, ginkgo biloba, horse chestnut
- hormones such as prednisone or cortisone
- medicines used to treat or prevent blood clots
- medicines for diabetes that are taken by mouth
- medicines for gout
- methotrexate
- other medicines that contain aspirin or aspirin-related ingredients (e.g., Pepto-Bismol®)
- seizure (convulsion) or epilepsy medicine

Tell your prescriber or health care professional about all other medicines you are taking, including non-prescription medicines, nutritional supplements, or herbal products. Also tell your prescriber or health care professional if you are a frequent user of drinks with caffeine or alcohol, if you smoke, or if you use illegal drugs. These may affect the way your medicine works. Check with your health care professional before stopping or starting any of your medicines.

What should I watch for while taking aspirin, ASA?

Check with your prescriber or health care professional if you are treating yourself for a pain that does not go away after 10 days; and for a fever that does not go away after 3 days or keeps coming back. Only take aspirin to prevent heart attacks or blood clotting if prescribed by your prescriber or health care professional. Many non-prescription products contain aspirin

A

or aspirin-like medicines as an ingredient. To prevent accidental aspirin overdose, read labels carefully. Do not take more than one product that contains aspirin or aspirin-like agents (e.g., Pepto-Bismol®). If you are taking oral medicines to decrease your blood sugar, large doses of aspirin may increase the levels of these drugs. Check with your prescriber or health care professional before you change your diet or the dose of your diabetic medicine. Aspirin can irritate your stomach. Do not smoke cigarettes or drink alcohol; these increase irritation in your stomach and may cause ulcers or bleeding problems. Do not lie down for 30 minutes after taking aspirin to prevent irritation to your throat. If you are receiving cancer chemotherapy or have had an organ transplant, do not take aspirin without checking with your prescriber or health care professional. Aspirin may hide the signs of an infection such as fever or pain and increase your risk of bleeding. Prior to and after surgery or dental procedures, you may need to avoid taking aspirin. However, in some cases your prescriber may tell you to continue taking aspirin for its heart protection effects. Aspirin can interfere with your body's ability to stop bleeding. Discuss your aspirin therapy with your surgeon or dentist at least 1 week prior to any procedures.

What side effects may I notice from taking aspirin, ASA?

Side effects that you should report to your prescriber or health care professional as soon as possible:

- signs or symptoms of bleeding from the stomach or intestine such as black, tarry stools, stomach pain, vomiting up blood, or what looks like coffee grounds
- confusion
- difficulty breathing, wheezing
- pain on swallowing
- redness, blistering, peeling or loosening of the skin, including inside the mouth or nose
- ringing in the ears or changes in hearing
- skin rash, hives
- unusual bleeding or bruising, red or purple spots on the skin

Side effects that usually do not require medical attention (report to your prescriber or health care professional if they continue or are bothersome):

- diarrhea or constipation
- nausea, vomiting
- stomach gas, heartburn

Where can I keep my medicine?

Keep out of the reach of children in a container that small children cannot open. Even small doses of aspirin can be dangerous to small children and pets. Store at room temperature, between 15 and 30 degrees C (59 and 86 degrees F). Heat and moisture can cause aspirin to break down, becoming inactive and possibly dangerous to use. Do not use products that have a strong vinegar smell; throw them away at once.

Aspirin, ASA; Butalbital; Caffeine tablets and capsules

FIORINAL®;
325 mg/50 mg/40 mg; Capsule
Novartis
Pharmaceuticals

FORTABS®;
325 mg/50 mg/40 mg; Tablet
Mutual/United
Research
Laboratories

What are aspirin-butalbital-caffeine tablets or capsules?

ASPIRN-BUTALBITAL-CAFFEINE (Fiorinal®, Fortabs, and others) is a combination product used to treat certain types of headaches and migraines as well as mild to moderate pain. Federal law prohibits the transfer of this medicine to any person other than the patient for whom it was prescribed. Do not share this medicine with any one else. Generic aspirin-butalbital-caffeine tablets and capsules are available.

What should my health care professional know before I take aspirin-butalbital-caffeine?

They need to know if you have any of these conditions:

- anemia
- asthma
- depression
- diabetes mellitus
- drink more than 3-alcohol containing drinks per day
- G6PD deficiency
- heart or circulation problems
- high or low blood pressure
- infection
- kidney disease
- liver disease
- lung disease or breathing difficulties
- nasal polyps
- peptic ulcer disease
- porphyria
- problems urinating
- thyroid disease
- an unusual or allergic reaction to aspirin or related drugs, butalbital or other barbiturates, caffeine, tartrazine dye, other medicines, foods, dyes, or preservatives
- pregnant or trying to get pregnant
- breast-feeding

How should I take this medicine?

Take aspirin-butalbital-caffeine tablets or capsules by mouth with a full glass of water. Follow the directions on the prescription label. If aspirin-butalbital-caffeine upsets your stomach, take it with food or milk. Do not take your medicine more often than directed. Contact your pediatrician or health care professional regarding the use of this medicine in children. Special care may be needed. Do not share this medicine with anyone.

What if I miss a dose?

If it is almost time for your next dose (within 2 hours), take only that dose. Do not take double or extra doses.

What may interact with aspirin-butalbital-caffeine?

- alcohol
- carbamazepine
- corticosteroids
- cyclosporine
- divalproex
- female hormones, including contraceptive or birth control pills
- grapefruit juice
- medicines for depression or other mental health problems
- medicines for high blood pressure or other heart problems
- medicines for pain
- medicines to control heart rhythm
- phenobarbital
- phenytoin
- quinine
- theophylline
- valproic acid
- warfarin

Because aspirin-butalbital-caffeine can cause drowsiness, other medicines that also cause drowsiness may increase this effect of aspirin-butalbital-caffeine. Some other medicines that cause drowsiness are:

- alcohol-containing medicines
- certain antidepressants or tranquilizers
- certain antihistamines used in cold medicines
- muscle relaxants

Tell your prescriber or health care professional about all other medicines that you are taking, including non-prescription medicines, nutritional supplements, or herbal products. Also, tell your prescriber or health care professional if you are a frequent user of drinks with caffeine or alcohol, if you smoke, or if you use illegal drugs. These may affect the way your medicine works. Check with your health care professional before stopping or starting any of your medicines.

What should I watch for while taking aspirin-butalbital-caffeine?

Visit your prescriber or health care professional for regular checks on your progress. After taking aspirin-butalbital-caffeine you may get a residual hangover effect that leaves you drowsy or dizzy. Do not drive, use machinery, or do anything that needs mental alertness until you know how this medicine affects you. To re-

duce dizzy or fainting spells, do not sit or stand up quickly, especially if you are an older patient. Avoid alcoholic drinks while you are taking this medicine. Alcohol can increase possible damage to your liver and can increase possible unpleasant effects. Aspirin-butalbital-caffeine can stop birth control pills (oral contraceptives) from working properly. You may need to use an additional method of birth control while you are taking this medicine. If you have been taking caffeine or butalbital (ingredients in this medicine) on a regular basis, you can get withdrawal symptoms if you stop taking them. Symptoms include tiredness, dizziness, headache, anxiety, or nervousness. Taking too much caffeine can also make you irritable or nervous. Try to avoid excessive caffeine from foods or beverages while taking this medicine. Grapefruit juice may increase the effects of the caffeine in this medicine. Do not take aspirin-butalbital-caffeine with other non-prescription medicines, especially cold and allergy medicines, without asking your prescriber or health care professional for advice. Many non-prescription medicines contain aspirin as an ingredient. Always read the labels carefully to avoid taking an accidental overdose, which can be dangerous. If you are receiving cancer chemotherapy or other immunosuppression medicine, do not take this medicine without checking with your prescriber or health care professional. Aspirin-butalbital-caffeine may hide the signs of an infection such as fever or pain. If you are going to have surgery, tell your prescriber or health care professional that you are taking aspirin-butalbital-caffeine.

What side effects may I notice from taking aspirin-butalbital-caffeine?

Side effects that you should report to your prescriber or health care professional as soon as possible:
- bone tenderness
- changes in behavior, mood, or mental ability
- difficulty breathing or shortness of breath
- eye problems, very small or enlarged centers to the eyes
- fever, sore throat
- hallucinations
- lightheadedness or fainting spells
- redness, blistering, peeling or loosening of the skin, including inside the mouth
- seizures
- skin rash, itching, hives
- slow or fast heartbeat
- swelling of the face or lips
- unusual bleeding or bruising, pinpoint red spots on the skin
- unusual tiredness or weakness

Side effects that usually do not require medical attention (report to your prescriber or health care professional if they continue or are bothersome):
- clumsiness, unsteadiness, or a "hang-over" effect
- confusion, agitation
- constipation

A

- difficulty sleeping or nightmares
- drowsiness, dizziness
- increased frequency passing urine
- irritability, nervousness
- nausea or vomiting
- trembling

Aspirin, ASA; Butalbital; Caffeine; Codeine capsules

FIORINAL®
with Codeine; 325 mg/50 mg/
40 mg/30 mg; Capsule
PD-RX Pharmaceuticals Inc

What are aspirin-butalbital-caffeine-codeine capsules?

ASPIRIN-BUTALBITAL-CAFFEINE-CODEINE (Fiorinal® with Codeine, and many others) is a combination product used to treat certain types of headaches and migraines as well as mild to moderate pain. Federal law prohibits the transfer of this medicine to any person other than the patient for whom it was prescribed. Do not share this medicine with any one else. Generic aspirin-butalbital-caffeine-codeine capsules are available.

What should my health care professional know before I take aspirin-butalbital-caffeine-codeine?

They need to know if you have any of these conditions:
- anemia
- asthma
- blood disorders or bleeding problems or taking 'blood thinners'
- depression, thoughts of suicide or other mental health disorders
- diabetes mellitus
- drink more than 3-alcohol containing drinks per day
- G6PD deficiency
- gout
- heart or circulation problems
- high or low blood pressure
- infection
- kidney disease
- liver disease
- lung disease, asthma, chronic obstructive pulmonary disease (COPD), sleep apnea, or other breathing difficulties
- nasal polyps
- peptic ulcer disease, constipation, or other stomach or intestinal problems
- porphyria
- problems urinating
- thyroid disease
- an unusual or allergic reaction to aspirin or related drugs, butalbital or other barbiturates, caffeine, codeine, other medicines, foods, dyes, or preservatives
- pregnant or trying to get pregnant
- breast-feeding

How should I take this medicine?

Take aspirin-butalbital-caffeine-codeine capsules by mouth with a full glass of water. Follow the directions on the prescription label. If this medicine upsets your stomach, take it with food or milk. Do not take your medicine more often than directed. Contact your pediatrician or health care professional regarding the use of this medicine in children. Special care may be needed. Do not share this medicine with anyone.

What if I miss a dose?

If it is almost time for your next dose (within 2 hours), take only that dose. Do not take double or extra doses.

What may interact with aspirin-butalbital-caffeine-codeine?

- alcohol
- carbamazepine
- corticosteroids
- cyclosporine
- divalproex
- female hormones, including contraceptive or birth control medications
- grapefruit juice
- medicines for depression or other mental health problems
- medicines for high blood pressure or other heart problems
- medicines to control heart rhythm
- phenobarbital
- phenytoin
- quinine
- theophylline
- valproic acid
- warfarin

Because this medicine can cause drowsiness, other medicines that also cause drowsiness may increase this effect of aspirin-butalbital-caffeine-codeine.
Some other medicines that cause drowsiness are:

- alcohol-containing medicines
- certain antidepressants or tranquilizers
- certain antihistamines used in cold medicines
- muscle relaxants
- other pain medicines

Tell your prescriber or health care professional about all other medicines that you are taking, including nonprescription medicines, nutritional supplements, or herbal products. Also, tell your prescriber or health care professional if you are a frequent user of drinks

Where can I keep my medicine?

Keep out of the reach of children in a container that small children cannot open. Store at room temperature between 15 and 30 degrees C (59 and 86 degrees F). Keep container tightly closed. Throw away any unused medicine after the expiration date.

with caffeine or alcohol, if you smoke, or if you use illegal drugs. These may affect the way your medicine works. Check with your health care professional before stopping or starting any of your medicines.

What should I watch for while taking aspirin-butalbital-caffeine-codeine?

Visit your prescriber or health care professional for regular checks on your progress. If you have been taking this medication regularly for a long time, do not suddenly stop taking it without your prescriber's advice. Your prescriber may want you to decrease your dose gradually. After taking this medicine you may get a residual hangover effect that leaves you drowsy or dizzy. Do not drive, use machinery, or do anything that needs mental alertness until you know how this medicine affects you. To reduce dizzy spells, do not sit or stand up quickly, especially if you are an older patient. Avoid alcoholic drinks while you are taking this medicine. Alcohol can increase possible damage to your liver and can increase possible unpleasant effects. Aspirin-butalbital-caffeine-codeine can stop birth control pills (oral contraceptives) from working properly. You may need to use an additional method of birth control while you are taking this medicine. If you have been taking caffeine or butalbital (ingredients in this medicine) on a regular basis, you can get withdrawal symptoms if you stop taking them. Symptoms include tiredness, dizziness, headache, anxiety, or nervousness. Taking too much caffeine can also make you irritable or nervous. Try to avoid excessive caffeine from foods or beverages while taking this medicine. Grapefruit juice may increase the effects of the caffeine in this medicine. Do not take this medicine with other non-prescription medicines, especially cold and allergy medicines, without asking your prescriber or health care professional for advice. Many non-prescription medicines contain aspirin as an ingredient. Always read the labels carefully to avoid taking an accidental overdose, which can be dangerous. If you are receiving cancer chemotherapy or other medicines that suppress the immune system, do not take this medicine without checking with your prescriber or health care professional. Aspirin-butalbital-caffeine-codeine may hide the signs of an infection such as fever or pain. If you are going to have surgery, tell your prescriber or health care professional that you are taking aspirin-butalbital-caffeine-codeine.

What side effects may I notice from taking aspirin-butalbital-caffeine-codeine?

Side effects that you should report to your prescriber or health care professional as soon as possible:
- bone tenderness
- changes in behavior, mood, or mental ability
- difficulty breathing or shortness of breath
- eye problems, very small or enlarged centers to the eyes
- fever, sore throat
- lightheadedness or fainting spells
- redness, blistering, peeling or loosening of the skin, including inside the mouth
- seizures
- skin rash, itching, hives
- slow or fast heartbeat
- swelling of the face or lips
- unusual bleeding or bruising, pinpoint red spots on the skin
- unusual tiredness or weakness

Side effects that usually do not require medical attention (report to your prescriber or health care professional if they continue or are bothersome):
- clumsiness, unsteadiness, or a "hang-over" effect
- confusion, agitation
- constipation
- difficulty sleeping or nightmares
- drowsiness, dizziness
- increased frequency passing urine
- irritability, nervousness
- nausea or vomiting
- trembling

Where can I keep my medicine?

Keep out of the reach of children in a container that small children cannot open. Store at room temperature between 15 and 30 degrees C (59 and 86 degrees F). Keep container tightly closed. Throw away any unused medicine after the expiration date.

Aspirin, ASA; Caffeine; Dihydrocodeine capsules

SYNALGOS® DC;
356.4 mg/30 mg/16 mg;
Capsule
Wyeth Laboratories Div
Wyeth Ayerst Pharmaceuticals
Inc

What are aspirin, ASA; caffeine; dihydrocodeine capsules?

ASPIRIN; CAFFEINE; DIHYDROCODEINE (Synalgos®-DC) is a combination product used to treat moderate to severe pain. Federal law prohibits the transfer of this medicine to any person other than the patient for whom it was prescribed. Do not share this medicine with any one else. Generic aspirin; caffeine; dihydrocodeine capsules are not available.

What should my health care professional know before I take aspirin, ASA; caffeine; dihydrocodeine?

They need to know if you have any of these conditions:
- adrenal gland disease (i.e., Addison's disease)
- alcoholism or alcohol consumption
- anemia
- asthma
- depression

A

- diabetes mellitus
- difficulty urinating or urinary tract disease
- G6PD deficiency
- gout
- heart or circulation problems
- high or low blood pressure
- infection
- kidney disease
- liver disease
- lung disease or breathing difficulties
- nasal polyps
- peptic ulcer disease
- prostate enlargement
- seizures or a seizure disorder
- thyroid disease
- ulcerative colitis or other intestinal diseases
- an unusual or allergic reaction to aspirin or related drugs, caffeine, dihydrocodeine, medicines, foods, dyes, or preservatives
- pregnant or trying to get pregnant
- breast-feeding

How should this medicine be used?

Take aspirin; caffeine; dihydrocodeine capsules by mouth. Follow the directions on the prescription label. Swallow the capsules with a drink of water. If the medicine upsets your stomach, take it with food or milk. Do not take your medicine more often than directed. Contact your pediatrician or health care professional regarding the use of this medicine in children. Special care may be needed. Do not share this medicine with anyone.

What if I miss a dose?

If you are taking aspirin; caffeine; dihydrocodeine on a regular basis and miss a dose, take it as soon as you can. If it is almost time for your next dose (within 2 hours), take only the next scheduled dose. Do not take double or extra doses.

What may interact with aspirin, ASA; caffeine; dihydrocodeine?

- alcohol
- alendronate
- blood thinners (aspirin, heparin, warfarin)
- clozapine
- cidofovir
- corticosteroids
- ginkgo biloba
- imatinib, STI-571
- lithium
- medicines for depression or other mental health problems
- medicines for pain
- methotrexate
- probenecid
- stimulants
- sulfinpyrazone
- varicella virus vaccine

Aspirin; caffeine; dihydrocodeine can cause drowsiness. If you take any of the below medicines with aspirin; caffeine; dihydrocodeine, you may have increased drowsiness.

- alcohol-containing medicines
- certain antidepressants or tranquilizers
- certain antihistamines used in cold medicines
- muscle relaxants

Tell your prescriber or health care professional about all other medicines that you are taking, including non-prescription medicines, nutritional supplements, or herbal products. Also, tell your prescriber or health care professional if you are a frequent user of drinks with caffeine or alcohol, if you smoke, or if you use illegal drugs. These may affect the way your medicine works. Check with your health care professional before stopping or starting any of your medicines.

What should I watch for while taking aspirin, ASA; caffeine; dihydrocodeine?

Visit your prescriber or health care professional for regular checks on your progress. If you have been taking this medication regularly for a long time, do not suddenly stop taking it without your prescriber's advice. Your prescriber may want you to decrease your dose gradually. Aspirin; caffeine; dihydrocodeine may cause drowsiness or dizziness. Do not drive, use machinery, or do anything that needs mental alertness until you know how this medicine affects you. To reduce dizzy spells, do not sit or stand up quickly, especially if you are an older patient. Avoid alcoholic drinks while you are taking aspirin; caffeine; dihydrocodeine. Alcohol can increase possible damage to your liver and can increase possible unpleasant effects. Aspirin; caffeine; dihydrocodeine may cause constipation. If your bowel habits (frequency and amount) change, tell your health care professional immediately. Try to avoid foods and drinks that contain caffeine while taking this medicine. Do not take aspirin; caffeine; dihydrocodeine with other non-prescription medicines, especially cold and allergy medicines without asking your prescriber or health care professional for advice. Many non-prescription medicines contain aspirin as an ingredient. Always read the labels carefully to avoid taking an accidental overdose, which can be dangerous. If you are receiving cancer chemotherapy or other immunosuppression medicine, do not take aspirin; caffeine; dihydrocodeine without checking with your prescriber or health care professional. Aspirin; caffeine; dihydrocodeine may hide the signs of an infection, such as fever or pain. If you are going to have surgery, tell your prescriber or health care professional that you are taking aspirin; caffeine; dihydrocodeine.

What side effects may I notice from taking aspirin, ASA; caffeine; dihydrocodeine?

Side effects that you should report to your prescriber or health care professional as soon as possible:

- changes in behavior, mood, or mental ability
- confusion
- difficulty breathing or shortness of breath

- hallucinations
- hearing loss or ringing in ears
- lightheadedness or fainting spells
- pinpoint pupils or change in vision
- redness, blistering, peeling or loosening of the skin, including inside the mouth
- seizures
- skin rash, itching, hives
- slow or fast heartbeat
- swelling of the face or lips
- unusual bleeding or bruising
- unusual tiredness or weakness

Side effects that usually do not require medical attention (report to your prescriber or health care professional if they continue or are bothersome):

- agitation
- changes in sexual function

- constipation
- diarrhea
- difficulty sleeping
- drowsiness, dizziness
- headache
- heartburn
- increased frequency passing
- irritability, nervousness
- nausea or vomiting
- trembling
- upset stomach

Where can I keep my medicine?

Keep out of the reach of children in a container that small children cannot open. Store at room temperature at 25 degrees C (77 degrees F). Keep container tightly closed. Throw away any unused medicine after the expiration date.

Aspirin, ASA; Carisoprodol tablets

SOMA®
COMPOUND;
325 mg/200 mg;
Tablet
Medpointe
Pharmaceuticals

ASPIRIN, ASA;
CARISOPRODOL;
325 mg/200 mg;
Tablet
Par Pharmaceutical
Inc

What are aspirin, ASA; carisoprodol tablets?

ASPIRIN, ASA; CARISOPRODOL tablets (Soma® Compound) contain a muscle relaxant, carisoprodol, with aspirin. Aspirin; carisoprodol is used to relieve muscle spasms and pains associated with acute injuries. The tablets should only be used for a short time and should be combined with rest, physcial therapy or other non-drug therapies. Generic aspirin; carisoprodol tablets are available.

What should my health care professional know before I take aspirin, ASA; carisoprodol tablets?

They need to know if you currently have or have a history of any of these conditions:

- anemia
- asthma
- bleeding or clotting problems
- drink more than 3 alcohol-containing beverages a day
- heart disease, including heart failure
- high blood pressure
- gout
- kidney disease
- liver disease
- nasal polyps
- porphyria
- smoke tobacco
- stomach ulcers, or other stomach problems
- systemic lupus erythematosus (SLE)
- thrombotic thrombocytopenic purpura (TTP)
- ulcerative colitis
- vitamin K deficiency
- an unusual or allergic reaction to carisoprodol, meprobamate, tartrazine, aspirin, non-steroidal drugs or any other substance.

- pregnant or trying to get pregnant
- breast-feeding

How should I take this medicine?

Take aspirin and carisoprodol compound tablets by mouth. Follow the directions on the prescription label. Swallow tablets whole with a full glass of water. Take tablets in an upright or sitting position. Taking a sip of water first, before taking the tablets, which may help you swallow them. If possible take bedtime doses at least 10 minutes before lying down. If tablets upset your stomach, take them with food or milk. Take your doses at regular intervals. Do not take your medicine more often than directed. This medication is not recommended for use in children under 12 years old or for individuals older than 65 years of age.

What if I miss a dose?

If you miss a dose, take it as soon as you can. If it is almost time for your next dose, take only that dose. Do not take double or extra doses.

What may interact with aspirin, ASA; carisoprodol?

- alcohol
- alendronate
- antacids
- barbiturate medicines for inducing sleep or treating seizures (convulsions), like phenobarbital
- cimetidine
- herbal products that contain feverfew, garlic, ginger, ginkgo biloba, horse chestnut, kava kava, or valerian
- hormones such as prednisone or cortisone
- isoniazid (INH)
- medicines for colds, hay fever or other allergies

are taken by mouth

...OS

...ression, anxiety, or emo-

...(convulsions) or epilepsy

...or prevent blood clots
...exate
...afinil
...neprazole
- other medicines that contain aspirin or aspirin-related ingredients (e.g., Pepto-Bismol®)
- other muscle relaxants
- rifampin, rifabutin, or rifapentine
- voriconazole

Tell your prescriber or health care professional about all other medicines you are taking, including non-prescription medicines, nutritional supplements, or herbal products. Also tell your prescriber or health care professional if you are a frequent user of drinks with caffeine or alcohol, if you smoke, or if you use illegal drugs. These may affect the way your medicine works. Check with your health care professional before stopping or starting any of your medicines.

What should I watch for while taking aspirin, ASA; carisoprodol?

You may get drowsy or dizzy. Do not drive, use machinery, or do anything that needs mental alertness until you know how this drug affects you. To reduce the risk of dizzy or fainting spells, do not sit or stand up quickly, especially if you are an older patient. Alcohol can make you more drowsy; avoid alcoholic drinks. Many non-prescription products contain aspirin or aspirin-like medicines as an ingredient. To prevent accidental aspirin overdose, read labels carefully. Do not take more than one product that contains aspirin or aspirin-like agents (e.g., Pepto-Bismol®).

What side effects may I notice from taking aspirin, ASA; carisoprodol?

Side effects that you should report to your prescriber or health care professional as soon as possible:
- signs or symptoms of bleeding from the stomach or intestine such as black, tarry stools, stomach pain, vomiting up blood, or what looks like coffee grounds
- confusion
- difficulty breathing, wheezing
- dizziness
- fainting spells
- intolerance to heat
- pain on swallowing
- redness, blistering, peeling or loosening of the skin, including inside the mouth or nose
- ringing in the ears or changes in hearing
- skin rash, hives
- trembling
- unsteadiness
- unusual bleeding or bruising, red or purple spots on the skin

Side effects that usually do not require medical attention (report to your prescriber or health care professional if they continue or are bothersome):
- drowsiness or dizziness
- flushing (reddening of skin)
- headache
- nausea, vomiting
- diarrhea
- constipation

Where can I keep my medicine?

Keep out of the reach of children in a container that small children cannot open. Store at room temperature between 15 and 30 degrees C (59 and 86 degrees F). Protect from moisture. Keep container tightly closed. Throw away any unused medicine after the expiration date.

Aspirin, ASA; Dipyridamole capsules

AGGRENOX®;
25 mg/200 mg; Capsule
Boehringer Ingelheim
Pharmaceuticals Inc

What are aspirin-dipyridamole capsules?

ASPIRIN-DIPYRIDAMOLE (Aggrenox®) decreases the risk of stroke in patients who have had a stroke or transient ischemic attack (known as a "TIA" or "mini-stroke"). Generic aspirin-dipyridamole combinations are not available.

What should my health care professional know before I take aspirin-dipyridamole?

They need to know if you have any of these conditions:
- anemia
- asthma
- bleeding or clotting problems
- drink more than 3 alcohol-containing beverages a day
- gout
- kidney disease
- liver disease
- lupus (SLE)
- nasal polyps
- skin problems
- smoke tobacco
- stomach ulcers, or other stomach problems
- thrombotic thrombocytopenic purpura (TTP)
- vitamin K deficiency
- an unusual or allergic reaction to aspirin, dipyridamole, tartrazine dye, other medicines, dyes, or preservatives

- pregnant or trying to get pregnant
- breast-feeding

How should I take this medicine?

Take the capsules by mouth with a glass of water. The capsules must be swallowed whole; do not crush or chew. Follow the directions on the label. Take your doses at regular intervals. Do not take your medicine more often than directed. This medicine is not intended for children.

What if I miss a dose?

If you are taking aspirin on a regular schedule and miss a dose, take it as soon as you can. If it is almost time for your next dose, take only that dose. Do not take double or extra doses.

What may interact with aspirin-dipyridamole?

- alcohol
- acetazolamide
- alendronate
- anti-inflammatory drugs (NSAIDs such as ibuprofen)
- aspirin-containing medicines or other salicylates
- blood thinners (anticoagulants), antiplatelet drugs, or other drugs which may affect bleeding
- fish oil (omega-3 fatty acids) supplements
- herbal medicines or dietary supplements like feverfew, garlic pills, ginger, gingko biloba, or horse chestnut
- hormones such as prednisone or cortisone
- medicines for diabetes that are taken by mouth
- medicines for high blood pressure (beta-blockers or ACE inhibitors)
- methotrexate
- medicines for seizures (phenytoin or valproic acid)
- porfimer
- probenecid
- steroids (such as dexamethasone)
- sulfinpyrazone
- vaccines for chickenpox (varicella virus vaccine live)
- water pills (diuretics)

Tell your prescriber or health care professional about all other medicines you are taking, including non-prescription medicines, nutritional supplements, or herbal products. Also tell your prescriber or health care professional if you are a frequent user of drinks with caffeine or alcohol, if you smoke, or if you use illegal drugs. These may affect the way your medicine works. Check with your health care professional before stopping or starting any of your medicines.

What should I watch for while taking aspirin-dipyridamole?

Only take other aspirin products if prescribed by your prescriber or health care professional. Many non-prescription medicines contain aspirin as an ingredient. To prevent accidental aspirin overdose, read labels carefully and do not take more than one product that contains aspirin. If you are diabetic, aspirin may alter your blood sugar levels. Check with your prescriber or health care professional before you change your diet or the dose of your diabetic medicine. Aspirin can irritate your stomach. Drinking alcohol and smoking cigarettes can make this irritation worse and may cause ulcers or bleeding problems. Ask your prescriber or health care professional for help to stop smoking or drinking. Do not lie down for 30 minutes after taking aspirin to prevent irritation to your throat. If you are receiving cancer chemotherapy or other immunosuppression medicine, do not take aspirin without checking with your prescriber or health care professional. Aspirin may hide the signs of an infection such as fever or pain and increase your risk of bleeding. Prior to and after surgery or dental procedures, you may need to avoid taking aspirin. However, in some cases your prescriber may tell you to continue taking aspirin for its heart protection effects. Aspirin can interfere with your body's ability to stop bleeding. Discuss your aspirin; dipyridamole therapy with your surgeon or dentist at least 1 week prior to any procedures.

What side effects may I notice from taking aspirin-dipyridamole?

Side effects that you should report to your prescriber or health care professional as soon as possible:
- black, tarry stools
- chest pain or palpitations
- confusion
- difficulty breathing, wheezing
- dizziness or fainting spells
- drowsiness or weakness
- pain on swallowing
- redness, blistering, peeling or loosening of the skin, including inside the mouth or nose
- ringing in the ears
- seizures
- skin rash
- stomach pain
- unusual bleeding or bruising, red or purple spots on the skin
- vomiting up blood, or what looks like coffee grounds

Side effects that usually do not require medical attention (report to your prescriber or health care professional if they continue or are bothersome):
- diarrhea
- flushing, reddening, or itching of the skin
- headache (if they occur, headaches may occur over time while receiving the drug)
- nausea, vomiting
- reduced amount of urine passed
- stomach gas, heartburn

Where can I keep my medicine?

Keep out of the reach of children in a container that small children cannot open. Even small doses of aspirin can be dangerous to small children and pets. Store at room temperature, between 15 and 30 degrees C (59 and 86 degrees F). Protect from excessive heat and moisture. Throw away any unused medicine after the expiration date.

A

Aspirin, ASA;
Oxycodone tablets

PERCODAN®;
325 mg/4.5 mg/0.38
mg; Tablet
Endo
Pharmaceuticals Inc

ASPIRIN, ASA;
OXYCODONE; 325
mg/4.5 mg/0.38 mg;
Tablet
Watson
Pharmaceuticals Inc

What are aspirin-ASA-oxycodone tablets?

ASPIRIN-ASA-OXYCODONE (Percodan®, Endodan®, Percodan®-Demi) is a combination of two different types of pain medicine and is used to treat moderate to severe pain. Federal law prohibits the transfer of aspirin; oxycodone to any person other than the patient for whom it was prescribed. Generic aspirin; oxycodone tablets are available.

What should my health care professional know before I take aspirin-oxycodone?

They need to know if you have any of these conditions:
- drink more than 3 alcohol-containing drinks per day
- infection
- heart or circulation problems
- lung disease or breathing difficulties
- kidney disease
- liver disease
- problems urinating
- seizures or other neurologic disorders
- constipation
- an unusual or allergic reaction to aspirin, oxycodone, other opioid analgesics, foods, dyes or preservatives
- pregnant or trying to get pregnant
- breast-feeding

How should I take this medicine?

Take aspirin-oxycodone tablets by mouth with a full glass of water. Follow the directions on the prescription label. You can take aspirin-oxycodone with food to prevent stomach upset. Do not take your medicine more often than directed. Do not share this medicine with anyone. Contact your pediatrician or health care professional regarding the use of this medicine in children. Special care may be needed.

What if I miss a dose?

If you miss a dose, take it as soon as you can. If it is almost time for your next dose, take only that dose. Do not take double or extra doses.

What may interact with aspirin-oxycodone?

- medicines for seizures
- medicines for high blood pressure
- alcohol
- warfarin
- Ginkgo biloba

Because aspirin-oxycodone can cause drowsiness, other medicines that also cause drowsiness may increase this effect of aspirin-oxycodone. Some other medicines that cause drowsiness are:

- alcohol-containing medicines
- barbiturates such as phenobarbital
- certain antidepressants or tranquilizers
- muscle relaxants
- certain antihistamines used in cold medicines

Tell your prescriber or health care professional about all other medicines you are taking, including non-prescription medicines, nutritional supplements, or herbal products. Also tell your prescriber or health care professional if you are a frequent user of drinks with caffeine or alcohol, if you smoke, or if you use illegal drugs. These may affect the way your medicine works. Check with your health care professional before stopping or starting any of your medicines.

What should I watch for while taking aspirin-oxycodone?

Tell your prescriber or health care professional if your pain does not go away, if it gets worse, or if you have new or different type of pain. Do not take other painkillers with aspirin-oxycodone without advice. Use exactly as directed by your prescriber or health care professional. If you get flu-like symptoms (fever, chills, muscle aches and pains), call your prescriber or health care professional; do not treat yourself. To reduce unpleasant effects on your throat and stomach, take aspirin-oxycodone with food or milk and never just before lying down. Aspirin-oxycodone may make you drowsy when you first start taking it or change doses. Do not drive, use machinery, or do anything that needs mental alertness until you know how aspirin-oxycodone affects you. Do not sit or stand up quickly. This reduces the risk of dizzy or fainting spells. These effects may be worse if you are an older patient. The drowsiness should decrease after taking aspirin-oxycodone for a couple of days. If you have not slept because of your pain, you may sleep more the first few days your pain is controlled to catch-up on missed sleep. Be careful taking other medicines that may also make you tired. This effect may be worse when taking these medicines with aspirin-oxycodone. Alcohol can increase possible drowsiness, dizziness, confusion and affect your breathing. Alcohol can increase possible damage to your liver. Avoid alcohol while taking aspirin-oxycodone. Aspirin-oxycodone can cause constipation. Make sure to take a laxative and/or a stool softener. Try to have a bowel movement at least every 2 to 3 days. If you do not have a bowel movement for 3 days or more call your prescriber or health care professional. They may recommend using an enema or suppository to help you move your bowels. Many non-prescription medicines contain aspirin as an ingredient. Always read the labels carefully to avoid taking an accidental overdose, which can be dangerous. Aspirin can affect your blood sugar. Check with your prescriber or health care professional before you change your diet or the dose of your diabetic medicine. If you are going to have surgery tell your prescriber or health care professional that you are taking oxycodone.

What side effects may I notice from taking aspirin-oxycodone?

Elderly patients are more likely to get side effects. Side effects that you should report to your prescriber or health care professional as soon as possible:
- chest pain or irregular heartbeat
- difficulty breathing, wheezing
- severe rash
- unusual weakness
- fever, chills, muscle aches and pains

Side effects that usually do not require medical attention (report to your prescriber or health care professional if they continue or are bothersome):

- constipation
- dizziness, drowsiness
- confusion
- gas or heartburn
- nausea, vomiting
- dry mouth
- itching
- pinpoint pupils

Where can I keep my medicine?

Keep out of the reach of children in a container that small children cannot open. Do not share or give this medicine to anyone else. Avoid accidental swallowing of aspirin-oxycodone by someone (especially children) other than for whom it was prescribed as this may result in severe side effects and possibly death. Store at room temperature between 15 and 30 degrees C (59 and 86 degrees F). Protect from light. Keep container tightly closed. Throw away any unused medicine after the expiration date.

Aspirin, ASA; Pravastatin tablets

PRAVIGARD™ PAC; 325 mg/40 mg; Tablet Bristol Myers Squibb Co

PRAVIGARD™ PAC; 81 mg/80 mg; Tablet Bristol Myers Squibb Co

What are aspirin, ASA; pravastatin tablets?

ASPIRIN, ASA; PRAVASTATIN (Pravigard™ PAC) blocks the body's ability to make cholesterol. This drug is discontinued in the United States. In addition to a low cholesterol diet, pravastatin helps to lower the blood cholesterol. Aspirin reduces the ability of the blood to clot. Both pravastatin and aspirin can decrease the risk of a heart attack or stroke in people who are at risk for these problems. Generic aspirin; pravastatin tablet packs are not yet available.

What should my health care professional know before I take aspirin, ASA; pravastatin?

They need to know if you have any of these conditions:
- anemia
- asthma
- bleeding or clotting problems
- blood salt imbalance
- diabetes
- drink more than 3 alcohol-containing beverages a day
- heart disease, including heart failure
- high or low blood pressure
- gout
- infection
- kidney disease
- liver disease
- lupus (systemic lupus erythematosus, SLE)
- muscle disorder or condition
- nasal polyps
- recent surgery
- seizures (convulsions)
- severe injury
- smoke tobacco

- stomach ulcers or other stomach problems
- thrombotic thrombocytopenic purpura (TTP)
- thyroid disease
- vitamin K deficiency
- an unusual or allergic reaction to aspirin, pravastatin, tartrazine dye, other medicines, foods, dyes, or preservatives
- pregnant or trying to get pregnant
- breast-feeding

How should this medicine be used?

Take aspirin; pravastatin tablets by mouth. Follow the directions on the label. Swallow the aspirin and pravastatin tablets whole with a sip of water. After taking the aspirin dose, drink a full glass of water. Take the tablets in an upright or sitting position. It is best to stand or sit upright for at least 10 minutes after taking the aspirin dose. Aspirin and pravastatin tablets may be taken with or without meals. Take your doses at regular intervals. Do not take your medicine more often than directed. This product is not intended for use in children.

What if I miss a dose?

If you miss a dose, take it as soon as you can. If it is almost time for your next dose, take only that dose. Do not take double or extra doses.

What may interact with aspirin, ASA; pravastatin?

- acetazolamide
- alcohol-containing beverages
- alendronate
- anti-inflammatory drugs (NSAIDs, such as ibuprofen)

A

- blood thinners (anticoagulants like warfarin) or other drugs which may affect bleeding
- fish oil (omega-3 fatty acids) supplements
- herbal medicines or dietary supplements like feverfew, garlic pills, ginger, gingko biloba, horse chestnut
- hormones such as prednisone or cortisone
- itraconazole
- medicines for high blood pressure (beta-blockers or ACE inhibitors)
- medicines for diabetes that are taken by mouth
- medicines to lower cholesterol or triglycerides (examples: cholestyramine, colestipol, fenofibrate, gemfibrozil, niacin)
- medicines that lower your immune response (cyclosporine)
- medicines for gout
- methazolamide
- methotrexate
- orlistat
- other medicines that contain aspirin or aspirin-like ingredients
- porfimer
- probenecid
- sulfinpyrazone
- vaccines for chickenpox (varicella virus vaccine live)
- valproic acid or divalproex
- water pills (diuretics)
- went yeast

Tell your prescriber or health care professional about all other medicines you are taking, including non-prescription medicines, nutritional supplements, or herbal products. Also tell your prescriber or health care professional if you are a frequent user of drinks with caffeine or alcohol, if you smoke, or if you use illegal drugs. These may affect the way your medicine works. Check with your health care professional before stopping or starting any of your medicines.

What should I watch for while taking aspirin, ASA; pravastatin?

Visit your prescriber or health care professional for regular checks on your progress. You will need to have regular tests to make sure your liver is working properly while you are taking pravastatin. Tell your prescriber or health care professional as soon as you can if you get any unexplained muscle pain, tenderness, or weakness, especially if you also have a fever and tiredness. Aspirin; pravastatin is only part of a total cholesterol-lowering program. Your physician or dietician can suggest a low-cholesterol and low-fat diet that will reduce your risk of getting heart and blood vessel disease. Avoid alcohol and smoking, and keep a proper exercise schedule. Many non-prescription products contain aspirin or aspirin-like medicines as an ingredient. To prevent accidental aspirin overdose, read labels carefully. Do not take more than one product that contains aspirin or aspirin-like agents (e.g., Pepto-Bismol®) unless approved by your prescriber. Aspirin can irritate your stomach. Drinking alcohol and smoking cigarettes can make this irritation worse and may cause ulcers or bleeding problems. Ask your prescriber or health care professional for help to stop smoking or drinking. If you are receiving cancer chemotherapy or have had an organ transplant, do not take aspirin without checking with your prescriber or health care professional. Aspirin may hide the signs of an infection such as fever or pain and increase your risk of bleeding. Prior to and after surgery or dental procedures, you may need to avoid taking aspirin. However, in some cases your prescriber may tell you to continue taking aspirin for its heart protection effects. Aspirin can interfere with your body's ability to stop bleeding. Discuss your aspirin therapy with your surgeon or dentist at least 1 week prior to any procedures.

What side effects may I notice from taking aspirin, ASA; pravastatin?

Side effects that you should report to your prescriber or health care professional as soon as possible:
Rare or uncommon:
- allergic-type reaction (hives, wheezing)
- dark yellow or brown urine
- decreased urination, difficulty passing urine
- difficulty breathing (troubled breathing)
- fever
- muscle pain, tenderness, cramps, or weakness
- pain on swallowing
- redness, blistering, peeling or loosening of the skin, including inside the mouth
- unusual tiredness or weakness
- yellowing of the skin or eyes

More common:
- black, tarry stools
- skin rash or redness, itching, flushing
- stomach pain
- unusual bleeding or bruising, red or purple spots on the skin
- vomiting up blood, or what looks like coffee grounds

Side effects that usually do not require medical attention (report to your prescriber or health care professional if they continue or are bothersome):
- diarrhea or constipation
- dizziness that does not go away
- drowsiness (mild)
- flu-like symptoms
- headache (mild)
- nausea, vomiting
- stomach gas, heartburn

Where can I keep my medicine?

Keep out of the reach of children in a container that small children cannot open. Even small doses of aspirin can be dangerous to small children and pets. Store at room temperature, between 20 and 25 degrees C (68 and 77 degrees F). Protect from heat and moisture. Throw away any unused medicine after the expiration date.

Atazanavir capsules

REYATAZ®;
150 mg; Capsule
Mead Johnson
Oncology Products

REYATAZ®;
200 mg; Capsule
Mead Johnson
Oncology Products

What are atazanavir capsules?

ATAZANAVIR (Reyataz®) is an antiviral drug called a protease inhibitor. Atazanavir is used to treat human immunodeficiency virus (HIV) infection. Atazanavir may reduce the amount of HIV in the blood and increase the number of CD4 cells (T-cells) in the blood. Atazanavir is used in combination with other drugs to treat HIV. For example, if you are taking atazanavir and efavirenz, you should also be taking ritonavir. Atazanavir will not cure or prevent HIV infection or AIDS. You may still develop other infections or conditions associated with HIV. Generic atazanavir capsules are not yet available.

What should my health care professional know before I take atazanavir?

They need to know if you have any of these conditions:
- hemophilia A or B
- high blood levels of bilirubin
- jaundice
- liver disease
- an unusual or allergic reaction to atazanavir, other medicines, foods, dyes, or preservatives
- breast-feeding
- pregnant or trying to get pregnant

How should this medicine be used?

Take atazanavir capsules by mouth. Do not open the capsules. Follow the directions on the prescription label. Take atazanavir with a light snack or meal. Avoid taking atazanavir on an empty stomach, with grapefruit or grapefruit juice, or with a high fat meal. Do not take within two hours of antacid or buffered didanosine (ddI) use. Take your doses at regular intervals. Do not take your medicine more often than directed. To help to make sure that your anti-HIV therapy works as well as possible, be very careful to take your medicine exactly as prescribed. Do not stop taking except on your prescriber's advice. Contact your pediatrician or health care professional regarding the use of this medicine in children. Special care may be needed.

What if I miss a dose?

If you miss a dose, take the dose immediately. Then, take your next dose at your regularly scheduled time. You need to take atazanavir every 24 hours. Do not take more or less than your prescribed dose. If you miss multiple doses in a row or miss doses on several occasions, contact your health care professional.

What may interact with atazanavir?

Many medicines may interact with atazanavir. If you have a question concerning other medicines you may be taking, talk with your pharmacist, prescriber or other health care professional. Tell your health care professional about all the medicines you take. Do not start a new medicine without talking to your health care professional.

Do not take atazanavir with any of these medicines:
- astemizole
- bepridil
- bromocriptine
- cisapride
- disopyramide
- dofetilide
- ergotamine, dihydroergotamine, ergonovine, or methylergonovine
- ibutilide
- indinavir
- irinotecan
- levomethadyl
- lovastatin
- midazolam
- pimozide
- proton pump inhibitors (such as esomeprazole, lansoprazole, omeprazole pantoprazole, rabeprazole)
- rifampin
- simvastatin
- St. John's wort
- terfenadine
- triazolam
- ziprasidone

Other medicines that may interact with atazanavir:
- amiodarone
- antacids
- aripiprazole
- atorvastatin
- bexarotene
- birth control pills or other hormonal birth control medicines (like the patch, ring, or injections)
- buffered didanosine (DDI)
- certain medicines for anxiety or difficulty sleeping
- certain medicines for high cholesterol (atorvastatin)
- clarithromycin
- cyclosporine
- digoxin
- diltiazem
- eplerenone
- felodipine
- fentanyl
- grapefruit juice
- H2-blockers (examples: ranitidine, cimetidine, famotidine, nizatidine)
- lidocaine
- medicines for diabetes
- methadone
- methysergide
- nicardipine

A

- nifedipine
- quinidine
- rifabutin
- rifapentine
- sildenafil
- sirolimus
- some medicines for seizures (examples: carbamazepine, phenobarbital, phenytoin, fosphenytoin, oxcarbazepine, primidone)
- tacrolimus
- theophylline or aminophylline
- tricyclic antidepressants (examples: amitriptyline, clomipramine, desipramine, doxepin, imipramine, nortriptyline, protriptyline, and trimipramine)
- verapamil
- warfarin

Tell your prescriber or health care professional about all other medicines you are taking, including non-prescription medicines, nutritional supplements, or herbal products. Also tell your prescriber or health care professional if you are a frequent user of drinks with caffeine or alcohol, if you smoke, or if you use illegal drugs. These may affect the way your medicine works. Check with your health care professional before stopping or starting any of your medicines.

What should I watch for while taking atazanavir?

Visit your prescriber or health care professional for regular checks on your progress. Discuss any new symptoms with your prescriber or health care professional. Atazanavir will not cure HIV and you can still get other illnesses or complications associated with your disease. Taking atazanavir does not reduce the risk of passing HIV infection to others through sexual or blood contact. It is best to avoid sexual contact so that you do not spread the disease to others. For any sexual contact, use a condom. Be careful about cuts, abrasions and other possible sources of blood contact. Never share a needle or syringe with anyone. If you are a woman of childbearing age and are using hormone contracep-

tives, then you should use another form of birth control while taking atazanavir. Atazanavir may decrease the effectiveness of hormone birth control agents, including birth control pills and injections. Do not take antacids or buffered didanosine, ddI, within 2 hours of taking atazanavir. These drugs may decrease the amount of atazanavir you may absorb. Know when you will run out of atazanavir. Fill your prescription before you run out of medicine. It is important to not miss even a single day of atazanavir.

What side effects may I notice from taking atazanavir?

Side effects that you should report to your prescriber or health care professional as soon as possible:
- muscle pain
- severe nausea and vomiting
- severe stomach pain
- skin rash or itchy skin
- sore throat, fever, or other sign or symptom of an infection
- unusual bleeding, black tarry stools, or coughing up blood
- unusual tiredness or weakness
- yellowing of the skin or whites of the eyes

Side effects that usually do not require medical attention (report to your prescriber or health care professional if they continue or are bothersome):
- changes in body appearance (such as weight gain or loss around the waist and/or face)
- diarrhea
- headache
- nausea
- stomach pain
- tingling or burning in your arms or legs

Where can I keep my medicine?

Keep out of the reach of children in a container that small children cannot open. Store tightly closed at controlled room temperature between 15 degrees and 30 degrees C (59 degrees and 86 degrees F). Protect from moisture. Throw away any unused medicine after the expiration date.

Atenolol tablets

TENORMIN®;
50 mg; Tablet
AstraZeneca
Pharmaceuticals LP

ATENOLOL;
25 mg; Tablet
Sandoz
Pharmaceuticals

What are atenolol tablets?

ATENOLOL (Tenormin®) belongs to a group of medicines called beta-blockers. Beta-blockers reduce the workload on the heart and help it to beat more regularly. Atenolol controls, but does not cure, high blood pressure (hypertension). Atenolol also relieves chest pain (angina), and can be helpful after a heart attack. Sometimes atenolol is used to help prevent migraine headaches. Generic atenolol tablets are available.

What should my health care professional know before I take atenolol?

They need to know if you have any of these conditions:
- asthma, bronchitis or bronchospasm
- circulation problems, or blood vessel disease (such as Raynaud's disease)
- depression
- diabetes
- emphysema
- history of heart attack or heart disease

- kidney disease
- muscle weakness or disease
- pheochromocytoma
- psoriasis
- thyroid disease
- an unusual or allergic reaction to atenolol, other beta-blockers, medicines, foods, dyes, or preservatives
- pregnant or trying to get pregnant
- breast-feeding

How should I take this medicine?

Take atenolol tablets by mouth. Follow the directions on the prescription label. Swallow the tablets with a drink of water. Atenolol may be taken with or without food. Take your doses at regular intervals. Do not take your medicine more often than directed. Do not stop taking except on your prescriber's advice. Contact your pediatrician or health care professional regarding the use of this medicine in children. Special care may be needed.

What if I miss a dose?

If you miss a dose, take it as soon as you can. If it is almost time for your next dose, take only that dose. Do not take double or extra doses. There should be at least 8 hours between doses.

What may interact with atenolol?

- antacids
- calcium salts
- cocaine
- hawthorn
- medicines for colds and breathing difficulties
- medicines for diabetes
- medicines for high blood pressure
- medicines to control heart rhythm
- water pills

Tell your prescriber or health care professional about all other medicines you are taking, including non-prescription medicines, nutritional supplements, or herbal products. Also tell your prescriber or health care professional if you are a frequent user of drinks with caffeine or alcohol, if you smoke, or if you use illegal drugs. These may affect the way your medicine works. Check with your health care professional before stopping or starting any of your medicines.

What should I watch for while taking atenolol?

Check your heart rate and blood pressure regularly while you are taking atenolol. Ask your prescriber or health care professional what your heart rate and blood pressure should be, and when you should contact him or her. Do not stop taking this medicine suddenly. This could lead to serious heart-related effects. You may get drowsy or dizzy. Do not drive, use machinery, or do anything that requires mental alertness until you know how atenolol affects you. To reduce the risk of dizzy or fainting spells, do not sit or stand up quickly. Alcohol can make you more drowsy, and increase flushing and rapid heartbeats. Therefore, it is best to avoid alcoholic drinks. Atenolol can affect blood sugar levels. If you have diabetes, check with your prescriber or health care professional before you change your diet or the dose of your diabetic medicine. If you are going to have surgery, tell your prescriber or health care professional that you are taking atenolol.

What side effects may I notice from taking atenolol?

Side effects that you should report to your prescriber or health care professional as soon as possible:
- changes in vision
- cold, tingling, or numb hands or feet
- confusion
- difficulty breathing, wheezing
- dizziness or fainting spells
- increased thirst
- increase in the amount of urine passed
- irregular heartbeat
- skin rash
- slow heart rate (fewer than recommended by your prescriber or health care professional)
- sweating
- swollen legs or ankles
- tremor, shakes
- vomiting
- weight loss

Side effects that usually do not require medical attention (report to your prescriber or health care professional if they continue or are bothersome):
- anxiety
- depression, nightmares
- diarrhea
- difficulty sleeping
- dry itching skin
- dry or burning eyes
- headache
- nausea
- sexual difficulties, impotence
- unusual tiredness

Where can I keep my medicine?

Keep out of the reach of children in a container that small children cannot open. Store at room temperature between 15 and 30 degrees C (59 and 86 degrees F). Protect from light. Throw away any unused medicine after the expiration date.

A

Atenolol; Chlorthalidone tablets

TENORETIC®;
100 mg/25 mg;
Tablet
AstraZeneca
Pharmaceuticals LP

ATENOLOL;
Chlorthalidone; 50
mg/25 mg; Tablet
Mylan
Pharmaceuticals Inc

What are atenolol; chlorthalidone tablets?

ATENOLOL; CHLORTHALIDONE (Tenoretic®) is a combination of two drugs used to lower blood pressure. Atenolol is a beta-blocker and chlorthalidone is a diuretic ("water pill"). Atenolol; chlorthalidone is used to control, but not cure, high blood pressure (hypertension). Generic atenolol; chlorthalidone tablets are available.

What should my health care professional know before I take atenolol; chlorthalidone?

They need to know if you have any of these conditions:
- asthma, bronchitis or bronchospasm
- autoimmune disease such as lupus (SLE)
- bradycardia (unusually slow heartbeat)
- chest pain (angina)
- circulation problems, or blood vessel disease (such as Raynaud's disease)
- depression
- diabetes
- electrolyte imbalance (such as low or high levels of potassium in the blood)
- emphysema, COPD, or other lung disease
- gout
- heart disease (such as heart failure or a history of heart attack)
- kidney disease
- liver disease
- muscle weakness or myasthenia gravis
- pancreatitis
- pheochromocytoma
- post-sympathectomy
- psoriasis
- thyroid disease
- sulfonamide (sulfa) or thiazide allergy
- an unusual or allergic reaction to chlorthalidone, atenolol, other beta-blockers, diuretics, sulfonamides, or other medicines, foods, dyes, or preservatives
- if you are on a special diet, such as a low-salt diet (using potassium substitutes)
- pregnant or trying to get pregnant
- breast-feeding

How should I take this medicine?

Take atenolol; chlorthalidone tablets by mouth. You can take atenolol; chlorthalidone tablets with or without food. Follow the directions on the prescription label. Swallow the tablets with a drink of water. Take your doses at regular intervals. Do not take your medicine more often than directed. Do not stop taking except on your prescriber's advice. Contact your pediatrician or health care professional regarding the use of this medicine in children. Special care may be needed.

Elderly patients over 65 years old may have a stronger reaction to this medicine and need smaller doses.

What if I miss a dose?

If you miss a dose, take it as soon as you can. If it is almost time for your next dose, take only that dose. Do not take double or extra doses.

What may interact with atenolol; chlorthalidone?

- allopurinol
- antacids
- anti-inflammatory drugs (NSAIDs, such as ibuprofen)
- calcium salts
- cevimeline
- clonidine
- cocaine or amphetamine
- dolasetron
- ginger, Zingiber officinale
- griseofulvin
- hawthorn
- lithium
- liothyronine
- mefloquine
- medicines for chest pain or angina
- medicines for colds and breathing difficulties
- medicines for diabetes
- medicines for high blood pressure or heart failure
- medicines known as MAO inhibitors, such as phenelzine (Nardil®), tranylcypromine (Parnate®), isocarboxazid (Marplan®), and selegiline (Carbex®, Eldepryl®)
- medicines to control heart rhythm (including amiodarone, digoxin, disopyramide, dofetilide, flecainide, propafenone, quinidine, and sotalol)
- porfimer
- prochlorperazine (Compazine®)
- rifampin
- some antibiotics which increase sensitivity to sunlight (sulfonamides, tetracyclines)
- some medicines for lowering cholesterol (colestipol or cholestyramine)
- some medicines for weight loss (including some herbal products, ephedrine, dextroamphetamine)
- vitamin A (retinol) creams or pills such as tretinoin Retin-A®, Renova®, Solage®, Atragen®, and others
- water pills (diuretics)

Tell your prescriber or health care professional about all other medicines you are taking, including non-prescription medicines, nutritional supplements, or herbal products. Also tell your prescriber or health care professional if you are a frequent user of drinks with caffeine or alcohol, if you smoke, or if you use illegal drugs. These may affect the way your medicine works. Check

with your health care professional before stopping or starting any of your medicines.

What should I watch for while taking atenolol; chlorthalidone?

Check your heart rate and blood pressure regularly while you are taking atenolol; chlorthalidone. Ask your prescriber or health care professional what your blood pressure should be and when you should contact him or her. When you check your blood pressure, write down the measurements to show your prescriber or health care professional. If you are taking this medicine for a long time you must visit your prescriber or health care professional for regular checks on your progress. Make sure you schedule appointments on a regular basis. Do not stop taking this medicine suddenly. This could lead to serious heart-related effects. You may get drowsy or dizzy. Do not drive, use machinery, or do anything that requires mental alertness until you know how atenolol; chlorthalidone affects you. To reduce the risk of dizzy or fainting spells, do not sit or stand up quickly. Alcohol can make you more drowsy, and increase the risk of flushing and rapid heartbeats. Therefore, it is best to avoid alcoholic drinks. Check with your health care professional if you get an attack of severe diarrhea, nausea and vomiting, or sweat a lot. The loss of too much body fluid while you are taking a diuretic can cause dehydration and lower the blood pressure below normal. Atenolol; chlorthalidone can affect blood sugar levels. If you have diabetes, check with your prescriber or health care professional before you change your diet or the dose of your diabetic medicine. Do not take medicines for appetite control, asthma, colds, cough, hay fever, or sinus problems without asking your prescriber or health care professional for advice. Do not treat yourself for a fever or sore throat; check with your prescriber or health care professional first. Avoid exposure to excessive sunlight (such as sunlamps, sunbathing) while taking this medicine. If you are going to have surgery, tell your prescriber or health care professional that you are taking atenolol; chlorthalidone.

What side effects may I notice from taking atenolol; chlorthalidone?

Side effects that you should report to your prescriber or health care professional as soon as possible:
- changes in vision (e.g., blurred vision)
- cold, tingling, or numb hands or feet
- confusion, dizziness, lightheadedness or fainting spells
- difficulty breathing, wheezing
- fever or chills
- increase or decrease in the amount of urine passed
- fast or uneven heart beat, palpitations, or chest pain
- slow heart rate
- muscle cramps
- redness, blistering, peeling or loosening of the skin, including inside the mouth
- stomach pain
- swollen legs or ankles
- unusual skin rash or bruising
- unusual tiredness or weakness
- vomiting
- worsened gout pain
- yellowing of the eyes or skin

Side effects that usually do not require medical attention (report to your prescriber or health care professional if they continue or are bothersome):
- depression, nightmares
- diarrhea
- dry eyes or dry mouth
- headache
- increased sensitivity to the sun
- nausea
- sexual difficulties, impotence
- tiredness or fatigue

Where can I keep my medicine?

Keep out of the reach of children in a container that small children cannot open. Store at room temperature at 20 to 25 degrees C (68 and 77 degrees F). Protect from light and moisture. Throw away any unused medicine after the expiration date.

Atomoxetine capsules

STRATTERA®;
10 mg; Capsule
Eli Lilly and Co

STRATTERA®;
40 mg; Capsule
Eli Lilly and Co

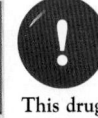
This drug requires an FDA medication guide. See page xxxvii.

What are atomoxetine capsules?

ATOMOXETINE (Strattera™) is a medication used to treat attention deficit/hyperactivity disorder, also known as ADHD. Atomoxetine does not have stimulant properties like those seen with other common drugs for ADHD. This drug can improve attention span, concentration, and emotional control, and reduce restless or overactive behavior. Atomoxetine is sometimes used for other purposes. Generic atomoxetine capsules are not yet available.

What should my health care professional know before I take atomoxetine?

They need to know if you have any of these conditions:
- dehydration
- glaucoma
- high or low blood pressure
- irregular heartbeat or other cardiac disease
- liver disease
- mania or bipolar disorder
- prostate enlargement
- recent weight loss

A

- seizures
- stroke
- suicidal thoughts
- trouble urinating
- an unusual or allergic reaction to atomoxetine, other medicines, foods, dyes, or preservatives
- pregnant or trying to get pregnant
- breast-feeding

How should this medicine be taken?

Take atomoxetine capsules by mouth. You may take this drug with food if it upsets your stomach. Follow the directions on the prescription label. If you find atomoxetine causes difficulty sleeping and you take more than 1 dose per day, take your last dose of the day before 6 PM. Do not take your medicine more often than directed. Contact your pediatrician or health care professional regarding the use of this medicine in children. Special care may be needed. Atomoxetine is used in children 6 years of age or older.

What if I miss a dose?

If you miss a dose, take it as soon as you can. If it is almost time for your next dose, take only that dose. Do not take double or extra doses.

What may interact with atomoxetine?

- alcohol
- amphetamines
- atropine
- breathing treatments, such as albuterol, formoterol or salmeterol
- cimetidine
- certain heart medications, such as amiodarone or quinidine
- decongestant or cold medications
- ephedra, *Ma huang* or ephedrine
- furazolidone
- linezolid
- medications for depression, anxiety or other mood problems
- medications for HIV infection or AIDS, such as ritonavir
- medications for weight loss
- monoamine oxidase inhibitors (MAOIs), such as isocarboxazid, phenelzine, or tranylcypromine
- procarbazine
- scopolamine
- selegiline
- thioridazine

Tell your prescriber or health care professional about all other medicines you are taking, including non-prescription medicines, nutritional supplements, or herbal products. Also tell your prescriber or health care professional if you are a frequent user of drinks with caffeine or alcohol, if you smoke, or if you use illegal drugs. These may affect the way your medicine works. Check with your health care professional before stopping or starting any of your medicines.

What should I watch for while taking atomoxetine?

It may take a week or more for this medicine to take effect. This is why it is very important to continue taking the medication and not miss any doses. Use caution while driving or while operating machinery or performing other tasks requiring concentration until you know how atomoxetine affects you. Do not drink alcohol while you take atomoxetine. Alcohol slows down the central nervous system and can worsen drowsiness. Atomoxetine is not habit-forming. There is no need to taper your dose; however, you should contact your doctor before you stop taking it. If you experience dry mouth while taking atomoxetine, make sure to drink plenty of water. It may also be helpful to suck on sugarless hard candy or crushed ice. If your dry mouth is severe, ask your doctor about a saliva substitute. If you are going to have surgery, tell your prescriber or health care professional that you are taking atomoxetine.

What side effects may I notice from taking atomoxetine?

Side effects that you should report to your prescriber or health care professional as soon as possible:

- changes in mood, such as agitation, irritability or excessive crying
- chest pain or irregular heart rhythm (too fast or slow)
- dark-colored urine
- difficulty breathing
- difficulty urinating
- "flu-like" symptoms, such as extreme tiredness (fatigue), body aches (muscle aches), chills
- increased blood pressure
- skin rash or hives, itching
- stomach pain or tenderness
- vomiting
- weight loss
- yellow color that appears in your skin or in the whites of your eyes

Side effects that usually do not require medical attention (report to your prescriber or health care professional if they continue or are bothersome):

- mild constipation or diarrhea
- decreased appetite
- dizziness
- drowsiness
- dry mouth
- headache
- menstrual period irregularities
- nausea
- sexual side effects, such as loss of interest in sex or impotence
- stomach upset
- sweating

Where can I keep my medicine?

Keep out of the reach of children in a container that small children cannot open. Store atomoxetine capsules at room temperature between 15 and 30 degrees C (59 and 86 degrees F). Discard any unused medication after the expiration date.

Atorvastatin tablets

LIPITOR®;
20 mg; Tablet
Parke Davis Division
of Pfizer Co.

LIPITOR®;
40 mg; Tablet
Parke Davis Division
of Pfizer Co.

What are atorvastatin tablets?

ATORVASTATIN (Lipitor®) blocks the body's ability to make cholesterol. Atorvastatin can help lower blood cholesterol for patients who are at risk of getting heart disease or a stroke. It is only for patients whose cholesterol level is not controlled by diet. It is not a cure. Generic atorvastatin tablets are not yet available.

What should my health care professional know before I take atorvastatin?

They need to know if you have any of these conditions:
- an alcohol problem
- any hormone disorder (such as diabetes, under-active thyroid)
- blood salt imbalance
- infection
- kidney disease
- liver disease
- low blood pressure
- muscle disorder or condition
- recent surgery
- seizures (convulsions)
- severe injury
- an unusual or allergic reaction to atorvastatin, other medicines, foods, dyes, or preservatives
- pregnant or trying to get pregnant
- breast-feeding

How should I take this medicine?

Take atorvastatin tablets by mouth. Follow the directions on the prescription label. Swallow the atorvastatin with a drink of water. Atorvastatin can be taken at anytime of the day with or without food. Take your doses at regular intervals. Do not take your medicine more often than directed. Contact your pediatrician or health care professional regarding the use of this medicine in children. Special care may be needed.

What if I miss a dose?

If you miss a dose, take it as soon as you can. If it is almost time for your next dose, take only that dose. Do not take double or extra doses.

What may interact with atorvastatin?

- alcohol-containing beverages
- amiodarone
- barbiturates (examples: phenobarbital, butalbital, primidone)
- antacids
- birth control pills
- bosentan
- carbamazepine
- certain antibiotics such as clarithromycin, erythromycin, or troleandomycin
- danazol
- digoxin
- diltiazem
- grapefruit juice
- herbal medicines such as went yeast (Cholestin™) or St. John's Wort
- medicines for fungal infections (examples: fluconazole, itraconazole, ketoconazole, voriconazole)
- medicines for treating HIV infections
- medicines that suppress your immune response (cyclosporine)
- medicines to lower cholesterol or triglycerides (examples: colestipol, fenofibrate, gemfibrozil, niacin)
- medicine used to stop early pregnancy (mifepristone, RU-486 or Mifeprex™)
- nefazodone
- nicardipine
- oxcarbazepine
- phenytoin
- pioglitazone
- rifampin, rifabutin, or rifapentine
- verapamil

Tell your prescriber or health care professional about all other medicines you are taking, including non-prescription medicines, nutritional supplements, or herbal products. Also tell your prescriber or health care professional if you are a frequent user of drinks with caffeine or alcohol, if you smoke, or if you use illegal drugs. These may affect the way your medicine works. Check with your health care professional before stopping or starting any of your medicines.

What should I watch for while taking atorvastatin?

Visit your prescriber or health care professional for regular checks on your progress. You will need to have regular tests to make sure your liver is working properly. Tell your prescriber or health care professional as soon as you can if you get any unexplained muscle pain, tenderness, or weakness, especially if you also have a fever and tiredness. Atorvastatin is only part of a total cholesterol-lowering program. Your physician or dietician can suggest a low-cholesterol and low-fat diet that will reduce your risk of getting heart and blood vessel disease. Avoid alcohol and smoking, and keep a proper exercise schedule. If you are going to have surgery tell your prescriber or health care professional that you are taking atorvastatin.

What side effects may I notice from taking atorvastatin?

Side effects that you should report to your prescriber or health care professional as soon as possible:

A

Rare or uncommon:
- dark yellow or brown urine
- decreased urination, difficulty passing urine
- fever
- muscle pain, tenderness, cramps, or weakness
- redness, blistering, peeling or loosening of the skin, including inside the mouth
- skin rash, itching
- unusual tiredness or weakness
- yellowing of the skin or eyes

Side effects that usually do not require medical attention (report to your prescriber or health care professional if they continue or are bothersome):

- diarrhea
- gas
- headache
- joint pain
- nausea, vomiting
- stomach upset or pain
- tiredness

Where can I keep my medicine?

Keep out of the reach of children in a container that small children cannot open. Store at controlled room temperature between 20 and 25 degrees C (68 and 77 degrees F). Keep container tightly closed. Throw away any unused medicine after the expiration date.

Atovaquone; Proguanil tablets

MALARONE®;
250 mg/100 mg;
Tablet
Glaxo Wellcome

MALARONE®
PEDIATRIC;
62.5 mg/25 mg;
Tablet
Glaxo Wellcome

What are atovaquone; proguanil tablets?

ATOVAQUONE; PROGUANIL (Malarone®, Malarone® Pediatric) is an antimalarial agent. Atovaquone; proguanil prevents and treats malaria infections. Generic atovaquone; proguanil tablets are not available.

What should my health care professional know before I take atovaquone; proguanil?

They need to know if you have any of these conditions:
- kidney or liver disease
- stomach or intestinal problems
- an unusual or allergic reaction to atovaquone, proguanil, other medicines, foods, dyes, or preservatives
- pregnant or trying to get pregnant
- breast-feeding

How should I take this medicine?

Take atovaquone; proguanil tablets by mouth. Follow the directions on the prescription label. You must take atovaquone; proguanil at the same time each day with food or a milky drink. If you vomit within 1 hour after taking, take another dose. If you are taking atovaquone; proguanil to prevent malaria, you should start taking it 1 or 2 days before entering the area, and continue for 7 days after leaving. Do not take your medicine more often than directed. For prolonged stays, consult your healthcare provider for proper dosing schedule.

What if I miss a dose?

If you miss a daily dose, take it as soon as you can and return to your normal dosing schedule. Only take one dose per day. Do not take double or extra doses.

What may interact with atovaquone; proguanil?

- bosentan
- metoclopramide
- rifabutin
- rifampin
- rifapentine
- sulfamethoxazole
- sulfamethoxazole-trimethoprim
- tetracycline
- trimethoprim
- zidovudine, ZDV

Tell your prescriber or health care professional about all other medicines you are taking, including non-prescription medicines, nutritional supplements, or herbal products. Also tell your prescriber or health care professional if you are a frequent user of drinks with caffeine or alcohol, if you smoke, or if you use illegal drugs. These may affect the way your medicine works. Check with your health care professional before stopping or starting any of your medicines.

What should I watch for while taking atovaquone; proguanil?

If you get a fever during or after you start taking atovaquone; proguanil, do not treat yourself. Contact your healthcare provider immediately. Tell your prescriber or health care professional if your symptoms do not improve in a few days. If you are taking atovaquone; proguanil for a long time, visit your prescriber or health care professional for regular checks. If you notice any changes in your vision see your ophthalmologist for an eye exam. Keep out of the sun, or wear protective clothing outdoors and use a sunscreen. Do not use sun lamps or sun tanning beds or booths. You may get dizzy. Do not drive, use machinery, or do anything that needs mental alertness until you know how atovaquone; proguanil affects you. While in areas where malaria is common, certain steps can be taken to prevent being bit by mosquitos. They include:
1) Stay in air-conditioned or well-screened rooms to reduce human-mosquito contact.
2) Sleep under mosquito netting, preferably one with pyrethrum-containing insecticide.

3) Wear long-sleeved shirts or blouses and long trousers to protect arms and legs.

4) Apply mosquito repellents containing DEET to uncovered areas of skin.

5) Use a pyrethrum-containing flying insect spray to kill mosquitos.

What side effects may I notice from taking atovaquone; proguanil?

Side effects that you should report to your prescriber or health care professional as soon as possible:
- difficulty breathing or increased shortness of breath
- fever or chills
- severe diarrhea
- skin rash, itching (there may be severe itching without a rash)
- unusual tiredness or weakness

- vomiting

Side effects that usually do not require medical attention (report to your prescriber or health care professional if they continue or are bothersome):
- dizziness
- loss of appetite
- mild diarrhea
- nausea
- stomach pain or upset

Where can I keep my medicine?

Keep out of the reach of children in a container that small children cannot open. It is important to keep atovaquone; proguanil out of reach of children; overdose is very dangerous. Store at room temperature between 15 and 30 degrees C (59 and 86 degrees F). Throw away any unused medicine after the expiration date.

Atropine tablets or soluble tablets

SAL-TROPINE®;
0.4 mg; Tablet
Hope Pharmaceuticals

What are atropine tablets?

ATROPINE (Sal-Tropine®) can help treat many conditions. Administration of atropine before surgery helps to reduce saliva and fluid in the respiratory tract (windpipe). Generic atropine sulfate tablets or soluble atropine sulfate tablets are available.

What should my health care professional know before I take atropine?

They need to know if you have any of these conditions:
- bleeding problems
- closed-angle glaucoma
- diarrhea
- difficulty passing urine
- heart disease, or previous heart attack
- hiatal hernia
- myasthenia gravis
- prostate trouble
- stomach infection
- stomach obstruction
- ulcerative colitis
- an unusual or allergic reaction to atropine, other medicines, foods, dyes, or preservatives
- pregnant or trying to get pregnant
- breast-feeding

How should I take this medicine?

Take atropine tablets by mouth. Follow the directions on the prescription label. Swallow the tablets with a drink of water, or if they are soluble tablets, dissolve in water before taking. Take the tablets 30 to 60 minutes before food. Do not take your medicine more often than directed.

What if I miss a dose?

If you miss a dose, take it as soon as you can. If it is almost time for your next dose, take only that dose. Do not take double or extra doses.

What may interact with atropine?

- amantadine
- benztropine
- cisapride
- digoxin
- donepezil
- galantamine
- glutethimide
- medicines for hay fever and other allergies
- medicines for mental depression
- medicines for mental problems and psychotic disturbances
- meperidine
- metoclopramide
- potassium salts
- quinidine
- rivastigmine
- tacrine
- tegaserod

Tell your prescriber or health care professional about all other medicines you are taking, including non-prescription medicines, nutritional supplements, or herbal products. Also tell your prescriber or health care professional if you are a frequent user of drinks with caffeine or alcohol, if you smoke, or if you use illegal drugs. These may affect the way your medicine works. Check with your health care professional before stopping or starting any of your medicines.

What should I watch for while taking atropine?

Side effects may occur even though you are no longer taking atropine. Contact your prescriber or health care professional if you are still getting side effects after several days. You may get dizzy or have blurred vision. Do not drive, use machinery, or do anything that requires mental alertness until you know how atropine affects you. To reduce the risk of dizzy or fainting spells, do not sit or stand up quickly, especially if you are an older patient. Alcohol can make you more dizzy, avoid alcoholic drinks. Stay out of bright light and wear sunglasses if atropine makes your eyes more sensitive to light. Your mouth may get dry. Chewing sugarless gum or sucking hard candy, and drinking plenty of water will help. Atropine may cause dry eyes and blurred vision. If you wear contact lenses you may feel some discomfort. Lubricating drops may help. See your ophthalmologist if the problem does not go away or is severe. Avoid extreme heat (e.g., hot tubs, saunas). Atropine can cause you to sweat less than normal. Your body temperature could increase to dangerous levels, which may lead to heat stroke.

What side effects may I notice from taking atropine?

Side effects that you should report to your prescriber or health care professional as soon as possible:
- anxiety, nervousness
- blurred vision or other eye problems
- confusion
- dizziness or fainting spells
- fast or slow heartbeat
- hallucinations (seeing or hearing things that are not really there)
- loss of memory
- redness, blistering, peeling or loosening of the skin, including inside the mouth
- slurred speech
- unusual weakness or tiredness
- vomiting

Side effects that usually do not require medical attention (report to your prescriber or health care professional if they continue or are bothersome):
- constipation
- dry mouth
- increased sensitivity of the eyes to sun or ultraviolet light
- nausea
- pain or difficulty passing urine

Where can I keep my medicine?

Keep out of the reach of children in a container that small children cannot open. Store at room temperature between 15 and 30 degrees C (59 and 86 degrees F). Do not freeze. Throw away any unused medicine after the expiration date.

Atropine; Hyoscyamine; Phenobarbital; Scopolamine capsules, tablets, or extended-release tablets

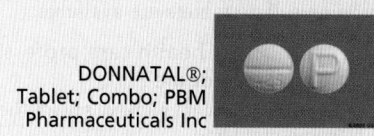

DONNATAL®;
Tablet; Combo; PBM
Pharmaceuticals Inc

What are atropine; hyoscyamine; phenobarbital; scopolamine capsules, tablets, or extended-release tablets?

ATROPINE; HYOSCYAMINE; PHENOBARBITAL; SCOPOLAMINE (Donnatal®) is used to treat different bowel problems including irritable bowel syndrome. It may also help in treating an intestinal ulcer (duodenal ulcer). Generic atropine; hyoscyamine; phenobarbital; scopolamine tablets are available. Generic capsules or extended-release tablets are not available.

What should my health care professional know before I take atropine; hyoscyamine; phenobarbital; scopolamine?

They need to know if you have any of these conditions:
- an alcohol or drug abuse problem
- closed-angle glaucoma
- diarrhea
- difficulty passing urine
- heart disease, or previous heart attack
- hiatal hernia (also known as esophageal reflux or GERD)
- kidney disease
- low blood pressure
- lung disease, chest infection or breathing difficulties
- mental depression or mental problems
- myasthenia gravis
- porphyria
- prostate trouble
- shock
- stomach infection
- stomach obstruction
- ulcerative colitis
- an unusual or allergic reaction to atropine; hyoscyamine; phenobarbital; scopolamine, other medicines, foods, dyes, or preservatives
- pregnant or trying to get pregnant
- breast-feeding

How should I take this medicine?

Take this drug by mouth. Follow the directions on the prescription label. Swallow the capsules or tablets whole with a drink of water 30 to 60 minutes before food. If you are taking the Donnatal Extentabs® or other extended-release dosage form, swallow the tablets whole; do not crush, cut, or chew them. Do not take your medicine more often than directed. Elderly patients over age 65 years may have a stronger reaction to this medicine and may need smaller doses. Contact your pediatrician or health care professional regarding the use of this medicine in children. Special care may be needed.

What if I miss a dose?

If it is almost time for your next dose, take only that dose. Do not take double or extra doses.

What may interact with atropine; hyoscyamine; phenobarbital; scopolamine?

- acetaminophen
- alcohol
- alosetron
- amantadine
- benztropine
- caffeine
- chloramphenicol
- cisapride
- cyclophosphamide
- cyclosporine
- digoxin
- doxorubicin
- doxycycline
- erythromycin
- female hormones, including contraceptive or birth control pills
- hormones such a prednisone or cortisone
- medicines for anxiety or sleeping problems
- medicines for high blood pressure or other heart problems
- medicines for hay fever and other allergies
- medicines for mental problems or psychotic disturbances
- medicines to control heart rhythm
- medicines for treating HIV infection or AIDS
- metronidazole
- opiates such as codeine, hydromorphone, and morphine
- potassium salts
- quinidine
- quinine
- seizure (convulsion) or epilepsy medicine
- theophylline
- warfarin

Tell your prescriber or health care professional about all other medicines you are taking, including non-prescription medicines, nutritional supplements, or herbal products. Also tell your prescriber or health care professional if you are a frequent user of drinks with caffeine or alcohol, if you smoke, or if you use illegal drugs. These may affect the way your medicine works. Check with your health care professional before stopping or starting any of your medicines.

What should I watch for while taking atropine; hyoscyamine; phenobarbital; scopolamine?

This medication can stop birth control pills (oral contraceptives) from working properly. Use another method of birth control while you are taking this medi-cation. If you are going to have surgery, tell your prescriber or health care professional that you are taking this medication. You may get dizzy or have blurred vision. Do not drive, use machinery, or do anything that needs mental alertness until you know how this medication affects you. To reduce the risk of dizzy or fainting spells, do not sit or stand up quickly, especially if you are an older patient. Alcohol can make you more dizzy, avoid alcoholic drinks. Stay out of bright light and wear sunglasses if this medication makes your eyes more sensitive to light. Your mouth may get dry. Chewing sugarless gum or sucking hard candy, and drinking plenty of water will help. This medication may cause dry eyes and blurred vision. If you wear contact lenses, you may feel some discomfort. Lubricating drops may help. See your ophthalmologist if the problem does not go away or is severe. Avoid extreme heat (e.g., hot tubs, saunas). This medication can cause you to sweat less than normal. Your body temperature could increase to dangerous levels, which may lead to heat stroke.

What side effects may I notice from taking atropine; hyoscyamine; phenobarbital; scopolamine?

Side effects that you should report to your prescriber or health care professional as soon as possible:
- anxiety, nervousness
- blurred vision or other eye problems
- bone tenderness
- changes in behavior, mood, or mental ability
- changes in the frequency or severity of seizures
- confusion, agitation
- difficulty breathing or shortness of breath
- dizziness or fainting spells
- eye problems, very small or enlarged centers to the eyes
- fast heartbeat
- fever, sore throat
- hallucinations
- lightheadedness or fainting spells
- pain or difficulty passing urine
- redness, blistering, peeling or loosening of the skin, including inside the mouth
- skin rash, itching, hives
- slow heartbeat
- swelling of the face or lips
- unusual bleeding or bruising, pinpoint red spots on the skin
- unusual tiredness or weakness
- vomiting
- weight loss
- yellowing of skin or eyes

Side effects that usually do not require medical attention (report to your prescriber or health care professional if they continue or are bothersome):
- altered taste
- clumsiness, unsteadiness, or a "hang-over" effect
- constipation
- difficulty sleeping or nightmares
- drowsiness

- dry mouth
- headache
- increased sensitivity of the eyes to sun or ultraviolet light
- irritability, nervousness
- nausea

Where can I keep my medicine?

Keep out of the reach of children in a container that small children cannot open. Store at room temperature between 15 and 30 degrees C (59 and 86 degrees F). Throw away any unused medicine after the expiration date.

Azithromycin tablets

ZITHROMAX®;
250 mg; Tablet
Pfizer Laboratories
Div Pfizer Inc

ZITHROMAX Z-PAK;
250 mg; Tablet
Pfizer

What are azithromycin tablets?

AZITHROMYCIN (Zithromax®, Zithromax Z-pak) is a macrolide antibiotic that interferes with the growth of bacterial cells. It is used to treat bacterial infections in many different parts of the body. Azithromycin also treats sexually transmitted vaginal or urinary tract infections caused by chlamydia. It will not work for colds, flu, or other virus infections. Generic azithromycin tablets are available.

What should my health care professional know before I take azithromycin?

They need to know if you have any of these conditions:
- kidney disease
- liver disease
- pneumonia
- stomach problems (especially colitis)
- other chronic illness
- an unusual or allergic reaction to azithromycin, other macrolide antibiotics (such as erythromycin), foods, dyes, or preservatives
- breast-feeding

How should I take this medicine?

Take azithromycin tablets by mouth. Follow the directions on the prescription label. Swallow tablets whole with a full glass of water. Azithromycin tablets can be taken with or without food. Take your doses at regular intervals. Do not take your medicine more often than directed. Finish the full course prescribed by your prescriber or health care professional even if you think your condition is better. Do not stop taking except on your prescriber's advice. Contact your pediatrician or health care professional regarding the use of this medicine in children. Special care may be needed.

What if I miss a dose?

If you miss a dose, take it as soon as you can. If it is almost time for your next dose, take only that dose. Do not take double or extra doses. There should be an interval of at least 12 hours between doses.

What may interact with azithromycin?

- antacids
- astemizole
- digoxin
- dihydroergotamine
- ergotamine
- magnesium salts
- terfenadine
- triazolam
- warfarin

Tell your prescriber or health care professional about all other medicines you are taking, including non-prescription medicines, nutritional supplements, or herbal products. Also tell your prescriber or health care professional if you are a frequent user of drinks with caffeine or alcohol, if you smoke, or if you use illegal drugs. These may affect the way your medicine works. Check with your health care professional before stopping or starting any of your medicines.

What should I watch for while taking azithromycin?

Tell your prescriber or health care professional if your symptoms do not improve in 2 to 3 days. Contact your prescriber or health care professional as soon as you can if you get an allergic reaction to azithromycin, such as rash, itching, difficulty swallowing, or swelling of the face, lips or tongue. Keep out of the sun, or wear protective clothing outdoors and use a sunscreen. Do not use sun lamps or sun tanning beds or booths. If you get severe or watery diarrhea, do not treat yourself. Call your prescriber or health care professional for advice. Antacids can stop azithromycin from working. If you get an upset stomach and want to take an antacid, make sure there is an interval of at least 2 hours since you last took azithromycin, or 4 hours before your next dose. If you are going to have surgery, tell your prescriber or health care professional that you are taking azithromycin.

What side effects may I notice from taking azithromycin?

Side effects that you should report to your prescriber or health care professional as soon as possible:
Rare or uncommon:
- dark yellow or brown urine
- difficulty breathing
- severe or watery diarrhea
- skin rash, itching
- irregular heartbeat, palpitations, or chest pain

- vomiting
- yellowing of the eyes or skin

Side effects that usually do not require medical attention (report to your prescriber or health care professional if they continue or are bothersome):
- diarrhea
- dizziness, drowsiness
- hearing loss
- headache
- increased sensitivity to the sun

- nausea
- stomach pain or cramps
- tiredness
- vaginal irritation, itching or discharge

Where can I keep my medicine?

Keep out of the reach of children in a container that small children cannot open. Store at room temperature between 15 and 30 degrees C (59 and 86 degrees F). Throw away any unused medicine after the expiration date.

A

Baclofen tablets and disintegrating tablets

 BACLOFEN; 10 mg; Tablet Upsher-Smith Laboratories Inc

 BACLOFEN; 20 mg; Tablet Ivax Pharmaceuticals Inc

What are baclofen tablets and disintegrating tablets?

BACLOFEN (Lioresal®, Kemstro®) is a muscle relaxant. It relieves spasms and cramping of muscles in conditions such as multiple sclerosis. Generic baclofen tablets are available. Generic baclofen disintegrating tablets are not available.

What should my health care professional know before I take baclofen?

They need to know if you have any of these conditions:

- bleeding disorders
- diabetes
- mental illness
- kidney disease
- recent stroke
- seizures (convulsions)
- an unusual or allergic reaction to baclofen, other medicines, foods, dyes, or preservatives
- pregnant or trying to get pregnant
- breast-feeding

How should I take this medicine?

Follow the directions on the prescription label. Take your doses at regular intervals. Do not take your medicine more often than directed. Do not stop taking your medicine suddenly. Contact your pediatrician or health care professional regarding the use of this medicine in children. Special care may be needed.
Tablets: Take baclofen tablets by mouth. Swallow with a drink of water.
Disintegrating Tablets: Take baclofen disintegrating tablets by mouth. With dry hands, place the tablet on your tongue. The tablet will dissolve rapidly and be swallowed in your saliva. It is not necessary to drink any water to take this medicine.

What if I miss a dose?

If you miss a dose, take it as soon as you can. If it is almost time for your next dose, take only that dose. Do not take double or extra doses.

What may interact with baclofen?

- medicines for high blood pressure

Because baclofen can cause drowsiness, other medicines that also cause drowsiness may increase this effect of baclofen. Some medicines that cause drowsiness are:

- alcohol-containing medicines
- barbiturates such as phenobarbital
- certain antidepressants or tranquilizers
- certain antihistamines used in cold medicines
- herbal products that contain kava kava or valerian

- other muscle relaxants
- tramadol or other strong medicines for pain

Ask your prescriber or health care professional about other medicines that may increase the effect of baclofen.
Tell your prescriber or health care professional about all other medicines you are taking, including non-prescription medicines, nutritional supplements, or herbal products. Also tell your prescriber or health care professional if you are a frequent user of drinks with caffeine or alcohol, if you smoke, or if you use illegal drugs. These may affect the way your medicine works. Check with your health care professional before stopping or starting any of your medicines.

What should I watch for while taking baclofen?

Visit your prescriber or health care professional for regular checks on your progress. It may take several days of treatment before you see the full effects of baclofen. Do not suddenly stop taking baclofen. You must gradually reduce the dose to avoid side effects. Ask your prescriber or health care professional for advice. Baclofen can affect blood sugar levels. If you are diabetic check with your prescriber or health care professional before you change your diet or the dose of your diabetic medicine. You may get drowsy or dizzy. Do not drive, use machinery, or do anything that needs mental alertness until you know how baclofen affects you. To reduce the risk of dizzy or fainting spells, do not sit or stand up quickly, especially if you are an older patient. Alcohol can make you more drowsy; avoid alcoholic drinks.

What side effects may I notice from taking baclofen?

Side effects that you should report to your prescriber or health care professional as soon as possible:

- chest pain
- difficulty passing urine or increased need to urinate
- difficulty walking or moving
- fainting spells
- increased spasticity
- mood or mental changes
- rapid heart beat
- ringing or buzzing in the ears
- seeing or hearing things that are not there (hallucinations)
- seizures
- skin rash, hives
- slurred speech or problems talking
- unusual restlessness or nervousness
- vision changes (blurred vision, seeing double)

Side effects that usually do not require medical attention (report to your prescriber or health care professional if they continue or are bothersome):
- changes in taste
- confusion
- constipation
- diarrhea
- difficulty sleeping at night (insomnia)
- dizziness or lightheadedness
- drowsiness
- dry mouth

- headache
- increased passing of urine
- muscle weakness
- nausea, vomiting
- weakness or tiredness

Where can I keep my medicine?

Keep out of the reach of children in a container that small children cannot open. Store at room temperature between 15 and 30 degrees C (59 and 86 degrees F). Keep container tightly closed. Throw away any unused medicine after the expiration date.

Balsalazide capsules

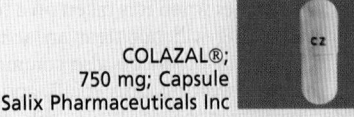

COLAZAL®;
750 mg; Capsule
Salix Pharmaceuticals Inc

What are balsalazide capsules?

BALSALAZIDE (Colazal®) is an anti-inflammatory agent. It reduces inflammation inside the bowel and pain associated with ulcerative colitis and helps to prevent recurring inflammation. Generic balsalazide capsules are not yet available.

What should my health care professional know before I take balsalazide?

They need to know if you have any of these conditions:
- kidney or liver disease
- an unusual or allergic reaction to balsalazide, aspirin, other medicines, foods, dyes, or preservatives
- pregnant or trying to get pregnant
- breast-feeding

How should I take this medicine?

Take balsalazide capsules by mouth. Follow the directions on the prescription label. Swallow the capsules whole with a drink of water. Take your doses at regular intervals. Do not take your medicine more often than directed. Contact your pediatrician or health care professional regarding the use of this medicine in children. Special care may be needed.

What if I miss a dose?

If you miss a dose, take it as soon as you can. If it is almost time for your next dose, take only that dose. Do not take double or extra doses.

What may interact with balsalazide?

Tell your prescriber or health care professional about all other medicines you are taking, including non-prescription medicines, nutritional supplements, or herbal products. Also tell your prescriber or health care professional if you are a frequent user of drinks with caffeine or alcohol, if you smoke, or if you use illegal drugs. These may affect the way your medicine works. Check with your health care professional before stopping or starting any of your medicines. Specific interactions between balsalazide capsules and other drugs have not been studied.

What should I watch for while taking balsalazide?

Tell your prescriber or health care professional if your symptoms do not start to improve after several days. There is usually an improvement in 3 to 21 days. You may need about 6 weeks of treatment to get good results. It is important that you go on taking your medicine and only stop taking it on your prescriber's advice.

What side effects may I notice from taking balsalazide?

Side effects that you should report to your prescriber or health care professional as soon as possible:
- chest pain
- difficulty breathing, wheezing
- fever, chills, sore throat
- skin rash or itching
- unusual bleeding or bruising
- unusual weakness or tiredness
- yellowing of the eyes or skin

Side effects that usually do not require medical attention (report to your prescriber or health care professional if they continue or are bothersome):
- diarrhea
- headache
- nausea, vomiting
- stomach pain or cramps

Where can I keep my medicine?

Keep out of the reach of children in a container that small children cannot open. Store at room temperature between 15 and 30 degrees C (59 and 86 degrees F). Throw away any unused medicine after the expiration date.

Belladonna Alkaloids; Ergotamine; Phenobarbital tablets

BELLERGAL-S®;
0.2 mg/0.6 mg/40 mg; Tablet
Novartis Pharmaceuticals

What are belladonna alkaloids; ergotamine; phenobarbital tablets?

BELLADONNA ALKALOIDS; ERGOTAMINE; PHENOBARBITAL (Bellamine S®, Bellaphen S®, Bellaspas™, Bellergal S®, Bel-Phen-Ergot S®, Spastrin™ and others) is a combination of several different drugs. This drug combination helps prevent migraine or cluster headaches when it is taken on a regular basis. However, this drug will not treat an acute migraine headache. This drug product is also commonly used to treat hot flashes, sweating, dizzy spells, and restlessness associated with menopause. While this drug may be used for other conditions, other uses are rare. Generic belladonna alkaloids; ergotamine; phenobarbital tablets are available.

What should my health care professional know before I take belladonna alkaloids; ergotamine; phenobarbital?

They need to know if you have any of these conditions:

- an alcohol or drug abuse problem
- blood clots or blood vessel disease
- chest pain
- diarrhea
- difficulty passing urine
- glaucoma
- heart disease, or previous heart attack
- hiatal hernia (also known as esophageal reflux or GERD)
- high blood pressure
- high cholesterol
- history of heart attacks
- infection
- kidney disease
- liver disease
- lung disease, chest infection or breathing difficulties
- mental depression or mental problems
- myasthenia gravis
- poor circulation
- porphyria
- prostate trouble
- stomach obstruction
- tobacco smoker
- ulcerative colitis
- an unusual or allergic reaction to atropine; belladonna; ergotamine; hyoscyamine; phenobarbital; scopolamine, other medicines, foods, dyes, or preservatives
- pregnant or trying to get pregnant
- breast-feeding (do not breast-feed while taking this medication)

How should I take this medicine?

Take this medication by mouth with a sip of water. Do not crush, chew or cut the tablets. If this medicine upsets your stomach, you may take it with food. Follow the directions on the prescription label. Do not take your medicine more often than directed. Contact your pediatrician or health care professional regarding the use of this medicine in children. Special care may be needed. This medication is not usually prescribed to children.

What if I miss a dose?

If it is almost time for your next dose, take only that dose. Do not take double or extra doses.

What may interact with belladonna alkaloids; ergotamine; phenobarbital?

This medication may interact with many other medications. Some of the important medications that might interact are listed. You should check with your pharmacist prior to taking any new medicine with this medicine.

Do not use any of the following migraine drugs within 24 hours of this medicine: almotriptan, eletriptan, frovatriptan, naratriptan, rizatriptan, sumatriptan, or zolmitriptan. Also, do not use this drug along with caffeine-ergotamine combinations (example: Cafergot® or Wigraine®); dihydroergotamine (DHE® or Migranal®); ergotamine (Ergomar®) or methysergide (Sansert®); ergonovine; or methylergonovine. *This medication may also interact with:*

- acetaminophen
- alcohol
- alosetron
- amantadine
- antibiotics such as erythromycin, clarithromycin, and troleandomycin
- antacids
- antifungal drugs like fluconazole, itraconazole, ketoconazole or voriconazole
- aprepitant
- benztropine
- bromocriptine
- cabergoline
- caffeine
- chloramphenicol
- cisapride
- cocaine
- cyclophosphamide
- cyclosporine
- danazol
- digoxin
- doxorubicin
- doxycycline
- ergoloid mesylates
- female hormones, including contraceptive or birth control pills

B

- grapefruit juice
- hormones such a prednisone or cortisone
- medicines for anxiety or sleeping problems
- medicines for colds, flu, or breathing difficulties
- medicines for hay fever and other allergies
- medicines for high blood pressure, chest pain or other heart problems
- medicines for mental depression, anxiety or other mood problems, especially fluoxetine, fluvoxamine and nefazodone
- medicines for treating HIV infection or AIDS
- medicines or herbal products for headaches
- medicines or herbal products for weight loss or appetite control
- medicines to control heart rhythm
- metronidazole
- nicotine
- prescription pain medications like codeine, hydromorphone, and morphine
- quinidine
- quinine
- seizure (convulsion) or epilepsy medicine
- tegaserod
- theophylline
- warfarin
- zileuton

Tell your prescriber or health care professional about all other medicines you are taking, including non-prescription medicines, nutritional supplements, or herbal products. Also tell your prescriber or health care professional if you are a frequent user of drinks with caffeine or alcohol, if you smoke, or if you use illegal drugs. These may affect the way your medicine works. Check with your health care professional before stopping or starting any of your medicines.

What should I watch for while taking belladonna alkaloids; ergotamine; phenobarbital?

Do not exceed the dosage on the label or take this medicine for longer than prescribed. Taking this medicine more often or longer than prescribed may lead to dependence on this drug or may result in unwanted side effects. If you take this medication to prevent headaches, check with your prescriber if you do not get relief from using this medication. It is important to tell your prescriber or health care professional as soon as possible if you get any of the following side effects: cold, numb, or painful hands or feet; leg cramps when walking; any type of pain around your chest; swelling; itching. This medication may decrease the circulation of blood to your skin, fingers, and toes. You may get more sensitive to the cold. Elderly patients are more likely to feel this effect. Avoid long exposure to the cold and dress warmly when appropriate to do so. Also avoid extreme heat (e.g., hot tubs, saunas). This medication can cause you to sweat less than normal, which may lead to heat stroke if your body temperature gets too high. You may get dizzy or have blurred vision.

Do not drive, use machinery, or do anything that needs mental alertness until you know how this medication affects you. To reduce the risk of dizzy or fainting spells, do not sit or stand up quickly, especially if you are an older patient. Alcohol can make you more dizzy, avoid alcoholic drinks. Because tobacco smoking could increase the risk of side effects of this drug, you should avoid smoking. This medication can reduce the ability of birth control pills to prevent pregnancy. Use another method of birth control while you are taking this medication or check with your prescriber regarding recommendations. Contact your prescriber for advice if you think you might be pregnant, as this medication may be harmful to an unborn baby. Stay out of bright light and wear sunglasses if this medication makes your eyes more sensitive to light. Your mouth may get dry. Chewing sugarless gum or sucking hard candy, and drinking plenty of water will help. This medication may cause dry eyes and blurred vision. If you wear contact lenses, you may feel some discomfort. Lubricating drops may help. See your ophthalmologist if the problem does not go away or is severe. If you are going to have any type of surgery, tell your prescriber or health care professional that you are taking this medication.

What side effects may I notice from taking belladonna alkaloids; ergotamine; phenobarbital?

Side effects that you should report to your prescriber or health care professional as soon as possible:
- anxiety, nervousness
- changes in behavior or mood
- chest pain or tightness
- cold hands or feet
- confusion
- decrease in the amount of urine passed
- difficulty breathing
- eye or vision problems
- fast, slow, or pounding heartbeat
- fever, chills or sore throat
- hallucinations
- leg or arm pain or cramps
- redness, blistering, peeling or loosening of the skin, including inside the mouth
- seizures
- skin rash, itching, hives
- stomach pain
- swelling of ankles, hands, face, or lips
- tingling, pain or numbness in feet or hands
- unusual bleeding or bruising, pinpoint red spots on the skin
- unusual tiredness or weakness
- vomiting
- weight loss
- yellowing of skin or eyes

Side effects that usually do not require medical attention (report to your prescriber or health care professional if they continue or are bothersome):

- altered taste
- constipation
- dizziness
- drowsiness
- dry mouth
- increased sensitivity of the eyes to sun or light
- nausea

Where can I keep my medicine?

Keep out of the reach of children in a container that small children cannot open. Store at room temperature between 15 and 30 degrees C (59 and 86 degrees F). Keep tightly closed and protect from heat and moisture. Throw away any unused medicine after the expiration date.

Benazepril tablets

LOTENSIN®;
10 mg; Tablet
Novartis
Pharmaceuticals
Corp Dba Ciba
Pharmaceuticals Co
Di

BENAZEPRIL;
20 mg; Tablet
Teva
Pharmaceuticals
USA Inc

What are benazepril tablets?

BENAZEPRIL (Lotensin®) is an antihypertensive (blood pressure lowering agent) known as an ACE inhibitor. Benazepril controls high blood pressure (hypertension) by relaxing blood vessels; it is not a cure. High blood pressure levels can damage your kidneys, and may lead to a stroke or heart failure. Generic benazepril tablets are available.

What should my health care professional know before I take benazepril?

They need to know if you have any of these conditions:
- autoimmune disease (such as lupus), or suppressed immune function
- previous swelling of the tongue, face, or lips with difficulty breathing, difficulty swallowing, hoarseness, or tightening of the throat (angioedema)
- bone marrow disease
- heart or blood vessel disease
- liver disease
- low blood pressure
- kidney disease
- if you are on a special diet, such as a low-salt diet
- an unusual or allergic reaction to benazepril, other ACE inhibitors, foods, dyes, or preservatives
- pregnant or trying to get pregnant
- breast-feeding

How should I take this medicine?

Take benazepril tablets by mouth. Follow the directions on the prescription label. Swallow the tablets with a drink of water. Take your doses at regular intervals. Do not take your medicine more often than directed. Do not stop taking benazepril except on your prescriber's advice. Contact your pediatrician or health care professional regarding the use of this medicine in children. Special care may be needed.

What if I miss a dose?

If you miss a dose, take it as soon as you can. If it is almost time for your next dose, take only that dose. Do not take double or extra doses. If you take only one dose a day and forget to take it that day, do not take a double dose the next day.

What may interact with benazepril?

- anti-inflammatory drugs (NSAIDs, such as ibuprofen)
- hawthorn
- heparin
- lithium
- medicines for high blood pressure
- potassium salts
- water pills

Tell your prescriber or health care professional about all other medicines you are taking, including non-prescription medicines, nutritional supplements, or herbal products. Also tell your prescriber or health care professional if you are a frequent user of drinks with caffeine or alcohol, if you smoke, or if you use illegal drugs. These may affect the way your medicine works. Check with your health care professional before stopping or starting any of your medicines.

What should I watch for while taking benazepril?

Visit your prescriber or health care professional for regular checks on your progress. Check your blood pressure regularly while you are taking benazepril. Ask your prescriber or health care professional what your blood pressure should be and when you should contact him or her. Call your prescriber or health care professional if you notice an uneven or fast heart beat. Check with your prescriber or health care professional if you get an attack of severe diarrhea, nausea and vomiting, or if you sweat a lot. The loss of body fluid can make it dangerous to take benazepril. You may get dizzy. Do not drive, use machinery, or do anything that needs mental alertness until you know how benazepril affects you. To avoid dizzy or fainting spells, do not stand or sit up quickly, especially if you are an older person. Alcohol can make you more dizzy. Avoid alcoholic drinks. If you are going to have surgery, tell your prescriber or health care professional that you are taking benazepril. Avoid salt substitutes or other foods or substances high in potassium salts. Do not treat yourself for coughs, colds, or pain while you are taking benazepril without asking your prescriber or health care professional for advice.

What side effects may I notice from taking benazepril?

Side effects that you should report to your prescriber or health care professional as soon as possible:

- decreased amount of urine passed
- difficulty breathing, or swallowing
- dizziness, lightheadedness or fainting spells
- redness, blistering, peeling or loosening of the skin, including inside the mouth
- skin rash, itching
- swelling of your face or tongue
- swelling of your legs or ankles
- uneven or fast heart beat

Side effects that usually do not require medical attention (report to your prescriber or health care professional if they continue or are bothersome):

- cough
- headache
- nausea
- tiredness

Where can I keep my medicine?

Keep out of the reach of children in a container that small children cannot open. Store at room temperature below 30 degrees C (86 degrees F). Protect from moisture. Keep container tightly closed. Throw away any unused medicine after the expiration date.

Benazepril; Hydrochlorothiazide, HCTZ tablets

LOTENSIN HCT®;
20 mg/25 mg; Tablet
Novartis
Pharmaceuticals
Corp Dba Ciba
Pharmaceuticals Co
Di

BENAZEPRIL;
HYDROCHLORO-
THIAZIDE, HCTZ;
20 mg/25 mg; Tablet
Mylan
Pharmaceuticals Inc

What are benazepril; hydrochlorothiazide tablets?

BENAZEPRIL-HYDROCHLOROTHIAZIDE (Lotensin® HCT) is a combination of two drugs used to lower blood pressure. Benazepril is an ACE inhibitor that controls high blood pressure (hypertension) by relaxing blood vessels. Hydrochlorothiazide is a diuretic. High blood pressure can damage the blood vessels of the brain, heart, and kidneys, resulting in a stroke, heart failure, or kidney failure. By lowering blood pressure, benazepril-hydrochlorothiazide can help reduce your risk of having damage to your kidneys, heart, or other organs. This medicine does not cure high blood pressure. Generic benazepril-hydrochlorothiazide tablets are available.

What should my health care professional know before I take benazepril-hydrochlorothiazide?

They need to know if you have any of these conditions:

- autoimmune disease (e.g., lupus), or suppressed immune function
- previous swelling of the tongue, face, or lips with difficulty breathing, difficulty swallowing, hoarseness, or tightening of the throat (angioedema)
- bone marrow disease
- diabetes mellitus
- gout
- heart or blood vessel disease
- liver disease
- recent heart attack or stroke
- kidney disease, (e.g., renal failure or renal artery stenosis)
- pancreatitis
- electrolyte imbalance (e.g., low or high levels of potassium in the blood)
- if you are on a special diet, such as a low-salt diet (e.g., using potassium substitutes)

- sulfonamide (sulfa) or thiazide allergy
- an unusual or allergic reaction to benazepril, hydrochlorothiazide, other medicines, foods, dyes, or preservatives
- pregnant or trying to get pregnant
- breast-feeding

How should I use this medicine?

Take benazepril-hydrochlorothiazide tablets by mouth. Follow the directions on the prescription label. You may take benazepril-hydrochlorothiazide with or without food. Swallow the tablets with a drink of water. Take your doses at regular intervals. Do not take your medicine more often than directed. Do not stop taking this medicine except on your prescriber's advice. Many patients with high blood pressure will not notice any signs of the problem. Therefore, it is very important that you take this medicine exactly as directed and that you keep your appointments with your prescriber or health care professional even if you feel well. Contact your pediatrician or health care professional regarding the use of this medicine in children. Special care may be needed.

What if I miss a dose?

If you miss a dose, take it as soon as you can. If it is almost time for your next dose, take only that dose. Do not take double or extra doses.

What may interact with benazepril-hydrochlorothiazide?

- anti-inflammatory drugs (NSAIDs, such as ibuprofen)
- blood pressure medications
- cholesterol-lowering medications (e.g., cholestyramine or colestipol)
- diabetic medications
- dofetilide

- hawthorn
- lithium
- potassium salts or potassium supplements
- water pills (especially potassium-sparing diuretics such as triamterene or amiloride)

Tell your prescriber or health care professional about all other medicines you are taking, including non-prescription medicines, nutritional supplements, or herbal products. Also tell your prescriber or health care professional if you are a frequent user of drinks with caffeine or alcohol, if you smoke, or if you use illegal drugs. These may affect the way your medicine works. Check with your health care professional before stopping or starting any of your medicines.

What should I watch for while taking benazepril-hydrochlorothiazide?

Check your blood pressure regularly while you are taking benazepril-hydrochlorothiazide. Ask your prescriber or health care professional what your blood pressure should be and when you should contact him or her. When you check your blood pressure, write down the measurements to show your prescriber or health care professional. You must not get dehydrated, ask your prescriber or health care professional how much fluid you need to drink a day. If you are taking this medicine for a long time you must visit your prescriber or health care professional for regular checks on your progress. Make sure you schedule appointments on a regular basis. Check with your prescriber or health care professional if you get an attack of severe diarrhea, nausea and vomiting, or if you sweat a lot. The loss of too much body fluid can make it dangerous for you to take benazepril-hydrochlorothiazide. You may get dizzy. Do not drive, use machinery, or do anything that requires mental alertness until you know how benazepril-hydrochlorothiazide affects you. To avoid dizzy or fainting spells, do not stand or sit up quickly. Alcohol may increase the possibility of dizziness. Avoid alcoholic drinks until you have discussed their use with your prescriber or health care professional. If you are going to have surgery tell your prescriber or health care professional that you are taking benazepril-hydrochlorothiazide. Benazepril-hydrochlorothiazide may affect your blood sugar level. If you have diabetes, check with your prescriber or health care professional before changing the dose of your diabetic medicine. Avoid salt substitutes unless you are told otherwise by your prescriber or health care professional. Do not take medicines for appetite control, asthma, colds, cough, hay fever, or sinus problems without asking your prescriber or health care professional for advice. Do not treat yourself for a fever or sore throat; check with your prescriber or health care professional first.

What side effects may I notice from taking benazepril-hydrochlorothiazide?

Side effects that you should report to your prescriber or health care professional as soon as possible:
Rare or uncommon:
- difficulty breathing, difficulty swallowing, hoarseness, or tightening of the throat
- redness, blistering, peeling or loosening of the skin, including inside the mouth
- swelling of your face, lips, tongue, hands, or feet
- unusual rash, bleeding or bruising, or pinpoint red spots on the skin

Other:
- confusion, dizziness, lightheadedness or fainting spells
- decreased amount of urine passed
- decreased sexual function
- fast or uneven heart beat, palpitations, or chest pain
- fever or chills
- irregular heartbeat
- muscle cramps
- stomach pain
- vomiting
- unusual tiredness or weakness
- worsened gout pain
- yellowing of the eyes or skin

Side effects that usually do not require medical attention (report to your prescriber or health care professional if they continue or are bothersome):
- cough
- diarrhea
- headache
- increased sensitivity to the sun
- nausea
- tiredness or fatigue

Where can I keep my medicine?

Keep out of the reach of children. Store at room temperature below 30 degrees C (86 degrees F). Protect from moisture and light. Keep container tightly closed. Throw away any unused medicine after the expiration date.

Bendroflumethiazide; Nadolol Tablets

CORZIDE®;
5 mg/40 mg; Tablet
Monarch
Pharmaceuticals Inc

CORZIDE®;
5 mg/80 mg; Tablet
Monarch
Pharmaceuticals Inc

What are bendroflumethiazide; nadolol tablets?

BENDROFLUMETHIAZIDE; NADOLOL (Corzide®) is a combination of two drugs used to lower blood pressure. Nadolol is a beta-blocker and bendroflumethiazide is a thiazide diuretic ("water pill"). Bendroflumethiazide; nadolol is used to control, but not cure, high blood pressure (hypertension). Generic bendroflumethiazide; nadolol tablets are available.

What should my health care professional know before I take bendroflumethiazide; nadolol?

They need to know if you have any of these conditions:

- asthma, bronchitis or bronchospasm
- autoimmune disease such as lupus (SLE)
- bradycardia (unusually slow heartbeat)
- chest pain (angina)
- circulation problems, or blood vessel disease (such as Raynaud's disease)
- depression
- diabetes
- electrolyte imbalance (such as low or high levels of potassium in the blood)
- emphysema, COPD, or other lung disease
- gout
- heart disease (such as heart failure or a history of heart attack)
- kidney disease
- liver disease
- muscle weakness or myasthenia gravis
- pancreatitis
- pheochromocytoma
- post-sympathectomy
- psoriasis
- thyroid disease
- an unusual reaction to bendroflumethiazide or other thiazides; nadolol, sulfonamide (sulfa) drugs, or other medicines, foods, dyes, or preservatives
- if you are on a special diet, such as a low-salt diet (using salt substitutes)
- pregnant or trying to get pregnant
- breast-feeding

How should this medicine be taken?

Take bendroflumethiazide; nadolol tablets by mouth. You can take the tablets with or without food. Follow the directions on the prescription label. Swallow the tablets with a drink of water. Take your doses at regular intervals. Do not take your medicine more often than directed. Do not stop taking except on your prescriber's advice. Contact your pediatrician or health care professional regarding the use of this medicine in children. Special care may be needed.

What if I miss a dose?

If you miss a dose, take it as soon as you can. If it is almost time for your next dose, take only that dose. Do not take double or extra doses.

What may interact with bendroflumethiazide; nadolol?

- allopurinol
- amphetamine
- anti-inflammatory drugs (NSAIDs, such as ibuprofen)
- cevimeline
- clonidine
- cocaine
- ginger, Zingiber officinale
- griseofulvin
- hawthorn
- lithium
- liothyronine
- mefloquine
- medicines for chest pain or angina
- medicines for colds and breathing difficulties
- medicines for diabetes
- medicines for high blood pressure or heart failure
- medicines known as MAO inhibitors, such as phenelzine (Nardil®), tranylcypromine (Parnate®), isocarboxazid (Marplan®), and selegiline (Carbex®, Eldepryl®)
- medicines to control heart rhythm (including amiodarone, digoxin, disopyramide, dofetilide, flecainide, propafenone, quinidine, and sotalol)
- porfimer
- prochlorperazine
- retinol creams or pills
- rifampin
- some antibiotics which increase sensitivity to sunlight (sulfonamides, tetracyclines)
- some medicines for lowering cholesterol (colestipol or cholestyramine)
- some medicines for weight loss (including some herbal products, ephedrine, dextroamphetamine)
- water pills (diuretics)

Tell your prescriber or health care professional about all other medicines you are taking, including non-prescription medicines, nutritional supplements, or herbal products. Also tell your prescriber or health care professional if you are a frequent user of drinks with caffeine or alcohol, if you smoke, or if you use illegal drugs. These may affect the way your medicine works. Check with your health care professional before stopping or starting any of your medicines.

What should I watch for while taking bendroflumethiazide; nadolol?

Check your heart rate and blood pressure regularly while you are taking bendroflumethiazide; nadolol. Ask

B

your prescriber or health care professional what your blood pressure should be and when you should contact him or her. When you check your blood pressure, write down the measurements to show your prescriber or health care professional. If you are taking this medicine for a long time you must visit your prescriber or health care professional for regular checks on your progress. Make sure you schedule appointments on a regular basis. Do not stop taking this medicine suddenly. This could lead to serious heart-related effects. You may get drowsy or dizzy. Do not drive, use machinery, or do anything that requires mental alertness until you know how this medicine affects you. To reduce the risk of dizzy or fainting spells, do not sit or stand up quickly. Alcohol can make you more drowsy, and increase the risk of flushing and rapid heartbeats. Therefore, it is best to avoid alcoholic drinks. Check with your health care professional if you get an attack of severe diarrhea, nausea and vomiting, or sweat a lot. The loss of too much body fluid while you are taking a diuretic can cause dehydration and lower the blood pressure below normal. This medicine can affect blood sugar levels. If you have diabetes, check with your prescriber or health care professional before you change your diet or the dose of your diabetic medicine. Do not take medicines for appetite control, asthma, colds, cough, hay fever, or sinus problems without asking your prescriber or health care professional for advice. Do not treat yourself for a fever or sore throat; check with your prescriber or health care professional first. Avoid exposure to excessive sunlight (such as sunlamps, sunbathing) while taking this medicine. If you are going to have surgery, tell your prescriber or health care professional that you are taking bendroflumethiazide; nadolol.

What side effects may I notice from taking bendroflumethiazide; nadolol?

Side effects that you should report to your prescriber or health care professional as soon as possible:

- changes in vision (e.g., blurred vision)
- cold, tingling, or numb hands or feet
- confusion, dizziness, lightheadedness or fainting spells
- difficulty breathing, wheezing
- fever or chills
- increased thirst or sweating
- increase or decrease in the amount of urine passed
- fast or uneven heart beat, palpitations, or chest pain
- slow heart rate
- muscle cramps
- redness, blistering, peeling or loosening of the skin, including inside the mouth
- stomach pain
- swollen legs or ankles
- unusual skin rash or bruising
- unusual tiredness or weakness
- vomiting
- worsened gout pain
- yellowing of the eyes or skin

Side effects that usually do not require medical attention (report to your prescriber or health care professional if they continue or are bothersome):

- depression, nightmares
- diarrhea or constipation
- dry eyes or dry mouth
- headache
- increased sensitivity to the sun
- nausea
- sexual difficulties, impotence
- tiredness or fatigue

Where can I keep my medicine?

Keep out of the reach of children in a container that small children cannot open. Store at room temperature at 15 to 30 degrees C (59 to 86 degrees F). Keep bottle tightly closed. Avoid excessive heat. Throw away any unused medicine after the expiration date.

Benzocaine lozenges

CEPACOL®
MAXIMUM
STRENGTH;
10 mg/2.6 mg;
Lozenge
Combe Inc

CEPACOL®
MAXIMUM
STRENGTH;
10 mg/4.5 mg;
Lozenge
Combe Inc

What are benzocaine lozenges?

BENZOCAINE (Cepacol®, Chloraseptic®) causes loss of feeling and decreases pain in the mouth and throat. Generic benzocaine lozenges are available.

What should my health care professional need to know before I take benzocaine lozenges?

They need to know if you have any of these conditions:
- mouth sores or infection
- an unusual or allergic reaction to benzocaine, para-
aminobenzoic acid (PABA), other medicines, foods, dyes, or preservatives
- pregnant or trying to get pregnant
- breast-feeding

How should I take this medicine?

Dissolve benzocaine lozenges slowly and completely in the mouth. Do not chew or swallow whole. Repeat as needed, but not more often than instructed. Do not use more than 12 lozenges per day. Contact your pediatrician or health care professional regarding the use of this medicine in children. Special care may be needed. Children should not repeat more often than once an hour.

What if I miss a dose?

If you miss a dose, take it as soon as you can. If it is almost time for your next dose, take only that dose. Do not take double or extra doses.

What may interact with benzocaine?

Benzocaine at regular doses does not interact with other medicines.

Tell your prescriber or health care professional about all other medicines you are taking, including non-prescription medicines, nutritional supplements, or herbal products. Also tell your prescriber or health care professional if you are a frequent user of drinks with caffeine or alcohol, if you smoke, or if you use illegal drugs. These may affect the way your medicine works. Check with your health care professional before stopping or starting any of your medicines.

What should I watch for while taking benzocaine?

Benzocaine lozenges are not for long-term use. Do not use for more than one week without checking with your prescriber or health care professional. Contact your prescriber or health care professional, or dentist if your condition does not improve within a few days

or if you notice redness, itching or swelling. Your mouth will be numb, try to avoid injury to the area. To avoid biting the tongue or cheek, or difficulty swallowing, do not chew gum or food until the numbness wears off.

What side effects may I notice from taking benzocaine?

Side effects that you should report to your prescriber or health care professional as soon as possible:
- itching, redness, swelling, pain, and rash

Very rare with benzocaine lozenges:
- difficulty breathing
- dizziness or drowsiness
- fast or slow heartbeat
- headache
- increased sweating
- restlessness, nervousness, anxiety
- seizures (convulsions)
- swelling of the face
- tremor

Where can I keep my medicine?

Keep out of the reach of children in a container that small children cannot open. Store at room temperature between 15 and 25 degrees C (59 and 77 degrees F). Keep container tightly closed; protect from moisture. Throw away any unused medicine after the expiration date.

Benzonatate capsules

TESSALON PERLES®; 100 mg; Capsule Forest Pharmaceuticals Inc

TESSALON®; 200 mg; Capsule Forest Pharmaceuticals Inc

What are benzonatate capsules?

BENZONATATE (Tessalon® Perles, Tessalon®) helps to relieve coughs caused by colds, flu or other lung conditions. Occasionally this medicine is prescribed for hiccups that do not stop. Generic benzonatate capsules are available.

What should my health care professional know before I take benzonatate?

They need to know if you have any of these conditions:
- kidney or liver disease
- an unusual or allergic reaction to benzonatate, anesthetics, other medicines, foods, dyes, or preservatives
- pregnant or trying to get pregnant
- breast-feeding

How should I take this medicine?

Take benzonatate by mouth. Follow the directions on the container. Swallow the capsules whole. Do not break, chew, or dissolve the capsules in the mouth as this could cause temporary numbness of the mouth and throat and could cause choking. Take your doses at regular intervals. Do not take your medicine more often than directed. Contact your pediatrician or health care

professional regarding the use of this medicine in children. Special care may be needed.

What if I miss a dose?

If you miss a dose, take it as soon as you can. If it is almost time for your next dose, take only that dose. Do not take double or extra doses.

What may interact with benzonatate?

- medicines called MAO inhibitors-phenelzine (Nardil®), tranylcypromine (Parnate®), isocarboxazid (Marplan®)
- pain medications (examples: codeine, hydrocodone, morphine or oxycodone)
- selegiline

Tell your prescriber or health care professional about all other medicines you are taking, including non-prescription medicines, nutritional supplements, or herbal products. Also tell your prescriber or health care professional if you are a frequent user of drinks with caffeine or alcohol, if you smoke, or if you use illegal drugs. These may affect the way your medicine works. Check with your health care professional before stopping or starting any of your medicines.

What should I watch for while taking benzonatate?

If you have a fever, skin rash, or persistent headache as well as a cough, see your prescriber or health care professional. Let your prescriber know if your cough does not get better after one week or if your problem gets worse. Let your prescriber or health care professional know you get a feeling of numbness in your mouth or throat. If a benzonatate capsule is chewed, the numbness may cause you to choke. Do not suck on the capsules. Never chew or open the capsules, always swallow them whole. You may get drowsy or dizzy. Do not drive, use machinery, or do anything that needs mental alertness until you know how benzonatate affects you.

What side effects may I notice from taking benzonatate?

Side effects that you should report to your prescriber or health care professional as soon as possible:

- difficulty breathing or swallowing
- confusion or feeling of restlessness
- itching or skin rash
- numbness of mouth or throat
- shakiness of hands, arms or legs

Side effects that usually do not require medical attention (report to your prescriber or health care professional if they continue or are bothersome):

- dizziness
- mild drowsiness
- headache

Where can I keep my medicine?

Keep out of the reach of children in a container that small children cannot open. Store at room temperature between 15 and 30 degrees C (59 and 86 degrees F). Keep tightly closed. Protect from moisture. Throw away any unused medicine after the expiration date.

Benztropine tablets

COGENTIN®;
0.5 mg; Tablet
Merck and Co Inc

BENZTROPINE;
1 mg; Tablet
Par Pharmaceutical
Inc

What are benztropine tablets?

BENZTROPINE (Cogentin®) is a medicine that prevents or controls movement-related side effects of antipsychotic medicines (medicines for treating mental disorders). It also treats symptoms of parkinsonism from unknown causes. Symptoms such as tremor, rigid muscles and difficulties in walking, talking, balancing and swallowing. Generic benztropine tablets are available.

What should my health care professional know before I take benztropine?

They need to know if you have any of these conditions:
- closed-angle glaucoma
- heart disease, or a rapid heartbeat
- prostate trouble
- muscle weakness
- uncontrollable movements of the hands, mouth or tongue
- an unusual or allergic reaction to benztropine, other medicines, foods, dyes, or preservatives
- pregnant or trying to get pregnant
- breast-feeding

How should I take this medicine?

Take benztropine tablets by mouth. Follow the directions on the prescription label. Swallow the tablets with a drink of water. Take with food, unless your prescriber or health care professional instructs you otherwise. If you have difficulty swallowing you can crush the tablets and mix with food. Take your doses at regular intervals. Do not take your medicine more often than directed. It may take several days to see the full effect of benztropine; do not stop taking except on your prescriber's advice. Contact your pediatrician or health care professional regarding the use of this medicine in children. Special care may be needed.

What if I miss a dose?

If you miss a dose, take it as soon as you can. If it is almost time for your next dose (less than 2 hours), take only that dose. Do not take double or extra doses.

What may interact with benztropine?

- alcohol
- amantadine
- levodopa
- medicines for diarrhea
- medicines for hay fever and other allergies
- medicines for mental depression
- medicines for mental problems and psychotic disturbances
- medicines for movement abnormalities as in Parkinson's disease, or for gastrointestinal problems
- medicines that help relieve anxiety or sleeping problems (such as diazepam or temazepam)
- metoclopramide

Tell your prescriber or health care professional about all other medicines you are taking, including non-prescription medicines, nutritional supplements, or herbal products. Also tell your prescriber or health care professional if you are a frequent user of drinks with caffeine or alcohol, if you smoke, or if you use illegal drugs. These may affect the way your medicine works. Check with your health care professional before stopping or starting any of your medicines.

What should I watch for while taking benztropine?

Visit your prescriber or health care professional for regular checks on your progress. Do not stop taking this medicine abruptly. Your prescriber or health care professional may want to gradually reduce the dose so that you do not get side effects or make your condition worse. Your prescriber or health care professional may want you to have an eye exam from time to time. You may get dizzy or have blurred vision. Do not drive, use machinery, or do anything that requires mental alertness until you know how benztropine affects you. To reduce the risk of dizzy or fainting spells, do not sit or stand up quickly, especially if you are an older patient. Alcohol can make you more dizzy, and increase flushing and rapid heartbeats. Avoid alcoholic drinks. Your mouth may get dry. Chewing sugarless gum or sucking hard candy, and drinking plenty of water will help. Benztropine may cause dry eyes and blurred vision. If you wear contact lenses, you may feel some discomfort. Lubricating drops may help. See your ophthalmologist if the problem does not go away or is severe. Stay out of bright light and wear sunglasses if benztropine makes your eyes more sensitive to light. You may sweat less than usual while you are taking benztropine. As a result your body temperature could rise to a dangerous level. Be careful not to get overheated during exercise or in hot weather; you could get heat stroke. Avoid taking hot baths, and using hot tubs and saunas.

What side effects may I notice from taking benztropine?

Side effects that you should report to your prescriber or health care professional as soon as possible:

- agitation, nervousness
- blurred vision, or other eye problems
- confusion, memory loss, slurred speech, hallucinations (seeing or hearing things that are not really there)
- decrease in sweating
- difficulty breathing
- difficulty swallowing
- dizziness or fainting
- fast, or irregular heartbeat (palpitations)
- pain or difficulty passing urine
- vomiting
- weakness or tiredness

Side effects that usually do not require medical attention (report to your prescriber or health care professional if they continue or are bothersome):

- anxiety
- constipation
- dry mouth
- nausea
- skin rash, itching

Where can I keep my medicine?

Keep out of the reach of children in a container that small children cannot open. Store at room temperature between 15 and 30 degrees C (59 and 86 degrees F). Keep container tightly closed. Throw away any unused medicine after the expiration date.

Bepridil tablets

This drug is no longer on the market.

VASCOR®;
300 mg; Tablet
OMP Div, Ortho-
McNeil
Pharmaceuticals

VASCOR®;
200 mg; Tablet
OMP Div, Ortho-
McNeil
Pharmaceuticals

What are bepridil tablets?

BEPRIDIL (Vascor®) is a calcium-channel blocker. It affects the amount of calcium found in your heart and muscle cells. This results in relaxation of blood vessels, which can reduce the amount of work the heart has to do. Bepridil relieves chest pain (angina). It is not a cure. NOTE: This drug is discontinued in the United States.

What should my health care professional know before I take bepridil?

They need to know if you have any of these conditions:

- heart problems, low blood pressure, slow heart rate
- kidney disease
- liver disease
- previous heart attack
- over 65 years old
- low blood potassium
- an unusual or allergic reaction to bepridil, other medicines, foods, dyes, or preservatives
- pregnant or trying to get pregnant
- breast-feeding

How should I take this medicine?

Take bepridil tablets by mouth. Follow the directions on the prescription label. Swallow the tablets with a drink of water. If bepridil upsets your stomach, take it with food or at bedtime. Do not significantly increase grapefruit juice intake while taking this drug, or avoid grapefruit juice if possible. Take your doses at regular intervals. Do not take your medicine more often then directed. Do not stop taking except on your prescriber's advice. Contact your pediatrician or health care professional regarding the use of this medicine in children. Special care may be needed.

What if I miss a dose?

If you miss a dose, take it as soon as you can. If it is almost time for your next dose, take only that dose. Do not take double or extra doses.

What may interact with bepridil?

Do not take bepridil with any of the following:

- arsenic trioxide
- astemizole
- certain medicines to control heart rhythm such as amiodarone, disopyramide, dofetilide, flecainide, procainamide, propafenone, quinidine, sotalol
- chloroquine
- chlorpromazine
- cisapride
- droperidol
- grapefruit juice
- halofantrine
- levomethadyl
- mesoridazine
- methadone
- pentamidine
- pimozide
- probucol
- some antibiotics (clarithromycin, erythromycin, gatifloxacin, levofloxacin, moxifloxacin, sparfloxacin, telithromycin, troleandomycin)
- terfenadine
- thioridazine
- ziprasidone

Bepridil may also interact with the following medications:

- acetazolamide
- alfuzosin
- amphotericin B
- anti-inflammatory drugs (NSAIDs, such as ibuprofen)
- aprepitant
- barbiturates such as phenobarbital
- bosentan
- cimetidine
- fentanyl
- herbal or dietary supplements such as gingko biloba, ginseng, hawthorn, ma huang (ephedra), melatonin, St. John's wort, went yeast
- hormones such as prednisone or cortisone
- imatinib, STI-571
- local anesthetics or general anesthetics
- medicines for asthma or breathing difficulties
- medicines for depression or mental problems
- medicines for fungal infections (fluconazole, itraconazole, ketoconazole, voriconazole)
- medicines for heart-rhythm problems
- medicines for high blood pressure
- medicines for HIV infection or AIDS
- medicines for prostate problems
- medicines for seizures (carbamazepine, phenobarbital, phenytoin, primidone)
- methazolamide
- rifampin, rifapentine, or rifabutin
- sodium phosphate
- tacrolimus
- water pills (diuretics)
- yohimbine
- zafirlukast
- zileuton

Tell your prescriber or health care professional about all other medicines you are taking, including non-prescription medicines, nutritional supplements, or herbal products. Also tell your prescriber or health care professional if you are a frequent user of drinks with caffeine or alcohol, if you smoke, or if you use illegal drugs. These may affect the way your medicine works. Check with your health care professional before stopping or starting any of your medicines.

What should I watch for while taking bepridil?

Check your blood pressure and pulse rate regularly; this is important while you are taking bepridil. Ask your prescriber or health care professional what your blood pressure and pulse rate should be and when you should contact him or her. It is important to keep up your potassium level while you are taking bepridil. Serious heart problems can develop if you are short of potassium. Bananas and orange juice are high-potassium foods. You may need to take a potassium supplement. Visit your prescriber or health care professional for regular checks on your progress. You may feel dizzy or lightheaded. Do not drive, use machinery, or do anything that needs mental alertness until you know how bepridil affects you. To reduce the risk of dizzy or fainting spells, do not sit or stand up quickly, especially if you are an older patient. Avoid alcoholic drinks; they can make you more dizzy, increase flushing and rapid heartbeats. Do not suddenly stop taking bepridil. Ask your prescriber or health care professional how to gradually reduce the dose. If you are going to have surgery, tell your prescriber or health care professional that you are taking bepridil.

What side effects may I notice from taking bepridil?

Side effects that you should report to your prescriber or health care professional as soon as possible:

- blurred vision
- difficulty breathing, wheezing
- fainting spells, lightheadedness
- fast heartbeat or pounding heart
- irregular heartbeat
- mental depression
- nervousness or agitation, confusion, tremors
- slow heartbeat (fewer than 50 beats per minute)
- swelling of the feet and ankles
- unusual weakness or tiredness

Side effects that usually do not require medical attention (report to your prescriber or health care professional if they continue or are bothersome):

- constipation or diarrhea
- drowsiness or dizziness
- dry mouth
- flu-like symptoms, muscle aches and pains
- headache
- increased appetite
- nausea, vomiting
- sexual difficulties (impotence or decreased sexual urges)
- stomach pain, stomach upset, heartburn

Where can I keep my medicine?

Keep out of the reach of children in a container that small children cannot open. Store at room temperature between 15 and 25 degrees C (59 and 77 degrees F). Protect from light. Throw away any unused medicine after the expiration date.

Betamethasone tablets

CELESTONE®;
0.6 mg; Tablet
Schering Corp

What are betamethasone tablets?

BETAMETHASONE (Celestone®) is a corticosteroid. It helps to reduce swelling, redness, itching, and allergic reactions. Betamethasone treats allergies, skin problems, asthma, arthritis, Crohn's disease, ulcerative colitis, and many other conditions. Generic betamethasone tablets are not yet available.

What should my health care professional know before I take betamethasone?

They need to know if you have any of these conditions:

- diabetes
- blood clotting problems
- heart, liver, or kidney disease
- high blood pressure
- infection; measles, tuberculosis, herpes or chickenpox
- mental problems or psychosis
- myasthenia gravis
- osteoporosis
- previous heart attack
- seizures (convulsions)
- stomach or intestinal disease
- under-active thyroid
- an unusual or allergic reaction to betamethasone, corticosteroids, other medicines, foods, dyes, or preservatives
- pregnant or trying to get pregnant
- breast-feeding

How should I take this medicine?

Take betamethasone tablets by mouth. Follow the directions on the prescription label. Swallow the tablets with a drink of water. Take with milk or food to avoid stomach upset. If you are only taking betamethasone once a day, take it in the morning, which is the time your body normally secretes cortisol. Take your doses at regular intervals. Do not take your medicine more often than directed. Do not stop taking betamethasone except on your prescriber's advice. Contact your pediatrician or health care professional regarding the use of this medicine in children. Special care may be needed.

What if I miss a dose?

If you miss a dose, take it as soon as you can. If it is almost time for your next dose, consult your prescriber or health care professional. You may need to miss a dose or take a double dose, depending on your condition and treatment. Do not take double or extra doses without advice.

What may interact with betamethasone?

- anti-inflammatory drugs (NSAIDs, such as ibuprofen)
- aspirin
- barbiturate medicines for inducing sleep or treating seizures (convulsions)
- bosentan
- carbamazepine
- female hormones, including contraceptive or birth control pills
- heart medicines
- medicines for diabetes
- medicines that improve muscle tone or strength for conditions like myasthenia gravis
- phenytoin
- rifampin
- vaccines and other immunization products
- water pills

Tell your prescriber or health care professional about all other medicines you are taking, including non-prescription medicines, nutritional supplements, or herbal products. Also tell your prescriber or health care professional if you are a frequent user of drinks with caffeine or alcohol, if you smoke, or if you use illegal drugs. These may affect the way your medicine works. Check with your health care professional before stopping or starting any of your medicines.

What should I watch for while taking betamethasone?

Visit your prescriber or health care professional for regular checks on your progress. If you are taking corticosteroids for a long time, carry an identification card with your name, the type and dose of corticosteroid, and your prescriber's name and address. Do not suddenly stop taking betamethasone. You may need to gradually reduce the dose, so that your body can adjust. Follow the advice of your prescriber or health care professional. If you take corticosteroids for a long time, avoid contact with people who have an infection. You may be at an increased risk from infection while taking betamethasone. Tell your prescriber or health care professional if you are exposed to anyone with measles or chickenpox, or if you develop sores or blisters that do not heal properly. People who are taking certain dosages of betamethasone may need to avoid immunization with certain vaccines or may need to have changes in their vaccination schedules to ensure adequate protection from certain diseases. Make sure to tell your prescriber or health care professional that you

B

are taking betamethasone before receiving any vaccine. If you are diabetic, betamethasone can affect your blood sugar. Check with your prescriber or health care professional if you need help adjusting the dose of your diabetic medicine. If you take betamethasone tablets every day, you may need to watch your diet. Your body can also lose potassium while you take this medicine. Ask your prescriber or health care professional about your diet, especially about your salt intake. If you are going to have surgery tell your prescriber or health care professional that you are taking betamethasone, or have taken it within the last 12 months. Alcohol can increase the risk of getting serious side effects while you are taking betamethasone. Avoid alcoholic drinks. Elderly patients have an increased risk of side effects from betamethasone. Betamethasone can interfere with certain lab tests and can cause false skin test results.

What side effects may I notice from taking betamethasone?

Side effects that you should report to your prescriber or health care professional as soon as possible:
- bloody or black, tarry stools
- confusion, excitement, restlessness, a false sense of well-being
- eye pain, decreased or blurred vision, or bulging eyes
- fever, sore throat, sneezing, cough, or other signs of infection
- frequent passing of urine
- hallucinations (seeing and hearing things that are not really there)

- increased thirst
- irregular heartbeat
- menstrual problems
- mental depression, mood swings, mistaken feelings of self-importance, mistaken feelings of being mistreated
- muscle cramps or muscle weakness
- nausea, vomiting
- pain in hips, back, ribs, arms, shoulders, or legs
- rounding out of face
- skin problems, acne
- stomach pain
- swelling of feet or lower legs
- unusual bruising or red pinpoint spots on the skin
- unusual tiredness or weakness
- weight gain or weight loss
- wounds that will not heal

Side effects that usually do not require medical attention (report to your prescriber or health care professional if they continue or are bothersome):
- diarrhea or constipation
- headache
- increased appetite
- increased sweating
- nervousness, restlessness, or difficulty sleeping
- unusual increased growth of hair on the face or body
- upset stomach

Where can I keep my medicine?

Keep out of the reach of children in a container that small children cannot open. Store at room temperature between 2 and 30 degrees C (36 and 86 degrees F). Throw away any unused medicine after the expiration date.

Betaxolol tablets

 KERLONE®; 20 mg; Tablet Sanofi-Synthelabo Inc

 KERLONE®; 10 mg; Tablet Sanofi-Synthelabo Inc

What are betaxolol tablets?

BETAXOLOL (Kerlone®) belongs to a group of medicines called beta-blockers. Beta-blockers reduce the workload on the heart and help it to beat more regularly. Betaxolol controls, but does not cure, high blood pressure (hypertension). Generic betaxolol tablets are not yet available.

What should my health care professional know before I take betaxolol?

They need to know if you have any of these conditions:
- angina (chest pain)
- asthma, bronchitis or bronchospasm
- circulation problems, or blood vessel disease (such as Raynaud's disease)
- depression
- diabetes
- emphysema, or other lung disease
- history of heart attack or heart disease
- kidney disease

- muscle weakness or disease
- pheochromocytoma
- psoriasis
- thyroid disease
- an unusual or allergic reaction to betaxolol, other beta-blockers, medicines, foods, dyes, or preservatives
- pregnant or trying to get pregnant
- breast-feeding

How should I take this medicine?

Take betaxolol tablets by mouth. Follow the directions on the prescription label. Swallow the tablets with a drink of water. Take your doses at regular intervals. Do not take your medicine more often than directed. Do not stop taking except on your prescriber's advice. Contact your pediatrician or health care professional regarding the use of this medicine in children. Special care may be needed.

What if I miss a dose?

If you miss a dose, take it as soon as you can. If it is almost time for your next dose, take only that dose.

Do not take double or extra doses. There should be at least 8 hours between doses.

What may interact with betaxolol?

- anti-inflammatory drugs (NSAIDs, such as ibuprofen)
- cocaine
- hawthorn
- medicines for colds and breathing difficulties
- medicines for diabetes
- medicines for high blood pressure
- medicines to control heart rhythm
- water pills

Tell your prescriber or health care professional about all other medicines you are taking, including non-prescription medicines, nutritional supplements, or herbal products. Also tell your prescriber or health care professional if you are a frequent user of drinks with caffeine or alcohol, if you smoke, or if you use illegal drugs. These may affect the way your medicine works. Check with your health care professional before stopping or starting any of your medicines.

What should I watch for while taking betaxolol?

Check your heart rate and blood pressure regularly while you are taking betaxolol. Ask your prescriber or health care professional what your heart rate and blood pressure should be, and when you should contact him or her. Do not stop taking this medicine suddenly. This could lead to serious heart-related effects. You may get drowsy or dizzy. Do not drive, use machinery, or do anything that requires mental alertness until you know how betaxolol affects you. To reduce the risk of dizzy or fainting spells, do not sit or stand up quickly. Alcohol can make you more drowsy, and increase flushing and rapid heartbeats. Therefore, it is best to avoid alcoholic drinks. Betaxolol can affect blood sugar levels. If you have diabetes, check with your prescriber or health care professional before you change your diet or the dose of your diabetic medicine. If you are going to have

surgery, tell your prescriber or health care professional that you are taking betaxolol.

What side effects may I notice from taking betaxolol?

Side effects that you should report to your prescriber or health care professional as soon as possible:

- changes in vision
- cold, tingling, or numb hands or feet
- confusion
- difficulty breathing, wheezing
- dizziness or fainting spells
- increased thirst
- increase in the amount of urine passed
- irregular heartbeat
- joint pain
- skin rash
- slow heart rate (fewer than recommended by your prescriber or health care professional)
- sweating
- swollen legs or ankles
- tremor, shakes
- vomiting
- weight loss

Side effects that usually do not require medical attention (report to your prescriber or health care professional if they continue or are bothersome):

- anxiety
- depression, nightmares
- diarrhea
- difficulty sleeping
- dry itching skin
- dry or burning eyes
- headache
- nausea
- sexual difficulties, impotence
- unusual tiredness

Where can I keep my medicine?

Keep out of the reach of children in a container that small children cannot open. Store at room temperature below 30 degrees C (86 degrees F). Throw away any unused medicine after the expiration date.

Bethanechol tablets

URECHOLINE®;
25 mg; Tablet
Odyssey
Pharmaceuticals Inc

BETHANECHOL;
50 mg; Tablet
Ranbaxy
Pharmaceuticals Inc

What are bethanechol tablets?

BETHANECHOL (Urecholine®, Duvoid®) stimulates the bladder. It can help people who are having trouble passing urine to empty their bladder. Generic bethanechol tablets are available.

What should my health care professional know before I take bethanechol?

They need to know if you have any of these conditions:

- asthma
- bowel disease
- difficulty passing urine
- heart disease
- overactive thyroid
- Parkinson's disease
- seizures (convulsions)
- stomach disease, ulcers
- an unusual or allergic reaction to bethanechol, tartrazine dye, other medicines, foods, dyes, or preservatives
- pregnant or trying to get pregnant
- breast-feeding

How should I take this medicine?

Take bethanechol tablets by mouth. Follow the directions on the prescription label. Swallow the tablets with a drink of water. It is best to take bethanechol on an empty stomach, 1 hour before or 2 hours after meals. Take your doses at regular intervals. Do not take your medicine more often than directed. Do not stop taking except on your prescriber's advice. Contact your pediatrician or health care professional regarding the use of this medicine in children. Special care may be needed.

What if I miss a dose?

If you miss a dose, take it as soon as you can. If it is almost time for your next dose, take only that dose. Do not take double or extra doses.

What may interact with bethanechol?

- atropine
- procainamide
- quinidine
- medicines for colds and breathing difficulties
- medicines for mental depression
- other medicines that act in a similar way to bethanechol (such as pilocarpine, neostigmine)

Tell your prescriber or health care professional about all other medicines you are taking, including non-prescription medicines, nutritional supplements, or herbal products. Also tell your prescriber or health care professional if you are a frequent user of drinks with caffeine or alcohol, if you smoke, or if you use illegal drugs. These may affect the way your medicine works. Check with your health care professional before stopping or starting any of your medicines.

What should I watch for while taking bethanechol?

Visit your prescriber or health care professional for regular checks on your progress. You may get dizzy or lightheaded. Do not drive, use machinery, or do anything that needs mental alertness until you know how bethanechol affects you. To reduce the risk of fainting spells, do not stand or sit up quickly.

What side effects may I notice from taking bethanechol?

Side effects that you should report to your prescriber or health care professional as soon as possible:
- difficulty breathing
- lightheadedness or fainting spells
- vomiting

Side effects that usually do not require medical attention (report to your prescriber or health care professional if they continue or are bothersome):
- diarrhea
- flushing
- increased sweating
- increased saliva
- increase in tears
- nausea
- stomach pain, or gas
- urgent need to pass urine

Where can I keep my medicine?

Keep out of the reach of children in a container that small children cannot open. Store at room temperature below 40 degrees C (104 degrees F). Keep container tightly closed. Throw away any unused medicine after the expiration date.

Bicalutamide tablets

CASODEX®;
50 mg; Tablet
AstraZeneca Pharmaceuticals
LP

What are bicalutamide tablets?

BICALUTAMIDE (Casodex®) is an antiandrogen. An androgen is a male hormone. Bicalutamide blocks the effect of the male hormone called testosterone. Prostate cancer responds to the removal of androgens. Bicalutamide is used in combination with another medicine. Generic bicalutamide tablets are not yet available.

What should my health care professional know before I take bicalutamide?

They need to know if you have any of these conditions:
- liver disease
- an unusual or allergic reaction to bicalutamide, other chemotherapy, other medicines, foods, dyes, or preservatives
- trying to produce pregnancy

How should I take this medicine?

Take bicalutamide tablets by mouth at the same time each day. Follow the directions on the prescription label. Swallow the tablets with a drink of water. Do not take your medicine more often than directed. Finish the full course prescribed by your doctor or health care professional, even if the tablets make you feel unwell. Do not stop taking except on your prescriber's advice. Contact your pediatrician or health care professional regarding the use of this medicine in children. Special care may be needed.

What if I miss a dose?

If you miss a dose, take it as soon as you can. If it is almost time for your next dose, take only that dose. Do not take double or extra doses. If you vomit after taking a dose, call your prescriber or health care professional for advice.

What may interact with bicalutamide?

- warfarin

Tell your prescriber or health care professional about all other medicines you are taking, including non-pre-

scription medicines, nutritional supplements, or herbal products. Also tell your prescriber or health care professional if you are a frequent user of drinks with caffeine or alcohol, if you smoke, or if you use illegal drugs. These may affect the way your medicine works. Check with your health care professional before stopping or starting any of your medicines.

What should I watch for while taking bicalutamide?

Visit your prescriber or health care professional for regular checks on your progress. At first your condition can get worse, but it will then improve as you continue your treatment. Improvement in your condition can take several days.

What side effects may I notice from taking bicalutamide?

Side effects that you should report to your prescriber or health care professional as soon as possible:

- dark
- exces
- pain i
- severe
- yellowi

Side effects
tion (report
sional if they
- decreased ap
- diarrhea
- nausea
- hot flashes

Where can I keep

Keep out of the reach
small children cannot ope
degrees C (59 and 86 degrees F
Throw away any unused medicine
date.

Bisacodyl tablets

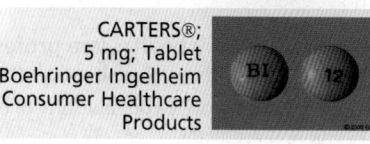

CARTERS®;
5 mg; Tablet
Boehringer Ingelheim
Consumer Healthcare
Products

What are bisacodyl tablets?

BISACODYL (Carters® Little Pills, Correctol®, Dulcolax®, Evac-U-Gen®, Feen-a-mint®, Fleets® Laxative and many others) is a stimulant laxative, a medicine that empties the bowel. Bisacodyl treats constipation and may be used to empty and prepare the colon (bowel) for rectal or colon exams (diagnostic tests) or surgery. Generic bisacodyl tablets are available.

What should my health care professional know before I take bisacodyl?

They need to know if you have any of these conditions
- appendicitis
- intestinal blockage
- persistent constipation
- rectal tears or fissures
- stomach pain
- ulcerative colitis
- an unusual or allergic reaction to bisacodyl, tartrazine dye, other medicines, foods, dyes, or preservatives
- pregnant or trying to get pregnant

How should I take this medicine?

Take bisacodyl tablets by mouth. Follow the directions on the prescription label. Swallow the tablets whole with a good drink of water; do not crush or chew. Take exactly as directed; do not exceed the recommended dose, and do not take more often than directed. Bisacodyl is not intended for long-term use. Contact your pediatrician or health care professional regarding the use of this medicine in children. Special care may be needed.

What if I miss a dose?

This does not apply. Bisacodyl tablets are not for regular use, but are taken on an as needed basis.

What may interact with bisacodyl?

- antacids

What should I watch for while taking bisacodyl?

Do not use bisacodyl for more than one week without consulting your prescriber or health care professional. Long-term use or use of large doses also can lead to laxative dependence and chronic constipation. Antacids and milk can destroy the protective coating on bisacodyl tablets and upset your stomach. Do not take antacids and milk within 1 to 2 hours of the bisacodyl dose.

What side effects may I notice from taking bisacodyl?

Side effects that you should report to your prescriber or health care professional as soon as possible:
- dehydration
- dizziness or lightheadedness
- severe diarrhea
- unusual tiredness
- vomiting

Side effects that usually do not require medical attention (report to your prescriber or health care professional if they continue or are bothersome):
- mild diarrhea
- nausea
- stomach cramps

degrees C (77 degrees F). Protect from mois-
...ray ... used medicine after the expi-

...OL®;
...ble
...mble
...inc Sub
...amble Co

...floxacin, ofloxacin, or other similar

...or diabetes
...exate
...ytoin
...benecid
- salicylates (choline salicylate, magnesium salicylate, or Trilisate®)
- sulfinpyrazone
- tetracyclines (demeclocycline, doxycycline, tetracycline, or minocycline)

Tell your prescriber or health care professional about all other medicines you are taking, including non-prescription medicines, nutritional supplements, or herbal products. Also tell your prescriber or health care professional if you are a frequent user of drinks with caffeine or alcohol, if you smoke, or if you use illegal drugs. These may affect the way your medicine works. Check with your health care professional before stopping or starting any of your medicines.

What should I watch for while taking bismuth subsalicylate?

Tell your prescriber or health care professional if your symptoms do not improve or get worse. Do not treat diarrhea for more than 2 days without talking to your prescriber or health care professional. Call your prescriber or health care professional as soon as you can if you get a fever, or nausea and vomiting. These could be symptoms of a more serious illness. Do not smoke cigarettes or drink alcohol; these increase irritation in your stomach. If you are diabetic you may get a false result for sugar in your urine, especially if you take a lot of bismuth subsalicylate. Check with your prescriber or health care professional before you change your diet or the dose of your diabetic medicine.

What side effects may I notice from taking bismuth subsalicylate?

Side effects with bismuth subsalicylate are uncommon if you only take the recommended dose. Serious side effects include:
- anxiety, confusion
- dizziness, drowsiness
- headache
- increased sweating
- increased thirst
- loss of hearing, ringing in the ears
- muscle weakness
- nausea, vomiting that does not go away

---

yellow or brown urir
...ive tiredness
...your upper righ...
...nausea and vom...
...g of the eyes
...that usua...
...to your
...conti...
...peti...

...ch, he...
...lets and caple...
...without a prescripti...
mu... ...te chewable tablets ...
not caplets.

What ar... caplets? BISMUT... Bismatrol® Bismatrol® ...out a fever ...tion, and ...hey are av... ...th subsali...

What should my health care profes... know before I take bismuth subsalicylate?

They need to know if you have any of these conditions:
- bleeding problems
- dehydration
- diabetes
- dysentery
- fever
- gout
- hemophilia
- kidney disease
- liver disease
- recent vaccination with chickenpox vaccine
- recent viral illness, such as the flu or chickenpox
- an unusual or allergic reaction to aspirin, other salicylates or medicines, foods, dyes, or preservatives
- pregnant or trying to get pregnant
- breast-feeding

How should I take this medicine?

Take bismuth subsalicylate tablets or caplets by mouth. Follow the directions on the label. Swallow the caplets whole with a glass of water, do not chew. Chew the tablets or let them dissolve in your mouth. Do not take your medicine more often than directed. Contact your pediatrician or health care professional regarding the use of this medicine in children. Special care may be needed.

What if I miss a dose?

If you miss a dose, take it as soon as you can. If it is almost time for your next dose, take only that dose. Do not take double or extra doses.

What may interact with bismuth subsalicylate?

- acetazolamide or methazolamide
- agents that treat or prevent blood clots such as warfarin (Coumadin®)
- aspirin or other medicines containing aspirin

- tiredness
- trembling, or uncontrollable movements

Side effects that usually do not require medical attention (report to your prescriber or health care professional if they continue or are bothersome):
- black stools
- blackened tongue
- constipation

Where can I keep my medicine?

Keep out of the reach of children in a container that small children cannot open. Store at room temperature between 15 and 30 degrees C (59 and 86 degrees F). Throw away any unused medicine after the expiration date.

Bismuth Subsalicylate; Metronidazole; Tetracycline tablets and capsules

HELIDAC®;
262 mg/250 mg/500 mg;
Therapy Kit
Prometheus Laboratories Inc

What are bismuth subsalicylate; metronidazole; tetracycline tablets and capsules?

BISMUTH SUBSALICYLATE; METRONIDAZOLE; TETRACYCLINE (Helidac®) is a combination of medications used to treat stomach and intestinal ulcers associated with *Helicobacter pylori*, a bacterial infection. The Helidac® kit contains bismuth subsalicylate chewable tablets, metronidazole tablets, and tetracycline capsules packaged together. Generic Helidac® therapy kits are not available.

What should my health care professional know before I take bismuth subsalicylate; metronidazole; tetracycline?

They need to know if you have any of these conditions:
- if you smoke or drink alcoholic beverages
- anemia, bleeding problems, or other blood disorders
- dental disease
- diabetes
- disease of the nervous system such as neuropathy
- disease of the esophagus, stomach, or bowel (like Crohn's disease)
- fungal infection
- gout
- kidney disease
- liver disease
- recent vaccination with chickenpox vaccine
- recent viral illness, such as the flu or chickenpox
- seizures (convulsions)
- other chronic illness
- an unusual or allergic reaction to aspirin or other salicylates, bismuth compounds, metronidazole, tetracycline antibiotics, or other medicines, foods, dyes, or preservatives
- pregnant or trying to get pregnant
- breast-feeding

How should I take this medicine?

Each "dose" of Helidac® contains four pills: two bismuth subsalicylate chewable tablets, one metronidazole tablet, and one tetracycline capsule. Each dose should be taken four times each day, at mealtimes and at bedtime. Follow the directions on the prescription label. The bismuth subsalicylate tablets (pink) should be chewed and swallowed. The metronidazole tablet (white) and the tetracycline capsule (orange/white) should be swallowed whole, with a full glass of water (8 ounces). Take the metronidazole tablets and tetracycline capsules in an upright or sitting position. If possible, take the bedtime dose at least 10 minutes before lying down. Take your doses at regular intervals. Do not take your medicine more often than directed. Finish the full course prescribed by your prescriber or health care professional even if you think your condition is better. Do not stop taking except on your prescriber's advice. You should not drink alcoholic beverages or take other alcohol-containing preparations while you are taking bismuth subsalicylate; metronidazole; tetracycline and for at least 1 day after stopping it. Alcohol may make you dizzy, feel sick, and flushed; or give you headaches and stomach pains while you are taking metronidazole, a component of Helidac®. Do not take antacids, milk, milk formulas, or other dairy products within 1 to 2 hours of the time you take the tetracycline capsule. These products may keep tetracycline from working properly. Products containing calcium, iron or zinc (including multivitamins), can stop tetracycline from working properly. Take these products at least 2 hours after your last dose of tetracycline, or at least 4 hours before your next dose.

What if I miss a dose?

If you miss a bismuth subsalicylate; metronidazole; tetracycline dose, take it as soon as you can. If it is almost time for your next dose, take only that dose. Do not take double or extra doses. Continuing the normal dosing schedule until the medication is gone can make up missed doses. If more than 4 doses are missed, your prescriber should be contacted.

What may interact with Helidac®?

- acetazolamide
- alcohol or alcohol-containing beverages or liquid medicines containing alcohol
- antacids
- aspirin or other salicylate pain relievers (choline salicylate, magnesium salicylate, or Trilisate®)
- atovaquone
- bismuth subsalicylate (Pepto-Bismol®)
- calcium supplements

- celecoxib
- cholestyramine or colestipol
- cimetidine
- ciprofloxacin, levofloxacin, ofloxacin, or other similar antibiotics
- didanosine, ddI
- disulfiram
- female hormones, including birth control pills
- ferrous sulfate or other iron supplements
- lithium
- magnesium supplements
- medicines for diabetes
- medicines to control heart rhythm such as digoxin or dofetilide
- medicines that increase your sensitivity to sunlight such as sulfa drugs, tretinoin, or porfimer
- methadone
- methazolamide
- multivitamins with minerals
- probenecid
- quinapril
- ritonavir or Kaletra®
- sevelamer
- sirolimus or tacrolimus
- sodium bicarbonate
- soy isoflavones
- sucralfate
- vitamin A
- warfarin
- zinc supplements or zinc lozenges

Tell your prescriber or health care professional about all other medicines you are taking, including non-prescription medicines, nutritional supplements, or herbal products. Also tell your prescriber or health care professional if you are a frequent user of drinks with caffeine or alcohol, if you smoke, or if you use illegal drugs. These may affect the way your medicine works. Check with your health care professional before stopping or starting any of your medicines.

What should I watch for while taking bismuth subsalicylate; metronidazole; tetracycline?

It can take several days of therapy with bismuth subsalicylate; metronidazole; tetracycline before your stomach pains improve. Check with your prescriber or health care professional if your condition does not improve, or if it gets worse. Call your prescriber or health care professional as soon as you can if you get a fever, watery diarrhea, stomach pain, or vomiting. These could be symptoms of a more serious illness. Do not treat yourself. Call your prescriber for advice. Do not take tetracycline just before going to bed. It may not dissolve properly when you are lying down and can cause pain in your throat. Keep out of the sun, or wear protective clothing outdoors and use a sunscreen. Do not use sun lamps or sun tanning beds or booths. Birth control pills (contraceptive pills) may not work properly while you are taking this medicine. Use an extra method of birth control for at least one month. If you become pregnant, contact your prescriber immediately. Bismuth subsali-

cylate; metronidazole; tetracycline should not be used during pregnancy. You may get drowsy or dizzy. Do not drive, use machinery, or do anything that needs mental alertness until you know how bismuth subsalicylate; metronidazole; tetracycline affects you. To reduce the risk of dizzy or fainting spells, do not sit or stand up quickly, especially if you are an older patient. Do not smoke cigarettes or drink alcohol; these increase irritation of your stomach. If you are diabetic, you may get a false result for sugar in your urine while you are taking bismuth subsalicylate. Check with your prescriber or health care professional before you change your diet or the dose of your diabetic medicine. In some patients, bismuth subsalicylate; metronidazole; tetracycline in this combination of medicines may cause dark tongue and/or grayish black stools. This is only temporary and will go away when you stop taking bismuth subsalicylate. Your mouth may get dry. Chewing sugarless gum or sucking hard candy, and drinking plenty of water will help. If you are going to have surgery, tell your prescriber or health care professional that you are taking bismuth subsalicylate; metronidazole; tetracycline.

What side effects may I notice from taking bismuth subsalicylate; metronidazole; tetracycline?

Side effects that you should report to your prescriber or health care professional as soon as possible:
Rare or uncommon:
- clumsiness or unsteadiness
- decrease in the amount of urine passed
- fever or chills, sore throat
- loss of hearing, ringing in the ears
- numbness, tingling, pain or weakness in the hands or feet
- unusual or persistent skin rash, redness, blistering, peeling or loosening of the skin, including inside the mouth
- seizures (convulsions)

More common:
- dizziness or headache
- increased sweating or flushing
- itching or burning in the rectal or genital area
- nervousness
- skin rash, itching
- stomach pain or cramps
- trouble sleeping
- trouble swallowing
- unusual tiredness or weakness
- vomiting, blood in vomit
- watery diarrhea
- yellowing of the eyes or skin

Side effects that usually do not require medical attention (report to your prescriber or health care professional if they continue or are bothersome):
- change in taste
- constipation
- dark yellow or reddish-brown urine
- diarrhea (mild)
- discolored tongue (dark or black)

- discolored stools (gray-black)
- dry mouth, mild irritation of the mouth or throat
- increased skin sensitivity to sunlight
- joint pain
- nausea or loss of appetite
- mild stomach pain or cramps

Where can I keep my medicine?
Keep out of the reach of children in a container that small children cannot open. Store at room temperature between 20 and 25 degrees C (68 and 77 degrees F). Protect from light and moisture. Throw away any unused medicine after the expiration date. Never use tetracycline if it is past the expiration date; it can make you seriously ill.

Bisoprolol tablets

ZEBETA®;
5 mg; Tablet
Duramed
Pharmaceuticals Inc
Sub Barr
Laboratories Inc

ZEBETA®;
10 mg; Tablet
Duramed
Pharmaceuticals Inc
Sub Barr
Laboratories Inc

What are bisoprolol tablets?
BISOPROLOL (Zebeta®) belongs to a group of medicines called beta-blockers. Beta-blockers reduce the workload on the heart and help it to beat more regularly. Bisoprolol controls, but does not cure, high blood pressure (hypertension). Bisoprolol may also be used to improve symptoms in patients with heart disease. Generic bisoprolol tablets are available.

What should my health care professional know before I take bisoprolol?
They need to know if you have any of these conditions:
- asthma, bronchitis or bronchospasm
- bradycardia (unusually slow heartbeat)
- chest pain (angina)
- circulation problems, or blood vessel disease (such as Raynaud's disease)
- depression
- diabetes
- emphysema, or other lung disease
- heart disease (such as heart failure or history of heart attack)
- kidney disease
- liver disease
- muscle weakness or myasthenia gravis
- psoriasis
- thyroid disease
- an unusual or allergic reaction to bisoprolol, other beta-blockers, medicines, foods, dyes, or preservatives
- pregnant or trying to get pregnant
- breast-feeding

How should I take this medicine?
Take bisoprolol tablets by mouth. You can take bisoprolol tablets with or without food. Follow the directions on the prescription label. Swallow the tablets with a drink of water. Take your doses at regular intervals. Do not take your medicine more often than directed. Do not stop taking except on your prescriber's advice.

What if I miss a dose?
If you miss a dose, take it as soon as you can. If it is almost time for your next dose, take only that dose. Do not take double or extra doses.

What may interact with bisoprolol?
- anti-inflammatory drugs (NSAIDs, such as ibuprofen)
- cocaine
- hawthorn
- medicines for colds and breathing difficulties
- medicines for diabetes
- medicines for high blood pressure
- medicines to control heart rhythm
- rifampin

Tell your prescriber or health care professional about all other medicines you are taking, including non-prescription medicines, nutritional supplements, or herbal products. Also tell your prescriber or health care professional if you are a frequent user of drinks with caffeine or alcohol, if you smoke, or if you use illegal drugs. These may affect the way your medicine works. Check with your health care professional before stopping or starting any of your medicines.

What should I watch for while taking bisoprolol?
Check your heart rate and blood pressure regularly while you are taking bisoprolol. Ask your prescriber or health care professional what your heart rate and blood pressure should be, and when you should contact him or her. Do not stop taking this medicine suddenly. This could lead to serious heart-related effects. You may get drowsy or dizzy. Do not drive, use machinery, or do anything that requires mental alertness until you know how bisoprolol affects you. To reduce the risk of dizzy or fainting spells, do not sit or stand up quickly. Alcohol can make you more drowsy, and increase flushing and rapid heartbeats. Therefore, it is best to avoid alcoholic drinks. Bisoprolol can affect blood sugar levels. If you have diabetes, check with your prescriber or health care professional before you change your diet or the dose of your diabetic medicine. If you are going to have surgery, tell your prescriber or health care professional that you are taking bisoprolol.

What side effects may I notice from taking bisoprolol?
Side effects that you should report to your prescriber or health care professional as soon as possible:

- changes in vision
- cold, tingling, or numb hands or feet
- confusion
- difficulty breathing, wheezing
- dizziness or fainting spells
- increased thirst
- increase in the amount of urine passed
- irregular heartbeat
- joint pain
- skin rash
- slow heart rate (fewer than recommended by your prescriber or health care professional)
- sweating
- swollen legs or ankles
- tremor, shakes

Side effects that usually do not require medical attention (report to your prescriber or health care professional if they continue or are bothersome):

- anxiety
- depression, nightmares
- diarrhea
- nausea
- sexual difficulties, impotence
- unusual tiredness

Where can I keep my medicine?

Keep out of the reach of children in a container that small children cannot open. Store at room temperature below 30 degrees C (86 degrees F). Throw away any unused medicine after the expiration date.

Bisoprolol; Hydrochlorothiazide, HCTZ tablets

ZIAC®;
5 mg/6.25 mg;
Tablet
Duramed
Pharmaceuticals Inc
Sub Barr
Laboratories Inc

ZIAC®;
10 mg/6.25 mg;
Tablet
Duramed
Pharmaceuticals Inc
Sub Barr
Laboratories Inc

What are bisoprolol-hydrochlorothiazide tablets?

BISOPROLOL-HYDROCHLOROTHIAZIDE (Ziac™) belongs to a group of medicines called beta-blockers. Hydrochlorothiazide is a diuretic (water pill). Bisoprolol-hydrochlorothiazide controls, but does not cure, high blood pressure (hypertension). Generic bisoprolol-hydrochlorothiazide tablets are available.

What should my health care professional know before I take bisoprolol-hydrochlorothiazide?

They need to know if you have any of these conditions:

- asthma, bronchitis or bronchospasm
- autoimmune disease such as lupus (SLE)
- bradycardia (unusually slow heartbeat)
- chest pain (angina)
- circulation problems, or blood vessel disease (such as Raynaud's disease)
- depression
- diabetes
- electrolyte imbalance (e.g., low or high levels of potassium in the blood)
- emphysema, COPD, or other lung disease
- gout
- heart disease (such as heart failure or a history of heart attack)
- kidney disease
- liver disease
- muscle weakness or myasthenia gravis
- pancreatitis
- pheochromocytoma
- post-sympathectomy
- psoriasis
- thyroid disease
- sulfonamide (sulfa) or thiazide allergy
- an unusual or allergic reaction to hydrochlorothia-

zide, bisoprolol, other beta-blockers, medicines, foods, dyes, or preservatives
- if you are on a special diet, such as a low-salt diet (e.g., using potassium substitutes)
- pregnant or trying to get pregnant
- breast-feeding

How should I take this medicine?

Take bisoprolol-hydrochlorothiazide tablets by mouth. You can take bisoprolol-hydrochlorothiazide tablets with or without food. Follow the directions on the prescription label. Swallow the tablets with a drink of water. Take your doses at regular intervals. Do not take your medicine more often than directed. Do not stop taking except on your prescriber's advice. Contact your pediatrician or health care professional regarding the use of this medicine in children. Special care may be needed. Elderly patients over 65 years old may have a stronger reaction to this medicine and need smaller doses.

What if I miss a dose?

If you miss a dose, take it as soon as you can. If it is almost time for your next dose, take only that dose. Do not take double or extra doses.

What may interact with bisoprolol-hydrochlorothiazide?

- allopurinol
- anti-inflammatory drugs (NSAIDs, such as ibuprofen)
- cevimeline
- clonidine
- cocaine or amphetamine
- dolasetron
- ginger, Zingiber officinale
- griseofulvin
- hawthorn

- lithium
- liothyronine
- mefloquine
- medicines for chest pain or angina
- medicines for colds and breathing difficulties
- medicines for diabetes
- medicines for high blood pressure or heart failure
- medicines known as MAO inhibitors, such as phenelzine (Nardil®), tranylcypromine (Parnate®), isocarboxazid (Marplan®), and selegiline (Carbex®, Eldepryl®)
- medicines to control heart rhythm (including amiodarone, digoxin, disopyramide, dofetilide, flecainide, propafenone, quinidine, and sotalol)
- porfimer
- prochlorperazine (Compazine®)
- rifampin
- some antibiotics which increase sensitivity to sunlight (sulfonamides, tetracyclines)
- some medicines for lowering cholesterol (colestipol or cholestyramine)
- some medicines for weight loss (including some herbal products, ephedrine, dextroamphetamine)
- vitamin A (retinol) creams or pills
- water pills (diuretics)

Tell your prescriber or health care professional about all other medicines you are taking, including non-prescription medicines, nutritional supplements, or herbal products. Also tell your prescriber or health care professional if you are a frequent user of drinks with caffeine or alcohol, if you smoke, or if you use illegal drugs. These may affect the way your medicine works. Check with your health care professional before stopping or starting any of your medicines.

What should I watch for while taking bisoprolol-hydrochlorothiazide?

Check your heart rate and blood pressure regularly while you are taking bisoprolol-hydrochlorothiazide. Ask your prescriber or health care professional what your blood pressure should be and when you should contact him or her. When you check your blood pressure, write down the measurements to show your prescriber or health care professional. If you are taking this medicine for a long time you must visit your prescriber or health care professional for regular checks on your progress. Make sure you schedule appointments on a regular basis. Do not stop taking this medicine suddenly. This could lead to serious heart-related effects. You may get drowsy or dizzy. Do not drive, use machinery, or do anything that requires mental alertness until you know how bisoprolol-hydrochlorothiazide affects you. To reduce the risk of dizzy or fainting spells, do not sit or stand up quickly. Alcohol can make you more drowsy, and increase flushing and rapid heartbeats. Therefore, it is best to avoid alcoholic drinks. Check with your health care professional if you get an attack of severe diarrhea, nausea and vomiting, or sweat a lot. The loss of too much body fluid while you are taking a diuretic can cause dehydration and lower the blood pressure below normal. Bisoprolol-hydrochlorothiazide can affect blood sugar levels. If you have diabetes, check with your prescriber or health care professional before you change your diet or the dose of your diabetic medicine. Do not take medicines for appetite control, asthma, colds, cough, hay fever, or sinus problems without asking your prescriber or health care professional for advice. Do not treat yourself for a fever or sore throat; check with your prescriber or health care professional first. If you are going to have surgery, tell your prescriber or health care professional that you are taking bisoprolol-hydrochlorothiazide.

What side effects may I notice from taking bisoprolol-hydrochlorothiazide?

Side effects that you should report to your prescriber or health care professional as soon as possible:
- changes in vision (e.g., blurred vision)
- cold, tingling, or numb hands or feet
- confusion, dizziness, lightheadedness or fainting spells
- difficulty breathing, wheezing
- fever or chills
- increased thirst or sweating
- increase or decrease in the amount of urine passed
- fast or uneven heart beat, palpitations, or chest pain
- slow heart rate (fewer than recommended by your prescriber or health care professional)
- joint pain
- muscle cramps
- redness, blistering, peeling or loosening of the skin, including inside the mouth
- stomach pain
- swollen legs or ankles
- tremor, shakes
- unusual skin rash or bruising
- unusual tiredness or weakness
- vomiting
- worsened gout pain
- yellowing of the eyes or skin

Side effects that usually do not require medical attention (report to your prescriber or health care professional if they continue or are bothersome):
- anxiety
- cough
- depression, nightmares
- diarrhea
- increased sensitivity to the sun
- nausea
- sexual difficulties, impotence
- tiredness or fatigue

Where can I keep my medicine?

Keep out of the reach of children in a container that small children cannot open. Store at room temperature at 15 to 30 degrees C (59 to 86 degrees F). Throw away any unused medicine after the expiration date.

Bosentan tablets

B

This drug requires an FDA medication guide. See page xxxvii.

What are bosentan tablets?

BOSENTAN (TRACLEER®) is used to treat a serious heart and lung disorder called primary pulmonary hypertension. While bosentan will not cure this disorder, it is used to improve symptoms. It may help to increase your ability to exercise and/or improve your breathing. Generic bosentan tablets are not yet available.

What should my health care professional know before I take bosentan?

They need to know if you have any of these conditions:
- blood disorders (such as anemia)
- liver problems
- low blood pressure
- an unusual or allergic reaction to bosentan, other medicines, foods, dyes, or preservatives
- pregnant or trying to get pregnant
- breast-feeding

How should I take this medicine?

Take bosentan tablets by mouth. Follow the directions on the prescription label. Swallow the tablets with a drink of water. This medicine may be taken with or without meals. Do not take more often than directed. This medicine is not for use in children ≤ 12 years old. Older patients (over 65 years old) may have a stronger reaction to this medicine and may need smaller doses.

What if I miss a dose?

Try not to miss your scheduled doses. Ask your prescriber what you should do in case of a missed dose. If it is almost time for your next dose, take only that dose. Do not take double or extra doses.

What may interact with bosentan?

Do not take bosentan with any of the following medications (discuss your drug regimen with your prescriber):

- cyclosporine
- glyburide

Bosentan may also interact with the following medications:

- antiviral protease inhibitors (used to treat HIV infection such as indinavir, ritonavir, saquinavir, and others)
- atovaquone
- certain allergy medicines (such as astemizole, terfenadine)
- certain antibiotics used to treat tuberculosis such as rifampin or rifabutin
- certain medicines for cancer (chemotherapy)
- certain medicines for anxiety or insomnia (such as alprazolam, diazepam, midazolam, triazolam)
- certain medicines for fungal infections such as itraconazole or ketoconazole
- certain medicines to control the heart rhythm (such as amiodarone, disopyramide, dofetilide, quinidine)
- certain medicines for high cholesterol (such as atorvastatin, cerivastatin, lovastatin, simvastatin)
- certain pain medicines
- cevimeline
- cisapride
- clarithromycin
- dapsone
- donepezil
- ergot medicines (such as Cafergot®, Migranal®, D.H.E. 45®, and others)
- erythromycin
- galantamine
- female hormones, such as estrogens or progestins, birth control pills, injections, or implants
- levomethadyl
- medicines for diabetes
- medicines for high blood pressure
- medicines for seizures
- ondansetron
- paclitaxel
- pimozide
- sertraline
- sibutramine
- sildenafil
- sirolimus
- steroid medicines such as prednisone or hydrocortisone
- St. John's wort or any herbal products containing St. John's wort
- tacrolimus
- tolterodine
- warfarin
- zileuton

Tell your prescriber or health care professional about all other medicines you are taking, including non-prescription medicines, nutritional supplements, or herbal products. Also tell your prescriber or health care professional if you are a frequent user of drinks with caffeine or alcohol, if you smoke, or if you use illegal drugs. These may affect the way your medicine works. Check with your health care professional before stopping or starting any of your medicines.

What should I watch for while taking bosentan?

Visit your prescriber or health care professional for checks on your progress. You will need to be seen regularly. Report any unusual or severe side effects promptly. Despite receiving bosentan, your condition may worsen and you may need your dose adjusted. Call your prescriber or health care professional if you experience any worsening of your condition. Pregnancy must be avoided during bosentan therapy due to the potential for serious side effects to an unborn child. If you are female of child-bearing potential, your physician will have to check urine or serum pregnancy tests regularly (at least monthly) while you are taking bosentan. Discuss options for effective contraception and other measures to prevent pregnancy with your physician. Bosentan may reduce the effectiveness of hormonal birth control methods, including birth control pills, patches, implanted hormonal products (example: Norplant®), or injections (examples: Depo-Provera®, Lunelle®). Your health care professional will have to check blood tests regularly (at least monthly) to assess the effect of this medication on your liver. Bosentan may cause changes in some of these measurements. If you are going to have surgery, tell your prescriber or health care professional that you are taking bosentan.

What side effects may I notice from taking bosentan?

Side effects that you should report to your prescriber or health care professional as soon as possible:
- abdominal pain, nausea, vomiting
- cool, pale skin
- dark yellow or brown urine, yellowing of the eyes or skin

- dizziness or fainting spells
- fast heartbeat or palpitations
- fever
- swelling of the body (such as swelling of the ankles or legs)
- unusual weakness or tiredness

Side effects that usually do not require medical attention (report to your prescriber or health care professional if they continue or are bothersome):
- flushing (red, warm skin)
- itching of the skin
- headache
- runny nose or sore throat
- tiredness or fatigue
- upset stomach

Where can I keep my medicine?

Keep out of the reach of children in a container that small children cannot open. Store at room temperature between 15 and 30 degrees C (59 and 86 degrees F). Keep container tightly closed and protect from moisture and humidity. Throw away any unused medicine after the expiration date.

Brimonidine eye solution

ALPHAGAN;
5 ml/0.2%; Ophthalmic
Solution
Allergan Inc.

What is brimonidine eye solution?

BRIMONIDINE (Alphagan®, Alphagan® P) helps to reduce pressure in the eye for patients with increased pressure or open-angle glaucoma. Generic brimonidine eye solution is available for Alphagan®. Generic Alphagan® P (contains Purite® as a preservative) is not yet available.

What should my health care professional know before I use brimonidine?

They need to know if you have any of these conditions:
- eye infection or damage
- wear contact lenses
- closed-angle glaucoma
- heart disease
- depression
- kidney disease
- liver disease
- an unusual or allergic reaction to brimonidine, other medicines, foods, dyes, or preservatives
- pregnant or trying to get pregnant
- breast-feeding

How should I use this medicine?

Brimonidine eye solution is only for use in the eye. Do not take by mouth. Follow the directions on the prescription label. Wash hands before and after use. Tilt the head back slightly and pull down the lower lid with the index finger to form a pouch. Try not to touch the tip of the dropper to your eye or any other surface. Squeeze one drop into the pouch. Close the eye gently; do not blink or rub your eyes. Apply pressure to the inside corner of your eye for a few minutes after placing the medicine to help it stay in your eye longer. Use your doses at regular intervals. Do not use your medicine more often than directed. Contact your pediatrician or health care professional regarding the use of this medicine in children. Special care may be needed.

What if I miss a dose?

If you miss a dose, use it as soon as you can. If it is almost time for your next dose, use only that dose. Do not use double or extra doses.

What may interact with brimonidine?

- medicines that cause drowsiness or tiredness - brimonidine may increase these effects
- medicines for high blood pressure or other heart problems - brimonidine may have additional effects.

Tell your prescriber or other health care professional about all other medicines you are taking including nonprescription medicines, nutritional supplements, or herbal products. Also, tell your prescriber or health care professional if you are a frequent user of drinks with caffeine or alcohol, if you smoke or if you use illegal drugs. These may affect the way your medicine works. Check before stopping or starting any of your medications.

What should I watch for while taking brimonidine?

Visit your prescriber or health care professional for regular checks on your progress. Report any serious side effects promptly. Stop using brimonidine if your eyes get inflamed, painful, or have a discharge, and see your prescriber or health care professional as soon as you can. Be careful not to touch the tip of the dispensing container onto the eye, or any other surface. Serious eye infections can result from contamination of eye solutions. Do not use eye cups. If you are using another eye medicine, wait at least 10 minutes in between using the medicines. If you wear contact lenses, take them out before using brimonidine and wait 15 minutes before putting them back into your eye. Brimonidine may cause drowsiness or tiredness. Be careful driving or operating machinery until you know how this medication affects you. If brimonidine makes your mouth dry, sucking on hard candy or using an artificial saliva product might lessen this effect. Wear dark glasses if brimonidine makes your eyes more sensitive to light.

What side effects may I notice from taking brimonidine?

Side effects that you should report to your prescriber or health care professional as soon as possible:
Rare:
- inflamed or infected eyes or eyelids
- bleeding in your eye

Side effects that usually do not require medical attention (report to your prescriber or health care professional if they continue or are bothersome):
- dry mouth
- blurred vision
- headache
- tiredness
- bitter taste in the mouth
- burning, stinging, or discomfort immediately after using the solution
- dry or itchy eyes
- sensitivity of the eyes to light

Where can I keep my medicine?

Keep out of the reach of children. Store at room temperature less than 77 degrees F (25 degrees C). Throw away any unused medicine after the expiration date.

Bromocriptine tablets or capsules

PARLODEL®;
5 mg; Capsule
Novartis Pharmaceuticals

What are bromocriptine tablets or capsules?

BROMOCRIPTINE (Parlodel®) comes from a group of medicines known as ergot alkaloids. It blocks the release of a hormone called prolactin that affects the menstrual cycle and breast milk production. Bromocriptine is useful in treating menstrual and fertility problems and symptoms caused by cancers (adenomas) that raise prolactin levels in the body. Bromocriptine can be used to treat Parkinson's disease. The drug is also helpful in treating acromegaly (excessive growth hormone). Generic bromocriptine tablets and capsules are available.

What should my health care professional know before I receive bromocriptine?

They need to know if you have any of these conditions:
- history of heart attack
- heart or vessel disease
- high or low blood pressure
- irregular heart rate
- liver disease
- mental disorders
- retroperitoneal fibrosis
- seizures (convulsions)
- ulcers or history of ulcers
- an unusual or allergic reaction to bromocriptine, ergot alkaloids, sulfites, other medicines, foods, dyes, or preservatives
- pregnant or trying to get pregnant
- breast-feeding

How should this medicine be used?

Take bromocriptine tablets or capsules by mouth. Follow the directions on the prescription label. Swallow the tablets or capsules with a drink of water. It is best to take bromocriptine with food to help with symptoms such as upset stomach. Take your doses at regular intervals. Do not take your medicine more often than directed. Do not stop taking except on your prescriber's advice. Contact your pediatrician or health care professional regarding the use of this medicine in children. Special care may be needed.

What if I miss a dose?

If you miss a dose, take it as soon as you can. If it is more than 4 hours since your dose was due, wait until your next dose. Do not take double or extra doses.

What may interact with bromocriptine?

- alcohol
- cabergoline
- cyclosporine
- dihydroergotamine
- ergoloid mesylates
- ergonovine or methylergonovine
- ergotamine
- erythromycin or related medicines such as clarithromycin, dirithromycin, and troleandomycin
- female hormones, including contraceptive or birth control pills
- imatinib

- levodopa
- medicines for HIV infection (such as amprenavir, delavirdine, efavirenz, indinavir, nelfinavir, ritonavir, saquinavir)
- medicines for high blood pressure
- medicines for mental depression
- medicines for mental problems and psychotic disturbances
- memantine
- methysergide
- metoclopramide
- sirolimus
- tacrolimus
- tamoxifen

Tell your prescriber or health care professional about all other medicines you are taking, including non-prescription medicines, nutritional supplements, or herbal products. Also tell your prescriber or health care professional if you are a frequent user of drinks with caffeine or alcohol, if you smoke, or if you use illegal drugs. These may affect the way your medicine works. Check with your health care professional before stopping or starting any of your medicines.

What should I watch for while taking bromocriptine?

Visit your prescriber or health care professional for regular checks on your progress. Ask your prescriber or health care professional if you should check your blood pressure regularly, especially if you get severe headaches, and report changes in blood pressure if they occur. Contact your provider promptly if you develop an unusual or severe headache or have changes in your vision. If you stop taking bromocriptine when it is being used for tumor treatment, the tumor may regrow quickly, and your original symptoms may return. Do not stop taking this medication unless your prescriber tells you to. You may get dizzy or drowsy. Do not drive, use machinery, or do anything that requires mental alertness until you know how bromocriptine affects you. To reduce the risk of dizzy or fainting spells, do not stand or sit up quickly, especially if you are an older patient. Alcohol can make you more dizzy, and increase flushing and rapid heartbeats. Avoid alcoholic drinks. Dizziness is more common after the first dose. Take it before bedtime if possible and be careful getting out of bed. Avoid exposure to cold. Contact your provider promptly if you experience tingling, burning, or numbness in your hands or feet. Your mouth may get dry. Chewing sugarless gum or sucking hard candy, and

drinking plenty of water, will help. If you are going to have surgery, tell your prescriber or health care professional that you are taking bromocriptine.

What side effects may I notice from taking bromocriptine?

Side effects that you should report to your prescriber or health care professional as soon as possible:
Rare or uncommon:
- unusual bleeding
- blurred vision
- difficulty breathing
- fainting spells, dizziness or lightheadedness
- unusual or severe headache
- irregular heartbeat, chest pain or palpitations
- numbness, tingling, or burning in hands or feet
- rash or hives
- seizures (convulsions)
- spasm in fingers or toes, or unusual muscle movements
- stomach pain
- vomiting

More common:
- changes in blood pressure
- confusion or hallucinations (seeing or hearing things that are not really there)
- persistent, watery nasal discharge
- severe weakness or tiredness

Side effects that usually do not require medical attention (report to your prescriber or health care professional if they continue or are bothersome):
- anxiety or nervousness
- diarrhea or constipation
- difficulty sleeping
- drowsiness
- dry mouth or metallic taste in mouth
- headache
- loss of appetite
- nausea
- ringing in ears
- runny nose, or stuffy nose
- mild stomach cramps
- mild swelling in feet
- tiredness
- mild weakness

Where can I keep my medicine?

Keep out of the reach of children in a container that small children cannot open. Store at room temperature below 25 degrees C (77 degrees F). Do not freeze. Protect from light. Keep container tightly closed. Throw away any unused medicine after the expiration date.

Brompheniramine tablets, extended-release tablets, or capsules

LODRANE® 12HR;
6 mg; Tablet, Extended
Release
ECR Pharmaceuticals

What are brompheniramine tablets, extended-release tablets, or capsules?

BROMPHENIRAMINE (Dimetane® Extentabs, Dimetapp® Allergy Liqui-Gels, Lodrane® 12HR) is an antihistamine. It is used to relieve or prevent the symptoms of hay fever (seasonal rhinitis), hives (rash and itching) and other types of allergy. It is also used to relieve symptoms of runny nose from colds (rhinitis). Generic brompheniramine capsules, tablets and extended-release tablets are available.

What should my health care professional know before I use brompheniramine?

They need to know if you have any of these conditions:
- asthma or other lung disease
- glaucoma or other eye disease
- heart disease
- high or low blood pressure
- liver disease
- pain or difficulty passing urine
- prostate trouble
- seizures
- stomach or intestinal problems
- thyroid disease
- wear contact lenses
- an unusual or allergic reaction to brompheniramine, other medicines, foods, dyes, or preservatives
- pregnant or trying to become pregnant
- breast-feeding

How should I use this medicine?

Take brompheniramine tablets or capsules by mouth. Follow the directions on the prescription label. Take with food or milk if brompheniramine upsets your stomach. Swallow extended-release tablets whole; do not crush or chew. Take your doses at regular intervals. Do not take your medicine more often than directed. Contact your pediatrician or health care professional regarding the use of this medicine in children. Special care may be needed.

What if I miss a dose?

If you miss a dose, use it as soon as you can. If it is almost time for your next dose, use only that dose. Do not use double or extra doses.

What may interact with brompheniramine?

- alcohol
- barbiturate medicines for inducing sleep or treating seizures (convulsions)
- medicines for anxiety or sleeping problems, such as diazepam or temazepam
- medicines for hay fever and other allergies
- medicines for mental depression
- medicines for mental problems and psychotic disturbances
- medicines for movement abnormalities as in Parkinson's disease
- medicines for pain such as codeine, hydrocodone, meperidine, methadone, morphine, oxycodone, propoxyphene, and tramadol
- some medicines for gastrointestinal problems (such as atropine, dicyclomine, glycopyrrolate, hyoscyamine, or propantheline)

Tell your prescriber or health care professional about all other medicines you are taking, including non-prescription medicines, nutritional supplements, or herbal products. Also tell your prescriber or health care professional if you are a frequent user of drinks with caffeine or alcohol, if you smoke, or if you use illegal drugs. These may affect the way your medicine works. Check with your health care professional before stopping or starting any of your medicines.

What should I watch for while taking brompheniramine?

Tell your prescriber or health care professional if your symptoms do not improve in 1 or 2 days. You may get drowsy or dizzy. Do not drive, use machinery, or do anything that needs mental alertness until you know how brompheniramine affects you. To reduce the risk of dizzy or fainting spells, do not stand or sit up quickly, especially if you are an older patient. Alcohol may increase dizziness and drowsiness. Avoid alcoholic drinks. Your mouth may get dry. Chewing sugarless gum or sucking hard candy, and drinking plenty of water will help. Brompheniramine may cause dry eyes and blurred vision. If you wear contact lenses you may feel some discomfort. Lubricating drops may help. See your ophthalmologist if the problem does not go away or is severe. If you are receiving skin tests for allergies, tell your physician you are using brompheniramine.

What side effects may I notice from taking brompheniramine?

Side effects that you should report to your prescriber or health care professional as soon as possible:
- agitation, nervousness, excitability, not able to sleep (these are more likely in children)
- blurred vision
- fainting spells
- irregular heartbeat, palpitations, or chest pain
- muscle or facial twitches
- pain or difficulty passing urine
- seizures (convulsions)

Side effects that usually do not require medical attention (report to your prescriber or health care professional if they continue or are bothersome):

- drowsiness, dizziness
- dry mouth
- headache
- loss of appetite
- stomach upset, nausea, vomiting, diarrhea or constipation

Where can I keep my medicine?

Keep out of the reach of children. Store upright at room temperature between 15 and 30 degrees C (59 and 86 degrees F) in a tight container; do not freeze. Throw away any unused medicine after the expiration date.

Brompheniramine; Pseudoephedrine extended-release capsules

BROMFENEX®;
12 mg/120 mg; Capsule,
Extended Release
Ethex Corporation

What are brompheniramine; pseudoephedrine extended-release capsules?

BROMPHENIRAMINE; PSEUDOEPHEDRINE capsules (Allent®, Bromadrine®, Bromfed®, Bromfenex®, and others) contain a decongestant and an antihistamine. It can help relieve runny nose, nasal or sinus congestion (stuffiness), sneezing, and itchy or watery eyes that may occur with hay fever (seasonal allergies). Generic brompheniramine; pseudoephedrine products are available.

What should my health care professional know before I take brompheniramine; pseudoephedrine?

They need to know if you have any of the following conditions:
- asthma, emphysema, or other lung disease
- blood vessel disease
- diabetes
- pain or difficulty passing urine (urinary retention)
- glaucoma or other eye disease
- heart disease or heart rhythm problems
- high or low blood pressure
- kidney disease
- liver disease
- overactive thyroid
- prostate trouble
- seizure disorder
- stomach or intestinal problems
- wear contact lenses
- an unusual or allergic reaction to brompheniramine, pseudoephedrine, other medicines, foods, dyes, or preservatives
- pregnant or trying to get pregnant
- breast-feeding

How should I take this medicine?

Take the brompheniramine; pseudoephedrine capsules by mouth. Follow the directions on the prescription label. Swallow the capsules with a drink of water. This medication may be taken with food if it upsets your stomach. Take your doses at regular intervals. Do not take your medicine more often than directed. Contact your pediatrician or health care professional regarding the use of this medicine in children. Special care may be needed. Elderly patients over 60 years old may have a stronger reaction to this medicine and need smaller doses.

What if I miss a dose?

If you miss a dose, and you are taking it on a regular schedule, take it as soon as you can. If it is almost time for your next dose (less than 12 hours), take only that dose. Do not take double or extra doses.

What may interact with brompheniramine; pseudoephedrine?

- alcohol
- ammonium chloride
- amphetamine or other stimulant drugs
- barbiturate medicines for inducing sleep or treating seizures (convulsions)
- bicarbonate, citrate, or acetate products (such as sodium bicarbonate, sodium acetate, sodium citrate, sodium lactate, and potassium citrate)
- bromocriptine
- caffeine
- cocaine
- furazolidone
- linezolid
- medicines for anxiety or sleeping problems, such as diazepam or temazepam (sleeping pills or tranquilizers)
- medicines for chest pain, heart disease, high blood pressure or heart rhythm problems
- medicines for colds and breathing difficulties
- medicines for diabetes
- medicines for hay fever and other allergies
- medicines known as MAO inhibitors, such as phenelzine (Nardil®), tranylcypromine (Parnate®), isocarboxazid (Marplan®), and selegiline (Carbex®, Eldepryl®)
- medicines for mental depression or other mental disturbances
- medicines for migraine
- medicines for movement abnormalities as in Parkinson's disease
- medicines for pain such as codeine, hydrocodone, meperidine, methadone, morphine, oxycodone, propoxyphene, and tramadol
- procarbazine
- some medicines for gastrointestinal problems (such as atropine, dicyclomine, glycopyrrolate, hyoscyamine, or propantheline)
- some medicines for weight loss (including some herbal products, ephedrine, dextroamphetamine)
- St. John's wort
- theophylline
- thyroid hormones

Tell your prescriber or health care professional about all other medicines you are taking, including non-prescription medicines, nutritional supplements, or herbal products. Also tell your prescriber or health care professional if you are a frequent user of drinks with caffeine or alcohol, if you smoke, or if you use illegal drugs. These may affect the way your medicine works. Check before starting or stopping any of your medicines.

What should I watch for while taking with brompheniramine; pseudoephedrine?

If nervousness, dizziness, sleeplessness, or palpitations occur, stop using this product and consult a health care professional. If brompheniramine-pseudoephedrine extended-release products make it difficult for you to sleep at night; take your last dose of the day at least 12 hours before bedtime. You may get drowsy or dizzy. Do not drive, use machinery, or do anything that needs mental alertness until you know how this medicine affects you. To reduce the risk of dizzy or fainting spells, do not stand or sit up quickly, especially if you are an older patient. Alcohol may increase dizziness and drowsiness. Avoid alcoholic drinks. Your mouth may get dry. Chewing sugarless gum or sucking hard candy, and drinking plenty of water will help. The brompheniramine component of this product may cause dry eyes and blurred vision. If you wear contact lenses you may feel some discomfort. Lubricating drops may help. See your ophthalmologist if the problem does not go away or is severe. If you are receiving skin tests for allergies, tell your physician you are using a product which contains brompheniramine (an antihistamine).

What side effects may I notice from taking with brompheniramine; pseudoephedrine?

Side effects that you should report to your prescriber or health care professional as soon as possible:

- agitation, anxiety, excitement, irritability, or nervousness
- blurred vision
- chest pain or palpitations
- confusion
- dizziness or fainting spells
- fast or irregular heartbeat
- increased blood pressure
- increased sweating
- numbness or tingling in the hands or feet
- pain or difficulty passing urine
- rapid or troubled breathing
- severe, persistent, or worsening headache
- sleeplessness (insomnia)
- tremor or muscle contractions
- vomiting

Side effects that usually do not require medical attention (report to your prescriber or health care professional if they continue or are bothersome):
diarrhea or constipation
- difficulty sleeping
- drowsiness or fatigue
- dry mouth
- headache (mild)
- loss of appetite
- rash or reddening of the skin
- restlessness
- stomach upset, nausea

Where can I keep my medicine?

Keep out of the reach of children in a container that small children cannot open. Store at room temperature, between 15 and 30 degrees C (59 and 86 degrees F), unless otherwise specified on the product label. Throw away any unused medicine after the expiration date.

Budesonide capsules

ENTOCORT® EC;
3 mg; Capsule
Prometheus Laboratories Inc

What are budesonide capsules?

BUDESONIDE (Entocort® EC) is a corticosteroid. It is used in the treatment of Crohn's disease, which is an inflammatory bowel disease. Generic budesonide capsules are not yet available.

What should my health care professional know before I take oral budesonide?

They need to know if you have any of these conditions:
- cataracts or glaucoma
- Cushing's syndrome
- diabetes
- heart problems, or previous heart attack
- high blood pressure
- infection, such as herpes, measles, tuberculosis or chickenpox
- liver disease
- myasthenia gravis
- osteoporosis
- psychosis, or other mental health problems
- recent surgery
- stomach or intestinal disease, including colitis
- an unusual or allergic reaction to budesonide, other corticosteroids, medicines, foods, dyes, or preservatives
- pregnant or trying to get pregnant
- breast-feeding

How should I take this medicine?

Take budesonide capsules by mouth. Follow the directions on the prescription label. Swallow the capsules with a drink of water. Do not chew, crush, or break open the capsules. The capsules need to be swallowed whole. If you are only taking budesonide once a day, take it in the morning, which is the time your body normally secretes cortisol. Take your doses at regular intervals. Do not take your medicine more often than directed.

Contact your pediatrician or health care professional regarding the use of this medicine in children. Special care may be needed.

What if I miss a dose?

If you miss a dose and remember within an hour or so, use it as soon as you remember. If it is almost time for your next dose, use only that dose and continue with your regular schedule. Do not use double or extra doses.

What may interact with oral budesonide?

- anastrozole
- antacids
- barbiturates, medicines used for inducing sleep or treating seizures
- bosentan
- certain antifungals, like fluconazole, griseofulvin, itraconazole, ketoconazole, miconazole and oxiconazole
- certain heart medicines like diltiazem, mibefradil, nicardipine and verapamil
- cyclosporine
- danazol
- diltiazem
- certain antibiotics like erythromycin, clarithromycin, nafcillin and troleandomycin
- dexamethasone
- ethosuximide
- grapefruit juice
- isoniazid, INH
- medicines used for seizures such as carbamazepine, ethosuximide, fosphenytoin, phenytoin or primidone
- medicines used for ulcers or stomach acid, such as cimetidine or omeprazole
- modafinil
- norfloxacin
- quinidine
- quinine
- rifabutin
- rifampin
- rifapentine
- some HIV medicines, for example indinavir, nelfinavir, ritonavir or saquinavir
- some medicines for depression, such as fluoxetine, fluvoxamine or nefazodone
- St. John's wort
- troglitazone
- vaccines
- zafirlukast

Tell your prescriber or health care professional about all other medicines you are taking, including non-prescription medicines, nutritional supplements, or herbal products. Also tell your prescriber or health care professional if you are a frequent user of drinks with caffeine or alcohol, if you smoke, or if you use illegal drugs. These may affect the way your medicine works. Check with your health care professional before stopping or starting any of your medicines.

What should I watch for while taking oral budesonide?

If you are taking budesonide regularly, avoid contact with people who have an infection. You may have an increased risk from infection while taking budesonide. Tell your prescriber or health care professional if you are exposed to anyone with measles or chickenpox, or if you develop sores or blisters that do not heal properly. People who are taking certain dosages of budesonide may need to avoid immunization with certain vaccines or may need to have changes in their vaccination schedules to ensure adequate protection from certain diseases. Make sure to tell your prescriber or health care professional that you are taking budesonide before receiving any vaccine. If you are going to have surgery, tell your prescriber or health care professional that you are taking oral budesonide. Your body may lose potassium while you are taking oral budesonide. Ask your prescriber or health care professional about your diet. Corticosteroids like budesonide may affect your blood sugar. If you are diabetic check with your prescriber or health care professional if you need help adjusting the dose of your diabetic medicine. Alcohol can increase the risk of getting serious side effects while you are taking budesonide. Avoid alcoholic drinks.

What side effects may I notice from taking oral budesonide?

Side effects that you should report to your prescriber or health care professional as soon as possible:
- bloody or black, tarry stools
- confusion, excitement, restlessness, a false sense of well-being
- eye pain, decreased or blurred vision
- fever, sore throat, sneezing, cough, or other signs of infection, wounds that will not heal
- frequent passing of urine or painful passing of urine
- hair loss
- hemorrhoids
- increased thirst
- irregular heartbeat, chest pain or high blood pressure
- menstrual problems
- severe mood swings
- muscle cramps or weakness
- numbness or tingling in fingers, toes or other areas
- pain in hips, back, ribs, arms, shoulders, or legs
- rounding out of face
- skin problems, acne, thin and shiny skin
- stomach pain
- swelling of feet or lower legs
- unusual bruising
- unusual tiredness or weakness
- vomiting
- weight gain or weight loss

Side effects that usually do not require medical attention (report to your prescriber or health care professional if they continue or are bothersome):

- dizziness or drowsiness
- headache
- increased or decreased appetite
- increased sweating
- nausea
- nervousness or difficulty sleeping
- upset stomach
- increased growth of hair on the face or body

Where can I keep my medicine?

Keep out of the reach of children in a container that small children cannot open. Store at room temperature between 15 and 30 degrees C (59 and 86 degrees F). Throw away any unused medicine after the expiration date.

Bumetanide tablets

BUMEX®;
1 mg; Tablet
Hoffmann La Roche
Inc

BUMEX®;
0.5 mg; Tablet
Hoffmann La Roche
Inc

What are bumetanide tablets?

BUMETANIDE (Bumex®) is a diuretic (water or fluid pill). Diuretics increase the amount of urine passed, which causes the body to lose water and salt. Bumetanide is a loop diuretic; "loop" refers to the part of the kidney where bumetanide works. Bumetanide is given as a diuretic in conditions that make the body retain water and produce swelling (edema), like heart failure, liver or kidney problems. It is not a cure. Generic bumetanide tablets are available.

What should my health care professional know before I take bumetanide?

They need to know if you have any of these conditions:
- diabetes
- diarrhea
- gout
- hearing problems
- heart disease, or previous heart attack
- kidney disease, small amounts of urine, or difficulty passing urine
- liver disease
- low blood levels of calcium, potassium, chloride, sodium or magnesium
- pancreatitis
- an unusual or allergic reaction to bumetanide, thiazides, sulfonamides, other medicines, foods, dyes, or preservatives
- pregnant or trying to get pregnant
- breast-feeding

How should I take this medicine?

Take bumetanide tablets by mouth. Follow the directions on the prescription label. Swallow the tablets with a drink of water. If bumetanide upsets your stomach, take it with food or milk. Take your doses at regular intervals. Do not take your medicine more often than directed. Remember that you will need to pass urine frequently after taking bumetanide. Do not take your doses at a time of day that will cause you problems. Do not take at bedtime. Contact your pediatrician or health care professional regarding the use of this medicine in children. Special care may be needed.

What if I miss a dose?

If you miss a dose, take it as soon as you can. If it is almost time for your next dose, take only that dose. Do not take double or extra doses.

What may interact with bumetanide?

- alcohol
- anti-inflammatory drugs (NSAIDs, such as ibuprofen)
- amphotericin B
- cisplatin
- dofetilide
- heart medicines such as digoxin
- hormones such as cortisone, fludrocortisone, hydrocortisone
- medicines for high blood pressure
- lithium
- water pills

Tell your prescriber or health care professional about all other medicines you are taking, including non-prescription medicines, nutritional supplements, or herbal products. Also tell your prescriber or health care professional if you are a frequent user of drinks with caffeine or alcohol, if you smoke, or if you use illegal drugs. These may affect the way your medicine works. Check with your health care professional before stopping or starting any of your medicines.

What should I watch for while taking bumetanide?

Visit your prescriber or health care professional for regular checks on your progress. Check your blood pressure regularly. Ask your prescriber or health care professional what your blood pressure should be, and when you should contact him or her. You must not get dehydrated, ask your prescriber or health care professional how much fluid you need to drink a day. Do not stop taking bumetanide except on your prescriber's advice. Watch your diet while you are taking bumetanide. Ask your prescriber or health care professional about both potassium and sodium intake. Bumetanide can make your body lose potassium and you may need an extra supply. Some foods have a high potassium content such as bananas, coconuts, dates, figs, prunes, apricots, peaches, grapefruit juice, tomato juice, and orange juice. You may get dizzy or lightheaded. Do not drive, use machinery, or do anything that needs mental alertness until you know how bumetanide affects you. To reduce the risk of dizzy or fainting spells, do not sit or stand up quickly, especially if you are an older patient. Alcohol can make you lightheaded, dizzy and increase confusion. Avoid or limit intake of alcoholic drinks. If you are going to have surgery, tell your prescriber or health care professional that you are taking bumetanide.

What side effects may I notice from taking bumetanide?

Side effects that you should report to your prescriber or health care professional as soon as possible:
- blood in the urine
- blurred vision
- dry mouth
- fever or chills
- hearing loss, ringing in the ears
- increased thirst

- irregular heartbeat, chest pain
- muscle cramps, pain or weakness
- nausea, vomiting
- skin rash
- stomach pain
- unusual bleeding or bruising
- unusual tiredness or weakness

Side effects that usually do not require medical attention (report to your prescriber or health care professional if they continue or are bothersome):
- diarrhea
- dizziness or lightheadedness
- headache
- loss of appetite
- sexual difficulties, difficulty keeping an erection

Where can I keep my medicine?

Keep out of the reach of children in a container that small children cannot open. Store at room temperature between 15 and 30 degrees C (59 and 86 degrees F). Throw away any unused medicine after the expiration date.

Bupropion extended-release tablets and sustained-release tablets

WELLBUTRIN® XL;
150 mg; Tablet,
Extended Release
Glaxo Wellcome

WELLBUTRIN® SR;
100 mg; Tablet,
Extended Release
Glaxo Wellcome

This drug requires an FDA medication guide. See page xxxvii.

What are bupropion extended-release tablets and sustained-release tablets?

BUPROPION (Wellbutrin® XL, Wellbutrin® SR) is an antidepressant, a medicine that helps to lift mental depression. Bupropion acts differently from other antidepressants and may be useful for treating patients who have had unusual or limiting effects from other antidepressants. Occasionally bupropion is prescribed for other behavioral or emotional problems. Generic bupropion extended-release tablets are not yet available; however, generic sustained-release tablets are not available.

What should my health care professional know before I take bupropion?

They need to know if you have any of these conditions:
- frequently drink alcoholic beverages
- an eating disorder, such as anorexia or bulimia
- bipolar disorder or psychosis
- diabetes or high blood sugar, treated with medication
- heart disease, previous heart attack, or irregular heart beat
- head injury or brain tumor
- high blood pressure
- kidney disease
- liver disease
- seizures (convulsions)
- suicidal thoughts or a previous suicide attempt

- Tourette's syndrome
- use of sedatives
- weight loss
- an unusual or allergic reaction to bupropion, other medicines, foods, dyes, or preservatives
- breast-feeding
- pregnant or trying to become pregnant

How should I take this medicine?

Take bupropion extended-release tablets by mouth. Follow the directions on the prescription label. Swallow the tablets whole with a drink of water. Do not crush or chew these tablets. Do not cut these tablets in half. It is important to take your doses at regular intervals; this medicine is taken once daily at the same time each day. Do not take your medicine more often than directed. Do not stop taking the tablets except on your prescriber's advice. If you take more than one dose of bupropion daily: To limit difficulty in sleeping, the second dose of the day should not be taken at bedtime; take it earlier in the day, but at least 8 hours after your morning dose. Contact your pediatrician or health care professional regarding the use of this medicine in children. Special care may be needed.

What if I miss a dose?

If you miss a dose, skip the missed dose and take your next tablet at the regular time. There should be 8 hours between doses. Do not take double or extra doses.

What may interact with bupropion?

NOTE: Do not take bupropion with other medicines containing bupropion, like Zyban®.

Other medicines that can interact with bupropion include:

- alcohol
- amphetamine
- carbamazepine
- cimetidine
- cocaine
- corticosteroids
- dextroamphetamine
- kava kava, Piper methysticum
- levodopa or combination drugs containing levodopa
- linezolid
- medications or herbal products for weight control or appetite
- medicines for mental depression, emotional, or psychotic disturbances
- medicines for difficulty sleeping
- medicines called MAO inhibitors-phenelzine (Nardil®), tranylcypromine (Parnate®), isocarboxazid (Marplan®), and selegiline (Eldepryl®)
- nicotine
- orphenadrine
- phenobarbital
- phenytoin
- rifampin
- ritonavir
- some medicines for heart rhythm or blood pressure
- some medicines for migraine headache (propranolol)
- some medicines for pain, such as codeine
- St. John's wort, Hypericum perforatum
- theophylline
- tramadol
- valerian, Valeriana officinalis
- valproic acid
- warfarin

Tell your prescriber or health care professional about all other medicines you are taking, including non-prescription medicines. Also, tell your prescriber or health care professional if you are a frequent user of drinks with caffeine or alcohol, if you smoke, or if you use illegal drugs. These may affect the way your medicine works. Check with your health care professional before stopping or starting any of your medicines.

What should I watch for while taking bupropion?

Visit your prescriber or health care professional for regular checks on your progress. You may have to take bupropion for several days before you see the effects. If you have been taking bupropion for some time, do not suddenly stop taking it. Your prescriber or health care professional may want you to gradually reduce the dose; ask for advice. Patients and their families should watch out for worsening depression or thoughts of suicide. Also watch out for sudden or severe changes in feelings such as feeling anxious, agitated, panicky, irritable, hostile, aggressive, impulsive, severely restless, overly excited and hyperactive, or not being able to sleep. If this happens, especially at the beginning of bupropion treatment or after a change in dose, call your doctor. Alcohol may increase dizziness or drowsiness; avoid alcoholic drinks while taking bupropion. Drinking excessive alcoholic beverages, using sleeping or anxiety medicines, or quickly stopping the use of these agents while taking bupropion may increase your risk for a seizure (convulsion). You may get dizzy or have blurred vision. Do not drive, use machinery, or do anything that needs mental alertness until you know how bupropion affects you. Do not stand or sit up quickly, especially if you are an older patient. This reduces the risk of dizzy or fainting spells. Bupropion can make your mouth dry. Chewing sugarless gum, sucking hard candy and drinking plenty of water will help. Do not treat yourself for coughs, colds, or allergies without asking your prescriber or health care professional for advice. Also do not take any herbal or non-prescription medicines for weight loss without your prescriber's advice. Some ingredients may increase possible side effects. If you are going to have surgery, tell your prescriber or health care professional well before your scheduled surgery that you are taking bupropion.

What side effects may I notice from taking bupropion?

Side effects that you should report to your prescriber or health care professional as soon as possible:

Uncommon:

- blurred vision
- difficulty breathing or wheezing
- fast or irregular heartbeat (palpitations)
- increased blood pressure
- hallucinations
- redness, blistering, peeling or loosening of the skin, including inside the mouth
- unusual tiredness or weakness

More common:

- agitation, anxiety, or restlessness, especially in the first week of treatment or when doses are changed
- confusion
- seizures
- skin rash, itching, hives
- vomiting

Side effects that usually do not require medical attention (report to your prescriber or health care professional if they continue or are bothersome):

Less common:

- loss of appetite
- loss of sexual drive
- menstrual changes

More common:

- change in taste
- constipation
- difficulty sleeping
- dizziness
- dry mouth
- headache
- increased sweating

- nausea
- tremor
- weight loss

Where can I keep my medicine?

Keep out of the reach of children in a container that small children cannot open. Store at room temperature between 20 and 25 degrees C (68 and 77 degrees F), away from direct sunlight and moisture. Keep tightly closed. Throw away any unused medicine after the expiration date.

Bupropion sustained-release tablets

ZYBAN®;
150 mg; Tablet, Extended Release
Glaxo Wellcome

What are bupropion sustained-release tablets?

BUPROPION (Zyban®) is a prescription medicine to help people quit smoking. Bupropion can reduce the symptoms caused by stopping smoking. Bupropion can also decrease the urge to smoke and decrease nicotine cravings. Bupropion is used with a patient support program recommended by your physician. Generic bupropion sustained-release tablets for Zyban® are not yet available. NOTE: You should only use Zyban® with nicotine skin patches or nicotine gum if these have been prescribed by your healthcare prescriber. Ask your prescriber for information and advice before purchasing any non-prescription nicotine products while you are on Zyban®. The use of the two medicines together requires special observation by your prescriber.

What should my health care professional know before I take bupropion?

They need to know if you have any of these conditions:
- frequently drink alcoholic beverages
- an eating disorder, such as anorexia or bulimia
- bipolar disorder or psychosis
- diabetes or high blood sugar, treated with medication
- heart disease, previous heart attack, or irregular heart beat
- head injury or brain tumor
- high blood pressure
- kidney disease
- liver disease
- seizures (convulsions)
- suicidal thoughts or a previous suicide attempt
- Tourette's syndrome
- use of sedatives
- weight loss
- an unusual or allergic reaction to bupropion, other medicines, foods, dyes, or preservatives
- breast-feeding
- pregnant or trying to become pregnant

How should I take this medicine?

NOTE: You should schedule to stop smoking during the second week of taking bupropion. You may smoke up until that day, bupropion takes about 1 week before it starts to control nicotine cravings. Choose your "quit date" and tell your prescriber. Stick to your plan; ask your prescriber about support groups or other ways to help you remain a "quitter." Take bupropion tablets by mouth. Follow the directions on the prescription label. Swallow the tablets whole with a drink of water. Do not crush or chew these tablets. Do not cut these tablets in half unless instructed to do so by your health care prescriber. It is important to take your doses at regular intervals. Do not take your medicine more often than directed. Do not stop taking the tablets except on your prescriber's advice. If you take more than one dose of bupropion daily: To limit difficulty in sleeping, the second dose of the day should not be taken at bedtime; take it earlier in the day but at least 8 hours after your morning dose. Contact your pediatrician or health care professional regarding the use of this medicine in children. Special care may be needed.

What if I miss a dose?

If you miss a dose, take it as soon as you can. If it is less than four hours to your next dose, skip the missed dose. Do not take double or extra doses.

What may interact with bupropion?

NOTE: Do not take bupropion with other medicines containing bupropion, like Wellbutrin® or Wellbutrin®SR.

Other medicines that can interact with bupropion include:

- alcohol
- amphetamine
- carbamazepine
- cimetidine
- cocaine
- corticosteroids
- dextroamphetamine
- kava kava, Piper methysticum
- levodopa or combination drugs containing levodopa
- linezolid
- medications or herbal products for weight control or appetite
- medicines for mental depression, emotional, or psychotic disturbances
- medicines for difficulty sleeping
- medicines called MAO inhibitors-phenelzine (Nardil®), tranylcypromine (Parnate®), isocarboxazid (Marplan®), and selegiline (Eldepryl®)
- nicotine
- orphenadrine

- phenobarbital
- phenytoin
- rifampin
- ritonavir
- some medicines for heart rhythm or blood pressure
- some medicines for migraine headache (propranolol)
- some medicines for pain, such as codeine
- St. John's wort, Hypericum perforatum
- theophylline
- tramadol
- valerian, Valeriana officinalis
- valproic acid
- warfarin

Tell your prescriber or health care professional about all other medicines you are taking, including non-prescription medicines. Also, tell your prescriber or health care professional if you are a frequent user of drinks with caffeine or alcohol, if you smoke, or if you use illegal drugs. These may affect the way your medicine works. Check with your health care professional before stopping or starting any of your medicines.

What should I watch for while taking bupropion?

The goal of taking medication for smoking cessation is to stop smoking or using tobacco. Ask for ongoing advice and encouragement from your prescriber, friends, and family to help you quit. If you smoke while on this medication, quit again. Visit your prescriber or health care professional for regular checks on your progress. You may have to take bupropion for several days before you see the effects. If you have been taking bupropion for some time, do not suddenly stop taking it. Your prescriber or health care professional may want you to gradually reduce the dose; ask for advice. Even though you are using bupropion to help you stop smoking or use of tobacco products, you and your family or caregivers should watch out for signs of depression or thoughts of suicide. Also watch out for sudden or severe changes in feelings such as feeling anxious, agitated, panicky, irritable, hostile, aggressive, impulsive, severely restless, overly excited and hyperactive, or not being able to sleep. If this happens, especially at the beginning of bupropion treatment or after a change in dose, call your doctor. Alcohol may increase dizziness or drowsiness; avoid alcoholic drinks while taking bupropion. Drinking excessive alcoholic beverages, using sleeping or anxiety medicines, or quickly stopping the use of these agents while taking bupropion may increase your risk for a seizure (convulsion). Do not use nicotine patches or chewing gum without the advice of your prescriber while on bupropion. You may need to have your blood pressure taken regularly if your prescriber recommends that you use both nicotine and bupropion together. You may get dizzy or have blurred vision. Do not drive, use machinery, or do anything that needs mental alertness until you know how bupropion affects you. Do not stand or sit up quickly,

especially if you are an older patient. This reduces the risk of dizzy or fainting spells. Bupropion can make your mouth dry. Chewing sugarless gum, sucking hard candy and drinking plenty of water will help. Do not treat yourself for coughs, colds, or allergies without asking your prescriber or health care professional for advice. Also do not take any herbal or non-prescription medicines for weight loss without your prescriber's advice. Some ingredients may increase possible side effects. If you are going to have surgery, tell your prescriber or health care professional well before your scheduled surgery that you are taking bupropion.

What side effects may I notice from taking bupropion?

Side effects that you should report to your prescriber or health care professional as soon as possible:
Uncommon:
- blurred vision
- difficulty breathing or wheezing
- fast or irregular heartbeat (palpitations)
- increased blood pressure
- hallucinations
- redness, blistering, peeling or loosening of the skin, including inside the mouth
- unusual tiredness or weakness

More common:
- agitation, anxiety, or restlessness, especially in the first week of treatment or when doses are changed
- confusion
- seizures
- skin rash, itching, hives
- vomiting

Side effects that usually do not require medical attention (report to your prescriber or health care professional if they continue or are bothersome):
Less common:
- loss of appetite
- loss of sexual drive
- menstrual changes

More common:
- change in taste
- constipation
- difficulty sleeping
- dizziness
- dry mouth
- headache
- increased sweating
- nausea
- tremor
- weight loss

Where can I keep my medicine?

Keep out of the reach of children in a container that small children cannot open. Store at room temperature between 20 and 25 degrees C (68 and 77 degrees F), away from direct sunlight and moisture. Keep tightly closed. Throw any unused medicine after the expiration date.

Bupropion tablets

WELLBUTRIN®;
100 mg; Tablet
Glaxo Wellcome

WELLBUTRIN®;
75 mg; Tablet
Glaxo Wellcome

What are bupropion tablets?

BUPROPION (Wellbutrin®) is an antidepressant, a medicine that helps to lift mental depression. Bupropion acts differently from other antidepressants and may be useful for treating patients who have had unusual or limiting effects from other antidepressants. Occasionally bupropion is prescribed for other behavioral or emotional problems. Generic bupropion tablets are available.

What should my health care professional know before I take bupropion?

They need to know if you have any of these conditions:
- frequently drink alcoholic beverages
- an eating disorder, such as anorexia or bulimia
- bipolar disorder or psychosis
- heart disease, previous heart attack, or irregular heart beat
- head injury or brain tumor
- high blood pressure
- kidney disease
- liver disease
- seizures (convulsions)
- suicidal thoughts or a previous suicide attempt
- Tourette's syndrome
- use of sedatives
- weight loss
- an unusual or allergic reaction to bupropion, other medicines, foods, dyes, or preservatives
- breast-feeding
- pregnant or trying to become pregnant

How should I take this medicine?

Take bupropion tablets by mouth. Follow the directions on the prescription label. Swallow the tablets with a drink of water. It is important to take your doses at regular intervals. Do not take your medicine more often than directed. Do not stop taking the tablets except on your prescriber's advice. Contact your pediatrician or health care professional regarding the use of this medicine in children. Special care may be needed.

What if I miss a dose?

If you miss a dose, take it as soon as you can. If it is less than four hours to your next dose, take only that dose and skip the missed dose. Do not take double or extra doses.

What may interact with bupropion?

NOTE: Do not take bupropion with other medicines containing bupropion, like Zyban®
Other medicines that can interact with bupropion include:

- alcohol
- amphetamine
- carbamazepine
- cimetidine
- cocaine
- corticosteroids
- dextroamphetamine
- kava kava, Piper methysticum
- levodopa or combination drugs containing levodopa
- linezolid
- medications or herbal products for weight control or appetite
- medicines for mental depression, emotional, or psychotic disturbances
- medicines for difficulty sleeping
- medicines called MAO inhibitors-phenelzine (Nardil®), tranylcypromine (Parnate®), isocarboxazid (Marplan®), and selegiline (Eldepryl®)
- nicotine
- orphenadrine
- phenobarbital
- phenytoin
- rifampin
- ritonavir
- some medicines for heart rhythm or blood pressure
- some medicines for migraine headache (propranolol)
- some medicines for pain, such as codeine
- St. John's wort, Hypericum perforatum
- theophylline
- tramadol
- valerian, Valeriana officinalis
- valproic acid
- warfarin

Tell your prescriber or health care professional about all other medicines you are taking, including non-prescription medicines. Also, tell your prescriber or health care professional if you are a frequent user of drinks with caffeine or alcohol, if you smoke, or if you use illegal drugs. These may affect the way your medicine works. Check with your health care professional before stopping or starting any of your medicines.

What should I watch for while taking bupropion?

Visit your prescriber or health care professional for regular checks on your progress. You may have to take bupropion for several days before you see the effects. If you have been taking bupropion for some time, do not suddenly stop taking it. Your prescriber or health care professional may want you to gradually reduce the dose; ask for advice. Patients and their families should watch out for worsening depression or thoughts of suicide. Also watch out for sudden or severe changes in feelings such as feeling anxious, agitated, panicky, irritable, hostile, aggressive, impulsive, severely restless, overly excited and hyperactive, or not being able to sleep. If this happens, especially at the beginning of bupropion treatment or after a change in dose, call your doctor. You may get dizzy or have blurred vision. Do not drive, use machinery, or do anything that needs mental alertness until you know how bupropion affects you. Do not stand or sit up quickly, especially if you are an older patient. This reduces the risk of dizzy or fainting spells. Alcohol may increase dizziness or drowsiness; avoid alcoholic drinks while taking bupropion. Drinking excessive alcoholic beverages, using sleeping or anxiety medicines, or quickly stopping the use of these agents while taking bupropion may increase your risk for a seizure (convulsion). Bupropion can make your mouth dry. Chewing sugarless gum, sucking hard candy and drinking plenty of water will help. Do not treat yourself for coughs, colds, or allergies without asking your prescriber or health care professional for advice. Also do not take any herbal or non-prescription medicines for weight loss without your prescriber's advice. Some ingredients may increase possible side effects. If you are going to have surgery, tell your prescriber or health care professional well before your scheduled surgery that you are taking bupropion.

What side effects may I notice from taking bupropion?

Side effects that you should report to your prescriber or health care professional as soon as possible:
Uncommon:
- blurred vision
- difficulty breathing or wheezing
- fast or irregular heartbeat (palpitations)
- increased blood pressure
- hallucinations

- redness, blistering, peeling or loosening of the skin, including inside the mouth
- unusual tiredness or weakness

More common:
- agitation, anxiety, or restlessness, especially in the first week of treatment or when doses are changed
- confusion
- seizures
- skin rash, itching, hives
- vomiting

Side effects that usually do not require medical attention (report to your prescriber or health care professional if they continue or are bothersome):
Less common:
- loss of appetite
- loss of sexual drive
- menstrual changes

More common:
- change in taste
- constipation
- difficulty sleeping
- dizziness
- dry mouth
- headache
- increased sweating
- nausea
- tremor
- weight loss

Where can I keep my medicine?

Keep out of the reach of children in a container that small children cannot open. Store at room temperature between 20 and 25 degrees C (68 and 77 degrees F), away from direct sunlight and moisture. Keep tightly closed. Throw away any unused medicine after the expiration date.

Buspirone tablets

BUSPAR®;
5 mg; Tablet
Bristol Myers Squibb
Co

BUSPAR®;
15 mg; Tablet
Bristol Myers Squibb
Co

What are buspirone tablets?

BUSPIRONE (Buspar®) helps to relieve certain states of anxiety. It is chemically different from other medicines that treat anxiety and has very little effect on mental alertness. Buspirone does not produce dependency problems. Generic buspirone tablets are available.

What should my health care professional know before I take buspirone?

They need to know if you have any of these conditions:
- if you are currently receiving other medications for the treatment of anxiety
- liver disease
- kidney disease
- an unusual or allergic reaction to buspirone, other medicines, foods, dyes, or preservatives
- pregnant or trying to get pregnant

- breast-feeding

How should I take this medicine?

Take buspirone tablets by mouth. Follow the directions on the prescription label. Swallow the tablets with a drink of water. You may take this medicine with or without food. However, to ensure that buspirone always works the same way for you, you should take buspirone either always with or always without food. Take your doses at regular intervals. Do not take your medicine more often than directed. Contact your pediatrician or health care professional regarding the use of this medicine in children. Special care may be needed.

What if I miss a dose?

If it is almost time for your next dose, take only that dose. Do not take double or extra doses.

What may interact with buspirone?

- alcohol
- aspirin
- carbamazepine
- clarithromycin
- digoxin
- diltiazem
- erythromycin
- furazolidone
- grapefruit juice (avoid drinking large amounts of grapefruit juice)
- haloperidol
- linezolid
- medicines called MAO inhibitors-phenelzine (Nardil®), tranylcypromine (Parnate®), isocarboxazid (Marplan®), selegiline (Eldepryl®)
- medicines for pain, like codeine or tramadol
- medicines for sleep
- other medications for anxiety
- phenobarbital
- phenytoin
- primidone
- procarbazine
- rifampin
- ritonavir
- some antifungal medicines (examples: itraconazole, ketoconazole, voriconazole)
- various medicines for mental depression or mood problems, like citalopram, fluoxetine, fluvoxamine, nefazodone, paroxetine, sertraline, trazodone or venlafaxine
- verapamil
- warfarin

Tell your prescriber or health care professional about all other medicines you are taking, including non-prescription medicines, nutritional supplements, or herbal products. Also tell your prescriber or health care professional if you are a frequent user of drinks with caffeine or alcohol, if you smoke, or if you use illegal drugs. These may affect the way your medicine works. Check with your health care professional before stopping or starting any of your medicines.

What should I watch for while taking buspirone?

Visit your prescriber or health care professional for regular checks on your progress. It may be one or two weeks before your anxiety goes away. Do not stop taking buspirone except on your prescriber's advice. You may get drowsy or dizzy. Do not drive, use machinery, or do anything that needs mental alertness until you know how buspirone affects you. Alcohol can increase possible drowsiness and dizziness and may make you more anxious. Avoid alcoholic drinks.

What side effects may I notice from taking buspirone?

Side effects that you should report to your prescriber or health care professional as soon as possible:
- blurred vision or other vision changes
- difficulty breathing
- chest pain
- confusion
- feelings of hostility or anger
- muscle aches and pains
- numbness or tingling in hands or feet
- ringing in the ears
- skin rash and itching (hives)
- sore throat
- vomiting
- weakness

Side effects that usually do not require medical attention (report to your prescriber or health care professional if they continue or are bothersome):
- disturbed dreams, nightmares
- dizziness
- drowsiness
- headache
- nasal congestion
- nausea
- restlessness or nervousness
- stomach upset

Where can I keep my medicine?

Keep out of the reach of children in a container that small children cannot open. Store at room temperature between 15 and 30 degrees C (59 and 86 degrees F). Protect from light. Keep container tightly closed. Throw away any unused medicine after the expiration date.

Butabarbital tablets

BUTISOL®;
30 mg; Tablet
Medpointe
Pharmaceuticals

BUTISOL®;
50 mg; Tablet
Medpointe
Pharmaceuticals

What are butabarbital tablets?

BUTABARBITAL (Butisol®) is a barbiturate that slows down activity of the brain and nervous system. Butabarbital has both sedative and hypnotic properties which means it will help you to relax and sleep. Butabarbital is only for short-term use of two weeks or less for treatment of insomnia (difficulty sleeping). Butabarbital can help produce relaxation and drowsiness before surgery. Federal law prohibits the transfer of butabarbital to any person other than the patient for whom it was prescribed. Do not share your medicine with anyone else. Generic butabarbital tablets are available.

B

What should my health care professional know before I take butabarbital?

They need to know if you have any of these conditions:
- an alcohol or drug abuse problem
- breathing difficulties or lung disease
- attempted suicide
- heart disease
- liver disease
- low blood pressure
- mental depression or mental problems
- porphyria
- an unusual or allergic reaction to butabarbital, other barbiturates, other medicines, foods, dyes (such as tartrazine), or preservatives
- pregnant or trying to get pregnant
- breast-feeding

How should I take this medicine?

Take butabarbital tablets by mouth. Follow the directions on the prescription label. Swallow the tablets with a drink of water. If butabarbital upsets your stomach, take it with food or milk. Do not take your medicine more often than directed. Elderly patients over age 65 years may have a stronger reaction to this medicine and need smaller doses.

What if I miss a dose?

Butabarbital should only be taken as needed to induce sleep or relaxation. If you are on a regular schedule and miss a dose, take it as soon as you can. Do not take double or extra doses.

What may interact with butabarbital?

- alcohol
- caffeine
- chloramphenicol
- chlorpromazine
- cyclophosphamide
- cyclosporine
- digitoxin
- doxorubicin
- doxycycline
- female hormones, including contraceptive or birth control pills
- methoxyflurane
- metronidazole
- medicines for anxiety or sleeping problems
- medicines for hay fever and other allergies
- medicines for high blood pressure
- medicines for mental depression
- medicines for pain
- medicines that help the heart to beat regularly
- quinine
- seizure (convulsion) or epilepsy medicine
- steroid medicines such as prednisone or cortisone
- theophylline
- warfarin

Tell your prescriber or health care professional about all other medicines you are taking, including non-prescription medicines, nutritional supplements, or herbal products. Also tell your prescriber or health care professional if you are a frequent user of drinks with caffeine or alcohol, if you smoke, or if you use illegal drugs. These may affect the way your medicine works. Check with your health care professional before stopping or starting any of your medicines.

What should I watch for while taking butabarbital?

Visit your prescriber or health care professional for regular checks on your progress. If sleep medicine is taken every night for a long time it may no longer help you to sleep. In most cases butabarbital should not be taken for longer than 1 or 2 weeks. Consult your prescriber or health care professional if you still have difficulty in sleeping. If you have been taking butabarbital regularly and suddenly stop taking it, you may get unpleasant withdrawal symptoms. Your prescriber or health care professional may want to gradually reduce the dose. Do not stop taking except on your prescriber's advice. After taking butabarbital you may get a residual hangover effect that leaves you drowsy or dizzy. Do not drive, use machinery, or do anything that needs mental alertness until you know how butabarbital affects you. To reduce dizzy or fainting spells, do not sit or stand up quickly, especially if you are an older patient. Alcohol can increase possible unpleasant effects. Avoid alcoholic drinks. Butabarbital can stop birth control pills (oral contraceptives) from working properly. Use another method of birth control while you are taking butabarbital. If you are going to have surgery, tell your prescriber or health care professional that you are taking butabarbital.

What side effects may I notice from taking butabarbital?

Side effects that you should report to your prescriber or health care professional as soon as possible:
- bone tenderness
- confusion, agitation, changes in mood, or mental ability
- depression
- eye problems, very small or enlarged centers to the eyes
- lightheadedness, fainting spells
- fever, sore throat
- hallucinations
- redness, blistering, peeling or loosening of the skin, including inside the mouth
- shortness of breath, or difficulty breathing
- skin rash, itching, hives
- slow heartbeat
- swelling of the face or lips
- unusual bleeding or bruising; pinpoint red spots on the skin
- unusual tiredness or weakness
- weight loss
- yellowing of skin or eyes

Side effects that usually do not require medical attention (report to your prescriber or health care professional if they continue or are bothersome):

- clumsiness, unsteadiness, or a "hangover" effect
- constipation
- difficulty sleeping or nightmares
- drowsiness, dizziness
- headache
- irritability, nervousness
- nausea or vomiting

Where can I keep my medicine?

Keep out of the reach of children in a container that small children cannot open. Store at room temperature between 15 and 30 degrees C (59 and 85 degrees F). Keep container tightly closed. Throw away any unused medicine after the expiration date.

Cabergoline tablets

DOSTINEX®;
0.5 mg; Tablet
Pharmacia and Upjohn Div
Pfizer

What are cabergoline tablets?

CABERGOLINE (Dostinex®) is used to treat high levels of prolactin, a hormone made by the body that affects such things as the menstrual cycle, breast milk production, fertility, and sexual function. Cabergoline also treats high levels of prolactin which occur with certain tumors such as adenomas. This medication is sometimes used for the treatment of Parkinson's disease or restless-legs syndrome. Generic cabergoline tablets are available.

What should my health care professional know before I take cabergoline?

They need to know if you have any of these conditions:
- anxiety
- depression
- heart disease
- high or low blood pressure
- liver disease
- lung disease
- memory disorder
- schizophrenia
- an unusual or allergic reaction to cabergoline, other medicines, foods, dyes, or preservatives
- pregnant or trying to get pregnant
- breast-feeding

How should I take this medicine?

Take cabergoline tablets by mouth. Depending on your illness, you may take as little as one pill twice per week to as much as one pill daily. This medicine may be taken with or without food. Follow the directions on the prescription label. Do not take your medicine more often than directed. Contact your pediatrician or health care professional regarding the use of this medicine in children. Special care may be needed.

What if I miss a dose?

If you miss a dose, take it as soon as you can. If it is almost time for your next dose, take only that dose. Do not take double or extra doses.

What may interact with cabergoline?

- blood pressure medications
- chlorpromazine
- cimetidine
- clozapine
- dihydroergotamine
- ergoloid mesylates
- ergotamine
- fluphenazine
- haloperidol
- levodopa
- loxapine
- mesoridazine
- methyldopa
- methysergide
- metoclopramide
- molindone
- olanzapine
- perphenazine
- pimozide
- prochlorperazine
- promethazine
- quetiapine
- risperidone
- thiethylperazine
- thioridazine
- thiothixene

Tell your physician or health care provider about all other medicines you are taking, including non-prescription medicines, if you are a frequent user of drinks with caffeine or alcohol, if you smoke, or if you use illegal drugs. These may affect the way your medicine works. Check with your health care professional before stopping or starting any of your medicines.

What should I watch for while taking cabergoline?

If you are going to have surgery, tell your prescriber or health care professional that you are taking cabergoline. It may be helpful to take cabergoline with food if you experience nausea, stomach pain, or indigestion after taking it. If you experience dry mouth while taking cabergoline, make sure to drink plenty of water. It may also be helpful to suck on sugarless hard candy or crushed ice. If your dry mouth is severe, ask your doctor about a saliva substitute. Cabergoline can sometimes cause the blood pressure to temporarily drop. This may happen suddenly causing dizziness or lightheadedness if you try to stand up too quickly. Make sure to get up slowly from a lying or sitting position while taking cabergoline. Cabergoline may make you drowsy or dizzy. Do not drive, use machinery, or do anything that needs mental alertness until you know how cabergoline affects you. Avoid alcoholic beverages while taking cabergoline. Alcohol may add to side effects such as drowsiness or dizziness.

What side effects may I notice from taking cabergoline?

Side effects that you should report to your prescriber as soon as possible:
- confusion
- nausea/vomiting
- shortness of breath, wheezing

- skin rash, skin lumps, or hives
- tingling or numbness in hands or feet
- weakness

Stop using cabergoline and call your prescriber as soon as you can if you get any of these side effects.

Side effects that usually do not require medical attention (report to your prescriber or health care professional if they continue or are bothersome):
- constipation
- diarrhea
- dizziness
- drowsiness
- dry mouth
- headache

- indigestion
- low blood pressure
- nervousness
- pain in stomach or abdomen
- pain with menstruation
- swelling in ankles
- tiredness

Where can I keep my medicine?

Keep out of the reach of children in a container that small children cannot open. Store at room temperature between 20 and 25 degrees C (68 and 77 degrees F). Protect from light and moisture. Throw away any unused medicine after the expiration date.

Caffeine tablets or caplets

MAXIMUM STRENGTH STAY AWAKE™; 200 mg; Tablet Walgreens Health Initiatives

ALERTNESS AID®; 200 mg; Tablet Leader Brand Products

What are caffeine tablets or caplets?

CAFFEINE (Alertness Aid®, Enerjets®, Maximum Strength Stay Awake™, NoDoz®, Snap-Back®, Stay-Alert®, Vivarin®) acts as a central nervous system (CNS) or brain stimulant, increasing alertness in people who are tired or sleepy. Caffeine occurs naturally in tea, coffee, cocoa, and chocolate, and is added to many soft drinks. Generic forms of caffeine are available, and can be obtained without a prescription.

What should my health care professional know before I take caffeine?

They need to know if you have any of these conditions:
- anxiety
- diabetes
- heart disease or irregular heartbeat
- high blood pressure
- kidney disease
- liver disease
- panic attacks
- peptic ulcer disease or colitis
- seizure disorder
- thyroid disease
- trouble sleeping
- an unusual or allergic reaction to caffeine, aminophylline, theophylline, other medicines, foods, dyes, or preservatives
- pregnant or trying to get pregnant
- breast-feeding

How should I take this medicine?

Take caffeine tablets or caplets by mouth. Follow the directions on the prescription label. Swallow with a drink of water; do not take with grapefruit juice. If you are taking an extended-release form of caffeine, swallow whole, do not crush or chew. If you are taking chewable tablets, chew well and swallow. Do not take your medicine more often than directed. Do not stop taking except on your prescriber's advice. Contact your pediatrician or health care professional regarding the use of this medicine in children. Special care may be needed.

What if I miss a dose?

If you miss a dose, take it as soon as you can. If it is almost time for your next dose, take only that dose. Do not take double or extra doses.

What may interact with caffeine?

- cimetidine
- ciprofloxacin
- clarithromycin
- clozapine
- ephedra, *Ma huang*
- erythromycin
- female hormones, like estrogen or birth control pills
- fluvoxamine
- grapefruit juice
- guarana
- ketoconazole
- lithium
- medicines called MAO inhibitors-phenelzine, tranylcypromine, isocarboxazid, selegiline
- medicines for colds and breathing difficulties
- medicines for sleep
- medicines for weight loss
- phenobarbital
- phenytoin
- rifampin
- stimulants like amphetamine, dextroamphetamine, methylphenidate
- tacrine
- terbinafine
- theophylline

Tell your prescriber or health care professional about all other medicines you are taking, including non-prescription medicines, nutritional supplements, or herbal

products. Also tell your prescriber or health care professional if you are a frequent user of drinks with caffeine or alcohol, if you smoke, or if you use illegal drugs. These may affect the way your medicine works. Check with your health care professional before stopping or starting any of your medicines.

What should I watch for while taking caffeine?

Caffeine is not intended for long-term use. Do not use caffeine products regularly to make up for lost sleep. Do not increase the dose if tolerance develops; your body will not develop a tolerance to the harmful side effects of caffeine. See your prescriber or health care professional if you continue to experience tiredness or constant sleepiness; this may indicate a problem needing medical attention. Do not take caffeine close to bedtime. It may prevent you from sleeping. If you have been a regular caffeine user you can get withdrawal symptoms if you stop taking caffeine. Symptoms include tiredness, dizziness, headache, anxiety, or nervousness. This can be a weekend effect for people who drink a lot of coffee during their working week. If you are taking caffeine as a part of a medical treatment, avoid food and drinks that contain additional caffeine, like coffee, tea, colas and chocolate. Do not take caffeine with other non-prescription medicines, especially cold and allergy medicines, without asking your prescriber or health care professional for advice. Do not take caffeine with grapefruit juice, this can increase the effects of caffeine.

What side effects may I notice from taking caffeine?

Side effects that you should report to your prescriber or health care professional as soon as possible:
- anxiety or panic reactions
- confusion
- dizziness, lightheadedness, or fainting spells
- fast or irregular breathing or heartbeat (palpitations)
- muscle twitching
- nausea and vomiting
- seizures (convulsions)
- trembling

Side effects that usually do not require medical attention (report to your prescriber or health care professional if they continue or are bothersome):
- diarrhea
- frequent passing of urine
- headache
- nervousness, restlessness
- stomach upset

Reduce your intake of caffeine if you get any of these side effects. Let your prescriber or health care professional know about them if they do not go away or if they annoy you.

Where can I keep my medicine?

Keep out of the reach of children in a container that small children cannot open. Store at room temperature between 15 and 30 degrees C (59 and 86 degrees F). Throw away any unused medicine after the expiration date.

Caffeine; Ergotamine tablets

CAFERGOT®;
100 mg/1 mg; Tablet
Novartis Pharmaceuticals

What are caffeine; ergotamine tablets?

CAFFEINE; ERGOTAMINE (Cafergot®) is one of a group of medicines known as ergot alkaloids. Caffeine; ergotamine preparations help to prevent certain kinds of throbbing headaches such as migraine and cluster headaches. This medication should be used as soon as you know a headache is starting. Generic caffeine; ergotamine tablets are available.

What should my health care professional know before I take caffeine; ergotamine?

They need to know if you have any of these conditions:
- blood clots
- chest pain
- history of heart attacks
- heart or blood vessel disease
- high blood pressure
- high cholesterol
- infection
- kidney disease
- liver disease

- lung disease
- poor circulation
- stroke
- tobacco smoker
- an unusual or allergic reaction to caffeine, ergotamine, other medicines, foods, dyes, or preservatives
- pregnant or trying to get pregnant
- breast-feeding

How should I take this medicine?

Take caffeine; ergotamine tablets by mouth. Follow the directions on the prescription label. Swallow the tablets with a drink of water. Do not take your medicine more often than directed. Do not stop taking except on your prescriber's advice. Contact your pediatrician or health care professional regarding the use of this medicine in children. Special care may be needed.

What if I miss a dose?

This does not apply since you only take caffeine; ergotamine tablets when you have a headache. Do not take double or extra doses.

What may interact with caffeine; ergotamine?

Do not use any of the following migraine drugs within 24 hours of this medicine:

- almotriptan
- eletriptan
- frovatriptan
- naratriptan
- rizatriptan
- sumatriptan
- zolmitriptan

Also, do not use this drug with:

- ergotamine (Ergomar®)
- dihydroergotamine (DHE® or Migranal®)
- methysergide (Sansert®)
- ergonovine
- methylergonovine (Methergine®)

Caffeine; ergotamine may also interact with:

- antibiotics such as erythromycin, clarithromycin, and troleandomycin
- antifungal drugs like fluconazole, itraconazole, ketoconazole or voriconazole
- aprepitant
- bromocriptine
- cabergoline
- cocaine
- danazol
- ergoloid mesylates (Hydergine®)
- herbal products like feverfew or guarana
- fluoxetine
- fluvoxamine
- grapefruit juice
- imatinib, STI-571
- medicines for colds, flu, or breathing difficulties
- medicines for high blood pressure
- medicines or herbal products to decrease weight or appetite
- metronidazole
- nefazodone
- nicotine
- some medications for the treatment of HIV infection or AIDS
- zileuton

Tell your prescriber or health care professional about all other medicines you are taking, including non-prescription medicines, nutritional supplements, or herbal products. Also tell your prescriber or health care professional if you are a frequent user of drinks with caffeine or alcohol, if you smoke, or if you use illegal drugs. These may affect the way your medicine works. Check with your health care professional before stopping or starting any of your medicines.

What should I watch for while taking caffeine; ergotamine?

Check with your prescriber or health care professional if you do not get relief from your headaches after using this medication. You may need to be changed to a different kind of medicine to treat your migraines. It is important to tell your prescriber or health care professional as soon as possible if you get any of the following side effects: cold, numb, or painful hands or feet; leg cramps when walking; any type of pain around your chest; swelling; itching. Caffeine; ergotamine tablets decrease the circulation of blood to your skin, fingers, and toes. You may get more sensitive to the cold. Elderly patients are more likely to feel this effect. Dress warmly and avoid long exposure to the cold. Because this medicine contains caffeine, you may wish to limit your intake of caffeinated beverages on the days that you use this medicine. Alcohol can make headaches worse or bring on a new headache. Therefore, you should avoid alcoholic drinks. Because smoking can increase side effects of caffeine; ergotamine combinations, you should avoid smoking. If you are going to have any type of surgery, tell your prescriber or health care professional that you are taking caffeine; ergotamine.

What side effects may I notice from taking caffeine; ergotamine?

Side effects that you should report to your prescriber or health care professional as soon as possible:

- blurred vision
- chest pain or tightness
- cold hands or feet
- confusion
- decrease in the amount of urine passed
- difficulty breathing
- fast, slow, or pounding heartbeat
- fever or chills
- itching
- leg or arm pain or cramps
- seizures
- stomach pain
- swelling of hands, ankles, or feet
- tingling, pain or numbness in feet or hands
- vomiting
- weakness

Side effects that usually do not require medical attention (report to your prescriber or health care professional if they continue or are bothersome):

- increased urination
- nausea

Where can I keep my medicine?

Keep out of the reach of children in a container that small children cannot open. Store at room temperature between 15 and 30 degrees C (59 and 86 degrees F). Protect from light and moisture. Throw away any unused medicine after the expiration date. Keep container tightly closed.

Calcifediol capsules

CALDEROL®;
20 mcg; Capsule
Organon USA Inc

What are calcifediol capsules?

CALCIFEDIOL (Calderol®) is a man-made form of vitamin D. Vitamin D is necessary to maintain the right amount of calcium in the body for strong bones and teeth. Calcifediol helps your body keep the proper levels of calcium and phosphorus and maintain healthy bones. Generc calcifediol capsules are not yet available.

What should my health care professional know before I take calcifediol?

They need to know if you have any of the following conditions:

- kidney disease
- too much calcium or vitamin D in the blood
- parathyroid disease
- other chronic illness
- an unusual or allergic reaction to vitamin D, other medicines, foods, dyes, or preservatives
- pregnant or trying to get pregnant
- breast-feeding

How should I take this medicine?

Take calcifediol capsules by mouth. Follow the directions on the prescription label. Swallow the capsules with a drink of water. Take exactly as directed. Do not exceed the prescribed dose because calcifediol is stored in the body.

What if I miss a dose?

If you miss a dose, take it as soon as you can. If it is almost time for your next dose, take only that dose. Do not take double or extra doses.

What may interact with calcifediol?

- cholestyramine
- colestipol
- digoxin
- ketoconazole
- orlistat
- mineral oil
- seizure (convulsion) or epilepsy medicine
- water pills

Talk to your prescriber or other health care professional before taking any of these medicines:

- antacids
- calcium supplements
- magnesium supplements
- vitamin D

Tell your prescriber or health care professional about all other medicines you are taking, including non-prescription medicines, nutritional supplements, or herbal products. Also tell your prescriber or health care professional if you are a frequent user of drinks with caffeine or alcohol, if you smoke, or if you use illegal drugs. These may affect the way your medicine works. Check with your health care professional before stopping or starting any of your medicines.

What should I watch for while taking calcifediol?

Visit your prescriber or health care professional for regular checks on your progress. You may need a special diet and to take calcium supplements. Do not take any non-prescription medicines that contain vitamin D, phosphorus, magnesium, or calcium including antacids while taking calcifediol, unless your prescriber or health care professional says you can. The extra calcium, phosphorus, magnesium, or vitamin D can lead to side effects. Do not take more calcium, magnesium, or vitamin D than your prescriber or health care professional recommends.

What side effects may I notice from taking calcifediol?

The recommended daily allowance of calcifediol does not usually cause any side effects.

Early side effects related to overdose include:

- bone pain
- constipation
- dry mouth
- headache
- metallic taste
- nausea, vomiting
- unusual tiredness, or weakness

Late side effects include:

- increased thirst
- increase in the need to pass urine (especially at night)
- irregular heartbeat, high blood pressure
- loss of appetite
- seizures (convulsions)
- stomach pain
- weight loss

Where can I keep my medicine?

Keep out of the reach of children in a container that small children cannot open. Store at room temperature between 15 and 30 degrees C (59 and 86 degrees F). Protect from light. Keep container tightly closed. Throw away any unused medicine after the expiration date.

Calcitonin injection

MIACALCIN®;
200 unit/ml; Injection
Novartis Pharmaceuticals

What is calcitonin injection?

CALCITONIN (Miacalcin®) controls the amount of calcium in your body and helps maintain proper bone density. Calcitonin is used to treat diseases of the bone such as Paget's disease and osteoporosis. Calcitonin is used to treat excess amounts of calcium in the blood. Generic calcitonin injection is available.

What should my health care professional know before I receive calcitonin?

They need to know if you have any of these conditions:
- low level of blood calcium
- an unusual or allergic reaction to calcitonin, fish, other medicines, foods, dyes, or preservatives
- pregnant or trying to get pregnant
- breast-feeding

How should I use this medicine?

Calcitonin is for injection into a muscle or under the skin. If you have been instructed to give yourself calcitonin injections, make sure that you understand how to prepare and inject the dose. Use exactly as directed. Do not exceed the prescribed dose, and do not use more or less often than prescribed. Contact your pediatrician or health care professional regarding the use of this medicine in children. Special care may be needed.

What if I miss a dose?

If you use two doses per day, give the missed dose only if you remember within 2 hours. Otherwise, skip the dose and resume your regular schedule with the next dose. Do not use double doses. If you use one dose per day, give the missed dose as soon as you remember on the day the dose was due. If you do not remember until the next day, skip the dose and resume your regular schedule with the next dose. Do not use double doses. If you use one dose every other day, give the missed dose as soon as you remember on the day the dose was due. If you do not remember until the next day, use the dose and skip a day to resume an every-other-day schedule. Do not use double doses. If you use three doses per week (Monday, Wednesday, Friday), give the missed dose as soon as you remember on the day the dose was due. If you do not remember until the next day, give the missed dose and give the rest of the doses a day later than normal. Do not use double doses or use doses two days in a row. Return to your regular schedule the following week.

What drug(s) may interact with calcitonin?

- lithium

Tell your prescriber or health care professional about all other medicines you are taking, including non-prescription medicines, nutritional supplements, or herbal products. Also tell your prescriber or health care professional if you are a frequent user of drinks with caffeine or alcohol, if you smoke, or if you use illegal drugs. These may affect the way your medicine works. Check with your health care professional before stopping or starting any of your medicines.

What should I watch for while taking calcitonin?

Visit your prescriber or health care professional for regular checks on your progress. Calcitonin can make your blood calcium level dangerously low. You will need regular blood tests while using calcitonin. Ask your prescriber or health care professional about calcium in your diet. You may also need to take supplements of calcium and vitamin D while you are receiving calcitonin, unless you are being treated for high calcium levels. Discuss whether calcium and vitamin D supplements are right for you with your prescriber or health care provider. Store needles and syringes out of the reach of children. Make sure you receive a puncture-resistant container to dispose of the needles and syringes once you have finished with them. Do not reuse these items. Return the container to your prescriber or health care professional for proper disposal.

What side effects may I notice from taking calcitonin?

Side effects that you should report to your prescriber or health care professional as soon as possible:
- chest pain, fast or irregular heartbeat (palpitations)
- difficulty breathing, wheezing
- dizziness
- fever, chills
- rash or itching (hives)
- swelling of the tongue, difficulty swallowing
- tingling in the hands or feet

Side effects that usually do not require medical attention (report to your prescriber or health care professional if they continue or are bothersome):
- diarrhea
- flushing (reddening of the face, ears, or hands)
- headache
- heartburn
- loss of appetite
- nausea, vomiting
- pain, redness, irritation or swelling at the injection site
- stomach pain

Where can I keep my medicine?

Keep out of the reach of children. Store in a refrigerator between 2 and 8 degrees C (36 and 46 degrees F); do not freeze. Throw away any unused medicine after the expiration date.

Candesartan tablets

ATACAND®;
16 mg; Tablet
AstraZeneca LP

ATACAND®;
32 mg; Tablet
AstraZeneca LP

What are candesartan tablets?

CANDESARTAN (Atacand®) lowers elevated blood pressure. High blood pressure levels can cause you to have a stroke, get heart failure, or damage your kidneys. Candesartan helps prevent these things from happening. Generic candesartan tablets are not yet available.

What should my health care professional know before I take candesartan?

They need to know if you have any of these conditions:

- heart failure
- kidney disease
- liver disease
- electrolyte imbalance (e.g. low or high levels of potassium in the blood)
- if you are on a special diet, such as a low-salt diet (e.g. using potassium substitutes)
- an unusual or allergic reaction to candesartan, other medicines, foods, dyes, or preservatives
- pregnant or trying to get pregnant
- breast-feeding

How should I take this medicine?

Take candesartan tablets by mouth. Follow the directions on the prescription label. Swallow the tablets with a drink of water. Candesartan can be taken with or without food. Take your doses at regular intervals. Do not take your medicine more often than directed. Do not stop taking candesartan except on your prescriber's advice.

What if I miss a dose?

If you miss a dose, take it as soon as you can. If it is almost time for your next dose, take only that dose. Do not take double or extra doses.

What may interact with candesartan?

- blood pressure medications
- hawthorn
- lithium
- potassium salts or potassium supplements
- water pills (especially potassium-sparing diuretics such as triamterene or amiloride)

Tell your prescriber or health care professional about all other medicines you are taking, including non-prescription medicines, nutritional supplements, or herbal products. Also tell your prescriber or health care professional if you are a frequent user of drinks with caffeine or alcohol, if you smoke, or if you use illegal drugs. These may affect the way your medicine works. Check with your health care professional before stopping or starting any of your medicines.

What should I watch for while taking candesartan?

Check your blood pressure regularly while you are taking candesartan. Ask your prescriber or health care professional what your blood pressure should be and when you should contact him or her. Call your prescriber or health care professional if you notice an uneven or fast heart beat. It is very important that you take this medicine exactly as prescribed by your prescriber or health care professional. Many patients who have high blood pressure will not notice any signs of the problem. Therefore, it is important that you keep regular appointments with your prescriber or health care professional even if you feel well. If you are going to have surgery tell your prescriber or health care professional that you are taking candesartan.

What side effects may I notice from taking candesartan?

Side effects that you should report to your prescriber or health care professional as soon as possible:
Rare or uncommon:

- difficulty breathing or swallowing, hoarseness, or tightening of the throat
- swelling of your face, lips, tongue, hands, or feet

Other:

- confusion, dizziness, lightheadedness or fainting spells
- decreased amount of urine passed
- fast or uneven heart beat or palpitations

Side effects that usually do not require medical attention (report to your prescriber or health care professional if they continue or are bothersome):

- back pain
- cough
- dizziness or lightheadedness
- headache
- sore throat
- nasal congestion or runny nose

Where can I keep my medicine?

Keep out of the reach of children in a container that small children cannot open. Store at room temperature between 15 and 30 degrees C (59 and 86 degrees F). Protect from light. Keep container tightly closed. Throw away any unused medicine after the expiration date.

Candesartan; Hydrochlorothiazide, HCTZ tablets

ATACAND® HCT;
16 mg/12.5 mg;
Tablet
AstraZeneca LP

ATACAND® HCT;
Tablet; 32 mg/
12.5 mg
AstraZeneca LP

What are candesartan-hydrochlorothiazide tablets?

CANDESARTAN-HYDROCHLOROTHIAZIDE (Atacand® HCT) is a combination of two drugs used to lower blood pressure. Candesartan controls high blood pressure (hypertension) by relaxing blood vessels. Hydrochlorothiazide is a diuretic. High blood pressure can damage the blood vessels of the brain, heart, and kidneys, resulting in a stroke, heart failure, or kidney failure. This medicine does not cure high blood pressure. By lowering blood pressure, candesartan-hydrochlorothiazide can help reduce your risk of having damage to your kidneys, heart, or other organs. Generic candesartan-hydrochlorothiazide tablets are not yet available.

What should my health care professional know before I take candesartan-hydrochlorothiazide?

They need to know if you have any of these conditions:
- autoimmune disease (like lupus), or suppressed immune function
- diabetes mellitus
- gout
- heart or blood vessel disease (such as heart failure)
- liver disease
- recent heart attack or stroke
- kidney disease (such as renal failure or renal artery stenosis)
- pancreatitis
- electrolyte imbalance (e.g. low or high levels of potassium in the blood)
- if you are on a special diet, such as a low-salt diet (e.g. using potassium substitutes)
- sulfonamide (sulfa) or thiazide allergy
- an unusual or allergic reaction to candesartan, hydrochlorothiazide, other medicines, foods, dyes, or preservatives
- pregnant or trying to get pregnant
- breast-feeding

How should I take this medicine?

Take candesartan-hydrochlorothiazide tablets by mouth. Follow the directions on the prescription label. Swallow the tablets with a drink of water. This medicine can be taken with or without food. Take your doses at regular intervals. Do not take your medicine more often than directed. Contact your pediatrician or health care professional regarding the use of this medicine in children. Special care may be needed. Elderly patients over 65 years old may have a stronger reaction to this medicine and need smaller doses.

What if I miss a dose?

If you miss a dose, take it as soon as you can. If it is almost time for your next dose, take only that dose. Do not take double or extra doses.

What may interact with candesartan-hydrochlorothiazide?

- allopurinol
- anti-inflammatory drugs (NSAIDs, such as ibuprofen)
- diabetic medications
- blood pressure medications
- dofetilide
- griseofulvin
- hawthorn or horse chestnut
- lithium
- potassium salts or potassium supplements
- prochlorperazine
- some cholesterol-lowering medications (e.g. cholestyramine or colestipol)
- some medicines for mental disorders (phenothiazine)
- some antibiotics which increase sensitivity to sunlight (sulfonamide, tetracycline)
- vitamin A (retinol) creams or pills such as tretinoin Retin-A®, Renova®, Solage®, Atragen®, and others
- water pills (especially potassium-sparing diuretics such as triamterene or amiloride)

Tell your prescriber or health care professional about all other medicines you are taking, including non-prescription medicines, nutritional supplements, or herbal products. Also tell your prescriber or health care professional if you are a frequent user of drinks with caffeine or alcohol, if you smoke, or if you use illegal drugs. These may affect the way your medicine works. Check with your health care professional before stopping or starting any of your medicines.

What should I watch for while taking candesartan-hydrochlorothiazide?

Check your blood pressure regularly while you are taking this medicine. Ask your prescriber or health care professional what your blood pressure should be and when you should contact him or her. When you check your blood pressure, write down the measurements to show your prescriber or health care professional. You must not get dehydrated. Ask your prescriber or health care professional how much fluid you need to drink a day. If you are taking this medicine for a long time you must visit your prescriber or health care professional for regular checks on your progress. Make sure you schedule appointments on a regular basis. Check with your prescriber or health care professional if you get an attack of severe diarrhea, nausea and vomiting, or if you sweat a lot. The loss of too much body fluid can make it dangerous for you to take this medicine. You may get dizzy. Do not drive, use machinery, or do anything that requires mental alertness until you know how candesartan-hydrochlorothiazide affects you. To avoid dizzy or fainting spells, do not stand or sit up

C

quickly. Alcohol may increase the possibility of dizziness. Avoid alcoholic drinks until you have discussed their use with your prescriber or health care professional. If you are going to have surgery tell your prescriber or health care professional that you are taking candesartan; hydrochlorothiazide. Candesartan-hydrochlorothiazide may affect your blood sugar level. If you have diabetes, check with your prescriber or health care professional before changing the dose of your diabetic medicine. Avoid salt substitutes unless you are told otherwise by your prescriber or health care professional. Do not take medicines for appetite control, asthma, colds, cough, hay fever, or sinus problems without asking your prescriber or health care professional for advice. Do not treat yourself for a fever or sore throat; check with your prescriber or health care professional first.

What side effects may I notice from taking candesartan-hydrochlorothiazide?

Side effects that you should report to your prescriber or health care professional as soon as possible:
Rare or uncommon:
- difficulty breathing, difficulty swallowing, hoarseness, or tightening of the throat
- redness, blistering, peeling or loosening of the skin, including inside the mouth
- swelling of your face, lips, tongue, hands, or feet

- unusual rash, bleeding or bruising, or pinpoint red spots on the skin

Other:
- confusion, dizziness, lightheadedness or fainting spells
- decreased amount of urine passed
- decreased sexual function
- fast or uneven heart beat, palpitations, or chest pain
- fever or chills
- irregular heartbeat
- muscle cramps or pain
- stomach pain
- vomiting
- unusual tiredness or weakness
- worsened gout pain
- yellowing of the eyes or skin

Side effects that usually do not require medical attention (report to your prescriber or health care professional if they continue or are bothersome):
- cough
- increased sensitivity to the sun

Where can I keep my medicine?

Keep out of the reach of children in a container that small children cannot open. Store at room temperature between 15 and 30 degrees C (59 and 86 degrees F). Protect from light. Keep container tightly closed. Throw away any unused medicine after the expiration date.

Capecitabine tablets

| XELODA®; 150 mg; Tablet Hoffmann La Roche Inc | | XELODA®; 500 mg; Tablet Hoffmann La Roche Inc | |

What are capecitabine tablets?

CAPECITABINE (Xeloda®) is a type of chemotherapy for treating cancer. Capecitabine interferes with the growth of cancer cells and decreases the size of the tumor. It is used for treating breast cancer, and colon or rectal cancer. Generic capecitabine tablets are not yet available.

What should my health care professional know before I take capecitabine?

They need to know if you have any of these conditions:
- bleeding or blood disorders
- decreased kidney function
- heart disease such as angina or coronary artery disease
- infection (especially virus infection such as chickenpox or herpes)
- irregular heart beat
- liver disease
- recent radiation therapy
- an unusual or allergic reaction to capecitabine, 5-fluorouracil, other medicines, foods, dyes, or preservatives
- pregnant or trying to get pregnant
- breast-feeding

How should I take this medicine?

Take capecitabine tablets by mouth within 30 minutes after the end of a meal (usually breakfast and dinner). Follow the directions on the prescription label. Swallow the tablets with a drink of water. Do not take your medicine more often than directed. Finish the full course prescribed by your doctor or health care professional, even if the tablets make you feel unwell. Do not stop taking except on your prescriber's advice. Your prescriber or health care professional may want you to take a combination of 150 mg and 500 mg tablets for each dose. If a combination of tablets is prescribed, it is very important that you correctly identify the tablets. Taking the wrong tablets could result in an overdose (too much medication) or underdose (too little medication).

What if I miss a dose?

If you miss a dose, skip that dose and do not take double or extra doses. Instead, continue your regular dosing schedule and check with your prescriber or health care professional. If you vomit after taking a dose, call your prescriber or health care professional for advice.

What may interact with capecitabine?

- aluminum hydroxide or magnesium hydroxide (Maalox®)
- digoxin
- folic acid
- leucovorin
- phenytoin
- warfarin

Tell your prescriber or health care professional about all other medicines you are taking, including non-prescription medicines, nutritional supplements, or herbal products. Also tell your prescriber or health care professional if you are a frequent user of drinks with caffeine or alcohol, if you smoke, or if you use illegal drugs. These may affect the way your medicine works. Check with your health care professional before stopping or starting any of your medicines.

What should I watch for while taking capecitabine?

Visit your prescriber or health care professional for checks on your progress. You will need to have regular blood checks. The side effects of capecitabine can continue after you finish your treatment; report side effects right away. Capecitabine may make you feel generally unwell. This is not uncommon because capecitabine affects good cells as well as cancer cells. Report any side effects as below, but continue your course of medicine even though you feel ill, unless your prescriber or health care professional tells you to stop. Capecitabine will decrease your body's ability to fight infections. Call your prescriber or health care professional if you have a fever, chills, sore throat or other symptoms of a cold or flu. Do not treat these symptoms yourself. Try to avoid being around people who are sick. Capecitabine may increase your risk to bruise or bleed. Call your prescriber or health care professional if you notice any unusual bleeding. Be careful not to cut, bruise or injure yourself because you may get an infection and bleed more than usual. Capecitabine may harm your unborn baby. You should contact your prescriber immediately if you believe or suspect you or your partner have become pregnant while you are taking capecitabine. If you are going to have surgery, tell your prescriber or health care professional that you are taking capecitabine.

What side effects may I notice from taking capecitabine?

The side effects you may experience with capecitabine therapy depend upon the dose, other types of chemotherapy or radiation therapy given, and the disease being treated. Not all of these effects occur in all patients. Discuss any concerns or questions with your prescriber or health care professional.

Side effects that you should report to your prescriber or health care professional as soon as possible:

- low blood counts—capecitabine may decrease the number of white blood cells, red blood cells and platelets. You may be at increased risk for infections and bleeding.
- signs of infection—fever (100.5 degrees F or greater) or chills, cough, sore throat, pain or difficulty passing urine
- signs of decreased platelets or bleeding—bruising, pinpoint red spots on the skin, black, tarry stools, blood in the urine
- signs of decreased red blood cells—unusual weakness or tiredness, fainting spells, lightheadedness
- dehydration (excessive water loss from the body)
- hand-and-foot syndrome: pain, swelling, redness, or tingling of the hands and/or feet
- pain, redness, swelling, or sores in your mouth or throat
- severe diarrhea (more than 4 bowel movements a day or any diarrhea at night)
- severe nausea/vomiting (if you lose your appetite and eat much less than usual or vomit more than once in a 24 hour period)
- yellow color of skin or eyes

Side effects that usually do not require medical attention (report to your prescriber or health care professional if they continue or are bothersome):

- bone pain
- constipation
- difficulty sleeping
- dry or itchy skin
- eye irritation
- headache
- heart burn or indigestion
- loss of appetite or decreased appetite
- mild nausea or stomach upset
- mild diarrhea
- muscle aches
- tiredness
- weakness

Where can I keep my medicine?

Keep out of the reach of children in a container that small children cannot open. Store at room temperature between 15 and 30 degrees C (59 and 86 degrees F). Protect from moisture. Keep container tightly closed. Throw away any unused medicine after the expiration date.

C

Captopril tablets

CAPOTEN®;
25 mg; Tablet
Par Pharmaceutical
Inc

CAPOTEN®;
50 mg; Tablet
Par Pharmaceutical
Inc

What are captopril tablets?

CAPTOPRIL (Capoten®) is an antihypertensive (blood pressure lowering agent) known as an ACE inhibitor. Captopril controls high blood pressure (hypertension) by relaxing blood vessels; it is not a cure. High blood pressure levels can damage your kidneys, and may lead to a stroke or heart failure. Captopril also can help to treat heart failure (heart does not pump strongly enough) and certain kidney disorders. Generic captopril tablets are available.

What should my health care professional know before I take captopril?

They need to know if you have any of these conditions:

- autoimmune disease or collagen-vascular disease (such as lupus)
- suppressed immune function
- previous swelling of the tongue, face, or lips with difficulty breathing, difficulty swallowing, hoarseness, or tightening of the throat (angioedema)
- bone marrow disease
- heart or blood vessel disease
- liver disease
- low blood pressure
- kidney disease
- if you are on a special diet, such as a low-salt diet
- an unusual or allergic reaction to captopril, other ACE inhibitors, foods, dyes, or preservatives
- pregnant or trying to get pregnant
- breast-feeding

How should I take this medicine?

Take captopril tablets by mouth. Follow the directions on the prescription label. Swallow the tablets with a drink of water. Take captopril on an empty stomach, at least 1 hour before or 2 hours after meals. Take your doses at regular intervals. Do not take your medicine more often than directed. Do not stop taking captopril except on your prescriber's advice. Contact your pediatrician or health care professional regarding the use of this medicine in children. Special care may be needed.

What if I miss a dose?

If you miss a dose, take it as soon as you can. If it is almost time for your next dose, take only that dose. Do not take double or extra doses.

What may interact with captopril?

- antacids
- anti-inflammatory drugs (NSAIDs, such as ibuprofen)
- aspirin and aspirin-like medicines
- digoxin
- heparin
- lithium
- medicines for diabetes
- medicines for high blood pressure
- potassium salts
- probenecid
- water pills

Tell your prescriber or health care professional about all other medicines you are taking, including non-prescription medicines, nutritional supplements, or herbal products. Also tell your prescriber or health care professional if you are a frequent user of drinks with caffeine or alcohol, if you smoke, or if you use illegal drugs. These may affect the way your medicine works. Check with your health care professional before stopping or starting any of your medicines.

What should I watch for while taking captopril?

Visit your prescriber or health care professional for regular checks on your progress. Check your blood pressure regularly while you are taking captopril. Ask your prescriber or health care professional what your blood pressure should be and when you should contact him or her. Call your prescriber or health care professional if you notice an uneven or fast heart beat. Do not treat yourself for a fever or sore throat; check with your prescriber or health care professional as these may be the result of a captopril side effect. Check with your prescriber or health care professional if you get an attack of severe diarrhea, nausea and vomiting, or if you sweat a lot. The loss of body fluid can make it dangerous to take captopril. You may get dizzy. Do not drive, use machinery, or do anything that needs mental alertness until you know how captopril affects you. To avoid dizzy or fainting spells, do not stand or sit up quickly, especially if you are an older person. Alcohol can make you more dizzy. Avoid alcoholic drinks. If you are going to have surgery, tell your prescriber or health care professional that you are taking captopril. Avoid salt substitutes or other foods or substances high in potassium salts. Do not treat yourself for coughs, colds, or pain while you are taking captopril without asking your prescriber or health care professional for advice. Antacid can stop captopril working. If you want to take antacid for an upset stomach, make sure there is an interval of at least 2 hours since you last took captopril, or 4 hours before your next dose. Captopril can alter certain lab test results, giving a false-positive for urine ketone tests.

What side effects may I notice from taking captopril?

Side effects that you should report to your prescriber or health care professional as soon as possible:

- chest pain, uneven or fast heart beat, palpitations
- decreased or increased amount of urine passed
- difficulty breathing, or difficulty swallowing
- dizziness, lightheadedness or fainting spells
- fever or chills
- numbness or tingling in your fingers or toes
- skin rash, itching
- swelling of your face, lips, or tongue
- swelling of your legs or ankles

Side effects that usually do not require medical attention (report to your prescriber or health care professional if they continue or are bothersome):

- cough
- loss of taste
- fatigue or tiredness
- increased sensitivity to the sun

Where can I keep my medicine?

Keep out of the reach of children in a container that small children cannot open. Store at room temperature below 30 degrees C (86 degrees F). Protect from moisture. Keep container tightly closed. Throw away any unused medicine after the expiration date.

Captopril; Hydrochlorothiazide, HCTZ tablets

CAPOZIDE®;
25 mg/25 mg;
Tablet
Bristol Myers Squibb Co

CAPOZIDE®;
50 mg/15 mg;
Tablet
Bristol Myers Squibb Co

What are captopril-hydrochlorothiazide tablets?

CAPTOPRIL-HYDROCHLOROTHIAZIDE (Capozide®) is a combination of two drugs used to lower blood pressure. Captopril is an ACE inhibitor that controls high blood pressure (hypertension) by relaxing blood vessels. Hydrochlorothiazide is a diuretic. High blood pressure can damage the blood vessels of the brain, heart, and kidneys, resulting in a stroke, heart failure, or kidney failure. By lowering blood pressure, captopril-hydrochlorothiazide can help reduce your risk of having damage to your kidneys, heart, or other organs. This medicine does not cure high blood pressure. Generic captopril-hydrochlorothiazide tablets are available.

What should my health care professional know before I take captopril-hydrochlorothiazide?

They need to know if you have any of these conditions:
- autoimmune disease (such as lupus), or suppressed immune function
- previous swelling of the tongue, face, or lips with difficulty breathing, difficulty swallowing, hoarseness, or tightening of the throat (angioedema)
- bone marrow disease
- diabetes mellitus
- gout
- heart or blood vessel disease
- liver disease
- recent heart attack or stroke
- kidney disease, (such as renal failure or renal artery stenosis)
- pancreatitis
- electrolyte imbalance (such as low or high levels of potassium in the blood)
- if you are on a special diet, or using salt substitutes
- sulfonamide (sulfa) or thiazide allergy
- an unusual or allergic reaction to captopril, hydrochlorothiazide, other medicines, foods, dyes, or preservatives
- pregnant or trying to get pregnant
- breast-feeding

How should I use this medicine?

Take captopril-hydrochlorothiazide tablets by mouth. Follow the directions on the prescription label. Take captopril-hydrochlorothiazide tablets on an empty stomach (one hour before meals). Swallow the tablets with a drink of water. Take your doses at regular intervals. Do not take your medicine more often than directed. Do not stop taking this medicine except on your prescriber's advice. Many patients with high blood pressure will not notice any signs of the problem. Therefore, it is very important that you take this medicine exactly as directed and that you keep your appointments with your prescriber or health care professional even if you feel well. Contact your pediatrician or health care professional regarding the use of this medicine in children. Special care may be needed.

What if I miss a dose?

If you miss a dose, take it as soon as you can. If it is almost time for your next dose, take only that dose. Do not take double or extra doses.

What may interact with captopril-hydrochlorothiazide?

- allopurinol
- antacids
- anti-inflammatory drugs (NSAIDs such as ibuprofen)
- aspirin and aspirin-like medicines
- blood pressure medications
- cholesterol-lowering medications (such as cholestyramine or colestipol)
- diabetic medications
- digoxin
- dofetilide
- lithium
- porfimer
- potassium salts or potassium supplements
- probenecid
- water pills (especially potassium-sparing diuretics such as triamterene or amiloride)

Tell your prescriber or health care professional about all other medicines you are taking, including non-prescription medicines, nutritional supplements, or herbal products. Also tell your prescriber or health care professional if you are a frequent user of drinks with caffeine or alcohol, if you smoke, or if you use illegal drugs. These may affect the way your medicine works. Check with your health care professional before stopping or starting any of your medicines.

What should I watch for while taking captopril-hydrochlorothiazide?

Check your blood pressure regularly while you are taking captopril-hydrochlorothiazide. Ask your prescriber or health care professional what your blood pressure should be and when you should contact him or her. When you check your blood pressure, write down the measurements to show your prescriber or health care professional. You must not get dehydrated, ask your prescriber or health care professional how much fluid you need to drink a day. If you are taking this medicine for a long time you must visit your prescriber or health care professional for regular checks on your progress. Make sure you schedule appointments on a regular basis. Check with your prescriber or health care professional if you get an attack of severe diarrhea, nausea and vomiting, or if you sweat a lot. The loss of too much body fluid can make it dangerous for you to take captopril-hydrochlorothiazide. You may get dizzy. Do not drive, use machinery, or do anything that requires mental alertness until you know how captopril-hydrochlorothiazide affects you. To avoid dizzy or fainting spells, do not stand or sit up quickly. Alcohol may increase the possibility of dizziness. Avoid alcoholic drinks until you have discussed their use with your prescriber or health care professional. If you are going to have surgery tell your prescriber or health care professional that you are taking captopril-hydrochlorothiazide. Captopril-hydrochlorothiazide may affect your blood sugar level. If you have diabetes, check with your prescriber or health care professional before changing the dose of your diabetic medicine. Avoid too much sun or the use of a sun lamp. Avoid salt substitutes unless you are told otherwise by your prescriber or health care professional. Do not take medicines for appetite control, asthma, colds, cough, hay fever, or sinus problems without asking your prescriber or health care professional for advice. Do not treat yourself for a fever or sore throat; check with your prescriber or health care professional first.

What side effects may I notice from taking captopril-hydrochlorothiazide?

Side effects that you should report to your prescriber or health care professional as soon as possible:
Rare or uncommon:
- difficulty breathing, difficulty swallowing, hoarseness, or tightening of the throat
- redness, blistering, peeling or loosening of the skin, including inside the mouth
- swelling of your face, lips, tongue, hands, or feet
- unusual rash, bleeding or bruising, or pinpoint red spots on the skin

Other:
- confusion, dizziness, lightheadedness or fainting spells
- decreased amount of urine passed
- decreased sexual function
- fast or uneven heart beat, palpitations, or chest pain
- fever or chills
- irregular heartbeat
- muscle cramps
- stomach pain
- vomiting
- unusual tiredness or weakness
- worsened gout pain
- yellowing of the eyes or skin

Side effects that usually do not require medical attention (report to your prescriber or health care professional if they continue or are bothersome):
- cough
- diarrhea
- headache
- increased sensitivity to the sun
- loss of taste
- nausea
- tiredness or fatigue

Where can I keep my medicine?

Keep out of the reach of children. Store at room temperature at or below 30 degrees C (86 degrees F). Protect from moisture and light. Keep container tightly closed. Throw away any unused medicine after the expiration date.

Carbamazepine extended-release tablets or capsules

TEGRETOL®-XR; 200 mg; Tablet, Extended Release Novartis Pharmaceuticals Corp Dba Ciba Pharmaceuticals Co Di

CARBATROL®; 200 mg; Capsule, Extended Release Shire US Inc

What are carbamazepine extended-release tablets or capsules?

CARBAMAZEPINE (Carbatrol®, Tegretol®-XR) can help with seizure (convulsion) control in certain types of epilepsy. Carbamazepine also treats nerve-related pain such as trigeminal neuralgia, or the pain associated with shingles. This medications is not for common aches and pains. Carbamazepine may also be used to control certain mood problems, and is used for manic-depressive illness in some people. Generic extended-release carbamazepine tablets or capsules are not yet available.

What should my health care professional know before I take carbamazepine?

They need to know if you have any of these conditions:
- frequently drink alcohol containing beverages
- anemia or other blood disorders or disease, like
- glaucoma
- heart disease
- irregular heartbeat
- kidney disease
- liver disease
- low sodium level in the blood
- psychotic disorders
- seizures (convulsions)
- an unusual or allergic reaction to carbamazepine, tricyclic antidepressants, phenytoin, phenobarbital or other medicines, foods, dyes, or preservatives
- pregnant or trying to get pregnant
- breast-feeding

How should I take this medicine?

Take carbamazepine tablets or capsules by mouth. Follow the directions on the prescription label. Take your doses at regular intervals. Do not take your medicine more often than directed. Tegretol®-XR tablets must be swallowed whole and should not be cut, crushed or chewed. Carbatrol® capsules can be swallowed whole or they can be opened and the beads sprinkled over food such as applesauce or other similar food product. The capsules (Carbatrol®) or the beads inside the capsules should not be crushed or chewed. Contact your pediatrician or health care professional regarding the use of this medicine in children. Special care may be needed. Carbamazepine is often prescribed to children to treat seizures.

What if I miss a dose?

If you miss a dose, take it as soon as you can. If it is almost time for your next dose, take only that dose. Do not take double or extra doses.

What may interact with carbamazepine?

Carbamazepine can interact with many different types of medications. You should check with your prescriber or pharmacist before taking other medications with carbamazepine. The following list includes many of the types of medications that may interact:
- barbiturate medicines for inducing sleep or treating seizures (convulsions), like phenobarbital
- bosentan
- cancer-treating medications
- charcoal
- cefixime
- cimetidine
- clarithromycin
- colestipol
- cyclosporine
- danazol
- doxycycline
- erythromycin
- female hormones, including estrogens and birth control pills
- grapefruit juice
- herbal medicines like St. John's wort
- influenza virus vaccine
- isoniazid, INH
- levothyroxine and other thyroid hormones
- lithium and other medicines to treat mood problems or psychotic disturbances
- medicines for angina or high blood pressure
- medicines for rheumatoid or other inflammatory arthritis conditions
- medicines for depression or anxiety
- medicines for sleep
- medicines to treat fungal infections, like fluconazole, itraconazole or ketoconazole
- medicines used to treat HIV infection or AIDS
- metronidazole
- omeprazole
- propoxyphene
- quinidine
- rifampin
- rifabutin
- riluzole
- seizure (convulsion) or epilepsy medicine
- sirolimus
- steroid medicines such as prednisone or cortisone
- tacrolimus
- tamoxifen
- terfenadine
- theophylline
- toremifene

C

- tramadol
- troleandomycin
- warfarin
- zafirlukast

Tell your prescriber or health care professional about all other medicines you are taking, including non-prescription medicines. Also tell your prescriber or health care professional if you are a frequent user of drinks with caffeine or alcohol, if you smoke, or if you use illegal drugs. These may affect the way your medicine works. Check with your health care professional before stopping or starting any of your medicines.

What should I watch for while taking carbamazepine?

Visit your prescriber or health care professional for a regular check on your progress. Report any unusual side effects to your prescriber promptly. Do not change brands or dosage forms of carbamazepine without discussing the change with your prescriber or healthcare professional. If you are taking carbamazepine for epilepsy (seizures) do not stop taking it suddenly. This increases the risk of seizures. Wear a Medic Alert bracelet or necklace. Carry an identification card with information about your condition, medications, and prescriber or health care professional. You may get drowsy, dizzy, or have blurred vision. Do not drive, use machinery, or do anything that needs mental alertness until you know how carbamazepine affects you. To reduce dizzy or fainting spells, do not sit or stand up quickly, especially if you are an older patient. Alcohol can increase drowsiness and dizziness. Avoid alcoholic drinks. If you are female and are taking birth control pills (contraceptive pills) or other hormonal birth control methods (like injections), you should know that the birth control may not work as well while you are taking carbamazepine. You may need to talk to your prescriber about effective ways to prevent pregnancy. Let your prescriber know if you experience any unusual menstrual-type bleeding or spotting or if you think you might be pregnant while on this medicine. Carbamazepine may make your skin more sensitive to the sun or ultraviolet light. Keep out of the sun, or wear protective clothing outdoors and use a sunscreen (at least SPF 15). Do not use sun lamps or sun tanning beds or booths. If you are going to have surgery, tell your prescriber or health care professional that you are taking carbamazepine.

What side effects may I notice from taking carbamazepine?

Side effects that you should report to your prescriber or health care professional as soon as possible:
Less common:
- blurred or double vision, uncontrollable eye movements
- chest pain or tightness
- dark yellow or brown urine
- difficulty breathing or shortness of breath
- fainting spells
- fast or irregular heartbeat (palpitations)
- fever or chills, sore throat
- increased thirst
- mouth ulcers
- pain or difficulty passing urine
- redness, blistering, peeling or loosening of the skin, including inside the mouth
- ringing in the ears
- seizures (convulsions)
- shortness of breath, wheezing
- skin rash, hives, itching
- sore throat
- stomach pain
- swollen joints or muscle/joint aches and pains
- unusual bleeding or bruising
- unusual swelling
- vomiting
- yellowing of the eyes or skin

More common:
- confusion
- lightheadedness
- mood changes, nervousness, or hostility
- unusual tiredness or weakness

Side effects that usually do not require medical attention (report to your prescriber or health care professional if they continue or are bothersome):
- clumsiness or unsteadiness
- diarrhea or constipation
- mild dizziness or drowsiness
- headache
- increased sensitivity to the sun
- increased sweating
- nausea

Where can I keep my medicine?

Keep out of reach of children in a container that small children cannot open. Store at room temperature below 30 degrees C (86 degrees F). Keep container tightly closed. Protect from moisture. Throw away any unused medicine after the expiration date.

Carbamazepine tablets or chewable tablets

TEGRETOL®;
100 mg; Tablet, Chewable
Novartis Pharmaceuticals Corp Dba Ciba Pharmaceuticals Co
Di

TEGRETOL®;
200 mg; Tablet
Novartis Pharmaceuticals Corp Dba Ciba Pharmaceuticals Co
Di

What are carbamazepine tablets or chewable tablets?

CARBAMAZEPINE (Epitol®, Tegretol®, Teril®, and others) can help with seizure (convulsion) control in certain types of epilepsy. Carbamazepine also treats nerve-related pain such as trigeminal neuralgia, or the pain associated with shingles. This medication is not for common aches and pains. Carbamazepine may also be used to control certain mood problems, and is used for manic-depressive illness in some people. Generic carbamazepine tablets and chewable tablets are available.

What should my health care professional know before I take carbamazepine?

They need to know if you have any of these conditions:
- frequently drink alcohol containing beverages
- anemia or other blood disorders or disease, like
- glaucoma
- heart disease
- irregular heartbeat
- kidney disease
- liver disease
- low sodium level in the blood
- psychotic disorders
- seizures (convulsions)
- an unusual or allergic reaction to carbamazepine, tricyclic antidepressants, phenytoin, phenobarbital or other medicines, foods, dyes, or preservatives
- pregnant or trying to get pregnant
- breast-feeding

How should I take this medicine?

Take carbamazepine tablets by mouth. Follow the directions on the prescription label. Swallow the tablets with a drink of water. Chewable tablets may be chewed first or swallowed whole. Take your doses at regular intervals. Do not take your medicine more often than directed. Contact your pediatrician or health care professional regarding the use of this medicine in children. Special care may be needed. Carbamazepine is often prescribed to children of all ages to treat seizures.

What if I miss a dose?

If you miss a dose, take it as soon as you can. If it is almost time for your next dose, take only that dose. Do not take double or extra doses.

What may interact with carbamazepine?

Carbamazepine can interact with many different types of medications. You should check with your prescriber or pharmacist before taking other medications with carbamazepine. The following list includes many of the types of medications that may interact:

- barbiturate medicines for inducing sleep or treating seizures (convulsions), like phenobarbital
- bosentan
- cancer-treating medications
- charcoal
- cefixime
- cimetidine
- clarithromycin
- colestipol
- cyclosporine
- danazol
- doxycycline
- erythromycin
- female hormones, including estrogens and birth control pills
- grapefruit juice
- herbal medicines like St. John's wort
- influenza virus vaccine
- isoniazid, INH
- levothyroxine and other thyroid hormones
- lithium and other medicines to treat mood problems or psychotic disturbances
- medicines for angina or high blood pressure
- medicines for rheumatoid or other inflammatory arthritis conditions
- medicines for depression or anxiety
- medicines for sleep
- medicines to treat fungal infections, like fluconazole, itraconazole or ketoconazole
- medicines used to treat HIV infection or AIDS
- metronidazole
- omeprazole
- propoxyphene
- quinidine
- rifampin
- rifabutin
- riluzole
- seizure (convulsion) or epilepsy medicine
- sirolimus
- steroid medicines such as prednisone or cortisone
- tacrolimus
- tamoxifen
- terfenadine
- theophylline
- toremifene
- tramadol
- troleandomycin
- warfarin
- zafirlukast

Tell your prescriber or health care professional about all other medicines you are taking, including non-

prescription medicines, nutritional supplements, or herbal products. Also tell your prescriber or health care professional if you are a frequent user of drinks with caffeine or alcohol, if you smoke, or if you use illegal drugs. These may affect the way your medicine works. Check with your health care professional before stopping or starting any of your medicines.

What should I watch for while taking carbamazepine?

Visit your prescriber or health care professional for a regular check on your progress. Report any unusual side effects to your prescriber promptly. Do not change brands or dosage forms of carbamazepine without discussing the change with your prescriber or healthcare professional. If you are taking carbamazepine for epilepsy (seizures) do not stop taking it suddenly. This increases the risk of seizures. Wear a Medic Alert bracelet or necklace. Carry an identification card with information about your condition, medications, and prescriber or health care professional. You may get drowsy, dizzy, or have blurred vision. Do not drive, use machinery, or do anything that needs mental alertness until you know how carbamazepine affects you. To reduce dizzy or fainting spells, do not sit or stand up quickly, especially if you are an older patient. Alcohol can increase drowsiness and dizziness. Avoid alcoholic drinks. If you are female and are taking birth control pills (contraceptive pills) or other hormonal birth control methods (like injections), you should know that the birth control may not work as well while you are taking carbamazepine. You may need to talk to your prescriber about effective ways to prevent pregnancy. Let your prescriber know if you experience any unusual menstrual-type bleeding or spotting or if you think you might be pregnant while on this medicine. Carbamazepine may make your skin more sensitive to the sun or ultraviolet light. Keep out of the sun, or wear protective clothing outdoors and use a sunscreen (at least SPF 15). Do not use sun lamps or sun tanning beds or booths. If you are going to have surgery, tell your prescriber or health care professional that you are taking carbamazepine.

What side effects may I notice from taking carbamazepine?

Side effects that you should report to your prescriber or health care professional as soon as possible:

Less common:
- blurred or double vision, uncontrollable eye movements
- chest pain or tightness
- dark yellow or brown urine
- difficulty breathing or shortness of breath
- fainting spells
- fast or irregular heartbeat (palpitations)
- fever or chills, sore throat
- increased thirst
- mouth ulcers
- pain or difficulty passing urine
- redness, blistering, peeling or loosening of the skin, including inside the mouth
- ringing in the ears
- seizures (convulsions)
- shortness of breath, wheezing
- skin rash, hives, itching
- sore throat
- stomach pain
- swollen joints or muscle/joint aches and pains
- unusual bleeding or bruising
- unusual swelling
- vomiting
- yellowing of the eyes or skin

More common:
- confusion
- lightheadedness
- mood changes, nervousness, or hostility
- unusual tiredness or weakness

Side effects that usually do not require medical attention (report to your prescriber or health care professional if they continue or are bothersome):
- clumsiness or unsteadiness
- diarrhea or constipation
- mild dizziness or drowsiness
- headache
- increased sensitivity to the sun
- increased sweating
- nausea

Where can I keep my medicine?

Keep out of reach of children in a container that small children cannot open. Store at room temperature below 30 degrees C (86 degrees F). Keep container tightly closed. Protect from moisture. Throw away any unused medicine after the expiration date.

Carbenicillin tablets

GEOCILLIN®;
382 mg; Tablet
Roerig Division of Pfizer

What are carbenicillin tablets?

CARBENICILLIN (Geocillin®) is a penicillin antibiotic. Carbenicillin kills certain bacteria that cause infection, or stops their growth. It treats infections of the urinary tract and prostate gland. Generic carbenicillin tablets are not yet available.

What should my health care professional know before I take carbenicillin?

They need to know if you have any of these conditions:
- asthma
- bleeding problems
- eczema

- kidney disease
- mononucleosis
- stomach problems (especially colitis)
- other chronic illness
- an unusual or allergic reaction to carbenicillin, other penicillins, cephalosporin antibiotics, imipenem, foods, dyes, or preservatives
- breast-feeding

How should I take this medicine?

Carbenicillin tablets are taken by mouth. Follow the directions on the prescription label. Take carbenicillin 1 to 2 hours before or at least 2 hours after eating; taking it with food can make it less effective. Take with a full glass of water. Take your doses at regular intervals. Do not take your medicine more often than directed. Finish the full course prescribed by your prescriber or health care professional even if you think your condition is better. Do not stop taking except on your prescriber's advice. Contact your pediatrician or health care professional regarding the use of this medicine in children. Special care may be needed.

What if I miss a dose?

If you miss a dose, take it as soon as you can. If it is almost time for your next dose, take only that dose. Do not take double or extra doses.

What may interact with carbenicillin?

- blood thinners
- certain antibiotics given by injection
- clavulanic acid
- methotrexate
- probenecid

Tell your prescriber or health care professional about all other medicines you are taking, including non-prescription medicines, nutritional supplements, or herbal products. Also tell your prescriber or health care professional if you are a frequent user of drinks with caffeine or alcohol, if you smoke, or if you use illegal drugs. These may affect the way your medicine works. Check with your health care professional before stopping or starting any of your medicines.

What should I watch for while taking carbenicillin?

Tell your prescriber or health care professional if your symptoms do not improve in 2 or 3 days. If you get severe or watery diarrhea, do not treat yourself. Call your prescriber or health care professional for advice. If you get a skin rash, do not treat yourself. Call your prescriber or health care professional for advice. If you are diabetic and taking large doses of carbenicillin, you may get a false-positive result for sugar in your urine. Check with your prescriber or health care professional before you change your diet or the dose of your diabetic medicine.

What side effects may I notice from taking carbenicillin?

Side effects that you should report to your prescriber or health care professional as soon as possible:
- difficulty breathing, wheezing
- fever
- muscle cramps
- redness, blistering, peeling or loosening of the skin, including inside the mouth
- seizures (convulsions)
- skin rash, itching
- stomach pain or cramps
- swelling
- severe or watery diarrhea
- unusual bleeding

Side effects that usually do not require medical attention (report to your prescriber or health care professional if they continue or are bothersome):
- diarrhea
- gas or heartburn
- nausea, vomiting

Where can I keep my medicine?

Keep out of the reach of children in a container that small children cannot open. Store at room temperature between 15 and 30 degrees C (59 and 86 degrees F). Throw away any unused medicine after the expiration date.

Carbetapentane; Chlorpheniramine tablets

TANNIC-12®;
60 mg/5 mg;
Tablet
Cypress
Pharmaceutical Inc

TUSSIZONE 12 RF®;
60 mg/5 mg;
Tablet
Mallinckrodt Inc
Pharmaceuticals
Group

What are carbetapentane; chlorpheniramine tablets?

CARBETAPENTANE; CHLORPHENIRAMINE (Tussizone-12®, Tannic-12®, Trionate®, Tussi-12® and others) is used to decrease the symptoms caused by colds or allergies. Carbetapentane helps to stop cough. Chlorpheniramine is an antihistamine that relieves runny nose, sneezing, and watery eyes. This product is not intended to treat chronic cough caused by smoking, asthma, emphysema, heart failure, or problems in which there is a large amount of phlegm. Generic carbetapentane; chlorpheniramine products are not available.

What should my health care professional know before I receive carbetapentane; chlorpheniramine?

They need to know if you have any of these conditions:
- asthma or other lung disease
- chronic bronchitis
- emphysema
- glaucoma or other eye disease
- heart disease
- high or low blood pressure
- liver disease
- pain or difficulty passing urine
- prostate trouble
- seizures
- stomach or intestinal problems
- thyroid disease
- wear contact lenses
- an unusual reaction to carbetapentane, chlorpheniramine, other medicines, foods, dyes, or preservatives
- pregnant or trying to get pregnant
- breast-feeding

How should this medicine be used?

Take the tablets by mouth. Follow the directions on your prescription label. Swallow the tablets whole with a glass of water; do not chew. May take with food, water, or milk to minimize stomach upset. Do not take your medicine more often than directed. Contact your pediatrician or health care professional regarding the use of this medicine in children. Special care may be needed.

What if I miss a dose?

If you miss a dose, take it as soon as you can. If it is almost time for your next dose, take only that dose. Do not take double or extra doses.

What may interact with carbetapentane; chlorpheniramine?

- alcohol
- barbiturate medicines for inducing sleep or treating seizures (convulsions)
- medicines for anxiety or sleeping problems, such as diazepam or temazepam
- medicines for hay fever and other allergies
- medicines for mental depression
- medicines for mental problems and psychotic disturbances
- medicines for movement abnormalities as in Parkinson's disease, or for gastrointestinal problems
- muscle relaxers
- prescription pain medicines

Tell your prescriber or health care professional about all other medicines you are taking, including non-prescription medicines, nutritional supplements, or herbal products. Also tell your prescriber or health care professional if you are a frequent user of drinks with caffeine or alcohol, if you smoke, or if you use illegal drugs. These may affect the way your medicine works. Check with your health care professional before stopping or starting any of your medicines.

What should I watch for while taking carbetapentane; chlorpheniramine?

Tell your prescriber or health care professional if your symptoms do not improve in 1 or 2 days. You may get drowsy or dizzy. Do not drive, use machinery, or do anything that needs mental alertness until you know how this medicine affects you. To reduce the risk of dizzy or fainting spells, do not stand or sit up quickly, especially if you are an older patient. Alcohol may increase dizziness and drowsiness. Avoid alcoholic drinks. Your mouth may get dry. Chewing sugarless gum or sucking hard candy, and drinking plenty of water will help. This medicine may cause dry eyes and blurred vision. If you wear contact lenses you may feel some discomfort. Lubricating drops may help. See your ophthalmologist if the problem does not go away or is severe.

What side effects may I notice from taking carbetapentane; chlorpheniramine?

Side effects that you should report to your prescriber or health care professional as soon as possible:
- agitation, nervousness, excitability, not able to sleep (these are more likely in children)
- blurred vision
- fainting spells
- irregular heartbeat, palpitations, or chest pain
- muscle or facial twitches
- pain or difficulty passing urine
- seizures (convulsions)

Side effects that usually do not require medical attention (report to your prescriber or health care professional if they continue or are bothersome):
- drowsiness, dizziness
- dry mouth
- headache
- loss of appetite
- stomach upset, nausea, vomiting, diarrhea, or constipation

Where can I keep my medicine?

Keep out of the reach of children in a container that small children cannot open. Store at controlled room temperature 15 and 30 degrees C (59 and 86 degrees F); do not freeze. Keep container tightly closed. Keep away from heat and light. Throw away any unused medicine after the expiration date.

Carbetapentane;
Phenylephrine;
Pyrilamine tablets

TUSSI 12™ D;
60 mg/10 mg/40 mg;
Tablet
Medpointe Pharmaceuticals

What are carbetapentane; phenylephrine; pyrilamine tablets?

CARBETAPENTANE; PHENYLEPHRINE; PY-RILAMINE (Tussi-12 D®) is used to relieve cough and congestion due to colds, acute respiratory infections, including bronchitis and allergies and may help to relieve sneezing and itching associated with allergies. Generic carbetapentane; phenylephrine; pyrilamine tablets are not available.

What should my health care professional know before I take carbetapentane; phenylephrine; pyrilamine?

They need to know if you have any of these conditions:
- asthma
- diabetes
- difficulty passing urine
- chronic cough
- emphysema
- enlarged prostrate
- heart disease including angina
- high blood pressure
- history of stroke or mini-strokes (TIAs)
- irregular heart beat
- liver disease
- thyroid disease
- an unusual reaction to carbetapentane, phenylephrine, pyrilamine, other medicines, foods, dyes, or preservatives
- pregnant or trying to get pregnant
- breast-feeding

How should this medicine be used?

Take carbetapentane; phenylephrine; pyrilamine by mouth. Follow the directions on the bottle. Take your doses at regular intervals. Do not take your medicine more often than directed. Contact your pediatrician or health care professional regarding the use of this medicine in children. Special care may be needed.

What if I miss a dose?

If you miss a dose, take it as soon as you can. If it is almost time for your next dose, take only that dose. Do not take double or extra doses.

What may interact with carbetapentane; phenylephrine; pyrilamine?

- caffeine
- cocaine
- furazolidone
- linezolid
- medicines for chest pain, heart disease, high blood pressure, or heart rhythm problems
- medicine for diabetes
- medicines known as MAO inhibitors, such as phenelzine (Nardil®), tranylcypromine (Parnate®), isocarboxazid (Marplan®), and selegiline (Carbex®, Eldepryl®)
- medicines for mental depression
- medicines for mental problems and psychotic disturbances
- medicines for movement abnormalities as in Parkinson's disease, or for gastrointestinal problems
- medicines for weight loss
- St. John's wort
- thyroid hormones

Because this product can cause drowsiness, other medicines that also cause drowsiness may increase this effect. Some medicines that cause drowsiness are:

- alcohol and alcohol-containing medicines
- barbiturate medicines for inducing sleep or treating seizures (convulsions)
- medicines for anxiety or sleeping problems, such as diazepam or temazepam
- medicines for hay fever and other allergies
- muscle relaxers
- prescription pain medicines

Tell your prescriber or health care professional about all other medicines you are taking, including non-prescription medicines, nutritional supplements, or herbal products. Also tell your prescriber or health care professional if you are a frequent user of drinks with caffeine or alcohol, if you smoke, or if you use illegal drugs. These may affect the way your medicine works. Check with your health care professional before stopping or starting any of your medicines.

What should I watch for while taking carbetapentane; phenylephrine; pyrilamine?

If you have a fever, skin rash, or persistent headache as well as a cough, see your prescriber or health care professional. Do not treat yourself for a cough for more than one week without consulting your prescriber or health care professional. You may get drowsy or dizzy. Do not drive, use machinery, or do anything that needs mental alertness until you know this medicine affects you. Alcohol can increase the risk of getting drowsy, dizzy, or confused. Avoid alcoholic drinks.

What side effects may I notice from taking carbetapentane; phenylephrine; pyrilamine?

Side effects that you should report to your prescriber or health care professional as soon as possible:
- agitation, nervousness, excitability, not able to sleep (these are more likely in children)
- confusion
- headache, especially if severe or gets worse

C

- high blood pressure
- seizures
- severe nausea, vomiting
- slow or troubled breathing
- slurred speech
- tremors

Side effects that usually do not require medical attention (report to your prescriber or health care professional if they continue or are bothersome):
- dizziness, drowsiness

- nausea, vomiting
- stomach ache
- tremors
- weakness

Where can I keep my medicine?

Keep out of the reach of children in a container that small children cannot open. Store at room temperature between 15 and 30 degrees C (59 and 86 degrees F). Throw away any unused medicine after the expiration date.

Carbidopa tablets

LODOSYN®;
25 mg; Tablet
Bristol Myers Squibb Pharma
Co

What are carbidopa tablets?

CARBIDOPA (Lodosyn®) is a used to treat Parkinson's disease. Carbidopa is always given with levodopa (e.g., Dopar® or Laridopa®) or carbidopa-levodopa combination products (e.g., Sinemet®). Carbidopa is added to levodopa to increase its therapeutic effects and reduce the risk of certain side effects, such as nausea. Generic carbidopa tablets are not available.

What should my health care professional know before I take carbidopa?

They need to know if you have any of these conditions:
- an unusual or allergic reaction to carbidopa, other medicines, foods, dyes, or preservatives
- pregnant or trying to get pregnant
- breast-feeding

Make sure to tell your health care provider about any other chronic conditions you may have that could affect your Parkinson's therapy.

How should I take this medicine?

Take carbidopa tablets by mouth. Swallow the tablets with a glass of water. You will take carbidopa at the same time as your levodopa or carbidopa-levodopa medicine, as directed by your prescriber. Follow the directions on the label. Do not take your medicine more often than directed. Do not stop taking this medicine without talking with your health care provider. Contact your pediatrician or health care professional regarding the use of this medicine in children. This medicine is not recommended for children less than 18 years of age.

What if I miss a dose?

If you miss a dose, take it as soon as you can. If it is less than 2 hours to your next dose, take only that dose. Do not take double or extra doses. Try not to miss a dose.

What may interact with carbidopa?

There are no drug interactions with carbidopa however, many drugs may interact with levodopa. Some of the drugs that interact with levodopa include:

- cocaine
- droperidol
- linezolid
- medicines for high blood pressure
- medicines for depression, avoid those called MAO inhibitors-phenelzine (Nardil®), tranylcypromine (Parnate®), isocarboxazid (Marplan®)
- medicines for movement abnormalities as in Parkinson's disease
- metoclopramide
- papaverine
- medicines for mental problems and psychotic disturbances
- phenytoin
- s-adenosyl-l-methionine, SAM-e
- water pills

Tell your prescriber or health care professional about all other medicines that you are taking, including non-prescription medicines, nutritional supplements, or herbal products. Also tell your prescriber or health care professional if you are a frequent user of drinks with caffeine or alcohol, if you smoke, or if you use illegal drugs. These may affect the way your medicine works. Check with your health care professional before stopping or starting any of your medicines.

What should I watch for while taking carbidopa?

Visit your prescriber or health care professional for regular checks on your progress. The addition of carbidopa to your regimen may decrease the amount of nausea and vomiting you may have been experiencing while taking levodopa alone or carbidopa-levodopa combination products. This may allow your prescriber to better adjust your Parkinson's therapy to control your symptoms. Until your dosage is adjusted properly, you may experience more muscle twitches or other uncontrolled movements. Make sure to tell your prescriber or health care professional if these occur.

What side effects may I notice from taking carbidopa?

There are no known side effects to carbidopa. You may notice side effects due to combination therapy with levodopa and carbidopa including some of the following effects.

Side effects that you should report to your prescriber or health care professional as soon as possible:

- difficulty passing urine
- dizziness, lightheadedness, or fainting spells
- fast or irregular heartbeat (palpitations)
- mental depression
- mood changes such as aggressive behavior or hallucinations
- stomach pain
- uncontrolled movements of the mouth, head, hands, feet, shoulders, eyelids or other unusual muscle movements

Side effects that usually do not require medical attention (report to your prescriber or health care professional if they continue or are bothersome):

- anxiety, confusion, or nervousness
- dark color (brown, red, or black) of saliva, urine or sweat
- headache
- loss of appetite
- muscle twitches
- nausea/vomiting
- nightmares, trouble sleeping
- unusual tiredness or weakness

Where can I keep my medicine?

Keep out of the reach of children in a container that small children cannot open. Store at room temperature between 15 and 30 degrees C (59 and 86 degrees F). Protect from light. Keep container tightly closed. Throw away any unused medicine after the expiration date.

Carbidopa; Levodopa sustained-release tablets

SINEMET® CR; 50 mg/200 mg; Tablet, Extended Release Bristol Myers Squibb Pharma Co

SINEMET® CR; Tablet, Extended Release; 25 mg/ 100 mg Bristol Myers Squibb Pharma Co

What are carbidopa-levodopa sustained-release tablets?

CARBIDOPA-LEVODOPA (Sinemet® CR) is used to treat Parkinson's disease. Levodopa can help correct an imbalance of chemicals in the brain caused by Parkinson's disease. Levodopa will not cure Parkinson's disease, but will help to control the symptoms. Carbidopa helps levodopa work better, and this can decrease some side effects, such as nausea. Sustained-release tablets slowly release the medicine over 4 to 6 hours. Generic carbidopa-levodopa sustained-release tablets are available.

What should my health care professional know before I take carbidopa-levodopa?

They need to know if you have any of these conditions:

- asthma or lung disease
- depression or other mental illness
- diabetes
- glaucoma
- heart disease, including history of a heart attack
- irregular heart beat
- kidney disease
- liver disease
- melanoma or suspicious skin lesions
- seizure disorder
- stomach or intestinal ulcers
- an unusual or allergic reaction to levodopa, carbidopa, other medicines, foods, dyes, or preservatives
- pregnant or trying to get pregnant
- breast-feeding

How should I take this medicine?

Take carbidopa-levodopa tablets by mouth. Follow the directions on the prescription label. Swallow the tablets (either whole or half) with a glass of water; do not crush or chew the tablets. It is best to take carbidopa-levodopa on an empty stomach, either 30 minutes before you eat or 1 hour after you eat. If the medicine upsets your stomach, you can take it with a cracker or fruit. Take your doses at regular intervals. Do not take your medicine more often than directed. Do not stop taking this medicine without talking with your health care provider. Contact your pediatrician or health care professional regarding the use of this medicine in children. Special care may be needed.

What if I miss a dose?

If you miss a dose, take it as soon as you can. If it is less than 2 hours to your next dose, take only that dose. Do not take double or extra doses. Try not to miss a dose; it is important to keep your regular dosing schedule.

What may interact with carbidopa-levodopa?

- cocaine
- droperidol
- furazolidone
- isoniazid, INH
- iron supplements
- kava kava
- linezolid
- medicines for high blood pressure
- medicines for depression, avoid those called MAO inhibitors-phenelzine (Nardil®), tranylcypromine (Parnate®), isocarboxazid (Marplan®)
- medicines for mental problems and psychotic disturbances
- metoclopramide
- papaverine

- phenytoin
- procarbazine
- s-adenosyl-l-methionine, SAM-e
- water pills

Tell your prescriber or health care professional about all other medicines that you are taking, including non-prescription medicines, nutritional supplements, or herbal products. Also tell your prescriber or health care professional if you are a frequent user of drinks with caffeine or alcohol, if you smoke, or if you use illegal drugs. These may affect the way your medicine works. Check with your health care professional before stopping or starting any of your medicines.

What should I watch for while taking carbidopa-levodopa?

Visit your prescriber or health care professional for regular checks on your progress. It may be several weeks or months before you feel the full benefits of carbidopa-levodopa. Continue to take your medicine on a regular schedule and do not stop taking except on your prescriber's advice. Do not take any additional medicines for Parkinson's disease without first consulting with your health care provider. You may experience a "wearing off" effect prior to the time for your next dose of carbidopa-levodopa. You may also experience an "on-off" effect where the medicine apparently stops working for anything from a minute to several hours, then suddenly starts working again. Tell your prescriber or health care professional if any of these symptoms happen to you, as he/she may need to adjust your dosage. A high-protein diet can slow or prevent absorption of levodopa. Avoid high protein foods near the time of taking carbidopa-levodopa to help to prevent these problems. Take carbidopa-levodopa at least 30 minutes before eating or one hour after meals. You may want to eat higher protein foods later in the day or in small amounts. Discuss your diet with your prescriber or health care professional or nutritionist. Do not take iron supplements within 2 hours of taking levodopa. The iron may decrease the amount of levodopa in your system and decrease the effectiveness of the drug. Do not sit or stand up quickly. This reduces the risk of dizzy or fainting spells. The dizziness should decrease after taking carbidopa-levodopa for a couple of days. Alcohol can increase possible dizziness; avoid alcoholic drinks. If you are going to have surgery, tell your prescriber or health care professional that you are taking carbidopa-levodopa. If you are diabetic, carbidopa-levodopa may interfere with the accuracy of some tests for sugar or ketones in the urine (does not interfere with blood tests). Check with your prescriber or health care professional before changing the dose of your diabetic medicine. Carbidopa-levodopa may discolor the urine or sweat, making it look darker or red in color; this is of no cause for concern. However, this may stain clothing or fabrics.

What side effects may I notice from taking carbidopa-levodopa?

Side effects that you should report to your prescriber or health care professional as soon as possible:
- difficulty passing urine
- dizziness, lightheadedness, or fainting spells
- fast or irregular heartbeat (palpitations)
- mental depression
- mood changes such as aggressive behavior or hallucinations
- stomach pain
- uncontrolled movements of the mouth, head, hands, feet, shoulders, eyelids or other unusual muscle movements

Side effects that usually do not require medical attention (report to your prescriber or health care professional if they continue or are bothersome):
- anxiety, confusion, or nervousness
- dark color (brown, red, or black) of saliva, urine or sweat
- headache
- loss of appetite
- muscle twitches
- nausea/vomiting
- nightmares, trouble sleeping
- unusual tiredness or weakness

Where can I keep my medicine?

Keep out of the reach of children in a container that small children cannot open. Store at room temperature between 15 and 30 degrees C (59 and 86 degrees F). Protect from light. Keep container tightly closed. Throw away any unused medicine after the expiration date.

Carbidopa; Levodopa; Entacapone tablets

STALEVO™ 100;
25 mg/100 mg/
200 mg; Tablet
Novartis
Pharmaceuticals

STALEVO™ 150;
37.5 mg/150 mg/
200 mg; Tablet
Novartis
Pharmaceuticals

What are carbidopa; levodopa; entacapone tablets?

CARBIDOPA; LEVODOPA; ENTACAPONE (Stalevo™) is used to treat Parkinson's disease. Levodopa can help correct an imbalance of chemicals in the brain caused by Parkinson's disease. Levodopa will not cure Parkinson's disease, but will help to control the symptoms. Carbidopa and entacapone help levodopa to work better, and this can decrease some side effects, such as nausea. Generic carbidopa; levodopa; entacapone tablets are not available yet.

What should my health care professional know before I receive carbidopa; levodopa; entacapone?

They need to know if you have any of these conditions:
- asthma or lung disease
- depression or other mental illness
- diabetes
- dizzy or fainting spells
- glaucoma
- heart disease, including history of a heart attack
- irregular heart beat
- kidney disease
- liver disease
- low blood pressure
- melanoma or suspicious skin lesions
- seizure disorder
- stomach or intestinal ulcers
- an unusual or allergic reaction to levodopa, carbidopa, entacapone, other medicines, foods, dyes, or preservative
- pregnant or trying to get pregnant
- breast-feeding

How should this medicine be used?

Take your carbidopa; levodopa; entacapone tablets by mouth. Follow the directions on the prescription label. Do not crush or split the tablet; leave it whole. Swallow the tablet with a glass of water. It is best to take this medicine on an empty stomach, 30 minutes before you eat or 1 hour after you eat. If this medicine upsets your stomach, you can take it with a cracker or fruit. Take your doses at regular intervals. Do not take your medicine more often than directed. Do not change your dosage regimen and do not add additional Parkinson's medications while taking this medication, unless under your provider's care. Do not stop taking this medicine without talking with your health care provider. Contact your pediatrician or health care professional regarding the use of this medicine in children. Special care may be needed.

What if I miss a dose?

If you miss a dose, take it as soon as you can. If it is almost time for your next dose, take only that dose. Do not take double or extra doses.

What may interact with carbidopa; levodopa; entacapone?

- ampicillin
- apomorphine
- cholestyramine
- cocaine
- droperidol
- epinephrine
- erythromycin
- furazolidone
- iron supplements, such as those found in vitamins
- isoniazid, INH
- isoproterenol
- kava kava
- linezolid
- medicines for high blood pressure, including methyldopa
- medicines for depression, do not take those called MAO inhibitors-phenelzine (Nardil®), tranylcypromine (Parnate®), isocarboxazid (Marplan®)
- medicines for mental problems and psychotic disturbances
- metoclopramide
- papaverine
- phenytoin
- probenecid
- procarbazine
- s-adenosyl-l-methionine, SAM-e
- water pills

Tell your prescriber or health care professional about all other medicines you are taking, including non-prescription medicines, nutritional supplements, or herbal products. Also tell your prescriber or health care professional if you are a frequent user of drinks with caffeine or alcohol, if you smoke, or if you use illegal drugs. These may affect the way your medicine works. Check with your health care professional before stopping or starting any of your medicines.

What should I watch for while taking carbidopa; levodopa; entacapone?

Visit your prescriber or health care professional for regular checks on your progress. Continue to take your medicine on a regular schedule and do not stop taking except on your prescriber's advice. Do not take any additional medicines for Parkinson's disease without first consulting with your health care provider. Entacapone may increase the side effects caused by levodopa-carbidopa such as nausea or restless movements. If you notice an increase in or the appearance of certain side effects that occurred only while you are taking levodopa; carbidopa, contact your physician. The dose of levodopa-carbidopa may need to be lowered. Do not decrease your medicine dose without your prescriber's advice. You may get dizzy or have difficulty controlling your movements. Do not drive, use machinery, or do anything that needs mental alertness until you know how this medicine affects you. Do not stand or sit up quickly, especially if you are older. This reduces the risk of dizzy or fainting spells. Alcohol or other medicines that make you tired can increase possible dizziness; avoid alcoholic drinks. This medicine may make your mouth dry. Chewing sugarless gum, sucking hard candy, or drinking plenty of water may help. You may experience a "wearing off" effect prior to the time for your next dose of this medicine. You may also experience an "on-off" effect where the medicine apparently stops working for anything from a minute to several hours, then suddenly starts working again. Tell your prescriber or health care professional if any of these symptoms happen to you, your dosage may need adjustment. A high-protein diet can slow or prevent absorption of levodopa. Avoid high protein foods near the time of taking this medicine to help prevent this problem. Take this medicine at least 30 minutes before eating or 1 hour after meals. You may want to eat higher protein foods later in the day or in small amounts. Discuss your diet with your prescriber or nutritionist. Do not take iron supplements within 2 hours of taking this medicine. The iron may decrease the amount of levodopa in your system and decrease the effectiveness of the drug If you are diabetic, this medicine may interfere with the accuracy of some tests for sugar or ketones in the urine (does not interfere with blood tests). Check with your prescriber or health care professional before changing the dose of your diabetic medicine. This medicine may discolor your urine, saliva or sweat, making it look darker or red in color; this is of no cause for concern. However, this may stain clothing or fabrics. If you are going to have surgery, tell your prescriber or health care professional that you are taking carbidopa; levodopa; entacapone.

What side effects may I notice from taking carbidopa; levodopa; entacapone?

Side effects that you should report to your prescriber or health care professional as soon as possible:

- confusion
- decrease in urination
- difficulty passing urine
- dizziness, lightheadedness, or fainting spells
- fainting spells or lightheadedness
- fast or irregular heartbeat (palpitations)
- fever
- hallucinations
- involuntary muscle movements
- mental depression, crying, extreme sadness
- mood changes such as aggressive behavior or hallucinations
- severe diarrhea
- sore muscles
- stomach pain
- uncontrolled movements of the mouth, head, hands, feet, shoulders, eyelids or other unusual muscle movements
- vomiting or nausea that does not go away

Side effects that usually do not require medical attention (report to your prescriber or health care professional if they continue or are bothersome):

- anxiety, confusion, or nervousness
- constipation
- diarrhea
- dizziness
- drowsiness
- dry mouth
- fatigue
- headache
- muscle twitches
- nausea
- nightmares, trouble sleeping
- unusual tiredness or weakness
- upset stomach or loss of appetite
- urine, sweat or saliva that is dark yellow to orange or brown in color (entacapone can change the color of your urine)

Where can I keep my medicine?

Keep out of the reach of children in a container that small children cannot open. Store at room temperature between 15 and 30 degrees C (59 and 86 degrees F). Protect from light. Keep container tightly closed. Throw away any unused medicine after the expiration date.

Carbinoxamine tablets and capsules

HISTEX™ I/E;
2 mg/8 mg;
Capsule Release
Teamm
Pharmaceuticals Inc

HISTEX™ CT;
Tablet, Extended
Release; 8 mg
Teamm
Pharmaceuticals

What are carbinoxamine tablets and capsules?

CARBINOXAMINE (Clistin®, Histex™ IE, Histek™ CT) is an antihistamine that is used to relieve symptoms of hay fever (also known as allergic rhinitis), hives (rash or itching), and other allergic reactions. Generic carbinoxamine tablets and capsules are available.

What should my health care professional know before I take carbinoxamine?

They need to know if you have any of these conditions:
- asthma or congestive lung disease
- glaucoma
- high blood pressure or heart disease
- liver disease
- other chronic illness
- prostate trouble
- pain or difficulty passing urine
- ulcers or other stomach problems
- an unusual or allergic reaction to carbinoxamine, other medicines, foods, dyes, or preservatives such as sulfites
- pregnant or trying to get pregnant
- breast-feeding

How should I take this medicine?

Take carbinoxamine tablets or capsules by mouth. Follow the directions on the product label. Take with food or milk if this medicine upsets your stomach. Take your doses at regular intervals. Do not take your medicine more often than directed. Contact your pediatrician or health care professional regarding the use of this medicine in children. Special care may be needed.

What if I miss a dose?

If you miss a dose, take it as soon as you can. If it is almost time for your next dose, take only that dose. Do not take double or extra doses.

What may interact with carbinoxamine?

- alcohol
- barbiturate medicines for inducing sleep or treating seizures (convulsions)
- medicines for anxiety or sleeping problems, such as alprazolam, diazepam or temazepam
- medicines for gastrointestinal or bladder problems
- medicines for hay fever and other allergies
- medicines for mental depression
- medicines for mental problems and psychotic disturbances
- medicines for movement abnormalities as in Parkinson's disease

Tell your prescriber or health care professional about all other medicines you are taking, including non-prescription medicines, nutritional supplements, or herbal products. Also tell your prescriber or health care professional if you are a frequent user of drinks with caffeine or alcohol, if you smoke, or if you use illegal drugs. These may affect the way your medicine works. Check with your health care professional before stopping or starting any of your medicines.

What should I watch for while taking carbinoxamine?

Tell your prescriber or health care professional if your symptoms do not improve in 2 or 3 days. You may get drowsy or dizzy. Do not drive, use machinery, or do anything that needs mental alertness until you know how this medicine affects you. Be careful taking other medicines that may also make you tired. To reduce the risk of dizzy or fainting spells, do not stand or sit up quickly, especially if you are an older patient. Alcohol may increase dizziness and drowsiness. Avoid alcoholic drinks. Your skin may become more sensitive to the sun. While taking carbinoxamine avoid prolonged sun exposure and use sunscreen. Your mouth may get dry. Chewing sugarless gum or sucking hard candy, and drinking plenty of water will help. Carbinoxamine may cause you to have an upset stomach. If this happens, take the medicine with food. Carbinoxamine may cause you to experience dry eyes and blurred vision. If you wear contact lenses you may feel some discomfort. Lubricating drops may help. See your ophthalmologist if the problem does not go away or is severe.

What side effects may I notice from taking carbinoxamine?

Side effects that you should report to your prescriber or health care professional as soon as possible:
- agitation, nervousness, excitability, not able to sleep (these are more likely in children or the elderly)
- blurred vision
- fainting spells
- irregular heartbeat, palpitations, or chest pain
- muscle or facial twitches
- pain or difficulty passing urine
- seizures (convulsions)

Side effects that usually do not require medical attention (report to your prescriber or health care professional if they continue or are bothersome):
- constipation or diarrhea
- dizziness

- drowsiness
- dry mouth
- headache
- insomnia
- loss of appetite
- nervousness
- stomach upset, nausea, or vomiting

Where can I keep my medicine?

Keep out of the reach of children in a container that small children cannot open. Store at room temperature, between 15 and 30 degrees C (59 and 86 degrees F); do not freeze. Keep in a tightly closed, light-resistant container. Keep away from heat. Throw away any unused medicine after the expiration date.

Carbinoxamine; Pseudoephedrine tablets and extended-release tablets

RONDEC® TR; 8 mg/120 mg; Tablet, Extended Release Alliant Pharmaceuticals	COLDEC TR; 8 mg; 120 mg; Tablet Breckenridge Pharmaceutical

What are carbinoxamine; pseudoephedrine tablets and extended-release tablets?

CARBINOXAMINE; PSEUDOEPHEDRINE (Carbodec-TR®, Coldec-D, Coldec TR, Rondec-TR®, and others) is used to relieve congestion due to colds or allergies. Generic carbinoxamine; pseudoephedrine tablets and extended-release tablets are available.

What should my health care professional know before I take carbinoxamine; pseudoephedrine?

They need to know if you have any of these conditions:
- asthma or lung disease
- diabetes mellitus
- glaucoma
- high blood pressure
- heart disease
- intestinal problems
- kidney disease
- liver disease
- pain or difficulty passing urine
- prostate trouble
- thyroid disease
- vision problems
- an unusual reaction to carbinoxamine, pseudoephedrine, other medicines, foods, dyes, or preservatives
- pregnant or trying to get pregnant
- breast-feeding

How should this medicine be used?

Take carbinoxamine; pseudoephedrine tablets by mouth. Follow the directions on the prescription label. Swallow whole with a drink of water; do not bite, crush or chew. If the tablet has a groove in it, the tablet may be divided in half for a smaller dose by breaking the tablet along the groove. The tablet piece (one-half tablet) should be swallowed whole (do not bite or chew). Take your doses at regular intervals. Do not take your medicine more often than directed. Contact your pe-

diatrician or health care professional regarding the use of this medicine in children. Special care may be needed. Elderly patients over 60 years old may have a stronger reaction to this medicine.

What if I miss a dose?

If you miss a dose, take it as soon as you can. If it is almost time for your next dose, take only that dose. Do not take double or extra doses.

What may interact with carbinoxamine; pseudoephedrine?

- caffeine
- cocaine
- furazolidone
- linezolid
- medicines for chest pain, heart disease, high blood pressure, or heart rhythm problems
- medicine for diabetes
- medicines known as MAO inhibitors, such as phenelzine (Nardil®), tranylcypromine (Parnate®), isocarboxazid (Marplan®), and selegiline (Carbex®, Eldepryl®)
- medicines for mental depression
- medicines for mental problems and psychotic disturbances
- medicines for movement abnormalities as in Parkinson's disease, or for gastrointestinal problems
- medicines for weight loss
- St. John's wort
- terbinafine
- thyroid hormones

Because this product can cause drowsiness, other medicines that also cause drowsiness may increase this effect. Some medicines that cause drowsiness are:

- alcohol and alcohol-containing medicines
- barbiturates such as phenobarbital
- certain antidepressants or tranquilizers
- certain antihistamines used in cold medicines

- certain narcotics or pain medicines (for example, codeine, hydrocodone, meperidine, methadone, morphine, oxycodone, propoxyphene, or tramadol)
- medicines for anxiety or sleeping problems, such as diazepam or temazepam
- muscle relaxers

Tell your prescriber or health care professional about all other medicines that you are taking, including nonprescription medicines, nutritional supplements, or herbal products. Also tell your prescriber or health care professional if you are a frequent user of drinks with caffeine or alcohol, if you smoke, or if you use illegal drugs. These may affect the way your medicine works. Check with your health care professional before stopping or starting any of your medicines.

What should I watch for while taking carbinoxamine; pseudoephedrine?

Tell your prescriber or health care professional if your symptoms do not improve in 2 or 3 days. You may get drowsy or dizzy. Do not drive, use machinery, or do anything that needs mental alertness until you know how this medicine affects you. Be careful taking other medicines that may also make you tired. This effect may be worse when taking these medicines with products containing carbinoxamine. To reduce the risk of dizzy or fainting spells, do not stand or sit up quickly, especially if you are an older patient. Alcohol may increase dizziness and drowsiness. Avoid alcoholic drinks. If carbinoxamine; pseudoephedrine extended-release products make it difficult for you to sleep at night, avoid taking the medicine for about 8 to 10 hours before bedtime. If nervousness, dizziness, or sleeplessness occur, stop using carbinoxamine; pseudoephedrine and consult a physician. When carbinoxamine; pseudoephedrine is used you may experience dry eyes and blurred vision. If you wear contact lenses you may feel some discomfort. Lubricating drops may help. See your ophthalmologist if the problem does not go away or is severe.

What side effect may I notice from taking carbinoxamine; pseudoephedrine?

Side effects that you should report to your prescriber or health care professional as soon as possible:
- agitation, nervousness, excitability, not able to sleep
- difficulty breathing, wheezing, shortness of breath
- dizziness or fainting spells
- irregular heartbeat, palpitations, or chest pain
- pain or difficulty passing urine
- rash
- severe diarrhea
- severe vomiting
- swelling of the face, tongue, throat, hands or feet
- vision problems

Side effects that usually do not require medical attention (report to your prescriber or health care professional if they continue or are bothersome):
- difficulty sleeping
- dizziness
- drowsiness
- dry eyes
- mild diarrhea
- nausea, vomiting
- restlessness
- stomach upset
- tiredness

Where can I keep my medicine?

Keep out of the reach of children in a container that small children cannot open. Store at room temperature, between 15 and 30 degrees C (59 and 86 degrees F); do not freeze. Keep in a tightly closed, light-resistant container. Keep away from heat. Throw away any unused medicine after the expiration date.

Carisoprodol tablets

SOMA®;
350 mg; Tablet
Medpointe Pharmaceuticals

What are carisoprodol tablets?

CARISOPRODOL (Rela®, Soma®) is a muscle relaxant. Carisoprodol is used to relieve muscle spasms and pains associated with acute injuries. It should only be used for a short time and should be combined with rest, physical therapy or other non-drug therapies. Generic carisoprodol tablets are available.

What should my health care professional know before I take carisoprodol?

They need to know if you have any of these conditions:
- kidney disease
- liver disease
- porphyria
- an unusual or allergic reaction to carisoprodol, carbamate, sulfite, tartrazine, or any other substance
- pregnant or trying to get pregnant
- breast-feeding

How should I take this medicine?

Take carisoprodol tablets by mouth. Follow the directions on the prescription label. Swallow the tablets with a drink of water. If carisoprodol upsets your stomach, take the tablets with food or milk. Take your doses at regular intervals. Do not take your medicine more often than directed. Contact your pediatrician or health care professional regarding the use of this medicine in children. Special care may be needed. Elderly patients over 65 years old may have a stronger reaction to this medicine and need smaller doses.

What if I miss a dose?

If you miss a dose, take it as soon as you can. If it is almost time for your next dose, take only that dose. Do not take double or extra doses.

What may interact with carisoprodol?

- alcohol
- barbiturate medicines for inducing sleep or treating seizures (convulsions), like phenobarbital
- cimetidine
- isoniazid (INH)
- medicines for colds, hay fever or other allergies
- medicines for HIV or AIDS
- medicines for mental depression, anxiety, or emotional disturbances
- medicines for pain
- medicines for seizures (convulsions) or epilepsy
- medicines for sleep
- modafinil
- omeprazole
- other muscle relaxants
- rifampin, rifabutin, or rifapentine
- voriconazole

Tell your prescriber or health care professional about all other medicines you are taking, including non-prescription medicines, nutritional supplements, or herbal products. Also tell your prescriber or health care professional if you are a frequent user of drinks with caffeine or alcohol, if you smoke, or if you use illegal drugs. These may affect the way your medicine works. Check with your health care professional before stopping or starting any of your medicines.

What should I watch for while taking carisoprodol?

You may get drowsy or dizzy. Do not drive, use machinery, or do anything that needs mental alertness until you know how carisoprodol affects you. To reduce the risk of dizzy or fainting spells, do not sit or stand up quickly, especially if you are an older patient. Alcohol can make you more drowsy; avoid alcoholic drinks.

What side effects may I notice from taking carisoprodol?

Side effects that you should report to your prescriber or health care professional as soon as possible:

- confusion
- difficulty breathing
- fainting spells
- skin rash or redness
- trembling
- unsteadiness
- unusual weakness or tiredness

Side effects that usually do not require medical attention (report to your prescriber or health care professional if they continue or are bothersome):

- dizziness
- drowsiness
- flushing (reddening of the skin)
- headache
- nausea, vomiting

Where can I keep my medicine?

Keep out of the reach of children in a container that small children cannot open. Store at room temperature between 15 and 30 degrees C (59 and 86 degrees F). Protect from moisture. Keep container tightly closed. Throw away any unused medicine after the expiration date.

Carteolol tablets

Oral tablets no longer on the market.

CARTROL®;
5 mg; Tablet
Abbott
Pharmaceutical
Product Division

CARTROL®;
2.5 mg; Tablet
Abbott
Pharmaceutical
Product Division

What are carteolol tablets?

CARTEOLOL (Cartrol®) belongs to a group of medicines called beta-blockers. Carteolol controls, but does not cure, high blood pressure (hypertension). High blood pressure may not make you feel sick, but it can lead to serious problems. NOTE: Carteolol tablets are no longer available in the US.

What should my health care professional know before I take carteolol?

They need to know if you have any of these conditions:

- asthma, bronchitis or bronchospasm
- circulation problems, or blood vessel disease (such as Raynaud's disease)
- depression
- diabetes
- emphysema, or other lung disease
- history of heart attack or heart failure
- kidney disease
- low blood pressure
- muscle weakness or disease
- pheochromocytoma
- psoriasis
- thyroid disease
- an unusual or allergic reaction to carteolol, other beta-blockers, medicines, foods, dyes, or preservatives
- pregnant or trying to get pregnant
- breast-feeding

How should I take this medicine?

Take carteolol tablets by mouth. Follow the directions on the prescription label. Swallow the tablets with a drink of water. Take your doses at regular intervals. Do not take your medicine more often than directed. Do not stop taking except on your prescriber's advice. This medicine is not for use in children.

What if I miss a dose?

If you miss a dose, take it as soon as you can. If it is almost time for your next dose (less than 4 hours), take only that dose. Do not take double or extra doses.

What may interact with carteolol?

- anti-inflammatory drugs (NSAIDs, such as ibuprofen)
- atropine
- clonidine
- ergotamine
- hawthorn
- levodopa
- medicines for high blood pressure
- medicines for colds and breathing difficulties
- medicines for diabetes
- medicines for mental depression
- medicines for mental problems and psychotic disturbances
- medicines to control heart rhythm
- theophylline

Tell your prescriber or health care professional about all other medicines you are taking, including non-prescription medicines, nutritional supplements, or herbal products. Also tell your prescriber or health care professional if you are a frequent user of drinks with caffeine or alcohol, if you smoke, or if you use illegal drugs. These may affect the way your medicine works. Check with your health care professional before stopping or starting any of your medicines.

What should I watch for while taking carteolol?

Check your heart rate and blood pressure regularly while you are taking carteolol. Ask your prescriber or health care professional what your heart rate and blood pressure should be while taking this drug. Do not stop taking this medicine suddenly. This could lead to serious heart-related effects. You may get drowsy or dizzy. Do not drive, use machinery, or do anything that requires mental alertness until you know how carteolol affects you. To reduce the risk of dizzy or fainting spells, do not sit or stand up quickly. Alcohol can make you more drowsy, and increase flushing and rapid heartbeats. Therefore, it is best to avoid alcoholic drinks. Carteolol can affect blood sugar levels. If you have diabetes, check with your prescriber or health care professional before you change your diet or the dose of your diabetic medicine. If you are going to have surgery, tell your prescriber or health care professional that you are taking carteolol.

What side effects may I notice from taking carteolol?

Side effects that you should report to your prescriber or health care professional as soon as possible:

- changes in blood sugar
- cold hands or feet
- difficulty breathing, wheezing
- difficulty sleeping, nightmares
- dizziness or fainting spells
- irregular heartbeat, palpitations, chest pain
- joint or muscle aches or pains
- ringing in the ears
- skin rash, itching, peeling skin
- slow heart rate (less than 50 beats per minute)
- swelling of the legs or ankles
- vomiting

Side effects that usually do not require medical attention (report to your prescriber or health care professional if they continue or are bothersome):

- constipation or diarrhea
- gas
- hair loss
- nausea
- sexual difficulties (impotence or decreased sexual urges)
- weakness or tiredness

Where can I keep my medicine?

Keep out of the reach of children. Store at room temperature between 15 and 25 degrees C (59 and 77 degrees F). Protect from light. Keep container tightly closed. Throw away any unused medicine after the expiration date.

Carvedilol tablets

COREG™;
12.5 mg; Tablet
Smithkline Beecham
Pharmaceuticals Div
Smithkline Beecham
Co

COREG™;
3.125 mg; Tablet
Smithkline Beecham
Pharmaceuticals Div
Smithkline Beecham
Co

What are carvedilol tablets?

CARVEDILOL (Coreg™) belongs to a group of medicines called beta-blockers. Beta-blockers have many actions on the heart and blood vessels. Carvedilol is used for high blood pressure (hypertension) and heart failure. Carvedilol controls, but does not cure, these conditions. High blood pressure may not make you feel sick, but it can lead to serious health problems. Generic carvedilol tablets are not yet available.

What should my health care professional know before I take carvedilol?

They need to know if you have any of these conditions:

- asthma, bronchitis or bronchospasm
- circulation problems
- depression
- diabetes
- emphysema, or other lung disease
- history of heart attack or heart disease
- liver disease

- muscle weakness or disease
- psoriasis
- thyroid disease
- an unusual or allergic reaction to carvedilol, other beta-blockers, medicines, foods, dyes, or preservatives
- pregnant or trying to get pregnant
- breast-feeding

How should I take this medicine?

Take carvedilol tablets by mouth. Follow the directions on the prescription label. Swallow the tablets with a drink of water. It is best to take the tablets with food. Take your doses at regular intervals. Do not take your medicine more often than directed. Do not stop taking except on your prescriber's advice. Contact your pediatrician or health care professional regarding the use of this medicine in children. Special care may be needed.

What if I miss a dose?

If you miss a dose, take it as soon as you can. If it is almost time for your next dose, take only that dose. Do not take double or extra doses. There should be at least 12 hours between doses.

What may interact with carvedilol?

- cimetidine
- digoxin
- diltiazem
- hawthorn
- medicines for colds and breathing difficulties
- medicines for diabetes
- medicines for high blood pressure
- rifampin
- verapamil
- water pills (diuretics)

Tell your prescriber or health care professional about all other medicines you are taking, including nonprescription medicines, nutritional supplements, or herbal products. Also tell your prescriber or health care professional if you are a frequent user of drinks with caffeine or alcohol, if you smoke, or if you use illegal drugs. These may affect the way your medicine works. Check with your health care professional before stopping or starting any of your medicines.

What should I watch for while taking carvedilol?

Check your heart rate and blood pressure regularly while you are taking carvedilol. Ask your prescriber or health care professional what your heart rate and blood pressure should be, and when you should contact him or her. Contact your prescriber or health care professional if you have difficulty breathing while taking this drug. Check your weight daily. Ask your prescriber or health care professional when you should notify him/her of any weight gain. Do not stop taking this medicine suddenly. This could lead to serious heart-related effects. You may get drowsy or dizzy. Do not drive, use machinery, or do anything that requires mental alertness until you know how carvedilol affects you. To reduce the risk of dizzy or fainting spells, do not sit or stand up quickly. Alcohol can make you more drowsy, and increase flushing and rapid heartbeats. Therefore, it is best to avoid alcoholic drinks. Carvedilol may affect blood sugar levels. If you have diabetes, check with your prescriber or health care professional before you change your diet or the dose of your diabetic medicine. If you are going to have surgery, tell your prescriber or health care professional that you are taking carvedilol.

What side effects may I notice from taking carvedilol?

Side effects that you should report to your prescriber or health care professional as soon as possible:

- continued loss of appetite
- difficulty breathing, wheezing
- dizziness or fainting spells
- dark urine
- flu-like symptoms
- irregular heartbeat
- skin rash
- slow heart rate (fewer than recommended by your prescriber or health care professional)
- swollen legs or ankles
- vomiting
- weight gain
- yellowing of the eyes or skin

Side effects that usually do not require medical attention (report to your prescriber or health care professional if they continue or are bothersome):

- back pain
- diarrhea
- dry eyes (especially if wearing contact lenses)
- dry, itching skin
- headache
- insomnia
- nausea
- sore throat
- unusual tiredness

Where can I keep my medicine?

Keep out of the reach of children in a container that small children cannot open. Store at room temperature between 15 degrees and 30 degrees C (59 degrees and 86 degrees F). Protect from moisture. Throw away any unused medicine after the expiration date.

Cefaclor capsules and extended-release tablets

CECLOR®;
250 mg; Capsule
Eli Lilly and Co

CECLOR® CD;
500 mg; Tablet,
Extended Release
Elan
Pharmaceuticals Inc

What are cefaclor capsules?

CEFACLOR (Ceclor®, Ceclor® CD, Ceclor® ER) is a cephalosporin antibiotic. It treats many kinds of infections including those of the skin, respiratory tract, sinuses, ear, and urinary tract. Generic cefaclor capsules and extended-release tablets are available.

What should my health care professional know before I take cefaclor?

They need to know if you have any of these conditions:
- bleeding problems
- diarrhea
- kidney disease
- stomach or intestinal problems (especially colitis)
- other chronic illness
- an unusual or allergic reaction to cefaclor, other cephalosporin antibiotics, penicillin, penicillamine, other foods, dyes or preservatives
- pregnant or trying to get pregnant
- breast-feeding

How should I take this medicine?

Take cefaclor capsules and extended-release tablets by mouth. Follow the directions on the prescription label. Take your doses at regular intervals. Do not take your medicine more often than directed. Finish the full course prescribed by your prescriber or health care professional even if you think your condition is better. Do not stop taking except on your prescriber's advice. Contact your pediatrician or health care professional regarding the use of this medicine in children. Special care may be needed.
Capsules: You can take the capsules with or without food. If cefaclor upsets your stomach it may help to take with food.
Extended-release tablets: Take the tablets with food or within 1 hour after eating a meal. Swallow the tablets whole; do not chew, crush, or cut the tablets.

What if I miss a dose?

If you miss a dose, take it as soon as you can. If it is almost time for your next dose, take only that dose. Do not take double or extra doses. There should be an interval of at least 4 hours between doses.

What may interact with cefaclor?

- other antibiotics
- probenecid

Tell your prescriber or health care professional about all other medicines you are taking, including non-prescription medicines, nutritional supplements, or herbal products. Also tell your prescriber or health care professional if you are a frequent user of drinks with caffeine or alcohol, if you smoke, or if you use illegal drugs. These may affect the way your medicine works. Check with your health care professional before stopping or starting any of your medicines.

What should I watch for while taking cefaclor?

Tell your prescriber or health care professional if your symptoms do not begin to improve in a few days. If you are diabetic you may get a false-positive result for sugar in your urine. Check with your prescriber or health care professional before you change your diet or the dose of your diabetic medicine. If you get severe or watery diarrhea, do not treat yourself. Call your prescriber or health care professional for advice. If you have to have surgery, tell your prescriber or health care professional that you are taking cefaclor.

What side effects may I notice from taking cefaclor?

Side effects that you should report to your prescriber or health care professional as soon as possible:
- difficulty breathing, wheezing
- dizziness
- fever or chills, sore throat
- reduced amount of urine
- redness, blistering, peeling or loosening of the skin, including inside the mouth
- seizures (convulsions)
- severe or watery diarrhea
- skin rash, itching
- stomach pain or cramps
- swollen joints
- unusual bleeding or bruising
- unusual tiredness or weakness

Side effects that usually do not require medical attention (report to your prescriber or health care professional if they continue or are bothersome):
- diarrhea
- gas or heartburn
- headache
- nausea, vomiting

Where can I keep my medicine?

Keep out of the reach of children in a container that small children cannot open. Store at room temperature between 15 and 30 degrees C (59 and 86 degrees F). Throw away any unused medicine after the expiration date.

Cefadroxil tablets or capsules

DURICEF®;
500 mg; Capsule
Warner Chilcott PLC

DURICEF®;
1 g; Tablet
Warner Chilcott PLC

What are cefadroxil tablets or capsules?

CEFADROXIL (Duricef®) is a cephalosporin antibiotic. It treats many kinds of infections including those of the skin, respiratory tract, sinuses, ears, and urinary tract. Generic cefadroxil tablets and capsules are available.

What should my health care professional know before I take cefadroxil?

They need to know if you have any of these conditions:
- bleeding problems
- kidney disease
- stomach or intestinal problems (especially colitis)
- other chronic illness
- an unusual or allergic reaction to cefadroxil, other cephalosporin antibiotics, penicillin, penicillamine, other foods, dyes or preservatives
- pregnant or trying to get pregnant
- breast-feeding

How should I take this medicine?

Take cefadroxil tablets or capsules by mouth. Follow the directions on the prescription label. Swallow the tablets or capsules with a drink of water. You can take cefadroxil with or without food. If cefadroxil upsets your stomach it may help to take it with food. Take your doses at regular intervals. Do not take your medicine more often than directed. Finish the full course prescribed by your prescriber or health care professional even if you think your condition is better. Do not stop taking except on your prescriber's advice. Contact your pediatrician or health care professional regarding the use of this medicine in children. Special care may be needed.

What if I miss a dose?

If you miss a dose, take it as soon as you can. If it is almost time for your next dose, take only that dose. Do not take double or extra doses. There should be an interval of at least 4 to 6 hours between doses.

What may interact with cefadroxil?

- other antibiotics
- probenecid

Tell your prescriber or health care professional about all other medicines you are taking, including non-prescription medicines, nutritional supplements, or herbal products. Also tell your prescriber or health care professional if you are a frequent user of drinks with caffeine or alcohol, if you smoke, or if you use illegal drugs. These may affect the way your medicine works. Check with your health care professional before stopping or starting any of your medicines.

What should I watch for while taking cefadroxil?

Tell your prescriber or health care professional if your symptoms do not begin to improve in a few days. If you are diabetic you may get a false-positive result for sugar in your urine. Check with your prescriber or health care professional before you change your diet or the dose of your diabetic medicine. If you get severe or watery diarrhea, do not treat yourself. Call your prescriber or health care professional for advice.

What side effects may I notice from taking cefadroxil?

Side effects that you should report to your prescriber or health care professional as soon as possible:
- difficulty breathing, wheezing
- dizziness
- fever or chills, sore throat
- headache
- reduced amount of urine
- redness, blistering, peeling or loosening of the skin, including inside the mouth
- seizures (convulsions)
- severe or watery diarrhea
- skin rash, itching
- swollen joints
- unusual weakness or tiredness

Side effects that usually do not require medical attention (report to your prescriber or health care professional if they continue or are bothersome):
- diarrhea
- gas or heartburn
- nausea, vomiting

Where can I keep my medicine?

Keep out of the reach of children in a container that small children cannot open. Store at room temperature between 15 and 30 degrees C (59 and 86 degrees F). Throw away any unused medicine after the expiration date.

Cefdinir capsules

OMNICEF®;
300 mg; Capsule
Abbott Pharmaceutical
Product Division

What are cefdinir capsules?

CEFDINIR (Omnicef®) is a cephalosporin antibiotic. It treats many kinds of infections including those of the skin, respiratory tract, sinuses, ears, and urinary tract. Generic cefdinir capsules are not available.

What should my health care professional know before I take cefdinir?

They need to know if you have any of these conditions:
- bleeding problems
- kidney disease
- stomach or intestinal problems (especially colitis)
- other chronic illness
- an unusual or allergic reaction to cefdinir, other cephalosporin antibiotics, penicillin, penicillamine, other foods, dyes or preservatives
- pregnant or trying to get pregnant
- breast-feeding

How should I take this medicine?

Take cefdinir capsules by mouth. Follow the directions on the prescription label. Swallow the capsules with a drink of water. You can take cefdinir with or without food. If cefdinir upsets your stomach, it may help to take it with food. Take your doses at regular intervals. Do not take your medicine more often than directed. Finish the full course prescribed by your prescriber or health care professional even if you think your condition is better. Do not stop taking except on your prescriber's advice. Contact your pediatrician or health care professional regarding the use of this medicine in children. Special care may be needed.

What if I miss a dose?

If you miss a dose, take it as soon as you can. If it is almost time for your next dose, take only that dose. Do not take double or extra doses. There should be an interval of at least 4 to 6 hours between doses.

What may interact with cefdinir?

- other antibiotics
- probenecid

Tell your prescriber or health care professional about all other medicines you are taking, including non-prescription medicines, nutritional supplements, or herbal products. Also tell your prescriber or health care professional if you are a frequent user of drinks with caffeine or alcohol, if you smoke, or if you use illegal drugs. These may affect the way your medicine works. Check with your health care professional before stopping or starting any of your medicines.

What should I watch for while taking cefdinir?

Tell your prescriber or health care professional if your symptoms do not begin to improve in a few days. If you are diabetic, you may get a false-positive result for sugar in your urine. Check with your prescriber or health care professional before you change your diet or the dose of your diabetic medicine. If you get severe or watery diarrhea, do not treat yourself. Call your prescriber or health care professional for advice.

What side effects may I notice from taking cefdinir?

Side effects that you should report to your prescriber or health care professional as soon as possible:
- difficulty breathing, wheezing
- redness, blistering, peeling or loosening of the skin, including inside the mouth
- seizures (convulsions)
- severe or watery diarrhea
- skin rash, hives, or itching
- swelling of the lips, tongue or face
- swollen joints
- unusual weakness or tiredness
- vaginal itching
- vomiting

Side effects that usually do not require medical attention (report to your prescriber or health care professional if they continue or are bothersome):
- constipation, diarrhea, or other stool changes
- dizziness or drowsiness
- gas or heartburn
- insomnia
- loss of appetite
- nausea
- stomach pain

Where can I keep my medicine?

Keep out of the reach of children in a container that small children cannot open. Store at room temperature between 15 and 30 degrees C (59 and 86 degrees F). Throw away any unused medicine after the expiration date.

C

Cefditoren tablets

SPECTRACEF®;
200 mg; Tablet
Purdue Pharmaceutical
Products LP

C

What are cefditoren tablets?

CEFDITOREN (Spectracef®) is a cephalosporin antibiotic. It is used to treat bronchitis, pharyngitis, tonsillitis, and infections of the skin. Cefditoren may also be used to treat sinus infections. Generic cefditoren tablets are not yet available.

What should my health care professional know before I take cefditoren?

They need to know if you have any of these conditions:
- allergy to milk proteins (not lactose intolerant)
- bleeding problems
- carnitine deficiency
- kidney or liver disease
- stomach or intestinal problems (especially colitis)
- other chronic illness
- an unusual or allergic reaction to cefditoren, other cephalosporin antibiotics, penicillin, penicillamine, other medicines, foods, dyes or preservatives
- pregnant or trying to get pregnant
- breast-feeding

How should I take this medicine?

Take cefditoren tablets by mouth with food. Follow the directions on the prescription label. Take your doses at regular intervals. Do not take your medicine more often than directed. Finish the full course prescribed by your prescriber or health care professional even if you think your condition is better. Do not stop taking except on your prescriber's advice. Contact your pediatrician or health care professional regarding the use of this medicine in children. Special care may be needed.

What if I miss a dose?

If you miss a dose, take it as soon as you can. If it is almost time for your next dose, take only that dose. Do not take double or extra doses.

What may interact with cefditoren?

- antacids, including aluminum and magnesium salts
- probenecid
- stomach or ulcer drugs such as nizatidine (Axid®), cimetidine (Tagamet®), famotidine (Pepcid®), or ranitidine (Zantac®)

Tell your prescriber or health care professional about all other medicines you are taking, including non-prescription medicines, nutritional supplements, or herbal products. Also tell your prescriber or health care professional if you are a frequent user of drinks with caffeine or alcohol, if you smoke, or if you use illegal drugs. These may affect the way your medicine works. Check with your health care professional before stopping or starting any of your medicines.

What should I watch for while taking cefditoren?

Tell your prescriber or health care professional if your symptoms do not begin to improve in a few days. If you are diabetic you may get a false-positive result for sugar in your urine. Check with your prescriber or health care professional before you change your diet or the dose of your diabetic medicine. If you get severe or watery diarrhea, do not treat yourself. Call your prescriber or health care professional for advice.

What side effects may I notice from taking cefditoren?

Side effects that you should report to your prescriber or health care professional as soon as possible:
- difficulty breathing, wheezing
- fever or chills, sore throat
- redness, blistering, peeling or loosening of the skin, including inside the mouth
- severe or watery diarrhea
- skin rash, itching
- stomach pain or cramps
- unusual bleeding or bruising
- vaginal yeast infection
- vomiting

Side effects that usually do not require medical attention (report to your prescriber or health care professional if they continue or are bothersome):
- change in appetite
- constipation or diarrhea
- dry mouth
- gas or heartburn
- headache
- insomnia
- loss of appetite
- nausea

Where can I keep my medicine?

Keep out of the reach of children in a container that small children cannot open. Store at room temperature between 15 and 30 degrees C (59 and 86 degrees F). Throw away any unused medicine after the expiration date.

Cefixime tablets

SUPRAX®;
400 mg; Tablet
Lederle
Pharmaceutical

SURPAX®;
200 mg; Tablet
Lederle
Pharmaceutical

What are cefixime tablets?

CEFIXIME (Suprax®) is a cephalosporin antibiotic. It treats many kinds of infections, including those of the respiratory tract, sinuses, ears, and urinary tract. Cefixime also treats some sexually transmitted disease. Generic cefixime tablets are not yet available.

What should my health care professional know before I take cefixime?

They need to know if you have any of these conditions:

- bleeding problems
- diarrhea
- kidney disease
- stomach or intestinal problems (especially colitis)
- other chronic illness
- an unusual or allergic reaction to cefixime, other cephalosporin antibiotics, penicillin, penicillamine, other foods, dyes or preservatives
- pregnant or trying to get pregnant
- breast-feeding

How should I take this medicine?

Take cefixime tablets by mouth. Follow the directions on the prescription label. You can take cefixime with or without food. If cefixime upsets your stomach it may help to take it with food. Take your doses at regular intervals. Do not take your medicine more often than directed. Finish the full course prescribed by your prescriber or health care professional even if you think your condition is better. Do not stop taking except on your prescriber's advice. Contact your pediatrician or health care professional regarding the use of this medicine in children. Special care may be needed.

What if I miss a dose?

If you miss a dose, take it as soon as you can. If it is almost time for your next dose, take only that dose. Do not take double or extra doses. There should be an interval of at least 10 to 12 hours between doses.

What may interact with cefixime?

- aspirin and aspirin-like medicines
- probenecid

Tell your prescriber or health care professional about all other medicines you are taking, including non-prescription medicines, nutritional supplements, or herbal products. Also tell your prescriber or health care professional if you are a frequent user of drinks with caffeine or alcohol, if you smoke, or if you use illegal drugs. These may affect the way your medicine works. Check with your health care professional before stopping or starting any of your medicines.

What should I watch for while taking cefixime?

Tell your prescriber or health care professional if your symptoms do not begin to improve in a few days. If you are diabetic you may get a false-positive result for sugar in your urine. Check with your prescriber or health care professional before you change your diet or the dose of your diabetic medicine. If you get severe or watery diarrhea, do not treat yourself. Call your prescriber or health care professional for advice. If you are being treated for a sexually transmitted disease, avoid sexual contact until you have finished your treatment. Having sex can infect your sexual partner.

What side effects may I notice from taking cefixime?

Side effects that you should report to your prescriber or health care professional as soon as possible:

- difficulty breathing, wheezing
- dizziness
- fever or chills, sore throat
- pain or difficulty passing urine
- redness, blistering, peeling or loosening of the skin, including inside the mouth
- seizures (convulsions)
- severe or watery diarrhea
- skin rash, itching
- stomach pain or cramps
- swollen joints
- unusual bleeding or bruising
- unusual weakness or tiredness

Side effects that usually do not require medical attention (report to your prescriber or health care professional if they continue or are bothersome):

- diarrhea
- gas or heartburn
- genital and anal irritation
- headache
- loss of appetite
- nausea, vomiting

Let your prescriber or health care professional know about these side effects, if they do not go away or if they annoy you.

Where can I keep my medicine?

Keep out of the reach of children in a container that small children cannot open. Store at room temperature between 15 and 30 degrees C (59 and 86 degrees F). Throw away any unused medicine after the expiration date.

C

Cefpodoxime tablets

VANTIN®;
200 mg; Tablet
Pharmacia and
Upjohn Div Pfizer

VANTIN®;
100 mg; Tablet
Pharmacia and
Upjohn Div Pfizer

What are cefpodoxime tablets?

CEFPODOXIME (Vantin®) is a cephalosporin antibiotic. It treats many kinds of infections, including those of the respiratory tract, skin, and ears. Generic cefpodoxime tablets are available.

What should my health care professional know before I take cefpodoxime?

They need to know if you have any of these conditions:
- bleeding problems
- kidney disease
- stomach or intestinal problems (especially colitis)
- other chronic illness
- an unusual or allergic reaction to cefpodoxime, other cephalosporin antibiotics, penicillin, penicillamine, other foods, dyes or preservatives
- pregnant or trying to get pregnant
- breast-feeding

How should I take this medicine?

Take cefpodoxime tablets by mouth with food. Follow the directions on the prescription label. Do not take your medicine more often than directed. Finish the full course prescribed by your prescriber or health care professional even if you think your condition is better. Do not stop taking except on your prescriber's advice. Contact your pediatrician or health care professional regarding the use of this medicine in children. Special care may be needed.

What if I miss a dose?

If you miss a dose, take it as soon as you can. If it is almost time for your next dose, take only that dose. Do not take double or extra doses. There should be an interval of at least 10 to 12 hours between doses.

What may interact with cefpodoxime?

- antacids
- didanosine
- probenecid
- stomach or ulcer drugs such as cimetidine (Tagamet®), famotidine (Pepcid®), lansoprazole (Prevacid®), nizatidine (Axid®), omeprazole (Prilosec®), or ranitidine (Zantac®)

Tell your prescriber or health care professional about all other medicines you are taking, including nonprescription medicines, nutritional supplements, or herbal products. Also tell your prescriber or health care professional if you are a frequent user of drinks with caffeine or alcohol, if you smoke, or if you use illegal drugs. These may affect the way your medicine works. Check with your health care professional before stopping or starting any of your medicines.

What should I watch for while taking cefpodoxime?

Tell your prescriber or health care professional if your symptoms do not begin to improve in a few days. If you get severe or watery diarrhea, do not treat yourself. Call your prescriber or health care professional for advice.

What side effects may I notice from taking cefpodoxime?

Side effects that you should report to your prescriber or health care professional as soon as possible:
- difficulty breathing, wheezing
- nosebleed
- redness, blistering, peeling or loosening of the skin, including inside the mouth
- seizures (convulsions)
- severe or watery diarrhea
- skin rash, hives, or itching
- swelling of the lips, tongue or face
- swollen joints
- unusual weakness or tiredness
- vaginal itching
- vomiting

Side effects that usually do not require medical attention (report to your prescriber or health care professional if they continue or are bothersome):
- constipation, diarrhea, or other stool changes
- dizziness or drowsiness
- gas or heartburn
- headache
- insomnia
- loss of appetite
- nausea
- nervousness
- stomach pain

Where can I keep my medicine?

Keep out of the reach of children in a container that small children cannot open. Store at room temperature between 15 and 30 degrees C (59 and 86 degrees F). Throw away any unused medicine after the expiration date.

C

Cefprozil tablets

CEFZIL®;
250 mg; Tablet
Bristol Myers Squibb
Co

CEFZIL®;
500 mg; Tablet
Bristol Myers Squibb
Co

What are cefprozil tablets?

CEFPROZIL (Cefzil®) is a cephalosporin antibiotic. It treats many kinds of infections, including those of the respiratory tract, skin, ears. Generic cefprozil tablets are available.

What should my health care professional know before I take cefprozil?

They need to know if you have any of these conditions:
- bleeding problems
- kidney disease
- phenylketonuria
- stomach or intestinal problems (especially colitis)
- other chronic illness
- an unusual or allergic reaction to cefprozil, other cephalosporin antibiotics, penicillin, penicillamine, other foods, dyes or preservatives
- pregnant or trying to get pregnant
- breast-feeding

How should I take this medicine?

Take cefprozil tablets by mouth. Follow the directions on the prescription label. You can take cefprozil with or without food. If cefprozil upsets your stomach it may help to take it with food. Do not take your medicine more often than directed. Finish the full course prescribed by your prescriber or health care professional even if you think your condition is better. Do not stop taking except on your prescriber's advice. Contact your pediatrician or health care professional regarding the use of this medicine in children. Special care may be needed.

What if I miss a dose?

If you miss a dose, take it as soon as you can. If it is almost time for your next dose, take only that dose. Do not take double or extra doses. There should be an interval of at least 10 to 12 hours between doses.

What may interact with cefprozil?

- other antibiotics
- probenecid

Tell your prescriber or health care professional about all other medicines you are taking, including non-prescription medicines, nutritional supplements, or herbal products. Also tell your prescriber or health care professional if you are a frequent user of drinks with caffeine or alcohol, if you smoke, or if you use illegal drugs. These may affect the way your medicine works. Check with your health care professional before stopping or starting any of your medicines.

What should I watch for while taking cefprozil?

Tell your prescriber or health care professional if your symptoms do not begin to improve in a few days. If you are diabetic you may get a false-positive result for sugar in your urine. Check with your prescriber or health care professional before you change your diet or the dose of your diabetic medicine. If you get severe or watery diarrhea, do not treat yourself. Call your prescriber or health care professional for advice.

What side effects may I notice from taking cefprozil?

Side effects that you should report to your prescriber or health care professional as soon as possible:
- difficulty breathing, wheezing
- dizziness
- fever or chills, sore throat
- pain or difficulty passing urine
- redness, blistering, peeling or loosening of the skin, including inside the mouth
- seizures (convulsions)
- severe or watery diarrhea
- skin rash, itching
- stomach pain or cramps
- swollen joints
- unusual bleeding or bruising
- unusual weakness or tiredness

Side effects that usually do not require medical attention (report to your prescriber or health care professional if they continue or are bothersome):
- diarrhea
- gas or heartburn
- nausea, vomiting

Where can I keep my medicine?

Keep out of the reach of children in a container that small children cannot open. Store at room temperature between 15 and 30 degrees C (59 and 86 degrees F). Throw away any unused medicine after the expiration date.

C

Ceftibuten capsules

CEDAX®;
400 mg; Capsule
Shionogi USA, Inc.

What are ceftibuten capsules?

CEFTIBUTEN (Cedax®) is a cephalosporin antibiotic. It treats infections of the respiratory tract and ears. Generic ceftibuten capsules are not yet available.

What should my health care professional know before I take ceftibuten?

They need to know if you have any of these conditions:
- kidney disease
- stomach or intestinal problems (especially colitis)
- other chronic illness
- an unusual or allergic reaction to ceftibuten, other cephalosporin antibiotics, penicillin, penicillamine, other foods, dyes or preservatives
- pregnant or trying to get pregnant
- breast-feeding

How should I take this medicine?

Take ceftibuten capsules by mouth on an empty stomach. Follow the directions on the prescription label. Do not take your medicine more often than directed. Finish the full course prescribed by your prescriber or health care professional even if you think your condition is better. Do not stop taking except on your prescriber's advice. Contact your pediatrician or health care professional regarding the use of this medicine in children. Special care may be needed.

What if I miss a dose?

If you miss a dose, take it as soon as you can. If it is almost time for your next dose, take only that dose. Do not take double or extra doses.

What may interact with ceftibuten?

- didanosine
- Stomach or ulcer drugs such as cimetidine (Tagamet®), famotidine (Pepcid®), lansoprazole (Prevacid®), nizatidine (Axid®), omeprazole (Prilosec®), or ranitidine (Zantac®)

Tell your prescriber or health care professional about all other medicines you are taking, including non-prescription medicines, nutritional supplements, or herbal products. Also tell your prescriber or health care professional if you are a frequent user of drinks with caffeine or alcohol, if you smoke, or if you use illegal drugs.

These may affect the way your medicine works. Check with your health care professional before stopping or starting any of your medicines.

What should I watch for while taking ceftibuten?

Tell your prescriber or health care professional if your symptoms do not begin to improve in a few days. If you get severe or watery diarrhea, do not treat yourself. Call your prescriber or health care professional for advice. Your mouth may get dry. Chewing sugarless gum or sucking hard candy, and drinking plenty of water will help. Brush and floss teeth regularly and carefully to avoid problems with the mouth and gums.

What side effects may I notice from taking ceftibuten?

Side effects that you should report to your prescriber or health care professional as soon as possible:
- difficult or painful urination
- difficulty breathing, wheezing
- redness, blistering, peeling or loosening of the skin, including inside the mouth
- severe or watery diarrhea
- skin rash, hives, or itching
- swelling of the lips, tongue or face
- unusual weakness or tiredness
- vaginal itching
- vomiting

Side effects that usually do not require medical attention (report to your prescriber or health care professional if they continue or are bothersome):
- constipation, diarrhea, or other stool changes
- dizziness or drowsiness
- dry mouth
- gas or heartburn
- headache
- loss of appetite or changes in taste
- nausea
- stomach pain

Where can I keep my medicine?

Keep out of the reach of children in a container that small children cannot open. Store at room temperature between 2 degrees and 25 degrees C (36 degrees and 77 degrees F). Throw away any unused medicine after the expiration date.

Cefuroxime tablets

CEFUROXIME;
500 mg; Tablet
Watson Pharmaceuticals Inc

What are cefuroxime tablets?

CEFUROXIME (Ceftin®) is a cephalosporin antibiotic. It treats many kinds of infections including those of the skin, respiratory tract (tonsillitis and bronchitis), sinuses, ear, and urinary tract. Cefuroxime also treats some sexually transmitted disease. Generic cefuroxime tablets are available.

What should my health care professional know before I take cefuroxime?

They need to know if you have any of these conditions:
- bleeding problems
- kidney disease
- stomach or intestinal problems (especially colitis)
- other chronic illness
- an unusual or allergic reaction to cefuroxime, other cephalosporin antibiotics, penicillin, penicillamine, other foods, dyes or preservatives
- pregnant or trying to get pregnant
- breast-feeding

How should I take this medicine?

Take cefuroxime tablets by mouth. Follow the directions on the prescription label. Cefuroxime works best if you take it with food. Do not take your medicine more often than directed. Finish the full course prescribed by your prescriber or health care professional even if you think your condition is better. Do not stop taking except on your prescriber's advice. Contact your pediatrician or health care professional regarding the use of this medicine in children. Special care may be needed.

What if I miss a dose?

If you miss a dose, take it as soon as you can. If it is almost time for your next dose, take only that dose. Do not take double or extra doses. There should be an interval of at least 10 to 12 hours between doses.

What may interact with cefuroxime?

- other antibiotics
- probenecid
- water pills

Tell your prescriber or health care professional about all other medicines you are taking, including non-prescription medicines, nutritional supplements, or herbal products. Also tell your prescriber or health care professional if you are a frequent user of drinks with caffeine or alcohol, if you smoke, or if you use illegal drugs.

These may affect the way your medicine works. Check with your health care professional before stopping or starting any of your medicines.

What should I watch for while taking cefuroxime?

Tell your prescriber or health care professional if your symptoms do not begin to improve in a few days. If you are diabetic you may get a false-positive result for sugar in your urine. Check with your prescriber or health care professional before you change your diet or the dose of your diabetic medicine. If you get severe or watery diarrhea, do not treat yourself. Call your prescriber or health care professional for advice. If you are being treated for a sexually transmitted disease, avoid sexual contact until you have finished your treatment. Having sex can infect your sexual partner.

What side effects may I notice from taking cefuroxime?

Side effects that you should report to your prescriber or health care professional as soon as possible:
- difficulty breathing, wheezing
- dizziness
- fever or chills, sore throat
- headache
- reduced amount of urine
- redness, blistering, peeling or loosening of the skin, including inside the mouth
- seizures (convulsions)
- severe or watery diarrhea
- skin rash, itching
- swollen joints
- unusual bleeding or bruising
- unusual weakness or tiredness

Side effects that usually do not require medical attention (report to your prescriber or health care professional if they continue or are bothersome):
- diarrhea
- gas or heartburn
- nausea, vomiting
- vaginal itching

Where can I keep my medicine?

Keep out of the reach of children in a container that small children cannot open. Store at room temperature between 15 and 30 degrees C (59 and 86 degrees F). Keep container tightly closed. Protect from moisture. Throw away any unused medicine after the expiration date.

C

Celecoxib capsules

CELEBREX®;
100 mg; Capsule
GD Searle LLC a
Subsidiary of
Pharmacia Company
Pfizer

CELEBREX®;
200 mg; Capsule
GD Searle LLC a
Subsidiary of
Pharmacia Company
Pfizer

This drug
requires an
FDA
medication
guide. See
page
xxxvii.

What are celecoxib capsules?

CELECOXIB (Celebrex®) used to reduce inflammation and ease mild to moderate pain for such conditions as arthritis or painful menstrual cycles. Celecoxib may also be used to treat certain other conditions such as familial adenomatous polyposis (FAP). Generic celecoxib capsules are not available.

What should my health care professional know before I take celecoxib?

They need to know if you have any of these conditions:
- anemia
- asthma, especially aspirin sensitive asthma
- bleeding problems or taking medicines that make bleed easily such as anticoagulants ('blood thinners')
- cigarette smoker
- dehydrated
- drink more than 3 alcohol-containing beverages a day
- heart or circulation problems such as heart failure or leg edema (fluid retention)
- high blood pressure
- kidney disease
- liver disease
- nasal polyps
- stomach bleeding or ulcers
- taking hormones such as prednisone (steroids)
- an unusual or allergic reaction to celecoxib, aspirin, other salicylates, other NSAIDs, sulfonamides, other drugs, foods, dyes or preservatives
- pregnant or trying to get pregnant
- breast-feeding

How should I take this medicine?

Take celecoxib capsules by mouth. Follow the directions on the prescription label. Swallow capsules whole with a full glass of water; take capsules in an upright or sitting position. Taking a sip of water first, before taking the capsules, may help you swallow them. If possible take bedtime doses at least 10 minutes before lying down. If celecoxib upsets your stomach, take it with food or milk. Take your doses at regular intervals. Do not take your medicine more often than directed. Contact your pediatrician or health care professional regarding the use of this medicine in children. Special care may be needed.

What if I miss a dose?

If you miss a dose, take it as soon as you can. If it is almost time for your next dose, take only that dose. Do not take double or extra doses.

What may interact with celecoxib?

- alcohol
- alendronate
- amiodarone
- bosentan
- cidofovir
- cimetidine
- clopidogrel
- cyclosporine
- delavirdine
- drospirenone; ethinyl estradiol (Yasmin®)
- fluconazole
- fluoxetine
- fluvoxamine
- herbal products that contain feverfew, garlic, ginger, or ginkgo biloba
- imatinib, STI-571
- isoniazid, INH
- ketoconazole (oral products)
- lithium
- medicines for high blood pressure
- methotrexate
- other anti-inflammatory drugs (such as ibuprofen or prednisone)
- pemetrexed
- rifampin
- ticlopidine
- warfarin
- water pills (diuretics)

Tell your prescriber or health care professional about all other medicines you are taking, including non-prescription medicines, nutritional supplements, or herbal products. Also tell your prescriber or health care professional if you are a frequent user of drinks with caffeine or alcohol, if you smoke, or if you use illegal drugs. These may affect the way your medicine works. Check with your health care professional before stopping or starting any of your medicines.

What should I watch for while taking celecoxib?

Let your prescriber or health care professional know if your pain continues; do not take with other pain-killers without advice. If you get flu-like symptoms (fever, chills, muscle aches and pains), call your prescriber or health care professional; do not treat yourself. To reduce unpleasant effects on your stomach, take celecoxib with a full glass of water. If you notice black, tarry stools or experience severe stomach pain and vomit blood or what looks like coffee grounds, notify your health care prescriber immediately. Celecoxib cannot take the place of aspirin for the prevention of heart attack or stroke. If you are taking medicines that affect the clotting of your blood, such as aspirin or blood thinners such as Coumadin®, talk to your health care provider or prescriber before taking this medicine. If you are currently taking aspirin for this purpose, you should not discontinue taking aspirin without checking with your prescriber or health care professional. Do not smoke cigarettes or drink alcohol; these increase irritation to your stomach and can make it more susceptible to damage from celecoxib. Avoid taking other prescription or over-the-counter non steroidal anti-inflammatory drugs (NSIADs), such as ibuprofen (Advil®), naprosyn (Aleve®), or ketoprofen (Orudis® KT), while taking celecoxib. Side effects including stomach upset, heartburn, nausea, vomiting or serious side effects such as ulcers are more likely if celecoxib is given with other NSAIDs. Many non-prescription products contain NSAIDs; closely read labels before taking any medicines with celecoxib.

What side effects may I notice from taking celecoxib?

Patients should seek immediate emergency help in the case of a serious allergic reaction. Side effects that you should report to your prescriber or health care professional as soon as possible:
Signs of bleeding from the stomach
- black tarry stools, blood in the urine, unusual tiredness or weakness, vomiting blood or vomit that looks like coffee grounds

Signs of an allergic reaction
- difficulty breathing or wheezing, skin rash, redness, blistering or peeling skin, hives, itching, swelling of eyelids, throat, lips
- blurred vision
- decrease in the amount of urine passed
- pain on swallowing, difficulty swallowing, severe heartburn or pain in throat
- stomach tenderness, pain, bleeding, or cramps
- unexplained weight gain or edema
- yellowing of eyes or skin

Side effects that usually do not require medical attention (report to your prescriber or health care professional if they continue or are bothersome):
- constipation or diarrhea
- difficulty swallowing
- dizziness
- gas or heartburn
- minor upset stomach
- nausea or vomiting

Where can I keep my medicine?

Keep out of the reach of children in a container that small children cannot open. Store at room temperature between 15 and 30 degrees C (59 and 86 degrees F). Protect from moisture. Keep container tightly closed. Throw away any unused medicine after the expiration date.

Cephalexin capsules

KEFLEX®; 500 mg; Capsule Advancis Pharmaceutical Corp.	
KEFLEX®; 250 mg; Capsule Advancis Pharmaceutical Corp.	

What are cephalexin tablets or capsules?

CEPHALEXIN (Keflex®, Keftab®) is a cephalosporin antibiotic. It treats many kinds of infections including those of the skin, respiratory tract, bone, sinuses, ears, and urinary tract. Generic cephalexin capsules are available.

What should my health care professional know before I take cephalexin?

They need to know if you have any of these conditions:
- bleeding problems
- diarrhea
- kidney disease
- stomach or intestinal problems (especially colitis)
- other chronic illness
- an unusual or allergic reaction to cephalexin, other cephalosporin antibiotics, penicillin, penicillamine, other foods, dyes or preservatives
- pregnant or trying to get pregnant
- breast-feeding

How should I take this medicine?

Take cephalexin capsules by mouth. Follow the directions on the prescription label. Swallow the capsules with a drink of water. You can take cephalexin with or without food. If cephalexin upsets your stomach it may help to take it with food. Take your doses at regular intervals. Do not take your medicine more often than directed. Finish the full course prescribed by your prescriber or health care professional even if you think your condition is better. Do not stop taking except on your prescriber's advice. Contact your pediatrician or health care professional regarding the use of this medicine in children. Special care may be needed.

What if I miss a dose?

If you miss a dose, take it as soon as you can. If it is almost time for your next dose, take only that dose. Do not take double or extra doses. There should be an interval of at least 4 to 6 hours between doses.

What may interact with cephalexin?

- other antibiotics
- diuretics ("water pills")
- probenecid

Tell your prescriber or health care professional about all other medicines you are taking, including non-prescription medicines, nutritional supplements, or herbal

products. Also tell your prescriber or health care professional if you are a frequent user of drinks with caffeine or alcohol, if you smoke, or if you use illegal drugs. These may affect the way your medicine works. Check with your health care professional before stopping or starting any of your medicines.

What should I watch for while taking cephalexin?

Tell your prescriber or health care professional if your symptoms do not begin to improve in a few days. If you are diabetic you may get a false-positive result for sugar in your urine. Check with your prescriber or health care professional before you change your diet or the dose of your diabetic medicine. If you get severe or watery diarrhea, do not treat yourself. Call your prescriber or health care professional for advice.

What side effects may I notice from taking cephalexin?

Side effects that you should report to your prescriber or health care professional as soon as possible:
- difficulty breathing, wheezing
- fever or chills, sore throat
- pain or difficulty passing urine
- redness, blistering, peeling or loosening of the skin, including inside the mouth
- seizures (convulsions)
- severe or watery diarrhea
- skin rash, itching
- stomach pain or cramps
- swollen or tender joints
- unusual bleeding or bruising
- unusual weakness or tiredness

Side effects that usually do not require medical attention (report to your prescriber or health care professional if they continue or are bothersome):
- diarrhea
- gas or heartburn
- genital or anal irritation
- nausea, vomiting

Where can I keep my medicine?

Keep out of the reach of children in a container that small children cannot open. Store at room temperature between 15 and 30 degrees C (59 and 86 degrees F). Throw away any unused medicine after the expiration date.

Cetirizine tablets and chewable tablets

ZYRTEC®;
10 mg; Tablet
Pfizer Laboratories
Div Pfizer Inc

ZYRTEC®;
10 mg; Tablet,
Chewable
Pfizer Laboratories
Div Pfizer Inc

What are cetirizine tablets and chewable tablets?

CETIRIZINE (Zyrtec®) is an antihistamine. Antihistamines work by preventing the effects of a substance called histamine, which is produced by the body. Cetirizine is used to relieve or prevent the symptoms of hay fever and other types of allergy. It is also used to help relieve itching and hives. Generic cetirizine tablets and chewable tablets are not yet available.

What should my health care professional know before I take cetirizine?

They need to know if you have any of these conditions:
- liver disease
- kidney disease
- an unusual or allergic reaction to cetirizine, other medicines, foods, dyes, or preservatives
- pregnant or trying to get pregnant
- breast-feeding

How should I take this medicine?

Take cetirizine tablets by mouth. Follow the directions on the prescription label. Take your doses at regular intervals. Do not take more often than directed. You may need to take cetirizine for several days before your symptoms improve. Contact your pediatrician or health care professional regarding the use of this medicine in children. Special care may be needed. Cetirizine has been used in children as young as 2 years old.
Tablets: Swallow the tablets with a drink of water. You can take this medicine with or without food.
Chewable tablets: Chew the tablets well before swallowing. You can take this medicine with or without food or water.

What if I miss a dose?

If you miss a dose, take it as soon as you can. If it is almost time for your next dose, take only that dose. Do not take double or extra doses.

What may interact with cetirizine?

Because cetirizine can cause drowsiness, other medicines that also cause drowsiness may increase this effect of cetirizine. Some medicines that cause drowsiness are:

- alcohol
- barbiturates such as phenobarbital
- certain antidepressants or tranquilizers (for example, amitriptyline, chlorpromazine, desipramine, doxepin, imipramine, nortriptyline, thioridazine, trifluoperazine)
- certain narcotics or pain medicines (for example, codeine, hydrocodone, meperidine, methadone, morphine, oxycodone, or propoxyphene)

- certain medicines used for anxiety or to help produce sleep (for example, alprazolam, chloral hydrate, diazepam, lorazepam, meprobamate)
- certain antihistamines used in cold medicines (for example, diphenhydramine or chlorpheniramine)

Ask your prescriber or health care professional about other medicines that may increase the effect of cetirizine.

Tell your prescriber or health care professional about all other medicines you are taking, including non-prescription medicines, nutritional supplements, or herbal products. Also tell your prescriber or health care professional if you are a frequent user of drinks with caffeine or alcohol, if you smoke, or if you use illegal drugs. These may affect the way your medicine works. Check with your health care professional before stopping or starting any of your medicines.

What should I watch for while taking cetirizine?

Tell your prescriber or health care professional if your symptoms do not start to improve in 2 or 3 days. You may get drowsy or dizzy. Do not drive, use machinery, or do anything that needs mental alertness until you know how cetirizine affects you. Your mouth may get dry. Chewing sugarless gum or sucking hard candy, and drinking plenty of water will help.

What side effects may I notice from taking cetirizine?

Serious side effects to cetirizine are rare. Side effects that you should report to your prescriber or health care professional as soon as possible:
- any unusual effects that are bothersome

Side effects that usually do not require medical attention (report to your prescriber or health care professional if they continue or are bothersome):
- diarrhea
- dizziness
- drowsiness
- dry mouth
- fatigue
- headache
- nausea or stomach upset
- sore throat

Where can I keep my medicine?

Keep out of the reach of children in a container that small children cannot open. Store at room temperature, between 15 and 30 degrees C (59 and 86 degrees F). Throw away any unused medicine after the expiration date.

Cetirizine; Pseudoephedrine extended-release tablets

ZYRTEC-D 12 HOUR®;
5 mg/120 mg; Tablet,
Extended Release
Pfizer Laboratories Div Pfizer
Inc

What are cetirizine; pseudoephedrine extended-release tablets?

CETIRIZINE; PSEUDOEPHEDRINE (Zyrtec-D®) is a combination of an antihistamine and decongestant. It relieves the symptoms of allergies like hay fever (seasonal rhinitis) including nasal and sinus congestion. A generic product is not yet available.

What should my health care professional know before I take cetirizine; pseudoephedrine?

They need to know if you have any of these conditions:
- blood vessel disease
- diabetes
- difficulty swallowing
- glaucoma
- heart disease
- high blood pressure
- kidney disease
- liver disease
- overactive thyroid
- stomach ulcer
- urinary tract or prostate trouble
- an unusual or allergic reaction to cetirizine or pseudoephedrine, hydroxyzine, other medicines, foods, dyes, or preservatives
- pregnant or trying to get pregnant
- breast-feeding

How should I take this medicine?

Take cetirizine; pseudoephedrine extended-release tablets by mouth. Follow the directions on the prescription label. Swallow the tablets whole with water. Do not break, crush or chew the tablets. Take your doses at regular intervals, no more than every 12 hours. You may take with or without food. Do not take your medicine more often than directed. Contact your pediatrician or health care professional regarding the use of this medicine in children. Special care may be needed. Older patients (> 60 years of age) may have a stronger reaction to this medicine, especially if they have kidney or liver disease.

What if I miss a dose?

If it is almost time for your next dose, take only that dose. Do not take double doses.

What may interact with cetirizine; pseudoephedrine?

- alcohol or illicit drugs such as cocaine
- barbiturate medicines for inducing sleep or treating seizures (convulsions), like phenobarbital
- bromocriptine
- caffeine
- furazolidone
- linezolid

- MAO inhibitors (examples: Eldepryl®, Marplan®, Nardil® and Parnate®)
- mecamylamine
- medicines for anxiety or sleeping problems, such as alprazolam, diazepam or temazepam
- medicines for colds, breathing difficulties or weight loss, such as ephedra
- medicines for hay fever and other allergies such as antihistamines
- medicines for heart disease such as digoxin or beta-blockers
- medicines for mental problems, including anxiety, depression and psychotic disturbances
- medicines for migraine headaches such as dihydroergotamine or ergotamine
- medicines for nasal congestion, such as more pseudoephedrine
- medicines for pain such as codeine or morphine
- procarbazine
- reserpine
- sodium bicarbonate
- theophylline

Tell your prescriber or health care professional about all other medicines you are taking, including non-prescription medicines, nutritional supplements, or herbal products. Also tell your prescriber or health care professional if you are a frequent user of drinks with caffeine or alcohol, if you smoke, or if you use illegal drugs. These may affect the way your medicine works. Check with your health care professional before stopping or starting any of your medicines.

What should I watch for while taking cetirizine; pseudoephedrine?

Do not drive, use machinery, or do anything that needs mental alertness until you know how cetirizine; pseudoephedrine affects you. To reduce the risk of dizzy or fainting spells, do not stand or sit up quickly, especially if you are an older patient. Alcohol may increase dizziness and drowsiness. Avoid alcoholic drinks. Your mouth may get dry. Chewing sugarless gum or sucking hard candy, and drinking plenty of water will help.

What side effects may I notice from taking cetirizine; pseudoephedrine?

Side effects that you should report to your prescriber or health care professional as soon as possible:
- abdominal pain or rectal bleeding
- chest pain
- confusion
- convulsions (seizures)
- difficulty breathing or wheezing
- difficulty swallowing or enlarged tongue
- difficulty urinating
- dizziness, or fainting spells
- fast or irregular heartbeat, palpitations
- high blood pressure
- numbness or tingling in the hands or feet
- rash
- severe, persistent, or worsening headache
- tremor, muscle contractions
- visual changes
- vomiting
- yellow tint to your skin or the whites of your eyes

Side effects that usually do not require medical attention (report to your prescriber or health care professional if they continue or are bothersome):
- dry mouth
- headache (mild)
- loss of appetite or nausea
- nervousness or difficulty sleeping
- tiredness

Where can I keep my medicine?

Keep out of the reach of children in a container that small children cannot open. Store at room temperature or between 15 to 30 degrees C (59 to 86 degrees F). Protect from moisture. Throw away any unused medicine after the expiration date.

Cevimeline capsules

EVOXAC™;
30 mg; Capsule
Daiichi Pharmaceutical Corp

What are cevimeline capsules?

CEVIMELINE (Evoxac™) capsules help to increase the amount of saliva and decrease dry mouth in patients with Sjogren's syndrome. Generic cevimeline capsules are not yet available.

What should my health care professional know before I use cevimeline?

They need to know if you have any of these conditions:
- angina
- asthma
- bronchitis
- chronic obstructive lung disease (COPD)
- glaucoma
- heart disease
- history of a heart attack (acute myocardial infarction)
- iritis
- irregular heart beat
- an unusual or allergic reaction to cevimeline, other medicines, foods, dyes, or preservatives
- pregnant or trying to get pregnant
- breast-feeding

How should I use this medicine?

Take cevimeline capsules by mouth. Follow the directions on the prescription label. Swallow the capsules with a drink of water. You may take this medication with food. Take your doses at regular intervals. Do not take your medicine more often than directed. Do not stop taking except on your doctor's advice. Contact your pediatrician or health care professional regarding the use of this medicine in children. Special care may be needed.

What if I miss a dose?

If it is almost time for your next dose, take only that dose. Do not take double or extra doses.

What may interact with cevimeline?

- bosentan
- certain medicines for depression (i.e., fluoxetine, amitriptyline)
- certain medicines for high blood pressure (i.e., propranolol)
- certain medicines for seizures (i.e., carbamazepine, phenytoin, phenobarbital)
- cimetidine
- clarithromycin
- erythromycin
- fluconazole
- itraconazole
- ketoconazole
- rifabutin
- rifampin
- ritonavir

Tell your prescriber or health care professional about all other medicines you that are taking, including non prescription medicines, nutritional supplements, or herbal products. Also tell your prescriber or health care professional if you are a frequent user of drinks with caffeine or alcohol, if you smoke, or if you use illegal drugs. These may affect the way your medicine works. Check before stopping or starting any of your medicines.

What should I watch for while taking cevimeline?

You may have visual changes, noticeable especially at night, while taking cevimeline. Do not drive, use machinery, or do anything that requires mental alertness until you know how cevimeline affects you. If you sweat a lot while taking cevimeline, you may become dehydrated. Drink plenty of fluids to avoid dehydration. Talk with your health care provider if you are sweating a lot.

What side effects may I notice from taking cevimeline?

Side effects that you should report to your doctor as soon as possible:
- changes in vision
- difficulty breathing
- irregular heartbeat
- tremors
- upper respiratory infections (i.e., sinus infections)

Side effects that usually do not require medical attention (report to your doctor if they continue or are bothersome):
- blurred vision
- diarrhea
- excessive sweating
- headache
- heartburn
- nausea
- runny nose
- stomach pain

Where can I keep my medicine?

Keep out of the reach of children. Store at room temperature between 15 and 30 degrees C (59 and 86 degrees F). Throw away any unused medicine after the expiration date.

Chloral Hydrate capsules

SOMNOTE™;
500 mg; Capsule
Breckenridge Inc

What are chloral hydrate capsules?

CHLORAL HYDRATE (Somnote™)has two main actions. As a sedative it can relieve tension or anxiety, and may be used with painkillers to reduce pain and anxiety after surgery. As a hypnotic chloral hydrate can help you to sleep, but should only be used as a short-term treatment for insomnia (difficulty sleeping). Chloral hydrate can be given before surgery or dental procedures, especially to children. Tolerance to the effects of chloral hydrate develops quickly, limiting treatment periods to two weeks or less. Federal law prohibits the transfer of chloral hydrate to any person other than the patient for whom it was prescribed. Generic chloral hydrate capsules are available.

What should my health care professional know before I take chloral hydrate?

They need to know if you have any of these conditions:
- a drug or alcohol abuse problem
- heart disease
- kidney disease
- liver disease
- mental depression
- porphyria
- stomach or intestinal disease or digestive problems
- an unusual or allergic reaction to chloral hydrate, other medicines, foods, dyes, or preservatives
- pregnant or trying to get pregnant
- breast-feeding

C

How should I take this medicine?

Take chloral hydrate capsules by mouth. Follow the directions on the prescription label. Swallow the capsules whole with a full glass of water or other liquid, such as fruit juice or ginger ale. Do not crush or chew the capsules because the contents may have an unpleasant taste. Take your doses at regular intervals. Do not take your medicine more often than directed.

What if I miss a dose?

This will not apply if you are taking chloral hydrate before a special procedure. If you are taking chloral hydrate regularly and miss a dose, skip the missed dose and return to your regular schedule with the next dose. Do not take double or extra doses.

What may interact with chloral hydrate?

- alcohol
- barbiturate medicines for inducing sleep or treating seizures (convulsions)
- disulfiram
- furosemide
- medicines for anxiety or sleeping problems, such as diazepam or temazepam
- medicines for hay fever and other allergies
- medicines for mental depression
- medicines for mental problems and psychotic disturbances
- medicines for pain
- warfarin

Tell your prescriber or health care professional about all other medicines you are taking, including non-prescription medicines, nutritional supplements, or herbal products. Also tell your prescriber or health care professional if you are a frequent user of drinks with caffeine or alcohol, if you smoke, or if you use illegal drugs. These may affect the way your medicine works. Check with your health care professional before stopping or starting any of your medicines.

What should I watch for while taking chloral hydrate?

Visit your prescriber or health care professional for regular checks on your progress. If you have been taking chloral hydrate regularly for a few weeks and suddenly stop taking it, you may get unpleasant withdrawal symptoms. Your prescriber or health care professional may want to gradually reduce the dose. Do not stop taking except on your prescriber's advice. After taking chloral hydrate you may get a residual hangover effect that leaves you drowsy or dizzy. Until you know how chloral hydrate affects you, do not drive, use machinery, or do anything that needs mental alertness. To reduce dizzy or fainting spells, do not sit or stand up quickly, especially if you are an older patient. Alcohol can increase possible unpleasant effects. It is not safe to drink alcohol while taking chloral hydrate. While you are taking chloral hydrate, do not take any medicines for hay fever, allergies, or pain without asking your prescriber or health care professional for advice.

What side effects may I notice from taking chloral hydrate?

Side effects that you should report to your prescriber or health care professional as soon as possible:
- confusion
- difficulty breathing or shortness of breath
- extreme irritability or unusual excitement
- fever, chills, or sore throat
- hallucinations, nightmares
- irregular heart beat
- skin rash and itching (hives)
- slurred speech
- slow reflexes
- staggering, tremors
- unusual weakness or tiredness

Side effects that usually do not require medical attention (report to your prescriber or health care professional if they continue or are bothersome):
- diarrhea
- dizziness, drowsiness, lightheadedness, or "hangover"
- nausea, vomiting
- stomach upset

Where can I keep my medicine?

Keep out of the reach of children in a container that small children cannot open. Store at room temperature between 15 and 30 degrees C (59 and 86 degrees F). Keep container tightly closed. Throw away any unused medicine after the expiration date.

Chlorambucil tablets

LEUKERAN®;
2 mg; Tablet
Glaxo Wellcome

What are chlorambucil tablets?

CHLORAMBUCIL (Leukeran®) is a type of chemotherapy for treating cancer. Chlorambucil interferes with the way cancer cells grow. Chlorambucil is used to treat cancers of the blood and certain other types of cancer. Generic chlorambucil tablets are not yet available.

What should my health care professional know before I take chlorambucil?

They need to know if you have any of these conditions:
- bleeding problems
- blood disorders
- dental disease
- gout

- head injury
- infection (especially virus infection such as chickenpox or herpes)
- kidney disease
- recent radiation therapy
- seizures (convulsions)
- an unusual or allergic reaction to chlorambucil, other chemotherapy, other medicines, foods, dyes, or preservatives
- pregnant or trying to get pregnant
- breast-feeding

How should I take this medicine?

Take chlorambucil tablets by mouth. Follow the directions on the prescription label. Swallow the tablets with a drink of water. Take your doses at regular intervals. Do not take your medicine more often than directed. Finish the full course prescribed by your doctor or health care professional, even if the tablets make you feel unwell. Do not stop taking except on your prescriber's advice.

What if I miss a dose?

If you miss a dose, take it as soon as you can. If it is almost time for your next dose, take only that dose. Do not take double or extra doses. If you are only taking one dose a day and miss a dose, do not take two doses on the next day.

What may interact with chlorambucil?

- barbiturate medicines for inducing sleep or treating seizures (convulsions)
- live virus vaccine

Tell your prescriber or health care professional about all other medicines you are taking, including nonprescription medicines, nutritional supplements, or herbal products. Also tell your prescriber or health care professional if you are a frequent user of drinks with caffeine or alcohol, if you smoke, or if you use illegal drugs. These may affect the way your medicine works. Check with your health care professional before stopping or starting any of your medicines.

What should I watch for while taking chlorambucil?

Visit your prescriber or health care professional for checks on your progress. You will need to have regular blood checks. The side effects of chlorambucil can continue after you finish your treatment; report side effects promptly. Chlorambucil may make you feel generally unwell. This is not uncommon because chlorambucil affects good cells as well as cancer cells. Report any side effects as above, but continue your course of medicine even though you feel ill, unless your prescriber or health care professional tells you to stop. While you are taking chlorambucil you will be more susceptible to infection. Try to avoid people with colds, flu, and bronchitis. Do not have any vaccinations without your prescriber's approval and avoid anyone who has recently had oral polio vaccine. Call your prescriber or health care professional for advice if you get a fever, chills or sore throat. Do not treat yourself. Chlorambucil can cause blood problems. This can mean slow healing and a risk of infection. Try to avoid cutting or injuring yourself. Problems can arise if you need dental work, and in the day to day care of your teeth. Try to avoid damage to your teeth and gums when you brush or floss your teeth. Drink several glasses of water a day. This will help to reduce possible kidney or gout problems. Chlorambucil can change male sperm or female eggs. Talk to your prescriber or health care professional about how this medicine can affect your ability to have normal babies.

What side effects may I notice from taking chlorambucil?

Side effects that you should report to your prescriber or health care professional as soon as possible:
- blood in the urine
- black tarry stools
- chest pain
- dark yellow or brown urine
- difficulty breathing, wheezing
- confusion, clumsiness
- fever or chills, cough or sore throat
- joint or muscle pains
- lower back pain
- mouth or throat sores
- pain or difficulty passing urine
- seizures (convulsions)
- skin rash, itching
- swollen feet or legs
- tingling, pain or numbness in the hands or feet
- tremors
- unusual bleeding or bruising, nose or gum bleeds, pinpoint red spots on the skin
- unusual tiredness or weakness
- vomiting
- yellowing of the eyes or skin

Side effects that usually do not require medical attention (report to your prescriber or health care professional if they continue or are bothersome):
- diarrhea
- missed menstrual periods
- nausea
- weight loss

Where can I keep my medicine?

Keep out of the reach of children in a container that small children cannot open.

Store refrigerated between 2 and 8 degrees C (36 and 46 degrees F). Protect from moisture and light. Throw away any unused medicine after the expiration date.

Chlordiazepoxide capsules

CHLORDIAZEPOXIDE; 10 mg; Capsule Barr Laboratories Inc

CHLORDIAZEPOXIDE; 25 mg; Capsule Barr Laboratories Inc

What are chlordiazepoxide capsules?

CHLORDIAZEPOXIDE (Librium®) is a benzodiazepine. Benzodiazepines belong to a group of medicines that slow down the central nervous system. Chlordiazepoxide relieves anxiety and nervousness. It can also help people with alcohol withdrawal. Federal law prohibits the transfer of chlordiazepoxide to any person other than the patient for whom it was prescribed. Do not share this medicine with anyone else. Generic chlordiazepoxide capsules are available.

What should my health care professional know before I take chlordiazepoxide?

They need to know if you have any of these conditions:
- an alcohol or drug abuse problem
- bipolar disorder, depression, psychosis or other mental health condition
- glaucoma
- kidney disease
- liver disease
- lung disease, such as chronic obstructive pulmonary disease (COPD), sleep apnea or other breathing difficulties
- myasthenia gravis
- porphyria
- Parkinson's disease
- seizures or a history of seizures
- shortness of breath
- snoring
- suicidal thoughts
- an unusual or allergic reaction to chlordiazepoxide, other benzodiazepines, foods, dyes, or preservatives
- pregnant or trying to get pregnant
- breast-feeding

How should I take this medicine?

Take chlordiazepoxide capsules by mouth. Follow the directions on the prescription label. Swallow the capsules with a drink of water. If chlordiazepoxide upsets your stomach, take it with food or milk. Take your doses at regular intervals. Do not take your medicine more often than directed. Do not stop taking except on your prescriber's advice. Contact your pediatrician or health care professional regarding the use of this medicine in children. Special care may be needed.

What if I miss a dose?

If you miss a dose, take it as soon as you can. If it is almost time for your next dose, take only that dose. Do not take double or extra doses.

What may interact with chlordiazepoxide?

- alcohol
- bosentan
- caffeine
- cimetidine
- disulfiram
- female hormones, including contraceptive or birth control pills
- herbal or dietary supplements such as kava kava, melatonin, St. John's Wort or valerian
- imatinib, STI-571
- isoniazid
- levodopa
- medicines for anxiety or sleeping problems, such as alprazolam, diazepam, lorazepam or triazolam
- medicines for depression, mental problems or psychiatric disturbances
- medicines for fungal infections (fluconazole, itraconazole, ketoconazole, voriconazole)
- medicines for HIV infection or AIDS
- nicardipine
- prescription pain medicines
- probenecid
- rifampin, rifapentine, or rifabutin
- some antibiotics (clarithromycin, erythromycin, troleandomycin)
- some medicines for colds, hay fever or other allergies
- some medicines for high blood pressure or heart-rhythm problems (amiodarone, digoxin, diltiazem, verapamil)
- some medicines for seizures (carbamazepine, phenobarbital, phenytoin, primidone)
- theophylline
- warfarin
- zafirlukast
- zileuton

Tell your prescriber or health care professional about all other medicines you are taking, including non-prescription medicines, nutritional supplements, or herbal products. Also tell your prescriber or health care professional if you are a frequent user of drinks with caffeine or alcohol, if you smoke, or if you use illegal drugs. These may affect the way your medicine works. Check with your health care professional before stopping or starting any of your medicines.

What should I watch for while taking chlordiazepoxide?

Visit your prescriber or health care professional for regular checks on your progress. Your body can become dependent on chlordiazepoxide, ask your prescriber or health care professional if you still need to take it. However, if you have been taking chlordiazepoxide regularly for some time, do not suddenly stop taking it. You must gradually reduce the dose or you may get severe side effects. Ask your prescriber or health care professional for advice. Even after you stop taking chlordiazepoxide it can still affect your body for several days. You may get drowsy or dizzy. Do not drive, use machinery, or do anything that needs mental alertness until you know how chlordiazepoxide affects you. To reduce the risk of dizzy and fainting spells, do not stand or sit up quickly, especially if you are an older patient. Alcohol may increase dizziness and drowsiness. Avoid alcoholic drinks. Do not treat yourself for coughs, colds or allergies without asking your prescriber or health care professional for advice. Some ingredients can increase possible side effects. If you are going to have surgery, tell your prescriber or health care professional that you are taking chlordiazepoxide.

What side effects may I notice from taking chlordiazepoxide?

Side effects that you should report to your prescriber or health care professional as soon as possible:
- confusion
- depression
- lightheadedness or fainting spells
- mood changes, excitability or aggressive behavior
- movement difficulty, staggering or jerky movements
- muscle cramps
- restlessness, tremors
- weakness or tiredness

Side effects that usually do not require medical attention (report to your prescriber or health care professional if they continue or are bothersome):
- constipation
- drowsiness
- menstrual changes
- nausea, vomiting
- sexual dysfunction

Where can I keep my medicine?

Keep out of the reach of children in a container that small children cannot open. Store at room temperature between 15 and 30 degrees C (59 and 86 degrees F). Protect from light. Throw away any unused medicine after the expiration date.

Chlordiazepoxide; Clidinium capsules

CHLORDIAZEPOXIDE; Clidinium; 5 mg/ 2.5 mg; Capsule Mutual/United Research Laboratories	CHLORDIAZEPOXIDE; Clidinium; 5 mg/ 2.5 mg; Capsule Qualitest Pharmaceuticals Inc

What are chlordiazepoxide; clidinium capsules?

CHLORDIAZEPOXIDE; CLIDINIUM is a combination of medicines that helps to relax your stomach and bowel. It may help to relieve spasms and decrease stomach acid. It may help to treat peptic ulcer disease or irritable bowel syndrome.

What should my health care professional know before I take chlordiazepoxide; clidinium?

They need to know if you have any of these conditions:
- an alcohol or drug abuse problem
- depression, bipolar disorder, psychosis or other mental health condition
- difficulty passing urine
- glaucoma
- heart disease or irregular heartbeat
- hiatal hernia
- high blood pressure
- kidney disease
- liver disease
- lung disease or breathing difficulties, shortness of breath
- myasthenia gravis
- nervous system disease
- overactive thyroid
- Parkinson's disease
- porphyria
- seizures or a history of seizures
- snoring
- stomach or intestinal problems (including ulcerative colitis)
- suicidal thoughts
- an unusual or allergic reaction to chlordiazepoxide, clidinium, other benzodiazepines, other medicines, foods, dyes, or preservatives
- pregnant or trying to get pregnant
- breast-feeding

How should I take this medicine?

Take chlordiazepoxide; clidinium capsules by mouth. Follow the directions on the prescription label. Swallow the capsules with a drink of water. It is best to take this medicine 1/2 to 1 hour before meals (on an empty stomach) and at bedtime or as directed by your health care professional. Take your medicine at about the same time each day. Do not take your medicine more often than directed. Do not stop taking your medicine except on your prescriber's advice. Contact your pediatrician or health care professional regarding the use of this medicine in children. Special care may be needed.

What if I miss a dose?

If it is almost time for your next dose, take only that dose. Do not take double or extra doses.

What may interact with chlordiazepoxide; clidinium?

- acetazolamide
- alcohol
- amantadine
- anticholinergic medicines, such as atropine, benztropine, bethanechol, flavoxate, hyoscyamine or scopolamine
- bosentan
- caffeine
- cimetidine

- cyclobenzaprine
- disulfiram
- female hormones, including contraceptive or birth control pills
- herbal or dietary supplements such as kava kava, melatonin, St. John's Wort or valerian
- imatinib, STI-571
- isoniazid
- levodopa
- medicines for anxiety or sleeping problems, such as alprazolam, diazepam, lorazepam or triazolam
- medicines for depression, mental problems or psychiatric disturbances
- medicines for fungal infections (fluconazole, itraconazole, ketoconazole, voriconazole)
- medicines for HIV infection or AIDS
- methazolamide
- nicardipine
- prescription pain medicines
- probenecid
- rifampin, rifapentine, or rifabutin
- some antibiotics (clarithromycin, erythromycin, troleandomycin)
- some medicines for colds, hay fever or other allergies
- some medicines for high blood pressure or heart-rhythm problems
- some medicines for seizures (carbamazepine, phenobarbital, phenytoin, primidone)
- some medicines for stomach problems (cisapride, dicyclomine, hyoscyamine, metoclopramide, tegaserod)
- theophylline
- warfarin
- zafirlukast
- zileuton

Tell your prescriber or health care professional about all other medicines you are taking, including non-prescription medicines, nutritional supplements, or herbal products. Also tell your prescriber or health care professional if you are a frequent user of drinks with caffeine or alcohol, if you smoke, or if you use illegal drugs. These may affect the way your medicine works. Check with your health care professional before stopping or starting any of your medicines.

What should I watch for while taking chlordiazepoxide; clidinium?

Visit your prescriber for regular checks on your progress. Your body may become dependent upon this drug and you need to ask your prescriber if you still need to take it. Do not suddenly stop taking chlordiazepoxide; clidinium. You must gradually reduce the dose or you may get severe side effects. Ask your health care professional for advice. Even after you stop taking this medicine it can still affect your body for several days. You may get drowsy, dizzy, or have blurred vision. Do not drive, use machinery, or do anything that needs

mental alertness until you know how this drug affects you. To reduce the risk of dizzy or fainting spells, do not sit or stand up quickly, especially if you are an older patient. Alcohol can make you more drowsy and you should avoid alcoholic drinks. Do not treat yourself for coughs, colds or allergies without asking your prescriber or health care professional for advice. Some ingredients can increase the risk for side effects. Avoid extreme heat (e.g., hot tubs, saunas). This drug can cause you to sweat less than normal. Your body temperature could increase to dangerous levels, which may lead to heat stroke. Your mouth may get dry. Chewing sugarless gum or sucking hard candy, and drinking plenty of water will help. If you get constipation while taking this drug, do not treat yourself. You may have a blockage in the intestine. Call your prescriber or health care professional for advice. If you are going to have surgery, tell your health care professional that you are taking chlordiazepoxide; clidinium.

What side effects may I notice from taking chlordiazepoxide; clidinium?

Side effects that you should report to your prescriber or health care professional as soon as possible:
- agitation, nervousness, confusion
- blurred vision and other eye problems
- constipation
- decreased sweating
- depression
- dizziness
- irregular heartbeat (palpitations)
- lightheadedness or fainting spells
- mood changes, excitability or aggressive behavior
- movement difficulty, staggering or jerky movements
- muscle cramps
- pain in your stomach or difficulty passing urine
- restlessness, tremors
- unusual weakness or tiredness
- vomiting

Side effects that usually do not require medical attention (report to your prescriber or health care professional if they continue or are bothersome):
- changes in your menstrual cycle (period)
- difficulty sleeping
- excessive drowsiness
- dry mouth, change in taste
- headache
- nausea
- sexual difficulty (impotence)
- swelling

Where can I keep my medicine?

Keep out of the reach of children in a container that small children cannot open. Store at room temperature between 15 and 30 degrees C (59 and 86 degrees F). Protect from light. Throw away any unused medicine after the expiration date.

Chlorothiazide tablets

CHLOROTHIAZIDE;
250 mg; Tablet
UDL Laboratories Inc

What are chlorothiazide tablets?

CHLOROTHIAZIDE (DIURIL®) is a diuretic. Diuretics increase the amount of urine passed, which causes the body to lose water and salt. Chlorothiazide helps to treat high blood pressure (hypertension). It is not a cure. This drug also reduces the swelling and water retention caused by various medical conditions, such as heart, liver, or kidney disease. Generic chlorothiazide tablets are available.

What should my health care professional know before I take chlorothiazide?

They need to know if you have any of these conditions:
- diabetes mellitus
- gout
- heart disease
- kidney disease, small amounts of urine, or difficulty passing urine
- liver disease
- lupus syndrome or systemic lupus erythematosus (SLE)
- pancreatitis
- electrolyte imbalance (e.g. low or high levels of potassium in the blood)
- if you are on a special diet, such as a low-salt diet (e.g. using potassium substitutes)
- an unusual or allergic reaction to chlorothiazide or other thiazides, sulfonamides, or other medicines, foods, dyes, or preservatives
- pregnant or trying to get pregnant
- breast-feeding

How should I take this medicine?

Take chlorothiazide tablets by mouth. Follow the directions on the prescription label. Swallow the tablets with a drink of water. This medicine can be taken with or without food. Take your doses at regular intervals. Do not take your medicine more often than directed. Remember that you will need to pass urine frequently after taking chlorothiazide. Do not take your doses at a time of day that will cause you problems. Avoid taking this medicine at bedtime. Contact your pediatrician or health care professional regarding the use of this medicine in children. Special care may be needed. Elderly patients over 65 years old may have a stronger reaction to this medicine and need smaller doses.

What if I miss a dose?

If you miss a dose, take it as soon as you can. If it is almost time for your next dose, take only that dose. Do not take double or extra doses.

What may interact with chlorothiazide?

- allopurinol
- amphotericin B
- anti-inflammatory drugs including NSAIDs (e.g., ibuprofen), aspirin, or salicylates
- blood pressure medications
- diabetic medications
- digoxin
- dofetilide
- griseofulvin
- hawthorn or horse chestnut
- hormones such as cortisone, hydrocortisone, prednisone
- lithium
- potassium salts or potassium supplements
- prochlorperazine
- some antibiotics which increase sensitivity to sunlight (sulfonamides, tetracyclines)
- some cholesterol-lowering medications (e.g. cholestyramine or colestipol)
- some medicines for mental disorders (phenothiazines)
- vitamin A (retinol) creams or pills such as tretinoin Retin-A®, Renova®, Solage®, Atragen®, and others
- water pills (especially potassium-sparing diuretics such as triamterene or amiloride)

Tell your prescriber or health care professional about all other medicines you are taking, including non-prescription medicines, nutritional supplements, or herbal products. Also tell your prescriber or health care professional if you are a frequent user of drinks with caffeine or alcohol, if you smoke, or if you use illegal drugs. These may affect the way your medicine works. Check with your health care professional before stopping or starting any of your medicines.

What should I watch for while taking chlorothiazide?

Check your blood pressure regularly while you are taking this medicine. Ask your prescriber or health care professional what your blood pressure should be and when you should contact him or her. When you check your blood pressure, write down the measurements to show your prescriber or health care professional. If you are taking this medicine for a long time you must visit your prescriber or health care professional for regular checks on your progress. Make sure you schedule appointments on a regular basis. Check with your prescriber or health care professional if you get an attack of severe diarrhea, nausea and vomiting, or if you sweat a lot. You must not get dehydrated. Ask your prescriber or health care professional how much fluid you need to drink a day. The loss of too much body fluid can make it dangerous for you to take this medicine. Watch your diet while you are taking chlorothiazide. Ask your prescriber or health care professional about both potassium and sodium intake. Chlorothiazide can make your body lose potassium and you may need an extra supply.

Too high or too low potassium can cause problems. Some foods have a high potassium content such as bananas, coconuts, dates, figs, prunes, apricots, peaches, grapefruit juice, tomato juice, and orange juice. You may get dizzy. Do not drive, use machinery, or do anything that requires mental alertness until you know how chlorothiazide affects you. To avoid dizzy or fainting spells, do not stand or sit up quickly. Alcohol may increase the possibility of dizziness. Avoid alcoholic drinks until you have discussed their use with your prescriber or health care professional. Chlorothiazide can make your skin more sensitive to sun or ultraviolet light. Keep out of the sun, or wear protective clothing outdoors and use a sunscreen (at least SPF 15). Do not use sun lamps or sun tanning beds or booths. If you are going to have surgery, tell your prescriber or health care professional that you are taking chlorothiazide. Do not treat yourself for a fever or sore throat; check with your prescriber or health care professional first. Chlorothiazide can increase the amount of sugar in blood or urine. If you are a diabetic keep a close check on blood and urine sugar and check with your prescriber or health care professional before changing the dose of your diabetic medicine.

What side effects may I notice from taking chlorothiazide?

Side effects that you should report to your prescriber or health care professional as soon as possible:
Rare or uncommon:
- confusion
- decreased sexual function
- lower back or side pain

- nausea, vomiting
- redness, blistering, peeling or loosening of the skin, including inside the mouth
- severe stomach upset, pain, or cramps
- unusual rash, bleeding or bruising, or pinpoint red spots on the skin
- yellowing of the eyes or skin

Other:
- decreased amount of urine passed
- dizziness, lightheadedness or fainting spells
- fast or uneven heart beat, palpitations, or chest pain
- fever or chills, sore throat
- muscle pain or weakness, cramps
- tingling or numbness in the hands or feet
- unusual tiredness or weakness
- worsened gout pain

Side effects that usually do not require medical attention (report to your prescriber or health care professional if they continue or are bothersome):
- constipation or diarrhea
- headache
- increased sensitivity to the sun
- increased thirst
- loss of appetite
- stomach upset

Where can I keep my medicine?

Keep out of the reach of children in a container that small children cannot open. Store at room temperature between 15 and 30 degrees C (59 and 86 degrees F). Protect from light and moisture. Keep container tightly closed. Throw away any unused medicine after the expiration date.

Chlorpheniramine tablets or capsules

CHLORPHENIRAMINE; 4 mg; Tablet Amide Pharmaceutical Inc

CHLORPHENIRAMINE; 12 mg; Capsule, Extended Release Time Cap Laboratories Inc

What are chlorpheniramine tablets or capsules?

CHLORPHENIRAMINE (Aller-Chlor®, Chlor-Trimeton®, or Teldrin® and others) is an antihistamine. It relieves symptoms of runny nose you get with colds (rhinitis) and hay fever (seasonal rhinitis) and moderate to severe allergic reactions. Generic chlorpheniramine tablets, extended-release tablets or capsules are available.

What should my health care professional know before I take chlorpheniramine?

They need to know if you have any of these conditions:
- asthma or congestive lung disease
- glaucoma
- high blood pressure or heart disease
- liver disease
- pain or difficulty passing urine

- prostate trouble
- ulcers or other stomach problems
- pregnant or trying to get pregnant
- breast-feeding

How should I take this medicine?

Take chlorpheniramine tablets or capsules by mouth. Follow the directions on the prescription label. Take with food or milk if chlorpheniramine upsets your stomach. Swallow extended-release tablets whole; do not crush or chew. Take your doses at regular intervals. Do not take your medicine more often than directed. Contact your pediatrician or health care professional regarding the use of this medicine in children. Children less than 6 years should not receive the 8-hour or 12-hour extended-release chlorpheniramine tablets. Children less than 2 years should not receive chlorpheniramine.

What if I miss a dose?

If you miss a dose, take it as soon as you can. If it is almost time for your next dose, take only that dose. Do not take double doses.

What may interact with chlorpheniramine?

- alcohol
- barbiturate medicines for inducing sleep or treating seizures (convulsions)
- medicines for anxiety or sleeping problems, such as diazepam or temazepam
- medicines for hay fever and other allergies
- medicines for mental depression
- medicines for mental problems and psychotic disturbances
- medicines for movement abnormalities as in Parkinson's disease, or for gastrointestinal problems

Tell your prescriber or health care professional about all other medicines that you are taking, including nonprescription medicines, nutritional supplements, or herbal products. Also tell your prescriber or health care professional if you are a frequent user of drinks with caffeine or alcohol, if you smoke, or if you use illegal drugs. These may affect the way your medicine works. Check with your health care professional before stopping or starting any of your medicines.

What should I watch for while taking chlorpheniramine?

Tell your prescriber or health care professional if your symptoms do not improve in 1 or 2 days. You may get drowsy or dizzy. Do not drive, use machinery, or do anything that needs mental alertness until you know how chlorpheniramine affects you. To reduce the risk of dizzy or fainting spells, do not stand or sit up quickly, especially if you are an older patient. Alcohol may increase dizziness and drowsiness. Avoid alcoholic drinks. Your mouth may get dry. Chewing sugarless gum or sucking hard candy, and drinking plenty of water will help. Chlorpheniramine may cause dry eyes and blurred vision. If you wear contact lenses you may feel some discomfort. Lubricating drops may help. See your ophthalmologist if the problem does not go away or is severe.

What side effects may I notice from taking chlorpheniramine?

Side effects that you should report to your prescriber or health care professional as soon as possible:

- agitation, nervousness, excitability, not able to sleep (these are more likely in children)
- blurred vision
- fainting spells
- irregular heartbeat, palpitations, or chest pain
- muscle or facial twitches
- pain or difficulty passing urine
- seizures (convulsions)

Side effects that usually do not require medical attention (report to your prescriber or health care professional if they continue or are bothersome):

- drowsiness, dizziness
- dry mouth
- headache
- loss of appetite
- stomach upset, nausea, vomiting, diarrhea, or constipation

Where can I keep my medicine?

Keep out of the reach of children in a container that small children cannot open. Store at room temperature, between 15 and 30 degrees C (59 and 86 degrees F). Keep container tightly closed. Throw away any unused medicine after the expiration date.

Chlorpheniramine; Dextromethorphan; Phenylephrine effervescent tablets

What are chlorpheniramine; dextromethorphan; phenylephrine effervescent tablets?

CHLORPHENIRAMINE, DEXTROMETHORPHAN, AND PHENYLEPHRINE (Alka-Seltzer Plus® Cold & Cough) are used together to decrease symptoms caused by colds or allergies. Chlorpheniramine is an antihistamine that relieves runny nose, sneezing, and watery eyes. Dextromethorphan helps to stop cough. Phenylephrine helps reduce nasal and sinus congestion. This product is not intended to treat chronic cough caused by smoking, asthma, emphysema, heart failure, or problems in which there is a large amount of phlegm. Generic chlorpheniramine; dextromethorphan; phenylephrine products are available.

What should my health care professional know before I take chlorpheniramine; dextromethorphan; phenylephrine?

They need to know if you have any of these conditions:

- asthma
- diabetes
- difficulty passing urine
- chronic cough
- emphysema
- enlarged prostrate
- heart disease including angina
- high blood pressure
- history of stroke or mini-strokes (TIAs)
- irregular heart beat
- liver disease

- phenylketonuria
- thyroid disease
- an unusual reaction to chlorpheniramine; dextromethorphan; phenylephrine, other medicines, foods, dyes, or preservatives
- pregnant or trying to get pregnant
- breast-feeding

How should this medicine be used?

Completely dissolve 2 chlorpheniramine; dextromethorphan; phenylephrine effervescent tablets in 4 ounces (1/2 cup) of water. Drink the water. Take your doses at regular intervals. Do not take your medicine more often than directed. Do not take more than 8 tablets in 24 hours or as directed by your physician. Contact your pediatrician or health care professional regarding the use of this medicine in children. Special care may be needed.

What if I miss a dose?

If you miss a dose, take it as soon as you can. If it is almost time for your next dose, take only that dose. Do not take double or extra doses.

What may interact with chlorpheniramine; dextromethorphan; phenylephrine?

- caffeine
- cocaine
- furazolidone
- linezolid
- medicines for chest pain, heart disease, high blood pressure, or heart rhythm problems
- medicine for diabetes
- medicines known as MAO inhibitors, such as phenelzine (Nardil®), tranylcypromine (Parnate®), isocarboxazid (Marplan®), and selegiline (Carbex®, Eldepryl®)
- medicines for mental depression
- medicines for mental problems and psychotic disturbances
- medicines for movement abnormalities as in Parkinson's disease, or for gastrointestinal problems
- medicines for weight loss
- St. John's wort
- thyroid hormones

Because this product can cause drowsiness, other medicines that also cause drowsiness may increase this effect. Some medicines that cause drowsiness are:

- alcohol and alcohol-containing medicines
- barbiturate medicines for inducing sleep or treating seizures (convulsions)
- medicines for anxiety or sleeping problems, such as diazepam or temazepam
- medicines for hay fever and other allergies

- muscle relaxers
- prescription pain medicines

Tell your prescriber or health care professional about all other medicines you are taking, including non-prescription medicines, nutritional supplements, or herbal products. Also tell your prescriber or health care professional if you are a frequent user of drinks with caffeine or alcohol, if you smoke, or if you use illegal drugs. These may affect the way your medicine works. Check with your health care professional before stopping or starting any of your medicines.

What should I watch for while taking chlorpheniramine; dextromethorphan; phenylephrine?

If you have a fever, skin rash, or persistent headache as well as a cough, see your prescriber or health care professional. Do not treat yourself for a cough for more than one week without consulting your prescriber or health care professional. You may get drowsy or dizzy. Do not drive, use machinery, or do anything that needs mental alertness until you know this medicine affects you. Alcohol can increase the risk of getting drowsy, dizzy, or confused. Avoid alcoholic drinks.

What side effects may I notice from taking chlorpheniramine; dextromethorphan; phenylephrine?

Side effects that you should report to your prescriber or health care professional as soon as possible:

- agitation, nervousness, excitability, not able to sleep (these are more likely in children)
- confusion
- headache, especially if severe or gets worse
- high blood pressure
- seizures
- severe nausea, vomiting
- slow or troubled breathing
- slurred speech
- tremors

Side effects that usually do not require medical attention (report to your prescriber or health care professional if they continue or are bothersome):

- dizziness, drowsiness
- nausea, vomiting
- stomach ache
- tremors
- weakness

Where can I keep my medicine?

Keep out of the reach of children in a container that small children cannot open. Store at room temperature between 15 and 30 degrees C (59 and 86 degrees F). Throw away any unused medicine after the expiration date.

Chlorpheniramine; Hydrocodone; Pseudoephedrine tablets

TUSSEND®;
4 mg/5 mg/60 mg; Tablet
Monarch Pharmaceuticals Inc

What are chlorpheniramine; hydrocodone; pseudoephedrine tablets?

CHLORPHENIRAMINE; HYDROCODONE; and PSEUDOEPHEDRINE (Tussend®) are used together to relieve cough and congestion due to colds, acute respiratory infections, including bronchitis and hay fever and may help to relieve sneezing and itching associated with hay fever. Generic chlorpheniramine-hydrocodone-pseudoephedrine tablets are not available.

What should my health care professional know before I take chlorpheniramine; hydrocodone; pseudoephedrine?

They need to know if you have any of these conditions:
- asthma or lung disease
- diabetes mellitus
- glaucoma
- high blood pressure or heart disease
- intestinal problems
- kidney or liver disease
- pain or difficulty passing urine
- prostate trouble
- thyroid disease
- vision problems
- an unusual or allergic reaction to chlorpheniramine, codeine, hydrocodone, morphine, pseudoephedrine, other pain medicines, foods, dyes or preservatives
- pregnant or trying to get pregnant
- breast-feeding

How should I take this medicine?

Take chlorpheniramine - hydrocodone - pseudoephedrine tablets by mouth with a glass of water. Follow the directions on the prescription label. Take with food or milk if this medicine upsets your stomach. Take your doses at regular intervals. Do not take your medicine more often than directed. Contact your pediatrician or health care professional regarding the use of this medicine in children. Special care may be needed. Do not share this medicine with anyone.

What if I miss a dose?

If you miss a dose, take it as soon as you can. If it is almost time for your next dose (less than 2 hours), take only that dose. Do not take double doses.

What may interact with chlorpheniramine; hydrocodone; pseudoephedrine?

- caffeine
- cocaine
- linezolid
- medicines for chest pain, heart disease, high blood pressure, or heart rhythm problems
- medicine for diabetes
- medicines known as MAO inhibitors, such as phenelzine (Nardil®), tranylcypromine (Parnate®), or isocarboxazid (Marplan®)
- medicines for mental depression
- medicines for mental problems and psychotic disturbances
- medicines for movement abnormalities as in Parkinson's disease, or for gastrointestinal problems
- medicines for weight loss
- St. John's wort
- thyroid hormones

Because this product can cause drowsiness, other medicines that also cause drowsiness may increase this effect. Some medicines that cause drowsiness are:

- alcohol and alcohol-containing medicines
- barbiturates such as phenobarbital
- certain antidepressants or tranquilizers
- certain antihistamines used in cold medicines
- medicines for anxiety or sleeping problems, such as diazepam or temazepam
- muscle relaxers

Tell your prescriber or health care professional about all other medicines that you are taking, including nonprescription medicines, nutritional supplements, or herbal products. Also tell your prescriber or health care professional if you are a frequent user of drinks with caffeine or alcohol, if you smoke, or if you use illegal drugs. These may affect the way your medicine works. Check with your health care professional before stopping or starting any of your medicines.

What should I watch for while taking chlorpheniramine; hydrocodone; pseudoephedrine?

Tell your prescriber or health care professional if your symptoms do not improve in 5 days or if you have a high fever. You may get drowsy or dizzy. Do not drive, use machinery, or do anything that needs mental alertness until you know how this medicine affects you. Be careful taking other medicines that may also make you tired. To reduce the risk of dizzy or fainting spells, do not stand or sit up quickly, especially if you are an older patient. Alcohol may increase dizziness and drowsiness. Avoid alcoholic drinks. When chlorpheniramine, hydrocodone, and pseudoephedrine are used together you may experience dry eyes and blurred vision. If you wear contact lenses you may feel some discomfort. Lubricating drops may help. See your ophthalmologist if the problem does not go away or is severe.

What side effects may I notice from taking chlorpheniramine; hydrocodone; pseudoephedrine?

Side effects that you should report to your prescriber or health care professional as soon as possible:

- agitation, anxiety, nervousness, excitability, not able to sleep
- chest pain
- confusion
- difficulty breathing, wheezing, shortness of breath
- dizziness or fainting spells
- excessive sweating
- fast or irregular heartbeat, palpitations
- high blood pressure
- numbness or tingling in the hands or feet
- pain or difficulty passing urine
- rash
- severe, persistent, or worsening headache
- swelling of the face, tongue, throat, hands or feet

- tremor or muscle contractions
- vision problems
- vomiting

Side effects that usually do not require medical attention (report to your prescriber or health care professional if they continue or are bothersome):

- constipation
- difficulty sleeping
- drowsiness or tiredness
- dry eyes
- headache (mild)
- itching
- mood changes
- stomach upset or nausea
- restlessness

Where can I keep my medicine?

Keep out of the reach of children in a container that small children cannot open. Store at room temperature, between 15 and 30 degrees C (59 and 86 degrees F). Keep container tightly closed. Keep away from heat and light. Throw away any unused medicine after the expiration date.

Chlorpromazine tablets

CHLORPROMAZINE;
50 mg; Tablet
UDL Laboratories
Inc

CHLORPROMAZINE;
25 mg; Tablet
Sandoz
Pharmaceuticals

What are chlorpromazine tablets?

CHLORPROMAZINE (Thorazine®, Thor-Prom®) has a number of uses in helping to treat emotional, nervous, or mental problems. Chlorpromazine reduces the symptoms of psychotic disorders like schizophrenia. It also can help children with severe behavioral problems. Chlorpromazine is also used for uncontrollable hiccups, control of nausea and vomiting, and relief of restlessness and apprehension before surgery. Chlorpromazine also helps patients with acute intermittent porphyria. Generic chlorpromazine tablets are available.

What should my health care professional know before I take chlorpromazine?

They need to know if you have any of these conditions:

- frequently drink alcoholic beverages
- asthma or other chronic lung disease
- blood disorders or disease
- breast cancer
- difficulty passing urine
- fever
- glaucoma
- head injury
- heart disease or irregular heartbeat
- liver disease
- low blood level of calcium
- Parkinson's disease
- prostate trouble
- recent fever or viral infection, especially in children
- Reye's syndrome

- seizures (convulsions)
- stomach problems or peptic ulcer
- uncontrollable movement disorder
- an unusual or allergic reaction to chlorpromazine, other medicines foods, dyes, or preservatives
- pregnant or trying to get pregnant
- breast-feeding

How should I take this medicine?

Take chlorpromazine tablets by mouth. Follow the directions on the prescription label. Swallow the tablets with a drink of water. Take chlorpromazine with food or milk if it upsets your stomach. Do not take with antacids. Take your doses at regular intervals. Do not take your medicine more often than directed. Contact your pediatrician or health care professional regarding the use of this medicine in children. Special care may be needed. Elderly patients over age 65 years may have a stronger reaction to this medicine and may need smaller doses.

What if I miss a dose?

If you miss a dose, take it as soon as you can. If it is almost time for your next dose, take only that dose. Try to take your doses at the same time(s) each day. Do not take double or extra doses.

What may interact with chlorpromazine?

- alcohol
- antacids

- some antibiotics
- antidiarrheal medications
- atropine
- bromocriptine
- cimetidine
- cisapride
- dextroamphetamine or amphetamine
- dronabinol or marijuana
- haloperidol or droperidol
- levodopa
- lithium
- medicines for an overactive thyroid gland
- medicines for colds and flu
- medicines for hay fever and other allergies
- medicines for mental depression
- medicines for movement abnormalities as in Parkinson's disease
- medicines to prevent or treat malaria
- medications for treating seizures (convulsions)
- medicines for pain or for use as muscle relaxants, including tramadol
- medicines to treat urine or bladder incontinence
- metoclopramide
- pimozide
- probucol
- some medications for high blood pressure or heart problems
- some weight loss medications

Tell your prescriber or health care professional about all other medicines you are taking, including non-prescription medicines, nutritional supplements, or herbal products. Also tell your prescriber or health care professional if you are a frequent user of drinks with caffeine or alcohol, if you smoke, or if you use illegal drugs. These may affect the way your medicine works. Check with your health care professional before stopping or starting any of your medicines.

What should I watch for while taking chlorpromazine?

Visit your prescriber or health care professional for regular checks on your progress. Do not stop taking chlorpromazine suddenly; this can cause nausea, vomiting, and dizziness. Ask your prescriber or health care professional for advice if you are to stop taking this medicine. You may get drowsy, dizzy, or have blurred vision. Do not drive, use machinery, or do anything that needs mental alertness until you know how chlorpromazine affects you. Do not stand or sit up quickly, especially if you are an older patient. This reduces the risk of dizzy or fainting spells. Alcohol can increase possible dizziness or drowsiness. Avoid alcoholic drinks. Chlorpromazine can reduce the response of your body to heat or cold. Try not to get overheated. Avoid temperature extremes, such as saunas, hot tubs, or very hot or cold baths or showers. Dress warmly in cold weather. Chlorpromazine can make your skin more sensitive to sun or ultraviolet light. Keep out of the sun, or wear protective

clothing outdoors and use a sunscreen (at least SPF 15). Do not use sun lamps or sun tanning beds or booths. Wear sunglasses to protect your eyes. Some medications taken with chlorpromazine may increase your sun sensitivity. Chlorpromazine may make your mouth dry, chewing sugarless gum or sucking hard candy and drinking plenty of water will help. Do not treat yourself for coughs, colds, sore throat, indigestion, diarrhea, or allergies. Ask your prescriber or health care professional for advice. If you are going to have surgery or will need an x-ray procedure that uses contrast agents, tell your prescriber or health care professional that you are taking this medicine.

What side effects may I notice from taking chlorpromazine?

Side effects that you should report to your prescriber or health care professional as soon as possible:
These following effects require that you contact your health care provider immediately if they occur:
- convulsions (seizures)
- chest pain, fast or irregular heartbeat
- difficulty breathing or swallowing or shortness of breath
- fever, chills, sore throat
- hot, dry, pale skin
- painful and prolonged erection (men)
- puffing cheeks, smacking lips, or worm-like movements of the tongue
- severe stiffness of the muscles
- shaking or uncontrolled/unusual movements of the arms, eyes, mouth, legs or tongue
- unusual weakness or tiredness
- unusual bleeding or bruising

Check with your health care provider as soon as possible for the following:
- blurred vision or other changes in vision
- breast enlargement, pain, or discharge in men or women
- confusion
- dark yellow or brown urine
- difficulty passing urine
- fainting spells, falls, or difficulty in balance
- nausea, vomiting, or diarrhea
- restlessness
- slurred speech
- stomach area pain
- twitching movements
- yellowing of skin or eyes

Side effects that usually do not require immediate medical attention (report to your prescriber or health care professional if they continue or are bothersome):
Common:
- constipation
- decreased perspiration or sweating
- dizziness or drowsiness
- dry mouth
- headache
- increased sensitivity to the sun or ultraviolet light

- menstrual changes
- stuffy nose

Less Common:
- sexual difficulties (decreased sexual desire or impotence in men)
- skin discoloration
- weight gain

Where can I keep my medicine?

Keep out of the reach of children in a container that small children cannot open. Store at room temperature between 15 and 30 degrees C (59 and 86 degrees F). Protect from light. Keep container tightly closed. Throw away any unused medicine after the expiration date.

Chlorpropamide tablets

DIABINESE®; 250 mg; Tablet Pfizer Laboratories Div Pfizer Inc

DIABINESE®; 100 mg; Tablet Pfizer Laboratories Div Pfizer Inc

What are chlorpropamide tablets?

CHLORPROPAMIDE (Diabinese®) helps to treat type 2 diabetes mellitus. Treatment is combined with a suitable diet and balanced exercise. Chlorpropamide increases the amount of insulin released from the pancreas and helps your body to use insulin more efficiently. Generic chlorpropamide tablets are available.

What should my health care professional know before I take chlorpropamide?

They need to know if you have any of these conditions:
- kidney disease
- liver disease
- major surgery
- porphyria
- severe infection or injury
- thyroid disease
- an unusual or allergic reaction to chlorpropamide, sulfonamides, other medicines, foods, dyes, or preservatives
- pregnant or trying to get pregnant
- breast-feeding

How should I take this medicine?

Take chlorpropamide tablets by mouth. Follow the directions on the prescription label. Swallow the tablets with a drink of water. If you take chlorpropamide once a day, take it with breakfast. Take your doses at the same time each day; do not take more often than directed. Contact your pediatrician or health care professional regarding the use of this medicine in children. Special care may be needed. Elderly patients over 65 years old may have a stronger reaction and need a smaller dose.

What if I miss a dose?

If you miss a dose, take it as soon as you can. If it is almost time for your next dose, take only that dose. Do not take double or extra doses.

What may interact with chlorpropamide?

- alcohol
- beta-blockers (used for high blood pressure or heart conditions)
- bosentan
- chloramphenicol
- cisapride
- clofibrate
- diazoxide
- medicines for fungal or yeast infections (examples: itraconazole, miconazole, voriconazole)
- metoclopramide
- rifampin
- warfarin (a blood thinner)

Many medications may cause changes (increase or decrease) in blood sugar, these include:
- alcohol containing beverages
- aspirin and aspirin-like drugs
- beta-blockers, often used for high blood pressure or heart problems (examples include atenolol, metoprolol, propranolol)
- chromium
- female hormones, such as estrogens or progestins, birth control pills
- isoniazid
- male hormones or anabolic steroids
- medications for weight loss
- medicines for allergies, asthma, cold, or cough
- niacin
- pentamidine
- phenytoin
- quinolone antibiotics (examples: ciprofloxacin, levofloxacin, ofloxacin)
- some herbal dietary supplements
- steroid medicines such as prednisone or cortisone
- thyroid hormones
- water pills (diuretics)

Tell your prescriber or health care professional about all other medicines you are taking, including non-prescription medicines, nutritional supplements, or herbal products. Also tell your prescriber or health care professional if you are a frequent user of drinks with caffeine or alcohol, if you smoke, or if you use illegal drugs. These may affect the way your medicine works. Check with your health care professional before stopping or starting any of your medicines.

What should I watch for while taking chlorpropamide?

Visit your prescriber or health care professional for regular checks on your progress. Learn how to monitor blood or urine sugar and urine ketones regularly. Check with your prescriber or health care professional if your blood sugar is high, you may need a change of dose of chlorpropamide. Do not skip meals. If you are exercising much more than usual you may need extra snacks to avoid side effects caused by low blood sugar. Alcohol can increase possible side effects of chlorpropamide. Ask your prescriber or health care professional if you should avoid alcohol. If you have mild symptoms of low blood sugar, eat or drink something containing sugar at once and contact your prescriber or health care professional. It is wise to check your blood sugar to confirm that it is low. It is important to recognize your own symptoms of low blood sugar so that you can treat them quickly. Make sure family members know that you can choke if you eat or drink when you have serious symptoms of low blood sugar, such as seizures or unconsciousness. They must get medical help at once. Chlorpropamide can increase the sensitivity of your skin to the sun. Keep out of the sun, or wear protective clothing outdoors and use a sunscreen. Do not use sun lamps or sun tanning beds or booths. If you are going to have surgery, tell your prescriber or health care professional that you are taking chlorpropamide. Wear a medical identification bracelet or chain to say you have diabetes, and carry a card that lists all your medications.

What side effects may I notice from taking chlorpropamide?

Side effects that you should report to your prescriber or health care professional as soon as possible:

- hypoglycemia (low blood glucose) which can cause symptoms such as anxiety or nervousness, confusion, difficulty concentrating, hunger, pale skin, nausea, fatigue, perspiration, headache, palpitations, numbness of the mouth, tingling in the fingers, tremors, muscle weakness, blurred vision, cold sensations, uncontrolled yawning, irritability, rapid heartbeat, shallow breathing, and loss of consciousness
- breathing difficulties, severe skin reactions or excessive phlegm, which may indicate that you are having an allergic reaction to the drug
- dark yellow or brown urine, or yellowing of the eyes or skin, indicating that the drug is affecting your liver
- fever, chills, sore throat; which means the drug may be affecting your immune system
- unusual bleeding or bruising; which occurs when the drug is affecting your blood clotting system

Side effects that usually do not require medical attention (report to your prescriber or health care professional if they continue or are bothersome):

- diarrhea
- headache
- heartburn
- increased sensitivity to the sun
- nausea, vomiting
- stomach discomfort
- skin rash, redness, swelling or itching

Let your prescriber or health care professional know if these side effects are severe, if they do not go away or if they annoy you.

Where can I keep my medicine?

Keep out of the reach of children in a container that small children cannot open. Store at room temperature below 30 degrees C. Throw away any unused medicine after the expiration date.

Chlorthalidone tablets

THALITONE®; 15 mg; Tablet Monarch Pharmaceuticals Inc	CHLORTHALIDONE; 25 mg; Tablet Mylan Pharmaceuticals Inc

What are chlorthalidone tablets?

CHLORTHALIDONE (Hygroton®, Thalitone®) is a diuretic (water or fluid pill). Diuretics increase the amount of urine passed, which causes the body to lose water and salt. Chlorthalidone helps to treat high blood pressure (hypertension). It is not a cure. It also reduces the swelling (edema) and water retention caused by various medical conditions, such as heart, liver, or kidney disease. Generic chlorthalidone tablets are available.

What should my health care professional know before I take chlorthalidone?

They need to know if you have any of these conditions:
- diabetes
- gout
- high blood levels of calcium
- kidney disease, small amounts of urine, or difficulty passing urine
- liver disease
- low blood levels of potassium, chloride, or sodium
- pancreatitis
- systemic lupus erythematosus (SLE)
- an unusual or allergic reaction to chlorthalidone, sulfonamides, carbonic anhydrase inhibitors, other medicines, foods, dyes, or preservatives
- pregnant or trying to get pregnant
- breast-feeding

How should I take this medicine?

Take chlorthalidone tablets by mouth. Follow the directions on the prescription label. Swallow the tablets with a drink of water. If chlorthalidone upsets your stomach, take it with food or milk. Take your doses at regular intervals. Do not take your medicine more often than directed. Remember that you will need to pass urine frequently after taking chlorthalidone. Do not take your doses at a time of day that will cause you problems. Do not take at bedtime. Contact your pediatrician or health care professional regarding the use of this medicine in children. Special care may be needed.

What if I miss a dose?

If you miss a dose, take it as soon as you can. If it is almost time for your next dose, take only that dose. Chlorthalidone tablets are often taken every other day. If you miss one day, take it the next and then return to the correct dosing interval. Do not take double or extra doses.

What may interact with chlorthalidone?

- amphotericin B
- anti-inflammatory drugs (NSAIDs, such as ibuprofen)
- cholestyramine
- colestipol
- diazoxide
- digoxin
- dofetilide
- hormones such as prednisone, cortisone, hydrocortisone, corticotropin
- lithium
- medicines for diabetes that are taken by mouth
- medicines for high blood pressure
- water pills

Tell your prescriber or health care professional about all other medicines you are taking, including non-prescription medicines, nutritional supplements, or herbal products. Also tell your prescriber or health care professional if you are a frequent user of drinks with caffeine or alcohol, if you smoke, or if you use illegal drugs. These may affect the way your medicine works. Check with your health care professional before stopping or starting any of your medicines.

What should I watch for while taking chlorthalidone?

Visit your prescriber or health care professional for regular checks on your progress. Check your blood pressure regularly. Ask your prescriber or health care professional what your blood pressure should be, and when you should contact him or her. You must not get dehydrated, ask your prescriber or health care professional how much fluid you need to drink a day. Do not stop taking chlorthalidone except on your prescriber's advice. Watch your diet while you are taking chlorthalidone. Ask your prescriber or health care professional about both potassium and sodium intake. Chlorthalidone can make your body lose potassium and you may need an extra supply. Some foods have a high potassium content such as bananas, coconuts, dates, figs, prunes, apricots, peaches, grapefruit juice, tomato juice, and orange juice. You may get dizzy or lightheaded. Do

not drive, use machinery, or do anything that needs mental alertness until you know how chlorthalidone affects you. To reduce the risk of dizzy or fainting spells, do not sit or stand up quickly, especially if you are an older patient. Alcohol can make you lightheaded, dizzy and increase confusion. Avoid or limit intake of alcoholic drinks. Your skin may be more sensitive to the sun. Keep out of the sun, or wear protective clothing outdoors and use a sunscreen. Do not use sun lamps or sun tanning booths or beds. If you are going to have surgery, tell your prescriber or health care professional that you are taking chlorthalidone.

What side effects may I notice from taking chlorthalidone?

Side effects that you should report to your prescriber or health care professional as soon as possible:

- black, tarry stools
- blood in the urine
- dark yellow or brown urine
- dry mouth
- fever, chills, sore throat
- increased thirst
- irregular heartbeat (palpitations)
- lower back pain
- mood changes
- muscle pain, cramps
- nausea, vomiting
- pain or difficulty passing urine
- redness, blistering, peeling or loosening of the skin, including inside the mouth
- skin rash or itching
- stomach pain
- tingling, pain or numbness in the hands or feet
- unusual tiredness or weakness
- unusual bleeding or bruising
- yellowing of the eyes or skin
- yellow vision (everything looks yellow)

Side effects that usually do not require medical attention (report to your prescriber or health care professional if they continue or are bothersome):

- diarrhea or constipation
- dizziness or lightheadedness
- headache
- increased sensitivity to the sun
- loss of appetite
- sexual difficulties (impotence)

Where can I keep my medicine?

Keep out of the reach of children in a container that small children cannot open. Store at room temperature between 15 and 30 degrees C (59 and 86 degrees F). Keep container tightly closed. Throw away any unused medicine after the expiration date.

Chlorzoxazone
tablets or caplets

PARAFON FORTE®
DSC;
500 mg; Tablet
Janssen Ortho, LLC

CHLORZOXAZONE;
500 mg; Tablet
Teva
Pharmaceuticals
USA Inc

What are chlorzoxazone tablets or caplets?

CHLORZOXAZONE (Parafon Forte® DSC, Para-flex®, Remular-S® and others) is a muscle relaxant that has sedative properties. It is used in combination with rest and physical therapy to relieve acute, painful muscle discomforts, like those caused by sprains, strains or other muscle injuries. Generic chlorzoxazone products are available.

What should my health care professional know before I take chlorzoxazone?

They need to know if you have any of these conditions:
- kidney disease
- liver disease or a history of liver disease
- porphyria
- an unusual or allergic reaction to chlorzoxazone, other medicines, foods, dyes, or preservatives
- pregnant or trying to get pregnant
- breast-feeding

How should I take this medicine?

Take chlorzoxazone tablets or caplets by mouth. Follow the directions on the prescription label. Swallow the tablets with a drink of water. If chlorzoxazone upsets your stomach, you may take it with food or milk. Take your doses at regular intervals. Do not take your medicine more often than directed. Contact your pediatrician or health care professional regarding the use of this medicine in children. Special care may be needed.

What if I miss a dose?

If it is almost time for your next dose, take only that dose. Do not take double or extra doses.

What may interact with chlorzoxazone?

- alcohol and alcoholic beverages
- baclofen
- barbiturate medicines for inducing sleep or treating seizures (convulsions), such as phenobarbital
- disulfiram
- dronabinol, THC
- entacapone
- isoniazid, INH
- kava kava
- medicines for hay fever and other allergies
- medicines for mental depression, anxiety or psychotic disturbances
- medicines to treat sleeping problems (insomnia)
- prescription medicines for pain
- simvastatin
- tolcapone
- valerian

Tell your prescriber or health care professional about all other medicines you are taking, including non-prescription medicines, nutritional supplements, or herbal products. Also tell your prescriber or health care professional if you are a frequent user of drinks with caffeine or alcohol, if you smoke, or if you use illegal drugs. These may affect the way your medicine works. Check with your health care professional before stopping or starting any of your medicines.

What should I watch for while taking chlorzoxazone?

Chlorzoxazone is usually used for a short period of time to relax muscles and relieve pain. Let your prescriber know if your condition does not improve. If you must take chlorzoxazone for a longer period of time, your prescriber may want to monitor your liver function by regularly taking a blood test. You may get drowsy or dizzy. Do not drive, use machinery, or do anything that needs mental alertness until you know how chlorzoxazone affects you. To reduce the risk of dizzy or fainting spells, do not sit or stand up quickly, especially if you are an older patient. Alcohol can make you more drowsy; avoid alcoholic drinks.

What side effects may I notice from taking chlorzoxazone?

Side effects that you should report to your prescriber or health care professional as soon as possible:
- abdominal pain
- darkened brown urine
- difficulty breathing
- nausea or vomiting
- skin rash, hives, itching
- unusual movements
- yellowing of the eyes or skin
- unusual tiredness or weakness

Side effects that usually do not require medical attention (report to your prescriber or health care professional if they continue or are bothersome):
- constipation
- dizziness
- drowsiness
- headache
- orange or purple-red color of the urine
- stomach upset

Where can I keep my medicine?

Keep out of the reach of children in a container that small children cannot open. Store at room temperature between 15 and 30 degrees C (59 and 86 degrees F). Throw away any unused medicine after the expiration date.

Choline Salicylate; Magnesium Salicylate tablets

SALICYLATE SALTS;
750 mg; Tablet
Amide
Pharmaceutical Inc

SALICYLATE SALTS;
750 mg; Tablet
Pliva Inc

What are choline salicylate; magnesium salicylate tablets?

CHOLINE SALICYLATE; MAGNESIUM SALI-CYLATE (CMT®, Tricosal®, Trilisate®) relieves the mild to moderate pain caused by a variety of conditions including arthritis, bursitis, tendinitis, headaches, menstrual cramps or pain, minor injuries, and others. Choline and magnesium salicylate reduces fever, pain, and inflammation (swelling and redness). Generic choline and magnesium salicylate tablets are available.

What should my health care professional know before I take choline salicylate; magnesium salicylate tablets?

They need to know if you have any of these conditions:
- anemia
- bleeding or clotting problems
- drink more than 3 alcohol-containing beverages a day
- gout
- heart disease, including heart failure
- high blood pressure
- kidney disease
- liver disease
- smoke tobacco
- stomach ulcers, or other stomach problems
- systemic lupus erythematosus (SLE)
- thrombotic thrombocytopenic purpura (TTP)
- ulcerative colitis
- vitamin K deficiency
- an unusual or allergic reaction to salicylates, aspirin, other medicines, dyes, or preservatives
- pregnant or trying to get pregnant
- breast-feeding

How should I take this medicine?

Take choline and magnesium salicylate tablets by mouth with a large glass of water. You may take the tablets with food to help decrease stomach upset. Follow the directions on the prescription label. Take your doses at regular intervals. Do not take your medicine more often than directed. Contact your pediatrician or health care professional regarding the use of this medicine in children. Special care may be needed.

What if I miss a dose?

If you are taking choline and magnesium salicylate on a regular schedule and miss a dose, take it as soon as you can. If it is almost time for your next dose, take only that dose. Do not take double or extra doses.

What may interact with choline salicylate; magnesium salicylate tablets?

- alcohol
- antacids (in large doses)
- anti-inflammatory drugs (NSAIDs, such as ibuprofen)
- hormones such as prednisone or cortisone
- itraconazole
- ketoconazole
- medicines used to treat or prevent blood clots
- medicines for diabetes that are taken by mouth
- medicines for gout
- methotrexate
- quinolone antibiotics (such as ciprofloxacin, levoflox-acin, ofloxacin)
- seizure (convulsion) or epilepsy medicine
- tetracyclines

Tell your prescriber or health care professional about all other medicines you are taking, including non-prescription medicines, nutritional supplements, or herbal products. Also tell your prescriber or health care professional if you are a frequent user of drinks with caffeine or alcohol, if you smoke, or if you use illegal drugs. These may affect the way your medicine works. Check with your health care professional before stopping or starting any of your medicines.

What should I watch for while taking choline salicylate; magnesium salicylate tablets?

Many non-prescription medicines contain aspirin as an ingredient. To prevent accidental overdose, read labels carefully and do not combine choline and magnesium salicylate with aspirin or other medicines unless your prescriber or health care professional tells you to do so. If you are taking choline and magnesium salicylate for arthritis or other types of pain, it can take up to 3 weeks to get the maximum effect. Do not stop taking without asking your prescriber or health care professional. If you are taking oral medicines to decrease your blood sugar, large doses of choline and magnesium salicylate may increase the levels of these drugs. Check with your prescriber or health care professional before you change your diet or the dose of your diabetic medicine. Choline and magnesium salicylate can irritate your stomach. Limit smoking and drinking of alcohol; these increase irritation in your stomach and may cause ulcers or bleeding problems. Do not lie down for 30 minutes after taking choline salicylate to prevent irritation to your throat.

What side effects may I notice from taking choline salicylate; magnesium salicylate tablets?

Side effects that you should report to your prescriber or health care professional as soon as possible:
- signs or symptoms of bleeding from the stomach or intestine such as black, tarry stools, stomach pain, vomiting up blood or what looks like coffee grounds
- confusion

- difficulty breathing, wheezing
- ringing in the ears or changes in hearing
- skin rash, hives
- unusual bleeding or bruising, red or purple spots on the skin

Side effects that usually do not require medical attention (report to your prescriber or health care professional if they continue or are bothersome):

- diarrhea or constipation

Chondroitin; Glucosamine tablets or capsules

- nausea, vomiting
- stomach gas, heartburn

Where can I keep my medicine?

Keep out of the reach of children in a container that small children cannot open. Even small doses of magnesium salicylate can be dangerous to small children and pets. Store at room temperature below 30 degrees C (86 degrees F). Throw away any unused medicine after the expiration date.

CHONDROITIN;
GLUCOSAMINE Capsules
400 mg/500 mg; Tablet/
Capsule
Walgreens Health Initiatives

What are chondroitin; glucosamine tablets or capsules?

CHONDROITIN; GLUCOSAMINE (Cosamin®-DS, Flexagen™, Osteo Bi-Flex®, and many others) is a non-prescription dietary supplement promoted for its ability to ease osteoarthritis symptoms, which may occur with aging as joints undergo "wear-and-tear." Chondroitin and glucosamine are two substances found naturally in our bodies that help maintain healthy joint cartilage. There is some proof that supplementing these two substances may help reduce symptoms associated with osteoarthritis. Chondroitin-glucosamine supplementation has not been shown to help rheumatoid arthritis, a different arthritic condition than osteoarthritis. Chondroitin; glucosamine is not officially endorsed by the FDA, but is under study by the National Institutes of Health (NIH).

What should my health care professional know before I take chondroitin; glucosamine?

It is important for you to tell your prescriber or other health care professional that you are using chondroitin; glucosamine. You should discuss this supplement with your health care professional BEFORE taking it if you have any of these conditions:

- diabetes mellitus
- heart problems
- kidney disease
- liver disease
- stomach or intestinal problems
- an unusual or allergic reaction to chondroitin or glucosamine, sulfates, other medicines, foods, dyes, or preservatives
- pregnant or trying to get pregnant
- breast-feeding

How should I take this medicine?

Chondroitin; glucosamine tablets and capsules should be taken orally (i.e., swallowed). Follow the directions on the product label or consult your health-care professional for advice. The effects of chondroitin; glucosamine take several weeks to appear so it should be taken daily for several weeks for best results. Take your doses at regular intervals. Do not take this supplement more often than directed. Contact your pediatrician or

health care professional regarding the use of this medicine in children. Special care may be needed.

What if I miss a dose?

Missing a dose is probably not harmful. If you miss a dose, simply resume taking it on your previous schedule. Do not take double or extra doses.

What may interact with chondroitin; glucosamine?

- warfarin

For many dietary supplements, interactions with other medications are unknown. That is why you should always be careful when mixing them with traditional medications. If you take any other medications, consult with your health care professional prior to taking chondroitin; glucosamine. Tell your prescriber or health care professional about all other medicines you are taking, including non-prescription medicines, nutritional supplements, or herbal products. Also tell your prescriber or health care professional if you are a frequent user of drinks with caffeine or alcohol, if you smoke, or if you use illegal drugs. These may affect the way your medicine works. Check with your health care professional before stopping or starting any of your medicines.

What should I watch for while taking chondroitin; glucosamine?

If you notice any changes in your physical health while taking chondroitin; glucosamine, you should contact your health care provider. Also, different brands of chondroitin; glucosamine might contain different amounts of active ingredient so try to use the same brand. Chondroitin; glucosamine may cause drowsiness. Driving or operating machinery, or performing other tasks that require mental alertness requires caution when taking chondroitin; glucosamine. You should not participate in these activities until you determine how chondroitin; glucosamine affects you. It is unclear if glucosamine may increase blood sugar if you have diabetes, some studies indicate that no significant change in blood sugar is expected. If you are diabetic, you may wish to monitor your blood sugar more frequently when you first start this supplement. Discuss any changes in your blood sugar control with your prescriber.

What side effects may I notice from taking chondroitin; glucosamine?

Side effects that you should report to your prescriber or health care professional as soon as possible:

- constipation or diarrhea
- difficulty sleeping
- drowsiness
- hair loss
- headache
- loss of appetite
- swelling of the face, feet or ankles
- skin rash or itching
- stomach pain

Side effects that usually do not require medical attention (report to your prescriber or health care professional if they continue or are bothersome):

- gas
- nausea
- upset stomach

Where can I keep my medicine?

Keep out of the reach of children. Store at room temperature; do not freeze. Throw away any unused medicine after the expiration date.

GENERAL INFORMATION REGARDING DIETARY SUPPLEMENTS:

Dietary supplements include amino acids, vitamins, minerals, herbs, and other plant-derived substances, and extracts of these substances. Products are easy to identify as they must state "Dietary Supplement" on the label. A "Supplement Facts" panel is provided on the label for most products. Supplements are not drugs and are not regulated like pharmaceuticals. You should note that rigid quality control standards are not required for dietary supplements. Differences in the potency and purity of these products can occur. Scientific data to support the use of a dietary supplement for a certain condition may not be available. This product is not intended to diagnose, treat, cure or prevent any disease. The Food and Drug Administration suggests the following to help consumers protect themselves:

- Always read product labels and follow directions.
- Look for products containing ingredients with the "USP" notation. This indicates the manufacturer followed the standards of the US Pharmacopoeia.
- "Natural" doesn't mean a product is safe for humans to consume.
- Supplements produced or distributed by a nationally known food or drug company are more likely to be made under tight controls as these companies have standards in place for their other products. You can write to the company or manufacturer for more information about the conditions under which the products are made.

Cilostazol tablets

PLETAL®;
50 mg; Tablet
Otsuka America
Pharmaceuticals Inc

PLETAL®;
100 mg; Tablet
Otsuka America
Pharmaceuticals Inc

What are cilostazol tablets?

CILOSTAZOL (Pletal®) is a medication that reduces the symptoms of intermittent claudication. This condition causes pain in the legs during walking, and goes away with rest. Cilostazol helps blood flow more smoothly through the blood vessels; this action improves oxygen flow to the tissues of the body. By improving blood flow, cilostazol helps people with claudication walk longer distances without pain. In some cases cilostazol may be prescribed for other health conditions where improved blood flow through the blood vessels is needed. Generic cilostazol tablets are available.

What should my health care professional know before I take cilostazol?

They need to know if you have any of the following conditions:

- angina
- bleeding disorder or hemophilia
- diabetes
- headaches
- history of heart failure, heart attack, or other heart disease
- low blood pressure

- an unusual or allergic reaction to cilostazol, other medicines, foods, dyes, or preservatives
- pregnant or trying to get pregnant
- breast-feeding

How should I take this medicine?

Take cilostazol tablets by mouth. Follow the directions on the prescription label. Swallow the tablets with plenty of water (at least a full glass) to avoid stomach upset. Take on an empty stomach, at least 1/2 hour before or 2 hours after a meal. Take your doses at regular intervals. Do not take your medicine more often than directed. Contact your pediatrician or health care professional regarding the use of this medicine in children. Special care may be needed.

What if I miss a dose?

If you miss a dose, take it as soon as you can. If it is almost time for your next dose, take only that dose. Do not take double or extra doses.

What may interact with cilostazol?

- agents that prevent or treat blood clots (such as enoxaparin or warfarin)
- anti-inflammatory drugs (NSAIDs, such as ibuprofen, naproxen, or ketoprofen)

- aspirin
- cimetidine (do not purchase non-prescription without prescriber advice)
- clopidogrel
- diltiazem
- erythromycin or clarithromycin
- fish oil (omega-3 fatty acids) supplements
- herbal medicines or dietary supplements like feverfew, garlic pills, ginger, gingko biloba, or horse chestnut
- grapefruit juice
- omeprazole
- pentoxifylline
- some medications for treating depression (examples: fluoxetine, fluvoxamine, nefazodone)
- some medications for treating fungal infections (examples: ketoconazole, fluconazole, itraconazole)
- ticlopidine

Tell your prescriber or health care professional about all other medicines you are taking, including non-prescription medicines, nutritional supplements, or herbal products. Also tell your prescriber or health care professional if you are a frequent user of drinks with caffeine or alcohol, if you smoke, or if you use illegal drugs. These may affect the way your medicine works. Check with your health care professional before stopping or starting any of your medicines.

What should I watch for while taking cilostazol?

After you start to take cilostazol, it may take 2 to 4 weeks for you to notice improvement in your condition. In some people, it can take as long as 3 months for claudication (leg pain) to improve. Visit your prescriber or health care professional for regular checks on your progress. Do not stop taking cilostazol except on your prescriber's advice. If you notice any unusual symptoms or side effects, contact your prescriber. You may get dizzy, especially when you sit or stand up quickly. Do not drive, use machinery or do anything that needs mental alertness until you know how cilostazol affects you. To reduce dizzy spells, do not sit or stand up quickly, especially if you are an older patient. Alcohol can increase dizziness, so try to avoid alcoholic drinks. Grapefruit juice can increase the levels of cilostazol in your body, which could increase the risk of

unwanted side effects. Try to avoid drinking grapefruit juice while on this medicine. Smoking tobacco may have effects on the circulation that may limit the benefits you receive from cilostazol. You may wish to discuss how to stop smoking with your prescriber or health care professional. Ask your prescriber or health care professional before you take certain non-prescription (OTC) pain relievers. These include aspirin, aspirin-containing products, and products that contain NSAIDs: like Motrin®, Aleve® and Orudis-KT®. These OTC medications could interfere with your cilostazol therapy. While taking aspirin with cilostazol may be beneficial for you, check with your prescriber prior to taking this combination on your own. If you are going to have surgery, tell your prescriber or health care professional that you are taking cilostazol.

What side effects may I notice from taking cilostazol?

Side effects that you should report to your prescriber or health care professional as soon as possible:
- fast, slow, or irregular heartbeat
- fluid (edema) in the legs or ankles
- palpitations, chest pain or tightness

Rare:
- black, tarry stools
- blood in urine or stools
- nosebleed or bleeding from gums
- skin rash or itching (hives)
- unusual bruising
- unusually heavy menstrual bleeding

Side effects that usually do not require medical attention (report to your prescriber or health care professional if they continue or are bothersome):
- dizziness
- diarrhea, or changes in stool appearance or frequency ("loose stools")
- headache
- nausea, or upset stomach

Where can I keep my medicine?

Keep out of the reach of children in a container that small children cannot open. Store at room temperature below 30 degrees C (86 degrees F). Throw away any unused medicine after the expiration date.

Cimetidine tablets

TAGAMET®; 300 mg; Tablet Smithkline Beecham Pharmaceuticals Div

TAGAMET®; 400 mg; Tablet Smithkline Beecham Pharmaceuticals Div

What are cimetidine tablets?

CIMETIDINE (Tagamet®) is a type of antihistamine that blocks the release of stomach acid. Cimetidine is used to treat gastric and duodenal ulcers. It can relieve ulcer pain and discomfort, and the heartburn from gastroesophageal reflux disease. Generic cimetidine tablets are available.

What should my health care professional know before I take cimetidine?

They need to know if you have any of these conditions:
- frequently drink alcoholic beverages or smoke
- kidney disease
- liver disease
- other chronic illness

- an unusual or allergic reaction to cimetidine, other medicines, foods, dyes, or preservatives
- pregnant or trying to get pregnant
- breast-feeding

How should I take this medicine?

Take cimetidine tablets by mouth. Follow the directions on the prescription label. Swallow the tablets with a drink of water. If you only take cimetidine once a day take it at bedtime. Take your doses at regular intervals. Do not take your medicine more often than directed. Contact your pediatrician or health care professional regarding the use of this medicine in children. Special care may be needed.

What if I miss a dose?

If you miss a dose, take it as soon as you can. If it is almost time for your next dose, take only that dose. Do not take double or extra doses.

What may interact with cimetidine?

- astemizole
- cisapride
- dofetilide
- pimozide
- terfenadine

Other drugs that can interact with cimetidine include:

- antacids
- beta blockers, often used for high blood pressure or heart problems
- caffeine
- carbamazepine
- carmustine
- cefditoren
- cefpodoxime
- cefuroxime
- clonazepam
- delavirdine
- fentanyl
- female hormones, including contraceptive or birth control pills
- flecainide
- guarana
- itraconazole
- ketoconazole
- meperidine
- metformin
- metronidazole
- nifedipine
- medicines for anxiety or sleeping problems, such as diazepam, triazolam, or temazepam
- medicines for heart rhythm problems
- medicines for mental depression
- phenytoin
- theophylline
- warfarin

Tell your prescriber or health care professional about all other medicines you are taking, including non-prescription medicines, nutritional supplements, or herbal products. Also tell your prescriber or health care professional if you are a frequent user of drinks with caffeine or alcohol, if you smoke, or if you use illegal drugs. These may affect the way your medicine works. Check with your health care professional before stopping or starting any of your medicines.

What should I watch for while taking cimetidine?

Tell your prescriber or health care professional if your ulcer pain does not improve or gets worse. You may need to take this medicine for several days as prescribed before your symptoms improve. Finish the full course of tablets prescribed by your prescriber or health care professional even if you feel better. Do not self-medicate with aspirin, ibuprofen or other anti-inflammatory medicines unless directed to do so by your health care professional; these can aggravate your condition. Do not smoke cigarettes or drink alcohol; these increase irritation in your stomach and can lengthen the time it will take for your ulcer to heal. If you get black, tarry stools or vomit up what looks like coffee grounds, call your prescriber or health care professional at once. You may have a bleeding ulcer. If you need to take an antacid you should take it at least 1 hour before or 1 hour after cimetidine. Cimetidine will not be as effective if taken at the same time as an antacid.

What side effects may I notice from taking cimetidine?

Side effects with cimetidine are infrequent but include:

- agitation, nervousness, depression, hallucinations
- breast swelling and tenderness, or sexual difficulties (impotence) in men
- dark yellow or brown urine
- diarrhea
- dizziness
- headache
- nausea, vomiting
- redness, blistering, peeling or loosening of the skin, including inside the mouth
- skin rash, itching
- sore throat, fever
- stomach pain
- unusual weakness or tiredness
- unusual bleeding or bruising
- yellowing of the skin or eyes

Let your prescriber or health care professional know if you get any of these side effects.

Where can I keep my medicine?

Keep out of the reach of children in a container that small children cannot open. Store at room temperature between 15 and 30 degrees C (59 and 86 degrees F). Protect from light. Keep container tightly closed. Throw away any unused medicine after the expiration date.

Cinacalcet tablets

What are cinacalcet tablets?

CINACALCET (Sensipar™) helps to slow the progression of bone disease in patients with chronic kidney disease who are on dialysis by decreasing the release of hormones from the parathyroid gland. This drug also helps to decrease high calcium blood levels in patients with cancer of the parathyroid gland. Generic cinacalcet tablets are not yet available.

What should my health care professional know before I take cinacalcet?

They need to know if you have any of these conditions:
- liver disease
- low serum calcium concentrations
- seizure disorder
- an unusual reaction to Cinacalcet, other medicines, foods, dyes, or preservatives
- pregnant or trying to get pregnant
- breast-feeding

How should this medicine be used?

Take cinacalcet tablets by mouth. Follow the directions on the prescription label. Take the tablets whole with a glass of water. Do not divide the tablets. Avoid taking this medication with grapefruit juice. This medication should be taken with food or shortly after a meal. Contact your pediatrician or health care professional regarding the use of this medicine in children. Special care may be needed.

What if I miss a dose?

If you miss a dose, take it as soon as you can. If it is almost time for your next dose, take only that dose. Do not take double or extra doses.

What may interact with cinacalcet?

- barbiturates such as phenobarbital
- grapefruit juice
- herbal or dietary supplements such as St. John's wort
- medicines for fungal infections (examples: fluconazole, itraconazole, ketoconazole, voriconazole)
- medicines for HIV infection or AIDS
- medicines for seizures (examples: carbamazepine, phenobarbital, phenytoin, primidone, zonisamide)
- rifampin, rifapentine, or rifabutin
- some medicines for pain, such as codeine
- some antibiotics (examples: clarithromycin, erythromycin, telithromycin, troleandomycin)
- some medicines for high blood pressure, chest pain, or heart-rhythm problems (examples: amiodarone, diltiazem, verapamil)
- some medicines for depression (examples: amitriptyline, fluoxetine, fluvoxamine, nefazodone)
- some medicines for mental problems (examples: clozapine, haloperidol, risperidone, thioridazine)
- zileuton

Tell your prescriber or health care professional about all other medicines you are taking, including non-prescription medicines, nutritional supplements, or herbal products. Also tell your prescriber or health care professional if you are a frequent user of drinks with caffeine or alcohol, if you smoke, or if you use illegal drugs. These may affect the way your medicine works. Check with your health care professional before stopping or starting any of your medicines.

What should I watch for while taking cinacalcet?

Visit your prescriber or health care professional for regular checks on your progress. Do not stop taking cinacalcet except on your prescriber's advice. You will receive regular blood tests to check the level of calcium in your blood. Cinacalcet alters the concentration of calcium in your blood. Tell your prescriber if your are taking any calcium supplements or vitamin or mineral products that contain calcium. Also tell your prescriber if you are taking any products that contain vitamin D. Follow your prescribers advice regarding the use of any vitamin, mineral or dietary supplement product.

What side effects may I notice from taking cinacalcet?

Side effects that you should report to your prescriber or health care professional as soon as possible:
- abdominal cramping or pain
- burning, numbness, pricking, tickling or tingling of the face, lips, tongue, hands or feet
- confusion
- cramps in the back or legs
- depression
- difficulty swallowing or breathing
- hallucinations
- irritability
- muscle spasms of the face
- muscle aches, pains
- seizures or convulsions

Side effects that usually do not require medical attention (report to your prescriber or health care professional if they continue or are bothersome):
- diarrhea
- nausea
- vomiting

Where can I keep my medicine?

Keep out of the reach of children in a container that small children cannot open. Store at room temperature between 15 and 30 degrees C (59 and 86 degrees F). Keep container tightly closed. Throw away any unused medicine after the expiration date.

Ciprofloxacin tablets and extended-release tablets

CIPRO®;
500 mg; Tablet
Schering Corp

CIPRO® XR;
500 mg; Tablet,
Extended Release
Schering Corp

What are ciprofloxacin tablets?

CIPROFLOXACIN (Cipro®, Cipro® XR) is an antibiotic. This drug treats many kinds of infections of the skin, bone, stomach, brain, blood, lungs, ear, and urinary tract. It also treats certain sexually transmitted diseases. Generic ciprofloxacin tablets are available. Generic ciprofloxacin extended-release tablets are not available.

What should my health care professional know before I take ciprofloxacin?

They need to know if you have any of these conditions:
- dehydration
- kidney disease
- liver disease
- seizures (convulsions)
- stomach problems (especially colitis)
- an unusual or allergic reaction to ciprofloxacin, other medicines, foods, dyes, or preservatives
- pregnant or trying to get pregnant
- breast-feeding

How should I take this medicine?

Take tablets by mouth. Follow the directions on the prescription label. Swallow ciprofloxacin tablets whole with a full glass of water. Do not split, crush or chew the extended-release tablets. Although this medicine can be taken with meals, it is best to take ciprofloxacin on an empty stomach. One hour before or two hours after meals is the preferred time. Do not take with magnesium/aluminum antacids, sucralfate, Videx® (didanosine) chewable/buffered tablets or pediatric powder, or with other products containing calcium, iron or zinc. Ciprofloxacin may be taken two hours before or six hours after taking these products. Ciprofloxacin should not be taken with dairy products (such as milk or yogurt) or calcium-fortified juices alone; however, ciprofloxacin may be taken with a meal that contains these products. Take your doses at regular intervals. Do not take your medicine more often than directed. Finish the full course prescribed by your prescriber or health care professional even if you think your condition is better. Do not stop taking except on your prescriber's advice. Contact your pediatrician or health care professional regarding the use of this medicine in children. Special care may be needed.

What if I miss a dose?

If you miss a dose, take it as soon as you can. If it is almost time for your next dose, take only that dose. Do not take double or extra doses. This medication should be taken at regular intervals.

What may interact with ciprofloxacin?

- acetazolamide
- aluminum salts
- antacids
- caffeine
- calcium salts
- citric acid; potassium citrate; sodium citrate products
- didanosine, ddI
- iron supplements
- magnesium salts
- manganese
- medicines for diabetes
- methazolamide
- multivitamins containing calcium, iron, magnesium, manganese, or zinc
- mexiletine
- NSAIDs such as Advil®, Aleve®, ibuprofen, Motrin®, naproxen
- phenytoin
- probenecid
- sodium bicarbonate
- sucralfate
- theophylline
- ursodiol
- warfarin
- zinc salts

Tell your prescriber or health care professional about all other medicines you are taking, including non-prescription medicines, nutritional supplements, or herbal products. Also tell your prescriber or health care professional if you are a frequent user of drinks with caffeine or alcohol, if you smoke, or if you use illegal drugs. These may affect the way your medicine works. Check with your health care professional before stopping or starting any of your medicines.

What should I watch for while taking ciprofloxacin?

Tell your prescriber or health care professional if your symptoms do not improve in 2 to 3 days. If you get severe or watery diarrhea, do not treat yourself. Call your prescriber or health care professional for advice. Make sure you stay well hydrated while taking ciprofloxacin. Drink several glasses of water a day. This helps to prevent crystals of the drug from developing in your urine. Cut down on drinks that contain caffeine. Ciprofloxacin can increase the stimulant effects of caffeine and cause heart, breathing and other problems. Keep out of the sun, or wear protective clothing outdoors and use a sunscreen. Do not use sun lamps or sun tanning beds or booths. You may get drowsy or dizzy. Do not drive, use machinery, or do anything that needs mental alertness until you know how ciprofloxacin affects you. To reduce the risk of dizzy or fainting spells, do not sit or stand up quickly, especially if you are an older patient. Antacids can make ciprofloxacin ineffective. If you get an upset stomach and want to take an antacid, make sure there is an interval of at least 2 hours since you last took ciprofloxacin, or 6 hours before your next dose. Iron and zinc preparations can also make ciprofloxacin ineffective. Do not take multivitamins at the same time you take your ciprofloxacin tablets. If you notice pain or swelling of a tendon or around a joint, stop taking ciprofloxacin. Call your healthcare provider. Rest the affected area. Do not exercise or take ciprofloxacin until your healthcare provider tells you to do so. If you notice pain, burning, tingling, numbness and/or weakness, discontinue ciprofloxacin and call your healthcare professional immediately. Stop taking ciprofloxacin if you develop a skin rash or other allergic reaction. Call your healthcare provider immediately. If you are going to have surgery, tell your prescriber or health care professional that you are taking ciprofloxacin.

What side effects may I notice from taking ciprofloxacin?

Side effects that you should report to your prescriber or health care professional as soon as possible:
- difficulty breathing
- fever
- hallucinations
- increased sensitivity to the sun or ultraviolet light
- irregular heartbeat, palpitations or chest pain
- joint, muscle or tendon pain
- nervousness, excitability, restlessness
- reduced amount of urine
- severe or watery diarrhea
- skin rash, itching
- seizures (convulsions)
- swelling of the face or neck
- unusual pain, numbness, tingling, or weakness
- vomiting

Side effects that usually do not require medical attention (report to your prescriber or health care professional if they continue or are bothersome):
- diarrhea
- difficulty sleeping
- dizziness, drowsiness
- headache
- nausea
- stomach upset

Where can I keep my medicine?

Keep out of the reach of children in a container that small children cannot open. Store at room temperature below 30 degrees C (86 degrees F). Keep container tightly closed. Throw away any unused medicine after the expiration date.

Citalopram tablets

CELEXA®;
20 mg; Tablet
Forest
Pharmaceuticals Inc

CELEXA®;
10 mg; Tablet
Forest
Pharmaceuticals Inc

This drug requires an FDA medication guide. See page xxxvii.

What are citalopram tablets?

CITALOPRAM (Celexa™) is a medicine for depression and other related problems. You may have to take citalopram for up to 4 weeks or longer before you begin to feel better. Generic citalopram tablets are available.

What should my health care professional know before I take citalopram?

They need to know if you have any of these conditions:
- diabetes
- heart disease
- kidney disease
- liver disease
- mania
- receive electroconvulsive therapy
- seizures (convulsions)
- suicidal thoughts or a previous suicide attempt
- an unusual or allergic reaction to citalopram, the related drug escitalopram, other medicines, foods, dyes, or preservatives
- pregnant or trying to become pregnant
- breast-feeding

How should I take this medicine?

Take citalopram tablets by mouth. Follow the directions on the prescription label. Swallow the tablets with a drink of water. Citalopram can be taken with or without food. Take your doses at regular intervals. Do not take your medicine more often than directed. Do not stop taking except on your prescriber or health care professional's advice.

What if I miss a dose?

If you miss a dose of citalopram, take it as soon as possible. However, if it is almost time for your next dose, skip the missed dose and go back to your regular dosing schedule. Follow your prescriber or health care professional's advice on missed doses. Do not take double or extra doses.

What may interact with citalopram?

Do not take citalopram with any of the following medications:

- cisapride
- escitalopram
- medicines called MAO inhibitors-phenelzine (Nardil®), tranylcypromine (Parnate®), isocarboxazid (Marplan®), selegiline (Eldepryl®)

Citalopram may also interact with the following medications:

- alosetron
- alprazolam
- amphetamine
- aspirin, warfarin, or nonsteroidal anti-inflammatory drugs (NSAIDs) such as ibuprofen or naproxen
- buspirone
- carbamazepine
- certain diet drugs (dexfenfluramine, fenfluramine, phentermine, sibutramine)
- clarithromycin
- cimetidine
- cyproheptadine
- dexamethasone
- dextromethorphan
- dextroamphetamine
- diazepam
- diltiazem
- erythromycin
- ethosuximide
- furazolidone
- grapefruit juice
- kava kava
- ketoconazole
- linezolid
- lithium
- medicines that treat depression or other mood problems
- medicines that treat HIV infection or AIDS
- methadone
- migraine headache medicines (almotriptan, eletriptan, frovatriptan, naratriptan, rizatriptan, sumatriptan, zolmitriptan)
- medicines for psychosis or severe mood problems
- modafinil
- nefazodone
- nicardipine
- phenobarbital
- phenytoin
- prescription pain relievers (codeine, hydrocodone, meperidine, morphine, tramadol, oxycodone)
- primidone
- procarbazine
- quinine
- rifabutin
- rifampin
- St. John's Wort
- troglitazone
- tryptophan
- valerian
- verapamil

Tell your prescriber or health care professional about all other medicines you are taking, including non-prescription medicines. Also tell your prescriber or health care professional if you are a frequent user of grapefruit juice, drinks with caffeine or alcohol, if you smoke, or if you use illegal drugs. These may affect the way your medicine works. Check with your health care professional before stopping or starting any of your medicines.

What should I watch for while taking citalopram?

Visit your prescriber or health care professional for regular checks on your progress. Continue to take your tablets even if you do not immediately feel better. It can take about 4 weeks before you feel the full effect of citalopram. Patients and their families should watch out for worsening depression or thoughts of suicide. Also watch out for sudden or severe changes in feelings such as feeling anxious, agitated, panicky, irritable, hostile, aggressive, impulsive, severely restless, overly excited and hyperactive, or not being able to sleep. If this happens, especially at the beginning of antidepressant treatment or after a change in dose, call your health care professional. If you have been taking citalopram regularly for some time, do not suddenly stop taking it. You must gradually reduce the dose, or your symptoms may get worse. Ask your prescriber or health care professional for advice. You may get drowsy or dizzy. Do not drive, use machinery, or do anything that needs mental alertness until you know how citalopram affects you. Do not stand or sit up quickly, especially if you are an older patient. This reduces the risk of dizzy or fainting spells. Alcohol may interfere with the effect of citalopram. Avoid alcoholic drinks. Do not treat yourself for coughs, colds, or allergies without asking your prescriber or health care professional for advice. Some ingredients can increase possible side effects. Your mouth may get dry. Chewing sugarless gum or sucking hard candy, and drinking plenty of water will help. If you are going to have surgery, tell your prescriber or health care professional that you are taking citalopram.

What side effects may I notice from taking citalopram?

Side effects that you should report to your prescriber or health care professional as soon as possible:
Rare or uncommon:
- confusion
- dizziness or lightheadedness
- skin rash, itching (hives)
- fast talking and excited feelings or actions that are out of control
- suicidal thoughts
- vomiting

More common:
- agitation, anxiety, or restlessness, especially in the first week of treatment or when doses are changed

Side effects that usually do not require medical attention (report to your prescriber or health care professional if they continue or are bothersome):
- blurred vision
- diarrhea
- difficulty sleeping
- drowsiness
- dry mouth

- fever
- frequent urination
- headache
- indigestion, nausea
- increased or decreased appetite
- increased sweating
- sexual difficulties (decreased sexual ability or desire)
- taste alterations

- tremor (shaking)
- weight changes

Where can I keep my medicine?

Keep out of reach of children in a container that small children cannot open. Store at room temperature between 15 and 30 degrees C (59 and 86 degrees F). Throw away any unused medicine after the expiration date.

Clarithromycin tablets and extended-release tablets

BIAXIN® XL;
500 mg; Tablet,
Extended Release
Abbott
Pharmaceutical
Product Division

BIAXIN®;
250 mg; Tablet
Abbott
Pharmaceutical
Product Division

What are clarithromycin tablets?

CLARITHROMYCIN (Biaxin® or Biaxin® XL) is an antibiotic. Clarithromycin kills certain bacteria or stops their growth. It treats ear, lung, sinus, throat and skin infections. This medicine is also is used to treat a certain bacteria that can cause stomach ulcers. Clarithromycin will not work for colds, flu, or other virus infections. Biaxin® XL is an extended-release form of clarithromycin that only needs to be taken once daily. Generic clarithromycin tablets are available.

What should my health care professional know before I take clarithromycin?

They need to know if you have any of these conditions:
- diarrhea
- irregular heart beat or abnormal heart beat
- kidney disease
- liver disease
- stomach problems (especially colitis)
- other chronic illness
- an unusual or allergic reaction to clarithromycin or other macrolide antibiotics (such as erythromycin), foods, dyes, or preservatives
- pregnant or trying to get pregnant
- breast-feeding

How should I take this medicine?

Take clarithromycin tablets by mouth. Follow the directions on the prescription label. Take the tablets with a full glass of water. You may take clarithromycin regular-release tablets with or without food, but be sure to take the extended-release tablets (Biaxin® XL) with food. Taking clarithromycin with food may reduce stomach upset. Do not crush or chew the Biaxin® XL tablets. Take your doses at regular intervals. Do not take your medicine more often than directed. Finish the full course prescribed by your prescriber or health care professional even if you think your condition is better. Do not stop taking except on your prescriber's advice. Contact your pediatrician or health care professional regarding the use of this medicine in children. Special care may be needed.

What if I miss a dose?

If you miss a dose, take it as soon as you can. If it is almost time for your next dose, take only that dose. Do not take double or extra doses. There should be an interval of at least 6 hours between Biaxin® doses, and at least 12 hours between Biaxin® XL doses.

What may interact with clarithromycin?

- astemizole
- birth control pills
- carbamazepine
- cisapride
- colchicine
- digoxin
- dofetilide
- ergot alkaloid medicines, like ergotamine
- other antibiotics, like grepafloxacin or sparfloxacin
- pimozide
- ritonavir
- some "statin" medicines for reducing cholesterol (examples: atorvastatin, lovastatin, simvastatin)
- terfenadine
- theophylline
- triazolam
- warfarin
- zidovudine

Tell your prescriber or health care professional about all other medicines that you are taking, including non-prescription medicines, nutritional supplements, or herbal products. Also tell your prescriber or health care professional if you are a frequent user of drinks with caffeine or alcohol, if you smoke, or if you use illegal drugs. These may affect the way your medicine works. Check with your health care professional before stopping or starting any of your medicines.

What should I watch for while taking clarithromycin?

Tell your prescriber or health care professional if your symptoms do not improve in 2 to 3 days. Make sure to take all of this medicine as prescribed, even if you begin to feel better. Clarithromycin may decrease the effectiveness of birth control pills. Women should use additional forms of birth control during the month they received clarithromycin. Depending on the length of clarithromycin treatment, additional birth control methods may be needed for at least one menstrual cycle after the antibiotic is finished. If you get severe or watery diarrhea, do not treat yourself. Call your prescriber or health care professional for advice. If you are going to have surgery, tell your prescriber or health care professional that you are taking clarithromycin.

What side effects may I notice from taking clarithromycin?

Side effects that you should report to your prescriber or health care professional as soon as possible:
- difficulty breathing
- redness, blistering, peeling or loosening of the skin, including inside the mouth
- severe or watery diarrhea
- skin rash, itching
- swelling of tongue or throat
- vomiting
- yellow color of eyes, skin, or urine

Side effects that usually do not require medical attention (report to your prescriber or health care professional if they continue or are bothersome):
- changes in taste or smell
- headache
- nausea
- stomach pains or cramps

Where can I keep my medicine?

Keep out of the reach of children in a container that small children cannot open. Store at room temperature between 15 and 30 degrees C (59 and 86 degrees F) degrees. Keep container tightly closed. Protect from light. Throw away any unused medicine after the expiration date.

Clemastine tablets

CLEMASTINE;
1.34 mg; Tablet
Sandoz
Pharmaceuticals

TAVIST;
2.68 mg; Tablet
Novartis
Pharmaceuticals

What are clemastine tablets?

CLEMASTINE (Tavist®) is an antihistamine. It relieves symptoms of runny nose from colds (rhinitis) and hay fever (seasonal rhinitis), hives (rash and itching), and other mild allergic conditions. Generic clemastine tablets are available.

What should my health care professional know before I take clemastine?

They need to know if you have any of these conditions:
- asthma or chronic obstructive lung disease (COPD)
- glaucoma
- high blood pressure or heart disease
- liver disease
- other chronic illness
- prostate trouble
- pain or difficulty passing urine
- ulcers or other stomach problems
- pregnant or trying to get pregnant
- breast-feeding

How should I take this medicine?

Take clemastine tablets by mouth. Follow the directions on the prescription label. Take with food or milk if clemastine upsets your stomach. Take your doses at regular intervals. Do not take your medicine more often than directed. Contact your pediatrician or health care professional regarding the use of this medicine in children. Special care may be needed.

What if I miss a dose?

If you miss a dose, take it as soon as you can. If it is almost time for your next dose, take only that dose. Do not take double doses.

What may interact with clemastine?

- alcohol
- barbiturate medicines for inducing sleep or treating seizures (convulsions)
- medicines for anxiety or sleeping problems, such as diazepam or temazepam
- medicines for hay fever and other allergies
- medicines for mental depression
- medicines for mental problems and psychotic disturbances
- medicines for movement abnormalities as in Parkinson's disease, or for gastrointestinal problems

Tell your prescriber or health care professional about all other medicines you are taking, including non-prescription medicines, nutritional supplements, or herbal products. Also tell your prescriber or health care professional if you are a frequent user of drinks with caffeine or alcohol, if you smoke, or if you use illegal drugs. These may affect the way your medicine works. Check with your health care professional before stopping or starting any of your medicines.

What should I watch for while taking clemastine?

Tell your prescriber or health care professional if your symptoms do not improve in 1 or 2 days. You may get drowsy or dizzy. Do not drive, use machinery, or do anything that needs mental alertness until you know how clemastine affects you. To reduce the risk of dizzy or fainting spells, do not stand or sit up quickly, especially if you are an older patient. Alcohol may increase dizziness and drowsiness. Avoid alcoholic drinks. Your mouth may get dry. Chewing sugarless gum or sucking hard candy, and drinking plenty of water will help. Clemastine may cause dry eyes and blurred vision. If you wear contact lenses you may feel some discomfort. Lubricating drops may help. See your ophthalmologist if the problem does not go away or is severe.

What side effects may I notice from taking clemastine?

Side effects that you should report to your prescriber or health care professional as soon as possible:

- agitation, nervousness, excitability, not able to sleep (these are more likely in children)
- blurred vision
- fainting spells
- irregular heartbeat, palpitations, or chest pain
- pain or difficulty passing urine

- seizures (convulsions)

Side effects that usually do not require medical attention (report to your prescriber or health care professional if they continue or are bothersome):

- drowsiness, dizziness
- dry mouth
- headache
- loss of appetite
- stomach upset, nausea, vomiting, constipation or diarrhea

Where can I keep my medicine?

Keep out of the reach of children in a container that small children cannot open. Store at room temperature, between 15 and 25 degrees C (59 and 77 degrees F). Keep away from heat and light. Throw away any unused medicine after the expiration date.

Clindamycin capsules

CLEOCIN®; 150 mg; Capsule Pharmacia and Upjohn Div Pfizer	CLEOCIN®; 300 mg; Capsule Pharmacia and Upjohn Div Pfizer

What are clindamycin capsules?

CLINDAMYCIN (Cleocin®) is an antibiotic or anti-infective. It treats serious blood, bone, joint, lung, urinary tract, or pelvic infections. Generic clindamycin capsules are available.

What should my health care professional know before I take clindamycin?

They need to know if you have any of these conditions:

- diarrhea
- inflammatory bowel disease
- kidney disease
- liver disease
- ulcerative colitis
- an unusual or allergic reaction to clindamycin, lincomycin, or other substances such as food, preservatives or dyes
- pregnant or trying to get pregnant
- breast-feeding

How should I take this medicine?

Take clindamycin capsules by mouth. Follow the directions on the prescription label. Take at regular intervals, every 6 or 8 hours, during the day and night. It is best to take clindamycin 1 hour before or 2 hours after eating; take the capsules with a full glass of water. Do not lie down for 1 to 2 hours after taking clindamycin to avoid irritation to your throat. If clindamycin upsets your stomach you can take it with food. Do not take your medicine more often than directed. Finish the full course of medicine prescribed by your prescriber or health care professional even if you feel better. Do not stop using except on your prescriber's advice.

What if I miss a dose?

If you miss a dose, take it as soon as you can. If it is almost time for your next dose, take only that dose. Do not take double or extra doses.

What may interact with clindamycin capsules?

- chloramphenicol
- erythromycin
- kaolin products
- medicines for pain
- oral contraceptives (birth control pills)

Tell your prescriber or health care professional about all other medicines you are taking, including non-prescription medicines, nutritional supplements, or herbal products. Also tell your prescriber or health care professional if you are a frequent user of drinks with caffeine or alcohol, if you smoke, or if you use illegal drugs. These may affect the way your medicine works. Check with your health care professional before stopping or starting any of your medicines.

What should I watch for while taking clindamycin?

Tell your prescriber or health care professional if your symptoms do not improve in a few days. Call your prescriber or health care professional if you get diarrhea. Do not treat yourself. Some diarrhea medicine will make the diarrhea worse. If you have to have surgery, tell your prescriber or health care professional that you are taking clindamycin.

What side effects may I notice from taking clindamycin?

Side effects that you should report to your prescriber or health care professional as soon as possible:

- diarrhea that is watery or severe
- pain on swallowing
- stomach pain or cramps
- skin rash
- unusual bleeding or bruising

Side effects that usually do not require medical attention (report to your prescriber or health care professional if they continue or are bothersome):

- itching in the rectal or genital area
- nausea, vomiting

Clomipramine capsules

ANAFRANIL®;
50 mg; Capsule
Mallinckrodt Inc
Pharmaceuticals
Group

ANAFRANIL®;
25 mg; Capsule
Mallinckrodt Inc
Pharmaceuticals
Group

This drug requires an FDA medication guide. See page xxxvii.

What are clomipramine capsules?
CLOMIPRAMINE (Anafranil®) is an antidepressant. Clomipramine can help patients with an obsessive compulsive disorder. It relieves the anxiety and unpleasant thoughts that make patients repeat everyday tasks (like hand-washing) many times. Clomipramine helps to maintain a normal lifestyle. Your prescriber or health care professional may prescribe clomipramine for other conditions. Generic clomipramine capsules are available.

What should my health care professional know before I take clomipramine?
They need to know if you have any of these conditions:

- an alcohol problem
- asthma, difficulty breathing
- blood disorders or disease
- diabetes
- difficulty passing urine, prostate trouble
- glaucoma
- having intramuscular injections
- heart disease, or recent heart attack
- liver disease
- overactive thyroid
- Parkinson's disease
- schizophrenia
- seizures (convulsions)
- stomach disease
- an unusual or allergic reaction to clomipramine, other medicines, foods, dyes, or preservatives
- pregnant or trying to get pregnant
- breast-feeding

How should I take this medicine?
Take clomipramine capsules by mouth. Follow the directions on the prescription label. Swallow the capsules with a drink of water. It is best to take the capsules with food to avoid stomach upset. Take your doses at regular intervals. Do not take your medicine more often than directed. Do not stop taking except on your prescriber's advice. Contact your pediatrician or health care professional regarding the use of this medicine in children. Special care may be needed. Elderly patients over 65 years old may have a stronger reaction to this medicine and need smaller doses.

What if I miss a dose?
If you miss a dose normally taken at bedtime to avoid daytime drowsiness, it may be better to miss that dose.

Where can I keep my medicine?
Keep out of the reach of children in a container that small children cannot open. Store at room temperature between 15 and 30 degrees C (59 and 86 degrees F) Throw away any unused medicine after the expiration date.

If you take more than one dose a day and miss a dose, take it as soon as you can. If it is almost time for your next dose, take only that dose. Follow your prescriber's advice on missed doses. Do not take double or extra doses.

What may interact with clomipramine?
Clomipramine can interact with many other medicines. Some interactions can be very important. Make sure your prescriber or health care professional knows about all other medicines you are taking. Many important interactions are listed below:
Do not take clomipramine with any of the following medications:

- astemizole (Hismanal®)
- cisapride (Propulsid®)
- probucol
- terfenadine (Seldane®)
- thioridazine (Mellaril®)
- medicines called MAO inhibitors-phenelzine (Nardil®), tranylcypromine (Parnate®), isocarboxazid (Marplan®), selegiline (Eldepryl®)
- other medicines for mental depression (may be duplicate therapies or cause additive side effects)

Clomipramine may also interact with any of the following medications:

- alcohol
- antacids
- atropine and related drugs like hyoscyamine, scopolamine, tolterodine and others
- barbiturate medicines for inducing sleep or treating seizures (convulsions), such as phenobarbital
- blood thinners, such as warfarin
- bromocriptine
- bupropion
- cimetidine
- clonidine
- cocaine
- delavirdine
- diphenoxylate
- disulfiram
- donepezil
- drugs for treating HIV infection
- female hormones, including contraceptive or birth control pills and estrogen
- galantamine

- herbs and dietary supplements like ephedra (*Ma huang*), kava kava, SAM-e, St. John's wort, valerian, or others
- imatinib, STI-571
- kaolin; pectin
- labetalol
- levodopa and other medicines for movement problems like Parkinson's disease
- lithium
- medicines for anxiety or sleeping problems
- medicines for colds, flu and breathing difficulties, like pseudoephedrine
- medicines for hay fever or allergies (antihistamines)
- medicines for weight loss or appetite control
- medicines used to regulate abnormal heartbeat or to treat other heart conditions (examples: amiodarone, bepridil, disopyramide, dofetilide, encainide, flecainide, ibutilide, mibefradil, procainamide, propafenone, quinidine, and others)
- metoclopramide
- muscle relaxants, like cyclobenzaprine
- other medicines for mental or mood problems and psychotic disturbances
- prescription pain medications like morphine, codeine, tramadol and others
- procarbazine
- seizure (convulsion) or epilepsy medicine such as carbamazepine or phenytoin
- stimulants like dexmethylphenidate or methylphenidate
- some antibiotics (examples: erythromycin, gatifloxacin, levofloxacin, linezolid, moxifloxacin, sotalol, sparfloxacin)
- tacrine
- thyroid hormones such as levothyroxine

Tell your prescriber or health care professional about all other medicines you are taking, including non-prescription medicines, nutritional supplements, or herbal products. Also tell your prescriber or health care professional if you are a frequent user of drinks with caffeine or alcohol, if you smoke, or if you use illegal drugs. These may affect the way your medicine works. Check with your health care professional before stopping or starting any of your medicines.

What should I watch for while taking clomipramine?

Visit your prescriber or health care professional for regular checks on your progress. It can take several days before you feel the full effect of clomipramine. If you have been taking clomipramine regularly for some time, do not suddenly stop taking it. You must gradually reduce the dose or you may get severe side effects. Ask your prescriber or health care professional for advice. Even after you stop taking clomipramine it can still affect your body for several days. You may get drowsy or dizzy. Do not drive, use machinery, or do anything that needs mental alertness until you know how clomipramine affects you. Do not stand or sit up quickly, especially if you are an older patient. This reduces the risk of dizzy or fainting spells. Alcohol may increase dizziness and drowsiness. Avoid alcoholic drinks. Do not treat yourself for coughs, colds or allergies without asking your prescriber or health care professional for advice. Some ingredients can increase possible side effects. Your mouth may get dry. Chewing sugarless gum or sucking hard candy, and drinking plenty of water will help. Clomipramine may cause dry eyes and blurred vision. If you wear contact lenses you may feel some discomfort. Lubricating drops may help. See your ophthalmologist if the problem does not go away or is severe. Clomipramine may make your skin more sensitive to the sun. Keep out of the sun, or wear protective clothing outdoors and use a sunscreen. Do not use sun lamps or sun tanning beds or booths. Clomipramine can affect blood glucose (sugar) levels. If you are a diabetic, check your blood sugar more often than usual, especially during the first few weeks of clomipramine treatment. Call your prescriber or health care professional for advice if you notice a change in the results of blood or urine glucose tests. If you are going to have surgery or will need an x-ray procedure that uses contrast agents, tell your prescriber or health care professional that you are taking this medicine.

What side effects may I notice from taking clomipramine?

Side effects that you should report to your prescriber or health care professional as soon as possible:
- abnormal production of milk in females
- blurred vision or eye pain
- breast enlargement in both males and females
- confusion, hallucinations (seeing or hearing things that are not really there)
- difficulty breathing
- fainting spells
- fever
- irregular or fast, pounding heartbeat, palpitations
- muscle stiffness, or spasms
- pain or difficulty passing urine, loss of bladder control
- seizures (convulsions)
- sexual difficulties (decreased sexual ability or desire, difficulty ejaculating)
- stomach pain
- swelling of the testicles
- tingling, pain, or numbness in the feet or hands
- tremor (shaking)
- unusual weakness or tiredness
- yellowing of the eyes or skin

Side effects that usually do not require medical attention (report to your prescriber or health care professional if they continue or are bothersome):
- anxiety
- constipation, or diarrhea
- drowsiness or dizziness
- dry mouth
- headache

- increased sensitivity of the skin to sun or ultraviolet light
- loss of appetite
- nausea, vomiting
- skin rash or itching
- weight gain or loss

Where can I keep my medicine?

Keep out of the reach of children in a container that small children cannot open. Store at room temperature below 30 degrees C (86 degrees F). Protect from moisture. Keep container tightly closed. Throw away any unused medicine after the expiration date.

Clonazepam tablets

KLONOPIN®;
2 mg; Tablet
Hoffmann La Roche
Inc

KLONOPIN®;
1 mg; Tablet
Hoffmann La Roche
Inc

What are clonazepam tablets?

CLONAZEPAM (Klonopin®) is a benzodiazepine. Benzodiazepines belong to a group of medicines that slow down the central nervous system. Clonazepam is effective in treating certain types of seizures (convulsions) and is also used for a mental health condition called Panic Disorder. Federal law prohibits the transfer of clonazepam to any person other than the patient for whom it was prescribed. Do not share this medicine with anyone else. Generic clonazepam tablets are available.

What should my health care professional know before I take clonazepam?

They need to know if you have any of these conditions:
- an alcohol or drug abuse problem
- bipolar disorder, depression, psychosis or other mental health condition
- glaucoma
- kidney disease
- liver disease
- lung disease, such as chronic obstructive pulmonary disease (COPD), sleep apnea or other breathing difficulties
- myasthenia gravis
- Parkinson's disease
- seizures or a history of seizures
- shortness of breath
- snoring
- suicidal thoughts
- an unusual or allergic reaction to clonazepam, other benzodiazepines, foods, dyes, or preservatives
- pregnant or trying to get pregnant
- breast-feeding

How should I take this medicine?

Take clonazepam tablets by mouth. Follow the directions on the prescription label. Swallow the tablets with a drink of water. If clonazepam upsets your stomach, take it with food or milk. Take your doses at regular intervals. Do not take your medicine more often than directed. Do not stop taking or change the dose except on your prescriber's advice. Contact your pediatrician or health care professional regarding the use of this medicine in children. Special care may be needed.

What if I miss a dose?

If you miss a dose and remember within an hour, take it as soon as you can. If it is more than an hour since you missed a dose, skip that dose and go back to your regular schedule. Do not take double or extra doses.

What may interact with clonazepam?

- alcohol
- bosentan
- caffeine
- cimetidine
- disulfiram
- female hormones, including contraceptive or birth control pills
- herbal or dietary supplements such as kava kava, melatonin, St. John's Wort or valerian
- imatinib, STI-571
- isoniazid
- medicines for anxiety or sleeping problems, such as alprazolam, diazepam, lorazepam or triazolam
- medicines for depression, mental problems or psychiatric disturbances
- medicines for fungal infections (fluconazole, itraconazole, ketoconazole, voriconazole)
- medicines for HIV infection or AIDS
- nicardipine
- prescription pain medicines
- probenecid
- rifampin, rifapentine, or rifabutin
- some antibiotics (clarithromycin, erythromycin, troleandomycin)
- some medicines for colds, hay fever or other allergies
- some medicines for high blood pressure or heart-rhythm problems (amiodarone, diltiazem, verapamil)
- some medicines for seizures (carbamazepine, phenobarbital, phenytoin, primidone)
- theophylline
- zafirlukast
- zileuton

Tell your prescriber or health care professional about all other medicines you are taking, including non-prescription medicines, nutritional supplements, or herbal products. Also tell your prescriber or health care professional if you are a frequent user of drinks with caffeine or alcohol, if you smoke, or if you use illegal drugs. These may affect the way your medicine works. Check with your health care professional before stopping or starting any of your medicines.

What should I watch for while taking clonazepam?

Visit your prescriber or health care professional for regular checks on your progress. Your body may become dependent on clonazepam. If you have been taking clonazepam regularly for some time, do not suddenly stop taking it. You must gradually reduce the dose or you may get severe side effects. Ask your prescriber or health care professional for advice before increasing or decreasing the dose. Even after you stop taking clonazepam it can still affect your body for several days. If you suffer from several types of seizures, clonazepam may increase the chance of grand mal seizures (epilepsy). Let your prescriber or health care professional know, he or she may want to prescribe an additional medicine. You may get drowsy or dizzy. Do not drive, use machinery, or do anything that needs mental alertness until you know how clonazepam affects you. To reduce the risk of dizzy and fainting spells, do not stand or sit up quickly, especially if you are an older patient. Alcohol may increase dizziness and drowsiness. Avoid alcoholic drinks. If you are a female patient with a newborn, it is not recommended that you breast-feed your infant while receiving clonazepam. Ask your health care professional for additional advice. Do not treat yourself for coughs, colds or allergies without asking your prescriber or health care professional for advice. Some ingredients can increase possible side effects. If you are going to have surgery, tell your prescriber or health care professional that you are taking clonazepam.

What side effects may I notice from taking clonazepam?

Side effects that you should report to your prescriber or health care professional as soon as possible:
- confusion
- depression
- double vision or abnormal eye movements
- hallucinations (seeing and hearing things that are not really there)
- lightheadedness or fainting spells
- mood changes, excitability or aggressive behavior
- movement difficulty, staggering or jerky movements
- muscle cramps
- restlessness
- tremors
- weakness or tiredness

Side effects that usually do not require medical attention (report to your prescriber or health care professional if they continue or are bothersome):
- constipation or diarrhea
- difficulty sleeping, nightmares
- dizziness, drowsiness, clumsiness, or unsteadiness; a "hangover" effect
- headache
- increased secretions or saliva from your mouth
- nausea, vomiting

Where can I keep my medicine?

Keep out of the reach of children in a container that small children cannot open. Store at room temperature between 15 and 30 degrees C (59 and 86 degrees F). Protect from light. Keep container tightly closed. Throw away any unused medicine after the expiration date.

Clonidine tablets

CATAPRES®;
0.2 mg; Tablet
Boehringer Ingelheim
Pharmaceuticals Inc

CATAPRES®;
0.1 mg; Tablet
Boehringer Ingelheim
Pharmaceuticals Inc

What are clonidine tablets?

CLONIDINE (Catapres®) is an antihypertensive. Clonidine relaxes blood vessels, relieving high blood pressure (hypertension). It is not a cure and has to be taken regularly. Untreated high blood pressure can cause a stroke, heart failure, or damage to your kidneys. Clonidine can be used to treat conditions other than hypertension, as determined by your health care professional. Generic clonidine tablets are available.

What should my health care professional know before I take clonidine?

They need to know if you have any of these conditions:
- depression
- diabetes
- heart or blood vessel disease
- kidney disease
- recent heart attack or stroke
- an unusual or allergic reaction to clonidine, other medicines, foods, dyes, or preservatives
- pregnant or trying to get pregnant
- breast-feeding

How should I take this medicine?

Take clonidine tablets by mouth. Follow the directions on the prescription label. Swallow the tablets with a drink of water. Take your doses at regular intervals. Do not take your medicine more often than directed. Do not stop taking except on your prescriber's advice. Contact your pediatrician or health care professional regarding the use of this medicine in children. Special care may be needed.

What if I miss a dose?

If you miss a dose, take it as soon as you can. If it is almost time for your next dose, take only that dose. Do not take double or extra doses. It is important not to miss a dose of clonidine. Even one or two missed doses can cause serious side effects. If you do miss more than one or two doses, check with your prescriber or health care professional.

What may interact with clonidine?

- alcohol
- anti-inflammatory drugs (NSAIDs, such as ibuprofen)
- barbiturate medicines for inducing sleep or treating seizures (convulsions)
- beta blockers, often used for high blood pressure or heart problems
- cyclosporine
- heart medicines such as digoxin or digitoxin
- fenfluramine
- guanethidine
- hawthorn
- medicines for colds and breathing difficulties
- medicine for mental depression
- medicine for pain
- verapamil
- water pills

Tell your prescriber or health care professional about all other medicines you are taking, including non-prescription medicines, nutritional supplements, or herbal products. Also tell your prescriber or health care professional if you are a frequent user of drinks with caffeine or alcohol, if you smoke, or if you use illegal drugs. These may affect the way your medicine works. Check with your health care professional before stopping or starting any of your medicines.

What should I watch for while taking clonidine?

Visit your prescriber or health care professional for regular checks on your progress. Check your heart rate and blood pressure regularly while you are taking clonidine. Ask your prescriber or health care professional what your heart rate should be and when you should contact him or her. Do not suddenly stop taking clonidine. You must gradually reduce the dose or you may get a dangerous increase in blood pressure. Ask your prescriber or health care professional for advice. You may get drowsy or dizzy. Do not drive, use machinery, or do anything that needs mental alertness until you know how clonidine affects you. To avoid dizzy or fainting spells, do not stand or sit up quickly, especially if you are an older person. Alcohol can make you more drowsy and dizzy. Avoid alcoholic drinks. Your mouth may get dry. Chewing sugarless gum or sucking hard candy, and drinking plenty of water will help. Do not treat yourself for coughs, colds or allergies without asking your prescriber or health care professional for advice. Some ingredients can affect your blood pressure control. If you are going to have surgery tell your prescriber or health care professional that you are taking clonidine.

What side effects may I notice from taking clonidine?

Stopping taking clonidine can produce some of these side effects. Ask your prescriber or health care professional before you reduce your dose, or stop taking clonidine.

Side effects that you should report to your prescriber or health care professional as soon as possible:

- anxiety, nervousness
- dizziness or fainting spells
- increased sweating
- irregular heartbeat or palpitations, chest pain
- pain or difficulty passing urine
- stomach pain
- swelling of feet or legs
- trembling, shakiness
- unusual tiredness or weakness

Side effects that usually do not require medical attention (report to your prescriber or health care professional if they continue or are bothersome):

- drowsiness
- dry mouth
- constipation
- difficulty sleeping (insomnia)
- headache
- sexual difficulties (decreased sexual desire and ability)

Where can I keep my medicine?

Keep out of the reach of children in a container that small children cannot open. Store at room temperature below 30 degrees C (86 degrees F). Protect from light. Keep container tightly closed. Throw away any unused medicine after the expiration date.

Clopidogrel tablets

PLAVIX®;
75 mg; Tablet
Bristol Myers Squibb
Sanofi
Pharmaceuticals
Partnership

PLAVIX®;
75 mg; Tablet
Bristol Myers Squibb
Sanofi
Pharmaceuticals
Partnership

What are clopidogrel tablets?

CLOPIDOGREL (Plavix®) helps to prevent blood clots. It reduces the chance of having a heart attack or a stroke in people who have already had a heart attack or a stroke. Clopidogrel can also decrease the chance of a heart attack or stroke in certain groups of people at high risk for these events. Generic clopidogrel tablets are not yet available.

What should my health care professional know before I take clopidogrel?

They need to know if you have any of the following conditions:

- bleeding disorder or hemophilia
- liver disease
- recent surgery or trauma
- stomach or intestinal ulcers

- an unusual or allergic reaction to clopidogrel, other medicines, foods, dyes, or preservatives
- pregnant or trying to get pregnant
- breast-feeding

How should I take this medicine?

Take clopidogrel tablets by mouth. Follow the directions on the prescription label. Swallow the tablets with a drink of water. Do not take your medicine more often than directed. Contact your pediatrician or health care professional regarding the use of this medicine in children. Special care may be needed.

What if I miss a dose?

If you miss a dose, take it as soon as you can. If it is almost time for your next dose, take only that dose. Do not take double or extra doses.

What may interact with clopidogrel?

- aspirin
- blood thinners such as warfarin or enoxaparin
- anti-inflammatory drugs such as NSAIDs (e.g., ibuprofen)
- cilostazol
- dipyridamole
- DHEA
- feverfew
- fish oil (omega-3 fatty acids) supplements
- garlic
- ginger
- ginkgo biloba
- horse chestnut
- fluvastatin
- phenytoin
- prasterone
- tamoxifen
- ticlopidine
- tolbutamide
- torsemide

Tell your prescriber or health care professional about all other medicines you are taking, including non-prescription medicines. Also tell your prescriber or health care professional if you are a frequent user of drinks with caffeine or alcohol, if you smoke, or if you use illegal drugs. These may affect the way your medicine works. Check with your physician or health care professional before stopping or starting any of your medicines.

What should I watch for while taking clopidogrel?

Visit your prescriber or health care professional for regular checks on your progress. Do not stop taking clopidogrel except on your prescriber's advice. You may bleed more easily and it may take longer to stop bleeding when taking clopidogrel. Report any unusual bleeding to your prescriber. Ask your prescriber or health care professional before you take non-prescription pain relievers. Do not take aspirin, aspirin-containing products, or anti-inflammatory drugs such as ibuprofen (e.g, Motrin), ketoprofen (Orudis(R)), naproxen (e.g., Aleve) unless directed to do so by your prescriber or health care professional. If you are going to have surgery or dental work, tell your prescriber or health care professional that you are taking clopidogrel.

What side effects may I notice from taking clopidogrel?

Side effects that you should report to your prescriber or health care professional as soon as possible:
More common:
- black, tarry stools
- blood from vomiting
- blood in urine or stools
- nosebleed
- red or purple spots on the skin
- skin rash or itching
- stomach pain

Rare:
- difficulty breathing, difficulty swallowing, hoarseness, or tightening of the throat
- fever
- sudden weakness
- swelling of your face, lips, tongue, hands, or feet
- unusual bleeding or bruising, or pinpoint red spots on the skin
- unusual rash, allergic reaction, or hives
- unusually heavy menstrual bleeding

Side effects that usually do not require medical attention (report to your prescriber or health care professional if they continue or are bothersome):
- diarrhea
- indigestion (heartburn)
- mild stomach upset

Where can I keep my medicine?

Keep out of the reach of children in a container that small children cannot open. Store at room temperature between 15 and 30 degrees C (59 and 86 degrees F). Throw away any unused medicine after the expiration date.

Clorazepate tablets

TRANXENE®;
3.75 mg; Tablet
Ovation
Pharmaceuticals, Inc

TRANXENE®;
15 mg; Tablet
Ovation
Pharmaceuticals, Inc

What are clorazepate tablets?

CLORAZEPATE (Tranxene®) is a benzodiazepine. Benzodiazepines belong to a group of medicines that slow down the central nervous system. Clorazepate relieves anxiety and nervousness, and can help patients cope with alcohol withdrawal. Clorazepate can also help to treat certain types of seizure (convulsive) disorders. Federal law prohibits the transfer of clorazepate to any person other than the patient for whom it was prescribed. Do not share this medicine with anyone else. Generic clorazepate tablets are available.

What should my health care professional know before I take clorazepate?

They need to know if you have any of these conditions:
- an alcohol or drug abuse problem
- bipolar disorder, depression, psychosis or other mental health condition
- glaucoma
- kidney disease
- liver disease
- lung disease, such as chronic obstructive pulmonary disease (COPD), sleep apnea or other breathing difficulties
- myasthenia gravis
- Parkinson's disease
- porphyria
- seizures or a history of seizures
- shortness of breath
- snoring
- suicidal thoughts
- an unusual or allergic reaction to clorazepate, other benzodiazepines, other medicines, foods, dyes, or preservatives
- pregnant or trying to get pregnant
- breast-feeding

How should I take this medicine?

Take clorazepate tablets by mouth. Follow the directions on the prescription label. Swallow the tablets with a drink of water. If clorazepate upsets your stomach, take it with food or milk. Take your doses at regular intervals. Do not take your medicine more often than directed. Do not stop taking except on your prescriber's advice. Contact your pediatrician or health care professional regarding the use of this medicine in children. Special care may be needed. Elderly patients over 65 years old may have a stronger reaction to this medicine and need smaller doses.

What if I miss a dose?

If you miss a dose, take it as soon as you can. If it is almost time for your next dose, take only that dose. Do not take double or extra doses.

What may interact with clorazepate?

- alcohol
- bosentan
- caffeine
- cimetidine
- disulfiram
- female hormones, including contraceptive or birth control pills
- herbal or dietary supplements such as kava kava, melatonin, St. John's Wort or valerian
- imatinib, STI-571
- isoniazid
- medicines for anxiety or sleeping problems, such as alprazolam, diazepam, lorazepam or triazolam
- medicines for depression, mental problems or psychiatric disturbances
- medicines for fungal infections (fluconazole, itraconazole, ketoconazole, voriconazole)
- medicines for HIV infection or AIDS
- nicardipine
- prescription pain medicines
- probenecid
- rifampin, rifapentine, or rifabutin
- some antibiotics (clarithromycin, erythromycin, troleandomycin)
- some medicines for colds, hay fever or other allergies
- some medicines for high blood pressure or heart-rhythm problems (amiodarone, diltiazem, verapamil)
- some medicines for seizures (carbamazepine, phenobarbital, phenytoin, primidone)
- theophylline
- zafirlukast
- zileuton

Tell your prescriber or health care professional about all other medicines you are taking, including non-prescription medicines, nutritional supplements, or herbal products. Also tell your prescriber or health care professional if you are a frequent user of drinks with caffeine or alcohol, if you smoke, or if you use illegal drugs. These may affect the way your medicine works. Check with your health care professional before stopping or starting any of your medicines.

What should I watch for while taking clorazepate?

Visit your prescriber or health care professional for regular checks on your progress. Your body can become dependent on clorazepate, ask your prescriber or health care professional if you still need to take it. However, if you have been taking clorazepate regularly for some time, do not suddenly stop taking it. You must gradually reduce the dose or you may get severe side effects. Ask your prescriber or health care professional for advice. Even after you stop taking clorazepate it can still affect your body for several days. You may get drowsy or dizzy. Do not drive, use machinery, or do anything that needs mental alertness until you know how clorazepate affects you. To reduce the risk of dizzy and fainting spells, do not stand or sit up quickly, especially if you are an older patient. Alcohol may increase dizziness and drowsiness. Avoid alcoholic drinks. Do not treat yourself for coughs, colds or allergies without asking your prescriber or health care professional for advice. Some ingredients can increase possible side effects. If you are going to have surgery, tell your prescriber or health care professional that you are taking clorazepate.

What side effects may I notice from taking clorazepate?

Side effects that you should report to your prescriber or health care professional as soon as possible:
- confusion
- depression
- lightheadedness or fainting spells
- mood changes, excitability or aggressive behavior
- movement difficulty, staggering or jerky movements
- muscle cramps
- restlessness
- tremors
- weakness or tiredness

Side effects that usually do not require medical attention (report to your prescriber or health care professional if they continue or are bothersome):
- blurred or double vision
- constipation
- difficulty sleeping, nightmares
- dizziness, drowsiness, clumsiness, or unsteadiness; a "hangover" effect
- dry mouth
- headache
- stomach upset

Where can I keep my medicine?

Keep out of the reach of children in a container that small children cannot open. Store at room temperature below 25 degrees C (77 degrees F). Protect from moisture and light; keep bottle tightly closed. Throw away any unused medicine after the expiration date.

Clotrimazole lozenges

MYCELEX® TROCHE;
10 mg; Troche
Ortho McNeil
Pharmaceutical Inc

CLOTRIMAZOLE;
10 mg; Troche
Roxane Laboratories
Inc

What are clotrimazole lozenges?

CLOTRIMAZOLE (Mycelex®) is an antifungal agent used to treat thrush infections of the mouth. Generic clotrimazole lozenges are available.

What should my health care professional know before I take clotrimazole?

They need to know if you have any of these conditions:
- an unusual or allergic reaction to clotrimazole, other medicines, foods, dyes or preservatives
- pregnant or trying to get pregnant
- breast-feeding

How should I take this medicine?

Let a clotrimazole lozenge dissolve in the mouth slowly and completely; do not swallow whole and do not chew. Follow the directions on the prescription label. Do not use your medicine more often than directed. Take at regular intervals. Finish the full course prescribed by your prescriber or health care professional even if you think your condition is better. Do not stop using except on your prescriber's advice. Contact your pediatrician or health care professional regarding the use of this medicine in children. Special care may be needed.

What if I miss a dose?

If you miss a dose, take it as soon as you can. If it is almost time for your next dose, take only that dose. Do not take double or extra doses.

What may interact with clotrimazole?

- amphotericin B

Tell your prescriber or health care professional about all other medicines you are taking, including non-prescription medicines, nutritional supplements, or herbal products. Also tell your prescriber or health care professional if you are a frequent user of drinks with caffeine or alcohol, if you smoke, or if you use illegal drugs. These may affect the way your medicine works. Check with your health care professional before stopping or starting any of your medicines.

What should I watch for while taking clotrimazole?

Tell your prescriber or health care professional if your symptoms do not improve within 1 week.

What side effects may I notice from taking clotrimazole?

Side effects that you should report to your prescriber or health care professional as soon as possible:
Minor side effects include:
- nausea and vomiting
- stomach pain, diarrhea

Where can I keep my medicine?

Keep out of the reach of children in a container that small children cannot open. Store at room temperature below 30 degrees C (86 degrees F); do not freeze. Throw away any unused medicine after the expiration date.

Clozapine tablets

CLOZARIL®;
100 mg; Tablet
Novartis
Pharmaceuticals

CLOZARIL®;
25 mg; Tablet
Novartis
Pharmaceuticals

What are clozapine tablets?

CLOZAPINE (Clozaril®) helps to treat emotional and mental problems like schizophrenia. Clozapine can help keep you in touch with reality and reduce your symptoms. It is not a cure. Clozapine is sometimes also used for the treatment of other severe emotional or mental problems. Clozapine is used to help people that have not responded to other medications. It is available only through a monitoring and dispensing system (special doctors, pharmacists, and laboratories). For the first several months of treatment, you will be required to have weekly or every-other-week blood testing before your doctor or pharmacist will be allowed to dispense the next supply of tablets. Generic clozapine tablets are available.

What should my health care professional know before I take clozapine?

They need to know if you have any of these conditions:
- being treated for cancer
- blood clots
- blood disease or disorder, like leukemia
- difficulty passing urine
- fever
- glaucoma
- heart disease or lung disease
- kidney disease
- liver disease
- Parkinson's disease
- prostate trouble
- receiving treatments for cancer
- seizure disorder (convulsions)
- uncontrollable movements, especially of the face and mouth
- an unusual or allergic reaction to clozapine, other medicines, foods, dyes, or preservatives
- pregnant or trying to get pregnant
- breast-feeding

How should I take this medicine?

Take clozapine tablets by mouth. Follow the directions on the prescription label. Swallow the tablets with a drink of water. If clozapine upsets your stomach, take it with food or milk. Take your doses at regular intervals. Do not take your medicine more often than directed. Do not stop taking except on your prescriber's advice. Contact your pediatrician or health care professional regarding the use of this medicine in children. Special care may be needed.

What if I miss a dose?

If you miss a dose, take it as soon as you can. If it is almost time for your next dose, take only that dose. Do not take double or extra doses. You will only be able to receive a 7 or 14 day supply of your medication at any one time, due to the rules of the clozapine medication watch system. It is important that you receive your blood tests on time so that your medication can be refilled by your pharmacist or health care provider before your supply has run out. Keep all appointments for these required tests.

What may interact with clozapine?

- alcohol
- caffeine
- carbamazepine
- cisapride
- digoxin
- divalproex sodium or valproic acid
- donepezil
- erythromycin or clarithromycin
- galantamine
- guarana
- haloperidol
- lithium
- medicines for anxiety or sleeping problems, such as diazepam or temazepam
- medicines for colds, hay fever, and other allergies
- medicines for high blood pressure
- medicines for mental depression, anxiety, or other mood problems
- medicines for muscle spasms such as gastrointestinal spasm or breathing difficulty
- medicines for pain
- olanzapine
- phenytoin
- rifampin or rifabutin
- risperidone
- ritonavir
- rivastigmine
- some medicines used to treat irregular heartbeats
- tacrine
- warfarin

Tell your prescriber or health care professional about all other medicines you are taking, including non-prescription medicines, nutritional supplements, or herbal products. Also tell your prescriber or health care professional if you are a frequent user of drinks with caffeine or alcohol, if you smoke, or if you use illegal drugs. These may affect the way your medicine works. Check with your health care professional before stopping or starting any of your medicines.

What should I watch for while taking clozapine?

Visit your prescriber or health care professional for regular checks on your progress. It may be several weeks before you see the full effects of clozapine. Do notify your prescriber if your symptoms get worse or you have new symptoms, if you are having an unusual effect from clozapine, or if you feel out of control, very discouraged or think you might harm yourself or others. You must have a weekly blood test when you first begin clozapine; if your blood counts stay in the right range, your tests may be reduced after 6 months to every other week. Your name will go on a national registry of patients that take this medicine, to make sure that you have never had a serious reaction to it. Do not suddenly stop taking clozapine. You may need to gradually reduce the dose. Only stop taking clozapine on your prescriber's advice. You may get dizzy or drowsy. Do not drive, use machinery, or do anything that needs mental alertness until you know how clozapine affects you. Do not stand or sit up quickly, especially if you are an older patient. This reduces the risk of dizzy or fainting spells. Alcohol can increase dizziness and drowsiness. Avoid alcoholic drinks. Do not treat yourself for colds, fever, diarrhea or allergies. Ask your prescriber or health care professional for advice, some non prescription medicines may increase possible side effects. Your mouth may get dry. Chewing sugarless gum or sucking hard candy, and drinking plenty of water will help. Be careful when brushing and flossing your teeth to avoid mouth infections or damage to your gums. See your dentist regularly. Sometimes clozapine can make your mouth water a lot, especially at night. If you are going to have surgery tell your prescriber or health care professional that you are taking clozapine.

What side effects may I notice from taking clozapine?

Side effects that you should report to your prescriber or health care professional as soon as possible:
More common:
- fainting spells, loss of balance
- fast heartbeat

Rare or Infrequent:
- changes in vision, inability to control eye movements
- chest pain or irregular heartbeat (palpitations)
- confusion
- difficulty breathing or shortness of breath
- difficulty in speaking or swallowing
- difficulty sleeping, nightmares
- difficulty passing urine
- fever, chills, sore throat, or mouth sores
- inability to control muscle movements in the face, hands, arms, or legs
- muscle and joint aches and pains
- restlessness or need to keep moving
- seizures (convulsions)
- stiffness, spasms, trembling
- uncontrollable tongue or chewing movements, smacking lips or puffing cheeks
- unusual tiredness or weakness

Side effects that usually do not require medical attention (report to your prescriber or health care professional if they continue or are bothersome):
Less common:
- changes in sexual desire or performance
- dry mouth
- heartburn
- increased sweating

More common:
- constipation
- dizziness, especially on standing from a sitting or lying position
- drowsiness
- headache
- increased watering of the mouth, drooling
- weight gain

Where can I keep my medicine?

Keep out of the reach of children in a container that small children cannot open. Store at room temperature below 30 degrees C (86 degrees F). Throw away any unused medicine after the expiration date.

Codeine tablets

CODEINE;
30 mg; Tablet
Roxane Laboratories
Inc

CODEINE;
60 mg; Tablet
Roxane Laboratories
Inc

What are codeine tablets?

CODEINE relieves mild to moderate pain, and helps to stop or reduce coughing. Federal law prohibits the transfer of codeine to any person other than the patient for whom it was prescribed. Do not share this medicine with anyone else. Generic codeine tablets are available.

What should my health care professional know before I take codeine?

They need to know if you have any of these conditions:
- diarrhea
- heart disease
- intestinal disease
- kidney disease
- liver disease
- lung disease or breathing difficulties
- seizures or other neurologic disorders
- an allergic or unusual reaction to codeine, morphine, methadone, other medicines, foods, dyes, or preservatives
- pregnant or trying to get pregnant
- breast-feeding

How should I take this medicine?

Take codeine tablets by mouth. Follow the directions on the prescription label. Swallow the tablets with a glass of water. If codeine upsets your stomach, take it with food or milk. Do not take your medicine more often than directed. Contact your pediatrician or health care professional regarding the use of this medicine in children. Special care may be needed. Do not share this medicine with anyone.

What if I miss a dose?

If you are taking codeine on a regular schedule and miss a dose, take it as soon as you can. If it is almost time for your next dose, take only that dose. Do not take double or extra doses.

What may interact with codeine?

- medicines for high blood pressure
- medicines for seizures

Because codeine can cause drowsiness, other medicines that also cause drowsiness may increase this effect of codeine. Some medicines that cause drowsiness are:

- alcohol and alcohol-containing medicines
- barbiturates such as phenobarbital
- certain antidepressants or tranquilizers
- certain antihistamines used in cold medicines

Tell your prescriber or health care professional about all other medicines you are taking, including non-prescription medicines, nutritional supplements, or herbal products. Also tell your prescriber or health care professional if you are a frequent user of drinks with caffeine or alcohol, if you smoke, or if you use illegal drugs. These may affect the way your medicine works. Check with your health care professional before stopping or starting any of your medicines.

What should I watch for while taking codeine?

Tell your prescriber or health care professional if your symptoms do not improve, get worse or if you have a new or different type of pain. Use exactly as directed by your prescriber or health care professional. If you are taking codeine on a regular basis, do not suddenly stop taking it. Your body becomes used to the codeine and when you suddenly stop taking it, you may develop a severe reaction. This DOES NOT mean you are "addicted" to codeine. Addiction is a behavior related to getting and using a drug for a non-medical reason. You may get drowsy or dizzy when you first start taking codeine or change doses. Do not drive, use machinery, or do anything that needs mental alertness until you know how codeine affects you. Stand or sit up slowly, this reduces the risk of dizzy or fainting spells. These effects may be worse if you are an older patient. The drowsiness should decrease after taking codeine for a couple of days. If you have not slept because of your pain, you may sleep more the first few days your pain is controlled to catch-up on missed sleep. Be careful taking other medicines which may also make you tired.

This effect may be worse when taking these medicines with codeine. Alcohol can increase possible drowsiness, dizziness, confusion and affect your breathing. Avoid alcohol while taking codeine. Codeine will cause constipation. Make sure to take a laxative and/or a stool softener while taking codeine. Try to have a bowel movement every 2 to 3 days, at least. If you do not have a bowel movement for 3 days or more call your prescriber or health care professional. They may recommend using an enema or suppository to help you move your bowels. Your mouth may get dry. Drinking plenty of water, chewing sugarless gum or sucking on hard candy may help to relieve dry mouth symptoms. Have regular dental checks. If you are going to have surgery, tell your prescriber or health care professional that you are taking codeine.

What side effects may I notice from taking codeine?

Side effects that you should report to your prescriber or health care professional as soon as possible:
Rare or uncommon:
- cold, clammy skin
- seizures
- slow or fast heart beat
- difficulty breathing, wheezing
- decreased ability to pass urine
- severe rash

More common:
- confusion
- lightheadedness or fainting spells
- nervousness or restlessness

Side effects that usually do not require medical attention (report to your prescriber or health care professional if they continue or are bothersome):
- blurred vision
- constipation
- dizziness or drowsiness
- dry mouth
- headache
- nausea, vomiting
- pinpoint pupils
- sweating

Where can I keep my medicine?

Keep out of the reach of children in a container that small children cannot open. Do not share or give this medicine to anyone else. Avoid accidental swallowing of codeine by someone (especially children) other than the person for whom it was prescribed as this may result in severe effects and possibly death. Store at room temperature between 15 and 30 degrees C (59 and 86 degrees F). Protect from light. Throw away any unused medicine after the expiration date.

Codeine;
Guaifenesin tablets

BRONTEX®;
10 mg/300 mg;
Tablet
Kenwood
Therapeutics Div
Bradley
Pharmaceuticals Inc

CODEINE;
Guaifenesin;
10 mg/300 mg;
Tablet
Ethex Corporation

What are codeine; guaifenesin tablets?

CODEINE; GUAIFENESIN (Brontex® Tablets) helps to stop or reduce coughing due to the common cold or inhaled irritants. Federal law prohibits the transfer of codeine to any person other than the patient for whom it was prescribed. Do not share this medicine with anyone else. Generic codeine; guaifenesin tablets are available.

What should my health care professional know before I take codeine; guaifenesin?

They need to know if you have any of these conditions:
- asthma or difficulties breathing
- chronic bronchitis
- constipation or diarrhea
- emphysema or other lung disease
- glaucoma
- heart disease
- intestinal or stomach problems
- kidney disease or a history of kidney stones
- liver disease
- other chronic illness
- pain or difficulty passing urine
- recent head trauma
- smoker
- stomach or intestinal disease
- an allergic or unusual reaction to codeine, hydromorphone, hydrocodone, oxycodone, morphine, guaifenesin, other medicines, foods, dyes, or preservatives
- pregnant or trying to get pregnant
- breast-feeding

How should I take this medicine?

Take codeine; guaifenesin tablets by mouth. Follow the directions on the prescription label. Swallow the tablets whole with a full glass of water. Take codeine; guaifenesin with food or milk if it upsets your stomach. Take your doses at regular intervals. Do not take your medicine more often than directed. Contact your pediatrician or health care professional regarding the use of this medicine in children. Special care may be needed. Do not share this medicine with anyone.

What if I miss a dose?

If it is almost time for your next dose, take only that dose. Do not take double doses.

What may interact with codeine; guaifenesin?

- alcohol and alcohol-containing medicines
- certain medicines used for pain
- certain medicines used for Parkinson's disease
- certain medicines used for sleep, anxiety or depression
- certain medicines used to control the heart's rhythm
- medicines for diarrhea
- medicines used for psychosis
- seizure medications
- some antibiotics
- some antihistamines

Tell your prescriber or health care professional about all other medicines you are taking, including non-prescription medicines, nutritional supplements, or herbal products. Also tell your prescriber or health care professional if you are a frequent user of drinks with caffeine or alcohol, if you smoke, or if you use illegal drugs. These may affect the way your medicine works. Check with your health care professional before stopping or starting any of your medicines.

What should I watch for while taking codeine; guaifenesin?

Tell your prescriber or health care professional if your cough does not improve in 7 days. If you have a high fever, skin rash, or persistent headache as well as a cough, see your prescriber or health care professional. Use exactly as directed by your prescriber or health care professional. If you are taking codeine; guaifenesin on a regular basis, do not suddenly stop taking it. Your prescriber may want to slowly lower your dose. You may get drowsy or dizzy when you first start taking this medicine. Be careful taking other medications that may also may you tired. Do not drive, use machinery, or do anything that needs mental alertness until you know how this medicine affects you. Stand or sit up slowly, this reduces the risk of dizzy or fainting spells. The drowsiness should decrease after taking this medicine for a couple of days. Alcohol can increase the possible drowsiness, dizziness or confusion from this medicine. Avoid alcoholic beverages while taking this medicine. Your mouth may get dry. Drinking plenty of water, chewing sugarless gum or sucking on hard candy may help to relieve dry mouth symptoms. Also, this medicine may cause dry eyes and blurred vision. If you wear contact lenses you may feel some discomfort. Lubricating drops may help. See your ophthalmologist if the problem does not go away or is severe. Higher doses of codeine; guaifenesin may cause constipation. You may need to take a laxative and/or a stool softener. Try to have a bowel movement at least every 2 to 3 days. If you do not have a bowel movement for 3 days or more call your prescriber or health care professional. They may recommend using an enema or suppository to help you move your bowels. If you are going to have surgery, tell your prescriber or health care professional that you are taking this medicine.

What side effects may I notice from taking codeine; guaifenesin?

Side effects that you should report to your prescriber or health care professional as soon as possible:
Rare or uncommon:
- side or back pain that extends to the groin (signs of kidney stones)
- confusion
- difficulty breathing
- decreased ability to pass urine
- feeling faint
- slow or fast heartbeat

Side effects that usually do not require medical attention (report to your prescriber or health care professional if they continue or are bothersome):

Common:
- blurred vision
- constipation or diarrhea
- drowsiness, dizziness
- dry mouth
- headache
- itching
- stomach upset, nausea

Where can I keep my medicine?

Keep out of the reach of children in a container that small children cannot open. Avoid accidental swallowing of codeine by someone (especially children) other than the person for whom it was prescribed as this may result in severe effects and possibly death. Store at room temperature between 15 and 30 degrees C (59 and 86 degrees F). Protect from light. Throw away any unused medicine after the expiration date.

Colchicine tablets

COLCHICINE;
0.6 mg; Tablet
Qualitest
Pharmaceuticals Inc

COLCHICINE;
0.6 mg; Tablet
West-Ward

What are colchicine tablets?

COLCHICINE treats joint pain and swelling. It helps to prevent gout and gouty attacks. Colchicine relieves pain and reduces the inflammation of acute gouty arthritis. Generic colchicine tablets are available.

What should my health care professional know before I take colchicine?

They need to know if you have any of these conditions:
- an alcohol abuse problem
- blood disorders
- dental disease
- having intramuscular injections
- heart disease
- kidney disease
- liver disease
- stomach or intestinal disease
- an unusual or allergic reaction to colchicine, other medicines, foods, dyes, or preservatives
- pregnant or trying to get pregnant
- breast-feeding

How should I take this medicine?

Take colchicine tablets by mouth. Follow the directions on the prescription label. Swallow the tablets with a drink of water. If you are taking colchicine regularly to prevent attacks of gout, take exactly as directed. Do not take colchicine more often or in higher doses than directed. If your prescriber or health care professional tells you to, increase the dose as directed when the first symptoms of a gouty attack occur. Reduce the dose as soon as the pain gets better or if nausea, vomiting, diarrhea, or stomach pains occur. Go back to your usual dose as soon as you can. If you only take colchi-

cine when you have a gouty attack, follow the above directions after the first symptoms appear. Contact your pediatrician or health care professional regarding the use of this medicine in children. Special care may be needed.

What if I miss a dose?

If you miss a dose, take it as soon as you can. If it is almost time for your next dose, take only that dose. Do not take double or extra doses.

What may interact with colchicine?

- alcohol
- anti-inflammatory drugs (NSAIDs, such as ibuprofen)
- clarithromycin
- cyanocobalamin, vitamin B_{12}
- cyclosporine
- erythromycin

Tell your prescriber or health care professional about all other medicines you are taking, including non-prescription medicines, nutritional supplements, or herbal products. Also tell your prescriber or health care professional if you are a frequent user of drinks with caffeine or alcohol, if you smoke, or if you use illegal drugs. These may affect the way your medicine works. Check with your health care professional before stopping or starting any of your medicines.

What should I watch for while taking colchicine?

Visit your prescriber or health care professional for regular checks on your progress. You may need periodic blood checks if you are taking colchicine regularly. Alcohol can increase the chance of getting stomach problems. It can also increase uric acid concentrations in the blood, which makes a gouty attack more likely. It is best to avoid alcoholic drinks. Do not treat yourself with non-prescription pain-relievers without consulting your prescriber or health care professional.

What side effects may I notice from taking colchicine?

Side effects that you should report to your prescriber or health care professional as soon as possible:

- blood in urine
- difficulty breathing
- fever, chills, or sore throat
- muscle weakness
- nausea, vomiting
- numbness or tingling in hands or feet
- pain or difficulty passing urine
- skin rash, itching

- stomach pain
- swelling of the face or mouth
- unusual bruising or bleeding
- unusual weakness or tiredness

Side effects that usually do not require medical attention (report to your prescriber or health care professional if they continue or are bothersome):

- diarrhea
- loss of appetite
- hair loss

Where can I keep my medicine?

Keep out of the reach of children in a container that small children cannot open. Store at room temperature between 15 and 30 degrees C (59 and 86 degrees F). Keep container tightly closed. Protect from light. Throw away any unused medicine after the expiration date.

Colesevelam tablets

WELCHOL®;
625 mg; Tablet
Sankyo Pharma Inc

What are colesevelam tablets?

COLESEVELAM (Welchol®) absorbs and combines with bile acids, which increases removal of cholesterol from the body through the stool. It lowers bad cholesterol for patients who are at risk of getting heart disease or a stroke. This medicine is only for patients whose cholesterol level is not controlled by diet. It is not a cure. Generic colesevelam tablets are not yet available.

What should my health care professional know before I take colesevelam?

They need to know if you have any of these conditions:

- bleeding problems
- constipation
- difficulty swallowing
- gall bladder disease
- hemorrhoids
- recent surgery
- stomach problems
- an unusual or allergic reaction to colesevelam, other medicines, foods, dyes, or preservatives
- pregnant or trying to get pregnant

How should I take this medicine?

Take colesevelam tablets by mouth. Follow the directions on the prescription label. Take the tablets with liquid and a meal. Swallow one tablet at a time whole with a drink of water; do not cut, crush or chew the tablets. Drink a total of at least 4 ounces (half a glass) of water with each dose of colesevelam. Take your doses at regular intervals. Do not take your medicine more often than directed. Contact your pediatrician or health care professional regarding the use of this medicine in children. Special care may be needed.

What if I miss a dose?

If you are taking colesevelam twice a day and miss the first dose, you can take the total daily dose with the next meal. If you miss an entire days dose of colesevelam, do not take double or extra doses the next day. Take only your normal dose for that day.

What may interact with colesevelam?

- ezetemibe
- ursodiol
- verapamil
- vitamin K products or phytonadione

Tell your prescriber or health care professional about all other medicines you are taking, including non-prescription medicines, nutritional supplements, or herbal products. Also tell your prescriber or health care professional if you are a frequent user of drinks with caffeine or alcohol, if you smoke, or if you use illegal drugs. These may affect the way your medicine works. Check with your health care professional before stopping or starting any of your medicines.

What should I watch for while taking colesevelam?

Colesevelam will not cure your condition, but taken regularly it will help lower your cholesterol level. Visit your prescriber or health care professional for regular checks on your progress. Do not stop taking colesevelam, except on your prescriber's advice. Colesevelam is only part of a total cholesterol-lowering program. Your physician or dietician can suggest a low-cholesterol and low-fat diet that will reduce your risk of getting heart and blood vessel disease. Avoid alcohol and smoking, and keep a proper exercise schedule. Drink plenty of water while you are taking colesevelam, to reduce the chance of getting constipated. Increase the amount of fiber in your diet. Ask your prescriber or health care professional for advice if you are constipated.

What side effects may I notice from taking colesevelam?

Side effects that you should report to your prescriber or health care professional as soon as possible:
- bloody or black, tarry stools
- severe stomach pain with nausea and vomiting

Side effects that usually do not require medical attention (report to your prescriber or health care professional if they continue or are bothersome):
- constipation
- heartburn or indigestion
- stomach upset

Where can I keep my medicine?

Keep out of the reach of children in a container that small children cannot open. Store at room temperature between 15 and 30 degrees C (59 and 86 degrees F). Protect from moisture. Throw away any unused medicine after the expiration date.

Colestipol tablets

COLESTID®;
1 g; Tablet
Pharmacia and Upjohn Div
Pfizer

What are colestipol tablets?

COLESTIPOL (Colestid®) absorbs and combines with bile acids, which increases removal of cholesterol from the body through the stool. It lowers blood fats and cholesterol for patients who are at risk of getting heart disease or a stroke. It is only for patients whose cholesterol level is not controlled by diet. It is not a cure. Generic colestipol tablets are not yet available.

What should my health care professional know before I take colestipol?

They need to know if you have any of these conditions:
- bleeding problems or blood vessel disease
- constipation
- gall bladder disease
- hemorrhoids
- kidney disease
- underactive thyroid
- an unusual or allergic reaction to cholestyramine, other medicines, foods, dyes, or preservatives
- pregnant or trying to get pregnant
- breast-feeding

How should I take this medicine?

Take colestipol tablets by mouth. Follow the directions on the prescription label. Swallow the tablets whole with a drink of water; do not cut, crush or chew. Drink at least 4 fluid ounces of water with each dose of colestipol. Take your doses at regular intervals. Do not take your medicine more often than directed. Contact your pediatrician or health care professional regarding the use of this medicine in children. Special care may be needed.

What if I miss a dose?

If you miss a dose, take it as soon as you can. If it is almost time for your next dose, take only that dose. Do not take double or extra doses.

What may interact with colestipol?

- carbamazepine
- heart medicines such as digoxin or digitoxin
- penicillin G
- phytonadione
- propranolol
- tetracycline antibiotics
- thyroid hormones
- ursodiol
- vancomycin
- vitamin A
- vitamin D
- warfarin
- water pills

In general, take other medicines at least 1 hour before, or 4 hours after a dose of colestipol, to avoid colestipol interfering with their absorption. Tell your prescriber or health care professional about all other medicines you are taking, including non-prescription medicines, nutritional supplements, or herbal products. Also tell your prescriber or health care professional if you are a frequent user of drinks with caffeine or alcohol, if you smoke, or if you use illegal drugs. These may affect the way your medicine works. Check with your health care professional before stopping or starting any of your medicines.

What should I watch for while taking colestipol?

Colestipol will not cure your condition, but taken regularly it will help keep down your cholesterol level. Visit your prescriber or health care professional for regular checks on your progress. Do not stop taking colestipol, except on your prescriber's advice. Colestipol is only part of a total cholesterol-lowering program. Your physician or dietician can suggest a low-cholesterol and low-fat diet that will reduce your risk of getting heart and blood vessel disease. Avoid alcohol and smoking, and keep a proper exercise schedule. Drink plenty of water while you are taking colestipol, to reduce the chance of getting constipated. Increase the amount of fiber in your diet. Ask your prescriber or health care professional for advice if you are constipated.

What side effects may I notice from taking colestipol?

Side effects that you should report to your prescriber or health care professional as soon as possible:
- bloody or black, tarry stools
- severe stomach pain with nausea and vomiting
- unusual bleeding
- weight loss

Side effects that usually do not require medical atten-

tion (report to your prescriber or health care professional if they continue or are bothersome):
- diarrhea
- dizziness
- headache
- indigestion
- nausea, vomiting
- stomach upset, belching, bloating

Where can I keep my medicine?

Keep out of the reach of children in a container that small children cannot open. Store at room temperature between 15 and 30 degrees C (59 and 86 degrees F). Protect from moisture. Throw away any unused medicine after the expiration date.

Conjugated Estrogens tablets

PREMARIN®;
0.625 mg; Tablet
Wyeth
Pharmaceuticals Inc

CENESTIN™;
0.3 mg; Tablet
Duramed
Pharmaceuticals Inc
Sub Barr
Laboratories Inc

What are conjugated estrogens tablets?

CONJUGATED ESTROGENS (Premarin®, Cenestin™) contains a mixture of estrogen hormones. Estrogens are essential for maintaining normal female functions. Conjugated estrogens can help relieve symptoms of the menopause (hot flashes, night sweats, mood changes, and vaginal dryness and irritation), and also help to prevent osteoporosis (thin weak bones). Conjugated estrogens can also help improve female functions in women with hormonal imbalance or problems with their ovaries. This drug may also be given to patients with inoperable breast cancers (in men or women) or prostate cancer (men). Estrogens are occasionally prescribed for other purposes. Generic conjugated estrogen tablets are not yet available.

What should my health care professional know before I take conjugated estrogens?

They need to know if you have any of these conditions:
- asthma
- blood vessel disease, blood clotting disorder, or suffered a stroke
- breast, cervical, endometrial, ovarian or uterine cancer
- diabetes
- endometriosis
- fibroids in the womb
- heart disease
- high blood lipids or cholesterol
- high blood pressure
- high level of calcium in the blood
- low level of calcium in the blood
- hysterectomy
- kidney disease
- liver disease
- mental depression
- migraine
- porphyria

- thyroid disease
- tobacco smoker
- vaginal bleeding
- an unusual or allergic reaction to estrogens, other hormones, medicines, foods, dyes, or preservatives
- pregnant or trying to get pregnant
- breast-feeding

How should I take this medicine?

Take conjugated estrogen tablets by mouth. Follow the directions on the prescription label. Swallow the tablet with a drink of water. Take the tablets with food. Take your doses at regular intervals, at the same time each day. Do not take your medicine more often than directed.

For all uses of this medicine:
Before starting this medication, read the paper on your prescription provided by your pharmacist or health care professional. This paper will tell you about the specific product you are taking. Make certain you understand the instructions.

Contact your pediatrician or health care professional regarding the use of this medicine in children. Special care may be needed.

What if I miss a dose?

If you miss a dose, take it as soon as you can. If it is almost time for your next dose, take only that dose. Do not take double or extra doses.

What may interact with conjugated estrogens?

- some antibiotics used to treat infections
- barbiturates or benzodiazepines used for inducing sleep or treating seizures (convulsions)
- bromocriptine
- carbamazepine
- cimetidine
- cyclosporine

- dantrolene
- medications for diabetes
- methotrexate
- griseofulvin
- hydrocortisone, cortisone, or prednisolone
- isoniazid (INH)
- methotrexate
- mineral oil
- phenytoin
- raloxifene or tamoxifen
- rifabutin, rifampin, or rifapentine
- thyroid hormones
- topiramate
- tricyclic antidepressants
- warfarin

Tell your prescriber or health care professional about all other medicines you are taking, including non-prescription medicines, nutritional supplements, or herbal products. Also tell your prescriber or health care professional if you are a frequent user of drinks with caffeine or alcohol, if you smoke, or if you use illegal drugs. These may affect the way your medicine works. Check with your health care professional before stopping or starting any of your medicines.

What should I watch for while taking conjugated estrogens?

Visit your prescriber or health care professional for regular checks on your progress. You should have a complete check-up every 6 months. You will need a regular breast and pelvic exam and 'Pap' smear while on conjugated estrogens therapy. You should also discuss the need for regular mammograms with your health care professional, and follow his or her guidelines for these tests. Conjugated estrogens can make your body retain fluid, making your fingers, hands, or ankles swell. Your blood pressure can go up. Contact your prescriber or health care professional if you feel you are retaining fluid. If you have any reason to think you are pregnant; stop taking conjugated estrogens at once and contact your prescriber or health care professional. Tobacco smoking increases the risk of getting a blood clot or having a stroke while you are taking conjugated estrogens, especially if you are more than 35 years old. You are strongly advised not to smoke. If you wear contact lenses and notice visual changes, or if the lenses begin to feel uncomfortable, consult your eye care specialist or health care professional. In women who still have their uterus, estrogens increase the risk of developing a condition (endometrial hyperplasia) that may lead to cancer of the lining of the uterus. Taking progestins,

another hormone drug, with estrogens lowers the risk of developing this condition. Therefore, if your uterus has not been removed (by a hysterectomy), your doctor may prescribe a progestin for you to take together with your estrogen. You should know, however, that taking estrogens with progestins may have additional health risks. You should discuss the use of estrogens and progestins with your health care professional to determine the benefits and risks for you. If you are going to have elective surgery, you may need to stop taking your estrogens one month beforehand. Consult your health care professional for advice prior to scheduling the surgery.

What side effects may I notice from taking conjugated estrogens?

Side effects that you should report to your prescriber or health care professional as soon as possible:
- breakthrough bleeding and spotting
- breast enlargement, tenderness, unusual discharge or milk production
- chest pain
- confusion, forgetfulness
- leg, arm or groin pain
- nausea, vomiting
- severe headaches
- stomach pain (severe)
- sudden shortness of breath
- swelling of the hands, feet or ankles, or rapid weight gain
- vision or speech problems
- yellowing of the eyes or skin

Side effects that usually do not require medical attention (report to your prescriber or health care professional if they continue or are bothersome):
- change in sexual desire
- mild stomach upset
- mood changes, anxiety, depression, frustration, anger, or emotional outbursts
- increased or decreased appetite
- skin rash, acne, or brown spots on the face
- tiredness
- urinary incontinence
- vaginal yeast infection (irritation and white discharge)
- weight gain

Where can I keep my medicine?

Keep out of the reach of children in a container that small children cannot open. Store at room temperature between 15 and 30 degrees C (59 and 86 degrees F). Throw away any unused medicine after the expiration date.

Conjugated Estrogens; Medroxyprogesterone tablets

PREMPRO®;
0.625 mg/5 mg;
Tablet
Wyeth
Pharmaceuticals Inc

PREMPHASE®;
0.625 mg/5 mg;
Tablet
Wyeth
Pharmaceuticals Inc

What are conjugated estrogens; medroxyprogesterone tablets?

CONJUGATED ESTROGENS; MEDROXY-PROGESTERONE (Prempro™, Premphase™) tablets are a mixture of estrogen hormones combined with a progestin hormone. Estrogens are essential for maintaining normal female functions. Conjugated estrogens can help relieve symptoms of the menopause (hot flashes, night sweats, mood changes, and vaginal dryness and irritation), and also help to prevent the onset of osteoporosis (weak thin bones). Medroxyprogesterone (a progestin) is helpful in reducing overgrowth of the lining of the uterus (the endometrium), which may help reduce your risk of endometrial cancer. Medroxyprogesterone is added to either all tablets in the prescription (Prempro™), or it is added only for days 15 to 28 of the prescription cycle (Premphase™). Medroxyprogesterone is effective either way. Generic conjugated estrogens; medroxyprogesterone tablets are not yet available.

What should my health care professional know before I take conjugated estrogens; medroxyprogesterone?

They need to know if you have any of these conditions:
- asthma
- blood vessel disease, blood clotting disorder, or suffered a stroke
- breast, cervical, endometrial, ovarian or uterine cancer
- diabetes
- endometriosis
- fibroids in the womb
- heart disease
- high blood lipids or cholesterol
- high blood pressure
- high level of calcium in the blood
- low level of calcium in the blood
- hysterectomy
- kidney disease
- liver disease
- mental depression
- migraine
- porphyria
- thyroid disease
- tobacco smoker
- vaginal bleeding
- an unusual or allergic reaction to estrogens, medroxyprogesterone, other hormones, medicines, foods, dyes, or preservatives
- pregnant or trying to get pregnant
- breast-feeding

How should I take this medicine?

Take conjugated estrogen; medroxyprogesterone tablets by mouth. Follow the directions on the prescription label. Swallow the tablet with a drink of water. Take the tablets with food. Take your doses at regular intervals, at the same time each day. Do not take your medicine more often than directed. For Premphase™: You will take one tablet daily. Your prescription will have two blister cards of 14 tablets each. The first card contains 14 maroon tablets that are taken on days 1 to 14. The second card contains 14 blue tablets that are taken on days 15 to 28 of each cycle. For Prempro™: You will take one tablet daily. Your prescription will have two blister cards of 14 tablets each. All tablets in the cards are of the same strength.

For all uses of this medicine:

Before starting this medication, read the paper on your prescription provided by your pharmacist or health care professional. This paper will tell you about the specific product you are taking. Make certain you understand the instructions.

Contact your pediatrician or health care professional regarding the use of this medicine in children. Special care may be needed.

What if I miss a dose?

If you miss a dose, take it as soon as you can. If it is almost time for your next dose, take only that dose. Do not take double or extra doses.

What may interact with conjugated estrogens; medroxyprogesterone?

- barbiturates or benzodiazepines used for inducing sleep or treating seizures (convulsions)
- bosentan
- bromocriptine
- carbamazepine
- cimetidine
- cyclosporine
- dantrolene
- medications for diabetes
- methotrexate
- griseofulvin
- hydrocortisone, cortisone, or prednisolone
- isoniazid (INH)
- methotrexate
- mineral oil
- phenytoin
- raloxifene or tamoxifen
- rifabutin, rifampin, or rifapentine
- thyroid hormones
- topiramate

- tricyclic antidepressants
- warfarin

Tell your prescriber or health care professional about all other medicines you are taking, including non-prescription medicines, nutritional supplements, or herbal products. Also tell your prescriber or health care professional if you are a frequent user of drinks with caffeine or alcohol, if you smoke, or if you use illegal drugs. These may affect the way your medicine works. Check with your health care professional before stopping or starting any of your medicines.

What should I watch for while taking conjugated estrogens; medroxyprogesterone?

Visit your prescriber or health care professional for regular checks on your progress. You should have a complete check-up every 6 months. You will need a regular breast and pelvic exam and "Pap" smear while on conjugated estrogens-medroxyprogesterone therapy. You should also discuss the need for regular mammograms with your health care professional, and follow his or her guidelines for these tests. Conjugated estrogens-medroxyprogesterone can make your body retain fluid, making your fingers, hands, or ankles swell. Your blood pressure can go up. Contact your prescriber or health care professional if you feel you are retaining fluid. If you have any reason to think you are pregnant; stop taking conjugated estrogens-medroxyprogesterone at once and contact your prescriber or health care professional. Tobacco smoking increases the risk of getting a blood clot or having a stroke while you are taking conjugated estrogens, especially if you are more than 35 years old. You are strongly advised not to smoke. If you wear contact lenses and notice visual changes, or if the lenses begin to feel uncomfortable, consult your eye care specialist. If you are going to have elective surgery, you may need to stop taking your estrogens one month beforehand. Consult your health care professional for advice prior to scheduling the surgery.

What side effects may I notice from taking conjugated estrogens; medroxyprogesterone?

Side effects that you should report to your prescriber or health care professional as soon as possible:
- breakthrough bleeding and spotting
- breast enlargement, tenderness, unusual discharge or milk production
- chest pain
- confusion, forgetfulness
- leg, arm or groin pain
- nausea, vomiting
- severe headaches
- stomach or abdominal pain (severe)
- sudden shortness of breath
- swelling of the hands, feet or ankles, or rapid weight gain
- vision or speech problems
- yellowing of the eyes or skin

Side effects that usually do not require medical attention (report to your prescriber or health care professional if they continue or are bothersome):
- change in sexual desire
- diarrhea
- mild stomach upset
- mood changes, anxiety, depression, frustration, anger, or emotional outbursts
- increased or decreased appetite
- skin rash, acne, or brown spots on the face
- tiredness
- urinary incontinence
- vaginal yeast infection (irritation and white discharge)
- weight gain

Where can I keep my medicine?

Keep out of the reach of children in a container that small children cannot open. Store at room temperature between 15 and 30 degrees C (59 and 86 degrees F). Throw away any unused medicine after the expiration date.

Cortisone tablets

CORTISONE;
25 mg; Tablet
West Ward Pharmaceutical
Corp

What are cortisone tablets?

CORTISONE (Cortone®) is a corticosteroid. It helps to reduce swelling, redness, itching, and allergic reactions and can be used to treat severe allergies, skin problems, asthma, arthritis and other conditions. Generic cortisone tablets are available.

What should my health care professional know before I take cortisone?

They need to know if you have any of these conditions:
- cataracts or glaucoma
- Cushing's syndrome
- diabetes
- heart problems, or previous heart attack
- high blood pressure or blood clotting disorder
- infection, such as herpes, measles, tuberculosis or chickenpox
- liver problems
- myasthenia gravis
- pschosis
- osteoporosis
- recent surgery
- seizures (convulsions)
- stomach or intestinal disease, including colitis
- underactive thyroid
- an unusual or allergic reaction to cortisone, other corticosteroids, medicines, foods, dyes, or preservatives

- pregnant or trying to get pregnant
- breast-feeding

How should I take this medicine?

Take cortisone tablets by mouth. Follow the directions on the prescription label. Swallow the tablets with a drink of water. Take with food or milk to avoid stomach upset. If you are only taking cortisone once a day, take it in the morning. This is the time your body normally secretes cortisol. Take your doses at regular intervals. Do not take your medicine more often than directed. Contact your pediatrician or health care professional regarding the use of this medicine in children. Special care may be needed.

What if I miss a dose?

If you miss a dose, take it a soon as you can. If it is almost time for your next dose, consult your prescriber or health care professional. You may need to miss a dose or take a double dose, depending on your condition and treatment. Do not take double or extra doses without advice.

What may interact with cortisone?

- acetazolamide
- anti-inflammatory drugs (NSAIDs, such as ibuprofen)
- barbiturate medicines for inducing sleep or treating seizures
- bosentan
- certain heart medicines
- female hormones, including contraceptives or birth control pills
- live virus vaccines, and other toxoids and vaccines
- medicines for diabetes
- phenytoin
- rifampin
- water pills
- warfarin

Tell your prescriber or health care professional about all other medicines you are taking, including non-prescription medicines, nutritional supplements, or herbal products. Also tell your prescriber or health care professional if you are a frequent user of drinks with caffeine or alcohol, if you smoke, or if you use illegal drugs. These may affect the way your medicine works. Check with your health care professional before stopping or starting any of your medicines.

What should I watch for while taking cortisone?

Visit your prescriber or health care professional for regular checks on your progress. If you are taking cortisone over a prolonged period, carry an identification card with your name and address, the type and dose of your medicine, and your prescriber's name and address. Do not suddenly stop taking cortisone. You may need to gradually reduce the dose, so that your body can adjust.

Follow the advice of your prescriber or health care professional. If you are taking cortisone regularly, avoid contact with people who have an infection. You will have an increased risk from infection while taking cortisone. Tell your prescriber or health care professional if you are exposed to anyone with measles or chickenpox, or if you develop sores or blisters that do not heal properly. People who are taking certain dosages of cortisone may need to avoid immunization with certain vaccines or may need to have changes in their vaccination schedules to ensure adequate protection from certain diseases. Make sure to tell your prescriber or health care professional that you are taking cortisone before receiving any vaccine. If you are going to have surgery, tell your prescriber or health care professional that you have taken cortisone within the last twelve months. If you take cortisone tablets every day, you may need to watch your diet. Your body can lose potassium while you are taking this medicine. Ask your prescriber or health care professional about your diet. Cortisone can affect your blood sugar. If you are diabetic check with your prescriber or health care professional if you need help adjusting the dose of your diabetic medicine. Alcohol can increase the risk of getting serious side effects while you are taking cortisone. Avoid alcoholic drinks. Cortisone can interfere with certain lab tests and can cause false skin test results.

What side effects may I notice from taking cortisone?

Side effects that you should report to your prescriber or health care professional as soon as possible:
- bloody or black, tarry stools
- confusion, excitement, restlessness, a false sense of well-being
- eye pain, decreased or blurred vision, or bulging eyes
- fever, sore throat, sneezing, cough, or other signs of infection, wounds that will not heal
- frequent passing of urine
- hallucinations (seeing and hearing things that are not really there)
- increased thirst
- irregular heartbeat
- menstrual problems
- mental depression, mood swings, mistaken feelings of self-importance or of being mistreated
- muscle cramps or weakness
- nausea, vomiting
- pain in hips, back, ribs, arms, shoulders, or legs
- rounding out of face
- skin problems, acne, thin and shiny skin
- stomach pain
- swelling of feet or lower legs
- unusual bruising, pinpoint red spots on the skin
- unusual tiredness or weakness
- weight gain

Side effects that usually do not require medical attention (report to your prescriber or health care professional if they continue or are bothersome):

- diarrhea or constipation
- headache
- increased appetite
- increased sweating
- nervousness, restlessness, or difficulty sleeping
- upset stomach
- unusual increased growth of hair on the face or body

Cyclobenzaprine tablets

FLEXERIL®;
5 mg; Tablet
McNeil Consumer
and Specialty
Pharmaceuticals

FLEXERIL®;
10 mg; Tablet
McNeil Consumer
and Specialty
Pharmaceuticals

What are cyclobenzaprine tablets?

CYCLOBENZAPRINE (Flexeril®) is a muscle relaxant. It helps to relieve pain and stiffness in muscles and can treat muscle spasms. Generic cyclobenzaprine tablets are available.

What should my health care professional know before I take cyclobenzaprine?

They need to know if you have any of these conditions:
- heart disease, irregular heartbeat, or previous heart attack
- cerebral palsy
- glaucoma
- overactive thyroid
- difficulty passing urine
- an unusual or allergic reaction to cyclobenzaprine, other medicines, foods, dyes, or preservatives
- pregnant or trying to get pregnant
- breast-feeding

How should I take this medicine?

Take cyclobenzaprine tablets by mouth. Follow the directions on the prescription label. Swallow the tablets with a drink of water. Take your doses at regular intervals. Do not take your medicine more often than directed. Contact your pediatrician or health care professional regarding the use of this medicine in children. Special care may be needed. Elderly patients over 65 years old may have a stronger reaction to this medicine and need smaller doses.

What if I miss a dose?

If you miss a dose, take it as soon as you can if you remember within an hour. If it is almost time for your next dose, take only the next dose. Do not take double or extra doses.

What may interact with cyclobenzaprine?

- atropine
- benztropine
- dicyclomine
- guanadrel
- guanethidine
- medicines for hay fever and other allergies
- medicines for mental depression
- medicines for mental problems and psychotic disturbances
- trihexyphenidyl

Tell your prescriber or health care professional about all other medicines you are taking, including non-prescription medicines, nutritional supplements, or herbal products. Also tell your prescriber or health care professional if you are a frequent user of drinks with caffeine or alcohol, if you smoke, or if you use illegal drugs. These may affect the way your medicine works. Check with your health care professional before stopping or starting any of your medicines.

What should I watch for while taking cyclobenzaprine?

Check with your prescriber or health care professional if your condition does not improve within 1 to 2 weeks. You may get drowsy or dizzy. Do not drive, use machinery, or do anything that needs mental alertness until you know how cyclobenzaprine affects you. To reduce the risk of dizzy or fainting spells, do not sit or stand up quickly, especially if you are an older patient. Alcohol can make you more drowsy; avoid alcoholic drinks. Your mouth may get dry. Chewing sugarless gum or sucking hard candy, and drinking plenty of water will help.

What side effects may I notice from taking cyclobenzaprine?

Side effects that you should report to your prescriber or health care professional as soon as possible:
- fast heartbeat
- hallucinations (seeing or hearing things that are not really there)
- lightheadedness, fainting spells
- pain or difficulty passing urine
- ringing in your ears
- seizures (convulsions)
- swelling of face, lips, or tongue
- unusual bleeding or bruising
- unusual weakness
- vomiting
- yellowing of eyes or skin

Side effects that usually do not require medical attention (report to your prescriber or health care professional if they continue or are bothersome):

Where can I keep my medicine?

Keep out of the reach of children in a container that small children cannot open. Store at room temperature between 15 and 30 degrees C (59 and 86 degrees F). Throw away any unused medicine after the expiration date.

- blurred vision
- constipation, or diarrhea
- drowsiness, dizziness
- dry mouth
- headache
- nausea
- nervousness or confusion
- trouble sleeping (insomnia)

Cyclophosphamide tablets

CYTOXAN®;
50 mg; Tablet
Mead Johnson and
Co Sub Bristol Myers
Co

CYTOXAN®;
25 mg; Tablet
Mead Johnson and
Co Sub Bristol Myers
Co

What are cyclophosphamide tablets?

CYCLOPHOSPHAMIDE (Cytoxan®) is a type of chemotherapy for treating various types of cancer. It also treats a number of immune-related diseases or conditions, such as systemic lupus erythematosus (SLE), lupus nephritis, rheumatoid arthritis or organ transplant rejection. Cyclophosphamide interferes with the growth of rapidly growing cancer cells and can suppress the immune system. Generic cyclophosphamide tablets are available.

What should my health care professional know before I take cyclophosphamide?

They need to know if you have any of these conditions:
- bleeding or blood disorders
- cystitis
- dehydration
- dental disease
- infection (especially virus infection such as chickenpox or cold sores)
- liver disease
- previous treatment with daunorubicin, doxorubicin, epirubicin, idarubicin, or mitoxantrone
- previous radiation therapy
- receiving dialysis
- an unusual or allergic reaction to cyclophosphamide, other chemotherapy agents, other medicines, foods, dyes, or preservatives
- pregnant or trying to get pregnant
- breast-feeding

How should I take this medicine?

Take cyclophosphamide tablets by mouth. Follow the directions on the prescription label. Swallow the tablets with a drink of water. Do not break or crush the tablets. Take your doses at regular intervals. Do not take your medicine more often than directed. Finish the full course prescribed by your doctor or health care professional, even if the tablets make you feel unwell. Do not stop taking except on your prescriber's advice.

What if I miss a dose?

If you miss a dose do not take that dose, or double the next dose. Continue with your regular schedule. If you vomit after taking a dose, call your prescriber or health care professional for advice.

Where can I keep my medicine?

Keep out of the reach of children in a container that small children cannot open. Store at room temperature between 15 and 30 degrees C (59 and 86 degrees F). Keep container tightly closed. Throw away any unused medicine after the expiration date.

What may interact with cyclophosphamide?

- agents that treat or prevent blood clots (such as warfarin)
- bupropion
- carbamazepine
- cocaine
- digoxin
- etanercept
- herbal products that contain St. John's wort
- orphenadrine
- other medications for chemotherapy or immunosuppression
- phenobarbital
- phenytoin
- rifabutin
- rifampin
- rifapentine
- select medications for fungal infections (fluconazole, itraconazole, ketoconazole, voriconazole)
- tamoxifen
- vaccines

Talk to your prescriber or health care professional before taking any of these medicines:

- acetaminophen
- aspirin
- ibuprofen
- naproxen
- ketoprofen

Tell your prescriber or health care professional about all other medicines you are taking, including nonprescription medicines, nutritional supplements, or herbal products. Also tell your prescriber or health care professional if you are a frequent user of drinks with caffeine or alcohol, if you smoke, or if you use illegal drugs. These may affect the way your medicine works. Check with your health care professional before stopping or starting any of your medicines.

What should I watch for while taking cyclophosphamide?

Visit your prescriber or health care professional for checks on your progress. You will need to have regular blood checks. The side effects of cyclophosphamide can continue after you finish your treatment; report side effects promptly. Cyclophosphamide may make you feel generally unwell. This is not uncommon because cyclophosphamide affects good cells as well as cancer cells. Report any side effects as above, but continue your course of medicine even though you feel ill, unless your prescriber or health care professional tells you to stop. Cyclophosphamide may decrease your body's ability to fight infections. Call your prescriber or health care professional if you have a fever, chills, sore throat, or other symptoms of a cold or flu. Do not treat these symptoms yourself. Try to avoid being around people who are sick. Cyclophosphamide may increase your risk to bruise or bleed. Call your prescriber or health care professional if you notice any unusual bleeding. Be careful not to cut, bruise or injure yourself because you may get an infection and bleed more than usual. Do not take your doses of cyclophosphamide in the evening or right before you go to bed. Drink several glasses of water a day while taking cyclophosphamide. Empty your bladder regularly, especially at night. This will help to reduce possible kidney and bladder problems. Avoid taking aspirin, acetaminophen (Tylenol®), ibuprofen (Advil®), naproxen (Aleve®), or ketoprofen (Orudis® KT) products as these may hide a fever, unless instructed to by your prescriber or health care professional. Be careful brushing and flossing your teeth or using a toothpick while receiving cyclophosphamide because you may get an infection or bleed more easily. If you have any dental work done, tell your dentist you are taking or have taken cyclophosphamide. Cyclophosphamide can decrease fertility in both men and women. Discuss options with your health care provider. In addition, cyclophosphamide can harm your unborn child if taken during pregnancy. Women who are able to have children should avoid becoming pregnant while taking cyclophosphamide. If you are going to have surgery, tell your prescriber or health care professional that you are taking or have taken cyclophosphamide.

What side effects may I notice from taking cyclophosphamide?

The side effects you may experience with cyclophosphamide therapy depend upon the dose, other types of chemotherapy or radiation therapy given, and the disease being treated. Not all of these effects occur in all patients. Discuss any concerns or questions with your prescriber or health care professional.

Side effects that you should report to your prescriber or health care professional as soon as possible:
- blood in the urine
- low blood counts—cyclophosphamide may decrease the number of white blood cells, red blood cells and platelets. You may be at increased risk for infections and bleeding.
- signs of infection—fever or chills, cough, sore throat, pain or difficulty passing urine
- signs of decreased platelets or bleeding—bruising, pinpoint red spots on the skin, black, tarry stools, nosebleeds
- signs of decreased red blood cells—unusual weakness or tiredness, fainting spells, lightheadedness
- confusion, agitation
- difficulty breathing, wheezing
- joint or muscle pains
- mouth or throat sores
- pain or difficulty passing urine
- swollen feet or legs
- weight gain

Side effects that usually do not require medical attention (report to your prescriber or health care professional if they continue or are bothersome):
- decreased appetite
- hair loss
- missed menstrual periods
- muscle pains
- nausea, vomiting
- skin rash
- stomach pain

Where can I keep my medicine?

Keep out of the reach of children in a container that small children cannot open. Store at room temperature below 25 degrees C (77 degrees F). Brief exposure up to 30 degrees C (86 degrees F) will be tolerated. Throw away any unused medicine after the expiration date.

Cyclosporine capsules

NEORAL®;
100 mg; Capsule
Novartis
Pharmaceuticals

SANDIMMUNE®;
100 mg; Capsule
Novartis
Pharmaceuticals

What are cyclosporine capsules?

CYCLOSPORINE (Sandimmune®, Neoral® Gengraf™) is a medication used to decrease the immune system's response to a transplanted organ, which the body would otherwise see as foreign. Cyclosporine is used to reduce immune responses and prevent rejection in patients who receive organ or bone marrow transplants. Cyclosporine is also used to treat severe rheumatoid arthritis, psoriasis, Crohn's disease or ulcerative colitis. Make sure you always use the same brand of cyclosporine unless your prescriber tells you to switch brands. Generic cyclosporine capsules are available.

What should my health care professional know before I take cyclosporine?

They need to know if you have any of these conditions:
- gout
- high blood pressure

- infection
- kidney disease
- liver disease
- previous coal tar, PUVA, ultraviolet, or radiation therapy
- recent vaccinations
- an unusual or allergic reaction to cyclosporine, alcohol, corn oil, castor oil, other medicines, foods, dyes, or preservatives
- pregnant or trying to get pregnant
- breast feeding

How should I take this medicine?

Take cyclosporine capsules by mouth with a glass of water. Swallow the capsules whole; do not chew or break the capsule. Follow the directions on the prescription label. Take the capsules in a regular manner at the same time each day and at the same time in relation to meals. This will help you keep a constant amount of cyclosporine in your body. Do not take with grapefruit juice. Do not take your medicine more often than directed.

What if I miss a dose?

If you miss a dose and if you are less than 2 hours late for your dose, take the dose immediately. If you are more than 2 hours late for your dose, call your prescriber or health care professional for advice. Do not take double or extra doses.

What may interact with cyclosporine?

- acyclovir
- antibiotics and other medicines for infections
- anti-inflammatory drugs (NSAIDs, such as ibuprofen)
- bosentan (NOTE: bosentan should not be taken with cyclosporine)
- female hormones, including contraceptive or birth control pills
- ganciclovir
- grapefruit juice
- hormones such as prednisone or cortisone
- lovastatin
- male hormones
- medicines for fungal infections
- medicines for high blood pressure
- misoprostol
- omeprazole
- orlistat
- other medicines that suppress the immune system
- probucol
- red wine
- seizure (convulsion) or epilepsy medicine
- sertraline
- St. John's wort
- vaccines
- water pills (diuretics)
- warfarin

Tell your prescriber or health care professional about all other medicines you are taking, including non-prescription medicines. Also tell your prescriber or health care professional if you are a frequent user of drinks with caffeine or alcohol, if you smoke, or if you use illegal drugs. These may affect the way your medicine works. Check with your health care professional before stopping or starting any of your medicines.

What should I watch for while taking cyclosporine?

Visit your prescriber or health care professional for regular checks on your progress. Your prescriber or health care professional may schedule regular blood checks. Do not change the brand of cyclosporine unless directed by your prescriber or health care professional. Cyclosporine can increase your blood pressure. Your prescriber or health care professional will want to monitor your blood pressure and you may have to take another medicine to keep your blood pressure under control. Cyclosporine can cause birth defects. Women should use effective birth control methods while taking cyclosporine. Women who become pregnant should discuss the potential risks and options with their physician. Cyclosporine will decrease your body's ability to fight infections. Call your prescriber or health care professional if you have a fever, chills, sore throat or other symptoms of a cold or flu. Do not treat these symptoms yourself. Try to avoid being around people who are sick. Discuss whether or not you should receive vaccinations with your prescriber or health care professional. After you stop taking this medication, some side effects can continue and some may not occur until years after the medicine was taken. These effects can include the development of certain types of cancer. Discuss this possibility with your prescriber or health care professional. Cyclosporine may increase your risk for certain types of skin cancer, especially if you have psoriasis. To decrease your risk, were protective clothing, including hats, and use sunscreen with a high protection factor when exposed to the sun. Avoid using tanning beds. Cyclosporine can cause unusual growth of gum tissue and can make your gums bleed. Practice good oral hygiene, and be careful when brushing and flossing your teeth. See your dentist regularly. Avoid drinking alcohol while taking cyclosporine. Do not drive or operate machinery until you know how cyclosporine will affect you. If you are going to have surgery, tell your prescriber or health care professional that you are taking cyclosporine.

What side effects may I notice from taking cyclosporine?

Side effects that you should report to your prescriber or health care professional as soon as possible:

- confusion, depression
- high blood pressure
- irregular heartbeat
- increased urge to urinate or frequent urination
- numbness, tingling in the hands and feet
- seizures (convulsions)
- signs and symptoms of an infection such as fever, chills, sore throat
- stomach pain

- wheezing or shortness of breath
- yellow-colored skin or eyes

Side effects that usually do not require medical attention (report to your prescriber or health care professional if they continue or are bothersome):
- acne
- bleeding or tender gums, overgrowth of gum tissue
- diarrhea
- excessive hair growth on the face or body
- headache

- leg cramps
- loss of appetite
- nausea, vomiting
- tremors

Where can I keep my medicine?

Keep out of the reach of children in a container that small children cannot open. Store at room temperature below 25 degrees C (77 degrees F). Keep doses in the original packaging. Throw away any unused medicine after the expiration date.

Cyproheptadine tablets

CYPROHEPTADINE;
4 mg; Tablet
Goldline Laboratories Inc/
IVAX Pharmaceuticals

What are cyproheptadine tablets?

CYPROHEPTADINE (Periactin®) is an antihistamine. It relieves symptoms of hay fever (seasonal rhinitis), hives (rash or itching), inflammation of the eyes (pink eye, allergic conjunctivitis), and other mild allergic conditions. Generic cyproheptadine tablets are available.

What should my health care professional know before I take cyproheptadine?

They need to know if you have any of these conditions:
- asthma or chronic obstructive lung disease (COPD)
- glaucoma
- high blood pressure or heart disease
- liver disease
- other chronic illness
- prostate disease
- pain or difficulty passing urine
- ulcers or other stomach problems
- pregnant or trying to get pregnant
- breast-feeding

How should I take this medicine?

Take cyproheptadine tablets by mouth. Follow the directions on the prescription label. Take cyproheptadine with food or milk if it upsets your stomach. Take your doses at regular intervals. Do not take your medicine more often than directed. Contact your pediatrician or health care professional regarding the use of this medicine in children. Special care may be needed.

What if I miss a dose?

If you miss a dose, take it as soon as you can. If it is almost time for your next dose, take only that dose. Do not take double doses.

What may interact with cyproheptadine?

- alcohol
- barbiturate medicines for inducing sleep or treating seizures (convulsions)
- medicines for anxiety or sleeping problems, such as alprazolam, diazepam or temazepam

- medicines for hay fever and other allergies
- medicines for mental depression
- medicines for mental problems and psychotic disturbances
- medicines for movement abnormalities as in Parkinson's disease, or for gastrointestinal problems

Tell your prescriber or health care professional about all other medicines you are taking, including non-prescription medicines, nutritional supplements, or herbal products. Also tell your prescriber or health care professional if you are a frequent user of drinks with caffeine or alcohol, if you smoke, or if you use illegal drugs. These may affect the way your medicine works. Check with your health care professional before stopping or starting any of your medicines.

What should I watch for while taking cyproheptadine?

Tell your prescriber or health care professional if your symptoms do not improve in 1 or 2 days. You may get drowsy or dizzy. Do not drive, use machinery, or do anything that needs mental alertness until you know how cyproheptadine affects you. To reduce the risk of dizzy or fainting spells, do not stand or sit up quickly, especially if you are an older patient. Alcohol may increase dizziness and drowsiness. Avoid alcoholic drinks. Your mouth may get dry. Chewing sugarless gum or sucking hard candy, and drinking plenty of water will help. Cyproheptadine may cause dry eyes and blurred vision. If you wear contact lenses you may feel some discomfort. Lubricating drops may help. See your ophthalmologist if the problem does not go away or is severe.

What side effects may I notice from taking cyproheptadine?

Side effects that you should report to your prescriber or health care professional as soon as possible:
- agitation, nervousness, excitability, not able to sleep (these are more likely in children)
- blurred vision
- dizziness or fainting spells

- irregular heartbeat, palpitations, or chest pain
- pain or difficulty passing urine
- seizures (convulsions)

Minor side effects from cyproheptadine include:
- drowsiness, dizziness
- dry mouth
- headache
- loss of appetite
- stomach upset, nausea, vomiting, constipation or diarrhea

Where can I keep my medicine?

Keep out of the reach of children in a container that small children cannot open. Store at room temperature, or below 40 degrees C (104 degrees F). Keep container tightly closed. Throw away any unused medicine after the expiration date.

C

Dapsone tablets

DAPSONE;
25 mg; Tablet
Jacobus
Pharmaceutical Co

DAPSONE;
100 mg; Tablet
Jacobus
Pharmaceutical Co

What are dapsone tablets?

DAPSONE (DDS) is an antiinfective medicine. Dapsone treats leprosy (Hansen's disease) and helps to control a skin problem called dermatitis herpetiformis. Certain other conditions may also respond to treatment with dapsone. Generic dapsone tablets are available.

What should my health care professional know before I take dapsone?

They need to know if you have any of these conditions:
- anemia
- glucose 6-phosphate dehydrogenase (G6PD) deficiency
- liver disease
- an unusual or allergic reaction to dapsone, sulfonamides, other medicines, foods, dyes, or preservatives
- pregnant or trying to get pregnant
- breast-feeding

How should I take this medicine?

Take dapsone tablets by mouth. Follow the directions on the prescription label. Swallow tablets with a drink of water. If dapsone upsets your stomach take it with food. Take your doses at regular intervals. Do not take your medicine more often than directed. Finish the full course prescribed by your prescriber or health care professional even if you think your condition is better. Do not stop taking except on your prescriber's advice.

What if I miss a dose?

If you miss a dose, take it as soon as you can. If it is almost time for your next dose, take only that dose. Do not take double or extra doses.

What may interact with dapsone?

- bosentan
- didanosine, ddI
- fluorouracil, 5-FU
- imatinib, STI-571
- methotrexate
- prilocaine
- probenecid
- pyrimethamine
- rifampin
- trimethoprim
- trimetrexate
- zidovudine, ZDV

Tell your prescriber or health care professional about all other medicines you are taking, including non-prescription medicines, nutritional supplements, or herbal products. Also tell your prescriber or health care professional if you are a frequent user of drinks with caffeine or alcohol, if you smoke, or if you use illegal drugs. These may affect the way your medicine works. Check with your health care professional before stopping or starting any of your medicines.

What should I watch for while taking dapsone?

You must visit your prescriber or health care professional for regular checks on your progress. If you are being treated for dermatitis herpetiformis tell your prescriber or health care professional if your symptoms do not improve in a few days. If you are being treated for leprosy your symptoms should start to improve in 2 to 3 months. The treatment for leprosy can take years, make sure you continue to take dapsone at regular intervals. If you get a fever or sore throat do not treat yourself. These symptoms can indicate a serious reaction. Call your prescriber or health care professional for advice. If you are taking dapsone for dermatitis herpetiformis you may need to have a gluten-free diet. Ask your prescriber or health care professional for advice about this diet. If your skin gets more sensitive to sunlight, keep out of the sun or wear protective clothing outdoors and use a sunscreen. Do not use sun lamps or sun tanning beds or booths. If your eyes are more sensitive to light wear sunglasses.

What side effects may I notice from taking dapsone?

Side effects that you should report to your prescriber or health care professional as soon as possible:
- blood in urine
- bluish fingernails or lips
- dark yellow or brown urine
- decrease or increase in the amount of urine passed
- difficulty breathing
- fever or chills, sore throat
- lower back pain
- pale skin
- skin rash, redness, blistering, peeling or loosening of skin
- stomach pain
- tingling, pain, or numbness in the hands or feet
- unusual bleeding or bruising
- unusual weakness or tiredness
- yellowing of they eyes or skin

Side effects that usually do not require medical attention (report to your prescriber or health care professional if they continue or are bothersome):
- nausea, vomiting
- loss of appetite
- increased sensitivity to sun or ultraviolet light

Where can I keep my medicine?

Keep out of the reach of children in a container that small children cannot open. Store at room temperature between 15 and 30 degrees C (59 and 86 degrees F). Protect from light. Keep container well closed. Throw away any unused medicine after the expiration date.

Darifenacin extended-release tablets

ENABLEX®; 7.5 mg; Tablet, Extended Release Novartis Pharmaceuticals	ENABLEX®; 15 mg; Tablet, Extended Release Novartis Pharmaceuticals

What are Darifenacin extended-release tablets?

DARIFENACIN (Enablex®) helps to control an overactive bladder, a chronic condition that can be improved with medication. Darifenacin may decrease the number of bathroom visits and help to control wetting accidents. Generic darifenacin extended-release tablets are not yet available.

What should my health care professional know before I take darifenacin?

They need to know if you have any of these conditions:
- difficulty passing urine
- glaucoma
- intestinal obstruction
- kidney disease
- liver disease
- stomach problems like pyloric stenosis or reflux, or other problems with proper emptying of the contents of the stomach
- an unusual or allergic reaction to darifenacin, other medicines, foods, dyes, or preservatives
- pregnant or trying to get pregnant
- breast-feeding

How should I take this medicine?

Take darifenacin extended-release tablets by mouth. Swallow the tablets with a drink of water. Do not chew, crush, or split the tablets. Darifenacin can be taken with or without food. Follow the directions on the prescription label. Take your doses at regular intervals. Do not take your medicine more often than directed. Do not stop taking except on your health care professional's advice. Contact your pediatrician or health care professional regarding the use of this medicine in children. Special care may be needed.

What if I miss a dose?

If you miss a dose, take it as soon as you can. If it is almost time for your next dose, take only that dose. Do not take double or extra doses.

What drug(s) may interact with darifenacin?

- alcohol-containing beverages
- amantadine
- aprepitant
- atropine
- bosentan
- caffeine
- chloroquine
- cimetidine
- cisapride
- cyclobenzaprine
- diltiazem
- donepezil
- duloxetine
- galantamine
- gefitinib
- grapefruit juice
- hydroxychloroquine
- hyoscyamine
- imatinib, STI-571
- memantine
- metoclopramide
- omeprazole
- quinine
- rifampin, rifapentine, or rifabutin
- rivastigmine
- scopolamine
- some antibiotics (clarithromycin, dalfopristin; quinupristin, erythromycin, norfloxacin, troleandomycin)
- some medicines for colds, hay fever, or allergies
- some medicines for fungal infections, like fluconazole, itraconazole, ketoconazole, or voriconazole
- some medicines for heart rhythm disturbances (amiodarone, digoxin, disopyramide, flecainide, propafenone, quinidine)
- some medicines for mental depression or psychotic disorders
- some medicines for seizures (carbamazepine, phenobarbital, phenytoin, primidone)
- some medicines for treating HIV infection or AIDS
- some medicines for treating pain (hydrocodone, morphine, oxycodone, propoxyphene)
- tacrine
- tegaserod
- tolterodine
- topiramate
- verapamil
- water pills (diuretics)
- zafirlukast
- zileuton

Tell your prescriber or health care professional about all other medicines you are taking, including non-prescription medicines, nutritional supplements, or herbal products. Also tell your prescriber or health care professional if you are a frequent user of drinks with caffeine or alcohol, if you smoke, or if you use illegal drugs. These may affect the way your medicine works. Check with your health care professional before stopping or starting any of your medicines.

What should I watch for while taking darifenacin?

Your health care professional may recommend techniques that may help improve control of your bladder and sphincter muscles. Such techniques will help train you to need the bathroom less frequently. You may need to limit your intake of tea, coffee, caffeinated sodas, and alcohol. These drinks may aggravate your symptoms. Keeping healthy bowel habits may lessen bladder symptoms. If you currently smoke, quitting smoking may help reduce irritation to the bladder muscle. You may get dizzy or have blurred vision. Do not drive, use machinery, or do anything that requires mental alertness until you know how darifenacin affects you. Your mouth may get dry. Chewing sugarless gum or sucking hard candy, and drinking plenty of water, will help. Darifenacin rarely causes dry eyes and blurred vision. If you wear contact lenses, you may feel some discomfort. Lubricating drops may help. See your ophthalmologist if the problem does not go away or is severe.

What side effects may I notice from taking darifenacin?

Serious side effects are not common. Side effects that you should report to your prescriber or health care professional as soon as possible:

- any signs of an allergic reaction, like skin itching or hives
- blurred vision or difficulty focusing vision
- confusion
- difficulty passing urine
- severe dizziness

Side effects that usually do not require medical attention (report to your prescriber or health care professional if they continue or are bothersome):

- constipation
- dry eyes
- dry mouth
- headache
- indigestion or stomach upset
- mild dizziness or drowsiness
- nausea

Where can I keep my medicine?

Keep out of the reach of children in a container that small children cannot open. Store at room temperature between 15 and 30 degrees C (59 and 86 degrees F). Protect from light. Throw away any unused medicine after the expiration date.

Delavirdine tablets

 RESCRIPTOR®;
200 mg; Tablet
Agouron
Pharmaceuticals Inc

RESCRIPTOR®;
100 mg; Tablet
Agouron
Pharmaceuticals Inc

What are delavirdine tablets?

DELAVIRDINE (Rescriptor®) is an antiviral drug called a nonnucleoside reverse transcriptase inhibitor or NNRTI. Delavirdine is used to treat human immunodeficiency virus (HIV) infection. Delavirdine may reduce the amount of HIV in the blood and increase the number of CD4 cells (T-cells) in the blood. Delavirdine is used in combination with other drugs to treat the HIV virus. Delavirdine will not cure or prevent HIV infection or AIDS. You may still develop other infections or conditions associated with HIV. Generic delavirdine tablets are not yet available.

What should my health care professional know before I take delavirdine?

They need to know if you have any of these conditions:
- achlorhydria (a condition associated with a decreased amount of stomach acid)
- liver disease
- an unusual or allergic reaction to delavirdine, other medicines, foods, dyes, or preservatives
- pregnant or trying to get pregnant
- breast-feeding

How should I take this medicine?

Take delavirdine tablets by mouth. Follow the directions on the prescription label. Swallow tablets with a drink of water. Delavirdine can be taken with or without food. Take your doses at regular intervals. Do not take your medicine more often than directed. Delavirdine 100 mg tablets may be dissolved in water, if you find them difficult to swallow. To dissolve, add four (4) 100 mg tablets to at least 3 ounces of water, allow to stand for a few minutes, and then stir. Take the liquid immediately. Rinse the glass thoroughly with water and drink the rinse to make sure you get the whole dose. Delavirdine 200 mg tablets do not dissolve in water and should be swallowed whole. Delavirdine 200 mg tablets are smaller than the 100 mg tablets. To make sure that your medication works as well as possible to treat your condition, take all of your medicine exactly as prescribed. Do not stop taking except on your prescriber's advice. Contact your pediatrician or health care professional regarding the use of this medicine in children. Special care may be needed.

What if I miss a dose?

If you miss a dose, take it as soon as you can. If it is almost time for your next dose, take only that dose. Do not take double or extra doses.

What may interact with delavirdine?

Delavirdine can interact with a large number of other drugs. Make sure to discuss all of your medicines with your health care prescriber before starting delavirdine or any other new medicine.
The following drugs should NOT be taken with delavirdine:

- alprazolam (Xanax®)
- astemizole (Hismanal®)

- carbamazepine (Tegretol®)
- cisapride (Propulsid®)
- ergotamine medicines (Cafergot®, Migranal®, D.H.E. 45®, and others)
- lovastatin (Mevacor®)
- midazolam (Versed®)
- phenobarbital
- phenytoin (Dilantin®)
- pimozide (Orap®)
- rifabutin (Mycobutin®)
- rifampin (Rimactane®, Rifadin®, Rifater®, Rifamate®)
- simvastatin (Zocor®)
- St. John's wort or products containing St. John's Wort
- terfenadine (Seldane®)
- triazolam (Halcion®)
- went yeast (Cholestin™)

As an interaction is possible, discuss your medicines with your prescriber before taking any these drugs with delavirdine:

- antacids
- anti-HIV medicines such as amprenavir, didanosine, ddI, indinavir, lopinavir, nelfinavir, ritonavir, or saquinavir
- birth control pills or other hormonal birth control medicines (like the patch, ring, or injections)
- certain strong medicines for pain (Demerol®, methadone, morphine, oxycodone, Vicodin®, etc.)
- clarithromycin
- cyclosporine
- dapsone
- dexamethasone
- dexfenfluramine
- dextroamphetamine
- dextromethorphan
- dronabinol, THC
- imatinib, STI-571
- itraconazole
- levomethadyl
- medicines for depression
- medicines for high cholesterol (e.g., atorvastatin, cerivastatin, fluvastatin)
- medicines for high blood pressure
- medicines for nerves or sleep
- medicines for stomach ulcers or heartburn (e.g., Nexium®, Prevacid®, Prilosec®, Tagamet®, or Zantac®)
- medicines to control heart rate
- ketoconazole
- sildenafil
- sirolimus
- tacrolimus
- warfarin

Tell your prescriber or health care professional about all other medicines you are taking, including non-prescription medicines, nutritional supplements, or herbal products. Also tell your prescriber or health care professional if you are a frequent user of drinks with caffeine or alcohol, if you smoke, or if you use illegal drugs.

These may affect the way your medicine works. Check with your health care professional before stopping or starting any of your medicines.

What should I watch for while taking delavirdine?

Visit your prescriber or health care professional for regular checks on your progress. Discuss any new symptoms with your prescriber or health care professional. The most common side effect of delavirdine is a skin rash. The rash occurs mainly on the upper body and arms, and sometimes on the neck and face. The rash appears as a red area with slight bumps, and it can be itchy. The rash is most common 1 to 3 weeks after you start taking delavirdine, and it usually lasts no more than 2 weeks. If you notice a severe rash or rash accompanied by symptoms such as fever, blisters, mouth sores, eye irritation, swelling, and/or muscle or joint pains, notify your prescriber immediately; these could be signs of a serious reaction. Patients who develop these symptoms may need to stop treatment with delavirdine. Delavirdine will not cure HIV and you can still get other illnesses or complications associated with your health condition. Taking delavirdine does not reduce the risk of passing HIV infection to others through sexual or blood contact. It is best to avoid sexual contact so that you do not spread the disease to others. For any sexual contact, use a condom. Be careful about cuts, abrasions and other possible sources of blood contact. Never share a needle or syringe with anyone. Delavirdine requires acid in the stomach to be absorbed into the body. Patients with achlorhydria (no or a decreased amount of stomach acid) should take delavirdine tablets with an acidic beverage (e.g., orange or cranberry juice). Do not take antacids or didanosine, ddI, within 1 hour of taking delavirdine.

What side effects may I notice from taking delavirdine?

Side effects that you should report to your prescriber or health care professional as soon as possible:

- signs of infection - fever or chills, cough, sore throat, pain or difficulty passing urine
- skin rash, itching, or rash with symptoms such as fever, blisters, eye irritation, edema, redness, peeling or loosening of the skin, including inside the mouth, and/or muscle and joint pain
- swelling of the eyelids, face, hands, or feet
- unusual tiredness or weakness
- yellowing of the skin

Side effects that usually do not require medical attention (report to your prescriber or health care professional if they continue or are bothersome):

- cough
- depression
- diarrhea
- difficulty sleeping
- headache
- nausea, vomiting
- stomach pain
- tiredness

Where can I keep my medicine?

Keep out of the reach of children in a container that small children cannot open. Store at room temperature 20 and 25 degrees C (68 and 77 degrees F). Keep container tightly closed. Protect from high humidity (keep away from moisture such as a sink or other damp places). Throw away any unused medicine after the expiration date.

Demeclocycline tablets

DECLOMYCIN®;
150 mg; Tablet
ESP Pharma Inc

DECLOMYCIN®;
300 mg; Tablet
ESP Pharma Inc

What are demeclocycline tablets?

DEMECLOCYCLINE (Declomycin®) is a tetracycline-type antibiotic. Demeclocycline kills certain bacteria that cause infection, or stops their growth. It treats many kinds of infections of the skin, bone, stomach, respiratory tract, sinuses, ear, and urinary tract. Demeclocycline also treats certain sexually transmitted diseases. Generic demeclocycline tablets are available.

What should my health care professional know before I take demeclocycline?

They need to know if you have any of these conditions:
- diabetes insipidus
- kidney disease
- liver disease
- long exposure to sunlight (working outdoors)
- an unusual or allergic reaction to demeclocycline, or other tetracyclines
- pregnant or trying to get pregnant
- breast-feeding

How should I take this medicine?

Take demeclocycline tablets by mouth. Follow the directions on the prescription label. Swallow tablets whole with a full glass of water; take tablets in an upright or sitting position. Taking a sip of water first, before taking the tablets, may help you swallow them. If possible take bedtime doses at least 10 minutes before lying down. Take demeclocycline 1 hour before or at least 2 hours after eating; taking it with food can make it less effective. Avoid having dairy products, such as yogurt, milk, or cheese with your medicine; they can reduce the effect of demeclocycline. Take your doses at regular intervals. Do not take your medicine more often than directed. Finish the full course prescribed by your prescriber or health care professional even if you think your condition is better. Do not stop taking except on your prescriber's advice. Contact your pediatrician or health care professional regarding the use of this medicine in children. Special care may be needed.

What if I miss a dose?

If you miss a dose, take it as soon as you can. If it is almost time for your next dose, take only that dose. Do not take double or extra doses. There should be an interval of at least 6 to 8 hours between doses.

What may interact with demeclocycline?

- antacids
- calcium salts
- cholestyramine
- colestipol
- desmopressin
- digoxin
- female hormones, including contraceptive or birth control pills
- ferrous sulfate
- magnesium salts
- methoxyflurane
- other antibiotics
- sodium bicarbonate
- vitamin A
- warfarin
- zinc salts

Tell your prescriber or health care professional about all other medicines you are taking, including non-prescription medicines, nutritional supplements, or herbal products. Also tell your prescriber or health care professional if you are a frequent user of drinks with caffeine or alcohol, if you smoke, or if you use illegal drugs. These may affect the way your medicine works. Check with your health care professional before stopping or starting any of your medicines.

What should I watch for while taking demeclocycline?

Tell your prescriber or health care professional if your symptoms do not improve in 2 to 3 days. Do not take demeclocycline just before going to bed. It may not dissolve properly when you are lying down and can cause pain in your throat. Keep out of the sun, or wear protective clothing outdoors and use a sunscreen. Do not use sun lamps or sun tanning beds or booths. You may get drowsy or dizzy. Do not drive, use machinery, or do anything that needs mental alertness until you know how demeclocycline affects you. To reduce the risk of dizzy or fainting spells, do not sit or stand up quickly, especially if you are an older patient. Make sure your diet provides vitamin B. Ask your prescriber or health care professional for advice if you think you are short of this vitamin. Birth control pills (contraceptive pills) may not work properly while you are taking this medicine. Use an extra method of birth control for at least one month. If you are being treated for a sexually transmitted disease, avoid sexual contact until you have finished your treatment. Your sexual partner may also need treatment. If you are going to have surgery, tell your prescriber or health care professional that you are taking demeclocycline. Antacid can stop demeclocycline from working. If you get an upset stomach and want to take an antacid, make sure there is an interval of at least 2 hours since you last took demeclocycline, or 4 hours before your next dose. Iron and zinc preparations can also stop demeclocycline from working properly. Never use demeclocycline if it is past the expiration date; it can make you seriously ill.

What side effects may I notice from taking demeclocycline?

Side effects that you should report to your prescriber or health care professional as soon as possible:
- blurred vision or other vision problems
- dark yellow or brown urine
- difficulty breathing
- dizziness
- frequent passing of urine
- headache
- increase in the amount of urine
- increased sensitivity to the sun or ultraviolet light
- increased thirst
- itching in the rectal or genital area

- pain on swallowing
- redness, blistering, peeling or loosening of the skin, including inside the mouth
- ringing in the ears (tinnitus)
- stomach pain or cramps
- skin rash or itching
- swelling of face or neck
- tingling or numbness of the hands or feet
- unusual bleeding or bruising
- unusual tiredness or weakness
- yellowing of eyes or skin

Side effects that usually do not require medical attention (report to your prescriber or health care professional if they continue or are bothersome):
- diarrhea
- discolored tongue
- loss of appetite
- nausea, vomiting
- sore mouth

Where can I keep my medicine?
Keep out of the reach of children in a container that small children cannot open. Store at room temperature between 15 and 30 degrees C (59 and 86 degrees F). Throw away any unused medicine after the expiration date.

Desipramine tablets

NORPRAMIN®;
75 mg; Tablet
Aventis
Pharmaceuticals Inc

NORPRAMIN®;
25 mg; Tablet
Aventis
Pharmaceuticals Inc

This drug requires an FDA medication guide. See page xxxvii.

What are desipramine tablets?
DESIPRAMINE (Norpramin®) is an antidepressant. Desipramine can help to lift your spirits by treating your depression. Generic desipramine tablets are available.

What should my health care professional know before I take desipramine?
They need to know if you have any of these conditions:
- an alcohol problem
- asthma, difficulty breathing
- blood disorders or disease
- diabetes
- difficulty passing urine, prostate trouble
- glaucoma
- having intramuscular injections
- heart disease, or recent heart attack
- liver disease
- overactive thyroid
- Parkinson's disease
- schizophrenia
- seizures (convulsions)
- stomach disease
- an unusual or allergic reaction to desipramine, other medicines, foods, dyes, or preservatives
- pregnant or trying to get pregnant
- breast-feeding

How should I take this medicine?
Take desipramine tablets by mouth. Follow the directions on the prescription label. Swallow the tablets with a drink of water. Take your doses at regular intervals. Do not take your medicine more often than directed. Do not stop taking except on your prescriber's advice. Contact your pediatrician or health care professional regarding the use of this medicine in children. Special care may be needed. Elderly patients over 65 years old and adolescents may have a stronger reaction to this medicine and need smaller doses.

What if I miss a dose?
If you take more than one dose a day and miss a dose, take it as soon as you can. If it is almost time for your next dose, take only that dose. If you miss a dose normally taken at bedtime to avoid daytime drowsiness, it may be better to miss that dose. Follow your prescriber's advice on missed doses. Do not take double or extra doses.

What may interact with desipramine?
Desipramine can interact with many other medicines. Some interactions can be very important. Make sure your prescriber or health care professional knows about all other medicines you are taking. Many important interactions are listed below:
Do not take desipramine with any of the following medications:

- astemizole (Hismanal®)
- cisapride (Propulsid®)
- probucol

- terfenadine (Seldane®)
- thioridazine (Mellaril®)
- medicines called MAO inhibitors-phenelzine (Nardil®), tranylcypromine (Parnate®), isocarboxazid (Marplan®), selegiline (Eldepryl®)
- other medicines for mental depression (may be duplicate therapies or cause additive side effects)

Desipramine may also interact with any of the following medications:

- alcohol
- antacids
- atropine and related drugs like hyoscyamine, scopolamine, tolterodine and others
- barbiturate medicines for inducing sleep or treating seizures (convulsions), such as phenobarbital
- blood thinners, such as warfarin
- bromocriptine
- bupropion
- cimetidine
- clonidine
- cocaine
- delavirdine
- diphenoxylate
- disulfiram
- donepezil
- drugs for treating HIV infection
- female hormones, including contraceptive or birth control pills and estrogen
- galantamine
- herbs and dietary supplements like ephedra (*Ma huang*), kava kava, SAM-e, St. John's wort, valerian, or others
- imatinib, STI-571
- kaolin; pectin
- labetalol
- levodopa and other medicines for movement problems like Parkinson's disease
- lithium
- medicines for anxiety or sleeping problems
- medicines for colds, flu and breathing difficulties, like pseudoephedrine
- medicines for hay fever or allergies (antihistamines)
- medicines for weight loss or appetite control
- medicines used to regulate abnormal heartbeat or to treat other heart conditions (examples: amiodarone, bepridil, disopyramide, dofetilide, encainide, flecainide, ibutilide, mibefradil, procainamide, propafenone, quinidine, and others)
- metoclopramide
- muscle relaxants, like cyclobenzaprine
- other medicines for mental or mood problems and psychotic disturbances
- prescription pain medications like morphine, codeine, tramadol and others
- procarbazine
- seizure (convulsion) or epilepsy medicine such as carbamazepine or phenytoin
- stimulants like dexmethylphenidate or methylphenidate
- some antibiotics (examples: erythromycin, gatifloxacin, levofloxacin, linezolid, moxifloxacin, sotalol, sparfloxacin)

- tacrine
- thyroid hormones such as levothyroxine

Tell your prescriber or health care professional about all other medicines you are taking, including non-prescription medicines, nutritional supplements, or herbal products. Also tell your prescriber or health care professional if you are a frequent user of drinks with caffeine or alcohol, if you smoke, or if you use illegal drugs. These may affect the way your medicine works. Check with your health care professional before stopping or starting any of your medicines.

What should I watch for while taking desipramine?

Visit your prescriber or health care professional for regular checks on your progress. It can take several days before you feel the full effect of desipramine. If you have been taking desipramine regularly for some time, do not suddenly stop taking it. You must gradually reduce the dose or you may get severe side effects. Ask your prescriber or health care professional for advice. Even after you stop taking desipramine it can still affect your body for several days. You may get drowsy or dizzy. Do not drive, use machinery, or do anything that needs mental alertness until you know how desipramine affects you. Do not stand or sit up quickly, especially if you are an older patient. This reduces the risk of dizzy or fainting spells. Alcohol can increase dizziness and drowsiness. Avoid alcoholic drinks. Do not treat yourself for coughs, colds or allergies without asking your prescriber or health care professional for advice. Some ingredients can increase possible side effects. Your mouth may get dry. Chewing sugarless gum or sucking hard candy, and drinking plenty of water will help. Desipramine may cause dry eyes and blurred vision. If you wear contact lenses you may feel some discomfort. Lubricating drops may help. See your ophthalmologist if the problem does not go away or is severe. Desipramine may make your skin more sensitive to the sun. Keep out of the sun, or wear protective clothing outdoors and use a sunscreen. Do not use sun lamps or sun tanning beds or booths. Desipramine can affect blood glucose (sugar) levels. If you are a diabetic, check your blood sugar more often than usual, especially during the first few weeks of desipramine treatment. Call your prescriber or health care professional for advice if you notice a change in the results of blood or urine glucose tests. If you are going to have surgery or will need an x-ray procedure that uses contrast agents, tell your prescriber or health care professional that you are taking this medicine.

What side effects may I notice from taking desipramine?

Side effects that you should report to your prescriber or health care professional as soon as possible:
- abnormal production of milk in females
- blurred vision or eye pain
- breast enlargement in both males and females
- confusion, hallucinations (seeing or hearing things that are not really there)

- difficulty breathing
- fainting spells
- fever
- irregular or fast, pounding heartbeat, palpitations
- muscle stiffness, or spasms
- pain or difficulty passing urine, loss of bladder control
- seizures (convulsions)
- sexual difficulties (decreased sexual ability or desire, difficulty ejaculating)
- stomach pain
- swelling of the testicles
- tingling, pain, or numbness in the feet or hands
- tremor (shaking)
- unusual weakness or tiredness
- yellowing of the eyes or skin

Side effects that usually do not require medical attention (report to your prescriber or health care professional if they continue or are bothersome):

- anxiety
- constipation, or diarrhea
- drowsiness or dizziness
- dry mouth
- headache
- increased sensitivity of the skin to sun or ultraviolet light
- loss of appetite
- nausea, vomiting
- skin rash or itching
- weight gain or loss

Where can I keep my medicine?

Keep out of the reach of children in a container that small children cannot open. Store at room temperature below 30 degrees C (86 degrees F). Throw away any unused medicine after the expiration date.

Desloratadine tablets

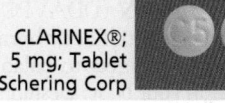

CLARINEX®;
5 mg; Tablet
Schering Corp

What are desloratadine tablets?

DESLORATADINE (Clarinex®) is an antihistamine. It relieves the symptoms of hay fever (sneezing, runny nose, and itchy, watery eyes), and may help treat hives and associated itching of the skin. Generic desloratadine tablets are not yet available.

What should my health care professional know before I take desloratadine?

They need to know if you have any of these conditions:
- asthma
- kidney disease
- liver disease or hepatitis
- an unusual or allergic reaction to desloratadine, other medicines, foods, dyes, or preservatives
- pregnant or trying to get pregnant
- breast-feeding

How should I use this medicine?

Take desloratadine tablets by mouth. Follow the directions on the prescription label. Swallow the tablets with a drink of water. Do not chew the tablets. Desloratadine is taken once daily. This drug may be taken at any time during the day, with or without food. Do not take your medicine more often than directed. Contact your pediatrician or health care professional regarding the use of this medicine in children. Special care may be needed.

What if I miss a dose?

If you miss a dose, take a dose as soon as you can, then go back to your regular dosing schedule the next day. Do not take double or extra doses.

What may interact with desloratadine?

- erythromycin
- ketoconazole

In addition, the following medicines can make you feel drowsy:

- alcohol
- barbiturate medicines for inducing sleep or treating seizures (convulsions)
- medicines for anxiety or sleeping problems, such as alprazolam, diazepam or temazepam
- medicines for hay fever and other allergies
- medicines for mental depression
- medicines for mental problems and psychotic disturbances
- medicines for pain

Tell your prescriber or health care professional about all other medicines you are taking, including non-prescription medicines, nutritional supplements, or herbal products. Also tell your prescriber or health care professional if you are a frequent user of drinks with caffeine or alcohol, if you smoke, or if you use illegal drugs. These may affect the way your medicine works. Check with your health care professional before stopping or starting any of your medicines.

What should I watch for while taking desloratadine?

Visit your prescriber or health care professional for checks on your progress. Tell your prescriber or health care professional if your symptoms do not improve within several days. Do not drive, use machinery, or do anything that needs mental alertness until you know how desloratadine affects you. To reduce the risk of dizzy or fainting spells, do not stand or sit up quickly, especially if you are an older patient. Alcohol may increase dizziness and drowsiness. Avoid alcoholic drinks. Your mouth may get dry. Chewing sugarless gum or sucking hard candy, and drinking plenty of water will help.

What side effects may I notice from taking desloratadine?

Side effects that you should report to your prescriber or health care professional as soon as possible.

- Severe side effects to desloratadine are rare. Side effects that usually do not require medical attention (report to your prescriber or health care professional if they continue or are bothersome):
- dizziness
- drowsiness or tiredness
- dry mouth
- muscle aches
- sore or dry throat

Where can I keep my medicine?

Keep out of the reach of children. Store at room temperature between 2 and 25 degrees C (36 and 77 degrees F). Avoid excessive heat temperatures greater than 30 degrees C (86 degrees F); do not freeze. Throw away any unused medicine after the expiration date.

Desmopressin tablets

D

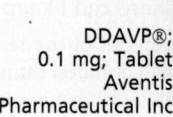
DDAVP®;
0.1 mg; Tablet
Aventis
Pharmaceutical Inc

DDAVP®;
0.2 mg; Tablet
Aventis
Pharmaceutical Inc

What are desmopressin tablets?

DESMOPRESSIN (DDAVP®) is a man-made form of vasopressin (antidiuretic hormone, or ADH). In the body, vasopressin acts to balance the amount of salt and water in your body. Desmopressin helps to prevent or control frequent urination, excessive thirst, and dehydration associated with decreased levels of vasopressin. Such problems occur with diabetes insipidus or certain brain injuries. Desmopressin is also used to help stop frequent night-time urination or bedwetting. Generic desmopressin tablets are not yet available.

What should my health care professional know before I take desmopressin?

They need to know if you have any of these conditions:
- blood clots
- cystic fibrosis
- heart disease, including history of a heart attack or heart failure
- high blood pressure
- an unusual or allergic reaction to desmopressin, vasopressin, other medicines, foods, dyes, or preservatives
- pregnant or trying to get pregnant
- breast-feeding

How should I take this medicine?

Take desmopressin tablets by mouth. Follow the directions on the prescription label. Swallow the tablets with a drink of water. Take doses at regular intervals. Do not take your medicine more often than directed. Contact your pediatrician or health care professional regarding the use of this medicine in children. Special care may be needed.

What if I miss a dose?

If you miss a dose, take it as soon as you can. If it is almost time for your next dose, take only that dose. Do not take double or extra doses.

What may interact with desmopressin?

- alcohol
- carbamazepine
- chlorpropamide
- cisplatin
- clofibrate
- cyclophosphamide
- demeclocycline
- fludrocortisone
- lithium
- vincristine

Tell your prescriber or health care professional: about all other medicines you are taking including non-prescription medicines; if you are a frequent user of drinks with caffeine or alcohol; if you smoke; or if you use illegal drugs. These can affect the way your medicine works. Check with your health care professional before stopping or starting any of your medicines.

What should I watch for while taking desmopressin?

Visit your prescriber or health care professional for regular checks on your progress. Desmopressin can prevent the loss of water. Only drink enough fluid to satisfy your thirst. Too much water in the body can cause confusion, drowsiness, or lethargy, which may lead to seizures or coma. The risk of too much water in the body is greater in young children and the elderly. Ask your prescriber or health care professional for advice about your fluid intake.

What side effects might I notice from taking desmopressin?

Side effects that you should report to your prescriber or health care professional as soon as possible:
- signs and symptoms of an allergic reaction: rash, itching, hives, difficulty breathing
- confusion
- drowsiness
- nausea, persistent or severe
- rapid weight gain
- retaining water
- severe or continuing headaches

- seizures
- weakness

Side effects that usually do not require medical attention (report to your prescriber or health care professional if they continue or are bothersome):
- flushing (reddening) of the skin
- headache

- nausea
- stomach pain or cramps

Where can I keep my medicine?

Keep out of the reach of children. Store at room temperature 20 and 25 degrees C (68 and 77 degrees F). Avoid exposure to excessive heat or light. Throw away any unused medicine after the expiration date.

Dexamethasone tablets

DEXAMETHASONE;
4 mg; Tablet
Par Pharmaceutical
Inc

DECADRON®;
0.5 mg; Tablet
Merck and Co Inc

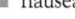

What are dexamethasone tablets?

DEXAMETHASONE (Decadron®, Dexone®, Hexadrol®) is a corticosteroid. It helps to reduce swelling, redness, itching, and allergic reactions. Dexamethasone is similar to natural steroid hormone produced by the adrenal gland. Dexamethasone treats severe allergies, skin problems, asthma, arthritis and other conditions. Generic dexamethasone tablets are available.

What should my health care professional know before I take dexamethasone?

They need to know if you have any of these conditions:
- diabetes
- blood clotting problems
- heart, liver, or kidney disease
- high blood pressure
- infection; measles, tuberculosis, herpes or chickenpox
- mental problems or psychosis
- myasthenia gravis
- osteoporosis
- previous heart attack
- seizures (convulsions)
- stomach or intestinal disease
- underactive thyroid
- an unusual or allergic reaction to dexamethasone, corticosteroids, other medicines, foods, dyes, or preservatives
- pregnant or trying to get pregnant
- breast-feeding

How should I take this medicine?

Take dexamethasone tablets by mouth. Follow the directions on the prescription label. Swallow the tablets with a drink of water. Take with milk or food to avoid stomach upset. If you are only taking dexamethasone once a day, take it in the morning, which is the time your body normally secretes cortisol. Take your doses at regular intervals. Do not take your medicine more often than directed. Do not stop taking dexamethasone except on your prescriber's advice. Contact your pediatrician or health care professional regarding the use of this medicine in children. Special care may be needed.

What if I miss a dose?

If you miss a dose, take it as soon as you can. If it is almost time for your next dose, consult your prescriber or health care professional. You may need to miss a dose or take a double dose, depending on your condition and treatment. Do not take double or extra doses without advice.

What may interact with dexamethasone?

- anti-inflammatory drugs (NSAIDs, such as ibuprofen)
- barbiturate medicines for inducing sleep or treating seizures (convulsions)
- bosentan
- certain heart medicines
- female hormones, including contraceptive or birth control pills
- medicines for diabetes
- medicines that improve muscle tone or strength for conditions like myasthenia gravis
- phenytoin
- rifampin
- vaccines and other immunization products
- water pills
- warfarin

Tell your prescriber or health care professional about all other medicines you are taking, including non-prescription medicines, nutritional supplements, or herbal products. Also tell your prescriber or health care professional if you are a frequent user of drinks with caffeine or alcohol, if you smoke, or if you use illegal drugs. These may affect the way your medicine works. Check with your health care professional before stopping or starting any of your medicines.

What should I watch for while taking dexamethasone?

Visit your prescriber or health care professional for regular checks on your progress. If you are taking corticosteroids for a long time, carry an identification card with your name, the type and dose of corticosteroid, and your prescriber's name and address. Do not suddenly stop taking dexamethasone. You may need to gradually reduce the dose, so that your body can adjust. Follow the advice of your prescriber or health care professional. If you take corticosteroids for a long time, avoid contact with people who have an infection. You may be at an increased risk from infection while taking dexamethasone. Tell your prescriber or health care professional if you are exposed to anyone with measles or chickenpox, or if you develop sores or blisters that do not heal properly. People who are taking certain dosages of dexamethasone may need to avoid immunization with certain vaccines or may need to have changes in their vaccination schedules to ensure adequate protection from certain diseases. Make sure to tell your prescriber or health care professional that you are taking dexamethasone before receiving any vaccine. If you are diabetic, dexamethasone can affect your blood sugar. Check with your prescriber or health care professional if you need help adjusting the dose of your diabetic medicine. If you take dexamethasone tablets every day, you may need to watch your diet. Your body can also lose potassium while you take this medicine. Ask your prescriber or health care professional about your diet, especially about your salt intake. If you are going to have surgery tell your prescriber or health care professional that you are taking dexamethasone, or have taken it within the last 12 months. Alcohol can increase the risk of getting serious side effects while you are taking dexamethasone. Avoid alcoholic drinks. Elderly patients have an increased risk of side effects from dexamethasone. Dexamethasone can interfere with certain lab tests and can cause false skin test results.

What side effects may I notice from taking dexamethasone?

Side effects that you should report to your prescriber or health care professional as soon as possible:

- bloody or black, tarry stools
- confusion, excitement, restlessness, a false sense of well-being
- eye pain, decreased or blurred vision, or bulging eyes
- fever, sore throat, sneezing, cough, or other signs of infection
- frequent passing of urine
- hallucinations (seeing and hearing things that are not really there)
- increased thirst
- irregular heartbeat
- menstrual problems
- mental depression, mood swings, mistaken feelings of self-importance, mistaken feelings of being mistreated
- muscle cramps or muscle weakness
- nausea, vomiting
- pain in hips, back, ribs, arms, shoulders, or legs
- rounding out of face
- skin problems, acne
- stomach pain
- swelling of feet or lower legs
- unusual bruising or red pinpoint spots on the skin
- unusual tiredness or weakness
- weight gain or weight loss
- wounds that will not heal

Side effects that usually do not require medical attention (report to your prescriber or health care professional if they continue or are bothersome):

- diarrhea or constipation
- change in taste
- headache
- increased appetite or loss of appetite
- increased sweating
- nervousness, restlessness, or difficulty sleeping
- unusual increased growth of hair on the face or body
- upset stomach

Where can I keep my medicine?

Keep out of the reach of children in a container that small children cannot open. Store at room temperature between 15 and 30 degrees C (59 and 86 degrees F). Throw away any unused medicine after the expiration date.

Dexmethylphenidate tablets

FOCALIN®;
5 mg; Tablet
Novartis
Pharmaceuticals

FOCALIN®;
2.5 mg; Tablet
Novartis
Pharmaceuticals

What are dexmethylphenidate tablets?

DEXMETHYLPHENIDATE (Focalin®) is a stimulant. It can improve attention span, concentration, and emotional control, and reduce restless or overactive behavior. This medicine treats attention-deficit hyperactivity disorder (ADHD). Federal law prohibits the transfer of dexmethylphenidate to any person other than the person for whom it was prescribed. Do not share this medicine with anyone else. Generic dexmethylphenidate tablets are not available.

What should my health care professional know before I take dexmethylphenidate?

They need to know if you have any of these conditions:

- regularly drink beverages containing alcohol
- a history of drug abuse
- glaucoma
- heart failure or other heart disease
- heart rhythm disturbance
- history of recent heart attack
- high blood pressure
- liver disease
- mental illness, including anxiety, bipolar disorder, depression, mania or schizophrenia
- overactive thyroid
- seizures (convulsions)
- Tourette's syndrome (speech repetition or involuntary use of obscene language)
- an unusual or allergic reaction to methylphenidate, other medicines, foods, dyes, or preservatives
- pregnant or trying to get pregnant
- breast-feeding

How should I take this medicine?

Take dexmethylphenidate tablets by mouth. Follow the directions on the prescription label. Swallow the tablets with a drink of water. You can take this medicine with or without food. Usually the last dose of the day will be taken at least 4 to 6 hours before your normal bedtime, so it will not interfere with sleep. Do not take your medicine more often than directed. Contact your pediatrician or health care professional regarding the use of this medicine in children. Special care may be needed. This medicine is commonly prescribed for children ≥ 6 years old.

What if I miss a dose?

If you miss a dose, take it as soon as you can. If it is almost time for your next dose, take only that dose. Do not take double or extra doses.

What may interact with dexmethylphenidate?

- amphetamine or dextroamphetamine
- bretylium
- caffeine
- carbamazepine
- clonidine
- furazolidone
- guarana
- linezolid
- lithium
- medicines for colds, sinus, and breathing difficulties
- medicines for high blood pressure
- medicines called MAO inhibitors- examples: phenelzine (Nardil®), tranylcypromine (Parnate®), isocarboxazid (Marplan®)
- other medicines for mental depression or anxiety
- medicines for mental problems and psychotic disturbances
- medicines to decrease appetite or cause weight loss
- methylphenidate
- modafinil
- pemoline
- procarbazine
- seizure (convulsion) or epilepsy medicine
- warfarin
- water pills

Tell your prescriber or health care professional about all other medicines you are taking, including non-prescription medicines, nutritional supplements, or herbal products. Also tell your prescriber or health care professional if you are a frequent user of drinks with caffeine or alcohol, if you smoke, or if you use illegal drugs. These may affect the way your medicine works. Check with your health care professional before stopping or starting any of your medicines.

What should I watch for while taking dexmethylphenidate?

Visit your prescriber or health care professional for regular checks on your progress. This prescription requires that you follow special procedures with your prescriber and pharmacy; you will need to have a new written prescription from your prescriber every time you need a refill. Dexmethylphenidate may affect your concentration, or hide signs of tiredness. Until you know how this drug affects you, do not drive, ride a bicycle, use machinery, or do anything that needs mental alertness. Tell your prescriber or health care professional if this medicine loses its effects, or if you feel you need to take more than the prescribed amount. Do not change the dosage without advice from your prescriber or health care professional. Do not suddenly stop your medication. You must gradually reduce the dose or you may feel withdrawal effects. Ask your prescriber or health care professional for advice. Decreased appetite is a common side effect when starting this medicine. Eating small, frequent meals or snacks can help. Talk to your prescriber if you continue to have poor eating habits. Height and weight growth of a child taking this medication will be monitored closely. If you are going to have surgery or other medical procedures, tell your health care professional that you are taking dexmethylphenidate.

What side effects may I notice from taking dexmethylphenidate?

Side effects that you should report to your prescriber or health care professional as soon as possible:
- anxiety or severe nervousness
- bruising
- changes in mood or behavior, including seeing or hearing things that are not really there or over-focused, staring-type behavior
- chest pain, fast or irregular heartbeat (palpitations)
- fever, or hot, dry skin
- increased blood pressure
- joint pain
- skin rash, itching
- uncontrollable head, mouth, neck, arm, or leg movements

Side effects that usually do not require medical attention (report to your prescriber or health care professional if they continue or are bothersome):
Less Common or Rare:
- a sense of well being
- blurred vision
- dizziness or lightheadedness
- stomach cramps

More Common, especially in the first few weeks of treatment:
- decreased appetite or loss of appetite
- headache
- mild stomach upset
- nervousness, restlessness, or difficulty sleeping
- weight loss

Where can I keep my medicine?

Keep out of the reach of children in a container that small children cannot open. Store at room temperature below 30 degrees C (86 degrees F). Protect from light and moisture. Keep container tightly closed. Throw away any unused medicine after the expiration date.

Dextroamphetamine tablets and extended-release capsules

DEXEDRINE®;
5 mg; Tablet
Smithkline Beecham
Pharmaceuticals Div
Smithkline Beecham
Co

DEXEDRINE®
SPANSULE®;
10 mg; Capsule,
Extended Release
Smithkline Beecham
Pharmaceuticals Div
Smithkline Beecham
Co

What are dextroamphetamine tablets?

DEXTROAMPHETAMINE (Dexedrine®, Dexedrine® Spansule®, Dextrostat® and others) is a stimulant. It can improve attention span, concentration, and emotional control, and reduce restless or overactive behavior. This medicine treats attention-deficit hyperactivity disorder (ADHD). It can also help a condition called narcolepsy, an illness that makes it difficult to stay awake during normal daytime hours. This medication is rarely used for weight loss. Federal law prohibits the transfer of this medicine to any person other than the patient for whom it was prescribed. Do not share this medicine with anyone else. Generic dextroamphetamine tablets and extended-release capsules are available.

What should my health care professional know before I take dextroamphetamine?

They need to know if you have any of these conditions:
- regularly drink alcohol-containing beverages
- diabetes or high blood sugar
- glaucoma
- hardening or blockages of the arteries or heart blood vessels
- heart disease
- high blood pressure
- overactive thyroid gland
- psychotic illness, depressed mood, or suicidal thoughts
- recent weight loss
- seizure disorder
- Tourette's syndrome
- an unusual or allergic reaction to dextroamphetamine, other amphetamines, other medicines, foods, dyes, or preservatives
- pregnant or trying to get pregnant
- breast-feeding

How should I take this medicine?

Take dextroamphetamine tablets or capsules by mouth. Follow the directions on the prescription label. Swallow the tablets with a drink of water. Take your last dose at least 6 hours before bedtime. Do not take your medicine more often than directed. Do not stop taking except on your prescriber's advice. Remember: The prescription for dextroamphetamine is only for the person for whom it was prescribed. Never share or give your prescription to anyone else. Contact your pediatrician or health care professional regarding the use of this medicine in children. Dextroamphetamine has been prescribed for children 3 years of age and older for the treatment of attention-deficit disorder. This medicine should not be used in children under the age of 12 years for weight loss.

What if I miss a dose?

If you miss a dose, take it as soon as you can. If it is almost time for your next dose, take only that dose. Do not take double or extra doses.

What may interact with dextroamphetamine?

- acetazolamide
- alcohol containing beverages
- bupropion
- caffeine
- furazolidone
- guarana
- insulin and other medicines for diabetes
- levodopa
- linezolid
- lithium
- medicines for colds, sinus, and breathing difficulties
- medicines for high blood pressure and heart medicines
- medicines called MAO inhibitors- examples: phenelzine (Nardil®), tranylcypromine (Parnate®), isocarboxazid (Marplan®)
- other medicines for mental depression or anxiety
- medicines for mental problems and psychotic disturbances
- some medicines for migraines (propranolol)
- medicines to decrease appetite or cause weight loss
- meperidine
- melatonin
- other stimulant medications (examples: dexmethylphenidate, methylphenidate, modafinil)
- pimozide
- propoxyphene
- seizure (convulsion) or epilepsy medicine
- selegiline
- sodium bicarbonate
- thyroid hormones

Tell your prescriber or health care professional about all other medicines you are taking, including non-prescription medicines, nutritional supplements, or herbal products. Also tell your prescriber or health care professional if you are a frequent user of drinks with caffeine or alcohol, if you smoke, or if you use illegal drugs. These may affect the way your medicine works. Check with your health care professional before stopping or starting any of your medicines.

What should I watch for while taking dextroamphetamine?

Visit your prescriber or health care professional for regular checks on your progress. This prescription requires that you follow special procedures with your prescriber and pharmacy; you will need to have a new written prescription from your prescriber every time you need a refill. Tell your prescriber or health care professional if this medicine loses its effects, or if you feel you need to take more than the prescribed amount. Do not change the dosage without advice from your prescriber or health care professional. If you suddenly stop taking this medicine you may get some unpleasant withdrawal effects. Ask your prescriber or health care professional for advice before you stop taking it. Decreased appetite is a common side effect when starting this medicine. Eating small, frequent meals or snacks can help. Talk to your prescriber if you continue to have poor eating habits. Height, weight and growth of a child taking this medication will be monitored closely. Do not take this medicine within 6 hours of bedtime. It can keep you from getting to sleep. Avoid drinks that contain caffeine and try to stick to a regular bedtime every night. Your mouth may get dry while on this medication. Sucking on hard candy, crushed ice, and drinking plenty of fluids will help. Do not take this medicine with other non-prescription medicines, especially cold and allergy medicines or weight-loss aides, without asking your prescriber or health care professional for advice. Dextroamphetamine can hide signs that you are tired, reduce your coordination, or make you dizzy. Do not drive, use machinery, or do anything that needs mental alertness until you know how this medicine affects you. Older adults may be more sensitive to these effects. If you are going to have surgery or will need an x-ray procedure that uses contrast agents, tell your prescriber or health care professional that you are taking this medicine.

What side effects may I notice from taking dextroamphetamine?

Side effects that you should report to your prescriber or health care professional as soon as possible:
- anxiety, or severe nervousness
- changes in mood or behavior, including seeing or hearing things that are not really there or over-focused, staring-type behavior
- chest pain, fast or irregular heartbeat (palpitations)
- fever, or hot, dry skin
- increased blood pressure
- muscle twitching
- skin rash and itching (hives)
- uncontrollable head, mouth, neck, arm, or leg movements

Side effects that usually do not require medical attention (report to your prescriber or health care professional if they continue or are bothersome):
Less Common or Rare:
- a sense of well being
- blurred vision
- changes in sexual ability or desire (adults and teenagers)
- constipation or diarrhea
- dizziness or lightheadedness
- increased sweating
- nausea, vomiting
- stomach cramps

More Common, especially in the first few weeks of treatment:
- decreased appetite or loss of appetite
- headache
- mild stomach upset
- nervousness, restlessness, or difficulty sleeping
- weight loss

Where can I keep my medicine?

Keep out of the reach of children in a container that small children cannot open. Store at room temperature between 15 and 30 degrees C (59 and 86 degrees F). Keep container tightly closed. Throw away any unused medicine after the expiration date.

Dextromethorphan all dosage forms

DEXALONE®;
30 mg; Capsules
Xanodyne Pharmacal Inc

What is dextromethorphan?

DEXTROMETHORPHAN (Benylin®, Delsym®, Pertussin®, Robitussin® and others) helps to relieve a persistent cough caused by colds or the flu. Do not use dextromethorphan for treatment of a chronic cough that is due to smoking, asthma, emphysema, or problems that cause a large amount of phlegm. Generic dextromethorphan is widely available in a variety of non-prescription medicines, in capsules, lozenges, syrups, extended-release oral suspensions, and chewable tablets.

What should my health care professional know before I take dextromethorphan?

They need to know if you have any of these conditions:
- asthma
- emphysema
- liver disease
- smoker
- an unusual or allergic reaction to dextromethorphan, other medicines, foods, dyes, or preservatives (some combination products contain bromides)
- pregnant or trying to get pregnant
- breast-feeding

How should I take this medicine?

Take dextromethorphan by mouth. Follow the directions on the container. Suck lozenges slowly or allow to dissolve in the mouth; do not swallow whole. For the oral syrup, use a specially marked spoon or container. Ask your pharmacist if you do not have one; household spoons are not always accurate. Take your doses at regular intervals. Do not take your medicine more often than directed. Contact your pediatrician or health care professional regarding the use of this medicine in children. Special care may be needed.

What if I miss a dose?

If you miss a dose, take it as soon as you can. If it is almost time for your next dose, take only that dose. Do not take double or extra doses.

What may interact with dextromethorphan?

- alcohol
- amiodarone
- barbiturates
- certain medicines for mental depression, anxiety, or other mental disturbances
- furazolidone
- medicines known as MAO inhibitors, such as phenelzine (Nardil®), tranylcypromine (Parnate®), isocarboxazid (Marplan®), and selegiline (Carbex®, Eldepryl®)
- linezolid
- quinidine
- sibutramine
- sleeping pills or tranquilizers
- terbinafine

Tell your prescriber or health care professional about all other medicines you are taking, including non-prescription medicines, nutritional supplements, or herbal products. Also tell your prescriber or health care professional if you are a frequent user of drinks with caffeine or alcohol, if you smoke, or if you use illegal drugs. These may affect the way your medicine works. Check with your health care professional before stopping or starting any of your medicines.

What should I watch for while taking dextromethorphan?

If you have a fever, skin rash, or persistent headache as well as a cough, see your prescriber or health care professional. Do not treat yourself for a cough for more than 7 days without consulting your prescriber or health care professional. You may get drowsy or dizzy. Do not drive, use machinery, or do anything that needs mental alertness until you know how dextromethorphan affects you. Alcohol can increase the risk of getting drowsy, dizzy or confused. Avoid alcoholic drinks.

What side effects may I notice from taking dextromethorphan?

Side effects that you should report to your prescriber or health care professional as soon as possible:
Rare, but serious side effects include:
- confusion
- excitement, nervousness, restlessness, or irritability
- severe nausea, vomiting
- slurred speech

Children may get the following side effects from an overdose:
- seizures (convulsions)
- shakey movements
- slow or troubled breathing

Side effects that usually do not require medical attention (report to your prescriber or health care professional if they continue or are bothersome):
- dizziness, drowsiness
- fatigue
- nausea, vomiting
- skin rash (not common)
- stomachache

Where can I keep my medicine?

Keep out of the reach of children in a container that small children cannot open. Store at room temperature between 15 and 30 degrees C (59 and 86 degrees F) unless otherwise directed. Protect liquid preparations from light; do not freeze. Throw away any unused medicine after the expiration date.

Dextromethorphan; Guaifenesin extended-release and regular-release tablets and capsules

MUCO-FEN® DM;
60 mg/1000 mg; Tablet,
Extended Release
Ivax Labs, Inc

What is dextromethorphan; guaifenesin extended-release and regular-release tablets and capsules?

DEXTROMETHORPHAN and GUAIFENESIN (Muco-Fen®, Silexin®, Tuss® DM and others) decrease a persistent cough caused by colds or flu. Generic dextromethorphan and guaifenesin products are available as prescription or non-prescription medicines, in capsules and tablets.

What should my health care professional know before I take dextromethorphan; guaifenesin?

They need to know if you have any of these conditions:
- asthma
- chronic bronchitis
- emphysema
- liver disease
- an unusual or allergic reaction to dextromethorphan,

guaifenesin, other medicines, foods, dyes, or preservatives (some combination products contain bromides)
- pregnant or trying to get pregnant
- breast-feeding

How should I take this medicine?

Take dextromethorphan; guaifenesin by mouth. Follow the directions on the container. Take your doses at regular intervals. Do not take your medicine more often than directed. Contact your pediatrician or health care professional regarding the use of this medicine in children. Special care may be needed.

What if I miss a dose?

If you miss a dose, take it as soon as you can. If it is almost time for your next dose, take only that dose. Do not take double or extra doses.

What may interact with dextromethorphan; guaifenesin?

- alcohol
- amiodarone
- furazolidone
- linezolid
- medicines known as MAO inhibitors, such as phenelzine (Nardil®), tranylcypromine (Parnate®), isocarboxazid (Marplan®), and selegiline (Carbex®, Eldepryl®)
- medicines for mental depression or other mental disturbances
- quinidine

Tell your prescriber or health care professional about all other medicines you are taking, including non-prescription medicines, nutritional supplements, or herbal products. Also tell your prescriber or health care professional if you are a frequent user of drinks with caffeine or alcohol, if you smoke, or if you use illegal drugs. These may affect the way your medicine works. Check with your health care professional before stopping or starting any of your medicines.

What should I watch for while taking dextromethorphan; guaifenesin?

If you have a fever, skin rash, or persistent headache as well as a cough, see your prescriber or health care professional. Do not treat yourself for a cough for more than one week without consulting your prescriber or health care professional. You may get drowsy or dizzy. Do not drive, use machinery, or do anything that needs mental alertness until you know how dextromethorphan and guaifenesin affects you. Alcohol can increase the risk of getting drowsy, dizzy or confused. Avoid alcoholic drinks. Drink plenty of water while taking dextromethorphan and guaifenesin products. This will help loosen mucus.

What side effects may I notice from taking dextromethorphan; guaifenesin?

Severe side effects from dextromethorphan; guaifenesin are usually only seen in patients who have taken very high doses. These side effects should be reported to your prescriber or health care professional as soon as possible:
- confusion
- excitement, nervousness, restlessness, or irritability
- severe nausea, vomiting
- slurred speech

Children may get the following side effects from an overdose:
- seizures
- shaky movements
- slow or troubled breathing

Side effects that usually do not require medical attention (report to your prescriber or health care professional if they continue or are bothersome):
Rare or uncommon:
- dizziness, drowsiness
- hives
- nausea, vomiting
- rash
- stomachache

Where can I keep my medicine?

Keep out of the reach of children in a container that small children cannot open. Store at room temperature between 15 and 30 degrees C (59 and 86 degrees F) unless otherwise directed. Throw away any unused medicine after the expiration date.

Dextromethorphan; Guaifenesin; Potassium Guaiacolsulfonate extended-release capsule

HUMIBID® DM;
50 mg / 400 mg / 200 mg ;
Capsule, Extended Release
Carolina Pharmaceuticals Inc.

What is dextromethorphan; guaifenesin; potassium guaiacolsulfonate extended-release capsule?

DEXTROMETHORPHAN; GUAIFENESIN; POTASSIUM GUAIACOLSULFONATE (Humibid® DM) decreases a persistent cough caused by colds or flu. Currently, no generic equivalent of this medication is available.

What should my health care professional know before I take dextromethorphan; guaifenesin; potassium guaiacolsulfonate?

They need to know if you have any of these conditions:
- asthma
- chronic bronchitis
- emphysema
- liver disease

- an unusual reaction to dextromethorphan; guaifenesin; potassium guaiacolsulfonate, medicines, foods, dyes, or preservatives
- pregnant or trying to get pregnant
- breast-feeding

How should this medicine be used?

Take dextromethorphan; guaifenesin; potassium guaiacolsulfonate capsules by mouth. Do not open or chew the capsule. Follow the directions on the container. Take your doses at regular intervals. Do not take your medicine more often than directed. Contact your pediatrician or health care professional regarding the use of this medicine in children. Special care may be needed.

What if I miss a dose?

If you miss a dose, take it as soon as you can. If it is almost time for your next dose, take only that dose. Do not take double or extra doses.

What may interact with dextromethorphan; guaifenesin; potassium guaiacolsulfonate?

- alcohol
- amiodarone
- furazolidone
- linezolid
- medicines known as MAO inhibitors, such as phenelzine (Nardil®), tranylcypromine (Parnate®), isocarboxazid (Marplan®), and selegiline (Carbex®, Eldepryl®)
- medicines for mental depression or other mental disturbances
- quinidine

Tell your prescriber or health care professional about all other medicines you are taking, including non-prescription medicines, nutritional supplements, or herbal products. Also tell your prescriber or health care professional if you are a frequent user of drinks with caffeine or alcohol, if you smoke, or if you use illegal drugs. These may affect the way your medicine works. Check with your health care professional before stopping or starting any of your medicines.

What should I watch for while taking dextromethorphan; guaifenesin; potassium guaiacolsulfonate?

If you have a fever, skin rash, or persistent headache as well as a cough, see your prescriber or health care professional. Do not treat yourself for a cough for more than one week without consulting your prescriber or health care professional. You may get drowsy or dizzy. Do not drive, use machinery, or do anything that needs mental alertness until you know how this medicine affects you. Alcohol can increase the risk of getting drowsy, dizzy or confused. Avoid alcoholic drinks. Drink plenty of water while taking this medicine. This will help loosen mucus.

What side effects may I notice from taking dextromethorphan; guaifenesin; potassium guaiacolsulfonate?

Severe side effects from this medicine are usually only seen in patients who have taken very high doses. These side effects should be reported to your prescriber or health care professional as soon as possible:
- confusion
- excitement, nervousness, restlessness, or irritability
- severe nausea, vomiting, or diarrhea
- slurred speech

Children may get the following side effects from an overdose:
- seizures
- shaky movements
- slow or troubled breathing

Side effects that usually do not require medical attention (report to your prescriber or health care professional if they continue or are bothersome):
Rare or uncommon:
- dizziness, drowsiness
- hives
- nausea, vomiting
- rash
- stomach ache

Where can I keep my medicine?

Keep out of the reach of children in a container that small children cannot open. Store at room temperature between 15 and 30 degrees C (59 and 86 degrees F) unless otherwise directed. Throw away any unused medicine after the expiration date.

Dextromethorphan; Guaifenesin; Pseudoephedrine regular-release and extended-release capsules or tablets

PROFEN® FORTE DM; 60 mg/800 mg/90 mg; Tablet, Extended Release
Ivax Labs, Inc

What are dextromethorphan; guaifenesin; pseudoephedrine regular-release and extended-release capsules or tablets?

DEXTROMETHORPHAN; GUAIFENESIN; PSEUDOEPHEDRINE (Contac® Cough and Chest Cold capsules or tablets, DayCare®, Dimacol®, Dimetapp® Cold and Congestion Caplet, Maxifed® DM, Profen® Forte DM, Protuss® DM, SYN RX® DM and others) products are used to treat cough, especially nonproductive coughs, and nasal congestion due to bronchitis, colds, or hay fever. Generic dextromethorphan, guaifenesin, and pseudoephedrine capsules or tablets are available.

What should my health care professional know before I take dextromethorphan, guaifenesin, pseudoephedrine?

They need to know if you have any of these conditions:
- asthma
- diabetes
- difficulty passing urine
- chronic cough
- emphysema
- enlarged prostrate
- heart disease including angina
- high blood pressure
- history of stroke or mini-strokes (TIAs)
- irregular heart beat
- liver disease
- thyroid disease
- an unusual or allergic reaction to dextromethorphan, guaifenesin, pseudoephedrine, other medicines, foods, dyes, or preservatives
- pregnant or trying to get pregnant
- breast-feeding

How should I take this medicine?

Take dextromethorphan, guaifenesin, pseudoephedrine capsules or tablets by mouth. Swallow capsules or tablets whole with a drink of water; do not crush or chew. Take your doses at regular intervals. Follow the directions on the prescription label, pack or on the product label. Take your doses at regular intervals. Do not take your medicine more often than directed. Contact your pediatrician or health care professional regarding the use of this medicine in children. Special care may be needed. Do not give to children less than 2 years of age without consulting your health care provider. Elderly patients over 60 years old may have a stronger reaction to this medicine and need smaller doses.

What if I miss a dose?

If you miss a dose, take it as soon as you can. If it is almost time for your next dose (within 2 hours), take only that dose. Do not take double or extra doses.

What may interact with dextromethorphan, guaifenesin, pseudoephedrine?

- alcohol
- amiodarone
- cocaine
- ergot drugs like dihydroergotamine or ergotamine
- herbal or dietary supplements like ephedra or St. John's wort
- medicines for depression
- medicines for high blood pressure
- medicines for weight loss, including dietary supplements
- other medicines for nasal congestion, cough or cold symptoms (may contain duplicate ingredients)
- quinidine
- ritonavir
- thyroid hormones like levothyroxine

Tell your prescriber or health care professional about all other medicines that you are taking, including non-prescription medicines, nutritional supplements, or herbal products. Also tell your prescriber or health care professional if you are a frequent user of drinks with caffeine or alcohol, if you smoke, or if you use illegal drugs. These may affect the way your medicine works. Check with your health care professional before stopping or starting any of your medicines.

What do I need to watch for while taking dextromethorphan, guaifenesin, pseudoephedrine?

If you have a fever, skin rash, or persistent headache as well as a cough, see your prescriber or health care professional. Do not treat yourself for a cough for more than one week without consulting your prescriber or health care professional. You may get drowsy or dizzy. Do not drive, use machinery, or do anything that needs mental alertness until you know this medicine affects you. Alcohol can increase the risk of getting drowsy, dizzy, or confused. Avoid alcoholic drinks. Drink plenty of water while taking dextromethorphan-guaifenesin-pseudoephedrine products. This will help loosen mucus.

What side effects may I notice from dextromethorphan, guaifenesin, pseudoephedrine?

Severe side effects from dextromethorphan, guaifenesin, pseudoephedrine are usually only seen in patients who have taken very high doses. These side effects should be reported to your prescriber or health care professional as soon as possible:
- agitation, anxiety, excitement, nervousness, restlessness, or irritability
- confusion
- dizziness or fainting spells
- excessive sweating
- high blood pressure
- numbness or tingling in the hands or feet
- seizures (convulsions)
- severe nausea, vomiting
- severe, persistent, or worsening headache
- slow or troubled breathing
- slurred speech
- tremor or muscle contractions

Side effects that usually do not require medical attention (report to your prescriber or health care professional if they continue or are bothersome):
- drowsiness
- headache (mild)
- nausea, stomach upset
- rash (mild)
- weakness

Where can I keep my medicine?

Keep out of the reach of children in a container that small children cannot open. Store at room temperature between 15 and 30 degrees C (59 and 86 degrees F) unless otherwise directed. Throw away any unused medicine after the expiration date.

D

Diazepam tablets

VALIUM®;
5 mg; Tablet
Roche Products Inc

VALIUM®;
10 mg; Tablet
Roche Products Inc

What are diazepam tablets?

DIAZEPAM (Valium®) is a benzodiazepine. Benzodiazepines belong to a group of medicines that slow down the central nervous system. Diazepam relieves anxiety and nervousness. It also can help patients cope with alcohol withdrawal, relax muscles, and treat certain types of seizures (convulsions). Federal law prohibits the transfer of diazepam to any person other than the patient for whom it was prescribed. Do not share this medicine with anyone else. Generic diazepam tablets are available.

What should my health care professional know before I take diazepam?

They need to know if you have any of these conditions:
- an alcohol or drug abuse problem
- bipolar disorder, depression, psychosis or other mental health condition
- glaucoma
- kidney disease
- liver disease
- lung disease, such as chronic obstructive pulmonary disease (COPD), sleep apnea or other breathing difficulties
- myasthenia gravis
- Parkinson's disease
- seizures or a history of seizures
- shortness of breath
- snoring
- suicidal thoughts
- an unusual or allergic reaction to diazepam, other benzodiazepines, foods, dyes, or preservatives
- pregnant or trying to get pregnant
- breast-feeding

How should I take this medicine?

Take diazepam tablets by mouth. Follow the directions on the prescription label. Swallow the tablets with a drink of water. If diazepam upsets your stomach, take it with food or milk. Take your doses at regular intervals. Do not take your medicine more often than directed. Do not stop taking except on your prescriber's advice. Contact your pediatrician or health care professional regarding the use of this medicine in children. Special care may be needed. Elderly patients over 65 years old may have a stronger reaction to this medicine and need smaller doses.

What if I miss a dose?

If you miss a dose, take it as soon as you can. If it is almost time for your next dose, take only that dose. Do not take double or extra doses.

What may interact with diazepam?

- alcohol
- bosentan
- caffeine
- cimetidine
- chloroquine
- disulfiram
- female hormones, including contraceptive or birth control pills
- grapefruit juice
- herbal or dietary supplements such as kava kava, melatonin, St. John's Wort or valerian
- imatinib, STI-571
- isoniazid
- levodopa
- medicines for anxiety or sleeping problems, such as alprazolam, lorazepam or triazolam
- medicines for depression, mental problems or psychiatric disturbances
- medicines for fungal infections (fluconazole, itraconazole, ketoconazole, voriconazole)
- medicines for HIV infection or AIDS
- omeprazole
- prescription pain medicines
- probenecid
- rabeprazole
- rifampin, rifapentine or rifabutin
- some antibiotics (clarithromycin, ciprofloxacin, erythromycin, troleandomycin)
- some medicines for colds, hay fever or other allergies
- some medicines for blood pressure or heart problems (amiodarone, digoxin, diltiazem, nicardipine, verapamil)
- some medicines for seizures (carbamazepine, phenobarbital, phenytoin, primidone)
- theophylline
- valproic acid
- zafirlukast
- zileuton

Tell your prescriber or health care professional about all other medicines you are taking, including non-prescription medicines, nutritional supplements, or herbal products. Also tell your prescriber or health care professional if you are a frequent user of drinks with caffeine or alcohol, if you smoke, or if you use illegal drugs. These may affect the way your medicine works. Check with your health care professional before stopping or starting any of your medicines.

What should I watch for while taking diazepam?

Visit your prescriber or health care professional for regular checks on your progress. Your body can become dependent on diazepam, ask your prescriber or health care professional if you still need to take it. However, if you have been taking diazepam regularly for some time, do not suddenly stop taking it. You must gradually reduce the dose or you may get severe side effects. Ask your prescriber or health care professional for advice. Even after you stop taking diazepam it can still affect your body for several days. You may get drowsy or dizzy. Do not drive, use machinery, or do anything that needs mental alertness until you know how diazepam affects you. To reduce the risk of dizzy and fainting spells, do not stand or sit up quickly, especially if you are an older patient. Alcohol may increase dizziness and drowsiness. Avoid alcoholic drinks. Do not treat yourself for coughs, colds or allergies without asking your prescriber or health care professional for advice. Some ingredients can increase possible side effects. If you are going to have surgery, tell your prescriber or health care professional that you are taking diazepam.

What side effects may I notice from taking diazepam?

Side effects that you should report to your prescriber or health care professional as soon as possible:
- confusion
- depression
- lightheadedness or fainting spells
- mood changes, excitability or aggressive behavior

- movement difficulty, staggering or jerky movements
- muscle cramps
- problems passing urine
- restlessness
- skin rash
- speech difficulty
- tremors
- weakness or tiredness

Side effects that usually do not require medical attention (report to your prescriber or health care professional if they continue or are bothersome):
- difficulty sleeping, nightmares
- dizziness, drowsiness, clumsiness, or unsteadiness; a "hangover" effect
- headache
- nausea, vomiting

Where can I keep my medicine?

Keep out of the reach of children in a container that small children cannot open. Store at room temperature between 15 and 30 degrees C (59 and 86 degrees F). Protect from light. Keep container tightly closed. Throw away any unused medicine after the expiration date.

D

Diclofenac delayed-release and extended-release tablets

VOLTAREN®;
50 mg; Tablet,
Delayed Release
Novartis
Pharmaceuticals

VOLTAREN®-XR;
100 mg; Tablet,
Extended Release
Novartis
Pharmaceuticals

This drug requires an FDA medication guide. See page xxxvii.

What are diclofenac delayed-release and extended-release tablets?

DICLOFENAC (Voltaren®, Voltaren® XR) is an anti-inflammatory drug. Diclofenac reduces the joint pain, stiffness, inflammation, or swelling caused by rheumatoid arthritis (rheumatism) and osteoarthritis. Generic diclofenac delayed-release and extended-release tablets are available.

What should my health care professional know before I take diclofenac?

They need to know if you have any of these conditions:
- asthma, especially aspirin sensitive asthma
- bleeding problems or taking medicines that make you bleed more easily such as anticoagulants ('blood thinners')
- cigarette smoker
- dental disease
- diabetes
- drink more than 3 alcohol-containing beverages a day
- heart or circulation problems such as heart failure or leg edema (fluid retention)
- high blood pressure
- kidney disease
- liver disease
- porphyria
- stomach or duodenal ulcers

- systemic lupus erythematosus
- ulcerative colitis
- an unusual or allergic reaction to aspirin, other salicylates, other NSAIDs, other medicines, foods, dyes or preservatives
- pregnant or trying to get pregnant
- breast-feeding

How should I take this medicine?

Take diclofenac tablets by mouth. Follow the directions on the prescription label. Swallow tablets whole with a full glass of water; take tablets in an upright or sitting position. Do not crush or chew tablets. Taking a sip of water first, before taking the tablets, may help you swallow them. It is better to take diclofenac with food. Take your doses at regular intervals. Do not take your medicine more often than directed. Contact your pediatrician or health care professional regarding the use of this medicine in children. Special care may be needed.

What if I miss a dose?

If you miss a dose, take it as soon as you can. If it is almost time for your next dose, take only that dose. Do not take double or extra doses.

What may interact with diclofenac?

- ACE inhibitors, often used to treat high blood pressure or heart problems

- alcohol
- alendronate
- aspirin and aspirin-like medicines
- cidofovir
- cyclosporine
- drospirenone; ethinyl estradiol (Yasmin®)
- entecavir
- herbal products that contain feverfew, garlic, ginger, or ginkgo biloba
- lithium
- medicines for high blood pressure
- medicines that affect platelets
- medicines that treat or prevent blood clots such as warfarin and other "blood thinners"
- methotrexate
- other anti-inflammatory drugs (such as ibuprofen or prednisone)
- pemetrexed
- water pills (diuretics)

Tell your prescriber or health care professional about all other medicines you are taking, including non-prescription medicines, nutritional supplements, or herbal products. Also tell your prescriber or health care professional if you are a frequent user of drinks with caffeine or alcohol, if you smoke, or if you use illegal drugs. These may affect the way your medicine works. Check with your health care professional before stopping or starting any of your medicines.

What should I watch for while taking diclofenac?

Let your prescriber or health care professional know if your pain continues, do not take with other pain-killers without advice. If you get flu-like symptoms (fever, chills, muscle aches and pains), call your prescriber or health care professional; do not treat yourself. To reduce unpleasant effects on your throat and stomach, take diclofenac with a full glass of water and never just before lying down. If you notice black, tarry stools or experience severe stomach pain and/or vomit blood or what looks like coffee grounds, notify your health care prescriber immediately. If you are taking medicines that affect the clotting of your blood, such as aspirin or blood thinners such as Coumadin®, talk to your health care provider or prescriber before taking this medicine. You may get dizzy. Do not drive, use machinery, or do anything that needs mental alertness until you know how diclofenac affects you. Do not sit or stand up quickly, especially if you are an older patient. This reduces the risk of dizzy or fainting spells. Do not smoke cigarettes or drink alcohol; these increase irritation to your stomach and can make it more susceptible to damage from diclofenac. If you are going to have surgery, tell your prescriber or health care professional that you are taking diclofenac. Diclofenac can cause you to bleed more easily. Problems can arise if you need dental work, and in the day to day care of your teeth. Try to avoid damage to your teeth and gums when you brush or floss your teeth. It is especially important not to use diclofenac during the last 3 months of pregnancy unless specifically directed to do so by your health care provider. Diclofenac may cause problems in the unborn child or complications during delivery.

What side effects may I notice from taking diclofenac?

Elderly patients are at increased risk for developing side effects.

Side effects that you should report to your prescriber or health care professional as soon as possible:

- signs of bleeding from the stomach—black tarry stools, blood in the urine, unusual tiredness or weakness, vomiting blood or vomit that looks like coffee grounds
- signs of an allergic reaction—difficulty breathing or wheezing, skin rash, redness, blistering or peeling skin, hives, or itching, swelling of eyelids, throat, lips
- change in the amount of urine passed
- difficulty swallowing, severe heartburn or burning, pain in throat
- pain or difficulty passing urine
- stomach pain or cramps
- swelling of feet or ankles
- yellowing and/or itching of eyes or skin, upper right abdominal/chest tenderness, fatigue

Side effects that usually do not require medical attention (report to your prescriber or health care professional if they continue or are bothersome):

- constipation or diarrhea
- dizziness
- gas or heartburn
- headache
- nausea, vomiting

Where can I keep my medicine?

Keep out of the reach of children in a container that small children cannot open. Store at room temperature below 30 degrees C (86 degrees F). Protect from moisture. Keep container tightly closed. Throw away any unused medicine after the expiration date.

Diclofenac immediate-release tablets

CATAFLAM®;
50 mg; Tablet
Novartis Pharmaceuticals

This drug requires an FDA medication guide. See page xxxvii.

What are diclofenac immediate-release tablets?

DICLOFENAC (Cataflam®) is an anti-inflammatory drug. Diclofenac reduces inflammation and eases mild to moderate pain, especially that associated with menstruation. Generic diclofenac immediate-release tablets are available.

What should my health care professional know before I take diclofenac?

They need to know if you have any of these conditions:
- asthma, especially aspirin sensitive asthma
- bleeding problems or taking medicines that make you bleed more easily such as anticoagulants ("blood thinners")
- cigarette smoker
- dental disease
- diabetes
- drink more than 3 alcohol-containing beverages a day
- heart or circulation problems such as heart failure or leg edema (fluid retention)
- high blood pressure
- kidney disease
- liver disease
- porphyria
- stomach or duodenal ulcers
- systemic lupus erythematosus
- ulcerative colitis
- an unusual or allergic reaction to aspirin, other salicylates, other anti-inflammatory drugs, foods, dyes or preservatives
- pregnant or trying to get pregnant
- breast-feeding

How should I take this medicine?

Take diclofenac tablets by mouth. Follow the directions on the prescription label. Swallow the tablets whole with a full glass of water. It is better to take diclofenac with food. Take your doses at regular intervals. Do not take your medicine more often than directed. Contact your pediatrician or health care professional regarding the use of this medicine in children. Special care may be needed.

What if I miss a dose?

If you miss a dose, take it as soon as you can. If it is almost time for your next dose, take only that dose. Do not take double or extra doses.

What may interact with diclofenac?

- ACE inhibitors, often used to treat high blood pressure or heart problems
- agents that treat or prevent blood clots such as warfarin or other "blood thinners"
- agents that affect platelets
- alcohol
- alendronate
- aspirin and aspirin-like medicines
- cidofovir
- cyclosporine
- drospirenone; ethinyl estradiol (Yasmin®)
- entecavir
- herbal products that contain feverfew, garlic, ginger, or ginkgo biloba
- lithium
- methotrexate
- other anti-inflammatory drugs (such as ibuprofen or prednisone)
- pemetrexed
- water pills (diuretics)

Tell your prescriber or health care professional about all other medicines you are taking, including non-prescription medicines, nutritional supplements, or herbal products. Also tell your prescriber or health care professional if you are a frequent user of drinks with caffeine or alcohol, if you smoke, or if you use illegal drugs. These may affect the way your medicine works. Check with your health care professional before stopping or starting any of your medicines.

What should I watch for while taking diclofenac?

Let your prescriber or health care professional know if your pain continues, do not take with other pain-killers without advice. If you get flu-like symptoms (fever, chills, muscle aches and pains), call your prescriber or health care professional; do not treat yourself. To reduce unpleasant effects on your throat and stomach, take diclofenac with a full glass of water and never just before lying down. If you notice black, tarry stools or experience severe stomach pain and/or vomit blood or what looks like coffee grounds, notify your health care prescriber immediately. If you are taking medicines that affect the clotting of your blood, such as aspirin or blood thinners such as Coumadin®, talk to your health care provider or prescriber before taking this medicine. You may get dizzy. Do not drive, use machinery, or do anything that needs mental alertness until you know how diclofenac affects you. Do not sit or stand up quickly, especially if you are an older patient. This reduces the risk of dizzy or fainting spells. Do not smoke cigarettes or drink alcohol; these increase irritation to your stomach and can make it more susceptible to damage from diclofenac. If you are going to have surgery, tell your prescriber or health care professional that you are taking diclofenac. Diclofenac can cause blood problems. This can mean slow healing and a risk of infec-

D

tion. Problems can arise if you need dental work, and in the day to day care of your teeth. Try to avoid damage to your teeth and gums when you brush or floss your teeth. It is especially important not to use diclofenac during the last 3 months of pregnancy unless specifically directed to do so by your health care provider. Diclofenac may cause problems in the unborn child or complications during delivery.

What side effects may I notice from taking diclofenac?

Elderly patients are at increased risk for developing side effects.

Side effects that you should report to your prescriber or health care professional as soon as possible:

- signs of bleeding—bruising, pinpoint red spots on the skin, black tarry stools, blood in the urine, unusual tiredness or weakness, vomiting blood or vomit that looks like coffee grounds
- signs of an allergic reaction—difficulty breathing or wheezing, skin rash, redness, blistering or peeling skin, hives, or itching, swelling of eyelids, throat, lips

- change in the amount of urine passed
- difficulty swallowing, severe heartburn or burning, pain in throat
- pain or difficulty passing urine
- stomach pain or cramps
- yellowing and/or itching of eyes or skin, upper right abdominal/chest tenderness, fatigue
- yellowing of eyes or skin

Side effects that usually do not require medical attention (report to your prescriber or health care professional if they continue or are bothersome):

- constipation or diarrhea
- dizziness
- gas or heartburn
- headache
- nausea, vomiting

Where can I keep my medicine?

Keep out of the reach of children in a container that small children cannot open. Store at room temperature below 30 degrees C (86 degrees F). Protect from moisture. Keep container tightly closed. Throw away any unused medicine after the expiration date.

This drug requires an FDA medication guide. See page xxxvii.

Diclofenac; Misoprostol tablets

ARTHROTEC®;
50 mg/200 mcg;
Tablet, Delayed
Release
GD Searle LLC a
Subsidiary of
Pharmacia Company
Pfizer

ARTHROTEC®;
75 mg/200 mcg;
Tablet, Delayed
Release
GD Searle LLC a
Subsidiary of
Pharmacia Company
Pfizer

What are diclofenac; misoprostol tablets?

DICLOFENAC; MISOPROSTOL (Arthrotec®) is a combination of two drugs. Diclofenac is an anti-inflammatory drug and reduces the joint pain, stiffness, inflammation, or swelling caused by rheumatoid arthritis (rheumatism) or osteoarthritis. Misoprostol is added to diclofenac to help prevent some of the adverse effects of diclofenac on the stomach. Generic diclofenac; misoprostol tablets are not yet available.

What should my health care professional know before I take diclofenac; misoprostol?

They need to know if you have any of these conditions:

- asthma, especially aspirin sensitive asthma
- bleeding problems or taking medicines that make you bleed more easily such as anticoagulants ("blood thinners")
- cigarette smoker
- dental disease
- diabetes
- drink more than 3 alcohol-containing beverages a day
- heart or circulation problems such as heart failure or leg edema (fluid retention)
- high blood pressure
- kidney disease
- liver disease

- porphyria
- stomach or duodenal ulcers
- systemic lupus erythematosus
- ulcerative colitis
- an unusual or allergic reaction to aspirin, other salicylates, other NSAIDs, misoprostol, other medicines, foods, dyes or preservatives
- pregnant or trying to get pregnant
- breast-feeding

How should I take this medicine?

Take diclofenac; misoprostol tablets by mouth. Follow the directions on the prescription label. Swallow tablets whole with a full glass of water; take tablets in an upright or sitting position. Do not crush or chew tablets. Taking a sip of water first, before taking the tablets, may help you swallow them. If possible take bedtime doses at least 10 minutes before lying down. It is better to take diclofenac; misoprostol with food. Take your doses at regular intervals. Do not take your medicine more often than directed. Contact your pediatrician or health care professional regarding the use of this medicine in children. Special care may be needed.

What if I miss a dose?

If you miss a dose, take it as soon as you can. If it is almost time for your next dose, take only that dose. Do not take double or extra doses.

What may interact with diclofenac; misoprostol?

- alcohol
- alendronate
- aspirin and aspirin-like medicines
- cidofovir
- cyclosporine
- drospirenone; ethinyl estradiol (Yasmin®)
- entecavir
- herbal products that contain feverfew, garlic, ginger, or ginkgo biloba
- lithium
- medicines for high blood pressure
- medicines that affect platelets
- medicines that treat or prevent blood clots such as warfarin and other 'blood thinners'
- methotrexate
- other anti-inflammatory drugs (such as ibuprofen or prednisone)
- pemetrexed
- water pills (diuretics)

Tell your prescriber or health care professional about all other medicines you are taking, including non-prescription medicines, nutritional supplements, or herbal products. Also tell your prescriber or health care professional if you are a frequent user of drinks with caffeine or alcohol, if you smoke, or if you use illegal drugs. These may affect the way your medicine works. Check with your health care professional before stopping or starting any of your medicines.

What should I watch for while taking diclofenac; misoprostol?

Let your prescriber or health care professional know if your pain continues, do not take with other pain-killers without advice. If you get flu-like symptoms (fever, chills, muscle aches and pains), call your prescriber or health care professional; do not treat yourself. To reduce unpleasant effects on your throat and stomach, take diclofenac; misoprostol with a full glass of water and never just before lying down. If you notice black, tarry stools or experience severe stomach pain and vomit blood or what looks like coffee grounds, notify your health care prescriber immediately. If you are taking medicines that affect the clotting of your blood, such as aspirin or blood thinners such as Coumadin®, talk to your health care provider or prescriber before taking this medicine. You may get dizzy. Do not drive, use machinery, or do anything that needs mental alertness until you know how diclofenac; misoprostol affects you. Do not sit or stand up quickly, especially if you are an older patient. This reduces the risk of dizzy or fainting spells. Do not smoke cigarettes or drink alcohol; these increase irritation to your stomach and can make it more susceptible to damage from diclofenac; misoprostol. If you are going to have surgery, tell your prescriber or health care professional that you are taking diclofenac; misoprostol. Diclofenac; misoprostol can cause you to bleed more easily. Problems can arise if you need dental work, and in the day to day care of your teeth. Try to avoid damage to your teeth and gums when you brush or floss your teeth. If you are female, you should not use diclofenac; misoprostol if you are pregnant. Females should avoid pregnancy while taking this medication and for at least one month (one full menstrual cycle) after discontinuing this medication. Misoprostol can cause contractions of the uterus that may cause abortion or the medication may harm an unborn baby. If you can still have children, you should use a reliable form of birth control while taking diclofenac; misoprostol; talk to your health care provider about birth control options. If you become pregnant, think you are pregnant, or want to become pregnant during diclofenac; misoprostol treatment, stop taking this drug immediately and contact your health care provider for advice.

What side effects may I notice from taking diclofenac; misoprostol?

Elderly patients are at increased risk for developing side effects.

Side effects that you should report to your prescriber or health care professional as soon as possible:

- signs of bleeding—bruising, pinpoint red spots on the skin, black tarry stools, blood in the urine, unusual tiredness or weakness, vomiting blood or vomit that looks like coffee grounds
- signs of an allergic reaction—difficulty breathing or wheezing, skin rash, redness, blistering or peeling skin, hives, or itching, swelling of eyelids, throat, lips
- blurred vision
- change in the amount of urine passed
- difficulty swallowing, severe heartburn or burning, pain in throat
- pain or difficulty passing urine
- stomach pain or cramps
- swelling of feet or ankles
- severe abdominal pain or diarrhea
- unusual vaginal bleeding
- yellowing of eyes or skin

Side effects that usually do not require medical attention (report to your prescriber or health care professional if they continue or are bothersome):

- diarrhea
- dizziness
- gas or heartburn
- headache
- menstrual irregularity or cramps
- nausea
- stomach pain or cramps

Where can I keep my medicine?

Keep out of the reach of children in a container that small children cannot open. Store below 25 degrees C (77 degrees F). Protect from moisture. Keep container tightly closed. Throw away any unused medicine after the expiration date.

Diclozacillin capsules

DICLOXACILLIN; 250 mg; Capsule Teva Pharmaceuticals USA Inc

DICLOXACILLIN; 500 mg; Capsule Sandoz Pharmaceuticals

What are diclozacillin capsules?

DICLOXACILLIN (Dynapen®, Pathocil®, Dyc-ill®) is a penicillin antibiotic. Diclozacillin kills certain bacteria that cause infection, or stops their growth. Diclozacillin treats infections of the skin and soft tissues, joints, urinary and respiratory tracts. Generic diclozacillin capsules are available.

What should my health care professional know before I take diclozacillin?

They need to know if you have any of these conditions:
- asthma
- eczema
- stomach problems (especially colitis)
- other chronic illness
- an unusual or allergic reaction to diclozacillin, other penicillins, cephalosporin antibiotics, foods, dyes, or preservatives
- breast-feeding

How should I take this medicine?

Take diclozacillin capsules by mouth. Follow the directions on the prescription label. Take diclozacillin 1 to 2 hours before or at least 2 hours after eating; taking it with food can make it less effective. Take with a full glass of water. Take your doses at regular intervals. Do not take your medicine more often than directed. Finish the full course prescribed by your prescriber or health care professional even if you think your condition is better. Do not stop taking except on your prescriber's advice.

What if I miss a dose?

If you miss a dose, take it as soon as you can. If it is almost time for your next dose, take only that dose. Do not take double or extra doses. There should be an interval of at least 4 to 6 hours between doses.

What may interact with diclozacillin?

- certain antibiotics given by injection
- probenecid

Tell your prescriber or health care professional about all other medicines you are taking, including non-prescription medicines, nutritional supplements, or herbal products. Also tell your prescriber or health care professional if you are a frequent user of drinks with caffeine or alcohol, if you smoke, or if you use illegal drugs. These may affect the way your medicine works. Check with your health care professional before stopping or starting any of your medicines.

What should I watch for while taking diclozacillin?

Tell your prescriber or health care professional if your symptoms do not improve in 2 or 3 days. If you get severe or watery diarrhea, do not treat yourself. Call your prescriber or health care professional for advice. If you get a skin rash, do not treat yourself. Call your prescriber or health care professional for advice. If you are diabetic and taking large doses of diclozacillin, you may get a false-positive result for sugar in your urine. Check with your prescriber or health care professional before you change your diet or the dose of your diabetic medicine.

What side effects may I notice from taking diclozacillin?

Side effects that you should report to your prescriber or health care professional as soon as possible:
- black, tarry stools
- difficulty breathing, wheezing
- fever or chills, sore throat
- headache
- red spots on the skin
- redness, blistering, peeling or loosening of the skin, including inside the mouth
- seizures (convulsions)
- severe or watery diarrhea
- skin rash, itching
- stomach pain or cramps
- swollen joints
- unusual bleeding or bruising
- unusual weakness or tiredness

Side effects that usually do not require medical attention (report to your prescriber or health care professional if they continue or are bothersome):
- diarrhea
- nausea, vomiting
- sore mouth

Where can I keep my medicine?

Keep out of the reach of children in a container that small children cannot open. Store at room temperature, approximately 25 degrees C (77 degrees F). Keep container tightly closed. Throw away any unused medicine after the expiration date.

Dicyclomine tablets or capsules

BENTYL®;
10 mg; Capsule
Aventis Pharmaceuticals
Inc

BENTYL®;
20 mg; Tablet
Aventis Pharmaceuticals
Inc

What are dicyclomine tablets or capsules?

DICYCLOMINE (Bentyl®) treats different bowel problems including irritable bowel syndrome. It is believed to be effective in reducing spasm of the bowel. Generic dicyclomine capsules and tablets are available.

What should my health care professional know before I take dicyclomine?

They need to know if you have any of these conditions:
- blood vessel disease
- difficulty passing urine
- esophagus problems or heartburn
- glaucoma
- heart disease, or previous heart attack
- hiatal hernia
- liver disease
- kidney disease
- myasthenia gravis
- nervous system disorder
- overactive thyroid
- prostate trouble
- stomach infection, or obstruction
- ulcerative colitis
- an unusual or allergic reaction to dicyclomine, other medicines, foods, dyes, or preservatives
- pregnant or trying to get pregnant
- breast-feeding

How should I take this medicine?

Take dicyclomine tablets or capsules by mouth. Follow the directions on the prescription label. Swallow the tablets or capsules with a drink of water. It is best to take dicyclomine on an empty stomach, 30 minutes to 1 hour before meals. Take your medicine at regular intervals. Do not take your medicine more often than directed. Contact your pediatrician or health care professional regarding the use of this medicine in children. Special care may be needed.

What if I miss a dose?

If you miss a dose, take it as soon as you can. If it is almost time for your next dose, take only that dose. Do not take double or extra doses.

What may interact with dicyclomine?

- amantadine
- antacids
- benztropine
- cisapride
- digoxin
- disopyramide
- donepezil
- erythromycin
- galantamine
- metoclopramide
- medicines for anxiety or sleeping problems (such as diazepam or temazepam)
- medicines for colds and breathing difficulties
- medicines for diarrhea
- medicines for hay fever and other allergies
- medicines for mental depression
- medicines for mental problems and psychotic disturbances
- medicines for pain
- rivastigmine
- tacrine
- tegaserod

Tell your prescriber or health care professional about all other medicines you are taking, including non-prescription medicines, nutritional supplements, or herbal products. Also tell your prescriber or health care professional if you are a frequent user of drinks with caffeine or alcohol, if you smoke, or if you use illegal drugs. These may affect the way your medicine works. Check with your health care professional before stopping or starting any of your medicines.

What should I watch for while taking dicyclomine?

You may get drowsy, dizzy, or have blurred vision. Do not drive, use machinery, or do anything that needs mental alertness until you know how dicyclomine affects you. To reduce the risk of dizzy or fainting spells, do not sit or stand up quickly, especially if you are an older patient. Alcohol can make you more drowsy, avoid alcoholic drinks. Stay out of bright light and wear sunglasses if dicyclomine makes your eyes more sensitive to light. Avoid extreme heat (e.g., hot tubs, saunas). Dicyclomine can cause you to sweat less than normal. Your body temperature could increase to dangerous levels, which may lead to heat stroke. Antacids can stop dicyclomine from working. If you get an upset stomach and want to take an antacid, make sure there is an interval of at least 1 to 2 hours since you took, or are due to take, dicyclomine. Your mouth may get dry. Chewing sugarless gum or sucking hard candy, and drinking plenty of water will help.

What side effects may I notice from taking dicyclomine?

Side effects that you should report to your prescriber or health care professional as soon as possible:
- agitation, nervousness, confusion
- blurred vision and other eye problems
- decreased sweating
- difficulty swallowing
- dizziness, drowsiness

- fast or slow heartbeat
- hallucinations (seeing or hearing things that are not really there)
- pain or difficulty passing urine
- slurred speech
- unusual weakness or tiredness
- vomiting

Side effects that usually do not require medical attention (report to your prescriber or health care professional if they continue or are bothersome):

- constipation
- difficulty sleeping

- dry mouth, change in taste
- headache
- increased sensitivity of the eyes to light
- nausea
- sexual difficulty (impotence)

Where can I keep my medicine?

Keep out of the reach of children in a container that small children cannot open. Store at room temperature below 30 degrees C (86 degrees F). Protect from light. Throw away any unused medicine after the expiration date.

Didanosine, ddI, chewable tablets, and delayed-release capsules

VIDEX® EC;
250 mg; Capsule,
Delayed Release
Pellets
Bristol Myers Squibb
Co

VIDEX®;
150 mg; Tablet,
Chewable
Bristol Myers Squibb
Co

What are didanosine, ddI, delayed-release capsules?

DIDANOSINE, ddI (Videx®, Videx® EC) is an antiviral drug called a nucleoside reverse transcriptase inhibitor or NRTI. Didanosine is used to treat human immunodeficiency virus (HIV) infection. Didanosine may reduce the amount of HIV in the blood and increase the number of CD4 cells (T-cells) in the blood. Didanosine is used in combination with other drugs to treat the HIV virus. Didanosine will not cure or prevent HIV infection or AIDS. You may still develop other infections or conditions associated with HIV. Generic didanosine delayed-release capsules are available; however, generic chewable tablets are not available.

What should my health care professional know before I take didanosine, ddI?

They need to know if you have any of these conditions:

- frequently drink alcoholic beverages
- gout
- high cholesterol
- kidney disease
- liver disease
- pancreatitis
- tingling or numbness in the hands or feet
- an unusual or allergic reaction to didanosine, other medicines, foods, dyes, or preservatives
- pregnant or trying to get pregnant
- breast-feeding

How should I take this medicine?

Take didanosine capsules by mouth. Follow the directions on the prescription label. Take your doses at regular intervals. Do not take your medicine more often than directed. To help to make sure that your anti-HIV therapy works as well as possible, be very careful to take all of your medicine exactly as prescribed. Do not stop taking except on your prescriber's advice.

Contact your pediatrician or health care professional regarding the use of this medicine in children. Special care may be needed.

Capsules: Swallow the capsule whole; do not open it. Take didanosine capsules at least 30 minutes before or 2 hours after eating; do not take with food.

Chewable tablets: You should take at least 2 tablets per dose. Do not swallow whole. Tablets should be chewed or dissolved in liquid before swallowing. If you chew tablets, make sure to chew completely and swallow with a drink of water. To dissolve tablets, drop tablets in at least 1 ounce (2 teaspoons) of water or clear apple juice only. Stir until tablets are completely dissolved, then drink solution. The solution must be used within 1 hour.

What if I miss a dose?

If you miss a dose, take it as soon as you can. If it is almost time for your next dose, take only that dose. Do not take double or extra doses.

What may interact with didanosine, ddI?

- alcohol
- allopurinol
- antacids that contain aluminum or magnesium
- delavirdine
- ganciclovir
- hydroxyurea
- methadone
- nelfinavir
- ribavirin
- stavudine, d4T
- tenofovir
- valganciclovir
- zalcitabine

Tell your prescriber or health care professional about all other medicines that you are taking, including nonprescription medicines, nutritional supplements, or herbal products. Also tell your prescriber or health care professional if you are a frequent user of drinks with caffeine or alcohol, if you smoke, or if you use illegal drugs. These may affect the way your medicine works. Check with your health care professional before stopping or starting any of your medicines.

What should I watch for while taking didanosine, ddI?

Visit your prescriber or health care professional for regular checks on your progress. Discuss any new symptoms with your prescriber or health care professional. Alcohol can increase the risk of developing severe side effects when taken with didanosine. Avoid alcoholic drinks while you are taking didanosine. Do not treat yourself for nausea, vomiting, or stomach pain. Call your prescriber or health care professional for advice. Tell your prescriber or health care professional if you get tingling, pain or numbness in your hands or feet. Didanosine will not cure HIV and you can still get other illnesses or complications associated with your disease. Taking didanosine does not reduce the risk of passing HIV infection to others through sexual or blood contact. It is best to avoid sexual contact so that you do not spread the disease to others. For any sexual contact, use a condom. Be careful about cuts, abrasions and other possible sources of blood contact. Never share a needle or syringe with anyone.

What side effects may I notice from taking didanosine, ddI?

Other drugs you are taking with didanosine may affect the severity and occurrence of side effects you experience. Not all the side effects listed occur in everyone. If you notice an unusual side effect, contact your health care provider.

Side effects that you should report to your prescriber or health care professional as soon as possible:
- changes in body appearance (such as weight gain or loss around the waist and/or face)
- changes in your eye sight
- fever or chills, sore throat
- nausea and vomiting
- stomach pain
- tingling, pain or numbness in the hands or feet
- rash, itching
- unusual bleeding or bruising
- unusual tiredness or weakness

Side effects that usually do not require medical attention (report to your prescriber or health care professional if they continue or are bothersome):
- diarrhea
- dry mouth or eyes
- gas
- headache
- heartburn
- muscle and joint pain
- stomach upset

Where can I keep my medicine?

Keep out of the reach of children in a container that small children cannot open. Store at room temperature between 15 and 30 degrees C (59 and 86 degrees F). Throw away any unused medicine after the expiration date.

Diflunisal tablets

DOLOBID®;
250 mg; Tablet
Merck and Co Inc

DOLOBID®;
500 mg; Tablet
Merck and Co Inc

What are diflunisal tablets?

DIFLUNISAL (Dolobid®) reduces the joint pain, stiffness, inflammation, or swelling caused by rheumatoid arthritis (rheumatism) and osteoarthritis. It also relieves mild to moderate pain. Generic diflunisal tablets are available.

What should my health care professional know before I take diflunisal?

They need to know if you have any of these conditions:
- anemia
- asthma, especially aspirin sensitive asthma
- bleeding disorders, such as hemophilia
- cigarette smoker
- dental disease
- diabetes
- heart or circulation problems, such as heart failure or leg edema (fluid retention)
- high blood pressure
- if you drink more than 3 alcohol-containing beverages a day

- kidney disease
- liver disease
- stomach or duodenal ulcers
- systemic lupus erythematosus
- taking medicines that make you bleed easily such as anticoagulants ("blood thinners")
- ulcerative colitis
- an unusual or allergic reaction to aspirin, other salicylates, other NSAIDs, other medicines, foods, dyes or preservatives
- pregnant or trying to get pregnant
- breast-feeding

How should I take this medicine?

Take diflunisal tablets by mouth. Follow the directions on the prescription label. Swallow the tablets whole with a full glass of water. You may take diflunisal with milk or food if it upsets your stomach. Take your doses at regular intervals. Do not take your medicine more often than directed. Contact your pediatrician or health care professional regarding the use of this medicine in children. Special care may be needed.

What if I miss a dose?

If you miss a dose, take it as soon as you can. If it is almost time for your next dose, take only that dose. Do not take double or extra doses.

What may interact with diflunisal?

- acetaminophen
- alcohol
- alendronate
- aspirin and aspirin-like medicines
- cidofovir
- cyclosporine
- drospirenone; ethinyl estradiol (Yasmin®)
- herbal products that contain feverfew, garlic, ginger, or ginkgo biloba
- lithium
- medicines for high blood pressure
- medicines that affect platelets
- medicines that treat or prevent blood clots such as warfarin and other "blood thinners"
- methotrexate
- other anti-inflammatory drugs (such as ibuprofen or prednisone)
- water pills (diuretics)

Tell your prescriber or health care professional about all other medicines you are taking, including non-prescription medicines, nutritional supplements, or herbal products. Also tell your prescriber or health care professional if you are a frequent user of drinks with caffeine or alcohol, if you smoke, or if you use illegal drugs. These may affect the way your medicine works. Check with your health care professional before stopping or starting any of your medicines.

What should I watch for while taking diflunisal?

Let your prescriber or health care professional know if your pain continues, do not take with other pain medicine without advice. If you get flu-like symptoms (fever, chills, muscle aches, and pains), call your prescriber or health care professional; do not treat yourself. To reduce unpleasant effects on your throat and stomach, take diflunisal with a full glass of water and never just before lying down. If you notice black, tarry stools or experience severe stomach pain and vomit blood or what looks like coffee grounds, notify your health care prescriber immediately. If you are taking medicines that affect the clotting of your blood, such as aspirin or blood thinners such as Coumadin®, talk to your health care provider or prescriber before taking this medicine.

Smoking cigarettes or drinking alcohol may increase irritation to your stomach and can make it more susceptible to adverse reactions from diflunisal. If you are going to have surgery or dental work, tell your prescriber or health care professional that you are taking diflunisal. It is especially important not to use diflunisal during the last 3 months of pregnancy unless specifically directed to do so by your health care provider. Diflunisal may cause problems in the unborn child or complications during delivery.

What side effects may I notice from taking diflunisal?

Elderly patients are at increased risk for developing side effects.

Side effects that you should report to your prescriber or health care professional as soon as possible:

- signs of bleeding from the stomach—black tarry stools, blood in the urine, unusual tiredness or weakness, vomiting blood or vomit that looks like coffee grounds
- signs of an allergic reaction—difficulty breathing or wheezing, skin rash, redness, blistering or peeling skin, hives, or itching, swelling of eyelids, throat, lips
- blurred vision
- change in the amount of urine passed
- difficulty swallowing, severe heartburn or burning, pain in throat
- pain or difficulty passing urine
- stomach pain or cramps
- swelling of feet or ankles
- yellowing of eyes or skin

Side effects that usually do not require medical attention (report to your prescriber or health care professional if they continue or are bothersome):

- constipation
- diarrhea
- dizziness
- drowsiness
- gas
- headache
- heartburn
- nausea, vomiting

Where can I keep my medicine?

Keep out of the reach of children in a container that small children cannot open. Store at room temperature between 15 and 30 degrees C (59 and 86 degrees F). Keep container tightly closed. Throw away any unused medicine after the expiration date.

D

Digoxin tablets or capsules

LANOXIN®;
0.25 mg; Tablet
Glaxo Wellcome

LANOXICAPS®;
0.2 mg; Capsule
Glaxo Wellcome

D

What are digoxin tablets or capsules?

DIGOXIN (Lanoxin®, Lanoxicaps®) is a cardiac gly-coside that can help a weakened heart to function properly. Digoxin increases the strength of the heart muscle, helps to maintain a normal heart rhythm, and helps to remove excess water from the body. Digoxin can relieve symptoms of congestive heart failure, a con-dition that reduces the ability of the heart to pump enough blood through the body. These symptoms in-clude swelling of the feet and legs, difficulty breathing, and extreme tiredness or weakness. It can also help to regulate heart rhythm problems. Generic digoxin tablets are available, but not generic digoxin capsules.

What should my health care professional know before I receive digoxin?

They need to know if you have any of these conditions:
- heart disease
- heart rhythm disorders such as slow heart rate or heart block, sick sinus syndrome, ventricular arrhyth-mias, Wolff-Parkinson-White syndrome, or Adams-Stokes syndrome
- kidney disease
- liver disease
- lung disease
- over- or underactive thyroid
- recent heart attack
- too much calcium, potassium, or magnesium in the body
- an unusual or allergic reaction to digoxin, other medi-cines, foods, dyes, or preservatives
- pregnant or trying to get pregnant
- breast-feeding

How should I take this medicine?

Take digoxin tablets or capsules by mouth. Follow the directions on the prescription label. Swallow the tab-lets or capsules with a drink of water. It is best to take digoxin on an empty stomach, at least 1 hour before, or 2 hours after meals. Take your doses at regular inter-vals. Do not take your medicine more often than di-rected. Contact your pediatrician or health care profes-sional regarding the use of this medicine in children. Special care may be needed. Do not administer adult preparations to children. Elderly patients over 65 years old may have a stronger reaction to this medicine and may need smaller doses.

What if I miss a dose?

If you miss a dose, take it as soon as you can (if you only take one dose a day, not more than 12 hours since your dose was due). If it is almost time for your next dose, take only that dose. Do not take double or extra doses.

What may interact with digoxin?

- acarbose
- agents used to treat cancer
- alprazolam, diazepam
- amphotericin B
- antacids
- barbiturate medicines for inducing sleep or treating seizures (convulsions)
- beta blockers, often used for high blood pressure or heart problems
- calcium, magnesium, or potassium salts
- captopril
- certain medicines used to decrease cholesterol (cholestyramine, colestipol, atorvastatin, fluvastatin, simvastatin)
- clarithromycin or erythromycin
- cyclosporine
- diet pills (stimulants) or drugs used to control weight
- diltiazem
- felodipine
- gatifloxacin
- herbal products such as flaxseed, ginger, ginseng, haw-thorn, St. John's wort
- hormones such as prednisone or cortisone
- indomethacin
- medicine for colds and breathing difficulties
- medicines to control heart rhythm (dofetilide, amio-darone, sotalol and others)
- metformin
- neomycin
- neomycin
- omeprazole
- phenytoin
- psyllium
- quinine
- rabeprazole
- rifampin
- sevelamer
- sodium polystyrene sulfonate
- spironolactone
- succinylcholine
- sulfasalazine
- tetracycline antibiotics (doxycycline, tetracycline)
- thyroid hormones
- tramadol
- trimethoprim
- verapamil
- water pills (diuretics)

Tell your prescriber or health care professional about all other medicines you are taking, including non-pre-scription medicines, nutritional supplements, or herbal products. Also tell your prescriber or health care profes-sional if you are a frequent user of drinks with caffeine or alcohol, if you smoke, or if you use illegal drugs.

These may affect the way your medicine works. Check with your health care professional before stopping or starting any of your medicines.

What should I watch for while taking digoxin?

Visit your prescriber or health care professional for regular checks on your progress. Do not stop taking your digoxin without your prescriber's advice, even if you feel better. Do not change the brand you are taking, other brands may affect you differently. Check your heart rate (pulse) and blood pressure regularly while you are taking digoxin. Ask your prescriber or health care professional what your heart rate and blood pressure should be, and when you should contact him or her. Your prescriber or health care professional also may schedule regular blood tests and electrocardiograms to check your progress. Digoxin tablets are easily confused with other look-alike tablets. This can have serious consequences. If you take other tablets that look similar, ask your pharmacist how to avoid mix-ups. Watch your diet. Less digoxin may be absorbed from the stomach if you have a diet high in bran fiber. If you are going to have surgery, tell your prescriber or health care professional that you are taking digoxin. Do not take antacids, or treat yourself with non-prescription medicines for pain, allergies, coughs or colds, without advice from your prescriber or health care professional. You will be able to take some of these medicines if you space doses several hours apart.

What side effects may I notice from taking digoxin?

Side effects that you should report to your prescriber or health care professional as soon as possible:

- anxiousness or nervousness
- changes in color vision (more yellow color), blurred vision, eyes sensitive to light, light flashes, or halos around bright lights
- changes in behavior, mood, or mental ability
- chest pain or palpitations
- confusion
- diarrhea, or constipation
- dizziness or drowsiness
- fainting spells
- fast heartbeat (more likely in children)
- headache
- irregular, slow heartbeat (less than 50 beats per minute)
- loss of appetite
- nausea, vomiting
- skin rash or itching
- stomach pain
- tingling or numbness in the hands or feet
- unusual bruising, or pinpoint red spots on the skin
- weakness or tiredness

Side effects that usually do not require medical attention (report to your prescriber or health care professional if they continue or are bothersome):

- breast enlargement in men and women
- sexual problems such as impotence

Where can I keep my medicine?

Keep out of the reach of children in a container that small children cannot open. Store at room temperature between 15 and 25 degrees C (59 and 77 degrees F). Protect from light. Throw away any unused medicine after the expiration date.

Diltiazem extended-release capsules or tablets

CARDIZEM® LA; 240 mg; Tablet, Extended Release Kos Pharmaceuticals Inc

CARTIA® XT; 120 mg; Capsule, Extended Release Andrx Pharmaceuticals Inc

What are diltiazem sustained-release capsules and tablets?

DILTIAZEM (Cardizem® CD, Cardizem® LA, Cartia XT™, Dilacor XR®, Diltia XT™, Tiazac®, Taztia XT™, and others) is a calcium-channel blocker. It affects the amount of calcium found in your heart and muscle cells. This results in relaxation of blood vessels, which can reduce the amount of work the heart has to do. Diltiazem reduces high blood pressure (hypertension). It is not a cure. Diltiazem may also be used to relieve angina (chest pain). Generic diltiazem extended-release capsules are available. Extended-release capsules from different companies do not always act the same way in the body. If you are used to one product, it is not a good idea to switch products without approval from your prescriber. Generic diltiazem sustained-release tablets are not available.

What should my health care professional know before I take diltiazem?

They need to know if you have any of these conditions:

- heart problems, low blood pressure, irregular heartbeat
- liver disease
- previous heart attack
- an unusual or allergic reaction to diltiazem, other medicines, foods, dyes, or preservatives
- pregnant or trying to get pregnant
- breast-feeding

How should I take this medicine?

Take diltiazem extended-release capsules or tablets by mouth. Follow the directions on the prescription label. Swallow the capsules or tablets whole with a drink of water, do not crush or chew. Most diltiazem extended-release products may be taken with or without food. However, Dilacor-XR® and Diltia XT™ extended-release capsules are recommended to taken on an empty stomach. Do not significantly increase grapefruit juice intake while taking this drug, or avoid grapefruit juice if possible. Take your doses at regular intervals. Do not take your medicine more often then directed. Do not stop taking except on your prescriber's advice. Contact your pediatrician or health care professional regarding the use of this medicine in children. Special care may be needed.

What if I miss a dose?

If you miss a dose, take it as soon as you can. If it is almost time for your next dose, take only that dose. Do not take double or extra doses.

What may interact with diltiazem?

Do not take Diltiazem with any of the following:

- astemizole
- cisapride
- grapefruit juice
- pimozide
- terfenadine

Diltiazem may also interact with the following medications:

- alfuzosin
- alosetron
- anti-inflammatory drugs (NSAIDs, such as ibuprofen)
- aspirin
- barbiturates such as phenobarbital
- bosentan
- certain antibiotics (clarithromycin, erythromycin, telithromycin, troleandomycin)
- certain medicines used to treat cancer
- certain medicines to treat migraine (ergotamine, dihydroergotamine, methysergide)
- cevimeline
- cilostazol
- cimetidine
- clonidine
- cyclosporine
- fentanyl
- galantamine
- herbal or dietary supplements such as ginger, gingko biloba, ginseng, hawthorn, ma huang (ephedra), melatonin, St. John's wort, went yeast
- lithium
- local anesthetics or general anesthetics
- medicines for anxiety or difficulty sleeping (examples: alprazolam, buspirone, midazolam, triazolam)
- medicines for depression or mental problems (imipramine, fluoxetine, fluvoxamine, nefazodone, ziprasidone)
- medicines for fungal infections (fluconazole, itraconazole, ketoconazole, voriconazole)
- medicines for heart-rhythm problems (amiodarone, digoxin, disopyramide, dofetilide, encainide, flecainide, moricizine, procainamide, quinidine)
- medicines for high cholesterol (atorvastatin, cerivastatin, colesevelam, lovastatin, simvastatin)
- medicines for high blood pressure or heart problems
- medicines for HIV infection or AIDS
- medicines for prostate problems
- medicines for seizures (carbamazepine, clonazepam, ethosuximide, phenobarbital, phenytoin, primidone, zonisamide)
- methadone
- rifampin, rifabutin, or rifapentine
- sildenafil
- sirolimus
- tacrolimus
- theophylline or aminophylline
- water pills (diuretics)
- yohimbine
- zafirlukast
- zileuton

Tell your prescriber or health care professional about all other medicines you are taking, including non-prescription medicines, nutritional supplements, or herbal products. Also tell your prescriber or health care professional if you are a frequent user of drinks with caffeine or alcohol, if you smoke, or if you use illegal drugs. These may affect the way your medicine works. Check with your health care professional before stopping or starting any of your medicines.

What should I watch for while taking diltiazem?

Check your blood pressure and pulse rate regularly; this is important while you are taking diltiazem. Ask your prescriber or health care professional what your blood pressure and pulse rate should be and when you should contact him or her. You may feel dizzy or lightheaded. Do not drive, use machinery, or do anything that needs mental alertness until you know how diltiazem affects you. To reduce the risk of dizzy or fainting spells, do not sit or stand up quickly, especially if you are an older patient. Avoid alcoholic drinks; they can make you more dizzy or increase flushing and rapid heartbeats. If you are going to have surgery, tell your prescriber or health care professional that you are taking diltiazem. Do not suddenly stop taking diltiazem. Ask your prescriber or health care professional how to gradually reduce the dose.

What side effects may I notice from taking diltiazem?

Side effects that you should report to your prescriber or health care professional as soon as possible:

- confusion, mental depression
- fainting spells, lightheadedness
- redness, blistering, peeling or loosening of the skin, including inside the mouth
- skin rash, itching
- slow heartbeat, irregular heartbeat
- swelling of the feet and ankles
- unusual weakness or tiredness
- unusual bleeding or bruising, pinpoint red spots on the skin

D

Side effects that usually do not require medical attention (report to your prescriber or health care professional if they continue or are bothersome):

- constipation or diarrhea
- difficulty sleeping
- drowsiness or dizziness
- facial flushing
- headache
- nausea, vomiting
- sexual dysfunction

Where can I keep my medicine?

Keep out of the reach of children in a container that small children cannot open. Store at room temperature between 15 and 30 degrees C (59 and 86 degrees F). Protect from humidity. Throw away any unused medicine after the expiration date.

Diltiazem tablets

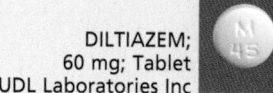

DILTIAZEM;
60 mg; Tablet
UDL Laboratories Inc

What are diltiazem tablets?

DILTIAZEM (Cardizem®) is a calcium-channel blocker. It affects the amount of calcium found in your heart and muscle cells. This results in relaxation of blood vessels, which can reduce the amount of work the heart has to do. Diltiazem relieves different types of chest pain (angina); it is not a cure. Generic diltiazem tablets are available.

What should my health care professional know before I take diltiazem?

They need to know if you have any of these conditions:

- heart problems, low blood pressure, irregular heartbeat
- liver disease
- previous heart attack
- an unusual or allergic reaction to diltiazem, other medicines, foods, dyes or preservatives
- pregnant or trying to get pregnant
- breast-feeding

How should I take this medicine?

Take diltiazem tablets by mouth. Follow the directions on the prescription label. Swallow the tablets with a drink of water. Take diltiazem tablets on an empty stomach, at least 1 hour before or 2 hours after food. Do not significantly increase grapefruit juice intake while taking this drug, or avoid grapefruit juice if possible. Take your doses at regular intervals. Do not take your medicine more often then directed. Do not stop taking except on your prescriber's advice. Contact your pediatrician or health care professional regarding the use of this medicine in children. Special care may be needed.

What if I miss a dose?

If you miss a dose, take it as soon as you can. If it is almost time for your next dose, take only that dose. Do not take double or extra doses.

What may interact with diltiazem?

Do not take Diltiazem with any of the following:

- astemizole
- cisapride
- grapefruit juice
- pimozide
- terfenadine

Diltiazem may also interact with the following medications:

- alfuzosin
- alosetron
- anti-inflammatory drugs (NSAIDs, such as ibuprofen)
- aspirin
- barbiturates such as phenobarbital
- bosentan
- certain antibiotics (clarithromycin, erythromycin, telithromycin, troleandomycin)
- certain medicines used to treat cancer
- certain medicines to treat migraine (ergotamine, dihydroergotamine, methysergide)
- cevimeline
- cilostazol
- cimetidine
- clonidine
- cyclosporine
- fentanyl
- galantamine
- herbal or dietary supplements such as ginger, gingko biloba, ginseng, hawthorn, ma huang (ephedra), melatonin, St. John's wort, went yeast
- lithium
- local anesthetics or general anesthetics
- medicines for anxiety or difficulty sleeping (examples: alprazolam, buspirone, midazolam, triazolam)
- medicines for depression or mental problems (imipramine, fluoxetine, fluvoxamine, nefazodone, ziprasidone)
- medicines for fungal infections (fluconazole, itraconazole, ketoconazole, voriconazole)
- medicines for heart-rhythm problems (amiodarone, digoxin, disopyramide, dofetilide, encainide, flecainide, moricizine, procainamide, quinidine)
- medicines for high cholesterol (atorvastatin, cerivastatin, colesevelam, lovastatin, simvastatin)
- medicines for high blood pressure or heart problems
- medicines for HIV infection or AIDS
- medicines for prostate problems
- medicines for seizures (carbamazepine, clonazepam, ethosuximide, phenobarbital, phenytoin, primidone, zonisamide)
- methadone
- rifampin, rifabutin or rifapentine

- sildenafil
- sirolimus
- tacrolimus
- theophylline or aminophylline
- water pills (diuretics)
- yohimbine
- zafirlukast
- zileuton

Tell your prescriber or health care professional about all other medicines you are taking, including non-prescription medicines, nutritional supplements, or herbal products. Also tell your prescriber or health care professional if you are a frequent user of drinks with caffeine or alcohol, if you smoke, or if you use illegal drugs. These may affect the way your medicine works. Check with your health care professional before stopping or starting any of your medicines.

What should I watch for while taking diltiazem?

Check your blood pressure and pulse rate regularly; this is important while you are taking diltiazem. Ask your prescriber or health care professional what your blood pressure and pulse rate should be and when you should contact him or her. You may feel dizzy or lightheaded. Do not drive, use machinery, or do anything that needs mental alertness until you know how diltiazem affects you. To reduce the risk of dizzy or fainting spells, do not sit or stand up quickly, especially if you are an older patient. Avoid alcoholic drinks; they can make you more dizzy or increase flushing and rapid heartbeats. If you are going to have surgery, tell your prescriber or health care professional that you are taking diltiazem. Do not suddenly stop taking diltiazem. Ask your prescriber or health care professional how to gradually reduce the dose.

What side effects may I notice from taking diltiazem?

Side effects that you should report to your prescriber or health care professional as soon as possible:
- confusion, mental depression
- fainting spells, lightheadedness
- redness, blistering, peeling or loosening of the skin, including inside the mouth
- skin rash, itching
- slow heartbeat, irregular heartbeat
- swelling of the feet and ankles
- unusual weakness or tiredness
- unusual bleeding or bruising, pinpoint red spots on the skin

Side effects that usually do not require medical attention (report to your prescriber or health care professional if they continue or are bothersome):
- constipation or diarrhea
- difficulty sleeping
- drowsiness or dizziness
- facial flushing
- headache
- nausea, vomiting
- sexual dysfunction

Where can I keep my medicine?

Keep out of the reach of children in a container that small children cannot open. Store at room temperature between 15 and 30 degrees C (59 and 86 degrees F). Protect from humidity. Throw away any unused medicine after the expiration date.

Dimenhydrinate capsules, tablets and chewable tablets

MOTION SICKNESS;
Tablet; 50 mg
Leader Brand
Products

DRAMAMINE®;
Tablet, Chewable;
50 mg
Pfizer Consumer
Healthcare

What are dimenhydrinate tablets and capsules?

DIMENHYDRINATE (Dramamine®, Motion Sickness) is an antihistamine. It helps to prevent nausea, vomiting, or dizziness associated with motion sickness, and to treat or prevent vertigo (extreme dizziness or a sensation that you or your surroundings are tilting or spinning around). Generic dimenhydrinate tablets and capsules are available.

What should my health care professional know before I take dimenhydrinate?

They need to know if you have any of these conditions:
- asthma or other lung disease
- constipation
- glaucoma or other eye disease
- head injury
- heart disease
- heart rhythm problems (irregular, fast, or slow heart rate)
- high or low blood pressure
- liver disease
- pain or difficulty passing urine (or other bladder problems)
- phenylketonuria
- porphyria
- prostate trouble
- seizure disorder (convulsions)
- stomach or intestinal problems
- wear contact lenses
- an unusual or allergic reaction to dimenhydrinate, aspirin, tartrazine dye, other medicines, foods, dyes, or preservatives
- pregnant or trying to get pregnant
- breast-feeding

How should I take this medicine?

Take dimenhydrinate tablets by mouth. Follow the directions on the prescription label. Swallow the tablets or capsules with a drink of water (chewable tablets can be chewed or swallowed whole). If you are using dimenhydrinate to prevent motion sickness, take the dose at least $1/2$ to 1 hour before travel. If dimenhydrinate upsets your stomach, take it with food or milk. Take your doses at regular intervals. Do not take your medicine more often than directed. Elderly patients over 65 years old may have a stronger reaction to this medicine and need smaller doses. Contact your pediatrician or health care professional regarding the use of this medicine in children. Special care may be needed.

What if I miss a dose?

If you miss a dose, use it as soon as you can. If it is almost time for your next dose, use only that dose. Do not use double or extra doses.

What may interact with dimenhydrinate?

- alcohol
- barbiturate medicines for inducing sleep or treating seizures (convulsions)
- medicines for anxiety or sleeping problems, such as diazepam or temazepam
- medicines for hay fever and other allergies
- medicines for mental depression
- medicines for mental problems and psychotic disturbances
- medicines for movement abnormalities as in Parkinson's disease
- some medicines for gastrointestinal problems

Tell your prescriber or health care professional about all other medicines you are taking, including non-prescription medicines, nutritional supplements, or herbal products. Also tell your prescriber or health care professional if you are a frequent user of drinks with caffeine or alcohol, if you smoke, or if you use illegal drugs. These may affect the way your medicine works. Check with your health care professional before stopping or starting any of your medicines.

What should I watch for while taking dimenhydrinate?

Tell your prescriber or health care professional if your symptoms do not improve in 1 or 2 days. If you are taking dimenhydrinate on a regular schedule, visit your prescriber or health care professional for regular checks on your progress. You may get drowsy or dizzy. Do not

drive, use machinery, or do anything that needs mental alertness until you know how dimenhydrinate affects you. To reduce the risk of dizzy or fainting spells, do not stand or sit up quickly, especially if you are an older patient. Alcohol may increase dizziness and drowsiness. Avoid alcoholic drinks. Your mouth may get dry. Chewing sugarless gum or sucking hard candy, and drinking plenty of water will help. Dimenhydrinate may cause dry eyes and blurred vision. If you wear contact lenses you may feel some discomfort. Lubricating drops may help. See your ophthalmologist if the problem does not go away or is severe. If you are receiving skin tests for allergies, tell your physician you are using dimenhydrinate.

What side effects may I notice from taking dimenhydrinate?

Side effects that you should report to your prescriber or health care professional as soon as possible:

- blurred vision
- confusion
- excitability, restlessness, nervousness, or not able to sleep (more likely in children)
- fainting spells
- incoordination
- irregular, slow or fast heartbeat, palpitations, or chest pain
- pain or difficulty passing urine
- ringing in the ears
- seizures (convulsions)
- persistent or unusual rash or hives
- wheezing

Side effects that usually do not require medical attention (report to your prescriber or health care professional if they continue or are bothersome):

- dizziness
- drowsiness, weakness, or tiredness
- dry mouth
- headache
- loss of appetite
- reddening of the skin
- sensitivity to light
- stomach upset, nausea, vomiting, diarrhea or constipation

Where can I keep my medicine?

Keep out of the reach of children. Store upright at room temperature between 20 and 25 degrees C (68 and 77 degrees F) in a tight container; do not freeze. Throw away any unused medicine after the expiration date.

Diphenhydramine tablets or capsules

BENADRYL®
ALLERGY
ULTRATAB®;
25 mg; Tablet
Pfizer Consumer
Healthcare

DIPHENHYDRAMINE;
50 mg; Capsule
Barr Laboratories
Inc

What are diphenhydramine tablets or capsules?

DIPHENHYDRAMINE (Banophen®, Benadryl®, Benadryl® Allergy Ultratab®) is an antihistamine that has many uses. It relieves irritant cough, symptoms of hay fever (allergic rhinitis), hives (rash or itching), and other allergic reactions, motion sickness and vertigo (dizziness and loss of balance), Parkinson's disease, and reduces some side effects associated with the use of antipsychotics. Generic diphenhydramine tablets or capsules are available, with or without a prescription.

What should my health care professional know before I take diphenhydramine?

They need to know if you have any of these conditions:
- asthma or chronic obstructive lung disease (COPD)
- glaucoma
- high blood pressure or heart disease
- liver disease
- other chronic illness
- prostate trouble
- pain or difficulty passing urine
- ulcers or other stomach problems
- an unusual or allergic reaction to diphenhydramine, other medicines foods, dyes, or preservatives such as sulfites
- pregnant or trying to get pregnant
- breast-feeding

How should I take this medicine?

Take diphenhydramine tablets or capsules by mouth. Follow the directions on the prescription label. Take diphenhydramine with food or milk if it upsets your stomach. Take your doses at regular intervals. Do not take your medicine more often than directed. If you are taking diphenhydramine to stop you from getting car (or travel) sick, take the first dose 30 to 60 minutes before you leave. Contact your pediatrician or health care professional regarding the use of this medicine in children. Special care may be needed.

What if I miss a dose?

If you miss a dose, take it as soon as you can. If it is almost time for your next dose, take only that dose. Do not take double doses.

What may interact with diphenhydramine?

- alcohol
- barbiturate medicines for inducing sleep or treating seizures (convulsions)
- medicines for anxiety or sleeping problems, such as diazepam or temazepam
- medicines for hay fever and other allergies
- medicines for mental depression
- medicines for mental problems and psychotic disturbances
- medicines for movement abnormalities as in Parkinson's disease, or for gastrointestinal problems

Tell your prescriber or health care professional about all other medicines you are taking, including non-prescription medicines, nutritional supplements, or herbal products. Also tell your prescriber or health care professional if you are a frequent user of drinks with caffeine or alcohol, if you smoke, or if you use illegal drugs. These may affect the way your medicine works. Check with your health care professional before stopping or starting any of your medicines.

What should I watch for while taking diphenhydramine?

Tell your prescriber or health care professional if your symptoms do not improve in 1 or 2 days. You may get drowsy or dizzy. Do not drive, use machinery, or do anything that needs mental alertness until you know how diphenhydramine affects you. To reduce the risk of dizzy or fainting spells, do not stand or sit up quickly, especially if you are an older patient. Alcohol may increase dizziness and drowsiness. Avoid alcoholic drinks. Your mouth may get dry. Chewing sugarless gum or sucking hard candy, and drinking plenty of water will help. Diphenhydramine may cause dry eyes and blurred vision. If you wear contact lenses you may feel some discomfort. Lubricating drops may help. See your ophthalmologist if the problem does not go away or is severe.

What side effects may I notice from taking diphenhydramine?

Side effects that you should report to your prescriber or health care professional as soon as possible:
- agitation, nervousness, excitability, not able to sleep (these are more likely in children)
- blurred vision
- dizziness or fainting spells
- irregular heartbeat, palpitations, or chest pain
- muscle or facial twitches
- pain or difficulty passing urine
- seizures (convulsions)

Call your prescriber or health care professional as soon as you can if you get any of these.

Side effects that usually do not require medical attention (report to your prescriber or health care professional if they continue or are bothersome):

- drowsiness, dizziness
- dry mouth
- headache
- loss of appetite
- stomach upset, nausea, vomiting, constipation or diarrhea

Where can I keep my medicine?

Keep out of the reach of children in a container that small children cannot open. Store at room temperature, between 15 and 30 degrees C (59 and 86 degrees F). Protect from moisture. Keep container tightly closed. Throw away any unused medicine after the expiration date.

Diphenoxylate tablets

DIPHENOXYLATE;
2.5 mg/0.025 mg;
Tablet
Ivax Pharmaceuticals
Inc

LOMOTIL®;
2.5 mg/0.025 mg;
Tablet
GD Searle LLC a
Subsidiary of
Pharmacia Company
Pfizer

What are diphenoxylate tablets?

DIPHENOXYLATE (Lomotil®) helps to control diarrhea. Small amounts of atropine are combined with diphenoxylate in available products. Generic diphenoxylate tablets are available.

What should my health care professional know before I take diphenoxylate?

They need to know if you have any of these conditions:
- bacterial food poisoning
- colitis
- dehydration
- Down's syndrome
- jaundice
- liver disease
- an unusual or allergic reaction to diphenoxylate, other medicines, foods, dyes, or preservatives
- pregnant or trying to get pregnant
- breast-feeding

How should I take this medicine?

Take diphenoxylate tablets by mouth. Follow the directions on the prescription label. Swallow the tablets with a drink of water. You can take the tablets with food. Take your doses at regular intervals. Do not take your medicine more often than directed. Once your diarrhea has been brought under control your prescriber or health care professional may reduce your doses. Contact your pediatrician or health care professional regarding the use of this medicine in children. Special care may be needed. Elderly patients may be more sensitive to the effects of diphenoxylate.

What if I miss a dose?

If you miss a dose, take it as soon as you can. If it is almost time for your next dose, take only that dose. Do not take double or extra doses.

What may interact with diphenoxylate?

- alcohol
- barbiturate medicines for inducing sleep or treating seizures (convulsions)
- medicines for anxiety or sleeping problems, such as diazepam or temazepam
- medicines for treating mental depression
- medicines for movement abnormalities as in Parkinson's disease, or for gastrointestinal problems
- naloxone
- naltrexone

Tell your prescriber or health care professional about all other medicines you are taking, including non-prescription medicines, nutritional supplements, or herbal products. Also tell your prescriber or health care professional if you are a frequent user of drinks with caffeine or alcohol, if you smoke, or if you use illegal drugs. These may affect the way your medicine works. Check with your health care professional before stopping or starting any of your medicines.

What should I watch for while taking diphenoxylate?

If your symptoms do not improve after taking diphenoxylate for two days, check with your prescriber or health care professional, you may have a problem that needs further evaluation. Check with your prescriber or health care professional at once if you develop a fever or bloody diarrhea. You may get drowsy or dizzy. Do not drive, use machinery, or do anything that needs mental alertness until you know how diphenoxylate affects you. Alcohol can increase possible drowsiness and dizziness; avoid alcoholic drinks. Your mouth may get dry. Sucking hard candy or chewing sugarless gum and drinking plenty of water can help. Drinking plenty of water can also help prevent dehydration that can occur with diarrhea. If you are going to have surgery, tell your prescriber or health care professional that you are taking diphenoxylate.

What side effects may I notice from taking diphenoxylate?

Serious side effects are rare at recommended doses; however, they can result from taking too large a dose; they include:
- bloated, swollen feeling
- blurred vision
- difficulty breathing, shortness of breath
- fast or irregular heartbeat
- stomach pain

Side effects that usually do not require medical attention (report to your prescriber or health care professional if they continue or are bothersome):

- drowsiness or dizziness
- dry mouth
- dry skin
- headache
- loss of appetite
- mood changes
- nausea, vomiting
- numbness or tingling in the hands and feet

Where can I keep my medicine?

Keep out of the reach of children in a container that small children cannot open. Accidental overdose can result in severe difficulty breathing, coma, permanent brain damage, and possibly death. Store at room temperature between 15 and 30 degrees C (59 and 86 degrees F). Protect from light. Keep container tightly closed. Throw away any unused medicine after the expiration date.

Dipyridamole tablets

PERSANTINE®;
50 mg; Tablet
Boehringer
Ingelheim
Pharmaceuticals Inc

PERSANTINE®;
75 mg; Tablet
Boehringer
Ingelheim
Pharmaceuticals Inc

What are dipyridamole tablets?

DIPYRIDAMOLE (Persantine®) helps to prevent blood clots and reduce the risk of related problems such as stroke, in patients who have had heart valve replacements. Generic dipyridamole tablets are available.

What should my health care professional know before I take dipyridamole?

They need to know if you have any of the following conditions:

- angina
- asthma
- low blood pressure
- an unusual or allergic reaction to dipyridamole, tartrazine dye, other medicines, foods, dyes, or preservatives
- pregnant or trying to get pregnant
- breast-feeding

How should I take this medicine?

Take dipyridamole tablets by mouth. Follow the directions on the prescription label. Swallow the tablets with a plenty of water (at least a full glass) to avoid stomach upset. Take on an empty stomach, at least 1 hour before or 2 hours after eating. Take your doses at regular intervals. Do not take your medicine more often than directed. Contact your pediatrician or health care professional regarding the use of this medicine in children. Special care may be needed.

What if I miss a dose?

If you miss a dose, take it as soon as you can. If it is almost time for your next dose, take only that dose. Do not take double or extra doses.

What may interact with dipyridamole?

- adenosine
- agents that dissolve blood clots
- anti-inflammatory drugs (NSAIDs, such as ibuprofen)
- aspirin
- cilostazol
- DHEA
- enoxaparin
- feverfew
- fish oil (omega-3 fatty acids) supplements
- garlic
- ginger
- ginkgo biloba
- horse chestnut
- pentoxifylline
- plicamycin
- ticlopidine
- valproic acid
- warfarin

Tell your prescriber or health care professional about all other medicines you are taking, including non-prescription medicines, nutritional supplements, or herbal products. Also tell your prescriber or health care professional if you are a frequent user of drinks with caffeine or alcohol, if you smoke, or if you use illegal drugs. These may affect the way your medicine works. Check with your health care professional before stopping or starting any of your medicines.

What should I watch for while taking dipyridamole?

Visit your prescriber or health care professional for regular checks on your progress. Do not stop taking dipyridamole except on your prescriber's advice. Check your heart rate and blood pressure regularly while you are taking dipyridamole. Ask your prescriber or health care professional what your heart rate and blood pressure should be, and when you should contact him or her. You may get dizzy, especially when you sit or stand up quickly. Do not drive, use machinery or do anything that needs mental alertness until you know how dipyridamole affects you. To reduce dizzy or fainting spells, do not sit or stand up quickly, especially if you are an older patient. Alcohol can increase dizziness and flushing. Avoid alcoholic drinks. Ask your prescriber

D

or health care professional before you take non-prescription pain relievers. Avoid aspirin and aspirin-containing products. If you are going to have surgery, tell your prescriber or health care professional that you are taking dipyridamole.

What side effects may I notice from taking dipyridamole?

Side effects that you should report to your prescriber or health care professional as soon as possible:
- fast, slow or irregular heartbeat
- palpitations, chest pain or tightness

Side effects that usually do not require medical attention (report to your prescriber or health care professional if they continue or are bothersome):

- dizziness
- diarrhea
- flushing
- headache
- muscle weakness
- nausea or vomiting
- skin rash
- stomach ache or cramps

Where can I keep my medicine?

Keep out of the reach of children in a container that small children cannot open. Store at room temperature below 30 degrees C (86 degrees F). Throw away any unused medicine after the expiration date.

Dirithromycin tablets

DYNABAC®; 250 mg; Tablet, Delayed Release Sanofi-Synthelabo Inc

D5-PAK DYNABAC; 250 mg; Tablet, Delayed Release Muro

What are dirithromycin tablets?

DIRITHROMYCIN (Dynabac®, D5-Pak Dynabac) is a macrolide antibiotic. Dirithromycin kills certain bacteria, or stops their growth. It treats respiratory (nose, throat, lung), and skin infections. It will not work for colds, flu, or other virus infections. Generic dirithromycin tablets are not yet available.

What should my health care professional know before I take dirithromycin?

They need to know if you have any of these conditions:
- liver disease
- stomach problems (especially colitis)
- other chronic illness
- an unusual or allergic reaction to dirithromycin or other macrolide antibiotics (such as erythromycin), foods, dyes, or preservatives
- pregnant or trying to get pregnant
- breast-feeding

How should I take this medicine?

Take dirithromycin tablets by mouth. Follow the directions on the prescription label. Swallow the tablets whole; do not break, crush, or chew. Take the tablets with a full glass of water. Take dirithromycin with food. Take your doses at regular intervals. Do not take your medicine more often than directed. Finish the full course prescribed by your prescriber or health care professional even if you think your condition is better. Do not stop taking except on your prescriber's advice.

What if I miss a dose?

If you miss a dose, take it as soon as you can. If it is almost time for your next dose, take only that dose. Do not take double or extra doses. There should be an interval of at least 6 hours between doses.

What may interact with dirithromycin?

- antacids
- digoxin
- cimetidine, nizatidine, famotidine or ranitidine
- oral contraceptives (birth control pills)
- pimozide

Tell your prescriber or health care professional about all other medicines you are taking, including non-prescription medicines, nutritional supplements, or herbal products. Also tell your prescriber or health care professional if you are a frequent user of drinks with caffeine or alcohol, if you smoke, or if you use illegal drugs. These may affect the way your medicine works. Check with your health care professional before stopping or starting any of your medicines.

What should I watch for while taking dirithromycin?

Tell your prescriber or health care professional if your symptoms do not improve in 2 to 3 days. If you get severe or bloody diarrhea, do not treat yourself. Call your prescriber or health care professional for advice. If you are going to have surgery, tell your prescriber or health care professional that you are taking dirithromycin.

What side effects may I notice from taking dirithromycin?

Side effects that you should report to your prescriber or health care professional as soon as possible:
- difficulty breathing
- fever
- severe or bloody diarrhea
- skin rash, hives, or itching
- swelling of the face, throat, or lips

Side effects that usually do not require medical attention (report to your prescriber or health care professional if they continue or are bothersome):

- diarrhea
- headache
- nausea, vomiting
- stomach pains or cramps

Where can I keep my medicine?

Keep out of the reach of children in a container that small children cannot open. Store at room temperature between 15 and 30 degrees C (59 and 86 degrees F). Keep container tightly closed. Protect from light. Throw away any unused medicine after the expiration date.

Disopyramide capsules or extended-release capsules

NORPACE® CR;
150 mg; Capsule,
Extended Release
GD Searle LLC a
Subsidiary of
Pharmacia Company
Pfizer

NORPACE®;
150 mg; Capsule
GD Searle LLC a
Subsidiary of
Pharmacia Company
Pfizer

What are disopyramide capsules or extended-release capsules?

DISOPYRAMIDE (Norpace®, Norpace® CR) is an antiarrhythmic agent. Disopyramide can help the heart to return to and maintain a normal heart rhythm. Disopyramide helps to slow rapid heartbeats (tachycardia). Generic disopyramide capsules are available.

What should my health care professional know before I take disopyramide?

They need to know if you have any of these conditions:

- abnormal levels of potassium in the blood
- bladder obstruction
- diabetes
- glaucoma
- heart disease or problems other than rhythm and heart rate problems
- kidney disease
- liver disease
- myasthenia gravis
- prostate trouble
- an unusual or allergic reaction to disopyramide, other medicines, foods, dyes, or preservatives
- pregnant or trying to get pregnant
- breast-feeding

How should I take this medicine?

Take disopyramide capsules or extended-release capsules by mouth. Follow the directions on the prescription label. Swallow the capsules with a drink of water; do not suck or chew the extended-release capsules. Take your doses at regular intervals. Do not take your medicine more often than directed.

What if I miss a dose?

If you miss a dose, take it as soon as you can. If it is almost time for your next dose, take only that dose. Leave an interval of at least 4 hours between doses of regular capsules and 6 to 8 hours between doses of extended-release capsules. Do not take double or extra doses.

What may interact with disopyramide?

- arsenic trioxide
- astemizole
- bepridil
- beta-blockers, often used for high blood pressure or heart problems
- bosentan
- certain antibiotics (such as clarithromycin, erythromycin, gatifloxacin, grepafloxacin, levofloxacin, moxifloxacin, sparfloxacin)
- cisapride
- cyclobenzaprine
- ginger
- hawthorn
- lidocaine
- medicines for colds or breathing difficulties (including asthma)
- medicines for mental depression such as tricyclic antidepressants
- medicines for anxiety, mental problems or psychotic disturbances
- medicines for movement abnormalities as in Parkinson's disease, or for gastrointestinal problems
- medicines for seizures such as phenytoin, phenobarbital, carbamazepine
- medicines to control heart rhythm (examples: amiodarone, digoxin, dofetilide, sotalol, procainamide, quinidine)
- mexiletine
- pimozide
- potassium salts
- probucol
- rifampin
- ritonavir
- terfenadine
- warfarin

Tell your prescriber or health care professional about all other medicines you are taking, including non-prescription medicines, nutritional supplements, or herbal products. Also tell your prescriber or health care professional if you are a frequent user of drinks with caffeine or alcohol, if you smoke, or if you use illegal drugs. These may affect the way your medicine works. Check with your health care professional before stopping or starting any of your medicines.

D

What should I watch for while taking disopyramide?

Visit your prescriber or health care professional for regular checks on your progress. Do not stop taking disopyramide suddenly; this may cause serious, heart-related side effects. Check your heart rate (pulse) and blood pressure regularly while you are taking disopyramide. Ask your prescriber or health care professional what your heart rate and blood pressure should be, and when you should contact him or her. Your prescriber or health care professional also may schedule regular blood tests and electrocardiograms to check your progress. You may feel dizzy, or have blurred vision. Do not drive, use machinery, or do anything that needs mental alertness until you know how disopyramide affects you. To reduce the risk of dizzy or fainting spells, do not sit or stand up quickly, especially if you are an older patient. Alcohol can make you more dizzy, increase flushing and rapid heartbeats. Avoid alcoholic drinks. Your mouth may get dry. Chewing sugarless gum or sucking hard candy and drinking plenty of water will help. Disopyramide may cause dry eyes and blurred vision. If you wear contact lenses you may feel some discomfort. Lubricating drops may help. See your ophthalmologist if the problem does not go away or is severe. Be careful in hot weather. Disopyramide can reduce sweating and lower your tolerance to heat. Disopyramide may affect your blood sugar level. Check with your prescriber or health care professional, especially if you have congestive heart disease or diabetes. If you are going to have surgery, tell your prescriber or health care professional that you are taking disopyramide.

What side effects may I notice from taking disopyramide?

Side effects that you should report to your prescriber or health care professional as soon as possible:
- change in the amount of urine passed, or difficulty passing urine
- chest pain, palpitations
- confusion
- cool, pale skin
- difficulty breathing
- fever, chills, or sore throat
- headache
- lightheadedness or fainting spells
- muscle weakness
- skin rash, itching
- swelling of feet or legs
- unusual weakness or tiredness
- unusual weight increase
- unusual hunger
- yellowing of the skin or eyes

Side effects that usually do not require medical attention (report to your prescriber or health care professional if they continue or are bothersome):
- dizziness, drowsiness
- blurred vision, dry eyes
- dry mouth and throat
- constipation, or less likely, diarrhea
- nausea, vomiting
- sexual difficulties
- stomach pain or bloating

Where can I keep my medicine?

Keep out of the reach of children in a container that small children cannot open. Store at room temperature below 30 degrees C (86 degrees F). Throw away any unused medicine after the expiration date.

Disulfiram tablets

ANTABUSE®;
250 mg; Tablet
Odyssey Pharmaceuticals Inc

What are disulfiram tablets?

DISULFIRAM (Antabuse®) can help patients with an alcohol abuse problem not to drink alcohol. It is not a cure for alcoholism. When taken with alcohol, disulfiram produces very unpleasant effects, such as severe headache, flushing, vomiting and chest pain. Taking disulfiram is part of a recovery program that includes medical supervision and counseling. Generic disulfiram tablets are available.

What should my health care professional know before I take disulfiram?

They need to know if you have any of the following conditions:
- blood disease
- diabetes
- heart, kidney or liver disease
- recent exposure to alcohol, or any medicines containing alcohol
- seizures (convulsions)
- underactive thyroid
- an unusual or allergic reaction to disulfiram, pesticides or rubber products, other medicines, foods, dyes, or preservatives
- pregnant or trying to get pregnant
- breast-feeding

How should I take this medicine?

Take disulfiram tablets by mouth. You must never take disulfiram within 12 hours of taking alcohol. Follow the directions on the prescription label. Swallow the tablets with a drink of water. The tablets can be crushed and mixed with liquid before taking. Disulfiram is usually taken in the morning, but if it makes you drowsy you can take it at bedtime. Take your doses regularly.

Do not take your medicine more often than directed and do not stop taking except on your prescriber's advice.

What if I miss a dose?

If you miss a dose, take it as soon as you can. If it is almost time for your next dose, take only that dose. Do not take double or extra doses.

What may interact with disulfiram?

- alcohol
- amprenavir
- carbamazepine
- certain antibiotics such as chloramphenicol, or imipenem; cilastatin
- chlorzoxazone
- cimetidine
- cocaine
- fluconazole
- isoniazid
- certain medicines for anxiety or difficulty sleeping
- metronidazole
- phenytoin
- propranolol
- quinidine
- rifampin
- sertraline
- theophylline
- verapamil
- voriconazole
- warfarin

Tell your prescriber or health care professional about all other medicines you are taking, including non-prescription medicines, nutritional supplements, or herbal products. Also tell your prescriber or health care professional if you are a frequent user of drinks with caffeine or alcohol, if you smoke, or if you use illegal drugs. These may affect the way your medicine works. Check with your health care professional before stopping or starting any of your medicines.

What should I watch for while taking disulfiram?

Visit your prescriber or health care professional or counselor for regular checks on your progress. Do not stop taking disulfiram except on your prescriber's advice. Never take alcohol or use toiletries that contain alcohol. Always read labels carefully. Many cough syrups, liquid pain medications, tonics, mouthwash, after-shave lotions, colognes, liniments, vinegars, or sauces contain alcohol. Avoid inhaling the fumes of paints, paint thinners, or other products that contain organic solvents. Reactions can occur for up to 2 weeks after you stop taking disulfiram. The following reactions can occur if you take alcohol with, or within 14 days of stopping disulfiram therapy: blurred vision; chest pain and fast or pounding heartbeat; dizziness, lightheadedness, or fainting; nervousness and confusion; severe nausea, vomiting; increased sweating; increased thirst; throbbing headache and neck pain; weakness. Make sure that family members or others in your household know about this medicine and what to do in an emergency. They must never give you disulfiram if you have been drinking alcohol. You may get drowsy, dizzy or have blurred vision. Do not drive, use machinery, or do anything that needs mental alertness until you know how disulfiram affects you. Carry an identification card with your name, name and dose of medicine being used, and name and phone number of your prescriber or health care professional and/or person to contact in an emergency. Do not treat yourself with medicines for coughs, colds, or allergies while you are taking disulfiram; they may add to its effects. Ask your prescriber or health care professional for advice.

What side effects may I notice from taking disulfiram?

Side effects that you should report to your prescriber or health care professional as soon as possible:
- changes in vision
- confusion, disorientation, irritability
- numbness, pain, tingling in the hands or feet
- unusual weakness or tiredness
- yellowing of the skin or eyes

Side effects that usually do not require medical attention (report to your prescriber or health care professional if they continue or are bothersome):
- dizziness, drowsiness
- headache
- tiredness
- sexual difficulty (impotence)
- skin reactions

Where can I keep my medicine?

Keep out of the reach of children in a container that small children cannot open. Store at room temperature, approximately 25 degrees C (77 degrees F). Throw away any unused medicine after the expiration date.

Docusate tablets or capsules

CORRECTOL®
SOFTGEL EXTRA
GENTLE;
100 mg; Capsule
Schering Plough
Products Inc

SURFAK®;
240 mg; Capsule
Pfizer Consumer
Healthcare

What are docusate tablets or capsules?

DOCUSATE (Colace®, Correctol® Softgel Extra Gentle, Surfak®) is an emollient laxative or stool softener that helps prevent constipation and straining or discomfort associated with hard or dry stools. Generic docusate capsules are available.

What should my health care professional know before I take docusate?

They need to know if you have any of these conditions:
- severe constipation
- an unusual or allergic reaction to docusate, other medicines, foods, dyes, or preservatives
- pregnant or trying to get pregnant

How should I take this medicine?

Take docusate tablets or capsules by mouth. Follow the directions on the label. Swallow the tablets or capsules with a drink of water. Do not take your medicine more often than directed. Contact your pediatrician or health care professional regarding the use of this medicine in children. Special care may be needed.

What if I miss a dose?

If you miss a dose, take it as soon as you can. If it is almost time for your next dose, take only that dose. Do not take double or extra doses. Do not take regularly for more than one week.

What may interact with docusate?

- mineral oil

Do not take docusate without your prescriber's advice if you are taking prescription medicines.

What should I watch for while taking docusate?

Do not use for more than one week without advice from your prescriber or health care professional. Long-term use can make your body depend on the laxative for regular bowel movements. If your constipation keeps returning, check with your prescriber or health care professional. Always drink plenty of water while taking docusate, to help fight constipation.

What side effects may I notice from taking docusate?

Serious reactions to docusate are unlikely. Call your prescriber or health care professional if you have any unexplained effects.

Side effects that usually do not require medical attention (report to your prescriber or health care professional if they continue or are bothersome):
- diarrhea
- skin rash
- stomach cramps
- throat irritation

Where can I keep my medicine?

Keep out of the reach of children in a container that small children cannot open. Store at room temperature, approximately 25 degrees C (77 degrees F). Throw away any unused medicine after the expiration date.

Dofetilide capsules

TIKOSYN®;
250 mcg; Capsule
Pfizer Laboratories
Div Pfizer Inc

TIKOSYN®;
500 mcg; Capsule
Pfizer Laboratories
Div Pfizer Inc

What are dofetilide capsules?

DOFETILIDE (Tikosyn®) is a medicine that is given to patients with atrial fibrillation (irregular heartbeats). Atrial fibrillation happens when certain parts of the heart (the chambers known as atria) beat too fast or irregularly. You may get an uncomfortable feeling in your chest and "fluttering" or "palpitations." Dofetilide may help your heart to beat more regularly and stay beating regularly for a longer period of time. Generic dofetilide is not yet available.

What should my health care professional know before I take dofetilide?

They need to know if you have any of these conditions:
- heart disease or heart failure
- heart rhythm problems
- heart valve problems
- history of low levels of potassium or magnesium
- kidney disease
- liver disease
- an unusual or allergic reaction to dofetilide, other medicines, foods, dyes, or preservatives
- pregnant or trying to get pregnant
- breast-feeding

How should I take this medicine?

Take dofetilide capsules by mouth. Swallow the capsules with a drink of water. Take the medicine with or without food. Follow the directions on the prescription label. Do not drink grapefruit juice with this medicine. Take dofetilide on a regular schedule as prescribed. Do not take your medicine more often than directed. Do not stop taking except on your prescriber's advice. Contact your pediatrician or health care professional regarding the use of this medicine in children. Special care may be needed.

Elderly patients over 65 years old may have a stronger reaction to this medicine and need smaller doses.

What if I miss a dose?

Never try to make up for a missed dose. If you miss a dose, skip it and get back on your regular dosage schedule. If it is almost time for your next dose, take only that dose at the next scheduled time. Do not take double or extra doses.

What may interact with dofetilide?

Do not take dofetilide with any of the following medications:

- amiloride
- arsenic trioxide
- astemizole
- bendroflumethiazide
- bepridil
- chlorothiazide
- chlorthalidone
- cimetidine (Tagamet®)
- cisapride
- entecavir
- grapefruit juice
- hydrochlorothiazide
- indapamide
- itraconazole
- ketoconazole
- megestrol
- methyclothiazide
- metolazone
- mibefradil
- metformin
- probucol
- prochlorperazine
- some antibiotics (gatifloxacin, grepafloxacin, levofloxacin, moxifloxacin, sparfloxacin)
- some medicines for treating heart-rhythm problems (amiodarone, encainide, flecainide, ibutilide, moricizine, procainamide, propafenone, quinidine, tocainide, sotalol)
- some medicines for treating depression or mental illness (amoxapine, maprotiline, pimozide, phenothiazines, tricyclic antidepressants)
- terfenadine
- triamterene
- trimethoprim
- trospium
- verapamil
- ziprasidone

Dofetilide may also interact with the following medications:

- amphotericin B
- aprepitant
- bosentan
- bumetanide
- certain antibiotics (erythromycin, clarithromycin, metronidazole, norfloxacin, Synercid®, troleandomycin)
- certain antidepressants (fluoxetine, fluvoxamine, nefazodone)
- certain medicines for fungal infections (fluconazole, voriconazole)
- medicines for treating HIV virus infection or AIDS (amprenavir, indinavir, nelfinavir, ritonavir, saquinavir)
- certain heart medicines (digoxin, diltiazem, nicardipine)
- cisplatin
- dronabinol, THC
- ethacrynic acid
- furosemide
- ginger
- hawthorn
- medicines for asthma or breathing difficulties (examples: formoterol, salmeterol)
- quinine
- torsemide
- zafirlukast

Tell your prescriber or health care professional about all other medicines you are taking, including non-prescription medicines, nutritional supplements, or herbal products. Also tell your prescriber or health care professional if you are a frequent user of drinks with caffeine or alcohol, if you smoke, or if you use illegal drugs. These may affect the way your medicine works. Tell your prescriber or health care professional before stopping or starting any of your medicines.

What should I watch for while taking dofetilide?

Visit your prescriber or health care professional for a regular check on your progress. Do not stop taking dofetilide suddenly; this may cause serious, heart-related problems. Because your condition and the use of dofetilide carry some risk, it is a good idea to carry an identification card, necklace or bracelet with details of your condition, medications, and prescriber or health care professional. Check your heart rate (pulse) and blood pressure regularly while you are taking dofetilide. Ask your prescriber or health care professional what your heart rate and blood pressure should be, and when you should contact him or her. Your prescriber or health care professional also may schedule regular blood tests and electrocardiograms to check your progress. If you have fast or irregular beating of the heart with light-headedness or fainting, contact your health care professional immediately for evaluation. You will be started on dofetilide in a specialized facility for at least three days to begin treating your heart rhythm problem. You will be monitored to find the right dose of the medicine for you. It is very important that you take your medication exactly as prescribed when you leave the hospital since the correct dosing of dofetilide is very important to effectively treat your heart rhythm and prevent possible serious side effects. Do not drink grapefruit juice while you are taking dofetilide. Grapefruit juice may interact with this medication. If you are going to have surgery, tell your prescriber or health care professional that you are taking dofetilide.

What side effects may I notice from taking dofetilide?

Stop taking this medication immediately and report these side effects to your prescriber or health care professional right away:

- chest pain
- fainting or falling spells
- fast or rapid beating of the heart, or irregular heartbeat
- swelling of the tongue, face, or lips with difficulty breathing, difficulty swallowing, hoarseness, or tightening of the throat

Contact your health care professional right away for evaluation.

Side effects that you should report to your prescriber or health care professional as soon as possible:

- difficulty breathing, shortness of breath
- dizziness
- unusual or persistent rash

- unusual weakness or tiredness
- swelling of the ankles
- vomiting

Side effects that usually do not require medical attention (report to your prescriber or health care professional if they continue or are bothersome):

- cough
- diarrhea
- difficulty sleeping
- headache
- nausea
- stomach pain

Where can I keep my medicine?

Keep out of the reach of children in a container that small children cannot open. Store in a cool, dry place at a controlled room temperature between 15 degrees and 30 degrees C (59 degrees and 86 degrees F). Protect the medicine from moisture or humidity. Throw away any unused medicine after the expiration date.

Dolasetron tablets

ANZEMET®;
100 mg; Tablet
Aventis
Pharmaceuticals Inc

ANZEMET®;
50 mg; Tablet
Aventis
Pharmaceuticals Inc

What are dolasetron tablets?

DOLASETRON (Anzemet®) helps to prevent nausea and vomiting, especially when associated with surgery or the treatment of cancer (chemotherapy). Generic dolasetron tablets are not yet available.

What should my health care professional know before I take dolasetron?

They need to know if you have any of these conditions:

- an unusual or allergic reaction to dolasetron, granisetron, ondansetron, other medicines, foods, dyes or preservatives
- pregnant or trying to get pregnant
- breast-feeding

How should I take this medicine?

Take dolasetron tablets by mouth. Swallow the tablets with a drink of water. The dose of dolasetron is given within 1 hour before chemotherapy. Contact your pediatrician or health care professional regarding the use of this medicine in children. Special care may be needed.

What if I miss a dose?

This does not apply.

What may interact with dolasetron?

- atenolol
- cimetidine
- rifampin

Tell your prescriber or health care professional about all other medicines you are taking, including non-pre-

scription medicines, nutritional supplements, or herbal products. Also tell your prescriber or health care professional if you are a frequent user of drinks with caffeine or alcohol, if you smoke, or if you use illegal drugs. These may affect the way your medicine works. Check with your health care professional before stopping or starting any of your medicines.

What should I watch for while taking dolasetron?

Check with your prescriber or health care professional as soon as you can if you have any sign of an allergic reaction. Do not drink alcohol while taking dolasetron.

What side effects may I notice from taking dolasetron?

Side effects that you should report to your prescriber or health care professional as soon as possible:

- difficulty breathing, wheezing, shortness of breath
- decrease in urine production
- slow, fast, or irregular heartbeat
- tightness in the chest
- swelling of the face, tongue, throat, hands and feet

Side effects that usually do not require medical attention (report to your prescriber or health care professional if they continue or are bothersome):

- change in blood pressure
- diarrhea
- dizziness
- fainting or lightheadedness
- fatigue
- fever, chills
- headache
- itching
- upset stomach

Where can I keep my medicine?

Keep out of the reach of children in a container that small children cannot open. Store between 20 and 25 degrees C (68 and 77 degrees F). Protect from light. Throw away any unused medicine after the expiration date.

Donepezil tablets

ARICEPT®;
5 mg; Tablet
Eisai Inc

ARICEPT®;
10 mg; Tablet
Eisai Inc

What are donepezil tablets?

DONEPEZIL (Aricept®) helps treat the symptoms associated with Alzheimer's disease or dementia. It is not a cure for Alzheimer's disease but offers improvement in memory, attention, reason, language, and the ability to perform simple tasks. Benefits are usually greater for mild to moderate symptoms seen in the early stages of the disease. Generic donepezil tablets are not yet available.

What should my health care professional know before I take donepezil?

They need to know if you have any of these conditions:
- asthma or other lung disease
- difficulty passing urine
- head injury
- heart disease, slow heartbeat
- liver disease
- low blood pressure
- Parkinson's disease
- seizures (convulsions)
- severe headaches
- stomach or intestinal disease, ulcers or stomach bleeding
- an unusual or allergic reaction to donepezil, other medicines, foods, dyes, or preservatives
- pregnant or trying to get pregnant
- breast-feeding

How should I take this medicine?

Take donepezil tablets by mouth. Follow the directions on the prescription label. Swallow the tablets with a drink of water. You may take donepezil with food. Take your doses at regular intervals; donepezil is usually taken before bedtime. Do not take your medicine more often than directed. Continue to take your medicine even if you feel better. Do not stop taking except on your prescriber's advice. Contact your pediatrician or health care professional regarding the use of this medicine in children. Special care may be needed.

What if I miss a dose?

If you miss a dose, take it as soon as you can. If it is almost time for your next dose, take only that dose, do not take double or extra doses.

What may interact with donepezil?

- some antibiotics (such as erythromycin and clarithromycin)
- some antidepressants (examples: fluoxetine, fluvoxamine, paroxetine, sertraline)
- some drugs for treating diabetes (pioglitazone, troglitazone)
- atropine
- benztropine
- bosentan
- carbamazepine
- dexamethasone
- dicyclomine
- digoxin
- galantamine
- glycopyrrolate
- hyoscyamine
- ipratropium
- itraconazole or ketoconazole
- medications for motion sickness (examples: dimenhydrinate, meclizine, scopolamine)
- medicines for treating HIV infection or AIDS
- medicines that relax your muscles for surgery
- modafinil
- non-steroidal anti-inflammatory drugs (NSAIDs, such as ibuprofen)
- oxybutynin
- phenytoin
- phenobarbital
- propantheline
- quinidine
- rifampin, rifabutin or rifapentine
- rivastigmine
- St. John's wort
- tacrine
- trihexyphenidyl

Tell your prescriber or health care professional about all other medicines you are taking, including non-prescription medicines, nutritional supplements, or herbal products. Also tell your prescriber or health care professional if you are a frequent user of drinks with caffeine or alcohol, if you smoke, or if you use illegal drugs. These may affect the way your medicine works. Check with your health care professional before stopping or starting any of your medicines.

What should I watch for while taking donepezil?

Visit your prescriber or health care professional for regular checks on your progress. Check with your prescriber or health care professional if there is no improvement in your symptoms or if they get worse. You may get dizzy or feel faint. Do not drive, use machinery, or do anything that needs mental alertness until you know how donepezil affects you. If you are going to have surgery tell your prescriber or health care professional that you are taking donepezil.

What side effects may I notice from taking donepezil?

Side effects that you should report to your prescriber or health care professional as soon as possible:
- changes in vision or balance
- diarrhea, if it is severe or does not stop
- dizziness, fainting spells, or falls
- increase in frequency of passing urine, or incontinence
- nervousness, agitation, or increased confusion
- skin rash or hives
- slow heartbeat, or palpitations
- stomach pain
- sweating
- uncontrollable movements
- unusual bleeding or bruising, red or purple spots on the skin

- vomiting
- weight loss

Side effects that usually do not require medical attention (report to your prescriber or health care professional if they continue or are bothersome):
- mild diarrhea, especially when starting treatment
- drowsiness
- headache
- indigestion or heartburn
- loss of appetite
- nausea
- joint pain
- muscle cramping

Where can I keep my medicine?

Keep out of reach of children in a container that small children cannot open. Store at room temperature between 15 degrees and 30 degrees C (59 degrees and 86 degrees F). Throw away any unused medicine after the expiration date.

Dorzolamide; Timolol eye solution

COSOPT™;
2%/0.5%; Solution
Merck and Co Inc

What is dorzolamide; timolol eye solution?

DORZOLAMIDE; TIMOLOL (Cosopt™) helps to reduce pressure in the eye for patients with increased pressure or open-angle glaucoma. Generic eye solution is not yet available.

What should my health care professional know before I use dorzolamide; timolol?

They need to know if you have any of these conditions:
- asthma, bronchitis or bronchospasm, emphysema, or other lung disease
- closed-angle glaucoma
- diabetes
- eye infection or damage
- heart or blood vessel disease
- kidney or liver disease
- thyroid disease
- wear contact lenses
- an unusual or allergic reaction to dorzolamide, acetazolamide, sulfonamides, timolol, other beta-blockers, medicines, foods, dyes, or preservatives
- pregnant or trying to get pregnant
- breast-feeding

How should I use this medicine?

Dorzolamide; timolol eye solution is only for use in the eye. Do not take by mouth. Follow the directions on the prescription label. Wash hands before and after use. Tilt the head back slightly and pull down the lower lid with the index finger to form a pouch. Try not to touch the tip of the dropper to your eye or any other surface. Squeeze the prescribed number of drops into the pouch. Close the eye gently; do not blink, and apply gentle finger pressure to the inner corner of the

eye (tear duct) for 1 to 2 minutes. Use your doses at regular intervals. Do not use your medicine more often than directed. If you use other topically applied ophthalmic medications, they should be used at least 10 minutes before or after dorzolamide; timolol. This medicine is not for use in children < 2 years old.

What if I miss a dose?

If you miss a dose, use it as soon as you can. If it is almost time for your next dose, use only that dose. Do not use double or extra doses.

What may interact with dorzolamide; timolol?

Do not use other eye products with dorzolamide; timolol without asking your prescriber or health care professional.

Tell your prescriber or health care professional about all other medicines you are taking or using, including non-prescription medicines; if you are a frequent user of drinks with caffeine or alcohol; if you smoke; or if you use illegal drugs. These may affect the way your medicine works. Check with your health care professional before stopping or starting any of your medicines.

What should I watch for while taking dorzolamide; timolol?

Visit your prescriber or health care professional for regular checks on your progress. Report any serious side effects promptly. Stop using this solution if your eyes get inflamed, painful, or have a discharge, and see your prescriber or health care professional as soon as you can. Ask your prescriber or health care professional if you should continue to use dorzolamide; timolol if you injure your eyes, get an eye infection, or need eye surgery. You may get dizzy while using this medicine. Do not drive, use machinery, or do anything that requires mental alertness until you know how this medicine affects you. To reduce the risk of dizzy or fainting spells, do not sit or stand up quickly. Alcohol can make you more drowsy, and increase flushing and rapid heartbeats. Therefore, it is best to avoid alcoholic drinks. Be careful not to touch the tip of the dispensing container onto the eye, or any other surface. Serious eye infections can result from contamination of eye solutions. If you are using another eye preparation, there should be an interval of at least ten minutes between use of dorzolamide; timolol and the other eye preparation. Wear dark glasses if this eye drop makes your eyes more sensitive to light. If you wear soft contact lenses, you should not put these eye drops in your eyes while wearing the lenses. After using the eye drops, wait about 15 minutes before putting lenses in your eyes.

What side effects may I notice from using dorzolamide; timolol?

Side effects that you should report to your prescriber or health care professional as soon as possible:
- blurred vision
- difficulty breathing, wheezing
- dizziness or fainting spells
- inflamed or infected eyes or eyelids
- irregular heartbeat, palpitations, chest pain
- redness, blistering, peeling or loosening of the skin, including inside the mouth
- slow heart rate (less than 50 beats per minute)
- skin rash
- unusual tiredness or weakness
- vomiting

Side effects that usually do not require medical attention (report to your prescriber or health care professional if they continue or are bothersome):
- bitter taste in the mouth
- burning, stinging, or discomfort immediately after using the solution
- dry eyes
- feeling as if there is something in the eye
- increased flow of tears
- nausea
- sensitivity of the eyes to light

Where can I keep my medicine?

Keep out of the reach of children. Store at room temperature between 15 and 25 degrees C (59 and 77 degrees F). Protect from light. Throw away any unused medicine after the expiration date.

Doxazosin tablets

CARDURA®;
2 mg; Tablet
Roerig Division of
Pfizer

CARDURA®;
1 mg; Tablet
Roerig Division of
Pfizer

What are doxazosin tablets?

DOXAZOSIN (Cardura®) is an antihypertensive. Doxazosin lowers, but does not cure, high blood pressure. It works by relaxing your blood vessels. It also can be used to treat enlargement of the prostate gland in men. Generic doxazosin tablets are available.

What should my health care professional know before I take doxazosin?

They need to know if you have any of the following conditions:
- kidney disease
- liver disease
- low blood pressure
- an unusual or allergic reaction to doxazosin, other medicines, foods, dyes or preservatives
- pregnant or trying to get pregnant
- breast-feeding

How should I take this medicine?

Take doxazosin tablets by mouth. Follow the directions on the prescription label. Swallow the tablets with a drink of water. Take your doses at regular intervals even if you feel better. Do not take your medicine more often than directed. Do not stop taking except on your prescriber's advice. Contact your pediatrician or health care professional regarding the use of this medicine in children. Special care may be needed.

What if I miss a dose?

If you miss a dose, take it as soon as you can. If it is almost time for your next dose, take only that dose. Do not take double or extra doses.

What may interact with doxazosin?

Do not take doxazosin if you are taking the following medications:

- other alpha-blockers such as alfuzosin, phentolamine, phenoxybenzamine, prazosin, tamsulosin, terazosin

Doxazosin may also interact with the following medications:

- anti-inflammatory drugs (NSAIDs, such as ibuprofen)
- dopamine
- female hormones, including contraceptive or birth control pills
- medicines for colds and breathing difficulties
- medicines for high blood pressure
- metaraminol
- methoxamine
- sildenafil (doses of sildenafil higher than 25 mg should be taken at least 4 hours apart from taking doxazosin)
- tadalafil
- vardenafil
- water pills

Tell your prescriber or health care professional about all other medicines you are taking, including non-

prescription medicines, nutritional supplements, or herbal products. Also tell your prescriber or health care professional if you are a frequent user of drinks with caffeine or alcohol, if you smoke, or if you use illegal drugs. These may affect the way your medicine works. Check with your prescriber or health care professional before stopping or starting any of your medicines.

What should I watch for while taking doxazosin?

Check your blood pressure regularly. Ask your prescriber or health care professional what your blood pressure should be and when you should contact him or her. You may feel drowsy or dizzy. Do not drive, use machinery, or do anything that requires mental alertness until you know how doxazosin affects you. To reduce the risk of dizzy or fainting spells, do not sit or stand up quickly. Avoid alcoholic drinks; they can make you more drowsy, and increase flushing and rapid heartbeats. Take doxazosin at bedtime to lessen the effects of drowsiness and dizziness, but be careful if you have to get up during the night. Drowsiness and dizziness are more likely to occur after the first dose, after an increase in dose, or during hot weather or exercise. Dizziness can decrease once your body adjusts to this medicine. Although extremely rare in men taking doxazosin, contact you health care provider immediately if you experience prolonged and painful erection of the penis which is unrelated to sexual activity (priapism). If not brought to immediate medical attention, priapism can lead to permanent erectile dysfunction (impotence). Do not take nonprescription medicine for weight-loss without asking your prescriber or health

care professional. Also, do not take cough and cold, hay fever or sinus medications without asking your prescriber or health care professional. If you are going to have surgery, tell your prescriber or health care professional that you are taking doxazosin.

What side effects may I notice from taking doxazosin?

Side effects that you should report to your prescriber or health care professional as soon as possible:
Rare or uncommon:
- difficulty breathing, shortness of breath
- prolonged painful erection of the penis (priapism)

More common:
- dizziness or drowsiness
- fainting spells
- numbness in hands or feet
- palpitations or pounding heart, irregular heartbeat
- swelling of the legs or ankles

Side effects that usually do not require medical attention (report to your prescriber or health care professional if they continue or are bothersome):
- headache
- nausea
- unusual tiredness

Where can I keep my medicine?

Keep out of the reach of children in a container that small children cannot open. Store at room temperature between 15 and 30 degrees C (59 and 86 degrees F). Throw away any unused medicine after the expiration date.

This drug requires an FDA medication guide. See page xxxvii.

Doxepin capsules

SINEQUAN®;
25 mg; Capsule
Roerig Division of
Pfizer

DOXEPIN;
50 mg; Capsule
Major
Pharmaceuticals Inc

What are doxepin capsules?

DOXEPIN (Sinequan®) belongs to a group of medicines called tricyclic antidepressants. Doxepin can lift your spirits and relieve your depression. Generic doxepin capsules are available.

What should my health care professional know before I take doxepin?

They need to know if you have any of these conditions:
- if you frequently drink alcohol-containing beverages
- asthma or breathing difficulties
- diabetes
- difficulty passing urine
- glaucoma
- heart disease, including a previous heart attack or abnormal heart beat/rhythm
- liver disease
- thyroid disease, including increased or decreased thyroid activity
- over 65 years old
- Parkinson's disease
- prostate trouble

- schizophrenia
- seizure disorder
- stomach disease, reflux or digestive disorders
- surgery scheduled
- an unusual or allergic reaction to doxepin, sulfites, tartrazine dye, other medicines, foods, dyes or preservatives
- pregnant or trying to get pregnant
- breast-feeding

How should I take this medicine?

Take doxepin capsules by mouth. Follow the directions on the prescription label. Swallow the capsules with a drink of water. Take your doses at regular intervals. Do not take your medicine more often than directed. Do not stop taking except on your prescriber's advice. Contact your pediatrician or health care professional regarding the use of this medicine in children. Special care may be needed. Elderly patients over 65 years old may have a stronger reaction to this medicine and need smaller doses.

What if I miss a dose?

If you miss a dose, take it as soon as you can. If it is almost time for your next dose, take only that dose. Do not take double or extra doses. If you are only taking doxepin once a day at bedtime and forget your dose, check with your prescriber or health care professional before taking it in the morning.

What may interact with doxepin?

Doxepin can interact with many other medicines. Some interactions can be very important. Make sure your prescriber or health care professional knows about all other medicines you are taking. Many important interactions are listed below:

Do not take doxepin with any of the following medications:

- astemizole (Hismanal®)
- cisapride (Propulsid®)
- probucol
- terfenadine (Seldane®)
- thioridazine (Mellaril®)
- medicines called MAO inhibitors-phenelzine (Nardil®), tranylcypromine (Parnate®), isocarboxazid (Marplan®), selegiline (Eldepryl®)
- other medicines for mental depression (may be duplicate therapies or cause additive side effects)

Doxepin may also interact with any of the following medications:

- alcohol
- antacids
- atropine and related drugs like hyoscyamine, scopolamine, tolterodine and others
- barbiturate medicines for inducing sleep or treating seizures (convulsions), such as phenobarbital
- blood thinners, such as warfarin
- bromocriptine
- bupropion
- cimetidine
- clonidine
- cocaine
- delavirdine
- diphenoxylate
- disulfiram
- donepezil
- drugs for treating HIV infection
- female hormones, including contraceptive or birth control pills and estrogen
- galantamine
- herbs and dietary supplements like ephedra (*Ma huang*), kava kava, SAM-e, St. John's wort, valerian, or others
- imatinib, STI-571
- kaolin; pectin
- labetalol
- levodopa and other medicines for movement problems like Parkinson's disease
- lithium
- medicines for anxiety or sleeping problems
- medicines for colds, flu and breathing difficulties, like pseudoephedrine
- medicines for hay fever or allergies (antihistamines)
- medicines for weight loss or appetite control
- medicines used to regulate abnormal heartbeat or to treat other heart conditions (examples: amiodarone, bepridil, disopyramide, dofetilide, encainide, flecainide, ibutilide, mibefradil, procainamide, propafenone, quinidine and others)
- metoclopramide
- muscle relaxants, like cyclobenzaprine
- other medicines for mental or mood problems and psychotic disturbances
- prescription pain medications like morphine, codeine, tramadol and others
- procarbazine
- seizure (convulsion) or epilepsy medicine such as carbamazepine or phenytoin
- stimulants like dexmethylphenidate or methylphenidate
- some antibiotics (examples: erythromycin, gatifloxacin, levofloxacin, linezolid, moxifloxacin, sotalol, sparfloxacin)
- tacrine
- thyroid hormones such as levothyroxine

Tell your prescriber or health care professional about all other medicines you are taking including non-prescription medicines; if you are a frequent user of drinks with caffeine or alcohol; if you smoke; or if you use illegal drugs. These can affect the way your medicine works. Check with your health care professional before stopping or starting any of your medicines.

What should I watch for while taking doxepin?

Visit your prescriber or health care professional for regular checks on your progress. It can take several days before you feel the full effect of doxepin. If you have been taking doxepin regularly for some time, do not suddenly stop taking it. Ask your prescriber or health care professional for advice. Even after you stop taking doxepin it can still affect your body for several days. If you are going to have surgery, tell your prescriber or health care professional that you are taking doxepin well before the scheduled date of surgery. You may get dizzy, drowsy or have blurred vision; until you know how doxepin affects you, do not drive, use machinery, or do anything that needs mental alertness. Do not stand or sit up quickly, especially if you are an older patient. This reduces the risk of dizzy or fainting spells. Alcohol can increase the side effects of doxepin; avoid alcoholic drinks. If you are diabetic, check your blood sugar levels more often than usual, especially during the first few weeks of treatment with doxepin. Doxepin can affect your blood sugar levels. Call your prescriber or health care professional for advice if you notice a change in the results of your urine or blood sugar tests.

What side effects might I notice from taking doxepin?

Side effects that you should report to your prescriber or health care professional as soon as possible:
- blurred vision or eye pain
- breast enlargement in both males and females
- fainting spells

- fast heartbeat
- fever or chills, with increased sweating
- hallucinations (seeing or hearing things that are not really there)
- muscle stiffness or problems with movement
- pain or difficulty passing urine, loss of bladder control
- seizures (convulsions)
- sexual difficulties
- stomach pain
- swelling of the testicles
- tingling in feet or hands
- unusual bleeding or bruising
- unusual weakness or tiredness

Side effects that usually do not require medical attention (report to your prescriber or health care professional if they continue or are bothersome):

- anxiety
- confusion or nervousness
- constipation or diarrhea
- difficulty sleeping (insomnia)
- drowsiness or dizziness
- dry mouth
- nausea, vomiting
- skin rash, itching, increased sensitivity to sun or UV light
- weight gain

Where can I keep my medicine?

Keep out of the reach of children in a container that small children cannot open. Store at room temperature between 15 and 30 degrees C (59 and 86 degrees F). Throw away any unused medicine after the expiration date.

Doxycycline tablets or capsules

DORYX®;
100 mg; Capsule
Warner Chilcott PLC

VIBRA-TABS®;
100 mg; Tablet
Pfizer Laboratories
Div Pfizer Inc

What are doxycycline tablets or capsules?

DOXYCYCLINE (Doryx®, Doxy®, Periostat®, Vibra-Tabs®, Vibramycin®) is a tetracycline-type antibiotic. Doxycycline kills certain bacteria that cause infection, or stops their growth. It treats many kinds of infections of the skin, bone, stomach, respiratory tract, sinuses, ear, and urinary tract. It also treats Lyme disease and certain sexually transmitted diseases. For travelers to certain areas doxycycline can be given to suppress malaria. Periostat® is a specific capsule and tablet form of doxycycline that helps to treat periodontitis. Generic regular doxycycline tablets and capsules are available. Generic Periostat® capsules and tablets are not available.

What should my health care professional know before I take doxycycline?

They need to know if you have any of these conditions:
- liver disease
- long exposure to sunlight (working outdoors)
- an unusual or allergic reaction to doxycycline or other tetracyclines
- pregnant or trying to get pregnant
- breast-feeding

How should I take this medicine?

Take doxycycline tablets or capsules by mouth. Follow the directions on the prescription label. Swallow tablets or capsules whole with a full glass of water; take tablets or capsules in an upright or sitting position. Taking a sip of water first, before taking the tablets or capsules, may help you swallow them. If possible take bedtime doses at least 10 minutes before lying down. It is best to take doxycycline without food, but if it upsets your stomach take it with food. Take your doses at regular intervals. Do not take your medicine more often than directed. Finish the full course prescribed by your prescriber or health care professional even if you think your condition is better. Do not stop taking except on your prescriber's advice. Contact your pediatrician or health care professional regarding the use of this medicine in children. Special care may be needed.

What if I miss a dose?

If you miss a dose, take it as soon as you can. If it is almost time for your next dose, take only that dose. Do not take double or extra doses. There should be an interval of at least 6 to 8 hours between doses.

What may interact with doxycycline?

- antacids
- barbiturate medicines for inducing sleep or treating seizures (convulsions)
- calcium salts
- carbamazepine
- cholestyramine
- colestipol
- digoxin
- female hormones, including contraceptive or birth control pills
- ferrous sulfate
- magnesium salts
- other antibiotics
- phenytoin
- sodium bicarbonate
- warfarin

Tell your prescriber or health care professional about all other medicines you are taking, including non-prescription medicines, nutritional supplements, or herbal products. Also tell your prescriber or health care professional if you are a frequent user of drinks with caffeine or alcohol, if you smoke, or if you use illegal drugs. These may affect the way your medicine works. Check

with your health care professional before stopping or starting any of your medicines.

What should I watch for while taking doxycycline?

Tell your prescriber or health care professional if your symptoms do not improve in 2 to 3 days. Do not take doxycycline just before going to bed. It may not dissolve properly when you are lying down and can cause pain in your throat. Keep out of the sun, or wear protective clothing outdoors and use a sunscreen. Do not use sun lamps or sun tanning beds or booths. Make sure your diet provides vitamin B. Ask your prescriber or health care professional for advice if you think you are short of this vitamin. Birth control pills (contraceptive pills) may not work properly while you are taking this medicine. Use an extra method of birth control for at least one month. If you are being treated for a sexually transmitted disease, avoid sexual contact until you have finished your treatment. Your sexual partner may also need treatment. If you are going to have surgery, tell your prescriber or health care professional that you are taking doxycycline. Antacids can stop doxycycline from working properly. If you get an upset stomach and want to take an antacid, make sure there is an interval of at least 2 hours since you last took doxycycline, or 4 hours before your next dose. Never use doxycycline if it is past the expiration date; it can make you seriously ill.

What side effects may I notice from taking doxycycline?

Side effects that you should report to your prescriber or health care professional as soon as possible:
- dark yellow or brown urine
- difficulty breathing
- increased sensitivity to the sun or ultraviolet light
- headache
- itching in the rectal or genital area
- pain on swallowing
- redness, blistering, peeling or loosening of the skin, including inside the mouth
- stomach pain or cramps
- skin rash or itching
- tingling or numbness of the hands or feet
- unusual bleeding or bruising
- unusual tiredness or weakness
- yellowing of eyes or skin

Side effects that usually do not require medical attention (report to your prescriber or health care professional if they continue or are bothersome):
- diarrhea
- discolored tongue
- loss of appetite
- nausea, vomiting
- sore mouth

Where can I keep my medicine?

Keep out of the reach of children in a container that small children cannot open. Store at room temperature, approximately 25 degrees C (77 degrees F). Protect from light.

Doxylamine tablets

SLEEP AID;
25 mg; Tablet
Leader Brand
Products

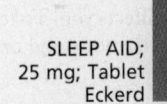

SLEEP AID;
25 mg; Tablet
Eckerd

What are doxylamine tablets?
DOXYLAMINE (Unisom® Sleep Aid, Sleeptabs™) is an antihistamine commonly used as a nighttime sleep aid. This drug is also used to relieve symptoms of hay fever (allergic rhinitis), hives (rash or itching), and other allergic reactions. Generic doxylamine tablets are available.

What should my health care professional know before I take doxylamine?
They need to know if you have any of these conditions:
- asthma or chronic obstructive lung disease (COPD)
- glaucoma
- high blood pressure or heart disease
- liver disease
- other chronic illness
- prostate trouble
- pain or difficulty passing urine
- ulcers or other stomach problems
- an unusual or allergic reaction to doxylamine, other medicines foods, dyes, or preservatives
- pregnant or trying to get pregnant
- breast-feeding

How should this medicine be used?
Take doxylamine tablets by mouth. Follow the directions on the label. Take doxylamine with food or milk if it upsets your stomach. Take your doses at regular intervals. Do not take your medicine more often than directed. If you take doxylamine to help you sleep, take the dose no more than once per day about 30 minutes before bedtime. If you continue to have trouble sleeping after 2 weeks of using doxylamine, contact your health care provider. Contact your pediatrician or health care professional regarding the use of this medicine in children. Special care may be needed.

What if I miss a dose?
If you miss a dose, take it as soon as you can. If it is almost time for your next dose, take only that dose. Do not take double or extra doses.

What may interact with doxylamine?

- alcohol
- barbiturate medicines for inducing sleep or treating seizures (convulsions)
- medicines for anxiety or sleeping problems, such as diazepam or temazepam
- medicines for hay fever and other allergies
- medicines for mental depression
- medicines for mental problems and psychotic disturbances
- muscle relaxers
- prescription pain medicines

Tell your prescriber or health care professional about all other medicines you are taking, including non-prescription medicines, nutritional supplements, or herbal products. Also tell your prescriber or health care professional if you are a frequent user of drinks with caffeine or alcohol, if you smoke, or if you use illegal drugs. These may affect the way your medicine works. Check with your health care professional before stopping or starting any of your medicines.

What should I watch for while taking doxylamine?

You should not take doxylamine to help you sleep for more than 2 weeks without first consulting your health care professional. Tell your prescriber or health care professional if you are taking doxylamine for cold or allergy symptoms and there is no improvement in 1 or 2 days, or if you develop a high fever, have difficulty breathing, or your symptoms worsen. You may get drowsy or dizzy. Do not drive, use machinery, or do anything that needs mental alertness until you know how doxylamine affects you. To reduce the risk of dizzy or fainting spells, do not stand or sit up quickly, espe-

cially if you are an older patient. Alcohol may increase dizziness and drowsiness. Avoid alcoholic drinks. Your mouth may get dry. Chewing sugarless gum or sucking hard candy, and drinking plenty of water will help. Doxylamine may cause dry eyes and blurred vision. If you wear contact lenses you may feel some discomfort. Lubricating drops may help. See your ophthalmologist if the problem does not go away or is severe.

What side effects may I notice from taking doxylamine?

Side effects that you should report to your prescriber or health care professional as soon as possible:

- agitation, nervousness, excitability, not able to sleep (these are more likely in children)
- blurred vision
- dizziness or fainting spells
- irregular heartbeat, palpitations, or chest pain
- muscle or facial twitches
- pain or difficulty passing urine
- seizures (convulsions)

Side effects that usually do not require medical attention (report to your prescriber or health care professional if they continue or are bothersome):

- drowsiness, dizziness
- dry mouth
- headache
- loss of appetite
- stomach upset, nausea, vomiting, diarrhea, or constipation

Where can I keep my medicine?

Keep out of the reach of children in a container that small children cannot open. Store at room temperature, between 15 and 30 degrees C (59 and 86 degrees F). Do not freeze. Protect from light. Throw away any unused medicine after the expiration date.

Dronabinol, THC capsules

MARINOL®; 5 mg; Capsule Solvay Pharmaceuticals Inc	MARINOL®; 2.5 mg; Capsule Solvay Pharmaceuticals Inc

What are dronabinol capsules?

DRONABINOL (Marinol®) helps to relieve the nausea and vomiting associated with the treatment of cancer, especially for those patients whose nausea and vomiting cannot be controlled with other medicines. Dronabinol can also help to stimulate appetite and overcome loss of appetite and weight loss in AIDS patients. Dronabinol is similar to one of the active substances found in marijuana. Federal law prohibits the transfer of dronabinol to any person other than the patient for whom it was prescribed. Generic dronabinol capsules are not yet available.

What should my health care professional know before I take dronabinol?

They need to know if you have any of these conditions:

- a history of drug or alcohol abuse
- heart disease, including angina or irregular heart rate
- high or low blood pressure
- dizziness or fainting spells on standing
- mental health problems (schizophrenia, mania, depression)
- an unusual or allergic reaction to dronabinol, marijuana, sesame oil, other medicines, foods, dyes or preservatives
- pregnant or trying to get pregnant
- breast-feeding

How should I take this medicine?

Take dronabinol capsules by mouth. Follow the directions on the prescription label. Take your doses at regular intervals. Do not take your medicine more often than directed. Contact your pediatrician or health care professional regarding the use of this medicine in children. Special care may be needed.

What if I miss a dose?

If you miss a dose, take it as soon as you can. If it is almost time for your next dose, take only that dose. Do not take double or extra doses.

What may interact with dronabinol?

- amphetamine or other stimulant drugs
- caffeine
- cocaine
- medicines for colds and breathing difficulties

Because dronabinol can cause drowsiness, other medicines that also cause drowsiness may increase this effect of dronabinol. Some medicines that cause drowsiness are:

- alcohol-containing medicines or alcoholic drinks
- barbiturates such as phenobarbital
- certain antidepressants or tranquilizers
- some medications for Parkinson's disease
- muscle relaxants
- certain antihistamines used in cold medicines

Ask your prescriber or health care professional about other medicines that may increase the effect of dronabinol.
Tell your prescriber or health care professional about all other medicines you are taking, including non-prescription medicines, nutritional supplements, or herbal products. Also tell your prescriber or health care professional if you are a frequent user of drinks with caffeine or alcohol, if you smoke, or if you use illegal drugs. These may affect the way your medicine works. Check with your health care professional before stopping or starting any of your medicines.

What should I watch for while taking dronabinol?

The first time you take dronabinol or have an increase in dose make sure there is a responsible person nearby. You may experience mood changes, easy laughter, or other changes in behavior. You may get drowsy or dizzy. Do not drive, use machinery, or do anything that needs mental alertness until you know how dronabinol affects you. To reduce the risk of dizzy or fainting spells, do not sit up or stand up quickly, especially if you have low blood pressure or are taking medicine to lower your blood pressure. Alcohol can increase possible drowsiness and dizziness and other side effects of dronabinol; avoid alcoholic drinks. If you are taking dronabinol to improve your appetite this is only part of your therapy. Discuss what you can eat and ways of improving your diet with your health care professional or nutritionist. Frequent small snacks as well as regular meals can help provide extra calories and protein. Do not smoke marijuana while you are taking dronabinol. Dronabinol is similar to one of the active substances found in marijuana. You are at increased risk of serious heart and/or nervous system side effects if these drugs are used together.

What side effects may I notice from taking dronabinol?

Side effects that you should report to your prescriber or health care professional as soon as possible:
- fast or irregular heartbeat (palpitations)
- fainting spells, lightheadedness
- hallucinations (seeing or hearing things that are not really there)
- panic reactions
- slurred speech

Side effects that usually do not require medical attention (report to your prescriber or health care professional if they continue or are bothersome):
- anxiety or nervousness
- confusion
- diarrhea
- drowsiness or dizziness
- impaired coordination
- irritability
- loss of memory
- mood changes (especially improved mood or euphoria)
- nightmares
- stomach upset

Where can I keep my medicine?

Keep out of the reach of children in a container that small children cannot open. Store in a cool place between 8 and 15 degrees C (46 and 59 degrees F) or in a refrigerator. Avoid freezing. Throw away any unused medicine after the expiration date.

Drospirenone; Ethinyl Estradiol tablets

YASMIN®;
3 mg/0.03 mg; Tablet
Berlex Laboratories Inc

What are drospirenone; ethinyl estradiol tablets?

DROSPIRENONE; ETHINYL ESTRADIOL (Yasmin®) is an oral contraceptive (birth control pill or "the pill"). This product combines an estrogen and progestin, similar to the natural sex hormones (estrogen and progesterone) produced in a woman's body. Ethinyl estradiol is the estrogen and drospirenone is the progestin. This product can prevent ovulation and pregnancy. In general, a combination of estrogen and progestin works better than a single-ingredient product. Drospirenone; ethinyl estradiol tablets can also help regulate menstrual flow, treat acne or may be used for other hormone-related problems in females. A generic product is not available for this birth control pill.

What should my health care professional know before I take drospirenone; ethinyl estradiol?

They need to know if you have or ever had any of these conditions:

- adrenal gland disease
- blood clots
- blood sugar problems, like diabetes
- cancer of the breast, cervix, ovary, uterus, vagina, or unusual vaginal bleeding that has not been evaluated by a health care professional
- depression
- fibroids
- gallbladder disease
- heart or circulation problems
- high blood pressure
- high potassium level
- kidney disease
- jaundice
- liver disease
- menstrual problems
- migraine headaches
- tobacco smoker
- stroke
- an unusual or allergic reaction to estrogen/progestin, other hormones, medicines, foods, dyes, or preservatives
- pregnant or trying to get pregnant
- breast-feeding

How should I take this medicine?

Take drospirenone; ethinyl estradiol pills by mouth. Before you start taking these pills decide what is a suitable time of day and always take them at the same time of day in the order directed on the pack. Swallow the pills with a drink of water. Take with food to reduce stomach upset. Do not take more often than directed. Most products contain a 21-day supply of pills containing the active ingredients. An additional 7 pills containing inactive ingredients may be included and are to be taken during the week of menstruation; this reduces the chance of missing the first day of the next cycle. Most products are to be started on the first Sunday after you start your period or on the first day of your period. You may need to ask your health care provider which day you should start your packet. Before starting this medication, read the paper on your prescription provided by your pharmacist. This paper will tell you about the specific product you are taking. Make certain you understand the instructions. Keep an extra month's supply of your pills available to ensure that you will not miss the first day of the next cycle. Contact your pediatrician or health care professional regarding the use of this medicine in children. Special care may be needed.

What if I miss a dose?

Try not to miss a dose. If you do, it may be necessary to consult your health care professional. 28 day schedule: If you miss one dose, take it as soon as you remember and then take the next pill at the regular time as usual.

You may take 2 tablets in one day. If you miss two doses (days) in a row, take 2 tablets for the next 2 days, then, continue with your regular schedule. Whenever 1 or 2 doses are missed, you should use a second method of contraception for the next 7 days in addition to taking the pills. If you miss three doses in a row, you should notify your physician or other health care professional for instructions. You will probably need to throw away the rest of the tablets in that cycle pack and start over. Another method of contraception should be used until at least 7 doses have been taken in the new cycle. Missing a pill can cause spotting or light bleeding. Make sure that no more than 7 days pass at the end of the 21 day cycle, before you start your next pack of pills. If you miss 1 of the 7 inactive pills, you can either double the inactive dose or skip it, but it is important to start the next month's cycle on the scheduled day.

What may interact with drospirenone; ethinyl estradiol?

- antibiotics or medicines for infections, especially rifampin, rifabutin, rifapentine, and griseofulvin
- aprepitant, a medicine used for chemotherapy-induced nausea and vomiting
- barbiturate medicines for producing sleep or treating seizures (convulsions)
- bosentan
- carbamazepine
- caffeine
- clofibrate
- cyclosporine
- dantrolene
- grapefruit juice
- hydrocortisone
- medicines for anxiety or sleeping problems, such as diazepam or temazepam
- medicines for mental depression
- medicines for diabetes, including troglitazone and pioglitazone
- mineral oil
- modafinil
- mycophenolate
- nefazodone
- oxcarbazepine
- phenytoin
- prednisolone
- ritonavir or other medicines for HIV infection or AIDS
- selegiline
- soy isoflavones supplements
- St. John's wort
- tamoxifen or raloxifene
- theophylline
- topiramate
- warfarin

Yasmin® is different from other birth control pills because it contains the progestin drospirenone. Drospirenone may increase potassium levels and interactions with other drugs that increase potassium may increase the chance you may get an elevated potassium level. You may need blood tests to check for this effect. Drugs that can increase your potassium level include:

- certain medications for high blood pressure or heart conditions (examples include ACE-inhibitors like Altace®, Capoten®, Lotensin®, Mavik®, Monopril®, Prinivil®, Univasc®, Vasotec®, Zestril®, and also Angiotensin-II receptor blockers like Atacand®, Avapro®, Cozaar®, Diovan®, Micardis®), as well as Eplerenone (Inspra™)
- dietary salt substitutes (these may contain potassium)
- heparin
- NSAIDs (anti-inflammatory drugs that include Advil®, Aleve®, Ansaid®, Cataflam®, Clinoril®, Daypro®, Feldene®, Indocin®, Lodine®, Naprosyn®, Orudis®, Motrin®, Voltaren®, and others) if they are taken long-term and daily, like for arthritis
- potassium supplements
- some "water pills" (diuretics like spironolactone or Aldactone®, Dyazide®, Midamor®, Moduretic®, and others)

Tell your prescriber or health care professional about all other medicines you are taking, including non-prescription medicines, nutritional supplements, or herbal products. Also tell your prescriber or health care professional if you are a frequent user of drinks with caffeine or alcohol, if you smoke, or if you use illegal drugs. These may affect the way your medicine works. Check before stopping or starting any of your medicines.

What should I watch for while taking drospirenone; ethinyl estradiol?

Visit your health care provider for regular checks on your progress. You should have a complete check-up every 6 to 12 months. If you have any unusual vaginal bleeding contact your prescriber or health care professional for advice. If you miss a period, the possibility of pregnancy must be considered. See your prescriber or health care provider as soon as you can. Use an additional method of contraception during the first cycle that you take these tablets. If you stop taking these tablets and want to get pregnant, a return to normal ovulation can take some time. You may not return to normal ovulation and fertility for 3 to 6 months. Discuss your pregnancy plans with your health care provider. If you are taking oral contraceptives for the treatment of acne, hirsutism (male-like hair growth), endometriosis or other hormone related problems, it may take several months of continued treatment to notice improvement in your symptoms or condition. Tobacco smoking increases the risk of getting a blood clot or having a stroke while you are taking birth control pills, especially if you are more than 35 years old. You are strongly advised not to smoke. Oral contraceptives can increase your sensitivity to the sun and you may burn more easily. Use sunscreen and protective clothing during long periods outdoors. Tanning booths should be used with caution. If you wear contact lenses and notice visual changes, or if the lenses begin to feel uncomfortable, consult your eye care specialist. In some women, tenderness, swelling, or minor bleeding of the gums may occur. Notify your dentist if this happens. Brushing and flossing your teeth regularly may help limit this. See your dentist regularly and inform your dentist of the medicines you are taking. You may get a vaginal yeast infection. If you have never had a yeast infection before, see your prescriber or other health care provider to confirm the problem. If you have had yeast infections in the past and are comfortable with self-medicating the problem, get and use a nonprescription medication to treat the yeast infection. If you are going to have elective surgery, you may need to stop taking your contraceptive pills one month beforehand. Consult your health care professional for advice prior to scheduling the surgery. Taking contraceptive pills does not protect you against HIV infection (AIDS) or any other sexually transmitted diseases.

What side effects may I notice from taking drospirenone; ethinyl estradiol?

Severe side effects are relatively rare in women who are healthy and do not smoke while they are taking oral contraceptives. On average, more women have problems due to complications from getting pregnant than have problems with oral contraceptives. Many of the minor side effects may go away as your body adjusts to the medicine. However, the potential for severe side effects does exist and you may want to discuss these with your health care provider.

The following symptoms or side effects may be related to blood clots and require immediate medical or emergency help:
- chest pain
- coughing up blood
- dizziness or fainting spells
- leg, arm or groin pain
- severe or sudden headaches
- stomach pain (severe)
- sudden shortness of breath
- sudden loss of coordination, especially on one side of the body
- swelling of the hands, feet or ankles, or rapid weight gain
- vision or speech problems
- weakness or numbness in the arms or legs, especially on one side of the body

Other serious side effects are rare. Contact your health care provider as soon as you can if the following side effects occur:
- breast tissue changes or discharge
- changes in vaginal bleeding during your period or between your periods
- headaches or migraines
- increases in blood sugar, especially if you have diabetes
- increases in blood pressure, especially if you are known to have high blood pressure
- symptoms of vaginal infection (itching, irritation or unusual discharge)

- tenderness in the upper abdomen
- vomiting
- yellowing of the eyes or skin

Side effects that usually do not require medical attention (report to your health care provider if they continue or are bothersome):

- breakthrough bleeding and spotting that continues beyond the 3 initial cycles of pills
- breast tenderness
- mild stomach upset
- mood changes, anxiety, depression, frustration, anger, or emotional outbursts

- increased or decreased appetite
- increased sensitivity to sun or ultraviolet light
- nausea
- skin rash, acne, or brown spots on the skin
- tiredness
- weight gain (slight)

Where can I keep my medicine?

Keep out of the reach of children. Store at room temperature between 15 and 30 degrees C (59 and 86 degrees F). Keep container tightly closed. Throw away any unused medicine after the expiration date.

Duloxetine capsules

CYMBALTA®;
30 mg; Capsule
Eli Lilly and Co

CYMBALTA®;
60 mg; Capsule
Eli Lilly and Co

This drug requires an FDA medication guide. See page xxxvii.

What are duloxetine capsules?

DULOXETINE (Cymbalta®) is an antidepressant, a medicine that helps to lift mental depression. Duloxetine may also be prescribed for the treatment of stress urinary incontinence. Duloxetine may also be prescribed for other uses as decided by your health care provider. Generic duloxetine capsules are not yet available.

What should my health care professional know before I take duloxetine?

They need to know if you have any of these conditions:

- anorexia or weight loss
- attempted suicide
- high blood pressure or heart problems
- kidney or liver disease
- mania or bipolar disorder
- an unusual reaction to duloxetine, other medicines, foods, dyes, or preservatives
- pregnant or trying to get pregnant
- breast-feeding

How should this medicine be used?

Take duloxetine capsules by mouth. Follow the directions on the prescription label. Swallow the capsules whole with a drink of water; do not open or chew the capsules. You may take the duloxetine capsules with food. Take your doses at regular intervals. Do not take your medicine more often than directed. Do not stop taking the capsules except on your prescriber's advice. Contact your pediatrician or health care professional regarding the use of this medicine in children. Special care may be needed.

What if I miss a dose?

If you miss a dose, take it as soon as you can. If it is almost time for your next dose, take only that dose and skip the missed dose. Do not take double or extra doses.

What may interact with duloxetine?

- alcohol

- amphetamine
- certain migraine headache medicines (almotriptan, eletriptan, frovatriptan, naratriptan, rizatriptan, sumatriptan, zolmitriptan)
- dextroamphetamine
- furazolidone
- linezolid
- lithium
- medicines for heart rhythm or blood pressure
- medications for weight control or appetite
- medicines called MAO inhibitors-phenelzine (Nardil®), tranylcypromine (Parnate®), isocarboxazid (Marplan®)
- other medicines for mental depression, mania, psychosis, or anxiety
- procarbazine
- selegiline
- St. John's wort, Hypericum perforatum

Tell your prescriber or health care professional about all other medicines you are taking, including non-prescription medicines. Also tell your prescriber or health care professional if you are a frequent user of drinks with caffeine or alcohol, if you smoke, or if you use illegal drugs. These may affect the way your medicine works. Check with your health care professional before stopping or starting any of your medicines.

What should I watch for while taking duloxetine?

Visit your prescriber or health care professional for regular checks on your progress. You may have to take duloxetine for 4 weeks before you feel better. If you have been taking duloxetine for some time, do not suddenly stop taking it. You must gradually reduce the dose to avoid side effects. Ask your prescriber or health care professional for advice. Duloxetine may cause an increase in blood pressure. Check with your prescriber or health care professional; you may be able to measure your own blood pressure and pulse. Find out what your blood pressure and heart rate should be and when you should contact him or her. You may get drowsy, dizzy or have blurred vision. Do not drive, use machinery, or do anything that needs mental alertness until you know how duloxetine affects you. Do not stand or sit up quickly, especially if you are an older patient. This reduces the risk of dizzy or fainting spells. Alcohol may increase dizziness or drowsiness; avoid alcoholic drinks. Duloxetine can make your mouth dry. Chewing sugarless gum, sucking hard candy and drinking plenty of water will help. Do not treat yourself for coughs, colds, or allergies without asking your prescriber or health care professional for advice. Some ingredients may increase possible side effects. If you are going to have surgery, tell your prescriber or health care professional that you are taking duloxetine.

What side effects may I notice from taking duloxetine?

Side effects that you should report to your prescriber or health care professional as soon as possible:
- difficulty breathing
- fainting spells
- mania (overactive behavior); inability to sleep
- rash
- thoughts of suicide or of harming yourself
- vomiting

Side effects that usually do not require medical attention (report to your prescriber or health care professional if they continue or are bothersome):
- dry mouth
- constipation
- dizziness
- drowsiness
- headache
- increased sweating or flushing
- loss of appetite, loss of weight
- loss of sexual desire, erectile or orgasm dysfunction
- nausea
- weakness or tiredness
- weight gain or weight loss

Where can I keep my medicine?

Keep out of the reach of children in a container that small children cannot open. Store at room temperature between 20 degrees and 25 degrees C (68 degrees and 77 degrees F), in a dry place. Throw away any unused medicine after the expiration date.

Dutasteride capsules

AVODART®;
0.5 mg; Capsule
Glaxo Wellcome

What are dutasteride capsules?

DUTASTERIDE (Avodart™) can reduce the size of the prostate gland in men with benign prostatic hyperplasia (BPH). The prostate is a part of the male reproductive system that produces a milky fluid for sperm. Over the age of 50 most men develop an enlarged prostate. As the prostate gets bigger it can restrict the flow of urine. Dutasteride can help to reduce symptoms caused by BPH such as a weak or interrupted urine flow; a feeling that the bladder is not completely empty; a need to pass urine more often, especially at night; an urgent feeling that you must pass urine right away; a delay or hesitation when you start to urinate. Dutasteride also reduces the risk of the need for BPH-related surgery. While some men have fewer problems and symptoms after 3 months of treatment, at least 6 months is usually necessary to see if dutasteride will work for you. Dutasteride is not for use in women. Generic dutasteride capsules are not yet available.

What should my health care professional know before I take dutasteride?

They need to know if you have any of these conditions:
- if you are female (dutasteride is not for use in women)
- liver disease
- prostate cancer
- an unusual or allergic reaction to dutasteride, finasteride (Proscar®, Propecia®), other medicines, foods, dyes, or preservatives

How should I take this medicine?

Take dutasteride capsules by mouth. Follow the directions on the prescription label. Swallow the capsules whole with a drink of water. You can take this medicine with or without food. Take your doses at regular intervals. Do not take your medicine more often than directed. Contact your pediatrician or health care professional regarding the use of this medicine in children. Special care may be needed.

What if I miss a dose?

If you miss a dose, you can take it later that day. If you do not remember until the next day, take only that day's dose. Do not take double or extra doses. Try taking the dose at the same time every day to help you remember to take your dose.

What may interact with dutasteride?

- amiodarone
- cimetidine
- clarithromycin, erythromycin, or troleandomycin
- diltiazem, nicardipine, or verapamil
- isoniazid
- male hormones (example: testosterone)
- quinine
- saw palmetto
- some antidepressants (examples: fluvoxamine, fluoxetine, nefazodone)
- some antifungal medicines (examples: ketoconazole, itraconazole, voriconazole)

D

- some medicines for HIV infection (examples: delavirdine, efavirenz, indinavir, ritonavir, saquinavir)
- soy isoflavones supplements
- zafirlukast

Tell your prescriber or health care professional about all other medicines you are taking, including non-prescription medicines. Also tell your prescriber or health care professional if you are a frequent user of drinks with caffeine or alcohol, if you smoke, or if you use illegal drugs. These may affect the way your medicine works. Check with your health care professional before stopping or starting any of your medicines.

What should I watch for while taking dutasteride?

Do not donate blood until at least 6 months after your final dose of dutasteride. This will prevent giving dutasteride to a pregnant female through a blood transfusion. Contact your prescriber or health care professional if there is no improvement in your symptoms. You may need to take dutasteride for 6 to 12 months to get the best results. Dutasteride is not for use in females. Females who are pregnant or may get pregnant must not handle dutasteride capsules. If a woman who is pregnant gets enough dutasteride into her body after swallowing it or through her skin after handling it, the medication could harm the unborn baby, particularly if the baby is male. If a pregnant woman comes into contact with dutasteride capsules she should check with her health care professional. Dutasteride may interfere with PSA laboratory tests for prostate cancer. If you are scheduled to have a lab test for prostate cancer, tell your prescriber or health care professional that you are taking dutasteride.

What side effects may I notice from taking dutasteride?

Side effects that usually do not require medical attention (report to your prescriber or health care professional if they continue or are bothersome):
- breast enlargement or tenderness
- sexual difficulties (less sexual desire or ability to get an erection)
- small amount of semen released during sex

Where can I keep my medicine?

Keep out of the reach of children in a container that small children cannot open. Avodart™ is a soft gelatin capsule that may become soft and leak or may stick to other capsules if kept at high temperatures. Store capsules at room temperature at or below 25 degrees C (77 degrees F). Keep container tightly closed. Throw away any unused medicine after the expiration date. If your capsules are cracked or leaking, do not use them, and contact your pharmacist.

Dyphylline tablets

LUFYLLIN®;
200 mg; Tablet
Medpointe
Pharmaceuticals

LUFYLLIN®;
400 mg; Tablet
Medpointe
Pharmaceuticals

What are dyphylline tablets?

DYPHYLLINE (Lufyllin®) is a bronchodilator. This medicine helps make breathing easier. It relaxes the bronchial airways, improving the flow of air through the lungs. Dyphylline helps to reduce coughing, wheezing, shortness of breath, or difficulty breathing in patients with chronic (long-term) lung disorders such as asthma, bronchitis, or emphysema. Generic dyphylline tablets are not yet available.

What should my health care professional know before I take dyphylline?

They need to know if you have any of these conditions:
- heart or blood vessel disease, or previous heart attack
- kidney disease
- seizures
- stomach disease, such as ulcers
- an unusual reaction to dyphylline, theophylline, aminophylline, caffeine, other medicines, foods, dyes, or preservatives
- pregnant or trying to get pregnant
- breast-feeding

How should this medicine be taken?

Take dyphylline tablets by mouth. Follow the directions on the prescription label. Swallow the tablets with a drink of water. It is best to take dyphylline on an empty stomach about 1 hour before or after a meal. If it upsets your stomach you can take it with food. Take your doses at regular intervals. Do not take your medicine more often than directed. Contact your pediatrician or health care professional regarding the use of this medicine in children. Special care may be needed.

What if I miss a dose?

If you miss a dose, take it as soon as you can. If it is almost time for your next dose, take only that dose. There should be at least 2 to 3 hours between your doses. Do not take double or extra doses.

What may interact with dyphylline?

- aminophylline
- caffeine
- ephedrine
- ephedra, *Ma huang*, or herbal products for weight loss or other purposes
- guarana
- medicines for colds and breathing difficulties (decongestants)
- probenecid
- theophylline

Tell your prescriber or health care professional about all other medicines you are taking, including non-prescription medicines, nutritional supplements, or herbal products. Also tell your prescriber or health care professional if you are a frequent user of drinks with caffeine or alcohol, if you smoke, or if you use illegal drugs. These may affect the way your medicine works. Check with your health care professional before stopping or starting any of your medicines.

What should I watch for while taking dyphylline?

Visit your prescriber or health care professional for regular checks on your progress. Your prescriber or health care professional may schedule blood tests to check how much dyphylline is in your blood. Tell your prescriber or health care professional if your symptoms do not improve. If your asthma or bronchitis gets worse while you are using dyphylline, call your prescriber or health care professional as soon as you can for advice. Do not treat yourself for coughs, colds and allergies. Some non-prescription medicines may interact with dyphylline. Also check with your prescriber or health care professional if you get diarrhea. This can mean that you are getting too much dyphylline. Watch your diet while you are taking dyphylline. Drinks with caffeine (like coffee, tea or cola) and food containing theobromine (like chocolate), can increase possible side effects of dyphylline. Avoid large amounts of these products. If you are going to have surgery, tell your prescriber or health care professional that you are taking dyphylline.

What side effects may I notice from taking dyphylline?

Side effects that you should report to your prescriber or health care professional as soon as possible:
- anxiety, nervousness, restlessness
- diarrhea
- fainting spells, lightheadedness
- fast or irregular heartbeat (palpitations)
- flushing of the face
- nausea, vomiting (especially if the vomit looks like coffee grounds)
- seizures (convulsions)
- skin rash and itching (hives)
- tremor
- unusual weakness or tiredness

Side effects that usually do not require medical attention (report to your prescriber or health care professional if they continue or are bothersome):
- difficulty sleeping
- dizziness
- headache
- irritability
- loss of appetite
- stomach cramps

Where can I keep my medicine?

Keep out of the reach of children in a container that small children cannot open. Store at room temperature between 15 and 30 degrees C (59 and 86 degrees F). Keep container tightly closed. Throw away any unused medicine after the expiration date.

Efavirenz capsules and tablets

SUSTIVA®;
200 mg; Capsule
Bristol Myers Squibb Pharma Co

What are efavirenz capsules?

EFAVIRENZ (Sustiva®) is an antiviral drug called a nonnucleoside reverse transcriptase inhibitor or NNRTI. Efavirenz is used to treat human immunodeficiency virus (HIV) infection. Efavirenz may reduce the amount of HIV in the blood and increase the number of CD4 cells (T-cells) in the blood. Efavirenz is used in combination with other drugs to treat the HIV virus. Efavirenz will not cure or prevent HIV infection or AIDS. You may still develop other infections or conditions associated with HIV. Generic efavirenz capsules or tablets are not yet available.

What should my health care professional know before I take efavirenz?

They need to know if you have any of these conditions:
- liver disease or hepatitis
- high levels of cholesterol or lipids in your blood
- history of mental illness (like depression), substance abuse, or alcohol abuse
- history of seizures or convulsions
- an unusual or allergic reaction to efavirenz, other medicines, foods, dyes, or preservatives
- pregnant or trying to get pregnant
- breast-feeding

How should I take this medicine?

Take efavirenz by mouth. Follow the directions on the prescription label. Swallow capsules or tablets with a drink of water. Efavirenz should be taken on an empty stomach at bedtime. Do not take your medicine more often than directed. If you can not swallow capsules, efavirenz capsules may be opened so the powder inside can be added to a small amount of liquid or food. Efavirenz has a peppery taste, some people disguise this taste by mixing efavirenz with grape jelly. Once mixed, eat or drink the full amount to make sure you get the entire dose. To make sure that your medication works as well as possible to treat your condition, take all of your medicine exactly as prescribed. Do not stop taking except on your prescriber's advice. Contact your pediatrician or health care professional regarding the use of this medicine in children. Special care may be needed.

What if I miss a dose?

If you miss a dose, take it as soon as you can. If it is almost time for your next dose, take only that dose. Do not take double or extra doses. If you need help in planning the best times to take your medicine, ask your prescriber or health care professional.

What may interact with efavirenz?

Efavirenz can interact with a large number of other drugs. Make sure to discuss all of your medicines with your health care prescriber before starting efavirenz or any other new medicine.

The following drugs should NOT be taken with efavirenz:
- alprazolam (Xanax®)
- astemizole (Hismanal®)
- cisapride (Propulsid®)
- ergotamine medicines (Cafergot®, Migranal®, D.H.E. 45®, and others)
- midazolam (Versed®)
- St. John's Wort or products containing St. John's Wort
- terfenadine (Seldane®)
- triazolam (Halcion®)

As an interaction is possible, discuss your medicines with your prescriber before taking any of these drugs with efavirenz:
- anti-HIV protease inhibitors (Agenerase®, Crixivan®, Fortovase®, Invirase®, Kaletra™, Norvir®, and Viracept™)
- amiodarone
- birth control pills or other hormonal birth control medicines (like the patch, ring, or injections)
- clarithromycin
- cyclosporine
- imatinib, STI-571
- itraconazole
- ketoconazole
- levomethadyl
- lovastatin
- certain medicines for anxiety or difficulty sleeping
- medicines to control seizures (e.g., Dilantin®, Tegretol®, phenobarbital, and others)
- methadone
- nelfinavir
- omeprazole
- pimozide
- rifabutin
- rifampin
- sildenafil
- simvastatin
- sirolimus
- tacrolimus
- tolbutamide
- tolterodine
- topiramate
- warfarin
- went yeast (Cholestin™)
- zonisamide

Tell your prescriber or health care professional about all other medicines you are taking, including nonprescription medicines, nutritional supplements, or herbal products. Also tell your prescriber or health care professional if you are a frequent user of drinks with caffeine or alcohol, if you smoke, or if you use illegal drugs. These may affect the way your medicine works. Check with your health care professional before stopping or starting any of your medicines.

What should I watch for while taking efavirenz?

Visit your prescriber or health care professional for regular checks on your progress. Discuss any new symptoms with your prescriber or health care professional. Efavirenz will not cure HIV and you can still get other illnesses or complications associated with your health condition. Taking efavirenz does not reduce the risk of passing HIV infection to others through sexual or blood contact. It is best to avoid sexual contact so that you do not spread the disease to others. For any sexual contact, use a condom. Be careful about cuts, abrasions and other possible sources of blood contact. Never share a needle or syringe with anyone. Skin rash is common in people taking efavirenz. The rash is most common 1 to 2 weeks after you start taking efavirenz, and it usually lasts no more than a month. If you notice a severe rash or a rash accompanied by fever, blisters, mouth sores, and/or eye irritation, contact your prescriber immediately. Patients who develop these symptoms may need to stop treatment with efavirenz. If any type of rash develops in a child taking efavirenz contact the prescriber immediately. Rash may be a serious problem in children. Efavirenz may cause dizziness, problems concentrating, and/or drowsiness. Therefore, do not drive or operate heavy machinery until you know how you will react to efavirenz. These symptoms may decrease or go away after 4 months. Drinking alcohol or alcohol-containing beverages may worsen these effects. Contact your health care prescriber if you experience side effects that affect your mood or concentration. Changes in body fat develop in some patients taking anti-HIV medicines. These changes may include an increased amount of fat in the upper back and neck ("buffalo hump"), in the breasts, and around the midsection of the body. Loss of fat from the legs, arms and face may also occur. The cause and long-term health effects of these changes is not known. If you are a woman of childbearing age and are using hormone contraceptives, then you should use another form of birth control while taking efavirenz. Efavirenz may decrease the effectiveness of hormone birth control agents, including pills, injections, and implants. When taking efavirenz, women must use a reliable form of barrier contraception, such as a condom or diaphragm, even if they also use other methods of birth control. For help in finding information on insurance coverage and reimbursement, the manufacturer has an assistance program that can be reached at 1-800-272-4878.

What side effects may I notice from taking efavirenz?

Side effects that you should report to your prescriber or health care professional as soon as possible:
- changes in behavior including severe depression, strange thoughts, thoughts of suicide, or angry behavior
- hallucinations (seeing things that are not there)
- skin rash, especially in children or if it is associated with redness, blistering, peeling or loosening of the skin, including inside the mouth

Side effects that usually do not require medical attention (report to your prescriber or health care professional if they continue or are bothersome):
- abnormal dreams
- diarrhea
- difficulty sleeping
- dizziness
- drowsiness
- nausea, vomiting
- trouble concentrating
- upset stomach

Many of these effects tend to improve after the first two weeks of taking efavirenz. Also, taking efavirenz at bedtime helps with some of the effects such as dizziness and drowsiness.

Where can I keep my medicine?

Keep out of the reach of children in a container that small children cannot open. Store at room temperature between 15 and 30 degrees C (59 and 86 degrees F). Throw away any unused medicine after the expiration date.

Eletriptan tablets

RELPAX®;
40 mg; Tablet
Roerig Division of Pfizer

What are eletriptan tablets?

ELETRIPTAN (Relpax®) helps to relieve a migraine attack (an intense, throbbing headache often accompanied by nausea, vomiting and increased sensitivity to light and noise). A migraine may start with or without aura (an unusual feeling or change in vision that warns you of an attack). Eletriptan works by reducing swelling around the blood vessels in your brain and by blocking release of a chemical from your nerve endings. Eletriptan is not used for migraine prevention. Generic eletriptan tablets are not yet available.

What should my health care professional know before I take eletriptan?

They need to know if you have any of these conditions:
- bowel disease or colitis
- diabetes
- family history of heart disease

- fast or irregular heartbeat
- headaches that are different from your usual migraine
- heart or blood vessel disease, angina (chest pain), or previous heart attack
- high blood pressure
- high cholesterol
- history of stroke, transient ischemic attacks (TIAs or "mini-strokes"), or intracranial bleeding
- liver disease
- overweight
- poor circulation
- postmenopausal or surgical removal of uterus and ovaries
- Raynaud's syndrome
- seizure disorder
- tobacco smoker
- unusual or allergic reaction to eletriptan, other medicines, foods, dyes, or preservatives
- pregnant or trying to get pregnant
- breast-feeding

How should I take this medicine?

Take eletriptan tablets by mouth with water. Follow the directions on the prescription label. Eletriptan is taken when the migraine attack starts; it is not for everyday use. Do not take your medicine more often than directed. Contact your pediatrician or health care professional regarding the use of this medicine in children. Special care may be needed.

What if I miss a dose?

This does not apply since eletriptan is not for regular use.

What may interact with eletriptan?

Do not take eletriptan with any of the following:

- amiodarone, cimetidine, dalfopristin; quinupristin, diltiazem, metronidazole, nicardipine, norfloxacin, quinine, verapamil, zafirlukast, and zileuton—do not take within 72 hours of taking eletriptan
- amphetamine
- certain antibiotics known as macrolides (clarithromycin, erythromycin, and troleandomycin)—do not take within 72 hours of taking eletriptan
- certain antidepressants (nefazodone, fluoxetine, or fluvoxamine)—do not take within 72 hours of taking eletriptan
- cocaine
- dihydroergotamine, ergotamine, ergoloid mesylates, methysergide, or ergot-type medication (examples: bromocriptine, pergolide)—do not take within 24 hours of taking eletriptan
- almotriptan, frovatriptan, naratriptan, rizatriptan, sumatriptan, zolmitriptan—do not take within 24 hours of taking eletriptan
- grapefruit juice
- imatinib, STI-571—do not take within 72 hours of taking eletriptan
- medicines for weight loss such as dexfenfluramine, dextroamphetamine, fenfluramine, or sibutramine
- monoamine oxidase inhibitors (MAOIs) such as phenelzine (Nardil®), tranylcypromine (Parnate®), isocarboxazid (Marplan®), and selegiline (Carbex®), Eldepryl®)—do not take eletriptan within 2 weeks of stopping MAOI therapy
- some antifungals (clotrimazole, fluconazole, itraconazole, ketoconazole, miconazole or voriconazole)—do not take within 72 hours of taking eletriptan
- some medicines used for HIV infection or AIDS (such as amprenavir, delavirdine, efavirenz, indinavir, nelfinavir, ritonavir, saquinavir)—do not take within 72 hours of taking eletriptan

Eletriptan may also interact with the following medications:

- cough syrup or other products containing dextromethorphan
- dextroamphetamine
- dopamine agonists
- feverfew
- lithium
- medicines for mental depression, anxiety or mood problems, or attention deficit hyperactivity disorder (such as buspirone, citalopram, duloxetine, mirtazapine, paroxetine, sertraline, trazodone, tricyclic antidepressants, or venlafaxine)
- meperidine
- St. John's wort
- tryptophan

Tell your physician or health care provider about all other medicines you are taking, including non-prescription medicines, if you are a frequent user of drinks with caffeine or alcohol, if you smoke, or if you use illegal drugs. These may affect the way your medicine works. Check with your health care professional before stopping or starting any of your medicines.

What should I watch for while taking eletriptan?

Only take eletriptan for a migraine headache. Take it if you get warning symptoms or at the start of a migraine attack. Eletriptan is not for regular use to prevent migraine attacks. Do not take it if your headache symptoms are different than your usual attacks; consult your doctor first. Do not take migraine products that contain ergotamine while you are taking eletriptan because this combination can affect your heart. Be sure to check with your health care professional about any other potential drug interactions with eletriptan before you take eletriptan for the first time. You may get drowsy or dizzy. Do not drive, use machinery, or do anything that needs mental alertness until you know how eletriptan affects you. To reduce dizzy or fainting spells, do not sit or stand up quickly. Alcohol can increase drowsiness, dizziness and flushing. Avoid alcoholic drinks. Smoking cigarettes may increase the risk of heart-related side effects from using eletriptan.

What side effects may I notice from taking eletriptan?

Side effects that you should report to your prescriber as soon as possible:

- a headache that is different or more severe than the usual migraines you have

- blurred vision
- chest, neck, or throat pain, tightness
- dizziness or faintness
- fast or irregular heart beat, palpitations
- feeling of chest heaviness or pressure
- seizures or convulsions
- severe stomach pain and cramping, bloody diarrhea
- shortness of breath, wheezing, or difficulty breathing
- tingling, pain, or numbness in the face, hands or feet
- unusual reaction or swelling of the skin, eyelids, face, or lips

Side effects that usually do not require medical attention (report to your prescriber or health care professional if they continue or are bothersome):

- back pain
- drowsiness
- dry mouth
- feeling warm or chilled, flushing, or redness of the face
- heartburn
- nausea, vomiting, or stomach upset
- tiredness or weakness

Where can I keep my medicine?

Keep out of the reach of children in a container that small children cannot open. Store at room temperature between 15 and 30 degrees C (59 and 86 degrees F). Protect from light and moisture. Throw away any unused medicine after the expiration date.

Emtricitabine capsules

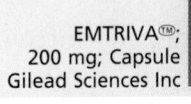

EMTRIVA™;
200 mg; Capsule
Gilead Sciences Inc

E

What are emtricitabine capsules?

EMTRICITABINE (Emtriva™) is an antiviral drug called a nucleoside reverse transcriptase inhibitor or NRTI. Emtricitabine is used to treat human immunodeficiency virus (HIV) infection. Emtricitabine may reduce the amount of HIV in the blood and increase the number of CD4 cells (T-cells) in the blood. Emtricitabine is used in combination with other drugs to treat the HIV virus. Emtricitabine will not cure or prevent HIV infection or AIDS. You may still develop other infections or conditions associated with HIV. Generic emtricitabine capsules are not yet available.

What should my health care professional know before I take emtricitabine?

They need to know if you have any of these conditions:
- if you have used the anti-HIV medicine lamivudine and developed resistance to it
- if you frequently drink alcohol-containing beverages
- kidney disease
- liver disease, including hepatitis B infection
- an unusual reaction to emtricitabine, other medicines, foods, dyes, or preservatives
- pregnant or trying to get pregnant
- breast-feeding

How should this medicine be used?

Take emtricitabine capsules by mouth. Follow the directions on the prescription label. Swallow the capsule with a drink of water. Emtricitabine can be taken with or without food. Do not take your medicine more often than directed. To help to make sure that your anti-HIV therapy works as well as possible, be very careful to take all of your medicine exactly as prescribed. Do not stop taking except on your prescriber's advice. Contact your pediatrician or health care professional regarding the use of this medicine in children. Special care may be needed.

What if I miss a dose?

If you miss a dose, take it as soon as you can. If it is almost time for your next dose, take only that dose. Do not take double or extra doses.

What may interact with emtricitabine?

No significant drug interactions have been reported with emtricitabine.

Tell your prescriber or health care professional about all other medicines you are taking, including non-prescription medicines, nutritional supplements, or herbal products. Also tell your prescriber or health care professional if you are a frequent user of drinks with caffeine or alcohol, if you smoke, or if you use illegal drugs. These may affect the way your medicine works. Check with your health care professional before stopping or starting any of your medicines.

What should I watch for while taking emtricitabine?

Visit your prescriber or health care professional for regular checks on your progress. Discuss any new symptoms with your prescriber or health care professional. Some people have worsening of hepatitis after stopping emtricitabine therapy. Alcohol can increase the risk of developing side effects. Avoid alcoholic drinks. Do not treat yourself for nausea, vomiting, or stomach pain. Call your prescriber or health care professional for advice. Emtricitabine will not cure HIV and you can still get other illnesses or complications associated with your disease. Taking emtricitabine does not reduce the risk of passing HIV infection to others through sexual or blood contact. It is best to avoid sexual contact so that you do not spread the disease to others. For any sexual contact, use a condom. Be careful about cuts, abrasions and other possible sources of blood contact. Never share a needle or syringe with anyone.

What side effects may I notice from taking emtricitabine?

Side effects that you should report to your prescriber or health care professional as soon as possible:
- breathing difficulties or shortness of breath
- changes in body appearance (weight gain around waist and/or face)
- fast or irregular heartbeat
- severe vomiting or diarrhea
- unusual muscle aches, pains, or weakness
- unusual weakness, fatigue or discomfort
- yellow eyes or skin or other signs of hepatitis

Side effects that usually do not require medical attention (report to your prescriber or health care professional if they continue or are bothersome):

- cough
- diarrhea
- dizziness
- nausea, vomiting
- difficulty sleeping
- headache
- runny or stuffy nose
- skin discoloration, usually seen on the palms of the hands or soles of the feet
- skin rash

Where can I keep my medicine?

Keep out of the reach of children in a container that small children cannot open. Store between 15 and 30 degrees C (59 and 86 degrees F). Keep the container tightly closed. Throw away any unused medicine after the expiration date.

Emtricitabine; Tenofovir tablets

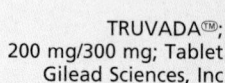

TRUVADA℠;
200 mg/300 mg; Tablet
Gilead Sciences, Inc

What are emtricitabine; tenofovir tablets?

EMTRICITABINE; TENOFOVIR, PMPA (Truvada℠) is a combination of 2 drugs used to treat human immunodeficiency virus (HIV) infection. Emtricitabine is an antiviral drug called a nucleoside reverse transcriptase inhibitor or NRTI. Tenofovir is an antiviral drug called a nucleotide reverse transcriptase inhibitor. This medicine may reduce the amount of HIV in the blood and increase the number of CD4 cells (T-cells) in the blood. This medicine is used in combination with other drugs to treat the HIV virus. This medicine will not cure or prevent HIV infection or AIDS. You may still develop other infections or conditions associated with HIV. Generic emtricitabine; tenofovir capsules are not yet available.

What should my health care professional know before I take emtricitabine; tenofovir?

They need to know if you have any of these conditions:
- if you have used the anti-HIV medicine lamivudine and developed resistance to it
- if you frequently drink alcohol-containing beverages
- bone disease or osteoporosis
- kidney disease
- liver disease, including hepatitis B infection
- an unusual reaction to emtricitabine; tenofovir, other medicines, foods, dyes, or preservatives
- pregnant or trying to get pregnant
- breast-feeding

How should this medicine be taken?

Take emtricitabine; tenofovir tablets by mouth. Follow the directions on the prescription label. Swallow the tablet with a drink of water. This medicine can be taken with or without food. Do not take your medicine more often than directed. To help to make sure that your anti-HIV therapy works as well as possible, be very careful to take all of your medicine exactly as prescribed. Do not stop taking except on your prescriber's advice. Contact your pediatrician or health care professional regarding the use of this medicine in children. Special care may be needed.

What if I miss a dose?

If you miss a dose, take it as soon as you can. If it is almost time for your next dose, take only that dose. Do not take double or extra doses.

What may interact with emtricitabine; tenofovir?

- amphotericin B
- antiviral agents (such as acyclovir, cidofovir, foscarnet, ganciclovir, valacyclovir, valganciclovir)
- cyclosporine
- didanosine, ddI
- hydroxyurea
- lopinavir
- probenecid
- tacrolimus

Tell your prescriber or health care professional about all other medicines you are taking, including non-prescription medicines, nutritional supplements, or herbal products. Also tell your prescriber or health care professional if you are a frequent user of drinks with caffeine or alcohol, if you smoke, or if you use illegal drugs. These may affect the way your medicine works. Check with your health care professional before stopping or starting any of your medicines.

What should I watch for while taking emtricitabine; tenofovir?

Visit your prescriber or health care professional for regular checks on your progress. Discuss any new symptoms with your prescriber or health care professional.

Some people have worsening of hepatitis after stopping emtricitabine; tenofovir therapy. Alcohol can increase the risk of developing side effects. Avoid alcoholic drinks. Do not treat yourself for nausea, vomiting, or stomach pain. Call your prescriber or health care professional for advice. Emtricitabine; tenofovir will not cure HIV and you can still get other illnesses or complications associated with your disease. Taking this medicine does not reduce the risk of passing HIV infection to others through sexual or blood contact. It is best to avoid sexual contact so that you do not spread the disease to others. For any sexual contact, use a condom. Be careful about cuts, abrasions and other possible sources of blood contact. Never share a needle or syringe with anyone.

What side effects may I notice from taking emtricitabine; tenofovir?

Side effects that you should report to your prescriber or health care professional as soon as possible:
- breathing difficulties or shortness of breath
- changes in body appearance (weight gain around waist and/or face)
- fast or irregular heartbeat
- passing out or fainting
- severe vomiting or diarrhea
- slow or irregular heartbeat
- symptoms of high blood sugar: dizziness, dry mouth, flushed dry-skin, fruit-like breath odor, loss of appetite, nausea, stomach ache, unusual thirst, frequent passing of urine
- unusual stomach pain or discomfort
- unusual muscle aches, pains, or weakness
- unusual weakness, fatigue or discomfort
- yellow eyes or skin or other signs of hepatitis

Side effects that usually do not require medical attention (report to your prescriber or health care professional if they continue or are bothersome):
- cough
- diarrhea
- difficulty sleeping
- dizziness
- headache
- gas
- loss of appetite
- nausea, vomiting
- runny or stuffy nose
- skin discoloration, usually seen on the palms of the hands or soles of the feet
- skin rash
- stomach pain
- tiredness

Where can I keep my medicine?

Keep out of the reach of children in a container that small children cannot open. Store between 15 and 30 degrees C (59 and 86 degrees F). Keep the container tightly closed. Throw away any unused medicine after the expiration date.

Enalapril, Enalaprilat tablets

VASOTEC®;
10 mg; Tablet
Biovail
Pharmaceuticals Inc

ENALAPRIL;
2.5 mg; Tablet
Par Pharmaceuticals Inc

What are enalapril tablets?

ENALAPRIL (Vasotec®, Enalapril) is an antihypertensive (blood pressure lowering agent) known as an ACE inhibitor. Enalapril controls high blood pressure (hypertension) by relaxing blood vessels; it is not a cure. High blood pressure levels can damage your kidneys, and may lead to a stroke or heart failure. Enalapril also helps to treat patients with congestive heart failure (heart does not pump strongly enough). Generic enalapril tablets are available.

What should my health care professional know before I take enalapril?

They need to know if you have any of these conditions:
- autoimmune disease (such as lupus), or suppressed immune function
- previous swelling of the tongue, face, or lips with difficulty breathing, difficulty swallowing, hoarseness, or tightening of the throat (angioedema)
- bone marrow disease
- heart or blood vessel disease
- liver disease
- low blood pressure
- kidney disease
- if you are on a special diet, such as a low-salt diet
- an unusual or allergic reaction to enalapril, other ACE inhibitors, foods, dyes, or preservatives
- pregnant or trying to get pregnant
- breast-feeding

How should I take this medicine?

Take enalapril tablets by mouth. Follow the directions on the prescription label. Swallow the tablets with a drink of water. Take your doses at regular intervals. Do not take your medicine more often than directed. Do not stop taking enalapril except on your prescriber's advice. Contact your pediatrician or health care professional regarding the use of this medicine in children. Special care may be needed.

What if I miss a dose?

If you miss a dose, take it as soon as you can. If it is almost time for your next dose, take only that dose. Do not take double or extra doses. If you take only one dose a day and forget to take it that day, do not take a double dose the next day.

What may interact with enalapril?

- anti-inflammatory drugs (NSAIDs, such as ibuprofen)
- hawthorn
- heparin
- lithium
- medicines for diabetes
- medicines for high blood pressure
- potassium salts
- water pills

Tell your prescriber or health care professional about all other medicines you are taking, including non-prescription medicines, nutritional supplements, or herbal products. Also tell your prescriber or health care professional if you are a frequent user of drinks with caffeine or alcohol, if you smoke, or if you use illegal drugs. These may affect the way your medicine works. Check with your health care professional before stopping or starting any of your medicines.

What should I watch for while taking enalapril?

Visit your prescriber or health care professional for regular checks on your progress. Check your blood pressure regularly while you are taking enalapril. Ask your prescriber or health care professional what your blood pressure should be and when you should contact him or her. Call your prescriber or health care professional if you notice an uneven or fast heart beat. Do not treat yourself for a fever or sore throat; check with your prescriber or health care professional as these may be the result of an enalapril side effect. Check with your prescriber or health care professional if you get an attack of severe diarrhea, nausea and vomiting, or if you sweat a lot. The loss of body fluid can make it dangerous to take enalapril. You may get dizzy. Do not drive, use machinery, or do anything that needs mental alertness until you know how enalapril affects you. To avoid dizzy or fainting spells, do not stand or sit up quickly, especially if you are an older person. Alcohol can make you more dizzy. Avoid alcoholic drinks. If you are going to have surgery, tell your prescriber or health care professional that you are taking enalapril. Avoid salt substitutes or other foods or substances high in potassium salts. Do not treat yourself for coughs, colds, or pain while you are taking enalapril without asking your prescriber or health care professional for advice.

What side effects may I notice from taking enalapril?

Side effects that you should report to your prescriber or health care professional as soon as possible:

- decreased amount of urine passed
- difficulty breathing, or difficulty swallowing
- dizziness, lightheadedness or fainting spells
- fast or uneven heart beat, palpitations, or chest pain
- fever or chills
- numbness or tingling in your fingers or toes
- skin rash, itching
- swelling of your face, lips, or tongue
- swelling of your legs or ankles

Side effects that usually do not require medical attention (report to your prescriber or health care professional if they continue or are bothersome):

- cough
- tiredness

Where can I keep my medicine?

Keep out of the reach of children in a container that small children cannot open. Store at room temperature below 30 degrees C (86 degrees F). Protect from moisture. Keep container tightly closed. Throw away any unused medicine after the expiration date.

Enalapril; Felodipine tablets

LEXXEL®; 5 mg/5 mg; Tablet, Extended Release AstraZeneca LP

LEXXEL®; 5 mg/2.5 mg; Tablet, Extended Release AstraZeneca LP

What are enalapril-felodipine tablets?

ENALAPRIL-FELODIPINE (Lexxel®) is a combination of two drugs used to lower blood pressure. They lower, but do not cure, high blood pressure. Generic enalapril-felodipine tablets are not yet available.

What should my health care professional know before I take enalapril-felodipine?

They need to know if you have any of these conditions:

- autoimmune disease (such as lupus), or suppressed immune function
- previous swelling of the tongue, face, or lips with difficulty breathing, difficulty swallowing, hoarseness, or tightening of the throat (angioedema)
- bone marrow disease
- heart or blood vessel disease
- liver disease
- low blood pressure
- kidney disease
- if you are on a special diet, such as a low-salt diet
- an unusual or allergic reaction to enalapril, felodipine, amlodipine, nifedipine, other medicines, foods, dyes, or preservatives
- pregnant or trying to get pregnant
- breast-feeding

How should I take this medicine?

Take enalapril; felodipine tablets by mouth. Follow the directions on the prescription label. Swallow the tablets whole with a drink of water, do not crush, break or chew. Take enalapril; felodipine regularly either on an empty stomach or with a light meal. Do not take enalapril; felodipine with grapefruit juice or grapefruit. Do not take your medicine more often than directed.

Do not stop taking except on your prescriber's advice. Contact your pediatrician or health care professional regarding the use of this medicine in children. Special care may be needed. Elderly patients over 65 years old may have a stronger reaction to this medicine and need smaller doses.

What if I miss a dose?

If you miss a dose, take it as soon as you can. If it is almost time for your next dose, take only that dose. Do not take double or extra doses.

What may interact with enalapril; felodipine?

Do not take enalapril; felodipine with any of the following:

- alfuzosin
- grapefruit juice

Enalapril; felodipine may also interact with the following medications:

- anti-inflammatory drugs (NSAIDs, such as ibuprofen)
- aspirin
- azathioprine
- barbiturates such as phenobarbital
- bosentan
- cimetidine
- cyclosporine
- drospirenone; ethinyl estradiol
- heparin
- herbal or dietary supplements such as ginkgo biloba, ginseng, hawthorn, *Ma huang* (ephedra), melatonin, St. John's wort, went yeast
- hymenoptera venom
- imatinib, STI-571
- lithium
- local anesthetics or general anesthetics
- medicines for diabetes
- medicines for fungal infections (fluconazole, itraconazole, ketoconazole, voriconazole)
- medicines for high blood pressure
- medicines for HIV infection or AIDS
- medicines for prostate problems
- medicines for seizures (carbamazepine, oxcarbazepine, phenobarbital, phenytoin, primidone, zonisamide)
- potassium salts (examples: potassium chloride, potassium gluconate)
- rifampin, rifapentine, or rifabutin
- sodium ferric gluconate complex
- some antibiotics (clarithromycin, erythromycin, telithromycin, trimethoprim, troleandomycin)
- some medicines for heart-rhythm problems (amiodarone, digoxin, diltiazem, verapamil)
- some medicines for depression or mental problems (fluoxetine, fluvoxamine, nefazodone)
- water pills or diuretics (especially amiloride, triamterene, or spironolactone)
- yohimbine
- zafirlukast
- zileuton

Tell your prescriber or health care professional about all other medicines you are taking, including non-prescription medicines, nutritional supplements, or herbal products. Also tell your prescriber or health care professional if you are a frequent user of drinks with caffeine or alcohol, if you smoke, or if you use illegal drugs. These may affect the way your medicine works. Check with your health care professional before stopping or starting any of your medicines.

What should I watch for while taking enalapril-felodipine?

Check your blood pressure and pulse rate regularly; this is important while you are taking enalapril-felodipine. Ask your prescriber or health care professional what your blood pressure and pulse rate should be and when you should contact him or her. You may feel dizzy or lightheaded. Do not drive, use machinery, or do anything that needs mental alertness until you know how enalapril-felodipine affects you. To reduce the risk of dizzy or fainting spells, do not sit or stand up quickly, especially if you are an older patient. Avoid alcoholic drinks; they can make you more dizzy, increase flushing and rapid heartbeats. Do not suddenly stop taking enalapril-felodipine. Ask your prescriber or health care professional how you can gradually reduce the dose. If you are going to have surgery, tell your prescriber or health care professional that you are taking enalapril-felodipine. Check with your prescriber or health care professional if you get an attack of severe diarrhea, nausea and vomiting, or if you sweat a lot. The loss of body fluid can make it dangerous to take enalapril-felodipine. Avoid salt substitutes or other foods or substances high in potassium salts. Do not treat yourself for coughs, colds, or pain while you are taking enalapril-felodipine without asking your prescriber for advice. This medicine can cause dental problems for some patients. Clean and floss your teeth carefully and regularly. Check with your dentist if your gums get swollen or inflamed and have the dentist clean your teeth regularly.

What side effects may I notice from taking enalapril-felodipine?

Side effects that you should report to your prescriber or health care professional as soon as possible:

- swelling of your face, lips, or tongue
- dizziness, lightheadedness, confusion, or fainting spells
- uneven or fast heartbeat, chest pain, palpitations
- swelling of your legs or ankles
- decreased amount of urine passed
- difficulty breathing, or swallowing
- redness, blistering, peeling or loosening of the skin, including inside the mouth
- skin rash, itching
- persistent dry cough
- sore throat with fever
- tingling, burning or numbness in the fingers and toes
- persistent muscle pain

Side effects that usually do not require medical atten-

E

tion (report to your prescriber or health care professional if they continue or are bothersome):

- occasional cough
- drowsiness or mild dizziness
- facial flushing
- headache
- nausea, vomiting or stomach pain
- weakness or tiredness, or mild muscle aches
- increased sensitivity to sunlight
- change in taste sensation

- overgrowth of the gums
- sexual dysfunction

Where can I keep my medicine?

Keep out of the reach of children in a container that small children cannot open. Store at room temperature between 15 and 30 degrees C (59 and 86 degrees F). Protect from moisture and light. Keep container tightly closed. Throw away any unused medicine after the expiration date.

Enalapril; Hydrochlorothiazide, HCTZ tablets

VASERETIC®;
10 mg/25 mg; Tablet
Biovail
Pharmaceuticals Inc

ENALAPRIL;
Hydrochloro-
thiazide, HCTZ; 10
mg/25 mg; Tablet
Mylan Pharmaceu-
ticals Inc

What are enalapril-hydrochlorothiazide tablets?

ENALAPRIL-HYDROCHLOROTHIAZIDE (Vaseretic®, Enalapril) is a combination of two drugs used to lower blood pressure. Enalapril is an ACE inhibitor that controls high blood pressure (hypertension) by relaxing blood vessels. Hydrochlorothiazide is a diuretic. High blood pressure can damage the blood vessels of the brain, heart, and kidneys, resulting in a stroke, heart failure, or kidney failure. By lowering blood pressure, enalapril-hydrochlorothiazide can help reduce your risk of having damage to your kidneys, heart, or other organs. This medicine does not cure high blood pressure. Generic enalapril-hydrochlorothiazide tablets are available.

What should my health care professional know before I take enalapril-hydrochlorothiazide?

They need to know if you have any of these conditions:

- autoimmune disease (e.g., lupus), or suppressed immune function
- previous swelling of the tongue, face, or lips with difficulty breathing, difficulty swallowing, hoarseness, or tightening of the throat (angioedema)
- bone marrow disease
- diabetes mellitus
- gout
- heart or blood vessel disease
- liver disease
- recent heart attack or stroke
- kidney disease
- pancreatitis
- electrolyte imbalance (e.g. low or high levels of potassium in the blood)
- if you are on a special diet, such as a low-salt diet (e.g. using potassium substitutes)
- sulfonamide (sulfa) or thiazide allergy
- an unusual or allergic reaction to enalapril, hydrochlorothiazide, other medicines, foods, dyes, or preservatives
- pregnant or trying to get pregnant
- breast-feeding

How should I take this medicine?

Take enalapril-hydrochlorothiazide tablets by mouth. Follow the directions on the prescription label. You may take enalapril-hydrochlorothiazide with or without food. Swallow the tablets with a drink of water. Take your doses at regular intervals. Do not take your medicine more often than directed. Do not stop taking this medicine except on your prescriber's advice. Many patients with high blood pressure will not notice any signs of the problem. Therefore, it is very important that you take this medicine exactly as directed and that you keep your appointments with your prescriber or health care professional even if you feel well. Contact your pediatrician or health care professional regarding the use of this medicine in children. Special care may be needed.

What if I miss a dose?

If you miss a dose, take it as soon as you can. If it is almost time for your next dose, take only that dose. Do not take double or extra doses.

What may interact with enalapril-hydrochlorothiazide?

- anti-inflammatory drugs (NSAIDs, such as ibuprofen)
- blood pressure medications
- cholesterol-lowering medications (e.g. cholestyramine or colestipol)
- diabetic medications
- dofetilide
- hawthorn
- lithium
- potassium salts or potassium supplements
- water pills (especially potassium-sparing diuretics such as triamterene or amiloride)

Tell your prescriber or health care professional about all other medicines you are taking, including non-prescription medicines, nutritional supplements, or herbal products. Also tell your prescriber or health care professional if you are a frequent user of drinks with caffeine or alcohol, if you smoke, or if you use illegal drugs. These may affect the way your medicine works. Check with your health care professional before stopping or starting any of your medicines.

What should I watch for while taking enalapril-hydrochlorothiazide?

Check your blood pressure regularly while you are taking enalapril-hydrochlorothiazide. Ask your prescriber or health care professional what your blood pressure should be and when you should contact him or her. When you check your blood pressure, write down the measurements to show your prescriber or health care professional. You must not get dehydrated, ask your prescriber or health care professional how much fluid you need to drink a day. If you are taking this medicine for a long time you must visit your prescriber or health care professional for regular checks on your progress. Make sure you schedule appointments on a regular basis. Check with your prescriber or health care professional if you get an attack of severe diarrhea, nausea and vomiting, or if you sweat a lot. The loss of too much body fluid can make it dangerous for you to take enalapril-hydrochlorothiazide. You may get dizzy. Do not drive, use machinery, or do anything that requires mental alertness until you know how enalapril-hydrochlorothiazide affects you. To avoid dizzy or fainting spells, do not stand or sit up quickly. Alcohol may increase the possibility of dizziness. Avoid alcoholic drinks until you have discussed their use with your prescriber or health care professional. If you are going to have surgery tell your prescriber or health care professional that you are taking enalapril-hydrochlorothiazide. Enalapril-hydrochlorothiazide may affect your blood sugar level. If you have diabetes, check with your prescriber or health care professional before changing the dose of your diabetic medicine. Avoid salt substitutes unless you are told otherwise by your prescriber or health care professional. Do not take medicines for appetite control, asthma, colds, cough, hay fever, or sinus problems without asking your prescriber or health care professional for advice. Do not treat yourself for a fever or sore throat; check with your prescriber or health care professional first.

What side effects may I notice from taking enalapril-hydrochlorothiazide?

Side effects that you should report to your prescriber or health care professional as soon as possible:
Rare or uncommon:
- difficulty breathing, difficulty swallowing, hoarseness, or tightening of the throat
- redness, blistering, peeling or loosening of the skin, including inside the mouth
- swelling of your face, lips, tongue, hands, or feet
- unusual rash, bleeding or bruising, or pinpoint red spots on the skin

Other:
- confusion, dizziness, lightheadedness or fainting spells
- decreased amount of urine passed
- decreased sexual function
- fast or uneven heart beat, palpitations, or chest pain
- fever or chills
- irregular heartbeat
- muscle cramps
- stomach pain
- vomiting
- unusual tiredness or weakness
- worsened gout pain
- yellowing of the eyes or skin

Side effects that usually do not require medical attention (report to your prescriber or health care professional if they continue or are bothersome):
- cough
- diarrhea
- headache
- increased sensitivity to the sun
- nausea
- tiredness or fatigue

Where can I keep my medicine?

Keep out of the reach of children. Store at room temperature below 30 degrees C (86 degrees F). Throw away any unused medicine after the expiration date.

Encainide capsules

What are encainide capsules?

ENCAINIDE (Enkaid®) is an antiarrhythmic agent. Encainide treats irregular heart rhythm and can slow rapid heartbeats (tachycardia). Encainide can help your heart to return to and maintain a normal rhythm. Generic encainide capsules are not available. It is no longer manufactured for general use but is available to patients who were taking and were stabilized on the medication before its removal from the market in 1991.

What should my health care professional know before I take encainide?

They need to know if you have any of these conditions:
- abnormal levels of potassium in the blood
- diabetes
- heart disease or problems other than rhythm and heart rate problems
- kidney disease
- liver disease
- previous heart attack
- an unusual or allergic reaction to encainide, local anesthetics, other medicines, foods, dyes, or preservatives
- pregnant or trying to get pregnant
- breast-feeding

How should I take this medicine?

Take encainide capsules by mouth. Follow the directions on the prescription label. Swallow the capsules with a drink of water. Take your doses at regular intervals. Do not take your medicine more often than directed. Contact your pediatrician or health care professional regarding the use of this medicine in children. Special care may be needed.

What if I miss a dose?

If you miss a dose, take it as soon as you can. If it is almost time for your next dose, take only that dose. Do not take the missed dose if it is more than 4 hours after the dose was due. Do not take double or extra doses.

What may interact with encainide?

- beta-blockers, often used for high blood pressure or heart problems
- cimetidine
- medicines for angina or high blood pressure
- medicines to control heart rhythm

Tell your prescriber or health care professional about all other medicines you are taking, including non-prescription medicines, nutritional supplements, or herbal products. Also tell your prescriber or health care professional if you are a frequent user of drinks with caffeine or alcohol, if you smoke, or if you use illegal drugs. These may affect the way your medicine works. Check with your health care professional before stopping or starting any of your medicines.

What should I watch for while taking encainide?

Visit your prescriber or health care professional for regular checks on your progress. Do not stop taking encainide suddenly; this may cause serious, heart-related side effects. Because your condition and the use of encainide carry some risk, it is a good idea to carry an identification card, necklace or bracelet with details of your condition, medications and prescriber or health care professional. Check your heart rate (pulse) and blood pressure regularly while you are taking encainide. Ask your prescriber or health care professional what your

heart rate and blood pressure should be, and when you should contact him or her. Your prescriber or health care professional also may schedule regular blood tests and electrocardiograms to check your progress. You may feel dizzy or faint. Do not drive, use machinery, or do anything that needs mental alertness until you know how encainide affects you. To reduce the risk of dizzy or fainting spells, do not sit or stand up quickly, especially if you are an older patient. Alcohol can make you more dizzy, increase flushing and rapid heartbeats. Avoid alcoholic drinks. If you are going to have surgery, tell your prescriber or health care professional that you are taking encainide.

What side effects may I notice from taking encainide?

Side effects that you should report to your prescriber or health care professional as soon as possible:
- changes in vision
- chest pain, continued irregular heartbeats
- difficulty breathing
- ringing in the ears
- swelling of the legs or feet
- trembling, shaking
- unusual weakness or tiredness

Side effects that usually do not require medical attention (report to your prescriber or health care professional if they continue or are bothersome):
- difficulty sleeping
- dizziness
- headache
- nausea, vomiting

Where can I keep my medicine?

Keep out of the reach of children in a container that small children cannot open. Store at room temperature below 30 degrees C (86 degrees F). Keep container tightly closed. Throw away any unused medicine after the expiration date.

Enfuvirtide injection

FUZEON℠;
90 mg; Injection
Roche

What is enfuvirtide injection?

ENFUVIRTIDE (Fuzeon™) is a medicine used to treat HIV, the virus that causes AIDS. Enfuvirtide blocks HIV's ability to infect healthy infection-fighting cells (CD4 cells or T-cells). Enfuvirtide must be taken with other anti-HIV medicines. When enfuvirtide is given with other anti-HIV medicine it lowers the amount of virus in your blood (the viral load) and increases the number of CD4 cells (or T-cells). Enfuvirtide will not cure HIV infection or AIDS. People taking enfuvirtide may still develop opportunistic infections or other conditions associated with HIV. Generic enfuvirtide injection is not available.

What should my health care professional know before I take enfuvirtide?

They need to know if you have any of these conditions:
- cigarette smoker
- lung disease or breathing difficulties
- use IV drugs
- an unusual reaction to enfuvirtide, mannitol, medicines, foods, dyes, or preservatives
- pregnant or trying to get pregnant
- breast-feeding

How should this medicine be used?

Enfuvirtide is for injection under the skin. You will be giving yourself 2 injections of enfuvirtide every day.

Your health care provider will give you instructions and show you and/or your caregiver how to give this medicine. Make sure that you and your caregiver understand how to prepare and inject the dose. Use twice daily exactly as directed. Rotate your injection site so that each site is not used more than once every 1 to 2 months. Do not give an injection into any are of skin that has an active injection site reaction. Do not use more enfuvirtide than prescribed. Do not use more or less often than prescribed. If you or your caregiver have any questions about how to give this medicine, call your health care provider before giving the medicine. Make sure you get a puncture-resistant container to take home for throwing away the used syringes and needles. Do not reuse any needles or syringes. Contact your pediatrician or health care professional regarding the use of this medicine in children. Special care may be needed.

What if I miss a dose?

If you miss a dose, use it as soon as you can. If it is almost time for your next dose, use only that dose. Do not use double or extra doses.

What may interact with enfuvirtide?

No interactions have been found.
Tell your prescriber or health care professional about all other medicines you are taking, including non-prescription medicines, nutritional supplements, or herbal products. Also tell your prescriber or health care professional if you are a frequent user of drinks with caffeine or alcohol, if you smoke, or if you use illegal drugs. These may affect the way your medicine works. Check with your health care professional before stopping or starting any of your medicines.

What should I watch for while taking enfuvirtide?

You must visit your prescriber or health care professional for regular checks on your progress. Taking enfuvirtide does not reduce the risk of passing HIV infection to others through sexual or blood contact. It is best to avoid sexual contact so that you do not spread the disease to others. For any sexual contact, use a condom. Be careful about cuts, abrasions and other possible sources of blood contact. Never share a needle or syringe with anyone. Skin reactions where you inject enfuvirtide are common during treatment. The injection site reactions are usually mild to moderate, but can be severe. Injection site reactions usually happen within the first week of using enfuvirtide and usually continue to happen as you keep using enfuvirtide. The reactions usually do not last longer than 7 days. The reactions may be worse when injections are given in the same place on the body or when the injection is given deeper than it should be (for example, into the muscle).

What side effects may I notice from taking enfuvirtide?

Enfuvirtide causes injection site reactions in almost every person who uses it. Reactions are usually mild to moderate, but they can be severe. Reactions on the skin where enfuvirtide is injected include:

- bumps
- hardened skin
- itching
- pain or tenderness
- swelling
- redness

Side effects that you should report to your prescriber or health care professional as soon as possible:

- an injections site reaction (see above) that is severe, infected, or in any way worrisome to you
- signs of infection—such as fever or chills, cough, difficulty breathing
- signs of allergic reaction including: difficulty breathing, fever with vomiting and skin rash, blood in the urine, swelling of the feet

Side effects that usually do not require medical attention (report to your prescriber or health care professional if they continue or are bothersome):

- constipation
- decreased appetite
- depression
- inability to sleep
- muscle pain
- pain or numbness in the feet or legs
- weakness or loss of strength

Where can I keep my medicine?

Keep out of the reach of children in a container that small children cannot open. Store vials of enfuvirtide that have not been mixed with sterile water at room temperature, 15 and 30 degrees C (59 and 86 degrees F). Enfuvirtide can also be stored in a refrigerator 2 and 8 degrees C (36 and 46 degrees F); do not freeze. After enfuvirtide has been mixed with sterile water, the vial should be stored in a refrigerator at 2 and 8 degrees C (36 and 46 degrees F) for up to 24 hours. Return individual vials to room temperature before use. Throw away any unused medicine after the expiration date. Do not inject the solution if it is not clear or if there are particles present. Return it to the pharmacy. Use the solution within 24 hours of dissolving the enfuvirtide powder with the sterile water. If you have not used the mixed medicine within 24 hours, throw it away. Store needles and syringes out of the reach of children. Make sure you receive a puncture-resistant container to dispose of the needles and syringes once you have finished with them. Do not reuse these items. Return the container to your prescriber or health care professional for proper disposal.

E

Entacapone tablets

COMTAN®;
200 mg; Tablet
Novartis Pharmaceuticals Corp
Dba Sandoz Pharmaceuticals
Corp

What are entacapone tablets?

ENTACAPONE (Comtan®) is used in combination with levodopa-carbidopa (Sinemet® or other brands) therapy to treat Parkinson's disease. Generic entacapone tablets are not yet available.

What should my health care professional know before I take entacapone?

They need to know if you have any of these conditions:
- dizzy or fainting spells
- liver disease
- low blood pressure
- an unusual or allergic reaction to entacapone, other medicines, foods, dyes, or preservatives
- pregnant or trying to get pregnant
- breast-feeding

How should I take this medicine?

Take entacapone tablets by mouth at the same time you take your levodopa-carbidopa. You may take entacapone with food. Follow the directions on the prescription label. Swallow the tablets with a drink of water. Do not stop taking entacapone except on your prescriber's advice.

What if I miss a dose?

If you miss a dose, take it as soon as you can. If it is almost time for your next dose, take only that dose. Do not take double or extra doses.

What may interact with entacapone?

- ampicillin
- apomorphine
- cholestyramine
- epinephrine
- erythromycin
- furazolidone
- isocarboxazid
- isoproterenol
- linezolid
- methyldopa
- phenelzine
- probenecid
- procarbazine
- tranylcypromine

Tell your prescriber or health care professional about all other medicines that you are taking, including nonprescription medicines. Also tell your prescriber or health care professional if you are a frequent user of drinks with caffeine or alcohol, if you smoke, or if you use illegal drugs. These may affect the way your medicine works. Check with your health care professional before stopping or starting any of your medicines.

What should I watch for while taking entacapone?

Entacapone may also increase the side effects caused by levodopa-carbidopa such as nausea or restless movements. If you notice an increase in or the appearance of certain side effects that occurred only while you are taking levodopa-carbidopa, contact your physician. The dose of levodopa-carbidopa may need to be lowered. Do not decrease your medicine dose without instruction by your prescriber. You may get dizzy or have difficulty controlling your movements. Do not drive, use machinery, or do anything that needs mental alertness until you know how entacapone affects you. Do not stand or sit up quickly, especially if you are older. This reduces the risk of dizzy or fainting spells. Other medicines that make you tired or alcohol can increase possible dizziness; avoid alcoholic drinks. Dizziness and sleepiness are more common at the beginning of treatment with entacapone. Entacapone may make your mouth dry. Chewing sugarless gum, sucking hard candy, or drinking plenty of water may help.

What side effects may I notice from taking entacapone?

Side effects that you should report to your prescriber or health care professional as soon as possible:
- abdominal pain
- confusion
- decrease in urination
- fainting spells or lightheadedness
- fever
- hallucinations
- involuntary muscle movements
- severe diarrhea
- sore muscles
- vomiting or nausea that does not go away

Side effects that usually do not require medical attention (report to your prescriber or health care professional if they continue or are bothersome):
- constipation
- diarrhea
- dizziness
- drowsiness
- dry mouth
- fatigue
- nausea
- upset stomach
- urine that is dark yellow to orange or brown in color (entacapone can change the color of your urine)

Where can I keep my medicine?

Keep out of the reach of children in a container that small children cannot open. Store at room temperature between 20 and 25 degrees C (68 and 77 degrees F) in tightly closed containers. Throw away any unused medicine after the expiration date.

Ephedrine tablets

What are ephedrine tablets?

EPHEDRINE is a medicine that opens up your air passages and makes breathing easier. It is a medicine for patients with various lung problems such as asthma or bronchitis. Generic ephedrine tablets are available.

What should my health care professional know before I take ephedrine?

They need to know if you have any of the following conditions:
- an anxiety disorder
- blood vessel disease
- diabetes
- glaucoma
- heart disease
- high blood pressure
- overactive thyroid
- prostate trouble
- an unusual or allergic reaction to ephedrine, other medicines, foods, dyes, or preservatives
- pregnant or trying to get pregnant
- breast-feeding

How should I take this medicine?

Take ephedrine tablets by mouth. Follow the directions on the prescription label. Swallow the tablets with a drink of water. Take your doses at regular intervals. Do not take your medicine more often than directed. Contact your pediatrician or health care professional regarding the use of this medicine in children. Special care may be needed.

What if I miss a dose?

If you miss a dose, and you are taking it on a regular schedule, take it as soon as you can. If it is almost time for your next dose (less than 2 hours), take only that dose. Do not take double or extra doses.

What may interact with ephedrine?

- atropine
- caffeine
- cocaine
- digoxin
- guarana
- linezolid
- medicines for colds and breathing difficulties
- medicines for mental depression
- medicines for migraine
- medicines for heart disease or high blood pressure
- sodium bicarbonate
- water pills

Tell your prescriber or health care professional about all other medicines you are taking, including non-prescription medicines, nutritional supplements, or herbal products. Also tell your prescriber or health care professional if you are a frequent user of drinks with caffeine or alcohol, if you smoke, or if you use illegal drugs. These may affect the way your medicine works. Check before starting or stopping any of your medicines.

What should I watch for while taking ephedrine?

Check with your prescriber or health care professional if your condition has not improved within 5 days, or if you have a high fever. Use ephedrine for asthma only if you are under the care of a physician. If ephedrine makes it difficult for you to sleep at night, take your last dose a few hours before bedtime.

What side effects may I notice from taking ephedrine?

Side effects that you should report to your prescriber or health care professional as soon as possible:
Rare or Uncommon:
- chest pain
- confusion
- dizziness or fainting spells
- hallucinations
- numbness or tingling in the hands or feet
- rapid or troubled breathing
- seizures (convulsions)
- severe, persistent, or worsening headache

More Common:
- anxiety
- excessive sweating or inability to cool down after strenuous exercise
- fast or irregular heartbeat, palpitations
- increased blood pressure
- pain or difficulty passing urine
- sleeplessness (insomnia)
- tremor
- vomiting

Side effects that usually do not require medical attention (report to your prescriber or health care professional if they continue or are bothersome):
- difficulty sleeping
- dry mouth
- headache (mild)
- loss of appetite
- nausea, stomach upset
- restlessness or nervousness

Where can I keep my medicine?

Keep out of the reach of children in a container that small children cannot open. Store at room temperature below 30 degrees C (86 degrees F). Throw away any unused medicine after the expiration date.

E

Epinephrine injection

EPIPEN 2-PAK;
0.3mg/injection; Injection
Dey

What is epinephrine injection?

EPINEPHRINE (Epipen®) can help to open up air passages and make breathing easier for people with various lung problems such as severe asthma. Epinephrine also treats extremely severe allergic reactions and certain heart problems. Generic epinephrine injections are available. Generic auto-injector devices are not yet available.

What should my health care professional know before I take epinephrine?

They need to know if you have any of the following conditions:

- blood vessel disease
- brain damage or disease
- diabetes
- glaucoma
- heart disease
- high blood pressure
- overactive thyroid
- an unusual or allergic reaction to epinephrine, sulfites, other medicines, foods, dyes, or preservatives
- pregnant or trying to get pregnant
- breast-feeding

How should I use this medicine?

Epinephrine is for injection under the skin, into a muscle or into a vein. Injections can be given by a health care professional in a clinic or hospital setting. An auto-injector form is available for self-administration by patients who suffer a severe allergic response to certain stimuli. Read the directions carefully so that you will know how to use the auto-injector properly. Do not remove the safety cap until you are ready to use the auto-injector. When you need to use it, remove the gray cap. Place the black tip on the thigh at a right angle to your leg. Press the tip hard into your leg until the automatic injection functions. Hold in place for several seconds and then remove and safely throw away. Massage your leg for 10 seconds. Do not use more often than directed.

What if I miss a dose?

If you miss a dose, use it as soon as you can. If it is almost time for your next dose, use only that dose. Do not use double or extra doses.

What may interact with epinephrine?

- beta-blockers, often used for high blood pressure or heart problems
- bromocriptine
- entacapone
- heart medicine (such as digoxin, digitoxin)
- linezolid

- medicines for colds and breathing difficulties
- medicines for hay fever and other allergies
- medicines for high blood pressure
- medicines for mental depression
- medicines for migraine
- medicines for mental problems and psychotic disturbances
- medicines that make the uterus contract
- thyroid hormones
- tolcapone

Tell your prescriber or health care professional about all other medicines you are taking, including non-prescription medicines, nutritional supplements, or herbal products. Also tell your prescriber or health care professional if you are a frequent user of drinks with caffeine or alcohol, if you smoke, or if you use illegal drugs. These may affect the way your medicine works. Check before starting or stopping any of your medicines.

What should I watch for while taking epinephrine?

Check with your prescriber or health care professional if your symptoms do not improve within 20 minutes of epinephrine use, or if they get worse. Keep an auto-injector handy if you need epinephrine ready for use to combat possible severe allergic reactions. Make sure that you have the phone number of your prescriber or health care professional and local hospital ready. Remember to check the expiration date regularly and replace the auto-injector when it becomes outdated. Do not use epinephrine products if you are pregnant, especially during labor, as epinephrine may delay contractions. If you have diabetes, epinephrine may increase your blood sugar. Check your blood sugar often and contact your prescriber or health care professional if you have any problems. Do not use an epinephrine solution that appears cloudy, pinkish, or brownish. Do not treat yourself for coughs, colds or allergies without checking with your prescriber or health care professional. Non-prescription medicines may contain ingredients that will increase the effects of your medicine.

What side effects may I notice from taking epinephrine?

Side effects that you should report to your prescriber or health care professional as soon as possible:

- difficulty breathing, wheezing
- flushing (reddening of the skin)
- irregular heartbeats, palpitations, or chest pain
- numbness in fingers or toes
- skin rash, hives
- swelling of the face
- vomiting

Side effects that usually do not require medical attention (report to your prescriber or health care professional if they continue or are bothersome):

- anxiety or nervousness
- dry mouth
- drowsiness or dizziness
- headache
- increased sweating
- nausea
- weakness or tiredness

Where can I keep my medicine?

Keep out of the reach of children. Store at room temperature between 15 and 30 degrees C (59 and 86 degrees F) unless otherwise indicated by the manufacturer. Protect from light. Store the suspension form of epinephrine injection in a refrigerator between 2 and 8 degrees C (36 and 46 degrees F); do not freeze. Throw away any unused medicine after the expiration date.

Eplerenone tablets

INSPRA℗;
25 mg; Tablet
GD Searle LLC a Subsidiary of
Pharmacia Company Pfizer

What are eplerenone tablets?

EPLERENONE (Inspra℗) helps to lower blood pressure. It controls high blood pressure, but it is not a cure. High blood pressure can damage your kidneys and can cause a stroke or heart failure. Blood pressure treatment might help prevent these complications. Eplerenone can also be used to improve symptoms of heart failure. Generic eplerenone tablets are not yet available.

What should my health care professional know before I take eplerenone?

They need to know if you have any of these conditions:

- diabetes
- high blood level of potassium
- kidney disease
- liver disease
- low blood level of sodium
- if you are on a special diet, such as a low-salt diet and are using dietary salt substitutes
- an unusual reaction to eplerenone, other medicines, foods, dyes, or preservatives
- pregnant or trying to get pregnant
- breast-feeding

How should this medicine be used?

Take eplerenone tablets by mouth. Follow the directions on the prescription label. Swallow the tablets with a drink of water. You may take this medicine with or without food. Take your doses at regular intervals. Do not take your medicine more often than directed. Contact your pediatrician or health care professional regarding the use of this medicine in children. Special care may be needed.

What if I miss a dose?

If you miss a dose, take it as soon as you can. However, if it is almost time for your next dose, take only that dose. Do not take double or extra doses.

What may interact with eplerenone?

Eplerenone has the potential to interact with many other drugs. Some of the possible interactions are listed:

- amiodarone
- anti-inflammatory drugs (NSAIDs, such as ibuprofen)
- certain antibiotics (examples: clarithromycin, erythromycin, penicillin, trimethoprim)
- dietary salt substitutes that contain potassium
- drospirenone; ethinyl estradiol
- fluconazole
- fluoxetine
- fluvoxamine
- grapefruit juice
- heparin
- imatinib, STI-571
- itraconazole
- ketoconazole
- lithium
- medicines for high blood pressure
- medicines for HIV infection
- omeprazole
- potassium salts or supplements
- some water pills (diuretics, especially amiloride, spironolactone or triamterene)
- St. John's wort
- voriconazole

Tell your prescriber or health care professional about all other medicines you are taking, including non-prescription medicines, nutritional supplements, or herbal products. Also tell your prescriber or health care professional if you are a frequent user of drinks with caffeine or alcohol, if you smoke, or if you use illegal drugs. These may affect the way your medicine works. Check with your health care professional before stopping or starting any of your medicines.

What should I watch for while taking eplerenone?

Visit your prescriber or health care professional for regular checks on your progress. Check your blood pressure regularly. Ask your prescriber or health care professional what your blood pressure should be, and when you should contact him or her. Do not stop taking eplerenone except on your prescriber's advice. Watch your diet while you are taking eplerenone. Ask your prescriber or health care professional about both potas-

E

sium and sodium intake. Eplerenone can make your body retain potassium and you may have too much. Elderly patients, the severely ill, or patients with diabetes and/or kidney problems are more likely to have too much potassium. Avoid salt-substitutes and nutritional supplements which contain potassium, unless your prescriber or health care professional tells you otherwise. Too much potassium can be very harmful. You may need to avoid or limit foods that are high in potassium such as bananas, coconuts, dates, figs, prunes, apricots, peaches, grapefruit juice, tomato juice, and orange juice. You may experience dizziness. Do not drive, use machinery, or do anything that requires mental alertness until you know how eplerenone affects you. To avoid dizziness, do not stand or sit up quickly.

What side effects may I notice from taking Eplerenone?

Side effects that you should report to your prescriber or health care professional as soon as possible:
- chest pain
- confusion
- deepening of voice in females
- enlarged breasts or breast pain in males
- fast or irregular heartbeat, palpitations
- increased hair growth in females
- irregular menstrual periods
- sexual difficulty
- unusual tiredness or weakness

Side effects that usually do not require medical attention (report to your prescriber or health care professional if they continue or are bothersome):
- abdominal pain
- cough
- diarrhea
- dizziness
- fatigue
- headache

Where can I keep my medicine?

Keep out of the reach of children in a container that small children cannot open. Store at room temperature between 15 and 30 degrees C (59 and 86 degrees F). Keep container tightly closed. Throw away any unused medicine after the expiration date.

Epoetin Alfa injection

EPOGEN®; 10000 unit/ml; Injection Angen Inc

PROCRIT®; 40000 unit/ml; Injection Ortho Biotech Products LP

What is epoetin alfa injection?

EPOETIN ALFA (Epogen®, Procrit®) is a man-made form of erythropoietin, which stimulates the production of red blood cells. Sometimes, your body does not make enough erythropoietin, and that may cause anemia. Epoetin alfa acts treats anemia associated with chronic kidney failure, cancer chemotherapy, or HIV-therapy. Epoetin alfa may also be used before surgery if you have anemia. Generic epoetin alfa injections are not available.

What should my health care professional know before I take epoetin alfa?

They need to know if you have any of these conditions:
- blood clotting disorders
- cystic fibrosis
- enlarged spleen
- heart disease, such as angina or heart failure
- high blood pressure
- infection
- leukemia
- low levels of folate, iron, or vitamin B_{12}
- overactive parathyroid gland
- porphyria
- seizures
- sickle cell disease
- an unusual or allergic reaction to erythropoietin, albumin, benzyl alcohol, hamster proteins, other medicines, foods, dyes, or preservatives
- pregnant or trying to get pregnant
- breast-feeding

How should I use this medicine?

Epoetin alfa is for injection into a vein or under the skin. A health-care professional in a hospital or clinic setting may give it to you. If you are given erythropoietin for home use, you will be instructed in the proper injection technique. Make sure you understand all the instructions before you or your caregiver attempt to give the first injection. Follow the directions exactly. Always wash your hands before use. Only use a disposable syringe once. Always change the site for the injection. Do not shake the solution before you withdraw a dose. Make sure you receive a puncture-resistant container to dispose of the needles and syringes once you have finished with them. Do not reuse these items. Return the container to your prescriber or health care professional for proper disposal. Contact your pediatrician or health care professional regarding the use of this medicine in children. Special care may be needed.

What if I miss a dose?

Try not to miss doses. Ask your prescriber or health care professional for instructions if you miss a dose.

What may interact with epoetin alfa?

- desmopressin
- iron supplements (you may need more iron while taking epoetin)

- male hormones (called androgens such as nandrolone or testosterone)

Tell your prescriber or health care professional about all other medicines you are taking, including non-prescription medicines, nutritional supplements, or herbal products. Also tell your prescriber or health care professional if you are a frequent user of drinks with caffeine or alcohol, if you smoke, or if you use illegal drugs. These may affect the way your medicine works. Check with your health care professional before stopping or starting any of your medicines.

What should I watch for while taking epoetin alfa?

Visit your prescriber or health care professional for regular checks on your progress (once or twice a week) and for blood tests and blood pressure measurements. It may take up to 6 weeks for you to notice the effects of epoetin alfa. Epoetin alfa can cause seizures, especially during the first 90 days of treatment; until you know how erythropoietin affects you, do not drive or use machinery. As your body makes more red blood cells, you may need to take iron, folic acid, or vitamin B supplements. Make sure to follow your prescribers instructions when taking these supplements. Ask your prescriber or health care provider which products are right for you. If you have kidney disease continue dietary restrictions, even though this medication can make you feel better. Talk with your prescriber or health care professional about individual nutritional requirements.

What side effects may I notice from taking epoetin alfa?

Side effects that you should report to your prescriber or health care professional as soon as possible:
- chest pain
- difficulty breathing
- headaches
- high blood pressure
- muscle aches or pains
- rapid weight gain
- seizures
- skin rash or hives
- swelling of feet or ankles
- unusual weakness

Side effects that usually do not require medical attention (report to your prescriber or health care professional if they continue or are bothersome):
- diarrhea
- fever, chills (flu-like symptoms)
- nausea, vomiting
- redness, stinging, or swelling at the injection site

Where can I keep my medicine?

Keep out of the reach of children. Store in a refrigerator between 2 and 8 degrees C (36 and 46 degrees F); do not freeze. Do not shake. Throw away any unused portion if using a single-dose vial. Multi-dose vials can be kept in the refrigerator for 21 days after the initial dose and between doses. Throw away unused portion.

Eprosartan tablets

TEVETEN®;
400 mg; Tablet
Kos
Pharmaceuticals

TEVETEN®;
600 mg; Tablet
Kos
Pharmaceuticals

What is eprosartan?

EPROSARTAN (Teveten®) helps lower blood pressure to normal levels. It controls high blood pressure, but it is not a cure. High blood pressure can damage your kidneys, and may lead to a stroke or heart failure. Eprosartan helps prevent these things from happening. Generic eprosartan is not yet available.

What should my health care professional know before I take eprosartan?

They need to know if you have any of these conditions:
- heart failure
- kidney disease
- liver disease
- electrolyte imbalance (e.g. low or high levels of potassium in the blood)
- if you are on a special diet, such as a low-salt diet (e.g. using potassium substitutes)
- an unusual or allergic reaction to eprosartan, other medicines, foods, dyes, or preservatives
- pregnant or trying to get pregnant
- breast-feeding

How should I take this medicine?

Take eprosartan by mouth. Follow the directions on the prescription label. Swallow the medicine with a drink of water. Eprosartan can be taken with or without food. Take your doses at regular intervals. Do not take your medicine more often than directed.

What if I miss a dose?

If you miss a dose, take it as soon as you can. If it is almost time for your next dose, take only that dose. Do not take double or extra doses.

What may interact with eprosartan?

- blood pressure medications
- hawthorn
- lithium
- potassium salts or potassium supplements
- water pills (especially potassium-sparing diuretics such as triamterene or amiloride)

Tell your prescriber or health care professional about all other medicines you are taking, including non-prescription medicines. Also tell your prescriber or health care professional if you are a frequent user of drinks with caffeine or alcohol, if you smoke, or if you use illegal drugs. These may affect the way your medicine works. Check with your health care professional before stopping or starting any of your medicines.

What should I watch for while taking eprosartan?

Check your blood pressure regularly while you are taking eprosartan. Ask your prescriber or health care professional what your blood pressure should be. When you check your blood pressure, write down the measurements to show your prescriber or health care professional. If you are taking this medicine for a long time you must visit your prescriber or health care professional for regular checks on your progress. Make sure you schedule appointments on a regular basis. If you are going to have surgery, tell your prescriber or health care professional that you are taking eprosartan.

What side effects may I notice from taking eprosartan?

Side effects that you should report to your prescriber or health care professional as soon as possible:

Rare or uncommon:

- difficulty breathing or swallowing, hoarseness, or tightening of the throat
- swelling of your face, lips, tongue, hands, or feet
- rash

Side effects that usually do not require medical attention (report to your prescriber or health care professional if they continue or are bothersome):

- aches in the joint or muscles
- cough
- dizziness or lightheadedness
- fatigue, weakness, or tiredness
- headache

Where can I keep my medicine?

Keep out of the reach of children and in a container that small children cannot open. Store your medicine at room temperature between 20 and 25 degrees C (68 and 77 degrees F). Keep your medicine container tightly closed. Throw away any unused medicine after the expiration date.

Eprosartan; Hydrochlorothiazide, HCTZ tablets

TEVETEN® HCT; 600 mg/12.5 mg; Tablet Solvay Pharmaceuticals BV

TEVETEN® HCT; 600 mg/25 mg; Tablet Solvay Pharmaceuticals BV

What are eprosartan-hydrochlorothiazide tablets?

EPROSARTAN-HYDROCHLOROTHIAZIDE (Teveten® HCT) is a combination of two drugs used to lower blood pressure. Eprosartan controls high blood pressure (hypertension) by relaxing blood vessels. Hydrochlorothiazide is a diuretic. High blood pressure can damage the blood vessels of the brain, heart, and kidneys, resulting in a stroke, heart failure, or kidney failure. This medicine does not cure high blood pressure. By lowering blood pressure, eprosartan-hydrochlorothiazide can help reduce your risk of having damage to your kidneys, heart, or other organs. Generic eprosartan-hydrochlorothiazide tablets are not yet available.

What should my health care professional know before I take eprosartan-hydrochlorothiazide?

They need to know if you have any of these conditions:

- autoimmune disease (like lupus), or suppressed immune function
- diabetes mellitus
- gout
- heart or blood vessel disease (such as heart failure)
- liver disease
- recent heart attack or stroke
- kidney disease (such as renal failure or renal artery stenosis)
- pancreatitis
- electrolyte imbalance (e.g. low or high levels of potassium in the blood)

- if you are on a special diet, such as a low-salt diet (e.g. using potassium substitutes)
- sulfonamide (sulfa) or thiazide allergy
- an unusual or allergic reaction to eprosartan, hydrochlorothiazide, other medicines, foods, dyes, or preservatives
- pregnant or trying to get pregnant
- breast-feeding

How should I take this medicine?

Take eprosartan-hydrochlorothiazide tablets by mouth. Follow the directions on the prescription label. Swallow the tablets with a drink of water. This medicine can be taken with or without food. Take your doses at regular intervals. Do not take your medicine more often than directed. Contact your pediatrician or health care professional regarding the use of this medicine in children. Special care may be needed. Elderly patients over 65 years old may have a stronger reaction to this medicine and need smaller doses.

What if I miss a dose?

If you miss a dose, take it as soon as you can. If it is almost time for your next dose, take only that dose. Do not take double or extra doses.

What may interact with eprosartan-hydrochlorothiazide?

- allopurinol
- anti-inflammatory drugs (NSAIDs, such as ibuprofen)
- diabetic medications

- blood pressure medications
- dofetilide
- griseofulvin
- hawthorn or horse chestnut
- lithium
- potassium salts or potassium supplements
- prochlorperazine
- some antibiotics which increase sensitivity to sunlight (sulfonamides, tetracyclines)
- some cholesterol-lowering medications (e.g. cholestyramine or colestipol)
- some medicines for mental disorders (phenothiazines)
- vitamin A (retinol) creams or pills such as tretinoin Retin-A®, Renova®, Solage®, Atragen®, and others
- water pills (especially potassium-sparing diuretics such as triamterene or amiloride)

Tell your prescriber or health care professional about all other medicines you are taking, including non-prescription medicines, nutritional supplements, or herbal products. Also tell your prescriber or health care professional if you are a frequent user of drinks with caffeine or alcohol, if you smoke, or if you use illegal drugs. These may affect the way your medicine works. Check with your health care professional before stopping or starting any of your medicines.

What should I watch for while taking eprosartan-hydrochlorothiazide?

Check your blood pressure regularly while you are taking this medicine. Ask your prescriber or health care professional what your blood pressure should be and when you should contact him or her. When you check your blood pressure, write down the measurements to show your prescriber or health care professional. You must not get dehydrated. Ask your prescriber or health care professional how much fluid you need to drink a day. If you are taking this medicine for a long time you must visit your prescriber or health care professional for regular checks on your progress. Make sure you schedule appointments on a regular basis. Check with your prescriber or health care professional if you get an attack of severe diarrhea, nausea and vomiting, or if you sweat a lot. The loss of too much body fluid can make it dangerous for you to take this medicine. You may get dizzy. Do not drive, use machinery, or do anything that requires mental alertness until you know how eprosartan-hydrochlorothiazide affects you. To avoid dizzy or fainting spells, do not stand or sit up quickly. Alcohol may increase the possibility of dizziness. Avoid alcoholic drinks until you have discussed their use with your prescriber or health care professional. If you are going to have surgery tell your prescriber or health care professional that you are taking eprosartan-hydrochlorothiazide. Eprosartan-hydrochlorothiazide may affect your blood sugar level. If you have diabetes, check with your prescriber or health care professional before changing the dose of your diabetic medicine. Avoid salt substitutes unless you are told otherwise by your prescriber or health care professional. Do not take medicines for appetite control, asthma, colds, cough, hay fever, or sinus problems without asking your prescriber or health care professional for advice. Do not treat yourself for a fever or sore throat; check with your prescriber or health care professional first.

What side effects may I notice from taking eprosartan-hydrochlorothiazide?

Side effects that you should report to your prescriber or health care professional as soon as possible:
Rare or uncommon:
- difficulty breathing, difficulty swallowing, hoarseness, or tightening of the throat
- redness, blistering, peeling or loosening of the skin, including inside the mouth
- swelling of your face, lips, tongue, hands, or feet
- unusual rash, bleeding or bruising, or pinpoint red spots on the skin

Other:
- confusion, dizziness, lightheadedness, or fainting spells
- decreased amount of urine passed
- decreased sexual function
- fast or uneven heart beat, palpitations, or chest pain
- fever or chills
- irregular heartbeat
- muscle cramps or joint pain
- stomach pain
- vomiting
- unusual tiredness or weakness
- worsened gout pain
- yellowing of the eyes or skin

Side effects that usually do not require medical attention (report to your prescriber or health care professional if they continue or are bothersome):
- cough
- increased sensitivity to the sun

Where can I keep my medicine?

Keep out of the reach of children in a container that small children cannot open. Store at room temperature between 20 and 25 degrees C (68 and 77 degrees F). Protect from light. Keep container tightly closed. Throw away any unused medicine after the expiration date.

E

Ergoloid Mesylates tablets

What are ergoloid mesylates tablets?

ERGOLOID MESYLATES (previously available with the brand name Hydergine®) is one of a group of medicines known as ergot alkaloids. Ergoloid mesylates are used to help to treat memory loss or confusion which can occur with aging, dementia, or Alzheimer's disease. Generic ergoloid mesylates products are available.

What should my health care professional know before I take ergoloid mesylates?

They need to know if you have any of these conditions:
- heart or blood vessel disease
- liver disease
- low blood pressure
- mental disorder
- an unusual or allergic reaction to ergot alkaloids (such as dihydroergotamine, ergoloid mesylates, or ergotamine), or other medicines, foods, dyes, or preservatives
- pregnant or trying to get pregnant
- breast-feeding

How should I take this medicine?

Take ergoloid mesylates tablets by mouth. Follow the directions on the prescription label. Swallow the tablets with a drink of water. Take this medicine at meal times or with food or milk to avoid upset stomach. Do not take your medicine more often than directed. Do not stop taking except on your prescriber's advice. This product should not be used in children. This medicine is commonly used in older patients.

What if I miss a dose?

Do not take the missed dose. Take only the next dose according to your normal schedule. Do not take double or extra doses.

What may interact with ergoloid mesylates?

Do not use any of the following migraine drugs within 24 hours of this medicine:

- almotriptan (Axert™)
- eletriptan (Relpax®)
- frovatriptan (Frova®)
- naratriptan (Amerge®)
- rizatriptan (Maxalt®)
- sumatriptan (Imitrex®)
- zolmitriptan (Zomig®)

Do not use any of the following medicines with ergoloid mesylates:

- bromocriptine (Ergoset®, Parlodel®)
- cabergoline (Dostinex®)
- ergonovine (Ergotrate®)
- methylergonovine (Methergine®)
- some medicines used to treat migraine such as caffeine-ergotamine (example: Cafergot® or Wigraine®), dihydroergotamine (DHE® or Migranal®), ergotamine (example: Ergomar®), or methysergide (Sansert®)
- some medications used to treat AIDS or HIV infection such as efavirenz (Sustiva™), delavirdine (Rescriptor®), indinavir (Crixivan®), lopinavir; ritonavir (Kaletra™), nelfinavir (Viracept™), ritonavir (Norvir®), or saquinavir (Fortovase®, Invirase®)

Tell your prescriber or health care professional about all other medicines you are taking, including non-prescription medicines, nutritional supplements, or herbal products. Also tell your prescriber or health care professional if you are a frequent user of drinks with caffeine or alcohol, if you smoke, or if you use illegal drugs. These may affect the way your medicine works. Check with your health care professional before stopping or starting any of your medicines.

What should I watch for while taking ergoloid mesylates?

Visit your prescriber or health care professional for regular checks on your progress. Ergoloid mesylates may cause sudden dizziness or lightheadedness if you try to stand up too quickly. Make sure to get up slowly from a lying or sitting position while taking ergoloid mesylates. You may get drowsy or dizzy. Do not drive, use machinery, or do anything that needs mental alertness until you know how this medicine affects you. Alcohol can make you more drowsy and dizzy. Avoid alcoholic drinks. If you are going to have surgery tell your prescriber or health care professional that you are taking ergoloid mesylates.

What side effects may I notice from taking ergoloid mesylates?

Side effects that you should report to your prescriber or health care professional as soon as possible:
- abdominal pain or cramping
- blurred vision or change in vision
- decrease in the amount of urine passed
- dizziness or fainting spells
- slow or fast heartbeat
- vomiting

Side effects that usually do not require medical attention (report to your prescriber or health care professional if they continue or are bothersome):
- loss of appetite
- mild headache
- nausea, upset stomach, or mild vomiting
- skin flushing or rash (mild)
- stuffy nose (nasal congestion)

Where can I keep my medicine?

Keep out of the reach of children in a container that small children cannot open. Store at room temperature between 15 and 30 degrees C (59 and 86 degrees F). Protect from heat, light, and moisture. Throw away any unused medicine after the expiration date.

Erlotinib tablets

What are erlotinib tablets?

ERLOTINIB (Tarceva™) targets a specific protein within cancer cells and stops the cancer cells from growing. Erlotinib is used to treat certain cancers including non-small cell lung cancer. This drug might be used to treat other cancers as well. Generic erlotinib tablets are not available.

What should my health care professional know before I take erlotinib?

They need to know if you have any of these conditions:
- liver disease
- lung fibrosis
- previous chemotherapy or radiation therapy
- an unusual reaction to erlotinib, other medicines, foods, dyes, or preservatives
- pregnant or trying to get pregnant
- breast-feeding

How should this medicine be used?

Take erlotinib tablets by mouth on an empty stomach, at least 1 hour before or 2 hours after food. Follow the directions on the prescription label. Do not take your medicine more often than directed. Contact your pediatrician or health care professional regarding the use of this medicine in children. Special care may be needed.

What if I miss a dose?

Take your missed dose as soon as you remember. If it is almost time for your next dose, take only that one, and skip your missed dose. Do not take extra or double doses.

What may interact with Erlotinib?

- amiodarone
- carbamazepine
- antiviral medicines for the treatment of HIV or AIDS
- bosentan
- certain medicines for fungal infections (such as fluconazole, itraconazole, ketoconazole, or voriconazole)
- certain medicines for high blood pressure
- clarithromycin
- erythromycin
- grapefruit juice
- medicines for depression
- non-steroidal anti-inflammatory drugs (NSAIDs such as ibuprofen or naproxen)
- phenobarbital
- phenytoin
- propafenone
- rifabutin
- rifampin
- risperidone
- St. John's wort or any herbal products containing St. John's wort
- warfarin

Tell your prescriber or health care professional about all other medicines you are taking, including non-prescription medicines, nutritional supplements, or herbal products. Also tell your prescriber or health care professional if you are a frequent user of drinks with caffeine or alcohol, if you smoke, or if you use illegal drugs. These may affect the way your medicine works. Check with your health care professional before stopping or starting any of your medicines.

What should I watch for while taking erlotinib?

Visit your prescriber or health care professional for checks on your progress. You will need to have regular blood checks. The side effects of erlotinib may continue after your finish your treatment; report side effects promptly. If you experience severe or continuing diarrhea, nausea, decreased appetite, or vomiting, contact your health care provider. Erlotinib has been associated with severe lung side effects. Contact your health care provider if your breathing gets worse and/or you develop any new symptoms, such as a cough. There is a risk of birth defects if erlotinib is given during pregnancy. Women should not become pregnant while being treated with erlotinib. Adequate birth control methods should be used during erlotinib therapy, and for at least two weeks after stopping therapy. Consult with your health care provider regarding appropriate options for birth control.

What side effects may I notice from taking erlotinib?

Side effects that you should report to your prescriber or health care professional as soon as possible:
- bleeding
- eye irritation
- eye pain
- fever
- mouth sores

- problems related to breathing including shortness of breath or cough
- severe or persistent diarrhea, nausea, vomiting, or loss of appetite

Side effects that usually do not require medical attention (report to your prescriber or health care professional if they continue or are bothersome):
- decreased appetite
- diarrhea
- dry skin
- itching

- nausea, vomiting
- skin rash, including acne
- weakness
- weight loss

Where can I keep my medicine?

Keep out of the reach of children in a container that small children cannot open. Store at room temperature between 15 and 30 degrees C (59 and 86 degrees F). Throw away any unused medicine after the expiration date on the label.

Erythromycin chewable tablets

ERYPED®;
200 mg; Tablet, Chewable
Abbott Pharmaceutical
Product Division

What are erythromycin chewable tablets?

ERYTHROMYCIN (Eryped®) is a macrolide antibiotic. Erythromycin kills certain bacteria or stops their growth. It treats many kinds of infection, including pneumonia (lung infections), skin infections, some sexually transmitted diseases, and Legionnaire's disease. Erythromycin also treats severe acne, and prevents heart problems in patients with rheumatic fever. Generic products are available; however, generic chewable tablets are not available.

What should my health care professional know before I take erythromycin?

They need to know if you have any of these conditions:
- hearing problems
- heart disease
- liver disease
- stomach problems (especially colitis)
- other chronic illness
- an unusual or allergic reaction to erythromycin, foods, dyes, or preservatives
- breast-feeding

How should I take this medicine?

Take erythromycin chewable tablets by mouth. Chew the tablet completely before swallowing. Follow the directions on the prescription label. Take tablets in an upright or sitting position. If possible take bedtime doses at least 10 minutes before lying down. As a general rule take 1 or 2 hours before food, or at least 2 hours after food. You can ask your prescriber or health care professional if you can take your brand with food. Take your doses at regular intervals. Do not take your medicine more often than directed. Finish the full course prescribed by your prescriber or health care professional even if you think your condition is better. Do not stop taking except on your prescriber's advice.

What if I miss a dose?

If you miss a dose, take it as soon as you can. If it is almost time for your next dose, take only that dose.

Do not take double or extra doses. There should be an interval of at least 4 to 6 hours between doses.

What may interact with erythromycin?

- astemizole
- carbamazepine
- cisapride
- colchicine
- cyclosporine
- digoxin
- dihydroergotamine
- dofetilide
- entacapone
- ergotamine
- certain medicines for anxiety or difficulty sleeping
- other antibiotics, like grepafloxacin or sparfloxacin
- oral contraceptives (birth control pills)
- pimozide
- "statin" medicines for reducing cholesterol (atorvastatin, cerivastatin, lovastatin, simvastatin and others)
- terfenadine
- theophylline
- warfarin

Tell your prescriber or health care professional about all other medicines you are taking, including non-prescription medicines, nutritional supplements, or herbal products. Also tell your prescriber or health care professional if you are a frequent user of drinks with caffeine or alcohol, if you smoke, or if you use illegal drugs. These may affect the way your medicine works. Check with your health care professional before stopping or starting any of your medicines.

What should I watch for while taking erythromycin?

Tell your prescriber or health care professional if your symptoms do not improve in 2 to 3 days. If you get severe or watery diarrhea, do not treat yourself. Call your prescriber or health care professional for advice. If you are going to have surgery, tell your prescriber or health care professional that you are taking erythromycin.

What side effects may I notice from taking erythromycin?

Side effects that you should report to your prescriber or health care professional as soon as possible:

- dark yellow or brown urine
- difficulty breathing
- hearing loss
- pain on swallowing
- ringing in the ears
- severe or watery diarrhea
- skin rash or itching
- swelling of face or neck
- yellowing of eyes or skin

Side effects that usually do not require medical attention (report to your prescriber or health care professional if they continue or are bothersome):

- diarrhea
- loss of appetite
- nausea, vomiting
- stomach pain

Where can I keep my medicine?

Keep out of the reach of children in a container that small children cannot open. Store at room temperature between 15 and 30 degrees C (59 and 86 degrees F). Keep container tightly closed. Throw away any unused medicine after the expiration date.

Erythromycin tablets or capsules, plain or extended-release

ERYTHROMYCIN; 250 mg; Tablet Abbott Pharmaceutical Product Division

ERYTHROMYCIN; 500 mg; Tablet Abbott Pharmaceutical Product Division

What are erythromycin tablets or capsules, plain or extended-release?

ERYTHROMYCIN (E.E.S.®, Ery-Tab®, Erythrocin®, PCE®, EryPed®, Ilosone®) is a macrolide antibiotic. Erythromycin kills certain bacteria or stops their growth. It treats many kinds of infection, including pneumonia (lung infections), skin infections, some sexually transmitted diseases, and Legionnaire's disease. Erythromycin also treats severe acne, and prevents heart problems in patients with rheumatic fever. Generic erythromycin tablets, extended-release tablets, capsules and extended-release capsules are available.

What should my health care professional know before I take erythromycin?

They need to know if you have any of these conditions:

- hearing problems
- heart disease
- liver disease
- stomach problems (especially colitis)
- other chronic illness
- an unusual or allergic reaction to erythromycin, foods, dyes, or preservatives
- breast-feeding

How should I take this medicine?

Take erythromycin tablets or capsules by mouth. Follow the directions on the prescription label. Swallow enteric-coated or sustained-release tablets or capsules whole, do not crush or chew them. Swallow tablets or capsules with a full glass of water; take tablets or capsules in an upright or sitting position. Taking a sip of water first, before taking the tablets or capsules, may help you swallow them. If possible take bedtime doses at least 10 minutes before lying down. The type of tablet or capsule you are taking decides if you can take it with or without food. As a general rule take 1 or 2 hours before food, or at least 2 hours after food. You can ask your prescriber or health care professional if you can take your brand with food. Take your doses at regular intervals. Do not take your medicine more often than directed. Finish the full course prescribed by your prescriber or health care professional even if you think your condition is better. Do not stop taking except on your prescriber's advice.

What if I miss a dose?

If you miss a dose, take it as soon as you can. If it is almost time for your next dose, take only that dose. Do not take double or extra doses. There should be an interval of at least 4 to 6 hours between doses.

What may interact with erythromycin?

- astemizole
- carbamazepine
- cisapride
- colchicine
- cyclosporine
- digoxin
- dihydroergotamine
- dofetilide
- entacapone
- ergotamine
- certain medicines for anxiety or difficulty sleeping
- other antibiotics, like grepafloxacin or sparfloxacin
- oral contraceptives (birth control pills)
- pimozide
- "statin" medicines for reducing cholesterol (atorvastatin, cerivastatin, lovastatin, simvastatin, and others)
- terfenadine
- theophylline
- warfarin

E

Tell your prescriber or health care professional about all other medicines you are taking, including non-prescription medicines, nutritional supplements, or herbal products. Also tell your prescriber or health care professional if you are a frequent user of drinks with caffeine or alcohol, if you smoke, or if you use illegal drugs. These may affect the way your medicine works. Check with your health care professional before stopping or starting any of your medicines.

What should I watch for while taking erythromycin?

Tell your prescriber or health care professional if your symptoms do not improve in 2 to 3 days. If you get severe or watery diarrhea, do not treat yourself. Call your prescriber or health care professional for advice. If you are going to have surgery, tell your prescriber or health care professional that you are taking erythromycin.

What side effects may I notice from taking erythromycin?

Side effects that you should report to your prescriber or health care professional as soon as possible:

- dark yellow or brown urine
- difficulty breathing
- hearing loss
- pain on swallowing
- ringing in the ears
- severe or watery diarrhea
- skin rash or itching
- swelling of face or neck
- yellowing of eyes or skin

Side effects that usually do not require medical attention (report to your prescriber or health care professional if they continue or are bothersome):

- diarrhea,
- loss of appetite
- nausea, vomiting
- stomach pain

Where can I keep my medicine?

Keep out of the reach of children in a container that small children cannot open. Store at room temperature between 15 and 30 degrees C (59 and 86 degrees F). Keep container tightly closed. Throw away any unused medicine after the expiration date.

This drug requires an FDA medication guide. See page xxxvii.

Escitalopram tablets

LEXAPRO®;
20 mg; Tablet
Forest Pharmaceuticals

LEXAPRO®;
10 mg; Tablet
Forest Pharmaceuticals

What are escitalopram tablets?

ESCITALOPRAM (Lexapro™) is a medicine for depression and other related problems. You may have to take escitalopram for up to 4 weeks or longer before you begin to feel better. Generic escitalopram tablets are not yet available.

What should my health care professional know before I take escitalopram?

They need to know if you have any of these conditions:
- diabetes
- heart disease
- kidney disease
- liver disease
- mania
- receive electroconvulsive therapy
- seizures (convulsions)
- suicidal thoughts or previous suicidal attempts
- an unusual or allergic reaction to escitalopram, the related drug citalopram, other medicines, foods, dyes, or preservatives
- pregnant or trying to become pregnant
- breast-feeding

How should I take this medicine?

Take escitalopram tablets by mouth. Follow the directions on the prescription label. Swallow the tablets with a drink of water. Escitalopram can be taken with or without food. If escitalopram upsets your stomach, taking it with food may help. Take your doses at regular intervals. Do not take your medicine more often than directed. Do not stop taking except on your prescriber or health care professional's advice.

What if I miss a dose?

If it is almost time for your next dose, take only that dose. Do not take double or extra doses. Follow your prescriber or health care professional's advice on missed doses.

What may interact with escitalopram?

Do not take escitalopram with any of the following medications:

- cisapride
- citalopram
- medicines called MAO inhibitors such as phenelzine (Nardil®), tranylcypromine (Parnate®), isocarboxazid (Marplan®), selegiline (Eldepryl®)

Escitalopram may also interact with the following medications:

- alosetron
- alprazolam
- amphetamine
- aspirin or nonsteroidal anti-inflammatory drugs (NSAIDs) such as ibuprofen or naproxen
- buspirone
- carbamazepine
- certain diet drugs (dexfenfluramine, fenfluramine, phentermine, sibutramine)
- clarithromycin

- cimetidine
- cyproheptadine
- dexamethasone
- dextromethorphan
- dextroamphetamine
- diazepam
- diltiazem
- erythromycin
- ethosuximide
- furazolidone
- grapefruit juice
- itraconazole
- kava kava
- ketoconazole
- linezolid
- lithium
- medicines that treat depression or other mood problems
- medicines that treat HIV infection or AIDS
- migraine headache medicines (almotriptan, eletriptan, frovatriptan, naratriptan, rizatriptan, sumatriptan, zolmitriptan)
- medicines for psychosis or severe mood problems
- methadone
- modafinil
- nefazodone
- phenobarbital
- phenytoin
- prescription pain relievers (codeine, hydrocodone, meperidine, morphine, tramadol, oxycodone)
- primidone
- procarbazine
- quinine
- rifabutin
- rifampin
- St. John's Wort
- troglitazone
- tryptophan
- valerian
- verapamil
- voriconazole
- warfarin

Tell your prescriber or health care professional about all other medicines you are taking, including non-prescription medicines. Also tell your prescriber or health care professional if you are a frequent user of grapefruit juice, drinks with caffeine or alcohol, if you smoke, or if you use illegal drugs. These may affect the way your medicine works. Check with your health care professional before stopping or starting any of your medicines.

What should I watch for while taking escitalopram?

Visit your prescriber or health care professional for regular checks on your progress. Continue to take your tablets even if you do not immediately feel better. It can take 1 to 2 weeks or longer before you feel the first effects of escitalopram. Patients and their families should watch out for worsening depression or thoughts of suicide. Also watch out for sudden or severe changes in feelings such as feeling anxious, agitated, panicky, irritable, hostile, aggressive, impulsive, severely restless, overly excited and hyperactive, or not being able to sleep. If this happens, especially at the beginning of antidepressant treatment or after a change in dose, call your health care professional. If you have been taking escitalopram regularly for some time, do not suddenly stop taking it. You must gradually reduce the dose, or your symptoms may get worse. Ask your prescriber or health care professional for advice. You may get drowsy or dizzy. Do not drive, use machinery, or do anything that needs mental alertness until you know how escitalopram affects you. Do not stand or sit up quickly, especially if you are an older patient. This reduces the risk of dizzy or fainting spells. Alcohol may interfere with the effect of escitalopram. Avoid alcoholic drinks. Do not treat yourself for coughs, colds, or allergies without asking your prescriber or health care professional for advice. Some ingredients can increase possible side effects. Your mouth may get dry. Chewing sugarless gum or sucking hard candy, and drinking plenty of water will help. If you are going to have surgery, tell your prescriber or health care professional that you are taking escitalopram.

What side effects may I notice from taking escitalopram?

Side effects that you should report to your prescriber or health care professional as soon as possible:
Rare or uncommon:
- confusion
- dizziness or lightheadedness
- skin rash, itching (hives)
- fast talking and excited feelings or actions that are out of control
- suicidal thoughts
- vomiting

More common:
- agitation, anxiety, or restlessness, especially in the first week of treatment or when doses are changed

Side effects that usually do not require medical attention (report to your prescriber or health care professional if they continue or are bothersome):
- blurred vision
- diarrhea
- difficulty sleeping
- drowsiness
- dry mouth
- fever
- frequent urination
- headache
- indigestion, nausea
- increased or decreased appetite
- increased sweating
- sexual difficulties (decreased sexual ability or desire)
- taste alterations
- tremor (shaking)
- weight changes

Where can I keep my medicine?

Keep out of reach of children in a container that small children cannot open. Store at room temperature between 15 and 30 degrees C (59 and 86 degrees F). Throw away any unused medicine after the expiration date.

Esomeprazole capsules

NEXIUM®;
20 mg; Capsule,
Extended Release
AstraZeneca LP

NEXIUM®;
40 mg; Capsule,
Extended Release
AstraZeneca LP

What are esomeprazole capsules?

ESOMEPRAZOLE (Nexium®) prevents the production of acid in the stomach. It reduces symptoms and prevents injury to the esophagus, stomach, or intestines in patients with gastroesophageal reflux disease (GERD) or ulcers and in those taking nonsteroidal anti-inflammatory (NSAID) drugs. Generic esomeprazole capsules are not available.

What should my health care professional know before I take esomeprazole?

They need to know if you have any of these conditions:
- liver disease
- an unusual or allergic reaction to esomeprazole, other medicines, foods, dyes, or preservatives
- pregnant or trying to get pregnant
- breast-feeding

How should I take this medicine?

Take esomeprazole capsules by mouth. Follow the directions on the prescription label. Swallow the capsules whole with a drink of water; do not crush, break or chew. The capsules can be opened and the contents sprinkled on applesauce or yogurt, given with fruit juices, or swallowed immediately with water. Do not crush the contents into the food. Esomeprazole works best if taken on an empty stomach at least one hour before a meal. Take your doses at regular intervals. Do not take your medicine more often than directed. Contact your pediatrician or health care professional regarding the use of this medicine in children. Special care may be needed.

What if I miss a dose?

If you miss a dose, just take your next scheduled dose when it is due. Do not use double or extra doses.

What may interact with esomeprazole?

- ampicillin
- atazanavir
- cilostazol
- delaviradine
- diazepam
- digoxin
- iron salts
- itraconazole, ketoconazole, voriconazole, or other prescription medicines for fungus or yeast infections
- other medicines for ulcers or heartburn
- phenytoin
- warfarin

Tell your prescriber or health care professional about all other medicines you are taking, including non-prescription medicines, nutritional supplements, or herbal products. Also tell your prescriber or health care professional if you are a frequent user of drinks with caffeine or alcohol, if you smoke, or if you use illegal drugs. These may affect the way your medicine works. Check with your health care professional before stopping or starting any of your medicines.

What should I watch for while taking esomeprazole?

It can take several days of therapy with esomeprazole before your stomach pains improve. Check with your prescriber or health care professional if your condition does not improve, or if it gets worse. You can take antacids for the occasional relief of pain unless your prescriber or health care professional tells you otherwise.

What side effects may I notice from taking esomeprazole?

Side effects that you should report to your prescriber or health care professional as soon as possible:
- chest pain or tightness
- dark yellow or brown urine
- shortness of breath
- skin rash
- unusual tiredness or fatigue

Side effects that usually do not require medical attention (report to your prescriber or health care professional if they continue or are bothersome):
- headache
- diarrhea or constipation
- flatulence (gas)
- nausea/vomiting
- dry mouth

Where can I keep my medicine?

Keep out of the reach of children in a container that small children cannot open. Store at room temperature between 15 and 30 degrees C (59 and 86 degrees F). Protect from light and moisture. Throw away any unused medicine after the expiration date.

Estazolam tablets

PROSOM®;
1 mg; Tablet
Abbott Pharmaceutical
Product Division

What are estazolam tablets?

ESTAZOLAM (ProSom™) is a medicine to help you sleep. Federal law prohibits the transfer of estazolam to any person other than the patient for whom it was prescribed. Do not share this medicine with anyone else. Generic estazolam tablets are available.

What should my health care professional know before I take estazolam?

They need to know if you have any of these conditions:
- an alcohol or drug abuse problem
- bipolar disorder, depression, psychosis or other mental health condition
- glaucoma
- kidney disease
- liver disease
- lung disease, such as chronic obstructive pulmonary disease (COPD), sleep apnea or other breathing difficulties
- myasthenia gravis
- porphyria
- Parkinson's disease
- seizures or a history of seizures
- shortness of breath
- snoring
- suicidal thoughts
- an unusual or allergic reaction to estazolam, other benzodiazepines, foods, dyes, or preservatives
- pregnant or trying to get pregnant
- breast-feeding

How should I take this medicine?

Take estazolam tablets by mouth. Use estazolam only at bedtime. Follow the directions on the prescription label. Swallow the capsules with a drink of water. Do not take your medicine more often than directed. Do not stop taking except on your prescriber's advice. Contact your pediatrician or health care professional regarding the use of this medicine in children. Special care may be needed.

What if I miss a dose?

If you miss a dose, take it as soon as you can. It can take up to 2 hours for drowsiness to occur. Do not take double or extra doses, unless specifically told to by your prescriber or health care professional.

What may interact with estazolam?

- alcohol
- bosentan
- caffeine
- cimetidine
- disulfiram
- female hormones, including contraceptive or birth control pills
- herbal or dietary supplements such as kava kava, melatonin, St. John's Wort or valerian
- imatinib, STI-571
- isoniazid
- medicines for anxiety or sleeping problems, such as alprazolam, diazepam, lorazepam or triazolam
- medicines for depression, mental problems or psychiatric disturbances
- medicines for fungal infections (fluconazole, itraconazole, ketoconazole, voriconazole)
- medicines for HIV infection or AIDS
- nicardipine
- prescription pain medicines
- probenecid
- rifampin, rifapentine, or rifabutin
- some antibiotics (clarithromycin, erythromycin, troleandomycin)
- some medicines for colds, hay fever or other allergies
- some medicines for high blood pressure or heart-rhythm problems, (amiodarone, diltiazem, verapamil)
- some medicines for seizures (carbamazepine, phenobarbital, phenytoin, primidone)
- theophylline
- zafirlukast
- zileuton

Tell your prescriber or health care professional about all other medicines that you are taking, including non-prescription medicines, nutritional supplements, or herbal products. Also tell your prescriber or health care professional if you are a frequent user of drinks with caffeine or alcohol, if you smoke, or if you use illegal drugs. These may affect the way your medicine works. Check with your health care professional before stopping or starting any of your medicines.

What should I watch for while taking estazolam?

Visit your prescriber or health care professional for regular checks on your progress. Your body can become used to estazolam, ask your prescriber or health care professional if you still need to take it. Estazolam should be used only for short time periods. However, if you have been taking estazolam regularly for some time, do not suddenly stop taking it. You must gradually reduce the dose or you may get severe side effects. Ask your prescriber or health care professional for advice. Even after you stop taking estazolam it can still affect your body for several days. Make sure to take estazolam on nights you know you will be able to get a full night of sleep; at least 8 hours. Sometimes the sleepy effects of estazolam may "hangover" to the next morning. If this occurs, contact your prescriber or health care professional. You may get drowsy or dizzy. Do not drive, use machinery, or do anything that needs mental alertness until you know how estazolam affects you. Alcohol may increase dizziness and drowsiness. Do not drink any alcoholic drinks or use any other medicines that contain alcohol while taking estazolam. Do not treat yourself for coughs, colds or allergies without asking your prescriber or health care professional for advice. Some ingredients can increase possible side effects. If you are going to have surgery, tell your prescriber or health care professional that you are taking estazolam. Women who may become pregnant should use appropriate birth control methods while taking estazolam. Estazolam may cause birth defects in the unborn child if taken during pregnancy.

What side effects may I notice from taking estazolam?

Side effects that you should report to your prescriber or health care professional as soon as possible:
- confusion
- depression
- difficulty with movements or coordination
- lightheadedness, fainting, or falls
- mood changes, excitability, or aggressive behavior
- restlessness
- weakness or tiredness

Side effects that usually do not require medical attention (report to your prescriber or health care professional if they continue or are bothersome):
- constipation or diarrhea
- dizziness, drowsiness, clumsiness, or unsteadiness; a "hangover" effect
- headache
- heartburn
- increased dreaming or strange dreams
- stomach upset or pain

Where can I keep my medicine?

Keep out of the reach of children in a container that small children cannot open. Store at room temperature between 15 and 30 degrees C (59 and 86 degrees F). Protect from light. Keep container tightly closed. Throw away any unused medicine after the expiration date.

Esterified Estrogens, Estrone, Estropipate tablets

MENEST®;
0.625 mg; Tablet
Monarch Pharmaceuticals Inc

What are esterified estrogens and estropipate tablets?

ESTERIFIED ESTROGENS (Estratab®, Menest®); and **ESTROPIPATE** (Ogen®, Ortho-Est®) contain estrogen hormones. Estrogens are essential for maintaining normal female functions and are normally produced by the ovaries. After menopause, the ovaries decrease their production of these hormones. Estrogens can help relieve symptoms of the menopause (hot flashes, night sweats, mood changes, and vaginal dryness and irritation), and help to prevent the onset of osteoporosis (a loss of bone mass, so that bones become brittle and easily broken). Estrogens can also help improve female functions in women with hormonal imbalance or problems with their ovaries. Estrogens may also be given to certain men or women with inoperable breast cancers or prostate cancer. Occasionally these medications are used for other purposes. Generic esterified estrogen and estropipate tablets are available.

What should my health care professional know before I take esterified estrogens or estropipate?

They need to know if you have any of these conditions:
- asthma
- blood vessel disease, blood clotting disorder, or suffered a stroke
- breast, cervical, endometrial, or uterine cancer
- diabetes
- fibroids in the womb, or endometriosis
- heart, kidney, or liver disease
- high blood lipids or cholesterol
- high blood pressure
- high level of calcium in the blood
- hysterectomy
- mental depression
- migraine
- porphyria
- tobacco smoker
- vaginal bleeding
- an unusual or allergic reaction to estrogens, other hormones, medicines, foods, dyes, or preservatives
- pregnant or trying to get pregnant
- breast-feeding

How should I take this medicine?

Take esterified estrogen or estropipate tablets by mouth. Follow the directions on the prescription label. Swallow the tablets with a drink of water. If the tablets upset your stomach, take them with food or milk. Take your doses at regular intervals; estrogens work best when taken at the same time each day. Do not take your medicine more often than directed.

For all uses of this medicine:

Before starting this medication, read the paper on your prescription provided by your pharmacist or health care professional. This paper will tell you about the specific product you are taking. Make certain you understand the instructions.

Contact your pediatrician or health care professional regarding the use of this medicine in children. Special care may be needed.

What if I miss a dose?

If you miss a dose, take it as soon as you can. If it is almost time for your next dose, take only that dose and resume your normal schedule. Do not take double or extra doses.

What may interact with esterified estrogens or estropipate?

- some antibiotics used to treat infections
- barbiturates or benzodiazepines used for inducing sleep or treating seizures (convulsions)
- bromocriptine
- carbamazepine
- cimetidine
- cyclosporine
- dantrolene
- medications for diabetes
- methotrexate
- griseofulvin
- hydrocortisone, cortisone, or prednisolone
- isoniazid (INH)
- methotrexate
- mineral oil
- phenytoin
- raloxifene or tamoxifen
- rifabutin, rifampin, or rifapentine
- thyroid hormones
- topiramate
- tricyclic antidepressants
- warfarin

Tell your prescriber or health care professional about all other medicines you are taking, including non-prescription medicines, nutritional supplements, or herbal products. Also tell your prescriber or health care professional if you are a frequent user of drinks with caffeine or alcohol, if you smoke, or if you use illegal drugs. These may affect the way your medicine works. Check with your health care professional before stopping or starting any of your medicines.

What should I watch for while taking esterified estrogens or estropipate?

Visit your prescriber or health care professional for regular checks on your progress. You should have a complete check-up every 6 months. You will also need a regular breast and pelvic exam and "Pap" smear while on estrogens therapy. You should also discuss the need for regular mammograms with your health care professional, and follow his or her guidelines for these tests. If you have any unusual bleeding contact your prescriber or health care professional for advice. Estrogens can make your body retain fluid, making your fingers, hands, or ankles swell. Your blood pressure can go up. Contact your prescriber or health care professional if you feel you are retaining fluid. If you have any reason to think you are pregnant, stop taking estrogens at once and contact your prescriber or health care professional. Tobacco smoking increases the risk of getting a blood clot or having a stroke while you are taking estrogens,

especially if you are more than 35 years old. You are strongly advised not to smoke. If you wear contact lenses and notice visual changes, or if the lenses begin to feel uncomfortable, consult your eye care specialist or health care professional. In women who still have their uterus, estrogens increase the risk of developing a condition (endometrial hyperplasia) that may lead to cancer of the lining of the uterus. Taking progestins, another hormone drug, with estrogens lowers the risk of developing this condition. Therefore, if your uterus has not been removed (by a hysterectomy), your doctor may prescribe a progestin for you to take together with your estrogen. You should know, however, that taking estrogens with progestins may have additional health risks. You should discuss the use of estrogens and progestins with your health care professional to determine the benefits and risks for you. If you are going to have elective surgery, you may need to stop taking your estrogens one month beforehand. Consult your health care professional for advice prior to scheduling the surgery.

What side effects may I notice from taking esterified estrogens or estropipate?

Side effects that you should report to your prescriber or health care professional as soon as possible:
- breakthrough bleeding and spotting
- breast enlargement, tenderness, unusual discharge or milk production
- chest pain
- leg, arm or groin pain
- nausea, vomiting
- severe headaches
- stomach pain (severe)
- sudden shortness of breath
- swelling of the hands, feet or ankles or rapid weight gain
- vision or speech problems
- yellowing of the eyes or skin

Side effects that usually do not require medical attention (report to your prescriber or health care professional if they continue or are bothersome):
- change in sexual desire
- mild stomach upset
- mood changes, anxiety, depression, frustration, anger, or emotional outbursts
- increased or decreased appetite
- skin rash, acne, or brown spots on the face
- tiredness
- vaginal yeast infection (irritation and white discharge)
- weight gain

Where can I keep my medicine?

Keep out of the reach of children in a container that small children cannot open. Store at room temperature between 15 and 30 degrees C (59 and 86 degrees F). Throw away any unused medicine after the expiration date.

E

Esterified Estrogens; Methyltestosterone tablets

ESTRATEST H.S.; 0.625 mg/1.25 mg; Tablet Solvay Pharmaceuticals

SYNTEST H.S.; 0.625 mg; 1.25 mg; Tablet Syntho Pharmaceuticals

What are esterified estrogens; methyltestosterone tablets?

ESTERIFIED ESTROGENS; METHYLTESTOS-TERONE (Estratest®, Estratest HS®, Menogen®, Menogen HS®, Syntest H.S.) tablets contain estrogen hormones in combination with an androgen hormone. Estrogens are essential for maintaining normal female functions and are normally produced by the ovaries. After menopause, the ovaries decrease their production of these hormones. Estrogens can help relieve symptoms of the menopause (hot flashes, night sweats, mood changes, and vaginal dryness and irritation), and help to prevent the onset of osteoporosis (a loss of bone mass, so that bones become brittle and easily broken). Methyltestosterone, which is an androgen or male-like hormone, is useful in women who have menopause symptoms that have not responded to estrogens alone. Women's bodies naturally contain small amounts of testosterone, and the natural levels of testosterone also decrease with menopause. Occasionally this medication is used for other purposes. Generic esterified estrogens; methyltestosterone tablets are available.

What should my health care professional know before I take esterified estrogens; methyltestosterone?

They need to know if you have any of these conditions:
- asthma
- blood vessel disease, blood clotting disorder, or suffered a stroke
- breast, cervical, endometrial, or uterine cancer
- diabetes
- fibroids in the womb, or endometriosis
- heart, kidney or liver disease
- high blood lipids or cholesterol
- high blood pressure
- high level of calcium in the blood
- hysterectomy
- mental depression
- migraine
- porphyria
- tobacco smoker
- vaginal bleeding
- an unusual or allergic reaction to estrogens, methyltestosterone, other medicines, foods, dyes, or preservatives
- pregnant or trying to get pregnant
- breast-feeding

How should I take this medicine?

Take esterified estrogens; methyltestosterone tablets by mouth. Follow the directions on the prescription label. Swallow the tablets with a drink of water. If the tablets upset your stomach, take them with food or milk. Take your doses at regular intervals; estrogen-methyltestosterone combinations work best when taken at the same time each day. Do not take your medicine more often than directed.

For all uses of this medicine:

Before starting this medication, read the paper on your prescription provided by your pharmacist or health care professional. This paper will tell you about the specific product you are taking. Make certain you understand the instructions.

Contact your pediatrician or health care professional regarding the use of this medicine in children. Special care may be needed.

What if I miss a dose?

If you miss a dose, take it as soon as you can. If it is almost time for your next dose, take only that dose and resume your normal schedule. Do not take double or extra doses.

What may interact with esterified estrogens; methyltestosterone?

- some antibiotics used to treat infections
- barbiturates or benzodiazepines used for inducing sleep or treating seizures (convulsions)
- carbamazepine
- cimetidine
- cyclosporine
- dantrolene
- medications for diabetes
- methotrexate
- grapefruit juice
- griseofulvin
- herbal remedies for menopause or female problems
- hydrocortisone, cortisone, or prednisolone
- isoniazid (INH)
- methotrexate
- mineral oil
- phenytoin
- raloxifene or tamoxifen
- rifabutin, rifampin, or rifapentine
- thyroid hormones
- topiramate
- tricyclic antidepressants, like amitriptyline or imipramine
- warfarin

Tell your prescriber or health care professional about all other medicines you are taking, including non-prescription medicines, nutritional supplements, or herbal

products. Also tell your prescriber or health care professional if you are a frequent user of drinks with caffeine or alcohol, if you smoke, or if you use illegal drugs. These may affect the way your medicine works. Check with your health care professional before stopping or starting any of your medicines.

What should I watch for while taking esterified estrogens; methyltestosterone?

Visit your prescriber or health care professional for regular checks on your progress. You should have a complete check-up every 6 months. You will also need a regular breast and pelvic exam and "Pap" smear while on estrogen therapy. You should also discuss the need for regular mammograms with your health care professional, and follow his or her guidelines for these tests. If you have any unusual bleeding contact your prescriber or health care professional for advice. These hormones can make your body retain fluid, making your fingers, hands, or ankles swell. Your blood pressure can go up. Contact your prescriber or health care professional if you feel you are retaining fluid. If you have any reason to think you are pregnant; stop taking this medication at once and contact your prescriber or health care professional. Tobacco smoking increases the risk of getting a blood clot or having a stroke while you are taking estrogen hormones, especially if you are more than 35 years old. You are strongly advised not to smoke. If you wear contact lenses and notice visual changes, or if the lenses begin to feel uncomfortable, consult your eye care specialist or health care professional. In women who still have their uterus, estrogens increase the risk of developing a condition (endometrial hyperplasia or overgrowth) that may lead to cancer of the lining of the uterus. Taking progestins, another hormone drug, with estrogens lowers the risk of developing this condition. Therefore, if your uterus has not been removed (by a hysterectomy), your doctor may prescribe a progestin for you to take together with your estrogen. You should know, however, that taking estrogens with progestins may have additional health risks. You should discuss the use of estrogens and progestins with your health care professional to determine the benefits and risks for you. If you are going to have elective surgery, you may need to stop taking your estrogen hormones one month beforehand. Consult your

health care professional for advice prior to scheduling the surgery.

What side effects may I notice from taking esterified estrogens; methyltestosterone?

Side effects that you should report to your prescriber or health care professional as soon as possible:
- breakthrough bleeding and spotting
- breast enlargement, tenderness, unusual discharge or milk production
- chest pain
- leg, arm or groin pain
- nausea, vomiting
- severe or frequent headaches
- stomach pain (severe)
- sudden shortness of breath
- swelling of the hands, feet or ankles, or rapid weight gain
- vision or speech problems
- yellowing of the eyes or skin

Side effects that may indicate a need for decrease in dosage of the hormone (report to your prescriber at the next appointment, or earlier if bothersome; do not change your dose without talking to your prescriber):
- change in sexual desire
- hair loss
- hoarseness of voice
- mood changes, anxiety, depression, frustration, anger, or emotional outbursts
- unusual hair growth
- weight gain

Side effects that usually do not require medical attention (report to your prescriber or health care professional if they continue or are bothersome):
- mild stomach upset
- increased or decreased appetite
- skin rash or brown spots on the face
- tiredness
- vaginal yeast infection (irritation and white discharge)—report to your prescriber if you have never had one before

Where can I keep my medicine?

Keep out of the reach of children in a container that small children cannot open. Store at room temperature between 15 and 30 degrees C (59 and 86 degrees F). Throw away any unused medicine after the expiration date.

Estradiol tablets

ESTRADIOL;
1 mg; Tablet
Watson Pharmaceuticals Inc

What are estradiol tablets?

ESTRADIOL (Estrace®) is an estrogen that is essential for maintaining normal female functions. Estradiol is normally produced by the ovaries. After menopause, the ovaries decrease their production of this hormone. Estrogens can help relieve symptoms of the menopause

(hot flashes, night sweats, mood changes, and vaginal dryness and irritation), and help to prevent the onset of osteoporosis (a loss of bone mass, so that bones become brittle and easily broken). Estrogens can also help improve female functions in women with hormonal imbalance or problems with their ovaries. Estrogens may also be given to certain men or women with inoperable breast cancers or prostate cancer. Occasionally these medications are used for other purposes. Generic estradiol tablets are available.

What should my health care professional know before I take estradiol?

They need to know if you have any of these conditions:
- asthma
- blood vessel disease, blood clotting disorder, or suffered a stroke
- breast, cervical, endometrial or uterine cancer
- diabetes
- fibroids in the womb, or endometriosis
- heart, kidney or liver disease
- high blood lipids or cholesterol
- high blood pressure
- high level of calcium in the blood
- hysterectomy
- mental depression
- migraine
- porphyria
- tobacco smoker
- vaginal bleeding
- an unusual or allergic reaction to estrogens, other hormones, medicines, foods, dyes, or preservatives
- pregnant or trying to get pregnant
- breast-feeding

How should I take this medicine?

Take estrogen tablets by mouth. Follow the directions on the prescription label. Swallow the tablets with a drink of water. If the tablets upset your stomach, take them with food or milk. Take your doses at regular intervals; estrogens work best when taken at the same time each day. Do not take your medicine more often than directed.

For all uses of this medicine:

Before starting this medication, read the paper on your prescription provided by your pharmacist or health care professional. This paper will tell you about the specific product you are taking. Make certain you understand the instructions.

Contact your pediatrician or health care professional regarding the use of this medicine in children. Special care may be needed.

What if I miss a dose?

If you miss a dose, take it as soon as you can. If it is almost time for your next dose, take only that dose and resume your normal schedule. Do not take double or extra doses.

What may interact with estradiol?

- some antibiotics used to treat infections
- some medications used to treat HIV (human immuno-deficiency virus) infection or AIDS
- ascorbic acid/vitamin C supplements
- barbiturates or benzodiazepines used for inducing sleep or treating seizures (convulsions)
- bromocriptine

- carbamazepine
- cimetidine
- clofibrate
- cyclosporine
- dantrolene
- grapefruit juice
- griseofulvin
- hormones
- hydrocortisone, cortisone, or prednisolone
- imipramine or some other antidepressants
- isoniazid (INH)
- medications for diabetes
- methotrexate
- mineral oil
- phenytoin
- raloxifene or tamoxifen
- rifabutin, rifampin, or rifapentine
- some medications for treating migraines
- theophylline
- thyroid hormones
- topiramate
- tricyclic antidepressants
- warfarin

Tell your prescriber or health care professional about all other medicines you are taking, including non-prescription medicines, nutritional supplements, or herbal products. Also tell your prescriber or health care professional if you are a frequent user of drinks with caffeine or alcohol, if you smoke, or if you use illegal drugs. These may affect the way your medicine works. Check with your health care professional before stopping or starting any of your medicines.

What should I watch for while taking estradiol?

Visit your prescriber or health care professional for regular checks on your progress. You should have a complete check-up every 6 months. You will also need a regular breast and pelvic exam and "Pap" smear while on estrogens therapy. You should also discuss the need for regular mammograms with your health care professional, and follow his or her guidelines for these tests. If you have any unusual bleeding contact your prescriber or health care professional for advice. Estrogens can make your body retain fluid, making your fingers, hands, or ankles swell. Your blood pressure can go up. Contact your prescriber or health care professional if you feel you are retaining fluid. If you have any reason to think you are pregnant, stop taking estrogens at once and contact your prescriber or health care professional. Tobacco smoking increases the risk of getting a blood clot or having a stroke while you are taking estrogens, especially if you are more than 35 years old. You are strongly advised not to smoke. If you wear contact lenses and notice visual changes, or if the lenses begin to feel uncomfortable, consult your eye care specialist or health care professional. In women who still have their uterus, estrogens increase the risk of developing a condition (endometrial hyperplasia) that may lead to cancer of the lining of the uterus. Taking progestins, another hormone drug, with estrogens lowers the risk of developing this condition. Therefore, if your uterus has not been removed (by a hysterectomy), your doctor may prescribe a progestin for you to take together with your estrogen. You should know, however, that taking estrogens with progestins may have additional health risks. You should discuss the use of estrogens and progestins with your health care professional to determine the benefits and risks for you. If you are going to have elective surgery, you may need to stop taking your estrogens one month beforehand. Consult your health care professional for advice prior to scheduling the surgery.

What side effects may I notice from taking estradiol?

Side effects that you should report to your prescriber or health care professional as soon as possible:
- breakthrough bleeding and spotting
- breast enlargement, tenderness, unusual discharge or milk production
- chest pain
- leg, arm or groin pain
- nausea, vomiting
- severe headaches
- stomach or abdominal pain (severe)
- sudden shortness of breath
- swelling of the hands, feet or ankles, or rapid weight gain
- vision or speech problems
- yellowing of the eyes or skin

Side effects that usually do not require medical attention (report to your prescriber or health care professional if they continue or are bothersome):
- change in sexual desire
- mild stomach upset
- mood changes, anxiety, depression, frustration, anger, or emotional outbursts
- increased or decreased appetite
- skin rash, acne, or brown spots on the face
- tiredness
- vaginal yeast infection (irritation and white discharge)
- weight gain

Where can I keep my medicine?

Keep out of the reach of children in a container that small children cannot open. Store at room temperature between 15 and 30 degrees C (59 and 86 degrees F). Throw away any unused medicine after the expiration date.

Estradiol; Levonorgestrel skin patches

CLIMARA®;
0.045 mg/24 hr/0.015 mg/
24 hr; Film, Extended Release
Berlex Laboratories Inc

What are estradiol; levonorgestrel skin patches?

ESTRADIOL; LEVONORGESTREL (Climara-Pro™, Climara®) skin patches contain a natural estrogen female hormone and a progestin. Estradiol is essential for maintaining normal female functions and is normally produced by the ovaries. After menopause, the ovaries make less of this hormone. Estradiol can help relieve symptoms of the menopause (hot flashes, night sweats, mood changes, and vaginal dryness and irritation), and may also help to prevent the onset of osteoporosis (a loss of bone mass, so that bones become brittle and easily broken). Levonorgestrel is a progestin that is helpful in reducing overgrowth of the lining of the uterus (the endometrium), which may help reduce your risk of endometrial cancer. Sometimes these patches are prescribed to women who need estrogens because they have ovaries that do not function properly, or because they have had their ovaries surgically removed. Generic estradiol; levonorgestrel skin patches are not yet available.

What should my health care professional know before I take estradiol; levonorgestrel?

They need to know if you have any of these conditions:
- blood vessel disease, blood clotting disorder, or suffered a stroke
- breast, cervical, endometrial, or uterine cancer
- diabetes
- fibroids in the womb, or endometriosis
- heart, kidney, or liver disease
- high blood lipids or cholesterol
- high blood pressure
- high level of calcium in the blood
- hysterectomy
- mental depression
- migraine
- porphyria
- skin reactions to bandages, tape, or adhesives
- tobacco smoker
- vaginal bleeding
- an unusual or allergic reaction to estrogens, progestins, other hormones, medicines, foods, dyes, or preservatives
- pregnant or trying to get pregnant
- breast-feeding

How should this medicine be used?

Estradiol; levonorgestrel skin patches are for external use only. Follow the directions on the prescription label. Use exactly as directed. Usually, women are prescribed to wear the estradiol; levonorgestrel patches every day of the monthly cycle. One estradiol; levonorgestrel patch contains enough medication for one week. It is worn continuously until it is time to replace with a new patch. Replace with a new patch once per week, or as directed by your prescriber. Make a schedule and keep to it, so that you always change your patch on the same day of the week. Tear open the pouch, do not use scissors. Remove the stiff protective liner covering the adhesive. Try not to touch the adhesive. Apply the patch, sticky side to the skin, to an area of the lower abdomen that is clean, dry and hairless; avoid injured, irritated, calloused, or scarred areas. Do not apply the skin patches to your breasts or around the waist area. Use a different site each time to prevent skin irritation. Do not cut or trim the patch. Do not stop using except on your prescriber's advice. Do not wear two patches at one time. You may bathe or participate in other activities while wearing your patch. If the patch pulls loose or falls off, you may reapply it if the patch is sticky enough to stay on the skin. You should reapply the patch in a different area. Otherwise use a fresh patch. You should change your patch on the same days each week. After removal of a patch, fold the used patch in half (sticky side in) and throw it away in an area where children or pets cannot reach it.

For all uses of this medicine:

Before starting this medication, read the paper on your prescription provided by your pharmacist or health care professional. This paper will tell you about the product you are using. Make certain you understand the instructions.

Contact your pediatrician or health care professional regarding the use of this medicine in children. Special care may be needed.

What if I miss a dose?

If you forget to change your patch as scheduled, remove the old patch and apply a new one as soon as possible. Remember to remove the old patch. If it is almost time to apply the next patch, skip the missed patch and get back on your normal schedule. Remember to remove the old patch. Do not wear more than one patch at a time unless you are told to do so by your prescriber.

What may interact with estradiol; levonorgestrel?

- barbiturates or benzodiazepines used for inducing sleep or treating seizures (convulsions)
- bosentan
- bromocriptine
- carbamazepine
- cimetidine
- cyclosporine
- dantrolene
- medications for diabetes
- methotrexate
- griseofulvin
- hydrocortisone, cortisone, or prednisolone
- isoniazid (INH)
- methotrexate
- phenytoin
- raloxifene or tamoxifen
- rifabutin, rifampin, or rifapentine
- thyroid hormones

- topiramate
- tricyclic antidepressants
- warfarin

Tell your prescriber or health care professional about all other medicines you are taking, including non-prescription medicines, nutritional supplements, or herbal products. Also tell your prescriber or health care professional if you are a frequent user of drinks with caffeine or alcohol, if you smoke, or if you use illegal drugs. These may affect the way your medicine works. Check with your health care professional before stopping or starting any of your medicines.

What should I watch for while taking estradiol; levonorgestrel?

Visit your prescriber or health care professional for regular checks on your progress. You should have a complete check-up every 6 months. You will need a regular breast and pelvic exam and "Pap" smear while on estradiol; levonorgestrel skin patches. You should also discuss the need for regular mammograms with your health care professional, and follow his or her guidelines for these tests. Estradiol; levonorgestrel skin patches can make your body retain fluid, making your fingers, hands, or ankles swell. Your blood pressure can go up. Contact your prescriber or health care professional if you feel you are retaining fluid. If you have any reason to think you are pregnant; stop wearing the skin patches at once and contact your prescriber or health care professional. Tobacco smoking increases the risk of getting a blood clot or having a stroke while you are wearing estradiol; levonorgestrel skin patches, especially if you are more than 35 years old. You are strongly advised not to smoke. If you wear contact lenses and notice visual changes, or if the lenses begin to feel uncomfortable, consult your eye care specialist. If you are going to have elective surgery, you may need to stop taking your estrogens one month beforehand. Consult your health care professional for advice prior to scheduling the surgery.

What side effects may I notice from taking estradiol; levonorgestrel?

Side effects that you should report to your prescriber or health care professional as soon as possible:
- breakthrough bleeding and spotting
- breast enlargement, tenderness, unusual discharge or milk production
- chest pain
- leg, arm or groin pain
- nausea, vomiting
- severe headaches
- stomach or abdominal pain (severe)
- sudden shortness of breath
- swelling of the hands, feet or ankles or rapid weight gain
- vision or speech problems
- yellowing of the eyes or skin

Side effects that usually do not require medical attention (report to your prescriber or health care professional if they continue or are bothersome):

- change in sexual desire
- mild stomach upset
- mood changes, anxiety, depression, frustration, anger, or emotional outbursts
- increased or decreased appetite
- skin rash, acne, or brown spots on the face
- tiredness

- vaginal yeast infection (irritation and white discharge)
- weight gain

Where can I keep my medicine?

Keep out of the reach of children in a container that small children cannot open. Store at room temperature between 15 and 30 degrees C (59 and 86 degrees F). Do not store any patches that have been removed from their protective pouch. Throw away any unused medicine after the expiration date.

Estradiol; Norethindrone skin patches

| COMBIPATCH®; 0.05 mg/24 hr/0.14 mg/24 hr; Film, Extended Release Novartis Pharmaceuticals | | COMBIPATCH®; 0.05 mg/24 hr/0.25 mg/24 hr; Film, Extended Release Novartis Pharmaceuticals | |

What are estradiol; norethindrone skin patches?

ESTRADIOL; NORETHINDRONE (CombiPatch™) skin patches are a mixture of a natural estrogen female hormone and a progestin. Estradiol is essential for maintaining normal female functions and is normally produced by the ovaries. After menopause, the ovaries decrease their production of this hormone. Estradiol can help relieve symptoms of the menopause (hot flashes, night sweats, mood changes, and vaginal dryness and irritation), and may also help to prevent the onset of osteoporosis (a loss of bone mass, so that bones become brittle and easily broken). Norethindrone is a progestin that is helpful in reducing overgrowth of the lining of the uterus (the endometrium), which may help reduce your risk of endometrial cancer. Sometimes these patches are prescribed to women who need estrogens because they have ovaries that do not function properly, or because they have had their ovaries surgically removed. Generic estradiol; norethindrone skin patches are not yet available.

What should my health care professional know before I use estradiol; norethindrone skin patches?

They need to know if you have any of these conditions:
- blood vessel disease, blood clotting disorder, or suffered a stroke
- breast, cervical, endometrial, or uterine cancer
- diabetes
- fibroids in the womb, or endometriosis
- heart, kidney or liver disease
- high blood lipids or cholesterol
- high blood pressure
- high level of calcium in the blood
- hysterectomy
- mental depression
- migraine
- porphyria
- skin reactions to bandages, tape, or adhesives
- tobacco smoker
- vaginal bleeding

- an unusual or allergic reaction to estrogens, other hormones, medicines, foods, dyes, or preservatives
- pregnant or trying to get pregnant
- breast-feeding

How should I use this medicine?

Estradiol; norethindrone skin patches are for external use only. Follow the directions on the prescription label. Use exactly as directed. Some women will only be prescribed the estradiol; norethindrone skin patches. Other women may be prescribed to wear a patch with estrogen only on certain days of the month, and will wear the estradiol; norethindrone patches on the rest of the days. One estradiol; norethindrone patch contains enough medication for several days. It is worn continuously until it is time to replace with a new patch. The system is worn continuously and replaced twice weekly, or as directed by your prescriber or health care professional. Make a schedule and keep to it, so that you always change your patch on the days you have marked. Tear open the pouch, do not use scissors. Remove the stiff protective liner covering the adhesive. Try not to touch the adhesive. Apply the patch, sticky side to the skin, to an area of the lower abdomen that is clean, dry and hairless; avoid injured, irritated, calloused, or scarred areas. Do not apply the skin patches to your breasts or around the waist area. Use a different site each time to prevent skin irritation. Do not cut or trim the patch. Do not stop using except on your prescriber's advice. Do not wear two patches at one time. You may bathe or participate in other activities while wearing your patch. If the patch pulls loose or falls off, you may reapply it if the patch is sticky enough to stay on the skin. You should reapply the patch in a different area. Otherwise use a fresh patch. You should change your patch on the same days each week. After removal of a patch, fold the used patch in half (sticky side in) and throw it away in an area where children or pets cannot reach it.

For all uses of this medicine:

Before starting this medication, read the paper on your prescription provided by your pharmacist or health care

E

professional. This paper will tell you about the product you are using. Make certain you understand the instructions.

Contact your pediatrician or health care professional regarding the use of this medicine in children. Special care may be needed.

What if I miss a dose?

If you forget to change your patch as scheduled, apply it as soon as possible. Remember to remove the old patch. If it is almost time to apply the next patch, skip the missed patch and get back on your normal schedule. Remember to remove the old patch. Do not wear more than one patch at a time unless you are told to do so by your prescriber.

What may interact with estradiol; norethindrone?

- barbiturates or benzodiazepines used for inducing sleep or treating seizures (convulsions)
- bosentan
- bromocriptine
- carbamazepine
- cimetidine
- cyclosporine
- dantrolene
- medications for diabetes
- methotrexate
- griseofulvin
- hydrocortisone, cortisone, or prednisolone
- isoniazid (INH)
- methotrexate
- phenytoin
- raloxifene or tamoxifen
- rifabutin, rifampin, or rifapentine
- thyroid hormones
- topiramate
- tricyclic antidepressants
- warfarin

Tell your prescriber or health care professional about all other medicines you are taking, including non-prescription medicines, nutritional supplements, or herbal products. Also tell your prescriber or health care professional if you are a frequent user of drinks with caffeine or alcohol, if you smoke, or if you use illegal drugs. These may affect the way your medicine works. Check with your health care professional before stopping or starting any of your medicines.

What should I watch for while taking estradiol; norethindrone?

Visit your prescriber or health care professional for regular checks on your progress. You should have a complete check-up every 6 months. You will need a regular breast and pelvic exam and "Pap" smear while on estradiol; norethindrone skin patches. You should also discuss the need for regular mammograms with your health care professional, and follow his or her guidelines for these tests. Estradiol; norethindrone skin patches can make your body retain fluid, making your

fingers, hands, or ankles swell. Your blood pressure can go up. Contact your prescriber or health care professional if you feel you are retaining fluid. If you have any reason to think you are pregnant, stop wearing the skin patches at once and contact your prescriber or health care professional. Tobacco smoking increases the risk of getting a blood clot or having a stroke while you are wearing estradiol; norethindrone skin patches, especially if you are more than 35 years old. You are strongly advised not to smoke. If you wear contact lenses and notice visual changes, or if the lenses begin to feel uncomfortable, consult your eye care specialist. If you are going to have elective surgery, you may need to stop taking your estrogens one month beforehand. Consult your health care professional for advice prior to scheduling the surgery. If you are going to have a MRI procedure, let your MRI technician know about the use of these patches. Some drug patches contain an aluminized backing that can become heated when exposed to MRI and may cause burns. You may need to temporarily remove the patch during the MRI procedure.

What side effects may I notice from using estradiol; norethindrone?

Side effects that you should report to your prescriber or health care professional as soon as possible:
- breakthrough bleeding and spotting
- breast enlargement, tenderness, unusual discharge or milk production
- chest pain
- leg, arm or groin pain
- nausea, vomiting
- severe headaches
- stomach or abdominal pain (severe)
- sudden shortness of breath
- swelling of the hands, feet or ankles or rapid weight gain
- vision or speech problems
- yellowing of the eyes or skin

Side effects that usually do not require medical attention (report to your prescriber or health care professional if they continue or are bothersome):
- change in sexual desire
- mild stomach upset
- mood changes, anxiety, depression, frustration, anger, or emotional outbursts
- increased or decreased appetite
- skin rash, acne, or brown spots on the face
- tiredness
- vaginal yeast infection (irritation and white discharge)
- weight gain

Where can I keep my medicine?

Keep out of the reach of children in a container that small children cannot open. Store at room temperature between 15 and 30 degrees C (59 and 86 degrees F). Do not store any patches that have been removed from their protective pouch. Throw away any unused medicine after the expiration date. The estradiol; norethindrone patches will expire 3 months after your pharmacist or health care professional dispenses them to you.

Estradiol; Norethindrone tablets

ACTIVELLA®;
1 mg/0.5 mg; Tablet
Novo Nordisk Pharmaceutical
Industries Inc

What are estradiol; norethindrone tablets?

ESTRADIOL; NORETHINDRONE (Activella™) tablets are a mixture of a natural estrogen female hormone and a progestin. Estradiol is essential for maintaining normal female functions and is normally produced by the ovaries. After menopause, the ovaries decrease their production of this hormone. Estradiol can help relieve symptoms of the menopause (hot flashes, night sweats, mood changes, and vaginal dryness and irritation), and also help to prevent the onset of osteoporosis (a loss of bone mass, so that bones become brittle and easily broken). Norethindrone is a progestin that is helpful in reducing overgrowth of the lining of the uterus (the endometrium), which may help reduce your risk of endometrial cancer. Generic estradiol; norethindrone tablets are not yet available.

What should my health care professional know before I take estradiol; norethindrone?

They need to know if you have any of these conditions:
- blood vessel disease, blood clotting disorder, or suffered a stroke
- breast, cervical, endometrial, or uterine cancer
- diabetes
- fibroids in the womb, or endometriosis
- heart, kidney or liver disease
- high blood lipids or cholesterol
- high blood pressure
- high level of calcium in the blood
- hysterectomy
- mental depression
- migraine
- porphyria
- skin reactions to bandages, tape, or adhesives
- tobacco smoker
- vaginal bleeding
- an unusual or allergic reaction to estrogens, other hormones, medicines, foods, dyes, or preservatives
- pregnant or trying to get pregnant
- breast-feeding

How should I take this medicine?

Take estradiol; norethindrone tablets by mouth. Follow the directions on the prescription label. You will take one tablet daily. Try to take your dose at the same time each day. Swallow the tablet with a drink of water. You may take the tablets with food. Do not take your medicine more often than directed.

For all uses of this medicine:

Before starting this medication, read the paper on your prescription provided by your pharmacist or health care professional. This paper will tell you about the product you are taking. Make certain you understand the instructions.

Contact your pediatrician or health care professional regarding the use of this medicine in children. Special care may be needed.

What if I miss a dose?

If you miss a dose, take it as soon as you can. If it is almost time for your next dose, take only that dose. Do not take double or extra doses.

What may interact with estradiol; norethindrone?

- barbiturates or benzodiazepines used for inducing sleep or treating seizures (convulsions)
- bosentan
- bromocriptine
- carbamazepine
- cimetidine
- cyclosporine
- dantrolene
- medications for diabetes
- grapefruit juice
- griseofulvin
- hydrocortisone, cortisone, or prednisolone
- isoniazid (INH)
- methotrexate
- mineral oil
- phenytoin
- raloxifene or tamoxifen
- rifabutin, rifampin, or rifapentine
- thyroid hormones
- topiramate
- tricyclic antidepressants
- warfarin

Tell your prescriber or health care professional about all other medicines you are taking, including non-prescription medicines, nutritional supplements, or herbal products. Also tell your prescriber or health care professional if you are a frequent user of drinks with caffeine or alcohol, if you smoke, or if you use illegal drugs. These may affect the way your medicine works. Check with your health care professional before stopping or starting any of your medicines.

What should I watch for while taking estradiol; norethindrone?

Visit your prescriber or health care professional for regular checks on your progress. You should have a complete check-up every 6 months. You will need a regular breast and pelvic exam and "Pap" smear while on estradiol; norethindrone. You should also discuss the need for regular mammograms with your health care professional, and follow his or her guidelines for these tests. Estradiol; norethindrone tablets can make your body retain fluid, making your fingers, hands, or ankles swell.

E

Your blood pressure can go up. Contact your prescriber or health care professional if you feel you are retaining fluid. If you have any reason to think you are pregnant; stop taking estradiol; norethindrone at once and contact your prescriber or health care professional. Tobacco smoking increases the risk of getting a blood clot or having a stroke while you are taking estradiol; norethindrone, especially if you are more than 35 years old. You are strongly advised not to smoke. If you wear contact lenses and notice visual changes, or if the lenses begin to feel uncomfortable, consult your eye care specialist. If you are going to have elective surgery, you may need to stop taking your estrogens one month beforehand. Consult your health care professional for advice prior to scheduling the surgery.

What side effects may I notice from taking estradiol; norethindrone?

Side effects that you should report to your prescriber or health care professional as soon as possible:
- breakthrough bleeding and spotting
- breast enlargement, tenderness, unusual discharge or milk production
- chest pain
- leg, arm or groin pain
- nausea, vomiting

- severe headaches
- stomach or abdominal pain (severe)
- sudden shortness of breath
- swelling of the hands, feet or ankles, or rapid weight gain
- vision or speech problems
- yellowing of the eyes or skin

Side effects that usually do not require medical attention (report to your prescriber or health care professional if they continue or are bothersome):
- change in sexual desire
- mild stomach upset
- mood changes, anxiety, depression, frustration, anger, or emotional outbursts
- increased or decreased appetite
- skin rash, acne, or brown spots on the face
- tiredness
- vaginal yeast infection (irritation and white discharge)
- weight gain

Where can I keep my medicine?

Keep out of the reach of children in a container that small children cannot open. Store at room temperature between 15 and 30 degrees C (59 and 86 degrees F). Throw away any unused medicine after the expiration date.

Estradiol; Norgestimate tablets

ORTHO-PREFEST(TM);
1 mg/0.09 mg; Tablet
Ortho McNeil Pharmaceutical
Inc

What are estradiol; norgestimate tablets?

ESTRADIOL; NORGESTIMATE (Ortho-Prefest(TM)) tablets are a mixture of a estrogen female hormone and a progestin. Estradiol is essential for maintaining normal female functions and is normally produced by the ovaries. After menopause, the ovaries decrease their production of this hormone. Estradiol can help relieve symptoms of the menopause (hot flashes, night sweats, mood changes, and vaginal dryness and irritation), and may also help to prevent the onset of osteoporosis (a loss of bone mass, so that bones become brittle and easily broken). Norgestimate is a progestin that is helpful in reducing overgrowth of the lining of the uterus (the endometrium), which may help reduce your risk of endometrial cancer. Generic estradiol-norgestimate tablets are available.

What should my health care professional know before I take estradiol-norgestimate?

They need to know if you have any of these conditions:
- blood vessel disease, blood clotting disorder, or suffered a stroke
- breast, cervical, endometrial, or uterine cancer
- diabetes
- fibroids in the womb, or endometriosis
- heart, kidney or liver disease
- high blood lipids or cholesterol

- high blood pressure
- high level of calcium in the blood
- hysterectomy
- mental depression
- migraine
- porphyria
- tobacco smoker
- vaginal bleeding
- an unusual or allergic reaction to estrogens, other hormones, medicines, foods, dyes, or preservatives
- pregnant or trying to get pregnant
- breast-feeding

How should I take this medicine?

Take estradiol-norgestimate tablets by mouth. Follow the directions on the prescription label. You will take one tablet daily, in the order indicated on the package. Take 1 pink tablet once daily for 3 days followed by 1 white tablet once daily for 3 days. Take in this order until package is complete, then start a new package. Try to take your dose at the same time each day. Swallow the tablet with a drink of water. You may take the tablets with food. Do not take your medicine more often than directed.

For all uses of this medicine:

Before starting this medication, read the paper on your prescription provided by your pharmacist or health care professional. This paper will tell you about the product you are taking. Make certain you understand the instructions.

Contact your pediatrician or health care professional regarding the use of this medicine in children. Special care may be needed.

What if I miss a dose?

If you miss a dose, take it as soon as you can. If it is almost time for your next dose, take only that dose. Do not take double or extra doses.

What may interact with estradiol-norgestimate?

- barbiturates or benzodiazepines used for inducing sleep or treating seizures (convulsions)
- bosentan
- bromocriptine
- carbamazepine
- cimetidine
- cyclosporine
- dantrolene
- medications for diabetes
- grapefruit juice
- griseofulvin
- hydrocortisone, cortisone, or prednisolone
- isoniazid (INH)
- methotrexate
- mineral oil
- phenytoin
- raloxifene or tamoxifen
- rifabutin, rifampin, or rifapentine
- thyroid hormones
- topiramate
- tricyclic antidepressants
- warfarin

Tell your prescriber or health care professional about all other medicines you are taking, including non-prescription medicines, nutritional supplements, or herbal products. Also tell your prescriber or health care professional if you are a frequent user of drinks with caffeine or alcohol, if you smoke, or if you use illegal drugs. These may affect the way your medicine works. Check with your health care professional before stopping or starting any of your medicines.

What should I watch for while taking estradiol-norgestimate?

Visit your prescriber for regular checks on your progress. You should have a complete check-up every 6 months. You will need a regular breast and pelvic exam and "Pap" smear while on estradiol-norgestimate. Regular breast examinations by a health professional and monthly self-examination are recommended for all women. You should also discuss the need for regular mammograms with you health care prescriber. Estradiol; norgestimate tablets can make your body retain fluid, making your fingers, hands, or ankles swell. Your blood pressure can go up. Contact your prescriber if you feel you are retaining fluid. If you have any reason to think you are pregnant; stop taking estradiol-norgestimate at once and contact your prescriber. Tobacco smoking increases the risk of getting a blood clot or having a stroke while you are taking estradiol-norgestimate, especially if you are more than 35 years old. You are strongly advised not to smoke. If you wear contact lenses and notice changes in vision, or if the lenses begin to feel uncomfortable, consult your eye care specialist. If you are going to have elective surgery, you may need to stop taking your estrogens one month beforehand. Consult your health care professional for advice prior to scheduling the surgery. In women who still have their uterus, taking a progestin with your estrogens lowers the risk of developing overgrowth of the uterine lining. You should know, however, that taking estrogens with progestins may have additional health risks. You should discuss the use of estrogens and progestins with your health care professional to determine the benefits and risks for you. This product contains both an estrogen and a progestin.

What side effects may I notice from taking estradiol-norgestimate?

Side effects that you should report to your prescriber or health care professional as soon as possible:
- breakthrough bleeding and spotting
- breast lumps or unusual discharge
- chest pain
- coughing up blood
- dizziness, fainting, or weakness
- leg, arm or groin pain
- nausea, vomiting
- severe headaches
- stomach or abdominal pain (severe), tenderness or swelling
- sudden loss of coordination, especially on one side of the body
- sudden shortness of breath
- swelling of the hands, feet or ankles, or rapid weight gain
- vision or speech problems
- yellowing of the eyes or skin
- weakness or numbness in the arms or legs, especially on one side of the body

Side effects that usually do not require medical attention (report to your prescriber or health care professional if they continue or are bothersome):
- breast tenderness
- change in sexual desire
- increased or decreased appetite
- mild stomach upset
- mood changes, anxiety, depression, frustration, anger, or emotional outbursts
- skin rash, acne, or brown spots on the face
- tiredness
- vaginal yeast infection (irritation and white discharge)
- weight gain

Where can I keep my medicine?

Keep out of the reach of children in a container that small children cannot open. Store at room temperature between 15 and 30 degrees C (59 and 86 degrees F). Throw away any unused medicine after the expiration date.

E

Estramustine capsules

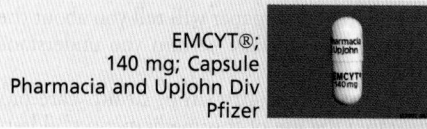

EMCYT®;
140 mg; Capsule
Pharmacia and Upjohn Div
Pfizer

What are estramustine capsules?

ESTRAMUSTINE (Emcyt®) is a chemotherapy agent for treating prostate cancer. Estramustine belongs to a group of medicines known as alkylating agents. Estramustine interferes with the growth of cancer cells, and eventually causes these cells to die. Estramustine may also be used to treat breast cancer and certain types of brain cancers. Generic estramustine capsules are not yet available.

What should my health care professional know before I take estramustine?

They need to know if you have any of these conditions:

- blood disorders (especially abnormal clotting)
- diabetes mellitus
- edema
- heart disease
- high levels of calcium
- hypertension
- infection (especially virus infections such as chickenpox or herpes)
- kidney disease
- liver disease
- migraine
- seizures
- stroke
- an unusual or allergic reaction to estramustine, estrogens, other chemotherapy, other medicines, foods, dyes, or preservatives
- pregnant or trying to get pregnant
- breast-feeding

How should I take this medicine?

Take estramustine capsules by mouth. Follow the directions on the prescription label. Swallow the capsules with a drink of water. Do not chew or open the capsules. Take the capsules at least one hour before or two hours after eating a meal. Do not take the capsules with food or any milk products including ice cream or cheese. Take your doses at regular intervals. Estramustine is usually taken in 3 or 4 divided daily doses. Do not take your medicine more often than directed. Finish the full course prescribed by your doctor or health care professional even if the capsules make you feel unwell. Do not stop taking except on your prescriber's advice.

What if I miss a dose?

It is important not to miss a dose. You will take one dose every day. If you vomit after taking a dose, call your prescriber or health care professional for advice.

What may interact with estramustine?

- antacid products such as Tums®, Mylanta® or Maalox®

- calcium supplements or vitamins containing calcium
- vaccines

Tell your prescriber or health care professional about all other medicines you are taking, including non-prescription medicines, nutritional supplements, or herbal products. Also tell your prescriber or health care professional if you are a frequent user of drinks with caffeine or alcohol, if you smoke, or if you use illegal drugs. These may affect the way your medicine works. Check with your health care professional before stopping or starting any of your medicines.

What should I watch for while taking estramustine?

Visit your prescriber or health care professional for checks on your progress. You will need to have regular blood checks. The side effects of estramustine can continue after you finish your treatment; report side effects promptly. Estramustine may make you feel generally unwell. This is not uncommon because estramustine affects good cells as well as cancer cells. Report any side effects as above, but continue your course of medicine even though you feel ill, unless your prescriber or health care professional tells you to stop. Call your prescriber or health care professional for advice if you get a fever, chills or sore throat. Do not treat yourself. Estramustine may harm your unborn baby. You should contact your prescriber immediately if you believe or suspect you or your partner have become pregnant while you are taking estramustine. Both men and women must use effective birth control continuously while taking estramustine. It is recommended that you use 2 reliable forms of contraception together. If you are going to have surgery, tell your prescriber or health care professional that you are taking estramustine.

What side effects may I notice from taking estramustine?

Side effects that you should report to your prescriber or health care professional as soon as possible:

- difficulty breathing, wheezing or shortness of breath
- numbness or tingling in arms or legs
- chest pain
- diarrhea
- fever or chills, cough or sore throat
- lower back pain
- vomiting
- soreness or swelling (knot) in legs

Side effects that usually do not require medical attention (report to your prescriber or health care professional if they continue or are bothersome):

- loss of appetite (this may last for several days)
- nausea
- trouble sleeping

- decreased interest in sex
- breast tenderness or enlargement

Where can I keep my medicine?

Keep out of the reach of children in a container that small children cannot open. Store in a refrigerator. The capsules may be stored outside of the refrigerator at normal room temperature, out of direct sunlight, for no more than 2 days without affecting the strength of the medicine. Keep container tightly closed and away from wet places. Throw away any unused medicine after the expiration date.

Eszopiclone tablets

LUNESTA™;
1 mg; Tablet
Sepracor Inc.

LUNESTA™;
2 mg; Tablet
Sepracor Inc.

What are Eszopiclone tablets?

ESZOPICLONE (Lunesta™) is a sedative-type drug that helps to relieve insomnia (sleeplessness). Trouble falling asleep, waking up too early in the morning, or waking up too often during the night are symptoms of insomnia. Eszopiclone helps treat these problems with sleep. Do not share your medicine with anyone else. Generic eszopiclone tablets are not yet available.

What should my health care professional know before I receive Eszopiclone?

They need to know if you have any of these conditions:
- frequently drink alcohol
- depression
- history of drug abuse
- liver disease
- lung or respiratory disease (breathing difficulties, like emphysema or sleep apnea)
- an unusual or allergic reaction to eszopiclone, other medicines, foods, dyes, or preservatives
- pregnant or trying to get pregnant
- breast-feeding

How should this medicine be used?

Take eszopiclone tablets by mouth. Follow the directions on the prescription label. Swallow the tablets with a drink of water. It is better to take eszopiclone on an empty stomach (without food). Only take eszopiclone when you are ready for bed. Do not take your medicine more often than directed. Do not share your medicine with anyone else. Contact your pediatrician or health care professional regarding the use of this medicine in children. Special care may be needed. Elderly patients over age 65 years may have a stronger reaction to this medicine and need smaller doses.

What if I miss a dose?

This does not apply. Eszopiclone should only be taken immediately before going to sleep. Do not take double or extra doses.

What may interact with Eszopiclone?

- caffeine
- flumazenil
- certain antidepressants, like citalopram, fluoxetine, fluvoxamine, or sertraline
- medications for fungal infections, like ketoconazole, fluconazole, or itraconazole
- some medicines used to treat HIV infection or AIDS, like ritonavir
- St. John's wort

Certain medications may cause additive drowsiness or decrease alertness with eszopiclone:

- alcohol
- allergy, cough, or cold medications (antihistamines)
- kava kava
- medicines for anxiety
- medicines for pain
- medicines for treating mental problems
- melatonin
- other sedatives given for sleep
- some medicines for Parkinson's disease or other movement disorders
- valerian

Tell your prescriber or health care professional about all other medicines you are taking, including non-prescription medicines, nutritional supplements, or herbal products. Also tell your prescriber or health care professional if you are a frequent user of drinks with caffeine or alcohol, if you smoke, or if you use illegal drugs. These may affect the way your medicine works. Check with your health care professional before stopping or starting any of your medicines.

What should I watch for while taking Eszopiclone?

Visit your prescriber or health care professional for regular checks on your progress. Keep a regular sleep schedule by going to bed at about the same time nightly. Avoid caffeine-containing drinks in the evening hours, as caffeine can cause trouble with falling asleep. Consult your prescriber or health care professional if you still have difficulty in sleeping. Sleep medicines sometimes cause a type of memory loss, in which the person may not remember what has happened in the several hours after taking the medication. This type of memory loss is usually not a problem since eszopiclone is taken right before bedtime. Be sure to talk to your doctor if you think you are having memory problems while on this medication. If you have been taking eszopiclone for several weeks and suddenly stop taking it, you may get unpleasant withdrawal symptoms. Your prescriber or health care professional may want to re-

E

duce the dose gradually. Do not stop taking eszopiclone on your own. Always follow your prescriber's advice. After you stop taking your eszopiclone prescription, you may notice some trouble with falling asleep. This is sometimes called 'rebound insomnia'. Do not get discouraged, because this problem usually goes away on its own after 1 or 2 nights. You may get drowsy or dizzy. Do not drive, use machinery, or do anything that needs mental alertness until you know how eszopiclone affects you. To reduce dizzy or fainting spells, do not sit or stand up quickly, especially if you are an older patient. Alcohol can increase possible unpleasant effects. Do not drink alcoholic drinks while taking medications to help you sleep. If you are going to have surgery, tell your prescriber or health care professional that you are taking eszopiclone.

What side effects may I notice from receiving Eszopiclone?

Side effects that you should report to your prescriber or health care professional as soon as possible:
- confusion

- depressed mood
- hallucinations (seeing, hearing, or feeling things that are not really there)
- lightheadedness, fainting spells, or falls
- slurred speech or difficulty with coordination
- vision changes
- restlessness, excitability, or feelings of agitation

Side effects that usually do not require medical attention (report to your prescriber or health care professional if they continue or are bothersome):
- dizziness, or daytime drowsiness, sometimes called a 'hangover' effect
- headache
- strange dreams
- slight stomach upset

Where can I keep my medicine?

Keep out of the reach of children in a container that small children cannot open. Store at controlled room temperature, 20 and 25 degrees C (68 and 77 degrees F). Throw away any unused medicine after the expiration date.

Ethacrynic Acid tablets

EDECRIN®;
25 mg; Tablet
Merck and Co Inc

EDECRIN®;
50 mg; Tablet
Merck and Co Inc

What are ethacrynic acid tablets?

ETHACRYNIC ACID (Edecrin®) is a diuretic (water or fluid pill). Diuretics increase the amount of urine passed, which causes the body to lose water and salt. Ethacrynic acid is a loop diuretic; "loop" refers to the part of the kidney where ethacrynic acid works. Ethacrynic acid is given as a diuretic in conditions that make the body retain water and produce swelling (edema), like heart failure, liver or kidney problems. It is not a cure. Generic ethacrynic acid tablets are not yet available.

What should my health care professional know before I take ethacrynic acid?

They need to know if you have any of these conditions:
- diabetes
- diarrhea
- gout
- hearing problems
- heart disease, or previous heart attack
- kidney disease, small amounts of urine, or difficulty passing urine
- liver disease
- low blood levels of calcium, potassium, chloride, sodium, or magnesium
- pancreatitis
- systemic lupus erythematosus (SLE)
- an unusual or allergic reaction to ethacrynic acid, other medicines, foods, dyes, or preservatives
- pregnant or trying to get pregnant
- breast-feeding

How should I take this medicine?

Take ethacrynic acid tablets by mouth. Follow the directions on the prescription label. Swallow the tablets with a drink of water. If ethacrynic acid upsets your stomach, take it with food or milk. Take your doses at regular intervals. Do not take your medicine more often than directed. Remember that you will need to pass urine frequently after taking ethacrynic acid. Do not take your doses at a time of day that will cause you problems. Do not take at bedtime. Contact your pediatrician or health care professional regarding the use of this medicine in children. Special care may be needed.

What if I miss a dose?

If you miss a dose, take it as soon as you can. If it is almost time for your next dose, take only that dose. Do not take double or extra doses.

What may interact with ethacrynic acid?

- alcohol
- anti-inflammatory drugs (NSAIDs, such as ibuprofen)
- certain antibiotics given by injection
- dofetilide
- heart medicines such as digoxin or digitoxin
- hormones such as cortisone, fludrocortisone, or hydrocortisone
- medicines for high blood pressure
- lithium
- warfarin
- water pills

Tell your prescriber or health care professional about all other medicines you are taking, including non-prescription medicines, nutritional supplements, or herbal products. Also tell your prescriber or health care professional if you are a frequent user of drinks with caffeine or alcohol, if you smoke, or if you use illegal drugs. These may affect the way your medicine works. Check with your health care professional before stopping or starting any of your medicines.

What should I watch for while taking ethacrynic acid?

Visit your prescriber or health care professional for regular checks on your progress. Check your blood pressure regularly. Ask your prescriber or health care professional what your blood pressure should be, and when you should contact him or her. You must not get dehydrated, ask your prescriber or health care professional how much fluid you need to drink a day. Do not stop taking ethacrynic acid except on your prescriber's advice. Watch your diet while you are taking ethacrynic acid. Ask your prescriber or health care professional about both potassium and sodium intake. Ethacrynic acid can make your body lose potassium and you may need an extra supply. Some foods have a high potassium content such as bananas, coconuts, dates, figs, prunes, apricots, peaches, grapefruit juice, tomato juice, and orange juice. You may get dizzy or lightheaded. Do not drive, use machinery, or do anything that needs mental alertness until you know how ethacrynic acid affects you. To reduce the risk of dizzy or fainting spells, do not sit or stand up quickly, especially if you are an older patient. Alcohol can make you lightheaded, dizzy and increase confusion. Avoid or limit intake of alcoholic drinks. If you are going to have surgery, tell your prescriber or health care professional that you are taking ethacrynic acid.

What side effects may I notice from taking ethacrynic acid?

Side effects that you should report to your prescriber or health care professional as soon as possible:
- blood in the urine
- blurred vision
- dry mouth
- fever or chills
- hearing loss, ringing in the ears
- increased thirst
- irregular heartbeat
- muscle cramps, pain or weakness
- nausea, vomiting
- skin rash
- stomach pain
- unusual bleeding or bruising
- unusual tiredness or weakness

Side effects that usually do not require medical attention (report to your prescriber or health care professional if they continue or are bothersome):
- confusion
- diarrhea
- difficulty swallowing
- dizziness or lightheadedness
- headache
- loss of appetite

Where can I keep my medicine?

Keep out of the reach of children in a container that small children cannot open. Store at room temperature between 15 and 30 degrees C (59 and 86 degrees F). Throw away any unused medicine after the expiration date.

Ethambutol tablets

ETHAMBUTOL;
400 mg; Tablet
Barr Laboratories
Inc

ETHAMBUTOL;
400 mg; Tablet
Versapharm
Incorporated

What are ethambutol tablets?

ETHAMBUTOL (Myambutol®) is an oral chemotherapeutic agent for the treatment and cure of tuberculosis. Ethambutol enters growing tubercular bacterial cells and interferes with their growth and multiplication. Ethambutol is not used alone, but always in combination with another medicine that treats tuberculosis. Generic ethambutol tablets are available.

What should my health care professional know before I take ethambutol?

They need to know if you have any of these conditions:
- eye problems or disease
- gout
- kidney disease
- other chronic illness
- an unusual or allergic reaction to ethambutol, other medicines, foods, dyes or preservatives
- pregnant or trying to get pregnant
- breast-feeding

How should I take this medicine?

Take ethambutol tablets by mouth. Follow the directions on the prescription label. Swallow tablets whole with a full glass of water. You can take ethambutol with food or milk. Take your doses at regular intervals and try not to miss any doses. Do not take your medicine more often than directed. Finish the full course prescribed by your prescriber or health care professional even if you think your condition is better. You may need to take this medicine for 1 or 2 years. Do not stop taking except on your prescriber's advice. Contact your pediatrician or health care professional regarding the use of this medicine in children. Special care may be needed.

What if I miss a dose?

If you miss a dose, take it as soon as you can. If it is almost time for your next dose, take only that dose. Do not take double or extra doses.

What may interact with ethambutol?

- antacids
- aluminum salts

Tell your prescriber or health care professional about all other medicines you are taking, including non-prescription medicines, nutritional supplements, or herbal products. Also tell your prescriber or health care professional if you are a frequent user of drinks with caffeine or alcohol, if you smoke, or if you use illegal drugs. These may affect the way your medicine works. Check with your health care professional before stopping or starting any of your medicines.

What should I watch for while taking ethambutol?

Tell your prescriber or health care professional as soon as you can if you notice any change in your eyesight; even if only one eye is affected. Antacid that contains aluminum can stop ethambutol working. If you get an upset stomach and want to take an antacid, make sure there is an interval of 3 to 4 hours between these two medicines.

What side effects may I notice from taking ethambutol?

Side effects that you should report to your prescriber or health care professional as soon as possible:
- fever or chills
- joint aches, pain, or swelling
- blurred vision
- changes in how you see color (especially seeing the difference between red and green)
- dizziness
- reduced amount of urine passed
- skin rash
- tingling, pain, or numbness in the hands or feet

Side effects that usually do not require medical attention (report to your prescriber or health care professional if they continue or are bothersome):
- fever
- headache
- loss of appetite
- nausea, vomiting
- stomach pain
- weakness or tiredness

Where can I keep my medicine?

Keep out of the reach of children in a container that small children cannot open. Store at room temperature between 15 and 30 degrees C (59 and 86 degrees F). Throw away any unused medicine after the expiration date.

Ethinyl Estradiol tablets

This drug is no longer on the market.

ESTINYL®;
0.05 mg; Tablet
Schering Corp

ESTINYL®;
0.02 mg; Tablet
Schering Corp

What are ethinyl estradiol tablets?

ETHINYL ESTRADIOL (Estinyl®) is an estrogen that is essential for maintaining normal female functions. Estrogens are normally produced by the ovaries. After menopause, the ovaries decrease their production of this hormone. Estrogens can help relieve symptoms of the menopause (hot flashes, night sweats, mood changes, and vaginal dryness and irritation), and help to prevent the onset of osteoporosis (a loss of bone mass, so that bones become brittle and easily broken). Estrogens can also help improve female functions in women with hormonal imbalance or problems with their ovaries. Estrogens may also be given to certain men or women with inoperable breast cancers or prostate cancer. Occasionally these medications are used for other purposes. NOTE: This drug is discontinued in the US.

What should my health care professional know before I take ethinyl estradiol?

They need to know if you have any of these conditions:
- asthma
- blood vessel disease, blood clotting disorder, or suffered a stroke
- breast, cervical, endometrial, or uterine cancer
- diabetes
- fibroids in the womb, or endometriosis
- heart, kidney, or liver disease
- high blood lipids or cholesterol
- high blood pressure
- high level of calcium in the blood
- hysterectomy
- mental depression
- migraine
- porphyria
- tobacco smoker
- vaginal bleeding
- an unusual or allergic reaction to estrogens, other hormones, other medicines, foods, dyes, or preservatives
- pregnant or trying to get pregnant
- breast-feeding

How should this medicine be taken?

Take estrogen tablets by mouth. Follow the directions on the prescription label. Swallow the tablets with a drink of water. If the tablets upset your stomach, take them with food or milk. Take your doses at regular intervals; estrogens work best when taken at the same time each day. Do not take your medicine more often than directed.

For all uses of this medicine:

Before starting this medication, read the paper on your prescription provided by your pharmacist or health care professional. This paper will tell you about the specific product you are taking. Make certain you understand the instructions.

Contact your pediatrician or health care professional regarding the use of this medicine in children. Special care may be needed.

What if I miss a dose?

If you miss a dose, take it as soon as you can. If it is almost time for your next dose, take only that dose and resume your normal schedule. Do not take double or extra doses.

What may interact with ethinyl estradiol?

- some antibiotics used to treat infections
- some medications used to treat HIV (human immuno-deficiency virus) infection or AIDS
- ascorbic acid/vitamin C supplements
- barbiturates or benzodiazepines used for inducing sleep or treating seizures (convulsions)
- bromocriptine
- carbamazepine
- cimetidine
- clofibrate
- cyclosporine
- dantrolene
- grapefruit juice
- griseofulvin
- hormones
- hydrocortisone, cortisone, or prednisolone
- imipramine or some other antidepressants
- isoniazid (INH)
- medications for diabetes
- methotrexate
- mineral oil
- phenytoin
- raloxifene or tamoxifen
- rifabutin, rifampin, or rifapentine
- some medications for treating migraines
- theophylline
- thyroid hormones
- topiramate
- tricyclic antidepressants
- warfarin

Tell your prescriber or health care professional about all other medicines you are taking, including non-prescription medicines, nutritional supplements, or herbal products. Also tell your prescriber or health care professional if you are a frequent user of drinks with caffeine or alcohol, if you smoke, or if you use illegal drugs. These may affect the way your medicine works. Check with your health care professional before stopping or starting any of your medicines.

What should I watch for while taking ethinyl estradiol?

Visit your prescriber or health care professional for regular checks on your progress. You should have a complete check-up every 6 months. You will also need a regular breast and pelvic exam and "Pap" smear while on estrogen therapy. You should also discuss the need for regular mammograms with your health care professional, and follow his or her guidelines for these tests. If you have any unusual bleeding contact your prescriber or health care professional for advice. Estrogens can make your body retain fluid, making your fingers, hands, or ankles swell. Your blood pressure can go up. Contact your prescriber or health care professional if you feel you are retaining fluid. If you have any reason to think you are pregnant; stop taking estrogens at once and contact your prescriber or health care professional. Tobacco smoking increases the risk of getting a blood clot or having a stroke while you are taking estrogens, especially if you are more than 35 years old. You are strongly advised not to smoke. If you wear contact lenses and notice visual changes, or if the lenses begin to feel uncomfortable, consult your eye care specialist or health care professional. In women who still have their uterus, estrogens increase the risk of developing a condition (endometrial hyperplasia) that may lead to cancer of the lining of the uterus. Taking progestins, another hormone drug, with estrogens lowers the risk of developing this condition. Therefore, if your uterus has not been removed (by a hysterectomy), your doctor may prescribe a progestin for you to take together with your estrogen. You should know, however, that taking estrogens with progestins may have additional health risks. You should discuss the use of estrogens and progestins with your health care professional to determine the benefits and risks for you. If you are going to have elective surgery, you may need to stop taking your estrogens one month beforehand. Consult your health care professional for advice prior to scheduling the surgery.

What side effects may I notice from taking ethinyl estradiol?

Side effects that you should report to your prescriber or health care professional as soon as possible:
- breakthrough bleeding and spotting
- breast enlargement, tenderness, unusual discharge or milk production
- chest pain
- leg, arm or groin pain
- nausea, vomiting
- severe headaches
- stomach or abdominal pain (severe)
- sudden shortness of breath
- swelling of the hands, feet or ankles, or rapid weight gain
- vision or speech problems
- yellowing of the eyes or skin

E

Side effects that usually do not require medical attention (report to your prescriber or health care professional if they continue or are bothersome):

- change in sexual desire
- mild stomach upset
- mood changes, anxiety, depression, frustration, anger, or emotional outbursts
- increased or decreased appetite
- skin rash, acne, or brown spots on the face
- tiredness

- vaginal yeast infection (irritation and white discharge)
- weight gain

Where can I keep my medicine?

Keep out of the reach of children in a container that small children cannot open. Store at room temperature between 15 and 30 degrees C (59 and 86 degrees F). Throw away any unused medicine after the expiration date.

Ethinyl Estradiol; Desogestrel tablets

ORTHO-CEPT™;
0.15 mg/0.03 mg; Tablet
Ortho McNeil Pharmaceutical
Inc

What are ethinyl estradiol; desogestrel tablets?

ETHINYL ESTRADIOL; DESOGESTREL (Orthocept™) products are effective as oral contraceptives (birth control pills or "the pill"). These products combine natural or synthetic estrogens and progestins, similar to the natural sex hormones (estrogen and progesterone) produced in a woman's body. Ethinyl estradiol is an estrogen and desogestrel is a progestin. These products can prevent ovulation and pregnancy. In general, a combination of estrogen and progestin works better than a single-ingredient product. Ethinyl estradiol/desogestrel tablets can also help regulate menstrual flow, treat acne or may be used for other hormone related problems in females. The type and amount of estrogen and/or progestin may be different from one product to another. For some formulations, a generic product is available.

What should my health care professional know before I take ethinyl estradiol; desogestrel?

They need to know if you have or ever had any of these conditions:

- blood clots
- blood sugar problems, like diabetes
- cancer of the breast, cervix, ovary, uterus, vagina, or unusual vaginal bleeding that has not been evaluated by a health care professional
- depression
- fibroids
- gallbladder disease
- heart or circulation problems
- high blood pressure
- jaundice
- liver disease
- menstrual problems
- migraine headaches
- tobacco smoker
- stroke
- an unusual or allergic reaction to estrogen/progestin, other hormones, medicines, foods, dyes, or preservatives
- pregnant or trying to get pregnant
- breast-feeding

How should I take this medicine?

Take ethinyl estradiol/desogestrel pills by mouth. Before you start taking these pills decide what is a suitable time of day and always take them at the same time of day and in the order directed. Swallow the pills with a drink of water. Take with food to reduce stomach upset. Do not take more often than directed. Most products (except Mircette™) contain a 21-day supply of pills containing the active ingredients. Some products contain an additional 7 pills containing iron or inactive ingredients to be taken during the week of menstruation; this reduces the chance of missing the first day of the next cycle. Most products are to be started on the first Sunday after you start your period or on the first day of your period. You may need to ask your health care provider which day you should start your packet. If you are taking the Mircette™ product, most of the 28 tablets contain active hormones. This product should be started on the first Sunday after you start your period or on the first day of your period. Before starting this medication, read the paper on your prescription provided by your pharmacist. This paper will tell you about the specific product you are taking. Make certain you understand the instructions. Keep an extra month's supply of your pills available to ensure that you will not miss the first day of the next cycle. Contact your pediatrician or health care professional regarding the use of this medicine in children. Special care may be needed.

What if I miss a dose?

Try not to miss a dose. If you do, it may be necessary to consult your health care professional, especially if you are taking Mircette™.
For all products (except Mircette™)
21-day schedule:
If you miss one dose, take it as soon as you remember and then take the next pill at the regular time as usual. You may take 2 tablets in one day. If you miss two doses (days) in a row, take 2 tablets for the next 2 days, then, continue with your regular schedule. Whenever 1 or 2 doses are missed, you should use a second method of contraception for the next 7 days in addition to

taking the pills. If you miss three doses in a row, you should notify your physician or other health care professional for instructions. You will probably need to throw away the rest of the tablets in that cycle pack and start over. Another method of contraception should be used until at least 7 doses have been taken in the new cycle. Missing a pill can cause spotting or light bleeding. Make sure that no more than 7 days pass at the end of the 21 day cycle, before you start your next pack of pills.

28-day schedule:

Follow the same directions as above for the first 21 days of the schedule. If you miss 1 of the last 7 pills, you can either double the dose or skip it, but it is important to start the next month's cycle on the scheduled day.

For Mircette™:

You will need to contact your health care provider for specific instructions based on which tablets have been missed, for how many days they have been missed, and based on what week of your current cycle you are currently taking tablets.

What may interact with ethinyl estradiol; desogestrel?

- antibiotics or medicines for infections, especially rifampin, rifabutin, rifapentine, and griseofulvin
- aprepitant, a medicine used for chemotherapy-induced nausea and vomiting
- barbiturate medicines for producing sleep or treating seizures (convulsions)
- bosentan
- carbamazepine
- caffeine
- clofibrate
- cyclosporine
- dantrolene
- grapefruit juice
- hydrocortisone
- medicines for anxiety or sleeping problems, such as diazepam or temazepam
- medicines for mental depression
- medicines for diabetes, including troglitazone and pioglitazone
- mineral oil
- modafinil
- mycophenolate
- nefazodone
- oxcarbazepine
- phenytoin
- prednisolone
- ritonavir or other medicines for the treatment of the HIV virus or AIDS
- selegiline
- soy isoflavone supplements
- St. John's wort
- tamoxifen or raloxifene
- theophylline
- topiramate
- warfarin

Tell your prescriber or health care professional about all other medicines you are taking, including non-prescription medicines, nutritional supplements, or herbal products. Also tell your prescriber or health care professional if you are a frequent user of drinks with caffeine or alcohol, if you smoke, or if you use illegal drugs. These may affect the way your medicine works. Check before stopping or starting any of your medicines.

What should I watch for while taking ethinyl estradiol; desogestrel?

Visit your health care provider for regular checks on your progress. You should have a complete check-up every 6 to 12 months. If you have any unusual vaginal bleeding contact your prescriber or health care professional for advice. If you miss a period, the possibility of pregnancy must be considered. See your prescriber or health care provider as soon as you can. Use an additional method of contraception during the first cycle that you take these tablets. If you stop taking these tablets and want to get pregnant, a return to normal ovulation can take some time. You may not return to normal ovulation and fertility for 3 to 6 months. Discuss your pregnancy plans with your health care provider. If you are taking oral contraceptives for the treatment of acne, hirsutism (male-like hair growth), endometriosis or other hormone related problems, it may take several months of continued treatment to notice improvement in your symptoms or condition. Tobacco smoking increases the risk of getting a blood clot or having a stroke while you are taking ethinyl estradiol/desogestrel, especially if you are more than 35 years old. You are strongly advised not to smoke. Oral contraceptives can increase your sensitivity to the sun and you may burn more easily. Use sunscreen and protective clothing during long periods outdoors. Tanning booths should be used with caution. If you wear contact lenses and notice visual changes, or if the lenses begin to feel uncomfortable, consult your eye care specialist. In some women, tenderness, swelling, or minor bleeding of the gums may occur. Notify your dentist if this happens. Brushing and flossing your teeth regularly may help limit this. See your dentist regularly and inform your dentist of the medicines you are taking. You may get a vaginal yeast infection. If you have never had a yeast infection before, see your prescriber or other health care provider to confirm the problem. If you have had yeast infections in the past and are comfortable with self-medicating the problem, get and use a non-prescription medication to treat the yeast infection. If you are going to have elective surgery, you may need to stop taking your contraceptive pills one month beforehand. Consult your health care professional for advice prior to scheduling the surgery. Taking contraceptive pills does not protect you against HIV infection (AIDS) or any other sexually transmitted diseases.

What side effects may I notice from taking ethinyl estradiol; desogestrel?

Severe side effects are relatively rare in women who are healthy and do not smoke while they are taking

E

oral contraceptives. On average, more women have problems due to complications from getting pregnant than have problems with oral contraceptives. Many of the minor side effects may go away as your body adjusts to the medicine. However, the potential for severe side effects does exist and you may want to discuss these with your health care provider.

The following symptoms or side effects may be related to blood clots and require immediate medical or emergency help:

- chest pain
- coughing up blood
- dizziness or fainting spells
- leg, arm or groin pain
- severe or sudden headaches
- stomach pain (severe)
- sudden shortness of breath
- sudden loss of coordination, especially on one side of the body
- swelling of the hands, feet or ankles, or rapid weight gain
- vision or speech problems
- weakness or numbness in the arms or legs, especially on one side of the body

Other serious side effects are rare. Contact your health care provider as soon as you can if the following side effects occur:

- breast tissue changes or discharge
- changes in vaginal bleeding during your period or between your periods

- headaches or migraines
- increases in blood sugar, especially if you have diabetes
- increases in blood pressure, especially if you are known to have high blood pressure
- symptoms of vaginal infection (itching, irritation or unusual discharge)
- tenderness in the upper abdomen
- vomiting
- yellowing of the eyes or skin

Side effects that usually do not require medical attention (report to your health care provider if they continue or are bothersome):

- breakthrough bleeding and spotting that continues beyond the 3 initial cycles of pills
- breast tenderness
- mild stomach upset
- mood changes, anxiety, depression, frustration, anger, or emotional outbursts
- increased or decreased appetite
- increased sensitivity to sun or ultraviolet light
- nausea
- skin rash, acne, or brown spots on the skin
- tiredness
- weight gain

Where can I keep my medicine?

Keep out of the reach of children. Store at room temperature between 15 and 30 degrees C (59 and 86 degrees F). Keep container tightly closed. Throw away any unused medicine after the expiration date.

Ethinyl Estradiol; Ethynodiol Diacetate tablets

DEMULEN® 1/35;
1 mg/35 mcg; Tablet
GD Searle LLC a Subsidiary of
Pharmacia Company Pfizer

What are ethinyl estradiol; ethynodiol diacetate tablets?

ETHINYL ESTRADIOL; ETHYNODIOL DIACE-TATE (Demulen® 1/35) products are effective as oral contraceptives (birth control pills or "the pill"). These products combine natural or synthetic estrogens and progestins, similar to the natural sex hormones (estrogen and progesterone) produced in a woman's body. Ethinyl estradiol is an estrogen and ethynodiol diacetate is a progestin. These products can prevent ovulation and pregnancy. In general, a combination of estrogen and progestin works better than a single-ingredient product. Ethinyl estradiol/ethynodiol diacetate tablets can also help regulate menstrual flow, treat acne, or may be used for other hormone related problems in females. The type and amount of estrogen and/or progestin may be different from one product to another.

What should my health care professional know before I take ethinyl estradiol; ethynodiol diacetate?

They need to know if you have or ever had any of these conditions:

- blood clots
- blood sugar problems, like diabetes
- cancer of the breast, cervix, ovary, uterus, vagina, or unusual vaginal bleeding that has not been evaluated by a health care professional
- depression
- fibroids
- gallbladder disease
- heart or circulation problems
- high blood pressure
- jaundice
- liver disease
- menstrual problems
- migraine headaches
- tobacco smoker
- stroke
- an unusual or allergic reaction to estrogen/progestin, other hormones, medicines, foods, dyes, or preservatives
- pregnant or trying to get pregnant
- breast-feeding

How should I take this medicine?

Take ethinyl estradiol/ethynodiol diacetate pills by mouth. Before you start taking these pills decide what is a suitable time of day and always take them at the same time of day and in the order directed. Swallow the pills with a drink of water. Take with food to reduce stomach upset. Do not take more often than directed. Most products contain a 21-day supply of pills containing the active ingredients. Some products contain an additional 7 pills containing iron or inactive ingredients to be taken during the week of menstruation; this reduces the chance of missing the first day of the next cycle. Most products are to be started on the first Sunday after you start your period or on the first day of your period. You may need to ask your health care provider which day you should start your packet. Before starting this medication, read the paper on your prescription provided by your pharmacist. This paper will tell you about the specific product you are taking. Make certain you understand the instructions. Keep an extra month's supply of your pills available to ensure that you will not miss the first day of the next cycle. Contact your pediatrician or health care professional regarding the use of this medicine in children. Special care may be needed.

What if I miss a dose?

Try not to miss a dose. If you do, it may be necessary to consult your prescriber or health care professional. 21-day schedule:
If you miss one dose, take it as soon as you remember and then take the next pill at the regular time as usual. You may take 2 tablets in one day. If you miss two doses (days) in a row, take 2 tablets for the next 2 days, then, continue with your regular schedule. Whenever 1 or 2 doses are missed, you should use a second method of contraception for the next 7 days in addition to taking the pills. If you miss three doses in a row, you should notify your physician or other health care professional for instructions. You will probably need to throw away the rest of the tablets in that cycle pack and start over. Another method of contraception should be used until at least 7 doses have been taken in the new cycle. Missing a pill can cause spotting or light bleeding. Make sure that no more than 7 days pass at the end of the 21 day cycle, before you start your next pack of pills.
28-day schedule:
Follow the same directions as above for the first 21 days of the schedule. If you miss 1 of the last 7 pills, you can either double the dose or skip it, but it is important to start the next month's cycle on the scheduled day.

What may interact with ethinyl estradiol; ethynodiol diacetate?

- antibiotics or medicines for infections, especially rifampin, rifabutin, rifapentine, and griseofulvin
- aprepitant
- barbiturate medicines for producing sleep or treating seizures (convulsions)
- bosentan
- carbamazepine
- caffeine
- clofibrate
- cyclosporine
- dantrolene
- grapefruit juice
- hydrocortisone
- medicines for anxiety or sleeping problems, such as diazepam or temazepam
- medicines for mental depression
- medicines for diabetes, including troglitazone and pioglitazone
- mineral oil
- modafinil
- mycophenolate
- nefazodone
- oxcarbazepine
- phenytoin
- prednisolone
- ritonavir or other medicines for the treatment of the HIV virus or AIDS
- selegiline
- soy isoflavone supplements
- St. John's wort
- tamoxifen or raloxifene
- theophylline
- topiramate
- warfarin

Tell your prescriber or health care professional about all other medicines you are taking, including non-prescription medicines, nutritional supplements, or herbal products. Also tell your prescriber or health care professional if you are a frequent user of drinks with caffeine or alcohol, if you smoke, or if you use illegal drugs. These may affect the way your medicine works. Check before stopping or starting any of your medicines.

What should I watch for while taking ethinyl estradiol; ethynodiol diacetate?

Visit your prescriber or health care provider for regular checks on your progress. You should have a complete check-up every 6 to 12 months. If you have any unusual vaginal bleeding contact your doctor or health care provider for advice. If you miss a period, the possibility of pregnancy must be considered. See your prescriber or health care professional as soon as you can. Use an additional method of contraception during the first cycle that you take these tablets. If you stop taking these tablets and want to get pregnant, a return to normal ovulation can take some time. You may not return to normal ovulation and fertility for 3 to 6 months. Discuss your pregnancy plans with your health care provider. If you are taking oral contraceptives for the treatment of acne, hirsutism (male-like hair growth), endometriosis or other hormone related problems, it may take several months of continued treatment to notice improvement in your symptoms or condition. Tobacco smoking increases the risk of getting a blood clot or having a stroke while you are taking oral contraceptives, especially if you are more than 35 years old. You are strongly advised not to smoke. Oral contraceptives can increase your sensitivity to the sun and you may burn more easily. Use sunscreen and protective clothing during long periods outdoors. Tanning booths should be used with caution. If you wear contact lenses and notice visual changes, or if the lenses begin to feel uncomfortable, consult your eye care specialist. In some women, tenderness, swelling, or minor bleeding of the gums may occur. Notify your dentist if this happens. Brushing and flossing your teeth regularly may help limit this. See your dentist regularly and inform your dentist of the medicines you are taking. You may get a vaginal yeast infection. If you have never had a yeast infection before, see your prescriber or other health care provider to confirm the problem. If you have had yeast infections in the past and are comfortable with self-medicating the problem, get and use a non-prescription medication to treat the yeast infection. If you are going to have elective surgery, you may need to stop taking your contraceptive pills one month beforehand. Consult your health care professional for advice prior to scheduling the surgery. Taking contraceptive pills does not protect you against HIV infection (AIDS) or any other sexually transmitted diseases.

What side effects may I notice from taking ethinyl estradiol; ethynodiol diacetate?

Severe side effects are relatively rare in women who are healthy and do not smoke while they are taking oral contraceptives. On average, more women have problems due to complications from getting pregnant than have problems with oral contraceptives. Many of the minor side effects may go away as your body adjusts to the medicine. However, the potential for severe side effects does exist and you may want to discuss these with your health care provider.

The following symptoms or side effects may be related to blood clots and require immediate medical or emergency help:

- chest pain
- coughing up blood
- dizziness or fainting spells
- leg, arm or groin pain
- severe or sudden headaches
- stomach pain (severe)

- sudden shortness of breath
- sudden loss of coordination, especially on one side of the body
- swelling of the hands, feet or ankles, or rapid weight gain
- vision or speech problems
- weakness or numbness in the arms or legs, especially on one side of the body

Other serious side effects are rare. Contact your health care provider as soon as you can if the following side effects occur:

- breast tissue changes or discharge
- changes in vaginal bleeding during your period or between your periods
- headaches or migraines
- increases in blood sugar, especially if you have diabetes
- increases in blood pressure, especially if you are known to have high blood pressure
- symptoms of vaginal infection (itching, irritation or unusual discharge)
- tenderness in the upper abdomen
- vomiting
- yellowing of the eyes or skin

Side effects that usually do not require medical attention (report to your health care provider if they continue or are bothersome):

- breakthrough bleeding and spotting that continues beyond the 3 initial cycles of pills
- breast tenderness
- mild stomach upset
- mood changes, anxiety, depression, frustration, anger, or emotional outbursts
- increased or decreased appetite
- increased sensitivity to sun or ultraviolet light
- nausea
- skin rash, acne, or brown spots on the skin
- tiredness
- weight gain

Where can I keep my medicine?

Keep out of the reach of children. Store at room temperature between 15 and 30 degrees C (59 and 86 degrees F). Keep container tightly closed. Throw away any unused medicine after the expiration date.

Ethinyl Estradiol; Levonorgestrel tablets

ALESSE®-28;
0.02 mg/0.1 mg; Tablet
Wyeth Div Wyeth
Pharmaceuticals Inc

What are ethinyl estradiol; levonorgestrel tablets?

ETHINYL ESTRADIOL; LEVONORGESTREL (Alesse®-28) products are effective as oral contraceptives (birth control pills or "the pill"). These products combine natural or synthetic estrogens and progestins, similar to the natural sex hormones (estrogen and progesterone) produced in a woman's body. Ethinyl estradiol is an estrogen and levonorgestrel is a progestin.

These products can prevent ovulation and pregnancy. In general, a combination of estrogen and progestin works better than a single-ingredient product. After consultation with a health care professional, this combination of products can be used under specific circumstances for emergency contraception after unprotected sex, contact your health care prescriber for information. Ethinyl estradiol/levonorgestrel tablets can also help regulate menstrual flow, treat acne, or may be used for other hormone related problems in females. The type and amount of estrogen and/or progestin may be different from one product to another.

What should my health care professional know before I take ethinyl estradiol; levonorgestrel?

They need to know if you have or ever had any of these conditions:

- blood clots
- blood sugar problems, like diabetes
- cancer of the breast, cervix, ovary, uterus, vagina, or unusual vaginal bleeding that has not been evaluated by a health care professional
- depression
- fibroids
- gallbladder disease
- heart or circulation problems
- high blood pressure
- jaundice
- liver disease
- menstrual problems
- migraine headaches
- tobacco smoker
- stroke
- an unusual or allergic reaction to estrogen/progestin, other hormones, medicines, foods, dyes, or preservatives
- pregnant or trying to get pregnant
- breast-feeding

How should I take this medicine?

For routine prevention of pregnancy:

Take ethinyl estradiol/levonorgestrel pills by mouth. Before you start taking these pills decide what is a suitable time of day and always take them at the same time of day and in the order directed. Swallow the pills with a drink of water. Take with food to reduce stomach upset. Do not take more often than directed.

Most products contain a 21-day supply of pills containing the active ingredients. Some products contain an additional 7 pills containing iron or inactive ingredients to be taken during the week of menstruation; this reduces the chance of missing the first day of the next cycle. One product (Seasonale®) contains a 91-day supply of pills. This product has 84 pills with active ingredients and 7 inactive pills to be taken during the week of menstruation. This product allows you to only have 4 menstrual cycles per year. Most products are to be started on the first Sunday after you start your period or on the first day of your period. You may need to ask your health care provider which day you should start your packet.

For emergency prevention of pregnancy:

Take ethinyl estradiol/levonorgestrel pills by mouth. You will need to follow the instructions provided by your health care provider exactly. You will be told what product and how many pills of that product you should take for each dose. Take the first dose as soon as you can after having unprotected sex, preferably in the first 24 hours, but no later than 72 hours (3 days) after the

event. You MUST take the second dose 12 hours after you take the first dose. Do not take any extra pills. Extra pills will not decrease your risk of pregnancy, but may increase your risk of side effects.

For all uses of this medicine:

Before starting this medication, read the paper on your prescription provided by your pharmacist. This paper will tell you about the specific product you are taking. Make certain you understand the instructions.

Keep an extra month's supply of your pills available to ensure that you will not miss the first day of the next cycle. Contact your pediatrician or health care professional regarding the use of this medicine in children. Special care may be needed.

What if I miss a dose?

If you miss a dose of an emergency contraceptive prescription, or vomit the dose within an hour of taking it, you MUST contact your health care professional for instructions. Try not to miss a dose of your regular birth control prescription. If you do, it may be necessary to consult your prescriber or health care professional. The following information describes only some of the ways that missed doses can be handled. For all cycles:

21-day schedule:

If you miss one dose, take it as soon as you remember and then take the next pill at the regular time as usual. You may take 2 tablets in one day. If you miss two doses (days) in a row, take 2 tablets the day you remember and 2 tablets the next day, then, continue with your regular schedule. Whenever 1 or 2 doses are missed, you should use a second method of contraception for the next 7 days in addition to taking the pills. If you miss three doses in a row, you should notify your physician or other health care professional for instructions. You will probably need to throw away the rest of the tablets in that cycle pack and start over. Another method of contraception should be used until at least 7 doses have been taken in the new cycle. Missing a pill can cause spotting or light bleeding. Make sure that no more than 7 days pass at the end of the 21 day cycle, before you start your next pack of pills.

28-day schedule:

Follow the same directions as above for the first 21 days of the schedule. If you miss 1 of the last 7 pills, you can either double the dose or skip it, but it is important to start the next month's cycle on the scheduled day.

91-day schedule:

If you miss one dose for the first 84 days of the schedule, take it as soon as you remember. Take the next pill at your regular time as usual, which means you may take 2 tablets in one day. If you miss 2 doses (days) in a row, take 2 tablets on the day you remember and 2 tablets the next day. Then, continue with your regular schedule. You could become pregnant if you have sex in the 7 days after you miss 2 doses in a row. You should use another method of birth control during the 7 days after you restart your pills. If you miss 3 doses (days) in a row, you will not take any of the 3 pills that you missed. Restart taking your pills for the actual day you restart. For example, if you resume taking the pill on Thursday, take the pill under "Thursday" and do not take the missed pills. Keep taking 1 pill every day until you have completed all of the remaining pills in the pack. You may experience bleeding during the week following the missed pills. You could become pregnant if you have sex in the 7 days after you miss 3 doses in a row. You should use another method of birth control during the 7 days after you restart your pills. If you miss any of the last 7 pills, throw away the missed pills. You will not need a back-up method of birth control. Keep taking the scheduled pills until the pack is finished.

What may interact with ethinyl estradiol; levonorgestrel?

- antibiotics or medicines for infections, especially rifampin
- aprepitant
- barbiturate medicines for producing sleep or treating seizures (convulsions)
- bosentan
- carbamazepine
- caffeine
- clofibrate
- cyclosporine
- dantrolene
- grapefruit juice
- hydrocortisone
- medicines for anxiety or sleeping problems, such as diazepam or temazepam
- medicines for mental depression
- medicines for diabetes, including troglitazone and pioglitazone
- mineral oil
- modafinil
- mycophenolate
- nefazodone
- oxcarbazepine
- phenytoin
- prednisolone
- ritonavir or other medicines for the treatment of the HIV virus or AIDS
- selegiline
- soy isoflavone supplements
- St. John's wort
- tamoxifen or raloxifene
- theophylline
- topiramate
- warfarin

Tell your prescriber or health care professional about all other medicines you are taking, including non-prescription medicines, nutritional supplements, or herbal products. Also tell your prescriber or health care professional if you are a frequent user of drinks with caffeine or alcohol, if you smoke, or if you use illegal drugs. These may affect the way your medicine works. Check before stopping or starting any of your medicines.

What should I watch for while taking ethinyl estradiol; levonorgestrel?

Visit your prescriber or health care provider for regular checks on your progress. You should have a complete check-up every 6 to 12 months. If you have any unusual vaginal bleeding contact your doctor or health care provider for advice. If you miss a period, the possibility of pregnancy must be considered. See your prescriber or health care professional as soon as you can. Use an additional method of contraception during the first 7 days that you take these tablets. If you stop taking these tablets and want to get pregnant, a return to normal ovulation can take some time. You may not return to normal ovulation and fertility for 3 to 6 months. Discuss your pregnancy plans with your health care provider. If you are taking oral contraceptives for the treatment of acne, hirsutism (male-like hair growth), endometriosis or other hormone related problems, it may take several months of continued treatment to notice improvement in your symptoms or condition. Tobacco smoking increases the risk of getting a blood clot or having a stroke while you are taking oral contraceptives, especially if you are more than 35 years old. You are strongly advised not to smoke. Oral contraceptives can increase your sensitivity to the sun and you may burn more easily. Use sunscreen and protective clothing during long periods outdoors. Tanning booths should be used with caution. If you wear contact lenses and notice visual changes, or if the lenses begin to feel uncomfortable, consult your eye care specialist. In some women, tenderness, swelling, or minor bleeding of the gums may occur. Notify your dentist if this happens. Brushing and flossing your teeth regularly may help limit this. See your dentist regularly and inform your dentist of the medicines you are taking. You may get a vaginal yeast infection. If you have never had a yeast infection before, see your prescriber or other health care provider to confirm the problem. If you have had yeast infections in the past and are comfortable with self-medicating the problem, get and use a non-prescription medication to treat the yeast infection. If you are going to have elective surgery, you may need to stop taking your contraceptive pills one month beforehand. Consult your health care professional for advice prior to scheduling the surgery. Taking contraceptive pills does not protect you against HIV infection (AIDS) or any other sexually transmitted diseases.

What side effects may I notice from taking ethinyl estradiol; levonorgestrel?

Severe side effects are relatively rare in women who are healthy and do not smoke while they are taking oral contraceptives. On average, more women have problems due to complications from getting pregnant than have problems with oral contraceptives. Many of the minor side effects may go away as your body adjusts to the medicine. However, the potential for severe side effects does exist and you may want to discuss these with your health care provider.

The following symptoms or side effects may be related to blood clots and require immediate medical or emergency help:

- chest pain
- coughing up blood
- dizziness or fainting spells
- leg, arm or groin pain
- severe or sudden headaches
- stomach pain (severe)
- sudden shortness of breath
- sudden loss of coordination, especially on one side of the body
- swelling of the hands, feet or ankles, or rapid weight gain
- vision or speech problems
- weakness or numbness in the arms or legs, especially on one side of the body

Other serious side effects are rare. Contact your health care provider as soon as you can if the following side effects occur:

- breast tissue changes or discharge
- changes in vaginal bleeding during your period or between your periods
- headaches or migraines
- increases in blood sugar, especially if you have diabetes
- increases in blood pressure, especially if you are known to have high blood pressure
- symptoms of vaginal infection (itching, irritation or unusual discharge)
- tenderness in the upper abdomen
- vomiting
- yellowing of the eyes or skin

Side effects that usually do not require medical attention (report to your health care provider if they continue or are bothersome):

- breakthrough bleeding and spotting that continues beyond the 3 initial cycles of pills
- breast tenderness
- mild stomach upset
- mood changes, anxiety, depression, frustration, anger, or emotional outbursts
- increased or decreased appetite
- increased sensitivity to sun or ultraviolet light
- nausea
- skin rash, acne, or brown spots on the skin
- tiredness
- weight gain

If you are taking this medicine for emergency prevention of pregnancy, it is common to have nausea, headache, abdominal pain or cramping, breast tenderness and dizziness. You may vomit. If you throw-up within 1 hour of taking your dose, you will need to contact your health care professional for instructions. If any of the other side effects are severe or continue, contact your health care professional. After you finish your prescription, it is common for you to have changes in your next period, or to have spotting. If you do not get a period within 21 days of taking your prescription, you should see your health care professional and get a pregnancy test.

Where can I keep my medicine?

Keep out of the reach of children. Store at room temperature between 15 and 30 degrees C (59 and 86 degrees F). Keep container tightly closed. Throw away any unused medicine after the expiration date.

Ethinyl Estradiol; Norelgestromin skin patches

ORTHO EVRA™;
20 mcg/24hr/150 mcg/24 hr;
Film, Extended Release
Ortho Pharmaceuticals

What are ethinyl estradiol; norelgestromin skin patches?

ETHINYL ESTRADIOL; NORELGESTROMIN (Ortho Evra™) is a skin patch that is effective as a contraceptive (birth control). This product combines natural or synthetic estrogens and progestins, similar to the natural sex hormones (estrogen and progesterone) produced in a woman's body. Ethinyl estradiol is an estrogen and norelgestromin is a progestin. This patch keeps you from becoming pregnant by delivering continuous levels of these hormones through the skin and into the bloodstream. This patch can also help regulate menstrual flow, treat acne or may be used for other hormone-related problems in females. A generic birth control patch is not available.

What should my health care professional know before I take ethinyl estradiol; norelgestromin?

They need to know if you have or ever had any of these conditions:

- blood clots
- blood sugar problems, like diabetes
- cancer of the breast, cervix, ovary, uterus, vagina, or unusual vaginal bleeding that has not been evaluated by a health care professional
- depression
- fibroids
- gallbladder disease
- heart disease or circulation problems
- high blood pressure
- jaundice
- liver disease
- menstrual problems
- migraine headaches
- tobacco smoker
- stroke
- an unusual or allergic reaction to estrogens, progestins, other hormones, medicines, foods, dyes, or preservatives
- pregnant or trying to get pregnant
- breast-feeding

How should I take this medicine?

Ortho Evra™ patches are for use on the skin. Follow carefully the directions that come with the patches. Use exactly as directed. Remove the patch from the sealed pouch. Do not try to cut or trim the patch. Apply the patch to a clean, dry, intact healthy skin area on the buttock, abdomen, upper outer arm or upper torso, in a place where it won't be rubbed by tight clothing. Do not place on skin that is red, irritated or cut, and do not place on the breasts. To prevent problems with the stickiness of the patch, no makeup, creams, lotions, oils, powders or other topical products should be applied to the skin area where the patch is or will be placed. Using your palm, press the patch firmly in place for 10 seconds to make sure that there is good contact with your skin. Change the patch every 7 days on the proper "patch change day," keeping to a regular schedule. When you apply a new patch, use a new area of skin. Wait at least 1 week before using the same area again. Keep an extra month's supply of your patches available to ensure that you will not miss the proper day you are to start your next cycle. Before starting this medication, read the paper on your prescription provided by your pharmacist. This paper will tell you about the specific product you are taking. Make certain you understand the instructions. Contact your pediatrician or health care professional regarding the use of this medicine in children. Special care may be needed.

What if I miss a dose?

Try not to miss your weekly patch change; your risk of pregnancy increases with each day in a row you have missed your patch. If you do miss a patch change, it may be necessary to consult your health care professional for instructions. The instructions may vary depending on when you have missed the patch (weeks 1, 2 or 3) during your monthly cycle. In some cases, you will also need to use a back-up method of birth control. If you forget to remove the patch on week 4, take it off as soon as you remember. However, it is important to start the next month's patch cycle on the scheduled day; there should not be more than a 7-day patch-free interval. If there are more than 7 patch-free days, there is a risk you could become pregnant and you should use a back-up birth control method for 7 days. If a patch is lost or falls off, it may be necessary to consult your health care professional for instructions. A replacement patch for your prescription may be needed to complete your monthly cycle and can be purchased from your pharmacist. In some cases, you will also need to use a back-up method of birth control if the patch has been off for more than 1 day.

What may interact with ethinyl estradiol; norelgestromin?

- antibiotics or medicines for infections, especially rifampin, rifapentine or rifabutin
- aprepitant
- atorvastatin
- barbiturate medicines for producing sleep or treating seizures (convulsions)
- bexarotene
- bosentan
- caffeine
- carbamazepine
- cimetidine
- clofibrate
- cyclosporine
- dantrolene
- exemestane
- felbamate
- griseofulvin
- growth hormone
- hydrocortisone
- isoniazid, INH
- medicines for anxiety or sleeping problems, such as diazepam or temazepam
- medicines for mental depression
- medicines for diabetes, including troglitazone and pioglitazone
- medicines for mental depression
- medicines for migraines
- methotrexate
- modafinil
- mycophenolate
- nefazodone
- oxcarbazepine
- phenytoin
- prednisolone
- ritonavir or other medicines for the treatment of the HIV virus or AIDS
- selegiline
- soy isoflavones supplements
- St. John's wort
- tamoxifen or raloxifene
- theophylline
- topiramate
- troleandomycin
- warfarin

Tell your prescriber or health care professional about all other medicines you are taking, including non-prescription medicines, nutritional supplements, or herbal products. Also tell your prescriber or health care professional if you are a frequent user of drinks with caffeine or alcohol, if you smoke, or if you use illegal drugs. These may affect the way your medicine works. Check before stopping or starting any of your medicines.

What should I watch for while taking ethinyl estradiol; norelgestromin?

Visit your health care provider for regular checks on your progress. You should have a complete check-up every 6 to 12 months. If you have any unusual vaginal bleeding contact your prescriber or health care professional for advice. If you miss a period, the possibility of pregnancy must be considered. See your prescriber or health care provider as soon as you can. To ensure adequate protection, use an additional method of contraception (like condoms, diaphragm or spermicide) during the first cycle that you use this patch. If you stop using this patch and want to get pregnant, a return to normal ovulation can take some time. You may not return to normal ovulation and fertility for 3 to 6 months. Discuss your pregnancy plans with your health care provider. If you are taking hormone-based contraceptives for the treatment of acne, hirsutism (male-like hair growth), endometriosis or other hormone related problems, it may take several months of continued treatment to notice improvement in your symptoms or condition. Tobacco smoking increases the risk of getting a blood clot or having a stroke while you are taking this medicine, especially if you are more than 35 years old. You are strongly advised not to smoke. This contraceptive can increase your sensitivity to the sun and you may burn more easily. Use sunscreen and protective clothing during long periods outdoors. Tanning booths should be used with caution. If you wear contact lenses and notice visual changes, or if the lenses begin to feel uncomfortable, consult your eye care specialist. In some women, tenderness, swelling, or minor bleeding of the gums may occur. Notify your dentist if this happens. Brushing and flossing your teeth regularly may help limit this. See your dentist regularly and inform your dentist of the medicines you are taking. You may get a vaginal yeast infection. If you have never had a yeast infection before, see your prescriber or other health care provider to confirm the problem. If you have had yeast infections in the past and are comfortable with self-medicating the problem, get and use a non-prescription medication to treat the yeast infection. If you are going to have elective surgery, you may need to stop using this contraceptive patch one month beforehand. Consult your health care professional for advice prior to scheduling the surgery. Using this contraceptive patch does not protect you against HIV infection (AIDS) or any other sexually transmitted diseases. If you are going to have a MRI procedure, let your MRI technician know about the use of these patches. Some drug patches contain an aluminized backing that can become heated when exposed to MRI and may cause burns. You may need to temporarily remove the patch during the MRI procedure.

What side effects may I notice from taking ethinyl estradiol; norelgestromin?

Severe side effects are relatively rare in women who are healthy and do not smoke while they are taking hormone-containing contraceptives. On average, more women have problems due to complications from getting pregnant than have problems with this contraceptive. Many of the minor side effects may go away as your body adjusts to the medicine. However, the potential for severe side effects does exist and you may want to discuss these with your health care provider.

The following symptoms or side effects may be related to blood clots and require immediate medical or emergency help:

- chest pain
- coughing up blood
- dizziness or fainting spells
- leg, arm or groin pain
- severe or sudden headaches
- stomach pain (severe)
- sudden shortness of breath
- sudden loss of coordination, especially on one side of the body
- swelling of the hands, feet or ankles, or rapid weight gain
- vision or speech problems
- weakness or numbness in the arms or legs, especially on one side of the body

Other serious side effects are rare. Contact your health care provider as soon as you can if the following side effects occur:

- breast tissue changes or discharge
- changes in vaginal bleeding during your period or between your periods
- headaches or migraines
- increases in blood sugar, especially if you have diabetes
- increases in blood pressure, especially if you are known to have high blood pressure
- symptoms of vaginal infection (itching, irritation or unusual discharge)
- tenderness in the upper abdomen
- vomiting
- yellowing of the eyes or skin

Side effects that usually do not require medical attention (report to your health care provider if they continue or are bothersome):

- breakthrough bleeding and spotting that continues beyond the 3 initial cycles
- breast tenderness
- mild stomach upset
- mood changes, anxiety, depression, frustration, anger, or emotional outbursts
- increased or decreased appetite
- increased sensitivity to sun or ultraviolet light
- nausea
- skin rash, acne, or brown spots on the skin
- tiredness
- weight gain

Where can I keep my medicine?

Keep out of the reach of children. Store unopened patches at room temperature between 15 and 30 degrees C (59 and 86 degrees F). Throw away any unused medicine after the expiration date. Once removed, a used patch should be folded to stick to itself and discarded in a waste receptacle out of the reach of children and pets (do not flush in toilet).

Ethinyl Estradiol; Norethindrone Acetate tablets

FEMHRT® 1/5;
0.05 mg/1 mg;
Tablet
Warner Chilcott PLC

FEMHRT® 1/5;
0.05 mg/1 mg;
Tablet
Physicians Total
Care Inc

What are ethinyl estradiol; norethindrone acetate tablets?

ETHINYL ESTRADIOL; NORETHINDRONE ACETATE (FemHRT®) products are usually used as oral contraceptives (birth control pills or "the pill"). Ethinyl estradiol/norethindrone acetate tablets can also help regulate menstrual flow, treat acne, or may be used for other hormone related problems in females. One ethinyl estradiol; norethindrone acetate product (FemHRT®1/5) is used as hormone replacement in women who still have their uterus and who are experiencing menopause. FEMHRT® 1/5 DOES NOT PREVENT PREGNANCY. When prescribed, this product helps to treat hot flashes, maintain healthy bones and prevent osteoporosis. Generic ethinyl estradiol; norethindrone tablets for hormone replacement are not available.

What should my health care professional know before I take ethinyl estradiol; norethindrone acetate?

They need to know if you have or ever had any of these conditions:
- blood clots
- blood sugar problems, like diabetes
- cancer of the breast, cervix, ovary, uterus, vagina, or unusual vaginal bleeding that has not been evaluated by a health care professional
- depression
- fibroids
- gallbladder disease
- heart or circulation problems
- high blood pressure
- jaundice
- liver disease
- menstrual problems
- migraine headaches
- tobacco smoker
- stroke
- an unusual or allergic reaction to estrogen/progestin, other hormones, medicines, foods, dyes, or preservatives
- pregnant or trying to get pregnant
- breast-feeding

How should I take this medicine?

Take ethinyl estradiol/norethindrone acetate pills by mouth. Before you start taking these pills decide what is a suitable time of day and always take them at the same time of day and in the order directed. Swallow the pills with a drink of water. Take with food to reduce stomach upset. Do not take more often than directed. Before starting this medication, read the paper on your prescription provided by your pharmacist. This paper will tell you about the specific product you are taking. Make certain you understand the instructions.

What if I miss a dose?

If you are taking this product for hormone replacement: If you miss a dose, take it as soon as you can. If it is almost time for your next dose, take only that dose. Do not take double or extra doses.

What may interact with ethinyl estradiol; norethindrone acetate?

- barbiturate medicines for producing sleep or treating seizures (convulsions)
- bosentan
- carbamazepine
- cyclosporine
- dantrolene
- medicines for anxiety or sleeping problems, such as diazepam or temazepam
- medicines for mental depression
- medicines for diabetes, including troglitazone and pioglitazone
- mycophenolate
- oxcarbazepine
- phenytoin
- soy isoflavone supplements
- tamoxifen or raloxifene
- warfarin

Tell your prescriber or health care professional about all other medicines you are taking, including non-prescription medicines, nutritional supplements, or herbal products. Also tell your prescriber or health care professional if you are a frequent user of drinks with caffeine or alcohol, if you smoke, or if you use illegal drugs. These may affect the way your medicine works. Check before stopping or starting any of your medicines.

What should I watch for while taking ethinyl estradiol; norethindrone acetate?

Visit your prescriber or health care provider for regular checks on your progress. You should have a complete check-up every 6 to 12 months. You will need a regular breast and pelvic exam and PAP smear while receiving FemHRT®. Regular breast examinations by a health professional and monthly exams are recommended for all women. You should also discuss the need for regular mammograms with your health care provider. You may retain water while taking this medicine, making your fingers, hands or ankles swell. Your blood pressure can go up. Contact your prescriber if you feel you are retaining water. If you think you may be pregnant, stop taking this medicine at once and contact your prescriber. Tobacco smoking increases the risk of getting a blood clot or having a stroke while you are taking estrogen hormones, especially if you are more than 35 years old. You are strongly advised not to smoke. If you wear contact lenses and notice visual changes, or if the lenses begin to feel uncomfortable, consult your eye care specialist. If you are going to have elective surgery, you may need to stop taking your estrogens one month beforehand. Consult your healthcare professional for advice prior to scheduling the surgery. In women who still have their uterus, taking a progestin with your estrogens lowers the risk of developing overgrowth of the uterine lining. You should know, however, that taking estrogens with progestins may have additional health risks. You should discuss the use of estrogens and progestins with your healthcare professional to determine the benefits and risks for you.

What side effects may I notice from taking ethinyl estradiol; norethindrone acetate?

Severe side effects are uncommon in women taking this combination in the low doses prescribed for hormone replacement during and after menopause. Many of the side effects listed below are for the use of this medicine in dosages used for birth control. However, if you notice any of these side effects while taking FemHRT®, you should report them.

The following symptoms or side effects may be related to blood clots and require immediate medical or emergency help:

- chest pain
- coughing up blood
- dizziness or fainting spells
- leg, arm or groin pain
- severe or sudden headaches
- stomach pain (severe)
- sudden shortness of breath
- sudden loss of coordination, especially on one side of the body
- swelling of the hands, feet or ankles, or rapid weight gain

- vision or speech problems
- weakness or numbness in the arms or legs, especially on one side of the body

Other serious side effects are rare. Contact your health care provider as soon as you can if the following side effects occur:

- breast tissue changes or discharge
- changes in vaginal bleeding during your period or between your periods
- headaches or migraines
- increases in blood sugar, especially if you have diabetes
- increases in blood pressure, especially if you are known to have high blood pressure
- symptoms of vaginal infection (itching, irritation or unusual discharge)
- tenderness in the upper abdomen
- vomiting
- yellowing of the eyes or skin

Side effects that usually do not require medical attention (report to your health care provider if they continue or are bothersome):

- breakthrough bleeding and spotting that continues beyond the 3 initial cycles of pills
- breast tenderness
- mild stomach upset
- mood changes, anxiety, depression, frustration, anger, or emotional outbursts
- increased or decreased appetite
- increased sensitivity to sun or ultraviolet light
- nausea
- skin rash, acne, or brown spots on the skin
- tiredness
- weight gain

Where can I keep my medicine?

Keep out of the reach of children. Store at room temperature between 15 and 30 degrees C (59 and 86 degrees F). Keep container tightly closed. Throw away any unused medicine after the expiration date.

Ethinyl Estradiol; Norethindrone tablets

TRI-NORINYL®;
Combo; Tablet
Watson Pharmaceuticals Inc

What are ethinyl estradiol; norethindrone tablets?

ETHINYL ESTRADIOL; NORETHINDRONE (Tri-Norinyl®) products are effective as oral contraceptives (birth control pills or "the pill"). These products combine natural or synthetic estrogens and progestins, similar to the natural sex hormones (estrogen and progesterone) produced in a woman's body. Ethinyl estradiol is an estrogen and norethindrone is a progestin. These products can prevent ovulation and pregnancy. In general, a combination of estrogen and progestin works better than a single-ingredient product. Ethinyl estradiol/norethindrone tablets can also help regulate menstrual flow, treat acne, or may be used for other

hormone related problems in females. On rare occasions, they may be prescribed for other purposes. The type and amount of estrogen and/or progestin may be different from one product to another.

What should my health care professional know before I take ethinyl estradiol; norethindrone?

They need to know if you have or ever had any of these conditions:

- blood clots
- blood sugar problems, like diabetes
- cancer of the breast, cervix, ovary, uterus, vagina, or unusual vaginal bleeding that has not been evaluated by a health care professional

- depression
- fibroids
- gallbladder disease
- heart or circulation problems
- high blood pressure
- jaundice
- liver disease
- menstrual problems
- migraine headaches
- tobacco smoker
- stroke
- an unusual or allergic reaction to estrogen/progestin, other hormones, medicines, foods, dyes, or preservatives
- pregnant or trying to get pregnant
- breast-feeding

How should I take this medicine?

Take ethinyl estradiol/norethindrone pills by mouth. Before you start taking these pills decide what is a suitable time of day and always take them at the same time of day and in the order directed. Swallow the pills with a drink of water. Take with food to reduce stomach upset. Do not take more often than directed. Most products contain a 21-day supply of pills containing the active ingredients. Some products contain an additional 7 pills containing iron or inactive ingredients to be taken during the week of menstruation; this reduces the chance of missing the first day of the next cycle. Most products are to be started on the first Sunday after you start your period or on the first day of your period. You may need to ask your health care provider which day you should start your packet. Before starting this medication, read the paper on your prescription provided by your pharmacist. This paper will tell you about the specific product you are taking. Make certain you understand the instructions. Keep an extra month's supply of your pills available to ensure that you will not miss the first day of the next cycle. Contact your pediatrician or health care professional regarding the use of this medicine in children. Special care may be needed.

What if I miss a dose?

Try not to miss a dose. If you do, it may be necessary to consult your prescriber or health care professional. The following information describes only some of the ways that missed doses can be handled.

For monophasic, biphasic or triphasic cycles:
21-day schedule:
If you miss one dose, take it as soon as you remember and then take the next pill at the regular time as usual. You may take 2 tablets in one day. If you miss two doses (days) in a row, take 2 tablets for the next 2 days, then, continue with your regular schedule. Whenever 1 or 2 doses are missed, you should use a second method of contraception for the next 7 days in addition to taking the pills. If you miss three doses in a row, you should notify your physician or other health care professional for instructions. You will probably need to

throw away the rest of the tablets in that cycle pack and start over. Another method of contraception should be used until at least 7 doses have been taken in the new cycle. Missing a pill can cause spotting or light bleeding. Make sure that no more than 7 days pass at the end of the 21 day cycle, before you start your next pack of pills.
28-day schedule:
Follow the same directions as above for the first 21 days of the schedule. If you miss 1 of the last 7 pills, you can either double the dose or skip it, but it is important to start the next month's cycle on the scheduled day.

What may interact with ethinyl estradiol; norethindrone?

- antibiotics or medicines for infections, especially rifampin, rifabutin, rifapentine, and griseofulvin
- aprepitant
- barbiturate medicines for producing sleep or treating seizures (convulsions)
- bosentan
- carbamazepine
- caffeine
- clofibrate
- cyclosporine
- dantrolene
- grapefruit juice
- hydrocortisone
- medicines for anxiety or sleeping problems, such as diazepam or temazepam
- medicines for mental depression
- medicines for diabetes, including troglitazone and pioglitazone
- mineral oil
- modafinil
- mycophenolate
- nefazodone
- oxcarbazepine
- phenytoin
- prednisolone
- ritonavir or other medicines for the treatment of the HIV virus or AIDS
- selegiline
- soy isoflavone supplements
- St. John's wort
- tamoxifen or raloxifene
- theophylline
- topiramate
- warfarin

Tell your prescriber or health care professional about all other medicines you are taking, including non-prescription medicines, nutritional supplements, or herbal products. Also tell your prescriber or health care professional if you are a frequent user of drinks with caffeine or alcohol, if you smoke, or if you use illegal drugs. These may affect the way your medicine works. Check before stopping or starting any of your medicines.

What should I watch for while taking ethinyl estradiol; norethindrone?

Visit your prescriber or health care provider for regular checks on your progress. You should have a complete check-up every 6 to 12 months. If you have any unusual vaginal bleeding contact your doctor or health care provider for advice. If you miss a period, the possibility of pregnancy must be considered. See your prescriber or health care professional as soon as you can. Use an additional method of contraception during the first cycle that you take these tablets. If you stop taking these tablets and want to get pregnant, a return to normal ovulation can take some time. You may not return to normal ovulation and fertility for 3 to 6 months. Discuss your pregnancy plans with your health care provider. If you are taking oral contraceptives for the treatment of acne, hirsutism (male-like hair growth), endometriosis or other hormone related problems, it may take several months of continued treatment to notice improvement in your symptoms or condition. Tobacco smoking increases the risk of getting a blood clot or having a stroke while you are taking oral contraceptives, especially if you are more than 35 years old. You are strongly advised not to smoke. Oral contraceptives can increase your sensitivity to the sun and you may burn more easily. Use sunscreen and protective clothing during long periods outdoors. Tanning booths should be used with caution. If you wear contact lenses and notice visual changes, or if the lenses begin to feel uncomfortable, consult your eye care specialist. In some women, tenderness, swelling, or minor bleeding of the gums may occur. Notify your dentist if this happens. Brushing and flossing your teeth regularly may help limit this. See your dentist regularly and inform your dentist of the medicines you are taking. You may get a vaginal yeast infection. If you have never had a yeast infection before, see your prescriber or other health care provider to confirm the problem. If you have had yeast infections in the past and are comfortable with self-medicating the problem, get and use a non-prescription medication to treat the yeast infection. If you are going to have elective surgery, you may need to stop taking your contraceptive pills one month beforehand. Consult your health care professional for advice prior to scheduling the surgery. Taking contraceptive pills does not protect you against HIV infection (AIDS) or any other sexually transmitted diseases.

What side effects may I notice from taking ethinyl estradiol; norethindrone?

Severe side effects are relatively rare in women who are healthy and do not smoke while they are taking oral contraceptives. On average, more women have problems due to complications from getting pregnant than have problems with oral contraceptives. Many of the minor side effects may go away as your body adjusts to the medicine. However, the potential for severe side effects does exist and you may want to discuss these with your health care provider.

The following symptoms or side effects may be related to blood clots and require immediate medical or emergency help:
- chest pain
- coughing up blood
- dizziness or fainting spells
- leg, arm or groin pain
- severe or sudden headaches
- stomach pain (severe)
- sudden shortness of breath
- sudden loss of coordination, especially on one side of the body
- swelling of the hands, feet or ankles, or rapid weight gain
- vision or speech problems
- weakness or numbness in the arms or legs, especially on one side of the body

Other serious side effects are rare. Contact your health care provider as soon as you can if the following side effects occur:
- breast tissue changes or discharge
- changes in vaginal bleeding during your period or between your periods
- headaches or migraines
- increases in blood sugar, especially if you have diabetes
- increases in blood pressure, especially if you are known to have high blood pressure
- symptoms of vaginal infection (itching, irritation or unusual discharge)
- tenderness in the upper abdomen
- vomiting
- yellowing of the eyes or skin

Side effects that usually do not require medical attention (report to your health care provider if they continue or are bothersome):
- breakthrough bleeding and spotting that continues beyond the 3 initial cycles of pills
- breast tenderness
- mild stomach upset
- mood changes, anxiety, depression, frustration, anger, or emotional outbursts
- increased or decreased appetite
- increased sensitivity to sun or ultraviolet light
- nausea
- skin rash, acne, or brown spots on the skin
- tiredness
- weight gain

Where can I keep my medicine?

Keep out of the reach of children. Store at room temperature between 15 and 30 degrees C (59 and 86 degrees F). Keep container tightly closed. Throw away any unused medicine after the expiration date.

Ethinyl Estradiol; Norgestimate tablets

ORTHO TRI-CYCLEN® LO;
Combo ; Tablet
Ortho McNeil Pharmaceutical
Inc

What are ethinyl estradiol; norgestimate tablets?

ETHINYL ESTRADIOL; NORGESTIMATE (OrthoCyclen®, Ortho Tri-Cyclen®, Ortho Tri-Cyclen Lo®, Previfem™, Sprintec™) products are effective as oral contraceptives (birth control pills or "the pill"). These products combine natural or synthetic estrogens and progestins, similar to the natural sex hormones (estrogen and progesterone) produced in a woman's body. Ethinyl estradiol is an estrogen and norgestimate is a progestin. These products can prevent ovulation and pregnancy. In general, a combination of estrogen and progestin works better than a single-ingredient product. Ethinyl estradiol/norgestimate tablets can also help regulate menstrual flow, treat acne, or may be used for other hormone related problems in females. The type and amount of estrogen and/or progestin may be different from one product to another.

What should my health care professional know before I take ethinyl estradiol; norgestimate?

They need to know if you have or ever had any of these conditions:

- blood clots
- blood sugar problems, like diabetes
- cancer of the breast, cervix, ovary, uterus, vagina, or unusual vaginal bleeding that has not been evaluated by a health care professional
- depression
- fibroids
- gallbladder disease
- heart or circulation problems
- high blood pressure
- jaundice
- liver disease
- menstrual problems
- migraine headaches
- tobacco smoker
- stroke
- an unusual or allergic reaction to estrogen/progestin, other hormones, medicines, foods, dyes, or preservatives
- pregnant or trying to get pregnant
- breast-feeding

How should I take this medicine?

Take ethinyl estradiol/norgestimate pills by mouth. Before you start taking these pills decide what is a suitable time of day and always take them at the same time of day and in the order directed. Swallow the pills with a drink of water. Take with food to reduce stomach upset. Do not take more often than directed. Most products contain a 21-day supply of pills containing the active ingredients. Some products contain an additional 7 pills containing iron or inactive ingredients to be taken during the week of menstruation; this reduces the chance of missing the first day of the next cycle. Most products are to be started on the first Sunday after you start your period or on the first day of your period. You may need to ask your health care provider which day you should start your packet. Before starting this medication, read the paper on your prescription provided by your pharmacist. This paper will tell you about the specific product you are taking. Make certain you understand the instructions. Keep an extra month's supply of your pills available to ensure that you will not miss the first day of the next cycle. Contact your pediatrician or health care professional regarding the use of this medicine in children. Special care may be needed.

What if I miss a dose?

Try not to miss a dose. If you do, it may be necessary to consult your prescriber or health care professional. The following information describes only some of the ways that missed doses can be handled.

For monophasic, biphasic or triphasic cycles:
21-day schedule:
If you miss one dose, take it as soon as you remember and then take the next pill at the regular time as usual. You may take 2 tablets in one day. If you miss two doses (days) in a row, take 2 tablets for the next 2 days, then, continue with your regular schedule. Whenever 1 or 2 doses are missed, you should use a second method of contraception for the next 7 days in addition to taking the pills. If you miss three doses in a row, you should notify your physician or other health care professional for instructions. You will probably need to throw away the rest of the tablets in that cycle pack and start over. Another method of contraception should be used until at least 7 doses have been taken in the new cycle. Missing a pill can cause spotting or light bleeding. Make sure that no more than 7 days pass at the end of the 21 day cycle, before you start your next pack of pills.
28-day schedule:
Follow the same directions as above for the first 21 days of the schedule. If you miss 1 of the last 7 pills, you can either double the dose or skip it, but it is important to start the next month's cycle on the scheduled day.

What may interact with ethinyl estradiol; norgestimate?

- antibiotics or medicines for infections, especially rifampin
- aprepitant

- barbiturate medicines for producing sleep or treating seizures (convulsions)
- bosentan
- carbamazepine
- caffeine
- clofibrate
- cyclosporine
- dantrolene
- grapefruit juice
- hydrocortisone
- medicines for anxiety or sleeping problems, such as diazepam or temazepam
- medicines for mental depression
- medicines for diabetes, including troglitazone and pioglitazone
- mineral oil
- modafinil
- mycophenolate
- nefazodone
- oxcarbazepine
- phenytoin
- prednisolone
- ritonavir or other medicines for the treatment of the HIV virus or AIDS
- selegiline
- soy isoflavones supplements
- St. John's wort
- tamoxifen or raloxifene
- theophylline
- topiramate
- warfarin

Tell your prescriber or health care professional about all other medicines you are taking, including non-prescription medicines, nutritional supplements, or herbal products. Also tell your prescriber or health care professional if you are a frequent user of drinks with caffeine or alcohol, if you smoke, or if you use illegal drugs. These may affect the way your medicine works. Check before stopping or starting any of your medicines.

What should I watch for while taking ethinyl estradiol; norgestimate?

Visit your prescriber or health care provider for regular checks on your progress. You should have a complete check-up every 6 to 12 months. If you have any unusual vaginal bleeding contact your doctor or health care provider for advice. If you miss a period, the possibility of pregnancy must be considered. See your prescriber or health care professional as soon as you can. Use an additional method of contraception during the first cycle that you take these tablets. If you stop taking these tablets and want to get pregnant, a return to normal ovulation can take some time. You may not return to normal ovulation and fertility for 3 to 6 months. Discuss your pregnancy plans with your health care provider. If you are taking oral contraceptives for the treatment of acne, hirsutism (male-like hair growth), endometriosis or other hormone related problems, it may take several months of continued treatment to notice improvement in your symptoms or con-

dition. Tobacco smoking increases the risk of getting a blood clot or having a stroke while you are taking oral contraceptives, especially if you are more than 35 years old. You are strongly advised not to smoke. Oral contraceptives can increase your sensitivity to the sun and you may burn more easily. Use sunscreen and protective clothing during long periods outdoors. Tanning booths should be used with caution. If you wear contact lenses and notice visual changes, or if the lenses begin to feel uncomfortable, consult your eye care specialist. In some women, tenderness, swelling, or minor bleeding of the gums may occur. Notify your dentist if this happens. Brushing and flossing your teeth regularly may help limit this. See your dentist regularly and inform your dentist of the medicines you are taking. You may get a vaginal yeast infection. If you have never had a yeast infection before, see your prescriber or other health care provider to confirm the problem. If you have had yeast infections in the past and are comfortable with self-medicating the problem, get and use a non-prescription medication to treat the yeast infection. If you are going to have elective surgery, you may need to stop taking your contraceptive pills one month beforehand. Consult your health care professional for advice prior to scheduling the surgery. Taking contraceptive pills does not protect you against HIV infection (AIDS) or any other sexually transmitted diseases.

What side effects may I notice from taking ethinyl estradiol; norgestimate?

Severe side effects are relatively rare in women who are healthy and do not smoke while they are taking oral contraceptives. On average, more women have problems due to complications from getting pregnant than have problems with oral contraceptives. Many of the minor side effects may go away as your body adjusts to the medicine. However, the potential for severe side effects does exist and you may want to discuss these with your health care provider.

The following symptoms or side effects may be related to blood clots and require immediate medical or emergency help:

- chest pain
- coughing up blood
- dizziness or fainting spells
- leg, arm or groin pain
- severe or sudden headaches
- stomach pain (severe)
- sudden shortness of breath
- sudden loss of coordination, especially on one side of the body
- swelling of the hands, feet or ankles, or rapid weight gain
- vision or speech problems
- weakness or numbness in the arms or legs, especially on one side of the body

Other serious side effects are rare. Contact your health care provider as soon as you can if the following side effects occur:

- breast tissue changes or discharge
- changes in vaginal bleeding during your period or between your periods

E

- headaches or migraines
- increases in blood sugar, especially if you have diabetes
- increases in blood pressure, especially if you are known to have high blood pressure
- symptoms of vaginal infection (itching, irritation or unusual discharge)
- tenderness in the upper abdomen
- vomiting
- yellowing of the eyes or skin

Side effects that usually do not require medical attention (report to your health care provider if they continue or are bothersome):

- breakthrough bleeding and spotting that continues beyond the 3 initial cycles of pills

- breast tenderness
- mild stomach upset
- mood changes, anxiety, depression, frustration, anger, or emotional outbursts
- increased or decreased appetite
- increased sensitivity to sun or ultraviolet light
- nausea
- skin rash, acne, or brown spots on the skin
- tiredness
- weight gain

Where can I keep my medicine?

Keep out of the reach of children. Store at room temperature between 15 and 30 degrees C (59 and 86 degrees F). Keep container tightly closed. Throw away any unused medicine after the expiration date.

Ethinyl Estradiol; Norgestrel tablets

LO/OVRAL®;
0.03 mg/0.3 mg; Tablet
Wyeth Div Wyeth
Pharmaceuticals Inc

What are ethinyl estradiol; norgestrel tablets?

ETHINYL ESTRADIOL/NORGESTREL (Low-Ogestrel®, Lo/Ovral®, Ovral®) products are effective as oral contraceptives (birth control pills or "the pill"). These products combine natural or synthetic estrogens and progestins, similar to the natural sex hormones (estrogen and progesterone) produced in a woman's body. Ethinyl estradiol is an estrogen and norgestrel is a progestin. These products can prevent ovulation and pregnancy. In general, a combination of estrogen and progestin works better than a single-ingredient product. After consultation with a health care professional, this combination of products can be used under specific circumstances for emergency contraception after unprotected sex. Ethinyl estradiol/norgestrel tablets can also help regulate menstrual flow, treat acne, or may be used for other hormone related problems in females. The type and amount of estrogen and/or progestin may be different from one product to another. For some formulations, a generic product is available.

What should my health care professional know before I take ethinyl estradiol; norgestrel?

They need to know if you have or ever had any of these conditions:

- blood clots
- blood sugar problems, like diabetes
- cancer of the breast, cervix, ovary, uterus, vagina, or unusual vaginal bleeding that has not been evaluated by a health care professional
- depression
- fibroids
- gallbladder disease
- heart or circulation problems
- high blood pressure
- jaundice
- liver disease
- menstrual problems

- migraine headaches
- tobacco smoker
- stroke
- an unusual or allergic reaction to estrogen/progestin, other hormones, medicines, foods, dyes, or preservatives
- pregnant or trying to get pregnant
- breast-feeding

How should I take this medicine?

For routine prevention of pregnancy:

Take ethinyl estradiol/norgestrel pills by mouth. Before you start taking these pills decide what is a suitable time of day and always take them at the same time of day and in the order directed. Swallow the pills with a drink of water. Take with food to reduce stomach upset. Do not take more often than directed.

Most products contain a 21-day supply of pills containing the active ingredients. Some products contain an additional 7 pills containing iron or inactive ingredients to be taken during the week of menstruation; this reduces the chance of missing the first day of the next cycle. Most products are to be started on the first Sunday after you start your period or on the first day of your period. You may need to ask your health care provider which day you should start your packet.

For emergency prevention of pregnancy:

Take ethinyl estradiol/norgestrel pills by mouth. You will need to follow the instructions provided by your health care provider exactly. Take the first dose as soon as you can after having unprotected sex, preferably in the first 24 hours, but no later than 72 hours (3 days) after the event. You MUST take the second dose 12 hours after you take the first dose. Do not take any extra pills. Extra pills will not decrease your risk of pregnancy, but may increase your risk of side effects. This type of birth control is not to be used as a regular means of preventing pregnancy. You should discuss birth control options with your health care provider to prevent future risk of pregnancy. Get started as soon as you can with a method of birth control you will be able to use every time you have sex. You should make a follow-up appointment to see your health care provider in 3 to 4 weeks.

For all uses of this medicine:

Before starting this medication, read the paper on your prescription provided by your pharmacist. This paper will tell you about the specific product you are taking. Make certain you understand the instructions.

Keep an extra month's supply of your pills available to ensure that you will not miss the first day of the next cycle. Contact your pediatrician or health care professional regarding the use of this medicine in children. Special care may be needed.

What if I miss a dose?

If you miss a dose of an emergency contraceptive prescription, or vomit the dose within an hour of taking it, you MUST contact your health care professional for instructions. Try not to miss a dose of your regular birth control prescription. If you do, it may be necessary to consult your prescriber or health care professional. The following information describes only some of the ways that missed doses can be handled. For all cycles:

21-day schedule:

If you miss one dose, take it as soon as you remember and then take the next pill at the regular time as usual. You may take 2 tablets in one day. If you miss two doses (days) in a row, take 2 tablets for the next 2 days, then, continue with your regular schedule. Whenever 1 or 2 doses are missed, you should use a second method of contraception for the next 7 days in addition to taking the pills. If you miss three doses in a row, you should notify your physician or other health care professional for instructions. You will probably need to throw away the rest of the tablets in that cycle pack and start over. Another method of contraception should be used until at least 7 doses have been taken in the new cycle. Missing a pill can cause spotting or light bleeding. Make sure that no more than 7 days pass at the end of the 21 day cycle, before you start your next pack of pills.

28-day schedule:

Follow the same directions as above for the first 21 days of the schedule. If you miss 1 of the last 7 pills, you can either double the dose or skip it, but it is important to start the next month's cycle on the scheduled day.

What may interact with ethinyl estradiol; norgestrel?

- antibiotics or medicines for infections, especially rifampin, rifabutin, rifapentine, and griseofulvin
- aprepitant, a medicine used for chemotherapy-induced nausea and vomiting
- barbiturate medicines for producing sleep or treating seizures (convulsions)
- bosentan

- carbamazepine
- caffeine
- clofibrate
- cyclosporine
- dantrolene
- grapefruit juice
- hydrocortisone
- medicines for anxiety or sleeping problems, such as diazepam or temazepam
- medicines for mental depression
- medicines for diabetes, including troglitazone and pioglitazone
- mineral oil
- modafinil
- mycophenolate
- nefazodone
- oxcarbazepine
- phenytoin
- prednisolone
- ritonavir or other medicines for the treatment of the HIV virus or AIDS
- selegiline
- soy isoflavone supplements
- St. John's wort
- tamoxifen or raloxifene
- theophylline
- topiramate
- warfarin

Tell your prescriber or health care professional about all other medicines you are taking, including non-prescription medicines, nutritional supplements, or herbal products. Also tell your prescriber or health care professional if you are a frequent user of drinks with caffeine or alcohol, if you smoke, or if you use illegal drugs. These may affect the way your medicine works. Check before stopping or starting any of your medicines.

What should I watch for while taking ethinyl estradiol; norgestrel?

Visit your prescriber or health care provider for regular checks on your progress. You should have a complete check-up every 6 to 12 months. If you have any unusual vaginal bleeding, contact your doctor or health care provider for advice. If you miss a period, the possibility of pregnancy must be considered. See your prescriber or health care professional as soon as you can. Use an additional method of contraception during the first cycle that you take these tablets. If you stop taking these tablets and want to get pregnant, a return to normal ovulation can take some time. You may not return to normal ovulation and fertility for 3 to 6 months. Discuss your pregnancy plans with your health care provider. If you are taking oral contraceptives for the treatment of acne, hirsutism (male-like hair growth), endometriosis or other hormone related problems, it may take several months of continued treatment to notice improvement in your symptoms or condition. Tobacco smoking increases the risk of getting a blood clot or having a stroke while you are taking oral contraceptives, especially if you are more than 35 years old. You are strongly advised not to smoke. Oral contraceptives can increase your sensitivity to the sun and you may burn more easily. Use sunscreen and protective clothing during long periods outdoors. Tanning booths should be used with caution. If you wear contact lenses and notice visual changes, or if the lenses begin to feel uncomfortable, consult your eye care specialist. In some women, tenderness, swelling, or minor bleeding of the gums may occur. Notify your dentist if this happens. Brushing and flossing your teeth regularly may help limit this. See your dentist regularly and inform your dentist of the medicines you are taking. You may get a vaginal yeast infection. If you have never had a yeast infection before, see your prescriber or other health care provider to confirm the problem. If you have had yeast infections in the past and are comfortable with self-medicating the problem, get and use a non-prescription medication to treat the yeast infection. If you are going to have elective surgery, you may need to stop taking your contraceptive pills one month beforehand. Consult your health care professional for advice prior to scheduling the surgery. Taking contraceptive pills does not protect you against HIV infection (AIDS) or any other sexually transmitted diseases.

What side effects may I notice from taking ethinyl estradiol; norgestrel?

Severe side effects are relatively rare in women who are healthy and do not smoke while they are taking oral contraceptives. On average, more women have problems due to complications from getting pregnant than have problems with oral contraceptives. Many of the minor side effects may go away as your body adjusts to the medicine. However, the potential for severe side effects does exist and you may want to discuss these with your health care provider.

The following symptoms or side effects may be related to blood clots and require immediate medical or emergency help:

- chest pain
- coughing up blood
- dizziness or fainting spells
- leg, arm or groin pain
- severe or sudden headaches
- stomach pain (severe)
- sudden shortness of breath
- sudden loss of coordination, especially on one side of the body
- swelling of the hands, feet or ankles, or rapid weight gain
- vision or speech problems

- weakness or numbness in the arms or legs, especially on one side of the body

Other serious side effects are rare. Contact your health care provider as soon as you can if the following side effects occur:

- breast tissue changes or discharge
- changes in vaginal bleeding during your period or between your periods
- headaches or migraines
- increases in blood sugar, especially if you have diabetes
- increases in blood pressure, especially if you are known to have high blood pressure
- symptoms of vaginal infection (itching, irritation or unusual discharge)
- tenderness in the upper abdomen
- vomiting
- yellowing of the eyes or skin

Side effects that usually do not require medical attention (report to your health care provider if they continue or are bothersome):

- breakthrough bleeding and spotting that continues beyond the 3 initial cycles of pills
- breast tenderness
- mild stomach upset
- mood changes, anxiety, depression, frustration, anger, or emotional outbursts
- increased or decreased appetite
- increased sensitivity to sun or ultraviolet light
- nausea
- skin rash, acne, or brown spots on the skin
- tiredness
- weight gain

If you are taking this medicine for emergency prevention of pregnancy, it is common to have nausea, headache, abdominal pain or cramping, breast tenderness and dizziness. You may vomit. If you throw-up within 1 hour of taking your dose, you will need to contact your health care professional for instructions. If any of the other side effects are severe or continue, contact your health care professional. After you finish your prescription, it is common for you to have changes in your next period, or to have spotting. If you do not get a period within 21 days of taking your prescription, you should see your health care professional and get a pregnancy test.

Where can I keep my medicine?

Keep out of the reach of children. Store at room temperature between 15 and 30 degrees C (59 and 86 degrees F). Keep container tightly closed. Throw away any unused medicine after the expiration date.

Ethosuximide capsules

ZARONTIN®;
250 mg; Capsule
Parke Davis Division
of Pfizer Co.

ETHOSUXIMIDE;
250 mg; Capsule
Pliva Inc

What are ethosuximide capsules?

ETHOSUXIMIDE (Zarontin®) can help with seizure (convulsion) control in those with absence (petit mal) epilepsy. Generic ethosuximide capsules are available.

What should my health care professional know before I take ethosuximide?

They need to know if you have any of these conditions:
- blood disorders or disease
- kidney disease
- liver disease
- an unusual or allergic reaction to ethosuximide, other medicines, foods, dyes, or preservatives
- pregnant or trying to get pregnant
- breast-feeding

How should I take this medicine?

Take ethosuximide capsules by mouth. Follow the directions on the prescription label. Swallow the capsules with a drink of water. If ethosuximide upsets your stomach, take it with food or milk. Take your doses at regular intervals. Do not take your medicine more often than directed. Contact your pediatrician or health care professional regarding the use of this medicine in children. Special care may be needed.

What if I miss a dose?

If you miss a dose, take it as soon as you can. If it is almost time for your next dose, take only that dose. Do not take double or extra doses.

What may interact with ethosuximide?

- alcohol
- bosentan
- medicines for mental depression
- medicines for mental problems and psychotic disturbances
- phenobarbital
- other seizure (convulsion) or epilepsy medicine
- pimozide
- some medications for the treatment of HIV infection
- some medicines for fungal or yeast infections (examples: fluconazole, itraconazole, ketoconazole, voriconazole)

Tell your prescriber or health care professional about all other medicines you are taking, including non-prescription medicines, nutritional supplements, or herbal products. Also tell your prescriber or health care professional if you are a frequent user of drinks with caffeine or alcohol, if you smoke, or if you use illegal drugs.

These may affect the way your medicine works. Check with your health care professional before stopping or starting any of your medicines.

What should I watch for while taking ethosuximide?

Visit your prescriber or health care professional for a regular check on your progress. Do not stop taking ethosuximide suddenly. This increases the risk of seizures. Wear a Medic Alert bracelet or necklace. Carry an identification card with information about your condition, medications, and prescriber or health care professional. You may get drowsy, dizzy, or have blurred vision. Do not drive, use machinery, or do anything that needs mental alertness until you know how ethosuximide affects you. To reduce dizzy or fainting spells, do not sit or stand up quickly, especially if you are an older patient. Alcohol can increase drowsiness and dizziness. Avoid alcoholic drinks. If you are going to have surgery, tell your prescriber or health care professional that you are taking ethosuximide.

What side effects may I notice from taking ethosuximide?

Side effects that you should report to your prescriber or health care professional as soon as possible:
- chest pain or tightness
- fever, sore throat, swollen glands
- mood changes, nervousness, or hostility
- mouth ulcers
- muscle aches and pain
- redness, blistering, peeling or loosening of the skin, including inside the mouth
- shortness of breath, or wheezing
- skin rash and itching
- unusual bleeding or bruising
- unusual tiredness or weakness

Side effects that usually do not require medical attention (report to your prescriber or health care professional if they continue or are bothersome):
- clumsiness or unsteadiness
- dizziness or drowsiness
- headache
- loss of appetite
- nausea, vomiting
- stomach cramps

Where can I keep my medicine?

Keep out of reach of children in a container that small children cannot open. Store at room temperature below 30 degrees C (86 degrees F). Throw away any unused medicine after the expiration date.

Ethotoin tablets

What are ethotoin tablets?

ETHOTOIN (Peganone®) helps to control seizures (convulsions) in certain types of epilepsy. Ethotoin is usually used in combination with another seizure medication. Generic ethotoin tablets are available.

What should my health care professional know before I take ethotoin?

They need to know if you have any of these conditions:
- an alcohol abuse problem
- blood disorders or disease
- diabetes
- fever
- liver disease
- porphyria
- an unusual reaction to Ethotoin, other medicines, foods, dyes, or preservatives
- pregnant or trying to get pregnant
- breast-feeding

How should this medicine be taken?

Take ethotoin tablets by mouth. Follow the directions on the prescription label. Swallow the tablet(s) whole with a drink of water. Take ethotoin with food if it upsets your stomach. Take your doses at regular intervals. Do not take your medicine more often than directed. Contact your pediatrician or health care professional regarding the use of this medicine in children. Special care may be needed.

What if I miss a dose?

If you miss a dose, take it as soon as you can. However, if it is almost time for your next dose, take only your next dose. Do not take double or extra doses.

What may interact with ethotoin?

Many medicines might interact with ethotoin; check with your prescriber or health care professional if you regularly take other medications or over-the-counter products. Some of the medicines that might interact are listed:

- alcohol
- amphetamines
- antacids
- barbiturate medicines for inducing sleep or treating seizures (convulsions)
- cimetidine
- female hormones, including contraceptive or birth control pills
- kava kava
- medicines for mental depression, anxiety or other mood problems
- medicines used to treat HIV infection or AIDS
- other medicines for seizures like carbamazepine, oxcarbazepine, ethosuximide, valproic acid, zonisamide

- rifampin, rifabutin or rifapentine
- St. John's wort
- sucralfate
- theophylline
- warfarin

Tell your prescriber or health care professional about all other medicines you are taking, including non-prescription medicines, nutritional supplements, or herbal products. Also tell your prescriber or health care professional if you are a frequent user of drinks with caffeine or alcohol, if you smoke, or if you use illegal drugs. These may affect the way your medicine works. Check with your health care professional before stopping or starting any of your medicines.

What should I watch for while taking ethotoin?

Visit your prescriber or health care professional for regular checks on your progress. Your prescriber or health care professional may schedule regular blood tests, because ethotoin therapy needs careful monitoring. Do not stop taking ethotoin suddenly. If you take ethotoin for seizures, it is a good idea to carry an identification card, necklace or bracelet with details of your condition, medications and prescriber or health care professional. You may feel dizzy or drowsy. Do not drive, use machinery, or do anything that needs mental alertness until you know how ethotoin affects you. To reduce the risk of dizzy or fainting spells, do not sit or stand up quickly, especially if you are an older patient. Alcohol can make you more dizzy, increase flushing and rapid heartbeats. Avoid alcoholic drinks. Birth control pills (contraceptive pills) may not work properly while you are taking ethotoin; talk with your prescriber about the use of other methods of birth control. Ethotoin can rarely cause unusual growth of gum tissues; visit your dentist regularly. Problems can arise if you need dental work, and in the day to day care of your teeth. Try to avoid damage to your teeth and gums when you brush or floss your teeth. Do not take antacids at the same time as ethotoin. If you get an upset stomach and want to take an antacid or medicine for diarrhea, make sure there is an interval of 2 to 3 hours before or after you take ethotoin. If you are going to have surgery, tell your prescriber or health care professional that you are taking ethotoin.

What side effects may I notice from taking ethotoin?

Side effects that you should report to your prescriber or health care professional as soon as possible:
- chest pain or tightness; fast or irregular heartbeat (palpitations)
- confusion, nervousness, hostility, or other behavioral changes (especially in children or elderly patients)

- dark yellow or brown urine
- a new onset of severe stomach pain
- difficulty breathing, wheezing or shortness of breath
- double vision or uncontrollable and rapid eye movement
- fainting spells or lightheadedness
- fever, sore throat
- headache
- loss of seizure control
- mouth ulcers
- poor control of body movements or difficulty walking
- redness, blistering, peeling or loosening of the skin, including inside the mouth
- skin rash, itching
- swollen or painful glands
- unusual bleeding or bruising, pinpoint red spots on skin
- unusual tiredness or weakness

- unusual swelling
- vomiting
- yellowing of the eyes or skin

Side effects that usually do not require medical attention (report to your prescriber or health care professional if they continue or are bothersome):

- clumsiness or unsteadiness
- constipation or diarrhea
- difficulty sleeping
- dizziness or drowsiness
- loss of appetite
- nausea
- stomach upset
- unusual growth of gum tissue

Where can I keep my medicine?

Keep out of the reach of children in a container that small children cannot open.

Etidronate tablets

DIDRONEL®;
200 mg; Tablet
Procter and Gamble
Pharmaceuticals Inc
Sub Procter and
Gamble Co

DIDRONEL®;
400 mg; Tablet
Procter and Gamble
Pharmaceuticals Inc
Sub Procter and
Gamble Co

E

What are etidronate tablets?

ETIDRONATE (Didronel®) reduces the release and breakdown of calcium from bone. This drug helps to reduce excess calcium in the blood (hypercalcemia) that you can get with certain cancers. This drug is also used to help prevent bone loss and to increase normal healthy bone production in patients with Paget's disease, in patients who have had hip surgery, or in those patients with osteoporosis. Generic etidronate tablets are available.

What should my health care professional know before I take etidronate?

They need to know if you have any of these conditions:
- kidney disease
- stomach, intestinal, or esophageal problems
- an unusual or allergic reaction to etidronate, other medicines, foods, dyes, or preservatives
- pregnant or trying to get pregnant
- breast-feeding

How should I take this medicine?

Take etidronate tablets by mouth. Follow the directions on the prescription label. Swallow the tablets with a full glass of water. Take etidronate on an empty stomach. Do not eat food for at least 30 minutes, and preferably not for 2 hours after taking etidronate. Do not take with milk or other calcium-rich foods. To avoid irritation of your throat, do not lay down for at least 30 minutes after taking etidronate. Do not take etidronate at the same time as iron supplements, vitamins with minerals (like iron or calcium), or antacids containing calcium, magnesium, or aluminum. Try to take your tablets at the same time each day. Do not

take your medicine more often than directed. Contact your pediatrician or health care professional regarding the use of this medicine in children. Special care may be needed.

What if I miss a dose?

If you miss a dose, take it as soon as you can if you have not already eaten. If you have already eaten, call your prescriber or health care professional for advice. Do not take double or extra doses.

What may interact with etidronate?

- aluminum hydroxide
- antacids
- calcium supplements
- iron supplements
- magnesium supplements
- parathyroid hormone
- teriparatide
- warfarin

Tell your prescriber or health care professional about all other medicines you are taking including non-prescription medicines; if you are a frequent user of drinks with caffeine or alcohol; if you smoke; or if you use illegal drugs. These can affect the way your medicine works. Check with your health care professional before stopping or starting any of your medicines.

What should I watch for while taking etidronate?

Visit your prescriber or health care professional for regular checks on your progress. If you have Paget's disease it may be some time before you see the benefit from etidronate. After your initial treatment period, you must have a 90-day treatment-free interval before re-treatment. Do not stop taking etidronate except on your prescriber's advice. High levels of phosphorus and low levels of calcium in the blood can occur but generally do not cause serious problems. Your prescriber or health care professional may order regular blood tests to check for these problems. Patients on calcium- and vitamin D-restricted diets are more sensitive to the effects of etidronate. You should maintain adequate amounts of calcium and vitamin D in your diet, unless directed otherwise by your health care provider. Discuss your dietary needs with your prescriber or health care professional or nutritionist. If you get bone pain or a worsening of bone pain, check with your prescriber or health care professional. If you want to take an antacid or a mineral supplement, make sure that there is an interval of at least 2 hours before or after taking etidronate. Do not take at the same time.

What side effects might I notice from taking etidronate?

Serious side effects from etidronate are rare. Patients using etidronate for more than 6 months at a time are at an increased risk of developing bone fractures (broken bones).

Side effects that you should report to your prescriber or health care professional as soon as possible:
- black or tarry stools
- broken bones
- difficulty passing urine or less frequent passing of urine
- increased bone pain
- redness, blistering, peeling or loosening of the skin, including inside the mouth
- skin rash, itching (hives)
- stomach or lower back pain
- swelling of the lips, arms, legs, face, tongue, or throat

Side effects that usually do not require medical attention (report to your prescriber or health care professional if they continue or are bothersome):
- diarrhea
- indigestion
- nausea, vomiting

Where can I keep my medicine?

Keep out of the reach of children in a container that small children cannot open. Store at room temperature below 40 degrees C (104 degrees F). Throw away any unused medicine after the expiration date.

This drug requires an FDA medication guide. See page xxxvii.

Etodolac extended-release tablets

LODINE® XL;
400 mg; Tablet,
Extended Release
Wyeth
Pharmaceuticals Inc

LODINE® XL;
500 mg; Tablet,
Extended Release
Wyeth
Pharmaceuticals Inc

What are etodolac extended-release tablets?

ETODOLAC (Lodine® XL) is a non-steroidal anti-inflammatory drug (NSAID). It is used to manage symptoms of osteoarthritis and rheumatoid arthritis. Generic etodolac extended-release tablets are available.

What should my health care professional know before I take etodolac?

They need to know if you have any of these conditions:
- asthma, especially aspirin sensitive asthma
- bleeding problems or taking medicines that make you bleed more easily such as anticoagulants ("blood thinners")
- cigarette smoker
- dental disease
- diabetes
- drink more than 3 alcohol-containing beverages a day
- heart or circulation problems such as heart failure or leg edema (fluid retention)
- high blood pressure
- kidney disease
- liver disease
- stomach or duodenal ulcers
- systemic lupus erythematosus
- ulcerative colitis
- an unusual or allergic reaction to aspirin, other salicylates, other NSAIDs, foods, dyes or preservatives

- pregnant or trying to get pregnant
- breast-feeding

How should I take this medicine?

Take etodolac extended-release tablets by mouth. Follow the directions on the prescription label. Swallow tablets or capsules whole with a full glass of water; take tablets or capsules in an upright or sitting position. Taking a sip of water first, before taking the tablets or capsules, may help you swallow them. If possible take bedtime doses at least 10 minutes before lying down. Etodolac may be taken with food to help decrease stomach upset. Take your doses at regular intervals. Do not take your medicine more often than directed. Contact your pediatrician or health care professional regarding the use of this medicine in children. Special care may be needed.

What if I miss a dose?

If you miss a dose, take it as soon as you can. If it is almost time for your next dose, take only that dose. Do not take double or extra doses.

What may interact with etodolac?

- alcohol
- alendronate
- aspirin and aspirin-like medicines
- cidofovir

- cyclosporine
- drospirenone; ethinyl estradiol (Yasmin®)
- entecavir
- herbal products that contain feverfew, garlic, ginger, or ginkgo biloba
- lithium
- medicines for high blood pressure
- medicines that affect platelets
- medicines that treat or prevent blood clots such as warfarin and other "blood thinners"
- methotrexate
- other anti-inflammatory drugs (such as ibuprofen or prednisone)
- pemetrexed
- water pills (diuretics)

Tell your prescriber or health care professional about all other medicines you are taking, including non-prescription medicines, nutritional supplements, or herbal products. Also tell your prescriber or health care professional if you are a frequent user of drinks with caffeine or alcohol, if you smoke, or if you use illegal drugs. These may affect the way your medicine works. Check with your health care professional before stopping or starting any of your medicines.

What should I watch for while taking etodolac?

Let your prescriber or health care professional know if your pain continues. Do not take with other pain-killers without advice. If you get flu-like symptoms (fever, chills, muscle aches and pains), call your prescriber or health care professional; do not treat yourself. To reduce unpleasant effects on your throat and stomach, take etodolac with a full glass of water and never just before lying down. If you notice black, tarry stools or experience severe stomach pain and vomit blood or what looks like coffee grounds, notify your health care prescriber immediately. If you are taking medicines that affect the clotting of your blood, such as aspirin or blood thinners such as Coumadin®, talk to your health care provider or prescriber before taking this medicine. You may get dizzy. Do not drive, use machinery, or do anything that needs mental alertness until you know how etodolac affects you. Do not sit or stand up quickly, especially if you are an older patient. This reduces the risk of dizzy or fainting spells. Do not smoke cigarettes or drink alcohol; these increase irritation to your stomach and can make it more susceptible to damage from etodolac. If you are going to have surgery, tell your prescriber or health care professional that you are taking etodolac. Etodolac can cause you to bleed more easily. Problems can arise if you need dental work, and in the day to day care of your teeth. Try to avoid damage to your teeth and gums when you brush or floss your teeth. It is especially important not to use etodolac during the last 3 months of pregnancy unless specifically directed to do so by your health care provider. Etodolac may cause problems in the unborn child or complications during delivery.

What side effects may I notice from taking etodolac?

Elderly patients are at increased risk for developing side effects.

Side effects that you should report to your prescriber or health care professional as soon as possible:

- signs of bleeding from the stomach—black tarry stools, blood in the urine, unusual tiredness or weakness, vomiting blood or vomit that looks like coffee grounds
- signs of an allergic reaction—difficulty breathing or wheezing, skin rash, redness, blistering or peeling skin, hives, or itching, swelling of eyelids, throat, lips
- blurred vision
- change in the amount of urine passed
- difficulty swallowing, severe heartburn or burning, pain in throat
- pain or difficulty passing urine
- stomach pain or cramps
- swelling of feet or ankles
- yellowing of eyes or skin

Side effects that usually do not require medical attention (report to your prescriber or health care professional if they continue or are bothersome):

- constipation or diarrhea
- dizziness, drowsiness
- gas or heartburn
- headache
- nausea, vomiting

Where can I keep my medicine?

Keep out of the reach of children in a container that small children cannot open. Store at room temperature between 20 and 25 degrees C (68 and 77 degrees F). Protect from moisture. Keep container tightly closed. Throw away any unused medicine after the expiration date.

E

Etodolac tablets or capsules

LODINE®;
500 mg; Tablet
Wyeth
Pharmaceuticals Inc

LODINE®;
300 mg; Capsule
Wyeth
Pharmaceuticals Inc

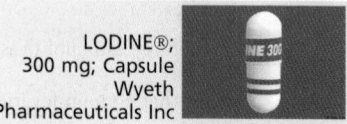

What are etodolac tablets and capsules?

ETODOLAC (Lodine®) is a non-steroidal anti-inflammatory drug (NSAID). It relieves mild to moderate pain and symptoms of osteoarthritis and rheumatoid arthritis. Generic etodolac tablets or capsules are available.

What should my health care professional know before I take etodolac?

They need to know if you have any of these conditions:
- asthma, especially aspirin sensitive asthma
- bleeding problems or taking medicines that make you bleed more easily such as anticoagulants ("blood thinners")
- cigarette smoker
- dental disease
- diabetes
- drink more than 3 alcohol-containing beverages a day
- heart or circulation problems such as heart failure or leg edema (fluid retention)
- high blood pressure
- kidney disease
- liver disease
- stomach or duodenal ulcers
- systemic lupus erythematosus
- ulcerative colitis
- an unusual or allergic reaction to aspirin, other salicylates, other NSAIDs, foods, dyes or preservatives
- pregnant or trying to get pregnant
- breast-feeding

How should I take this medicine?

Take etodolac tablets or capsules by mouth. Follow the directions on the prescription label. Swallow tablets or capsules whole with a full glass of water; take tablets or capsules in an upright or sitting position. Taking a sip of water first, before taking the tablets or capsules, may help you swallow them. If possible take bedtime doses at least 10 minutes before lying down. Etodolac may be taken with food to help decrease stomach upset. Take your doses at regular intervals. Do not take your medicine more often than directed. Contact your pediatrician or health care professional regarding the use of this medicine in children. Special care may be needed.

What if I miss a dose?

If you miss a dose, take it as soon as you can. If it is almost time for your next dose, take only that dose. Do not take double or extra doses.

What may interact with etodolac?

- ACE inhibitors, often used to treat high blood pressure or heart problems
- agents that treat or prevent blood clots such as warfarin or other "blood thinners"
- agents that affect platelets
- alcohol
- alendronate
- aspirin and aspirin-like medicines
- cyclosporine
- drospirenone; ethinyl estradiol (Yasmin®)
- entecavir
- herbal products that contain feverfew, garlic, ginger, or ginkgo biloba
- lithium
- methotrexate
- other anti-inflammatory drugs (such as ibuprofen or prednisone)
- pemetrexed
- water pills (diuretics)

Tell your prescriber or health care professional about all other medicines you are taking, including non-prescription medicines, nutritional supplements, or herbal products. Also tell your prescriber or health care professional if you are a frequent user of drinks with caffeine or alcohol, if you smoke, or if you use illegal drugs. These may affect the way your medicine works. Check with your health care professional before stopping or starting any of your medicines.

What should I watch for while taking etodolac?

Let your prescriber or health care professional know if your pain continues, do not take with other pain-killers without advice. If you get flu-like symptoms (fever, chills, muscle aches and pains), call your prescriber or health care professional; do not treat yourself. To reduce unpleasant effects on your throat and stomach, take etodolac with a full glass of water and never just before lying down. If you notice black, tarry stools or experience severe stomach pain and vomit blood or what looks like coffee grounds, notify your health care prescriber immediately. If you are taking medicines that affect the clotting of your blood, such as aspirin or blood thinners such as Coumadin®, talk to your health care provider or prescriber before taking this medicine. You may get dizzy. Do not drive, use machinery, or do anything that needs mental alertness until you know how etodolac affects you. Do not sit or stand up quickly, especially if you are an older patient. This reduces the risk of dizzy or fainting spells. Do not smoke cigarettes or drink alcohol; these increase irritation to your stomach and can make it more susceptible to damage from etodolac. If you are going to have surgery, tell your prescriber or health care professional that you are taking etodolac. Etodolac can cause you to bleed more easily. Problems can arise if you need dental work, and in the day to day care of your teeth. Try to avoid damage to your teeth and gums when you brush or floss your teeth. It is especially important not to use etodolac during the last 3 months of pregnancy unless specifically directed to do so by your health care provider. Etodolac may cause problems in the unborn child or complications during delivery.

What side effects may I notice from taking etodolac?

Elderly patients are at increased risk for developing side effects.

Side effects that you should report to your prescriber or health care professional as soon as possible:
- signs of bleeding from the stomach—black tarry stools, blood in the urine, unusual tiredness or weakness, vomiting blood or vomit that looks like coffee grounds
- signs of an allergic reaction—difficulty breathing or wheezing, skin rash, redness, blistering or peeling skin, hives, or itching, swelling of eyelids, throat, lips
- blurred vision

- change in the amount of urine passed
- difficulty swallowing, severe heartburn or burning, pain in throat
- pain or difficulty passing urine
- stomach pain or cramps
- swelling of feet or ankles
- yellowing of eyes or skin

Side effects that usually do not require medical attention (report to your prescriber or health care professional if they continue or are bothersome):
- constipation or diarrhea
- dizziness, drowsiness
- gas or heartburn
- headache
- nausea, vomiting

Where can I keep my medicine?

Keep out of the reach of children in the original container. Store at room temperature between 20 and 25 degrees C (68 and 77 degrees F). Protect from moisture and from light. Keep container tightly closed. Throw away any unused medicine after the expiration date.

E

Etoposide, VP-16 capsules

VEPESID®; 50 mg; Capsule Bristol Meyer Squibb Oncology Products		
ETOPOSIDE; 50 mg; Capsule UDL Laboratories Inc		

What are etoposide capsules?

ETOPOSIDE, VP-16 (VePesid®) is a type of chemotherapy for treating cancer. Etoposide interferes with the growth of cells. Etoposide is effective in treating cancer of the lung and testicles. Generic etoposide capsules are not yet available.

What should my health care professional know before I take etoposide?

They need to know if you have any of these conditions:
- bleeding problems
- blood disorders
- having intramuscular injections
- infection (bacterial, viral or fungal)
- an unusual or allergic reaction to etoposide, other chemotherapeutic agents, other medicines, foods, dyes, or preservatives
- pregnant or trying to get pregnant
- breast-feeding

How should I take this medicine?

Take etoposide capsules by mouth. Follow the directions on the prescription label. Swallow the capsules with a drink of water. Take your doses at regular intervals. Do not stop taking except on your prescriber's advice. After several days of treatment there is usually a break of 3 to 4 weeks before the treatment is repeated. Contact your pediatrician or health care professional regarding the use of this medicine in children. Special care may be needed.

What if I miss a dose?

If you miss a dose, skip that dose unless your prescriber or health care professional tells you otherwise. Do not take double or extra doses. If you vomit after taking a dose, call your prescriber or health care professional for advice.

What may interact with etoposide?

- bosentan
- cisplatin
- cyclosporine
- cytarabine
- ifosfamide
- live virus vaccines
- methotrexate
- verapamil
- voriconazole

Tell your prescriber or health care professional about all other medicines you are taking, including nonprescription medicines, nutritional supplements, or herbal products. Also tell your prescriber or health care professional if you are a frequent user of drinks with caffeine or alcohol, if you smoke, or if you use illegal drugs. These may affect the way your medicine works. Check with your health care professional before stopping or starting any of your medicines.

What should I watch for while taking etoposide?

Visit your prescriber or health care professional for regular checks on your progress. You will need to have regular blood checks. Etoposide may make you feel generally unwell. This is not uncommon because etoposide affects good cells as well as cancer cells. Report any side effects as above, but continue your course of medicine even though you feel ill, unless your prescriber or health care professional tells you to stop. Etoposide can cause blood problems. This can mean slow healing and a risk of infection. Try to avoid cutting or injuring yourself. Problems can arise if you need dental work, and in the day to day care of your teeth. Try to avoid damage to your teeth and gums when you brush or floss your teeth. While you are taking etoposide you will be more susceptible to infection. Try to avoid people with colds, flu, and bronchitis. Do not have any vaccinations without your prescriber's approval and avoid anyone who has recently had oral polio vaccine. Call your prescriber or health care professional for advice if you get a fever, chills or sore throat. Do not treat yourself.

What side effects may I notice from taking etoposide?

Side effects that you should report to your prescriber or health care professional as soon as possible:
- black, tarry stools
- blood in the urine

- difficulty breathing, wheezing
- fast heartbeat
- fever or chills, cough or sore throat
- lower back pain
- mouth or throat sores or ulcers
- pain or difficulty passing urine
- unusual bleeding or bruising, pinpoint red spots on your skin
- unusual tiredness or weakness
- vomiting

Side effects that usually do not require medical attention (report to your prescriber or health care professional if they continue or are bothersome):
- diarrhea
- hair loss
- headache
- loss of appetite
- nausea

Where can I keep my medicine?

Keep out of the reach of children in a container that small children cannot open. Store in a refrigerator between 2 and 8 degrees C (36 and 46 degrees F); do not freeze.

Exemestane tablets

AROMASIN®;
25 mg; Tablet
Pharmacia and Upjohn Div
Pfizer

What are exemestane tablets?

EXEMESTANE (Aromasin®) blocks the production of the hormone estrogen. Some types of breast cancer depend on estrogen to grow, and exemestane can stop tumor growth by blocking estrogen production. Exemestane is for the treatment of breast cancer in postmenopausal women only. Generic exemestane tablets are not available.

What should my health care professional know before I take exemestane?

They need to know if you have any of these conditions:
- an unusual or allergic reaction to exemestane, other medicines, foods, dyes, or preservatives
- pregnant or trying to get pregnant
- breast-feeding

How should I take this medicine?

Take exemestane tablets by mouth at the same time each day after a meal. Follow the directions on the prescription label. Swallow the tablets with a drink of water. Do not take your medicine more often than directed. Do not stop taking except on your prescriber's advice.

What if I miss a dose?

If you miss a dose, take it as soon as you can. If it is almost time for your next dose, take only that dose. Do not take double or extra doses. If you vomit after

taking a dose, call your prescriber or health care professional for advice.

What may interact with exemestane?

- androstenedione
- any medicine containing estrogens (this may include some herbal products and some birth control pills)
- DHEA

Tell your prescriber or health care professional about all other medicines that you are taking, including nonprescription medicines, nutritional supplements, or herbal products. Also tell your prescriber or health care professional if you are a frequent user of drinks with caffeine or alcohol, if you smoke, or if you use illegal drugs. These may affect the way your medicine works. Check with your health care professional before stopping or starting any of your medicines.

What should I watch for while taking exemestane?

Visit your prescriber or health care professional for regular checks on your progress. Do not treat yourself for diarrhea, nausea, vomiting or other side effects. Ask your prescriber or health care professional for advice.

What side effects may I notice from taking exemestane?

Side effects that you should report to your prescriber or health care professional as soon as possible:

- any new or unusual symptoms
- fever
- leg or arm swelling

Side effects that usually do not require medical attention (report to your prescriber or health care professional if they continue or are bothersome):

- anxiety
- constipation
- cough, or throat infection
- depression
- diarrhea
- difficulty sleeping
- dizziness
- headache

- hot flashes
- increase or decrease in appetite
- nausea
- stomach pain
- sweating
- weakness and tiredness
- weight gain

Where can I keep my medicine?

Keep out of the reach of children in a container that small children cannot open. Store at room temperature between 20 and 25 degrees C (68 and 77 degrees F). Throw away any unused medicine after the expiration date.

Ezetimibe Tablets

ZETIA®;
10 mg; Tablet
Merck/Schering Plough
Pharmaceuticals

E

What are ezetimibe tablets?

EZETIMIBE (Zetia®) blocks the absorption of cholesterol from the stomach. Ezetimibe can help lower blood cholesterol for patients who are at risk of getting heart disease or a stroke. It is only for patients whose cholesterol level is not controlled by diet. It is not a cure. Generic ezetimibe tablets are not yet available.

What should my health care professional know before I take ezetimibe?

They need to know if you have any of these conditions:

- an alcohol problem
- liver disease
- muscle disorder or condition
- an unusual reaction to ezetimibe, medicines, foods, dyes, or preservatives
- pregnant or trying to get pregnant
- breast-feeding

How should this medicine be used?

Take ezetimibe tablets by mouth. Follow the directions on the prescription label. Swallow the tablets with a drink of water. Ezetimibe can be taken with or without food. Take your doses at regular intervals. Do not take your medicine more often than directed. If you are taking a "statin" type medication (like atorvastatin, fluvastatin, lovastatin, pravastatin, rosuvastatin, or simvastatin) to lower your cholesterol, you can take ezetimibe once daily at the same time that you take the "statin" medication. If you are taking a "resin" type medication (like cholestyramine, colesevelam, or colestipol) to lower your cholesterol, you should take ezetimibe at least 2 hours before or 4 hours after you take the "resin" medication. Contact your pediatrician or health care professional regarding the use of this medicine in children. Special care may be needed.

What if I miss a dose?

If you miss a dose, take it as soon as you can. If it is almost time for your next dose, take only that dose. Do not take double or extra doses.

What may interact with ezetimibe?

- alcohol-containing beverages
- antacids
- cyclosporine
- herbal medicines such as went yeast (Cholestin™)
- other medicines to lower cholesterol or triglycerides

Tell your prescriber or health care professional about all other medicines you are taking, including non-prescription medicines, nutritional supplements, or herbal products. Also tell your prescriber or health care professional if you are a frequent user of drinks with caffeine or alcohol, if you smoke, or if you use illegal drugs. These may affect the way your medicine works. Check with your health care professional before stopping or starting any of your medicines.

What should I watch for while taking ezetimibe?

Visit your prescriber or health care professional for regular checks on your progress. Your prescriber may order regular tests to check your cholesterol and other plasma lipid levels. If you are also taking a "statin-type" drug (such as atorvastatin, fluvastatin, lovastatin, pravastatin, rosuvastatin, or simvastatin), you will also need to have regular tests to make sure your liver is working properly. Tell your prescriber or health care professional if you get any unexplained muscle pain, tenderness, or weakness, especially if you also have a fever and tiredness. Ezetimibe is only part of a total cholesterol-lowering program. Your physician or dietician can suggest a low-cholesterol and low-fat diet that will reduce your risk of getting heart and blood vessel disease. Avoid alcohol and smoking, and keep a proper exercise schedule.

What side effects may I notice from taking ezetimibe?

Side effects that you should report to your prescriber or health care professional as soon as possible:

Rare (possible increased risk if taking ezetimibe with other cholesterol-lowering drugs)
- dark yellow or brown urine
- muscle pain, tenderness, cramps, or weakness
- unusual tiredness or weakness
- yellowing of the skin or eyes

Side effects that usually do not require medical attention (report to your prescriber or health care professional if they continue or are bothersome):
- diarrhea
- dizziness

- headache
- joint pain
- stomach upset or pain
- tiredness

Where can I keep my medicine?

Keep out of the reach of children in a container that small children cannot open. Store at room temperature between 15 and 30 degrees C (59 and 86 degrees F). Protect from moisture. Keep container tightly closed. Throw away any unused medicine after the expiration date.

Ezetimibe; Simvastatin tablets

VYTORIN™; 10 mg/20 mg; Tablet Merck/Schering Plough Pharmaceuticals		VYTORIN™; 10 mg/10 mg; Tablet Merck/Schering Plough Pharmaceuticals	

What are ezetimibe; simvastatin tablets?

EZETIMIBE; SIMVASTATIN (Vytorin™) blocks the body's ability to absorb and make cholesterol. This product can help lower blood cholesterol. It helps patients whose cholesterol level is not controlled by diet alone. Generic ezetimibe; simvastatin tablets are not yet available.

What should my health care professional know before I take ezetimibe; simvastatin?

They need to know if you have any of these conditions:
- an alcohol problem
- any hormone disorder (such as diabetes, underactive thyroid)
- blood salt imbalance
- infection
- kidney disease
- liver disease
- low blood pressure
- muscle disorder or condition
- recent surgery
- seizures (convulsions)
- severe injury
- an unusual reaction to ezetimibe; simvastatin, other medicines, foods, dyes, or preservatives
- pregnant or trying to get pregnant
- breast-feeding

How should this medicine be used?

Take ezetimibe; simvastatin tablets by mouth. Follow the directions on the prescription label. Swallow the tablets with a drink of water. It is best to take your dose in the evening hours (like with the evening meal) or at bedtime. You may take this medicine with or without food. Do not take the tablet with grapefruit juice; orange juice may be used instead. Take your doses at regular intervals. Do not take your medicine more often than directed. Contact your pediatrician or health care professional regarding the use of this medicine in children. Special care may be needed.

What if I miss a dose?

If you miss a dose, take it as soon as you can. If it is almost time for your next dose, take only that dose. Take only one dose per day. Do not take double or extra doses.

What may interact with ezetimibe; simvastatin?

Do not take ezetimibe; simvastatin with any of the following:
- amprenavir
- atazanavir
- clarithromycin
- delavirdine
- erythromycin
- grapefruit juice
- indinavir
- itraconazole
- ketoconazole
- lopinavir; ritonavir
- mibefradil
- nefazodone
- nelfinavir
- ritonavir
- saquinavir
- went yeast

This medicine may also interact with the following medications:
- alcohol
- amiodarone
- barbiturates (examples: phenobarbital, butalbital, primidone)
- bosentan
- carbamazepine
- cyclosporine
- digoxin
- diltiazem
- efavirenz
- fluconazole
- medicines to lower cholesterol or triglycerides (examples: fenofibrate, gemfibrozil, niacin)

- medicine used to stop early pregnancy (mifepristone, RU-486)
- nicardipine
- oxcarbazepine
- phenytoin
- rifampin, rifabutin, or rifapentine
- St. John's wort
- telithromycin
- troleandomycin
- verapamil
- voriconazole
- warfarin

Tell your prescriber or health care professional about all other medicines you are taking, including non-prescription medicines, nutritional supplements, or herbal products. Also tell your prescriber or health care professional if you are a frequent user of drinks with caffeine or alcohol, if you smoke, or if you use illegal drugs. These may affect the way your medicine works. Check with your health care professional before stopping or starting any of your medicines.

What should I watch for while taking ezetimibe; simvastatin?

This drug is only part of a total cholesterol-lowering program. Your physician or dietician can suggest a low-cholesterol and low-fat diet that will reduce your risk of getting heart and blood vessel disease. Avoid alcohol and smoking, and keep a proper exercise schedule. Visit your prescriber or health care professional for regular checks on your progress. You will need to have regular tests to make sure your liver is working properly. Tell your prescriber or health care professional as soon as you can if you get any unexplained muscle pain, tenderness, or weakness, especially if you also have a fever and tiredness. Some medicines increase the risk of muscle side effects while taking simvastatin. Discuss your drug regimen with your health care provider if you are

prescribed certain antibiotics or antifungals (examples: clarithromycin, erythromycin, itraconazole, ketoconazole). Your prescriber may decide to temporarily stop taking ezetimibe; simvastatin while you are taking a short course of the antibiotic or antifungal therapy. Alternatively, your health care provider may prescribe another antibiotic or antifungal medicine for your condition. If you are going to have surgery tell your prescriber or health care professional that you are taking ezetimibe; simvastatin.

What side effects may I notice from taking ezetimibe; simvastatin?

Side effects that you should report to your prescriber or health care professional as soon as possible:
Rare or uncommon:
- dark yellow or brown urine
- decreased urination, difficulty passing urine
- fever
- muscle pain, tenderness, cramps, or weakness
- redness, blistering, peeling or loosening of the skin, including inside the mouth
- skin rash, itching
- unusual tiredness or weakness
- yellowing of the skin or eyes

Side effects that usually do not require medical attention (report to your prescriber or health care professional if they continue or are bothersome):
- constipation
- headache
- upset stomach, indigestion, gas, heartburn

Where can I keep my medicine?

Keep out of the reach of children in a container that small children cannot open. Store at room temperature between 20 and 25 degrees C (68 and 77 degrees F). Throw away any unused medicine after the expiration date.

E

Famciclovir tablets

FAMVIR®;
250 mg; Tablet
Novartis
Pharmaceuticals

FAMVIR®;
500 mg; Tablet
Novartis
Pharmaceuticals

F

What are famciclovir tablets?

FAMCICLOVIR (Famvir®) is an antiviral agent. Famciclovir relieves the symptoms of herpes zoster infection (shingles) or genital herpes infection. Famciclovir will not cure shingles or genital herpes; it will help the blisters heal faster and reduce the duration of pain and discomfort. Famciclovir is also used to reduce the number of episodes of genital herpes infection. Generic famciclovir tablets are not yet available.

What should my health care professional know before I take famciclovir?

They need to know if you have any of these conditions:
- kidney disease
- an unusual or allergic reaction to famciclovir, acyclovir, ganciclovir, valacyclovir, valganciclovir, other medicines, food, dyes, or preservatives
- pregnant or trying to get pregnant
- breast-feeding

How should I take this medicine?

Take famciclovir tablets by mouth. Follow the directions on the prescription label. Take the tablets with a full glass of water. Famciclovir may be taken with food or without food. Take your doses at regular intervals. Do not take your medicine more often than directed. Finish the full course prescribed by your prescriber or health care professional even if you think your condition is better. Do not stop taking except on your prescriber's advice. Contact your pediatrician or health care professional regarding the use of this medicine in children. Special care may be needed.

What if I miss a dose?

If you miss a dose, take it as soon as you can. If it is almost time for your next dose, take only that dose. Do not take double or extra doses.

What may interact with famciclovir?

- probenecid

Tell your prescriber or health care professional about all other medicines you are taking, including non-prescription medicines. Also tell your prescriber or health care professional if you are a frequent user of drinks with caffeine or alcohol, if you smoke, or if you use illegal drugs. These may affect the way your medicine works. Check with your health care professional before stopping or starting any of your medicines.

What should I watch for while taking famciclovir?

If famciclovir is used to treat (rather than prevent) an infection, it should be taken when you first notice symptoms of infection, such as tingling, itching, or pain in the affected area. Tell your prescriber or health care professional if your symptoms do not improve within a few days of starting famciclovir. Drink several glasses of water a day while taking this medicine. Keep affected area of blisters as clean and dry as possible. Wear loose-fitting clothing, and do not cover the area with an occlusive (plastic or waterproof) dressing. Famciclovir does not prevent the spread of genital herpes infection to others. Genital herpes is transmitted by sexual contact. You should avoid sex when lesions are present to avoid infecting your partner. Genital herpes can also be spread when symptoms are not present. Therefore, latex condoms should be used at all times during sexual intercourse.

What side effects may I notice from taking famciclovir?

Side effects that you should report to your prescriber or health care professional as soon as possible:
- confusion
- skin rash, itching, hives

Side effects that usually do not require medical attention (report to your prescriber or health care professional if they continue or are bothersome):
- diarrhea
- dizziness
- headache
- tiredness
- nausea, vomiting

Where can I keep my medicine?

Keep out of the reach of children in a container that small children cannot open. Store at room temperature between 15 and 30 degrees C (59 and 86 degrees F). Throw away any unused medicine after the expiration date.

Famotidine tablets or gelcaps

PEPCID®;
40 mg; Tablet
Merck and Co Inc

What are famotidine tablets or gelcaps?

FAMOTIDINE (Mylanta-AR®, Fluxid® Orally Disintegrating Tablets, Pepcid®, Pepcid® AC Gelcaps, Tablets or Chewable Tablets, Pepcid® RPD™ Orally Disintegrating Tablets) is a type of antihistamine that blocks the release of stomach acid. Famotidine is used to treat stomach and intestinal ulcers. It can relieve ulcer pain and discomfort. Famotidine is also used to control acid reflux (heartburn). Generic famotidine tablets are available; generic gelcaps are not available.

What should my health care professional know before I take famotidine?

They need to know if you have any of these conditions:
- an alcohol abuse problem
- bleeding, such as in your stool or any vomiting with blood
- kidney disease
- liver disease
- other chronic illness
- phenylketonuria
- trouble swallowing
- an unusual or allergic reaction to famotidine, other medicines, foods, dyes, or preservatives
- pregnant or trying to get pregnant
- breast-feeding

How should I take this medicine?

Take famotidine tablets or gelcaps by mouth. Follow the directions on the prescription label. Swallow the tablets or gelcaps with a drink of water. If you only take famotidine once a day, take it at bedtime. Take your doses at regular intervals. Do not take your medicine more often than directed. If you are taking Fluxid® or Pepcid® orally disintegrating tablets: Place the tablet on your tongue, allow to dissolve completely and then swallow. You can take the orally disintegrating tablets with or without water. Contact your pediatrician or health care professional regarding the use of this medicine in children. Special care may be needed.

What if I miss a dose?

If you miss a dose, take it as soon as you can. If it is almost time for your next dose, take only that dose. Do not take double or extra doses.

What may interact with famotidine?

- cefditoren
- cefpodoxime
- cefuroxime
- delavirdine
- itraconazole
- ketoconazole
- metformin
- theophylline

Tell your prescriber or health care professional about all other medicines you are taking, including non-prescription medicines, nutritional supplements, or herbal products. Also tell your prescriber or health care professional if you are a frequent user of drinks with caffeine or alcohol, if you smoke, or if you use illegal drugs. These may affect the way your medicine works. Check with your health care professional before stopping or starting any of your medicines.

What should I watch for while taking famotidine?

Tell your prescriber or health care professional if your condition does not improve or gets worse. Finish the full course of tablets prescribed, even if you feel better. Do not self-medicate with aspirin, ibuprofen or other anti-inflammatory medicines; these can aggravate your condition. Do not smoke cigarettes or drink alcohol; these increase irritation in your stomach and can lengthen the time it will take for ulcers to heal. Cigarettes and alcohol can also worsen acid reflux or heartburn. If you need to take an antacid, you should take it at least 1 hour before or 1 hour after famotidine. Famotidine will not be as effective if taken at the same time as an antacid. If you get black, tarry stools or vomit up what looks like coffee grounds, call your prescriber or health care professional at once. You may have a bleeding ulcer. If you have phenylketonuria you should not use Pepcid® AC chewable tablets as they contain 1.4 mg of phenylalanine per tablet.

What side effects may I notice from taking famotidine?

Side effects that you should report to your prescriber or health care professional as soon as possible:
Rare or uncommon:
- confusion
- hallucinations
- skin rash, itching

Side effects that usually do not require medical attention (report to your prescriber or health care professional if they continue or are bothersome):
- agitation, nervousness
- constipation
- diarrhea
- dizziness
- headache
- nausea

Where can I keep my medicine?

Keep out of the reach of children in a container that small children cannot open. Store at room temperatures below 40 degrees C (104 degrees F). Throw away any unused medicine after the expiration date.

Felbamate tablets

FELBATOL®;
400 mg; Tablet
MedPointe
Pharmaceuticals

What are felbamate tablets?

FELBAMATE (Felbatol®) can help with seizure (convulsion) control in certain types of epilepsy. Felbamate helps to control partial seizures in adults that have been unresponsive to other agents. Felbamate helps to maintain seizure control in children with Lennox-Gastaut syndrome, who have not responded to other therapy. Generic felbamate tablets are not yet available.

What should my health care professional know before I take felbamate?

They need to know if you have any of these conditions:
- blood disorders or disease
- having intramuscular injections
- liver disease
- an unusual or allergic reaction to felbamate, carbamate, other medicines, foods, dyes, or preservatives
- pregnant or trying to get pregnant
- breast-feeding

How should I take this medicine?

Take felbamate tablets by mouth. Follow the directions on the prescription label. Swallow the tablets with a drink of water. If felbamate upsets your stomach, take it with food or milk. Take your doses at regular intervals. Do not take your medicine more often than directed. Contact your pediatrician or health care professional regarding the use of this medicine in children. Special care may be needed.

What if I miss a dose?

If you miss a dose, take it as soon as you can. If it is almost time for your next dose, take only that dose. Do not take double or extra doses.

What may interact with felbamate?

- alcohol
- carbamazepine
- phenobarbital
- phenytoin
- valproic acid

Tell your prescriber or health care professional about all other medicines you are taking, including non-prescription medicines, nutritional supplements, or herbal products. Also tell your prescriber or health care professional if you are a frequent user of drinks with caffeine or alcohol, if you smoke, or if you use illegal drugs. These may affect the way your medicine works. Check with your health care professional before stopping or starting any of your medicines.

What should I watch for while taking felbamate?

Visit your prescriber or health care professional for a regular check on your progress. Do not stop taking felbamate suddenly. This increases the risk of seizures. Wear a Medic Alert bracelet or necklace. Carry an identification card with information about your condition, medications, and prescriber or health care professional. You may get drowsy, dizzy, or have blurred vision. Do not drive, use machinery, or do anything that needs mental alertness until you know how felbamate affects you. To reduce dizzy or fainting spells, do not sit or stand up quickly, especially if you are an older patient. Alcohol can increase drowsiness and dizziness. Avoid alcoholic drinks. Felbamate can make your skin more sensitive to the sun or ultraviolet light. Keep out of the sun, or wear protective clothing outdoors and use a sunscreen (at least SPF 15). Do not use sun lamps or sun tanning beds or booths. If you are going to have surgery, tell your prescriber or health care professional that you are taking felbamate.

What side effects may I notice from taking felbamate?

Children are especially sensitive to the effects of felbamate.

Side effects that you should report to your prescriber or health care professional as soon as possible:
- blood in urine
- confusion
- fever, chills, sore throat
- mood changes, nervousness, hostility
- mouth ulcers
- severe headache
- severe stomach pain
- shortness of breath, or wheezing
- skin rash and itching
- unusual bleeding or bruising, pinpoint red spots on skin
- unusual tiredness or weakness
- weight loss
- yellowing of the eyes or skin

Side effects that usually do not require medical attention (report to your prescriber or health care professional if they continue or are bothersome):
- diarrhea or constipation
- difficulty sleeping
- dizziness or drowsiness
- changes in taste
- changes in vision
- colds, runny nose, and upper respiratory infections
- headache
- loss of appetite
- nausea/vomiting
- tremor

Where can I keep my medicine?

Keep out of reach of children in a container that small children cannot open. Store at room temperature between 15 and 30 degrees C (59 and 86 degrees F). Keep container tightly closed. Throw away any unused medicine after the expiration date.

Felodipine extended-release tablets

PLENDIL®;
5 mg; Tablet,
Extended Release
AstraZeneca LP

PLENDIL®;
2.5 mg; Tablet,
Extended Release
AstraZeneca LP

What are felodipine extended-release tablets?

FELODIPINE (Plendil®) is a calcium-channel blocker. It affects the amount of calcium found in your heart and muscle cells. This results in relaxation of blood vessels, which can reduce the amount of work the heart has to do. Felodipine reduces high blood pressure (hypertension). It is not a cure. Generic felodipine extended-release tablets are available.

What should my health care professional know before I take felodipine?

They need to know if you have any of these conditions:

- heart problems, low blood pressure, irregular heartbeat
- liver disease
- previous heart attack
- an unusual or allergic reaction to felodipine, other medicines, foods, dyes, or preservatives
- pregnant or trying to get pregnant
- breast-feeding

How should I take this medicine?

Take felodipine tablets by mouth. Follow the directions on the prescription label. Swallow the tablets whole with a drink of water, do not crush or chew. Take felodipine tablets regularly either on an empty stomach or with a light meal. Do not take felodipine with grapefruit juice or grapefruit. Take your doses at regular intervals. Do not take your medicine more often then directed. Do not stop taking except on your prescriber's advice. Contact your pediatrician or health care professional regarding the use of this medicine in children. Special care may be needed. Elderly patients over 65 years old may have a stronger reaction to this medicine and need smaller doses.

What if I miss a dose?

If you miss a dose, take it as soon as you can. If it is almost time for your next dose, take only that dose. Do not take double or extra doses.

What may interact with felodipine?

Do not take felodipine with any of the following:

- grapefruit juice

Felodipine may also interact with the following medications:

- anti-inflammatory drugs (NSAIDs, such as ibuprofen)
- barbiturates such as phenobarbital
- bosentan
- cimetidine
- cyclosporine
- herbal or dietary supplements such as ginkgo biloba, ginseng, hawthorn, *Ma huang* (ephedra), melatonin, St. John's wort, went yeast
- imatinib, STI-571
- local anesthetics or general anesthetics
- medicines for fungal infections (fluconazole, itraconazole, ketoconazole, voriconazole)
- medicines for high blood pressure
- medicines for HIV infection or AIDS
- medicines for prostate problems
- medicines for seizures (carbamazepine, oxcarbazepine, phenobarbital, phenytoin, primidone, zonisamide)
- rifampin, rifapentine, or rifabutin
- some antibiotics (clarithromycin, erythromycin, telithromycin, troleandomycin)
- some medicines for heart-rhythm problems (amiodarone, digoxin, diltiazem, verapamil)
- some medicines for depression or mental problems (fluoxetine, fluvoxamine, nefazodone)
- water pills (diuretics)
- yohimbine
- zafirlukast
- zileuton

Tell your prescriber or health care professional about all other medicines you are taking, including non-prescription medicines, nutritional supplements, or herbal products. Also tell your prescriber or health care professional if you are a frequent user of drinks with caffeine or alcohol, if you smoke, or if you use illegal drugs. These may affect the way your medicine works. Check with your health care professional before stopping or starting any of your medicines.

What should I watch for while taking felodipine?

Check your blood pressure and pulse rate regularly; this is important while you are taking felodipine. Ask your prescriber or health care professional what your blood pressure and pulse rate should be and when you should contact him or her. You may feel dizzy or lightheaded. Do not drive, use machinery, or do anything that needs mental alertness until you know how felodipine affects you. To reduce the risk of dizzy or fainting spells, do not sit or stand up quickly, especially if you are an older patient. Avoid alcoholic drinks; they can make you more dizzy or increase flushing and rapid heartbeats. Felodipine can cause dental problems for some patients. Clean and floss your teeth carefully and regularly.

F

Check with your dentist if your gums get swollen or inflamed and have the dentist clean your teeth regularly. If you are going to have surgery, tell your prescriber or health care professional that you are taking felodipine. Do not suddenly stop taking felodipine. Ask your prescriber or health care professional how to gradually reduce the dose.

What side effects may I notice from taking felodipine?

Side effects that you should report to your prescriber or health care professional as soon as possible:
- chest infection
- fainting spells, lightheadedness
- fast heartbeat, irregular heartbeat
- swelling of the legs and ankles

Side effects that usually do not require medical attention (report to your prescriber or health care professional if they continue or are bothersome):
- diarrhea or constipation
- dizziness or drowsiness
- facial flushing
- headache
- nausea
- tingling, burning or numbness in the fingers and toes
- weakness or tiredness
- sexual dysfunction

Where can I keep my medicine?

Keep out of the reach of children in a container that small children cannot open. Store at room temperature below 30 degrees C (86 degrees F). Keep container tightly closed. Protect from light. Throw away any unused medicine after the expiration date.

Fenofibrate capsules

LOFIBRA™; 200 mg; Capsule Gate Pharmaceuticals		TRICOR®; 67 mg; Capsule Abbott Pharmaceutical Product Division	

What are fenofibrate capsules?

FENOFIBRATE capsules (Lofibra™, TriCor®) can help lower triglycerides and cholesterol for people who are at risk of getting inflammation of the pancreas (pancreatitis) from having very high amounts of fats in their blood. Inflammation of the pancreas is a painful condition of the abdomen that can sometimes cause serious health problems. Fenofibrate is only for patients whose blood fats are not controlled by diet. Fenofibrate can also help some persons who have high cholesterol and blood fats that have not responded well to other standard cholesterol lowering drugs. Fenofibrate is not a cure, and it is unclear at this time if this drug helps prevent heart disease. Generic fenofibrate capsules are available.

What should my health care professional know before I take fenofibrate?

They need to know if you have any of these conditions:
- if you are a frequent user of alcoholic beverages
- diabetes
- gallbladder disease
- heart disease
- kidney disease
- liver disease
- thyroid gland problems
- an unusual or allergic reaction to fenofibrate, gemfibrozil, other medicines, foods, dyes, or preservatives
- an unusual reaction to fenofibrate, medicines, foods, dyes, or preservatives
- pregnant or trying to get pregnant
- breast-feeding

How should this medicine be used?

Take fenofibrate capsules by mouth. Follow the directions on the prescription label. Swallow the capsules with a drink of water. Take your dose each day at a regular time during a meal. Take your doses at regular intervals. Do not take your medicine more often than directed. Contact your pediatrician or health care professional regarding the use of this medicine in children. Special care may be needed.

What if I miss a dose?

If you miss a dose, take it as soon as you can. If it is almost time for your next dose, take only that dose. Do not take double or extra doses.

What may interact with fenofibrate?

- cyclosporine
- medicines used to treat diabetes
- other medications used to lower cholesterol, like cholestyramine, atorvastatin, cerivastatin, fluvastatin, lovastatin, pravastatin or simvastatin
- ursodiol
- warfarin
- went yeast

Tell your prescriber or health care professional about all other medicines you are taking, including non-prescription medicines, nutritional supplements, or herbal products. Also tell your prescriber or health care professional if you are a frequent user of drinks with caffeine or alcohol, if you smoke, or if you use illegal drugs. These may affect the way your medicine works. Check with your health care professional before stopping or starting any of your medicines.

What should I watch for while taking fenofibrate?

Fenofibrate will not cure your condition but it will help lower your triglyceride and cholesterol levels. Visit your prescriber or health care professional for regular checks on your progress. Your blood fats and other tests will be measured from time to time. Do not stop taking fenofibrate except on the advice of your prescriber. Fenofibrate is only part of a total cholesterol-lowering program. Your health care professional or dietician can suggest a low-cholesterol and low-fat diet that will reduce your risk of getting heart and blood vessel disease. Avoid alcohol and smoking, and keep a proper exercise schedule. If you are diabetic, close regulation and monitoring of your blood sugars can help your blood fat levels. Fenofibrate may change the way your diabetic medication works, and sometimes will require that your prescriber change your medication dosages. Check with your prescriber or health care professional. Fenofibrate may cause drowsiness. Driving or operating machinery, or performing other tasks that require mental alertness requires caution when first starting fenofibrate. You should not participate in these activities until you determine how the medication affects you. Fenofibrate can increase your sensitivity to the sun and you may burn more easily. Use sunscreen and protective clothing during long periods outdoors. Tanning booths should be used with caution. If you are going to have surgery, tell your prescriber or health care professional that you are taking fenofibrate.

What side effects may I notice from taking fenofibrate?

Side effects that you should report to your prescriber or health care professional as soon as possible:

- abdominal pain
- cough or hoarseness
- dark yellow or brown urine
- fever or chills
- lower back or side pain
- muscle pain, tenderness, or weakness
- nausea and vomiting
- pain or difficulty passing urine
- skin rash or skin-bruising
- sore throat that does not go away
- unusual tiredness
- yellowing of the eyes or skin

Side effects that usually do not require medical attention (report to your prescriber or health care professional if they continue or are bothersome):

- blurred vision
- constipation or mild diarrhea
- dizziness
- drowsiness
- headache
- increased sensitivity to the sun or ultraviolet light
- sexual dysfunction (loss of sexual desire—rare)
- stomach gas, heartburn or upset

Where can I keep my medicine?

Keep out of the reach of children in a container that small children cannot open. Store at room temperature below 30 degrees C (86 degrees F). Keep container tightly closed. Throw away any unused medicine after the expiration date.

Fenoprofen tablets

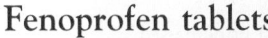

FENOPROFEN;
600 mg; Tablet
Ivax Pharmaceuticals
Inc

FENOPROFEN;
600 mg; Tablet
Mylan
Pharmaceuticals Inc

F

This drug requires an FDA medication guide. See page xxxvii.

What are fenoprofen tablets?

FENOPROFEN (Nalfon®) is a nonsteroidal anti-inflammatory drug (NSAID). It reduces inflammation and eases mild to moderate pain. Fenoprofen is used to treat the symptoms of rheumatoid arthritis, osteoarthritis, and to relieve mild to moderate pain including menstrual pain. Generic fenoprofen tablets are available.

What should my health care professional know before I take fenoprofen?

They need to know if you have any of these conditions:
- asthma, especially aspirin sensitive asthma
- bleeding problems or taking medicines that make you bleed more easily such as anticoagulants ("blood thinners")
- cigarette smoker
- dental disease
- diabetes
- drink more than 3 alcohol-containing beverages a day
- heart or circulation problems such as heart failure or leg edema (fluid retention)

- high blood pressure
- kidney disease
- liver disease
- stomach or duodenal ulcers
- systemic lupus erythematosus
- ulcerative colitis
- an unusual or allergic reaction to aspirin, other salicylates, other NSAIDs, foods, dyes or preservatives
- pregnant or trying to get pregnant
- breast-feeding

How should I take this medicine?

Take fenoprofen tablets by mouth. Follow the directions on the prescription label. Swallow tablets whole with a full glass of water; take tablets in an upright or sitting position. Taking a sip of water first, before taking the tablets, may help you swallow them. If possible take bedtime doses at least 10 minutes before lying down. It is better to take fenoprofen with food. Take your doses at regular intervals. Do not take your medicine more often than directed. Contact your pediatrician or health care professional regarding the use of this medicine in children. Special care may be needed.

What if I miss a dose?

If you miss a dose, take it as soon as you can. If it is almost time for your next dose, take only that dose. Do not take double or extra doses.

What may interact with fenoprofen?

- alcohol
- alendronate
- aspirin and aspirin-like medicines
- cidofovir
- cyclosporine
- drospirenone; ethinyl estradiol (Yasmin®)
- entecavir
- herbal products that contain feverfew, garlic, ginger, or ginkgo biloba
- lithium
- medicines for high blood pressure
- medicines that affect platelets
- medicines that treat or prevent blood clots such as warfarin and other "blood thinners"
- methotrexate
- other anti-inflammatory drugs (such as ibuprofen or prednisone)
- pemetrexed
- water pills (diuretics)

Tell your prescriber or health care professional about all other medicines you are taking, including non-prescription medicines, nutritional supplements, or herbal products. Also tell your prescriber or health care professional if you are a frequent user of drinks with caffeine or alcohol, if you smoke, or if you use illegal drugs. These may affect the way your medicine works. Check with your health care professional before stopping or starting any of your medicines.

What should I watch for while taking fenoprofen?

Let your prescriber or health care professional know if your pain continues, do not take with other pain-killers without advice. If you get flu-like symptoms (fever, chills, muscle aches and pains), call your prescriber or health care professional; do not treat yourself. To reduce unpleasant effects on your throat and stomach, take fenoprofen with a full glass of water and never just before lying down. If you notice black, tarry stools or experience severe stomach pain and vomit blood or what looks like coffee grounds, notify your health care prescriber immediately. If you are taking medicines that affect the clotting of your blood, such as aspirin or blood thinners such as Coumadin®, talk to your health care provider or prescriber before taking this medicine. You may get dizzy. Do not drive, use machinery, or do anything that needs mental alertness until you know how fenoprofen affects you. Do not sit or stand up quickly, especially if you are an older patient. This reduces the risk of dizzy or fainting spells. Do not smoke cigarettes or drink alcohol; these increase irritation to your stomach and can make it more susceptible to damage from fenoprofen. If you are going to have surgery, tell your prescriber or health care professional that you are taking fenoprofen. Fenoprofen can cause you to bleed more easily. Problems can arise if you need dental work, and in the day to day care of your teeth. Try to avoid damage to your teeth and gums when you brush or floss your teeth. It is especially important not to use fenoprofen during the last 3 months of pregnancy unless specifically directed to do so by your health care provider. Fenoprofen may cause problems in the unborn child or complications during delivery.

What side effects may I notice from taking fenoprofen?

Elderly patients are at increased risk for developing side effects.

Side effects that you should report to your prescriber or health care professional as soon as possible:

- signs of bleeding from the stomach—black tarry stools, blood in the urine, unusual tiredness or weakness, vomiting blood or vomit that looks like coffee grounds
- signs of an allergic reaction—difficulty breathing or wheezing, skin rash, redness, blistering or peeling skin, hives, or itching, swelling of eyelids, throat, lips
- blurred vision
- change in the amount of urine passed
- difficulty swallowing, severe heartburn or burning, pain in throat
- pain or difficulty passing urine
- stomach pain or cramps
- swelling of feet or ankles

Side effects that usually do not require medical attention (report to your prescriber or health care professional if they continue or are bothersome):

- constipation or diarrhea
- dizziness, drowsiness
- gas or heartburn
- headache
- nausea, vomiting

Where can I keep my medicine?

Keep out of the reach of children in a container that small children cannot open. Store at room temperature between 15 and 30 degrees C (59 and 86 degrees F). Keep container tightly closed. Throw away any unused medicine after the expiration date.

F

Fentanyl skin patches

DURAGESIC®;
50 mcg/hr; Film,
Extended Release
Janssen
Pharmaceutica Inc

DURAGESIC®;
75 mcg/hr; Film,
Extended Release
Janssen
Pharmaceutica Inc

What are fentanyl skin patches?

FENTANYL (Duragesic®, E-TRANS® Fentanyl) relieves moderate to severe chronic pain. Fentanyl patches are commonly used to treat pain associated with cancer. Do not use this medicine for pain that will go away in a few days such as pain from surgery, doctor or dentist visits or any other short-lasting pain. Once the patch is applied, the medicine is slowly absorbed through your skin into the bloodstream to help control your pain. Federal law prohibits the transfer of fentanyl to any person other than the patient for whom it was prescribed. Do not share this medicine with anyone else, it is only for you. Generic fentanyl skin patches are available.

What should my health care professional know before I use fentanyl?

They need to know if you have any of these conditions:
- diarrhea
- heart disease
- intestinal disease
- kidney disease
- liver disease
- lung disease or breathing difficulties
- seizures (convulsions)
- skin problems
- an allergic or unusual reaction to fentanyl, meperidine, other medicines, adhesives, sulfites, foods, dyes, or preservatives
- pregnant or trying to get pregnant
- breast-feeding

How should I use this medicine?

Fentanyl skin patches are for external use only. Follow the directions on the prescription label. Do not cut or damage the patch. Wash hands well before using. Select a clean, dry area of skin above your waist on your front or back. Do not apply the patch to oily, broken, burned, cut, or irritated skin. Use only water to clean the area. Do not use soap or alcohol because this can increase the effects of the medication. If the area is hairy, clip the hair with scissors, but do not shave it. Dry the area well before applying the patch. Take the patch out of its wrapper, and take off the protective strip over the adhesive. Do not touch the adhesive with your fingers. Press the adhesive surface to the skin using the palm of your hand and hold it for 30 seconds. Be sure the edges stick to the skin. Wash your hands at once. Apply each new patch to a different area of skin to avoid irritation. If a patch comes off or causes irritation, remove it and apply a new patch to different site. Do not take the patch out of its pouch before using, and do not use a patch if the packaging or backing has been damaged. To get rid of used patches, fold the patch in half with the sticky sides together. Then, flush it down the toilet. Replace the patch every 3 days (72 hours) or as directed by your prescriber or health care professional. Contact your pediatrician or health care professional regarding the use of this medicine in children. Fentanyl patches should not be used on children less than 12 years of age or in patients less than 18 years of age who weigh less than 110 pounds.

What if I miss a dose?

Change your patch as directed. Do not wear more than one patch at the same time unless directed to do so by your prescriber or health care professional.

What may interact with fentanyl?

- amiodarone
- antidepressant drugs called MAOIs
- anti-retroviral protease inhibitors, especially ritonavir
- bosentan
- butorphanol
- delavirdine
- efavirenz
- erythromycin
- fluconazole
- fluvoxamine
- fluoxetine
- imatinib, STI-571
- itraconazole
- herbal products containing St. John's wort
- ketoconazole
- medicines for diarrhea
- medicines for high blood pressure
- medicines for seizures
- mifepristone, RU-486
- nalbuphine
- nefazodone
- nevirapine
- other strong medicines for pain
- pentazocine
- rifabutin
- rifampin

Because fentanyl may cause drowsiness, other medications that also cause drowsiness may increase this effect of fentanyl. Some medicines that cause drowsiness are:
- alcohol and alcohol-containing medicines
- barbiturates, such as phenobarbital
- certain antidepressants or tranquilizers
- muscle relaxants
- certain antihistamines used in cold medicines

Ask your prescriber or health care professional about other medicines that may increase the effect of fentanyl.

Tell your prescriber or health care professional about all other medicines you that are taking, including nonprescription medicines, nutritional supplements, or herbal products. Also, tell your prescriber or health

F

care professional if you are a frequent user of drinks with caffeine or alcohol, if you smoke, or if you use illegal drugs. These may affect the way your medicine works. Check with your health care professional before stopping or starting any of your medicines.

What should I watch for while taking fentanyl?

Other pain relievers may be needed the first or two day you use the fentanyl patch, because it can take some time to start working. You should have medicine to take if you have occasional periods of "break-through" pain while using the fentanyl patch. Tell your prescriber or health care professional if fentanyl is not easing your pain. Visit your prescriber or health care professional for regular checks on your progress. Use exactly as directed by your prescriber or health care professional. If you are taking fentanyl on a regular basis, do not suddenly stop taking it. Your body becomes used to the fentanyl and when you suddenly stop taking it, you may develop a severe reaction. This DOES NOT mean you are "addicted" to fentanyl. Addiction is a behavior related to getting and using a drug for a non-medical reason. If you have pain, you have a medical reason to take pain medicine such as fentanyl to control your pain. Avoid exposing the application site to heat sources, such as heating pads, electric blankets, heat lamps, saunas, etc. Heat can increase the amount of fentanyl released from the patch. You can bathe or swim while using the skin patch. However, do not expose your fentanyl patch site to any source of direct heat, such as saunas, heated water beds, electric blankets, or hot tubs. You may get drowsy or dizzy when you first start taking fentanyl or change doses. Do not drive, use machinery, or do anything that needs mental alertness until you know how fentanyl affects you. Stand or sit up slowly, this reduces the risk of dizzy or fainting spells. These effects may be worse if you are an older patient. The drowsiness should decrease after taking fentanyl for a couple of days. If you have not slept because of your pain, you may sleep more the first few days your pain is controlled to catch-up on missed sleep. Be careful taking other medicines which may also make you tired. This effect may be worse when taking these medicines with fentanyl. Alcohol can increase possible drowsiness, dizziness, and confusion and may affect your breathing. Avoid alcohol while taking fentanyl. Fentanyl will cause constipation. Make sure to take a laxative and/or a stool softener while taking fentanyl. Try to have a bowel movement every 2 to 3 days, at least. If you do not have a bowel movement for 3 days or more call your prescriber or health care professional. They may recommend using an enema or suppository to help you move your bowels. Your mouth may get dry. Drinking plenty of water, chewing sugarless gum or sucking on hard candy may help to relieve dry mouth symptoms. Have regular dental checks. If you are going to have surgery, tell your prescriber or health care professional that you are taking fentanyl. Rarely, fentanyl may cause you to have hallucinations

(to see things that are not really there) or cause your legs or arms to "jerk" or have spasms. If you experience these effects, call your prescriber or health care professional. If you have a preexisting skin problem, you may get additional irritation when using the skin patches including redness, bumps, swelling, or itching at the site of application. If gel leaks from the fentanyl skin patch, wash your skin well with water only; do not use soap or cleansers containing alcohol. Throw the patch away.

What side effects may I notice from using fentanyl?

Side effects are more likely to occur if fentanyl skin patches are used over a prolonged period of time.
Side effects that you should report to your prescriber or health care professional as soon as possible:
Rare or uncommon:
- breathing difficulties, wheezing
- cold, clammy skin
- seizures
- slow or fast heartbeat
- severe rash
- unusual weakness

More common:
- confusion
- lightheadedness or fainting spells
- nervousness or restlessness

Side effects that usually do not require medical attention (report to your prescriber or health care professional if they continue or are bothersome):
- itching
- blurred vision
- clumsiness, unsteadiness
- constipation
- decrease or difficulty passing urine
- dizziness, drowsiness
- dry mouth
- flushing
- headache
- nausea/vomiting
- pinpoint pupils
- sweating

Where can I keep my medicine?

Keep out of the reach of children. Do not share or give this medicine to anyone else, it is for your use only. Fentanyl patches can cause injury or death in adults and children who are not already taking fentanyl to relieve chronic pain. Even after the patch has been removed, it still contains enough fentanyl to cause serious side effects and even death to children or pets. If someone accidentally uses a fentanyl patch and is not awake and alert, call 911 or for emergency help right away. If the person is awake and alert, call your prescriber or health care professional or the Poison Control Center. Store below 77 degrees F (25 degrees C). Do not use if the seal is broken. Once the patch is removed from the protective package, use it immediately. To dispose of used patches, fold the patch in half so it will stick together then flush it down the toilet.

Fexofenadine capsules or tablets

ALLEGRA®;
180 mg; Tablet
Aventis
Pharmaceuticals Inc

ALLEGRA®;
60 mg; Capsule
Aventis
Pharmaceuticals Inc

What are fexofenadine capsules or tablets?

FEXOFENADINE (Allegra®) is an antihistamine. It reduces allergy symptoms of hay fever (seasonal allergic rhinitis), and may reduced itching of the skin in those people with chronic itchy skin rashes. Generic fexofenadine capsules and tablets are available.

What should my health care professional know before I take fexofenadine?

They need to know if you have any of these conditions:
- kidney disease
- heart disease
- other chronic illness
- an unusual or allergic reaction to fexofenadine, terfenadine, other medicines, foods, dyes, or preservatives
- pregnant or trying to get pregnant
- breast-feeding

How should I take this medicine?

Take fexofenadine capsules by mouth, with a sip of water. you may take this medicine with food. Follow the directions on the prescription label. Take your doses at regular intervals. Do not take fexofenadine more often than directed. You may need to take it for several days as prescribed before your symptoms improve. Contact your pediatrician or health care professional regarding the use of this medicine in children. Special care may be needed. Fexofenadine is usually prescribed for children 6 years of age and older.

What if I miss a dose?

If you miss a dose, take it as soon as you can. If it is almost time for your next dose, take only that dose. Do not take double or extra doses.

What may interact with fexofenadine?

- antacids
- erythromycin
- grapefruit, apple, or orange juice
- ketoconazole
- rifampin
- St. John's wort

In addition, the following medicines can make you feel drowsy:

- alcohol
- barbiturate medicines for inducing sleep or treating seizures (convulsions)
- medicines for anxiety or sleeping problems, such as alprazolam, diazepam or temazepam
- medicines for hay fever and other allergies such as antihistamines
- medicines for mental depression (antidepressants)
- medicines for mental problems, anxieties and psychotic disturbances
- medicines for pain such as opiate analgesics (e.g. codeine)

Tell your prescriber or health care professional about all other medicines you are taking, including non-prescription medicines, nutritional supplements, or herbal products. Also tell your prescriber or health care professional if you are a frequent user of drinks with caffeine or alcohol, if you smoke, or if you use illegal drugs. These may affect the way your medicine works. Check with your health care professional before stopping or starting any of your medicines.

What should I watch for while taking fexofenadine?

Tell your prescriber or health care professional if your symptoms do not improve in 1 or 2 days. Fexofenadine causes less drowsiness than most other antihistamines. Until you know if it makes you drowsy or dizzy, do not drive, use machinery, or do anything that needs mental alertness. Do not sit or stand up quickly, especially if you are an older patient. This reduces the risk of dizzy or fainting spells.

What side effects may I notice from taking fexofenadine?

Side effects of fexofenadine include:
- menstrual changes
- stomach upset, nausea, vomiting
- tiredness or drowsiness

Where can I keep my medicine?

Keep out of the reach of children in a container that small children cannot open. Store at room temperature between 20 and 25 degrees C (68 and 77 degrees F). Protect from moisture. Throw away any unused medicine after the expiration date.

Fexofenadine; Pseudoephedrine tablets

ALLEGRA-D® 12-HOUR;
60 mg/120 mg; Tablet,
Extended Release
Aventis Pharmaceuticals Inc

What are fexofenadine; pseudoephedrine tablets?

FEXOFENADINE; PSEUDOEPHEDRINE (Allegra-D®, Allegra-D® 12-Hour, Allegra-D® 24-Hour) is an antihistamine and decongestant. It relieves the symptoms of hay fever (seasonal rhinitis) including nasal and sinus congestion. A generic tablet is not yet available.

What should my health care professional know before I take fexofenadine; pseudoephedrine?

They need to know if you have any of these conditions:
- blood vessel disease
- difficulty urinating (urinary retention)
- heart disease
- diabetes
- glaucoma
- high blood pressure
- kidney disease
- prostate trouble
- thyroid problems (overactive thyroid)
- an unusual or allergic reaction to fexofenadine, terfenadine, pseudoephedrine, other medicines, foods, dyes, or preservatives
- pregnant or trying to get pregnant
- breast-feeding

How should I take this medicine?

Take fexofenadine; pseudoephedrine tablets by mouth. Follow the directions on the prescription label. Swallow the tablet whole with water. Take the tablet on an empty stomach, one hour before a meal. Do not break, crush, or chew the tablets. Take your doses at regular intervals. Do not take your medicine more often than directed. Contact your pediatrician or health care professional regarding the use of this medicine in children. Special care may be needed. Older patients (> 60 years old) may have a stronger reaction to this medicine.

What if I miss a dose?

If you miss a dose, take it as soon as you can. If it is almost time for your next dose, take only that dose. Do not take double doses.

What may interact with fexofenadine; pseudoephedrine?

- alcohol or cocaine
- antacids
- caffeine
- barbiturate medicines for inducing sleep or treating seizures (convulsions)
- erythromycin
- furazolidone
- grapefruit, apple, or orange juice
- ketoconazole
- linezolid

- medicines known as MAO inhibitors, such as phenelzine (Nardil®), tranylcypromine (Parnate®), isocarboxazid (Marplan®), and selegiline (Carbex®, Eldepryl®)
- mecamylamine
- medicines for anxiety or sleeping problems, such as alprazolam, diazepam, or temazepam
- medicines for colds and breathing difficulties
- medicines for hay fever and other allergies such as antihistamines
- medicines for heart disease such as digoxin or beta-blockers
- medicines for mental depression (antidepressants)
- medicines for mental problems, anxieties and psychotic disturbances
- medicines for migraine headaches such as ergot alkaloids
- medicines for nasal congestion such as pseudoephedrine
- medicines for pain such as opiate analgesics (e.g. codeine)
- methyldopa
- procarbazine
- reserpine
- rifampin
- sodium bicarbonate, sodium acetate, sodium citrate, or sodium lactate
- St. John's wort

Tell your prescriber or health care professional about all other medicines you are taking, including non-prescription medicines, nutritional supplements, or herbal products. Also tell your prescriber or health care professional if you are a frequent user of drinks with caffeine or alcohol, if you smoke, or if you use illegal drugs. These may affect the way your medicine works. Check with your health care professional before stopping or starting any of your medicines.

What should I watch for while taking fexofenadine; pseudoephedrine?

Tell your prescriber or health care professional if your symptoms do not improve in 1 to 2 days or if you have a high fever. You may get drowsy or dizzy. Do not drive, use machinery, or do anything that needs mental alertness until you know how this drug affects you. To reduce the risk of dizzy or fainting spells, do not stand or sit up quickly, especially if you are an older patient. Alcohol may increase dizziness and drowsiness. Avoid alcoholic drinks. Your mouth may get dry. Chewing sugarless gum or sucking hard candy, and drinking plenty of water will help. This medicine may make it difficult for some people to sleep at night. If nervousness, dizziness, or sleeplessness occur, consult a health care professional to discuss your medications. If you are going to have surgery, tell your prescriber you are taking fexofenadine; pseudoephedrine.

What side effects may I notice from taking fexofenadine; pseudoephedrine?

Side effects that you should report to your prescriber or health care professional as soon as possible:
- abdominal pain or rectal bleeding
- chest pain
- confusion
- convulsions (seizures)
- difficulty breathing or wheezing
- difficulty urinating
- dizziness or fainting spells
- fast or irregular heartbeat, palpitations
- high blood pressure
- numbness or tingling in the hands or feet
- rash
- severe, persistent, or worsening headache
- tremor or muscle contractions
- visual changes
- vomiting

Side effects that usually do not require medical attention (report to your prescriber or health care professional if they continue or are bothersome):
- dry mouth
- headache (mild)
- loss of appetite or nausea
- nervousness or difficulty sleeping
- throat irritation
- tiredness or drowsiness

Where can I keep my medicine?

Keep out of the reach of children in a container that small children cannot open. Store at room temperature or between 20 and 25 degrees C (68 and 77 degrees F). Protect from moisture. Throw away any unused medicine after the expiration date.

Finasteride tablets

PROPECIA®;
1 mg; Tablet
Merck and Co Inc

PROSCAR®;
5 mg; Tablet
Merck and Co Inc

What are finasteride tablets?

FINASTERIDE (Propecia®, Proscar®) can reduce the size of the prostate gland in men with benign prostatic hyperplasia (BPH). The prostate is a part of the male reproductive system that produces a milky fluid for sperm. Over the age of 50 most men develop an enlarged prostate. As the prostate gets bigger it can restrict the flow of urine. Finasteride can help to reduce symptoms caused by BPH such as a weak or interrupted urine flow; a feeling that the bladder is not completely empty; a need to pass urine more often, especially at night; an urgent feeling that you must pass urine right away; or a delay or hesitation when you start to urinate. Finasteride is also used for the treatment of certain types of male hair loss. Finasteride is not for use in women. Generic finasteride tablets are available.

What should my health care professional know before I take finasteride?

They need to know if you have any of these conditions:
- if you are female (finasteride is not for use in women)
- kidney disease or infection
- liver disease
- prostate cancer
- an unusual or allergic reaction to finasteride, other medicines, foods, dyes, or preservatives

How should I take this medicine?

Take finasteride tablets by mouth. Follow the directions on the prescription label. Swallow the tablets with a drink of water. You can take this medicine with or without food. Take your doses at regular intervals. Do not take your medicine more often than directed. Contact your pediatrician or health care professional regarding the use of this medicine in children. Special care may be needed.

What if I miss a dose?

If you miss a dose, take it as soon as you can. If you do not remember until the next day, take only that day's dose. Do not take double or extra doses.

What may interact with finasteride?

- some blood pressure medications
- male hormones (example: testosterone)
- saw palmetto
- soy isoflavone supplements

Tell your prescriber or health care professional about all other medicines you are taking, including non-prescription medicines. Also tell your prescriber or health care professional if you are a frequent user of drinks with caffeine or alcohol, if you smoke, or if you use illegal drugs. These may affect the way your medicine works. Check with your health care professional before stopping or starting any of your medicines.

What should I watch for while taking finasteride?

Do not donate blood until at least 6 months after your final dose of finasteride. This will prevent giving finasteride to a pregnant female through a blood transfusion. Contact your prescriber or health care professional if there is no improvement in your symptoms. You may need to take finasteride for 6 to 12 months to get the best results. Women who are pregnant or may get pregnant must not handle broken or crushed finasteride tablets; the active ingredient could harm the unborn baby. If a pregnant woman comes into contact with broken or crushed finasteride tablets she should check

F

with her prescriber or health care professional. Exposure to whole tablets is not expected to cause harm as long as they are not swallowed. Finasteride can interfere with PSA laboratory tests for prostate cancer. If you are scheduled to have a lab test for prostate cancer, tell your prescriber or health care professional that you are taking finasteride.

What side effects may I notice from taking finasteride?

Side effects that usually do not require medical attention (report to your prescriber or health care professional if they continue or are bothersome):

- breast enlargement or tenderness
- skin rash
- sexual difficulties (less sexual desire or ability to get an erection)
- small amount of semen released during sex

Where can I keep my medicine?

Keep out of the reach of children in a container that small children cannot open. Store at room temperature between 15 and 30 degrees C (59 and 86 degrees F). Protect from light. Keep container tightly closed. Throw away any unused medicine after the expiration date.

Flecainide tablets

TAMBOCOR™;
150 mg; Tablet
3M Pharmaceuticals
Inc

TAMBOCOR™;
100 mg; Tablet
3M Pharmaceuticals
Inc

What are flecainide tablets?

FLECAINIDE (Tambocor®) is an antiarrhythmic agent. Flecainide treats irregular heart rhythm and can slow rapid heartbeats (tachycardia). Flecainide can help your heart to return to and maintain a normal rhythm. Generic flecainide tablets are available.

What should my health care professional know before I take flecainide?

They need to know if you have any of these conditions:
- abnormal levels of potassium in the blood
- heart disease including heart rhythm and heart rate problems
- kidney disease
- liver disease
- previous heart attack
- an unusual or allergic reaction to flecainide, local anesthetics, other medicines, foods, dyes, or preservatives
- pregnant or trying to get pregnant
- breast-feeding

How should I take this medicine?

Take flecainide tablets by mouth. Follow the directions on the prescription label. Swallow the tablets with a drink of water. Take your doses at regular intervals. Do not take your medicine more often than directed. Contact your pediatrician or health care professional regarding the use of this medicine in children. Special care may be needed.

What if I miss a dose?

If you miss a dose, take it as soon as you can. If it is almost time for your next dose, take only that dose. Do not take the missed dose if it is more than 4 hours after the dose was due. Do not take double or extra doses.

What may interact with flecainide?

- acetazolamide
- ammonium chloride
- arsenic trioxide
- astemizole
- bepridil
- beta-blockers, often used for high blood pressure or heart problems
- certain antibiotics (such as clarithromycin, erythromycin, gatifloxacin, gemifloxacin, grepafloxacin, levofloxacin, moxifloxacin, sparfloxacin)
- cimetidine
- citrate salts (examples: Bicitra®, Oracit®, Cytra-2, Polycitra®, Urocit®-K)
- cisapride
- ginger
- hawthorn
- medicines for angina or high blood pressure
- medicines for malaria
- medicines for asthma or breathing difficulties (such as formoterol or salmeterol)
- methazolamide
- some medicines for treating depression or mental illness (amoxapine, maprotiline, pimozide, phenothiazines, tricyclic antidepressants)
- medicines to control heart rhythm (examples: amiodarone, digoxin, disopyramide, dofetilide, procainamide, quinidine, sotalol)
- pimozide
- probucol
- quinine
- terfenadine
- sodium bicarbonate

Tell your prescriber or health care professional about all other medicines you are taking, including non-prescription medicines, nutritional supplements, or herbal products. Also tell your prescriber or health care professional if you are a frequent user of drinks with caffeine or alcohol, if you smoke, or if you use illegal drugs. These may affect the way your medicine works. Check with your health care professional before stopping or starting any of your medicines.

F

What should I watch for while taking flecainide?

Visit your prescriber or health care professional for regular checks on your progress. Do not stop taking flecainide suddenly; this may cause serious, heart-related side effects. Because your condition and the use of flecainide carry some risk, it is a good idea to carry an identification card, necklace or bracelet with details of your condition, medications and prescriber or health care professional. Check your heart rate (pulse) and blood pressure regularly while you are taking flecainide. Ask your prescriber or health care professional what your heart rate and blood pressure should be, and when you should contact him or her. Your prescriber or health care professional also may schedule regular blood tests and electrocardiograms to check your progress. You may feel dizzy or faint. Do not drive, use machinery, or do anything that needs mental alertness until you know how flecainide affects you. To reduce the risk of dizzy or fainting spells, do not sit or stand up quickly, especially if you are an older patient. Alcohol can make you more dizzy, increase flushing and rapid heartbeats. Avoid alcoholic drinks. If you are going to have surgery, tell your prescriber or health care professional that you are taking flecainide.

What side effects may I notice from taking flecainide?

Side effects that you should report to your prescriber or health care professional as soon as possible:
- chest pain, continued irregular heartbeats
- difficulty breathing
- swelling of the legs or feet
- trembling, shaking
- unusual weakness or tiredness

Side effects that usually do not require medical attention (report to your prescriber or health care professional if they continue or are bothersome):
- blurred vision
- constipation
- dizziness
- headache
- nausea, vomiting
- stomach pain

Where can I keep my medicine?

Keep out of the reach of children in a container that small children cannot open. Store at room temperature between 15 and 30 degrees C (59 and 86 degrees F). Protect from light. Keep container tightly closed. Throw away any unused medicine after the expiration date.

Fluconazole oral suspension or tablets

DIFLUCAN®;
150 mg; Tablet
Roerig Division of
Pfizer

DIFLUCAN®;
100 mg; Tablet
Roerig Division of
Pfizer

What are fluconazole oral suspension or tablets?

FLUCONAZOLE (Diflucan®) is an antifungal type of antibiotic. It treats serious fungal infections found throughout the body. These include oral candidiasis or thrush infections of the mouth or throat, vaginal yeast infections, candidal infection of the urinary tract, meningitis, and others. Generic fluconazole oral suspensions and tablets are available.

What should my health care professional know before I take fluconazole?

They need to know if you have any of these conditions:
- diabetes
- heart disease
- kidney disease
- liver disease
- other chronic illness
- an unusual or allergic reaction to fluconazole, other azole medicines (used to treat fungal or yeast infections), or other medicines, foods, dyes or preservatives
- pregnant or trying to get pregnant
- breast-feeding

How should I take this medicine?

Take fluconazole oral suspension or tablets by mouth. Follow the directions on the prescription label. If tak-ing the oral suspension, shake it well before using. Use a specially marked spoon or container to measure the oral suspension. Ask your pharmacist if you do not have one; household spoons are not always accurate. You can take the oral suspension or tablets with or without food. Take your doses at regular intervals. Do not take your medicine more often than directed. Finish the full course prescribed by your health care professional even if you feel better. Do not stop taking except on your prescriber's advice.

What if I miss a dose?

If you miss a dose, take it as soon as you can. If it is almost time for your next dose, take only that dose. Do not take double or extra doses.

What may interact with fluconazole?

- bosentan
- cilostazol
- cisapride
- cyclosporine
- dofetilide
- certain medicines for anxiety or difficulty sleeping
- medicines for diabetes that are taken by mouth
- medicines for high cholesterol such as atorvastatin, fluvastatin, lovastatin, or simvastatin
- medicines for yeast or fungal infections
- phenytoin

- pimozide
- rifabutin
- rifampin
- tacrolimus
- terfenadine
- warfarin
- water pills

Tell your prescriber or health care professional about all other medicines you are taking, including non-prescription medicines, nutritional supplements, or herbal products. Also tell your prescriber or health care professional if you are a frequent user of drinks with caffeine or alcohol, if you smoke, or if you use illegal drugs. These may affect the way your medicine works. Check with your health care professional before stopping or starting any of your medicines.

What should I watch for while taking fluconazole?

Tell your prescriber or health care professional if your symptoms do not improve in a few weeks. Some fungal infections need many weeks or months of treatment to cure. Keep taking your medicine regularly for as long as your prescriber or health care professional tells you to. If you are taking this medicine for a long time you must visit your prescriber or health care professional for regular blood and liver function tests. Alcohol can increase possible damage to your liver. Do not take alcoholic drinks while you take this medicine. If you have a vaginal infection, do not have sex until you have finished your treatment. Your clothing may get soiled if you have a vaginal discharge. You can wear a sanitary napkin; do not use tampons. Wear freshly washed cotton, not synthetic, panties. Fluconazole has been associated with birth defects when given at high doses early in a pregnancy. If you are pregnant or think you may be pregnant, tell you prescriber or health care professional immediately. Women who may become pregnant should use effective birth control while taking fluconazole.

What side effects may I notice from taking fluconazole?

Stop taking this medication immediately and report these side effects to your prescriber or health care professional right away:
- fainting or falling spells
- irregular heartbeat, palpitations, or chest pain

Side effects that you should report to your prescriber or health care professional as soon as possible:
- dark yellow or brown urine
- dizziness
- light-colored stools (bowel movements)
- redness, blistering, peeling or loosening of the skin, including inside the mouth
- skin rash, itching
- stomach pain
- unusual bruising or bleeding
- yellowing of the eyes or skin
- vomiting

Side effects that usually do not require medical attention (report to your prescriber or health care professional if they continue or are bothersome):
- diarrhea
- headache
- loss of appetite or changes in how food tastes
- nausea

Where can I keep my medicine?

Keep out of the reach of children in a container that small children cannot open. Store at room temperature below 30 degrees C (86 degrees F). Keep container tightly closed. Throw away any unused medicine after the expiration date.

Flucytosine capsules

ANCOBON®;
500 mg; Capsule
Valeant
Pharmaceuticals

What are flucytosine capsules?

FLUCYTOSINE (Ancobon®) is an antifungal type of antibiotic. It treats serious fungal infections found throughout the body. These include infections of the heart, blood, urinary tract, or lungs, and meningitis. Generic flucytosine capsules are not yet available.

What should my health care professional know before I take flucytosine?

They need to know if you have any of these conditions:
- anemia, blood disorders
- dental problems
- kidney disease
- liver disease
- other chronic illness
- an unusual or allergic reaction to flucytosine, other foods, dyes or preservatives
- pregnant or trying to get pregnant
- breast-feeding

How should I take this medicine?

Take flucytosine capsules by mouth. Follow the directions on the prescription label. Take the capsules at regular 6 hour intervals through the day and night. Do not take your medicine more often than directed. Finish the full course of capsules prescribed by your prescriber or health care professional even if you feel better. Do not stop taking except on your prescriber's advice. Contact your pediatrician or health care professional regarding the use of this medicine in children. Special care may be needed.

What if I miss a dose?

If you miss a dose, take it as soon as you can. If it is almost time for your next dose, take only that dose. Do not take double or extra doses.

What may interact with flucytosine?

- amphotericin B
- carbamazepine
- clozapine
- medicines for cancer chemotherapy
- medicines for mental problems and psychotic disturbances
- norfloxacin
- zidovudine (AZT)

Tell your prescriber or health care professional about all other medicines you are taking, including non-prescription medicines, nutritional supplements, or herbal products. Also tell your prescriber or health care professional if you are a frequent user of drinks with caffeine or alcohol, if you smoke, or if you use illegal drugs. These may affect the way your medicine works. Check with your health care professional before stopping or starting any of your medicines.

What should I watch for while taking flucytosine?

Tell your prescriber or health care professional if your symptoms do not improve in a few weeks. Some fungal infections need many weeks or months of treatment to cure. Use your medicine regularly for as long as your prescriber or health care professional tells you to. Flucytosine capsules may make you feel sick. If you are taking 2 or more capsules for each dose, take them 15 minutes apart with a drink of water. This will help to reduce stomach upset. Flucytosine can cause blood problems.

This can mean slow healing and a risk of infection. Problems can arise if you need dental work, or in the day to day care of your teeth. Try to avoid damage to your teeth and gums when you brush or floss your teeth. You may get dizzy; until you know how it affects you do not drive, use machinery, or do anything that needs mental alertness. Keep out of the sun, or wear protective clothing outdoors and use a sunscreen. Do not use sun lamps or sun tanning beds or booths.

What side effects may I notice from taking flucytosine?

Side effects that you should report to your prescriber or health care professional as soon as possible:
- dark yellow or brown urine
- increased sensitivity to the sun or ultraviolet light
- skin rash, redness, blistering, or peeling of skin
- stomach pain
- unusual weakness or tiredness
- unusual bleeding or bruising
- yellowing of the eyes or skin

Side effects that usually do not require medical attention (report to your prescriber or health care professional if they continue or are bothersome):
- diarrhea
- dizziness
- headache
- loss of appetite
- nausea, vomiting

Where can I keep my medicine?

Keep out of the reach of children in a container that small children cannot open. Store at room temperature between 15 and 30 degrees C (59 and 86 degrees F). Protect from light. Keep container tightly closed. Throw away any unused medicine after the expiration date.

Fludrocortisone tablets

FLUDROCORTISONE;
0.1 mg; Tablet
Global
Pharmaceuticals Div
of Impax Labs., Inc.

FLUDROCORTISONE;
0.1 mg; Tablet
Barr Laboratories
Inc

What are fludrocortisone tablets?

FLUDROCORTISONE (Florinef®) causes the body to retain salt and water. Fludrocortisone replaces the natural steroids that are lacking in patients with underactive adrenal glands. Fludrocortisone also treats a salt-losing condition called adrenogenital syndrome. Generic fludrocortisone tablets are available.

What should my health care professional know before I take fludrocortisone?

They need to know if you have any of these conditions:
- Cushing's syndrome
- diabetes mellitus
- heart problems, or previous heart attack
- high blood pressure or blood clotting disorder
- infection, such as herpes, measles, tuberculosis or chickenpox
- myasthenia gravis
- psychosis
- osteoporosis
- recent surgery
- seizures (convulsions)
- stomach or intestinal disease, including colitis
- kidney disease
- over- or underactive thyroid
- an unusual or allergic reaction to fludrocortisone, other corticosteroids, medicines, foods, dyes, or preservatives
- pregnant or trying to get pregnant
- breast-feeding

How should I take this medicine?

Take fludrocortisone tablets by mouth. Follow the directions on the prescription label. Swallow the tablets with a drink of water. Take with food or milk to avoid stomach upset. If you are only taking fludrocortisone once a day, take it in the morning, unless otherwise directed, which is the time your body normally secretes cortisol. Take your doses at regular intervals. Do not take your medicine more often than directed. Contact your pediatrician or health care professional regarding the use of this medicine in children. Special care may be needed.

What if I miss a dose?

If you miss a dose, take it a soon as you can. If it is almost time for your next dose, consult your prescriber or health care professional. You may need to miss a dose or take a double dose, depending on your condition and treatment. Do not take double or extra doses without advice.

What may interact with fludrocortisone?

- anti-inflammatory drugs (NSAIDs, such as ibuprofen)
- barbiturate medicines for inducing sleep or treating seizures (convulsions)
- bosentan
- certain heart medicines
- male hormones
- phenytoin
- rifampin
- water pills

Tell your prescriber or health care professional about all other medicines you are taking, including non-prescription medicines, nutritional supplements, or herbal products. Also tell your prescriber or health care professional if you are a frequent user of drinks with caffeine or alcohol, if you smoke, or if you use illegal drugs. These may affect the way your medicine works. Check with your health care professional before stopping or starting any of your medicines.

What should I watch for while taking fludrocortisone?

Visit your prescriber or health care professional for regular checks on your progress. If you are taking fludrocortisone over a prolonged period, carry an identification card with your name and address, the type and dose of your medicine, and your prescriber's name and address. Do not suddenly stop taking fludrocortisone. Follow the advice of your prescriber or health care professional. If you are receiving fludrocortisone for a long period of time, you may have an increased risk of infection while taking fludrocortisone. Tell your prescriber or health care professional if you are exposed to anyone with measles or chickenpox, or if you develop sores or blisters that do not heal properly. If you are going to have surgery, tell your prescriber or health care professional that you have taken fludrocortisone within the last twelve months. You may need to watch your diet. Your body can lose potassium while you are taking fludrocortisone. Ask your prescriber or health care professional about your diet. Alcohol can increase the risk of getting serious side effects while you are taking fludrocortisone. Avoid alcoholic drinks. Fludrocortisone can interfere with certain lab tests and can cause false skin test results.

What side effects may I notice from taking fludrocortisone?

Side effects that you should report to your prescriber or health care professional as soon as possible:
- difficulty breathing or shortness of breath
- headache, severe or continuing
- irregular heartbeat
- loss of appetite
- mental depression, mood swings
- muscle weakness, cramps or pain
- nausea, vomiting
- skin rash or itching
- sudden weight gain
- swelling of face, nasal passages or eyelids
- swelling of the feet or legs
- unusual tiredness

Side effects that usually do not require medical attention (report to your prescriber or health care professional if they continue or are bothersome):
- dizziness
- increased appetite
- restlessness
- trouble sleeping
- upset stomach

Where can I keep my medicine?

Keep out of the reach of children in a container that small children cannot open. Store at room temperature between 15 and 30 degrees C (59 and 86 degrees F). Protect from excessive heat. Throw away any unused medicine after the expiration date.

Fluoxetine
capsules or tablets

PROZAC®;
20 mg; Capsule
Dista Products Co
Div Eli Lilly and Co

PROZAC®
WEEKLY™;
90 mg; Capsule,
Extended Release
Eli Lilly and Co

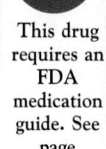

This drug requires an FDA medication guide. See page xxxvii.

What are fluoxetine capsules or tablets?

FLUOXETINE (Prozac®) belongs to a class of antidepressants known as selective serotonin reuptake inhibitors (SSRIs). It helps improve a person's mood. Fluoxetine can also help people with anxiety, obsessive compulsive disorder, eating disorders (bulimia), panic disorder, or post-traumatic stress. Generics are available for some products.

What should my health care professional know before I take fluoxetine?

They need to know if you have any of these conditions:
- diabetes
- heart disease
- kidney disease
- liver disease
- receiving electroconvulsive therapy
- seizures (convulsions)
- suicidal thoughts
- an unusual or allergic reaction to fluoxetine, other medicines, foods, dyes, or preservatives
- pregnant or trying to get pregnant
- breast-feeding

How should I take this medicine?

Take fluoxetine tablets or capsules by mouth. Follow the directions on the prescription label. Swallow with a drink of water. You can take fluoxetine with or without food. Take your doses at regular intervals. Do not take your medicine more often than directed. Do not stop taking except on your prescriber's advice. Contact your pediatrician or health care professional regarding the use of this medicine in children. Special care may be needed. While this drug may be prescribed for children as young as 7 years for selected conditions, precautions do apply. A special MedGuide will be given to you by the pharmacist with each prescription and refill. Be sure to read this information carefully each time.

What if I miss a dose?

If you miss a dose, take it as soon as you can. If it is almost time for your next dose, skip the missed dose and go back to your regular dosing schedule. Do not take double or extra doses.

What may interact with fluoxetine?

Fluoxetine has the potential to interact with a variety of medications, check with your healthcare professional. The following list contains some of these interactions.

Do not take fluoxetine with any of the following medications:

- astemizole (Hismanal®)
- cisapride (Propulsid®)
- pimozide (Orap®)
- terfenadine (Seldane®)
- thioridazine (Mellaril®)
- medicines called MAO inhibitors-phenelzine (Nardil®), tranylcypromine (Parnate®), isocarboxazid (Marplan®), selegiline (Eldepryl®)

Fluoxetine may also interact with the following medications:

- alcohol
- amphetamine
- aspirin
- benzodiazepines, commonly used for anxiety or sleeping problems, such as diazepam or alprazolam
- buspirone
- carbamazepine
- certain diet drugs (dexfenfluramine, fenfluramine, phentermine, sibutramine)
- certain medicines for migraine headache (almotriptan, eletriptan, frovatriptan, naratriptan, rizatriptan, sumatriptan, zolmitriptan, dihydroergotamine, ergotamine, methysergide)
- cimetidine
- cyproheptadine
- dextroamphetamine
- dextromethorphan
- dofetilide
- ergonovine
- furazolidone
- linezolid
- lithium
- metoprolol
- medicines for diabetes
- medicines for mental depression
- medicines for mental problems or psychotic disturbances
- methylergonovine
- nonsteroidal antiinflammatory drugs (NSAIDs, like ibuprofen)
- phenytoin
- propafenone
- propranolol
- St. John's wort
- warfarin

Tell your prescriber or health care professional about all other medicines you are taking, including non-prescription medicines, nutritional supplements, and herbal products. Also tell your prescriber or health care professional if you are a frequent user of drinks with caffeine or alcohol, if you smoke, or if you use illegal drugs. These may affect the way your medicine works.

F

Check with your health care professional before stopping or starting any of your medicines.

What should I watch for while taking fluoxetine?

Visit your prescriber or health care professional for regular checks on your progress. Continue to take your medicine even if you do not immediately feel better. It can take several weeks before you feel the full effect of fluoxetine. If you notice any unusual effects, such as restlessness, worsening of depression, agitation, difficulty sleeping, irritability, anger, acting on dangerous impulses, or thoughts of suicide or suicidal attempts, you should call your health care provider immediately. If you have been taking fluoxetine regularly for some time, do not suddenly stop taking it. You must gradually reduce the dose or your symptoms may get worse. Ask your prescriber or health care professional for advice. You may get drowsy or dizzy. Do not drive, use machinery, or do anything that needs mental alertness until you know how fluoxetine affects you. Do not stand or sit up quickly, especially if you are an older patient. This reduces the risk of dizzy or fainting spells. Alcohol can make you more drowsy and dizzy. Avoid alcoholic drinks. Do not treat yourself for coughs, colds or allergies without asking your prescriber or health care professional for advice. Some ingredients can increase possible side effects. Your mouth may get dry. Chewing sugarless gum or sucking hard candy, and drinking plenty of water will help. If you are going to have surgery, tell your prescriber or health care professional that you are taking fluoxetine.

What side effects may I notice from taking fluoxetine?

Side effects that you should report to your prescriber or health care professional as soon as possible:
- anxiety, agitation, panic attacks, inability to sleep, irritability, hostility or extreme anger, aggressiveness, engaging in unusual or dangerous activities, restlessness or inability to sit still, fast talking, actions that are out of control, extreme elation or feeling of happiness that may switch back and forth with a depressed or sad mood
- fast or irregular heart rate, palpitations
- difficulty breathing
- dizziness or lightheadedness
- fast or irregular heart rate, palpitations
- flu-like symptoms (fever, chills, cough, muscle or joint aches and pains)
- seizures (convulsions)
- skin rash, itching (hives)
- unusual tiredness or weakness
- vomiting

Side effects that usually do not require medical attention (report to your prescriber or health care professional if they continue or are bothersome):
- blurred vision
- difficulty sleeping
- daytime drowsiness
- diarrhea
- dry mouth
- flushing
- headache
- increased sweating
- indigestion
- increased or decreased appetite
- sexual difficulties (decreased sexual desire or ability)
- stuffy nose
- tremor (shaking)

Where can I keep my medicine?

Keep out of the reach of children in a container that small children cannot open. Store at room temperature between 15 and 30 degrees C (59 and 86 degrees F). Throw away any unused medicine after the expiration date.

Fluoxetine; Olanzapine capsules

SYMBYAX™; 6 mg/25 mg; Capsule Eli Lilly and Co		

SYMBYAX™; 12 mg/25 mg; Capsule Eli Lilly and Co		

What are fluoxetine; olanzapine capsules?

FLUOXETINE; OLANZAPINE (SYMBYAX®) is a combination of 2 drugs used to help control the depressive phase of a condition called bipolar disorder (also known as manic-depressive illness). Bipolar disorder is a mental condition where you may have fluctuations in your mood, energy level, and ability to function. This drug helps to control extreme mood swings, especially when you feel very sad and depressed. Your health care provider may decide that your bipolar disorder will require long-term medication treatment. Generic fluoxetine; olanzapine capsules are not yet available.

What should my health care professional know before I take fluoxetine; olanzapine?

They need to know if you have any of these conditions:
- a stomach problem called paralytic ileus
- Alzheimer's disease or dementia
- are currently taking another medication called fluoxetine or olanzapine; Prozac®, Prozac® Weekly™, Sarafem®, Zyprexa®, or Zyprexa® Zydis®. These medications also contain ingredients found in SYMBYAX®.
- breast cancer
- cigarette smoker
- diabetes mellitus, high blood sugar or a family history of diabetes

- difficulty passing urine
- difficulty swallowing
- frequently drink alcoholic beverages
- narrow or closed-angle glaucoma
- heart disease, irregular heartbeat, or previous heart attack
- high blood pressure treated with medication
- kidney or liver disease
- low blood pressure
- Parkinson's disease
- prostate trouble
- receiving electroconvulsive therapy
- seizures (convulsions)
- strokes, or mini-strokes called transient ischemic attacks (TIAs)
- suicidal thoughts
- an unusual reaction to fluoxetine, olanzapine, other medicines, foods, dyes, or preservatives
- pregnant or trying to get pregnant
- breast-feeding

How should this medicine be taken?

Take fluoxetine; olanzapine capsules by mouth. Follow the directions on the prescription label. Swallow the capsules with a drink of water. You can take fluoxetine; olanzapine with or without food. If it upsets your stomach, try taking your medicine after eating. Take your doses at regular intervals, the same time each day. Usually you will take fluoxetine; olanzapine at nighttime, but follow your prescriber's directions. Do not take your medicine more often than directed. Do not stop taking except on your prescriber's advice. Contact your pediatrician or health care professional regarding the use of this medicine in children. Special care may be needed.

What if I miss a dose?

If you miss a dose, take it as soon as you can. If it is almost time for your next dose, skip the missed dose and go back to your regular dosing schedule. Do not take double or extra doses.

What may interact with fluoxetine; olanzapine?

Fluoxetine; olanzapine has the potential to interact with a variety of medications; check with your health care professional. The following list contains some of these interactions.

Do not take fluoxetine; olanzapine with any of the following medications:

- astemizole (Hismanal®)
- cisapride (Propulsid®)
- pimozide (Orap®)
- terfenadine (Seldane®)
- thioridazine (Mellaril®); Do not take thioridazine for at least 5 weeks after you stop taking fluoxetine; olanzapine.
- medicines called MAO inhibitors—phenelzine (Nardil®), tranylcypromine (Parnate®), isocarboxazid (Marplan®), selegiline (Eldepryl®). Do not take MAO inhibitors for at least 5 weeks after you stop taking fluoxetine; olanzapine. If you have stopped

taking a MAO inhibitor, do not take fluoxetine; olanzapine for at least 2 weeks.

fluoxetine; olanzapine may also interact with the following medications:

- alcohol
- amphetamine
- aspirin; or other drugs often used for pain known as nonsteroidal anti-inflammatory drugs (NSAIDs)
- buspirone
- carbamazepine
- certain diet drugs (dexfenfluramine, fenfluramine, phentermine, sibutramine)
- certain medicines for migraine headache (almotriptan, eletriptan, frovatriptan, naratriptan, rizatriptan, sumatriptan, zolmitriptan, dihydroergotamine, ergotamine, methysergide)
- cimetidine
- clarithromycin
- clozapine
- cyproheptadine
- dextroamphetamine
- dextromethorphan
- dofetilide
- donepezil
- ergonovine
- erythromycin
- furazolidone
- kava kava
- ketoconazole
- levodopa and other medications for Parkinson's disease
- linezolid
- lithium
- medicines for anxiety or sleeping problems, such as diazepam or alprazolam
- medicines for colds, allergies or hay fever
- medicines for diabetes
- medicines for high blood pressure
- medicines for mental depression or psychotic disturbances
- methylergonovine
- phenobarbital
- phenytoin
- propafenone
- rifampin
- ritonavir
- some prescription pain medications
- some medicines for stomach cramping or irritable bowel syndrome
- St. John's wort
- tacrine
- tobacco in cigarettes
- voriconazole
- warfarin

Tell your prescriber or health care professional about all other medicines you are taking, including non-prescription medicines, nutritional supplements, or herbal products. Also tell your prescriber or health care professional if you are a frequent user of drinks with caffeine or alcohol, if you smoke, or if you use illegal drugs.

F

These may affect the way your medicine works. Check with your health care professional before stopping or starting any of your medicines.

What should I watch for while taking fluoxetine; olanzapine?

Visit your prescriber or health care professional for regular checks on your progress. Continue to take your capsules even if you do not immediately feel better. If you get suicidal thoughts, extreme agitation, inability to sleep or sit still call your prescriber or health care professional at once. Do notify your prescriber if your depression symptoms get worse, if you have new symptoms or if you are having an unusual effect from fluoxetine; olanzapine. Also notify your health care provider immediately if you feel out of control, very discouraged or think you might harm yourself or others. Your prescriber can help you manage these problems. You should not suddenly stop taking fluoxetine; olanzapine. You must gradually reduce the dose or your symptoms may get worse. Ask your prescriber or health care professional for advice; do not stop taking this medication unless you have discussed this with your prescriber. You may get drowsy or dizzy. Do not drive, use machinery, or do anything that needs mental alertness until you know how fluoxetine; olanzapine affects you. Do not stand or sit up quickly, especially if you are an older patient. This reduces the risk of dizzy or fainting spells. Alcohol can make you more drowsy and dizzy. Avoid alcoholic drinks. Do not treat yourself for coughs, colds diarrhea or allergies without asking your prescriber or health care professional for advice. Some ingredients can increase possible side effects. If you experience severe constipation contact your health care provider. Your mouth may get dry. Chewing sugarless gum or sucking hard candy, and drinking plenty of water will help. Be careful when brushing and flossing your teeth to avoid mouth infections or damage to your gums. See your dentist regularly. Fluoxetine; olanzapine can reduce the response of your body to heat or cold. Try not to get overheated or dehydrated from exercise. Avoid temperature extremes, such as saunas, hot tubs, or very hot or cold baths or showers. Dress warmly in cold weather. Fluoxetine; olanzapine may make your skin more sensitive to sun or ultraviolet light. Limit your sun exposure; wear protective clothing outdoors and use a sunscreen (at least SPF 15). Avoid using sun lamps or sun tanning beds or booths. If you notice you are bleeding more easily, for example, when you brush your teeth or floss your gums, or bruising very easily contact your prescriber. Some medicines including aspirin, ibuprofen or naproxen may increase the risk of bleeding if combined with fluoxetine; olanzapine. Aspirin, ibuprofen (for example Motrin®, Advil®) and naproxen (Aleve®) are found in many over-the-counter medications you can buy without a prescription. If you are going to have surgery, tell your prescriber or health care professional that you are taking fluoxetine; olanzapine.

What side effects may I notice from taking fluoxetine; olanzapine?

Side effects that you should report to your prescriber or health care professional as soon as possible:
- agitation, anger, hostility
- changes in vision
- changes in your period or menstrual cycle
- confusion
- difficulty breathing
- difficulty concentrating
- difficulty in swallowing
- excessive thirst
- dizziness, fainting, lightheadedness or loss of balance
- fast talking and excited feelings or actions that are out of control
- frequent need to urinate
- inability to control muscle movements in the face, hands, arms, or legs
- irregular, fast heartbeat (palpitations)
- lowered blood pressure
- painful erections
- seizures (convulsions)
- skin rash or itching (hives)
- stiffness or spasms
- tremors or trembling
- unable to sit still, extreme restlessness or inability to sleep
- uncontrollable tongue or chewing movements, smacking lips or puffing cheeks
- unusual tiredness or weakness
- severe or prolonged vomiting

Side effects that usually do not require medical attention (report to your prescriber or health care professional if they continue or are bothersome):
- minor agitation or restlessness
- minor anxiety or nervousness
- blurred vision
- constipation
- difficulty sleeping
- daytime drowsiness
- diarrhea
- dry mouth
- excessive watering or drooling from your mouth
- headache
- increased sweating
- indigestion
- increased or decreased appetite
- nausea or stomach upset
- sensitivity of skin to sunlight
- sexual difficulties (decreased sexual desire or ability)
- tremor (shaking)
- weight gain

Where can I keep my medicine?

Keep out of the reach of children in a container that small children cannot open. Store at room temperature between 15 and 30 degrees C (59 and 86 degrees F). Throw away any unused medicine after the expiration date.

Fluphenazine tablets

PROLIXIN®;
5 mg; Tablet
ER Squibb and Sons
Inc

PROLIXIN®;
10 mg; Tablet
ER Squibb and Sons
Inc

What are fluphenazine tablets?

FLUPHENAZINE (Prolixin®) helps to treat disordered thoughts and some other emotional, nervous, and mental problems. Generic fluphenazine tablets are available.

What should my health care professional know before I take fluphenazine?

They need to know if you have any of these conditions:
- blood disorders or disease
- difficulty passing urine
- glaucoma
- head injury
- heart or liver disease
- low blood level of calcium
- Parkinson's disease
- prostate trouble
- Reye's syndrome
- seizures (convulsions)
- stomach problems or peptic ulcer
- uncontrollable movement disorder
- an unusual or allergic reaction to fluphenazine, tartrazine dye, other medicines foods, dyes, or preservatives
- pregnant or trying to get pregnant
- breast-feeding

How should I take this medicine?

Take fluphenazine tablets by mouth. Follow the directions on the prescription label. Swallow the tablets with a drink of water. Take fluphenazine with food or milk if it upsets your stomach. Take your doses at regular intervals. Do not take your medicine more often than directed. Contact your pediatrician or health care professional regarding the use of this medicine in children. Special care may be needed. Elderly patients over age 65 years may have a stronger reaction to this medicine and need smaller doses.

What if I miss a dose?

If you miss a dose, take it as soon as you can. If it is almost time for your next dose, take only that dose. Try to take your doses at the same time each day. Do not take double or extra doses.

What may interact with fluphenazine?

- alcohol
- antacids
- some antibiotics
- antidiarrheal medications
- atropine
- bromocriptine
- cimetidine
- cisapride
- dextroamphetamine or amphetamine
- dronabinol or marijuana
- haloperidol or droperidol
- levodopa
- lithium
- medicines for an overactive thyroid gland
- medicines for colds and flu
- medicines for hay fever and other allergies
- medicines for mental depression
- medicines for movement abnormalities as in Parkinson's disease
- medicines to prevent or treat malaria
- medications for treating seizures (convulsions)
- medicines for pain or for use as muscle relaxants, including tramadol
- medicines to treat urine or bladder incontinence
- metoclopramide
- pimozide
- probucol
- some medications for high blood pressure or heart problems
- some weight loss medications

Tell your prescriber or health care professional about all other medicines you are taking, including non-prescription medicines, nutritional supplements, or herbal products. Also tell your prescriber or health care professional if you are a frequent user of drinks with caffeine or alcohol, if you smoke, or if you use illegal drugs. These may affect the way your medicine works. Check with your health care professional before stopping or starting any of your medicines.

What should I watch for while taking fluphenazine?

Visit your prescriber or health care professional for regular checks on your progress. Do not stop taking fluphenazine suddenly; this can cause nausea, vomiting, and dizziness. Ask your prescriber or health care professional for advice if you are to stop taking this medicine. You may get drowsy, dizzy, or have blurred vision. Do not drive, use machinery, or do anything that needs mental alertness until you know how fluphenazine affects you. Do not stand or sit up quickly, especially if you are an older patient. This reduces the risk of dizzy or fainting spells. Alcohol can increase possible dizziness or drowsiness. Avoid alcoholic drinks. Fluphenazine can reduce the response of your body to heat or cold. Try not to get overheated. Avoid temperature extremes, such as saunas, hot tubs, or very hot or cold baths or showers. Dress warmly in cold weather. Fluphenazine can make your skin more sensitive to sun or ultraviolet light. Keep out of the sun, or wear protective clothing outdoors and use a sunscreen (at least SPF 15). Do not use sun lamps or sun tanning beds or booths. Wear sunglasses to protect your eyes. Fluphenazine may make your mouth dry, chewing sugarless gum or sucking hard candy and drinking plenty of water will help. Do not treat yourself for coughs, colds, sore throat, indigestion, diarrhea, or allergies. Ask your prescriber or health care professional for advice. If you are going to have surgery or will need an x-ray procedure that uses contrast agents, tell your prescriber or health care professional that you are taking this medicine.

What side effects may I notice from taking fluphenazine?

Side effects that you should report to your prescriber or health care professional as soon as possible:

- blurred vision
- breast enlargement in men or women
- breast milk in women who are not breast-feeding
- chest pain, fast or irregular heartbeat
- confusion, restlessness
- dark yellow or brown urine
- difficulty breathing or swallowing
- dizziness or fainting spells
- drooling, shaking, movement difficulty (shuffling walk) or rigidity
- fever, chills, sore throat
- hot, dry skin, unable to sweat
- involuntary or uncontrollable movements of the eyes, mouth, head, arms, and legs
- menstrual changes
- puffing cheeks, smacking lips, or worm-like movements of the tongue
- seizures (convulsions)
- slurred speech
- stomach area pain
- sweating
- unusual weakness or tiredness
- unusual bleeding or bruising
- yellowing of skin or eyes

Side effects that usually do not require medical attention (report to your prescriber or health care professional if they continue or are bothersome):

- constipation
- difficulty passing urine
- difficulty sleeping, agitation or restlessness
- drowsiness
- dry mouth
- headache
- increased sensitivity to the sun or ultraviolet light
- sexual difficulties (impotence in men; increased sexual desire in women)
- skin rash, or itching
- stuffy nose
- weight gain

Where can I keep my medicine?

Keep out of the reach of children in a container that small children cannot open. Store at room temperature, approximately 25 degrees C (77 degrees F). Protect from light. Keep container tightly closed. Throw away any unused medicine after the expiration date.

Flurazepam capsules

DALMANE®;
15 mg; Capsule
Valeant
Pharmaceuticals

DALMANE®;
30 mg; Capsule
Valeant
Pharmaceuticals

What are flurazepam capsules?

FLURAZEPAM (Dalmane®) is a benzodiazepine. Benzodiazepines belong to a group of medicines that slow down the central nervous system. Flurazepam helps to treat insomnia (difficulty sleeping at night). Federal law prohibits the transfer of flurazepam to any person other than the patient for whom it was prescribed. Do not share this medicine with anyone else. Generic flurazepam capsules are available.

What should my health care professional know before I take flurazepam?

They need to know if you have any of these conditions:
- an alcohol or drug abuse problem
- bipolar disorder, depression, psychosis or other mental health condition
- glaucoma
- kidney disease
- liver disease
- lung disease, such as chronic obstructive pulmonary disease (COPD), sleep apnea or other breathing difficulties
- myasthenia gravis
- Parkinson's disease
- porphyria
- seizures or a history of seizures
- shortness of breath
- snoring
- suicidal thoughts
- an unusual or allergic reaction to flurazepam, other benzodiazepines, foods, dyes, or preservatives
- pregnant or trying to get pregnant
- breast-feeding

How should I take this medicine?

Take flurazepam capsules by mouth. Flurazepam is only for use at bedtime. Follow the directions on the prescription label. Swallow the capsules with a drink of water. Take your doses at regular intervals. Do not take your medicine more often than directed. Do not stop taking except on your prescriber's advice. Contact your pediatrician or health care professional regarding the use of this medicine in children. Special care may be needed.

What if I miss a dose?

If you miss a dose, take it as soon as you can. It can take up to 2 hours for drowsiness to occur; never repeat the dose before 2 hours have passed. Do not take double or extra doses.

What may interact with flurazepam?

- alcohol
- bosentan
- caffeine
- cimetidine
- disulfiram
- female hormones, including contraceptive or birth control pills
- herbal or dietary supplements such as kava kava, melatonin, St. John's Wort or valerian
- imatinib, STI-571
- isoniazid
- medicines for anxiety or sleeping problems, such as alprazolam, diazepam, lorazepam or triazolam
- medicines for depression, mental problems or psychiatric disturbances
- medicines for fungal infections (fluconazole, itraconazole, ketoconazole, voriconazole)
- medicines for HIV infection or AIDS
- nicardipine
- prescription pain medicines
- probenecid
- rifampin, rifapentine, or rifabutin
- some antibiotics (clarithromycin, erythromycin, troleandomycin)
- some medicines for colds, hay fever or other allergies
- some medicines for high blood pressure or heart-rhythm problems (amiodarone, diltiazem, verapamil)
- some medicines for seizures (carbamazepine, phenobarbital, phenytoin, primidone)
- theophylline
- zafirlukast
- zileuton

Tell your prescriber or health care professional about all other medicines you are taking, including non-prescription medicines, nutritional supplements, or herbal products. Also tell your prescriber or health care professional if you are a frequent user of drinks with caffeine or alcohol, if you smoke, or if you use illegal drugs. These may affect the way your medicine works. Check with your health care professional before stopping or starting any of your medicines.

What should I watch for while taking flurazepam?

Visit your prescriber or health care professional for regular checks on your progress. Your body can become dependent on flurazepam, ask your prescriber or health care professional if you still need to take it. Flurazepam should be used only for short time periods. However, if you have been taking flurazepam regularly for some time, do not suddenly stop taking it. You must gradually reduce the dose or you may get severe side effects. Ask your prescriber or health care professional for advice. Even after you stop taking flurazepam it can still affect your body for several days. You may get drowsy or dizzy. Do not drive, use machinery, or do anything that needs mental alertness until you know how flurazepam affects you. To reduce the risk of dizzy and fainting spells, do not stand or sit up quickly, especially if you are an older patient. Alcohol may increase dizziness and drowsiness. Avoid alcoholic drinks. Do not treat yourself for coughs, colds or allergies without asking your prescriber or health care professional for advice. Some ingredients can increase possible side effects. If you are going to have surgery, tell your prescriber or health care professional that you are taking flurazepam.

What side effects may I notice from taking flurazepam?

Side effects that you should report to your prescriber or health care professional as soon as possible:
- confusion
- depression
- lightheadedness or fainting spells
- mood changes, excitability or aggressive behavior
- movement difficulty, staggering or jerky movements
- muscle cramps
- restlessness
- tremors
- weakness or tiredness

Side effects that usually do not require medical attention (report to your prescriber or health care professional if they continue or are bothersome):
- blurred vision
- constipation or diarrhea
- dizziness, drowsiness, clumsiness, or unsteadiness; a "hangover" effect
- dry mouth
- headache
- heartburn
- increased dreaming
- stomach upset or pain

Where can I keep my medicine?

Keep out of the reach of children in a container that small children cannot open. Store at room temperature between 15 and 30 degrees C (59 and 86 degrees F). Protect from light. Keep container tightly closed. Throw away any unused medicine after the expiration date.

F

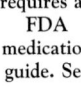

This drug requires an FDA medication guide. See page xxxvii.

Flurbiprofen tablets

ANSAID®; 100 mg; Tablet Pharmacia and Upjohn Div Pfizer	FLURBIPROFEN; 100 mg; Tablet UDL Laboratories Inc

What are flurbiprofen tablets?

FLURBIPROFEN (Ansaid®) is a nonsteroidal anti-inflammatory drug (NSAID). Flurbiprofen is used to relieve some symptoms caused by arthritis (rheumatism) such as inflammation, swelling, stiffness, and joint pain. Flurbiprofen is also used to treat other conditions associated with inflammation and/or pain (e.g., menstrual cramps, muscular pain). Generic flurbiprofen tablets are available.

What should my health care professional know before I take flurbiprofen?

They need to know if you have any of these conditions:

- anemia
- asthma
- bleeding problems
- cigarette smoker
- dental disease
- drink more than 3 alcohol-containing beverages a day
- heart or circulation problems
- high blood pressure
- kidney disease
- liver disease
- nasal polyps
- stomach or intestinal ulcers
- ulcerative colitis
- if you are on a special diet, such as a low-salt diet
- an unusual or allergic reaction to aspirin, other salicylates, other NSAIDs, foods, dyes or preservatives
- pregnant or trying to get pregnant
- breast-feeding

How should I take this medicine?

Take flurbiprofen tablets by mouth. To lessen stomach upset, take flurbiprofen tablets with food. Follow the directions on the prescription label. Swallow tablets whole with a full glass of water; take tablets in an upright or sitting position. Taking a sip of water first, before taking the tablets, may help you swallow them. If possible take bedtime doses at least 10 minutes before lying down. Take your doses at regular intervals. Do not take your medicine more often than directed.

What if I miss a dose?

If you miss a dose, take it as soon as you can. If it is almost time for your next dose, skip the missed dose and go back to your regular dosing schedule. Do not take double or extra doses.

What may interact with flurbiprofen?

- alcohol
- alendronate
- aspirin and aspirin-like medicines
- cidofovir
- cyclosporine
- entecavir
- herbal products that contain feverfew, garlic, ginger, or ginkgo biloba
- lithium
- medicines for high blood pressure
- medicines that affect platelets
- medicines that treat or prevent blood clots such as warfarin and other "blood thinners"
- methotrexate
- other anti-inflammatory drugs (such as ibuprofen or prednisone)
- pemetrexed
- water pills (diuretics)

Tell your prescriber or health care professional about all other medicines you are taking, including non-prescription medicines. Also tell your prescriber or health care professional if you are a frequent user of drinks with caffeine or alcohol, if you smoke, or if you use illegal drugs. These may affect the way your medicine works. Check with your health care professional before stopping or starting any of your medicines.

What should I watch for while taking flurbiprofen?

Let your prescriber or health care professional know if your pain or swelling continues. Do not take flurbiprofen with other pain-killers or anti-inflammatory drugs without advice. To reduce unpleasant effects on your throat and stomach, take flurbiprofen with a full glass of water and never just before lying down. You may get drowsy. Do not drive, use machinery, or do anything that needs mental alertness until you know how flurbiprofen affects you. Do not smoke cigarettes or drink alcohol; these increase irritation to your stomach and can make it more susceptible to damage from flurbiprofen. If you get black, tarry stools or vomit up what looks like coffee grounds, call your prescriber or health care professional at once. You may have a bleeding ulcer. If you are going to have surgery, tell your prescriber or health care professional that you are taking flurbiprofen. Flurbiprofen can cause you to bleed more easily. Problems can arise if you need dental work, and in the day to day care of your teeth. Try to avoid damage to your teeth and gums when you brush or floss your teeth.

What side effects may I notice from taking flurbiprofen?

Side effects that you should report to your prescriber or health care professional as soon as possible:

- blood in urine
- black, tarry stools
- change in the amount of urine passed

- confusion
- dark yellow or brown urine
- difficulty breathing
- pain on swallowing
- skin rash, redness, blistering, peeling or itching
- stomach pain or cramps
- swelling of eyelids, throat, or lips
- symptoms of bronchitis or other respiratory infection
- unusual bleeding or bruising
- unusual tiredness or weakness

Side effects that usually do not require medical attention (report to your prescriber or health care professional if they continue or are bothersome):
- constipation
- diarrhea

- difficulty sleeping
- dizziness
- drowsiness
- gas or heartburn
- headache
- increased sensitivity to the sun
- nausea, vomiting
- ringing in the ears
- weight gain

Where can I keep my medicine?

Keep out of the reach of children in a container that small children cannot open. Store at room temperature between 20 and 25 degrees C (66 and 77 degrees F). Keep container tightly closed. Throw away any unused medicine after the expiration date.

Flutamide capsules

EULEXIN®;
125 mg; Capsule
Schering Corp

What are flutamide capsules?

FLUTAMIDE (Eulexin®) is an antiandrogen. An androgen is a male hormone. Flutamide blocks the effect of the male hormone called testosterone. Prostate cancer responds to the removal of androgens. Flutamide is used in combination with another medicine. Generic flutamide capsules are available.

What should my health care professional know before I take flutamide?

They need to know if you have any of these conditions:
- lactose intolerance
- liver disease
- an unusual or allergic reaction to flutamide, other chemotherapy, other medicines, foods, dyes, or preservatives
- trying to produce pregnancy

How should I take this medicine?

Take flutamide capsules by mouth. Follow the directions on the prescription label. Swallow the capsules with a drink of water. Do not take your medicine more often than directed. Finish the full course prescribed by your doctor or health care professional, even if the capsules make you feel unwell. Do not stop taking except on your prescriber's advice. Contact your pediatrician or health care professional regarding the use of this medicine in children. Special care may be needed.

What if I miss a dose?

If you miss a dose, take it as soon as you can. If it is almost time for your next dose, take only that dose. Do not take double or extra doses. If you vomit after taking a dose, call your prescriber or health care professional for advice.

What may interact with flutamide?

- warfarin
- ritonavir

Tell your prescriber or health care professional about all other medicines you are taking, including non-prescription medicines, nutritional supplements, or herbal products. Also tell your prescriber or health care professional if you are a frequent user of drinks with caffeine or alcohol, if you smoke, or if you use illegal drugs. These may affect the way your medicine works. Check with your health care professional before stopping or starting any of your medicines.

What should I watch for while taking flutamide?

Visit your prescriber or health care professional for regular checks on your progress. At first your condition can get worse, but it will then improve as you continue your treatment. Improvement in your condition can take several days.

What side effects may I notice from taking flutamide?

Side effects that you should report to your prescriber or health care professional as soon as possible:
- dark yellow or brown urine
- vomiting
- yellowing of the eyes or skin

Side effects that usually do not require medical attention (report to your prescriber or health care professional if they continue or are bothersome):
- diarrhea
- nausea

Where can I keep my medicine?

Keep out of the reach of children in a container that small children cannot open. Store between 2 and 30 degrees C (36 and 86 degrees F). Protect from moisture. Throw away any unused medicine after the expiration date.

Fluticasone nasal spray

FLONASE®;
50 mcg/actuation; Spray,
Metered
Glaxo Wellcome

What is fluticasone nasal spray?

FLUTICASONE (Flonase®) is a corticosteroid. Fluticasone helps to relieve symptoms of allergic rhinitis such as runny or stuffy nose, sneezing, and itching of the nose. Generic fluticasone nasal spray is not yet available.

What should my health care professional know before I use fluticasone?

They need to know if you have any of these conditions:
- asthma
- infection, tuberculosis, herpes, or fungal infection
- nosebleeds
- an unusual or allergic reaction to fluticasone, other corticosteroids, medicines, foods, dyes, or preservatives
- pregnant or trying to get pregnant
- breast-feeding

How should I use this medicine?

Fluticasone nasal spray is only for use in the nose. Follow the directions on the prescription label. Shake inhaler well before using. Blow nose gently, without squeezing. With head upright, spray the medicine into each nostril. Sniff briskly while squeezing the bottle quickly and firmly. After use, rinse the tip of the spray bottle with hot water, taking care not to suck water into the bottle. Dry with a clean tissue. Replace the cap directly after cleaning. Do not use the inhaler for more than one person. Do not use extra doses or use more of this medicine than your prescriber or health care professional has prescribed. You may need to use this medicine for several days as prescribed before you start to feel better.

What if I miss a dose?

If you miss a dose and remember within an hour or so, use it as soon as you remember. If it is almost time for your next dose, use only that dose and continue with your regular schedule, spacing doses evenly. Do not use double or extra doses.

What may interact with fluticasone?

- ketoconazole

Tell your prescriber or health care professional about all other medicines you are taking, including non-prescription medicines, nutritional supplements, or herbal products. Also tell your prescriber or health care professional if you are a frequent user of drinks with caffeine or alcohol, if you smoke, or if you use illegal drugs. These may affect the way your medicine works. Check with your health care professional before stopping or starting any of your medicines.

What should I watch for while taking fluticasone?

Visit your prescriber or health care professional for regular checks on your progress. Carry an identification card with your name, the type and dose of corticosteroid you are taking, and your prescriber's name and address. It can take two or three days before your symptoms respond to fluticasone. Use the spray at regular intervals; effectiveness depends on regular use. Check with your prescriber or health care professional if there is no improvement in your condition after three weeks of use. Do not stop using fluticasone except on your prescriber's advice. This medicine may make your mouth dry. Chewing sugarless gum or sucking hard candy, and drinking plenty of water will help. Tell your prescriber or health care professional if you notice white patches or sores in your mouth while you are being treated with fluticasone.

What side effects may I notice from using fluticasone?

Side effects that you should report to your prescriber or health care professional as soon as possible:
- continuing runny nose, stuffy nose, or watering eyes
- coughing, hoarseness
- dizziness or lightheadedness
- nausea, vomiting
- nosebleeds
- stomach pain
- unusual tiredness or weakness

Side effects that usually do not require medical attention (report to your prescriber or health care professional if they continue or are bothersome):
- burning, dryness, or irritation inside the nose
- loss of taste, or unpleasant taste
- sneezing
- throat irritation

Where can I keep my medicine?

Keep out of the reach of children. Store at room temperature between 15 and 30 degrees C (59 and 86 degrees F). Protect from heat, and direct light. Throw away any unused medicine after the expiration date.

Fluvastatin capsules and extended-release tablets

LESCOL®;
40 mg; Capsule
Novartis
Pharmaceuticals

LESCOL® XL;
80 mg; Tablet,
Extended Release
Novartis
Pharmaceuticals

What are fluvastatin capsules?

FLUVASTATIN (Lescol®, Lescol® XL) blocks the body's ability to make cholesterol. Fluvastatin can help lower blood cholesterol for patients who are at risk of getting heart disease or a stroke. It is only for patients whose cholesterol level is not controlled by diet. It is not a cure. Generic fluvastatin capsules and extended-release tablets are not yet available.

What should my health care professional know before I take fluvastatin?

They need to know if you have any of these conditions:
- an alcohol problem
- any hormone disorder (such as diabetes, underactive thyroid)
- blood salt imbalance
- infection
- kidney disease
- liver disease
- low blood pressure
- muscle disorder or condition
- recent surgery
- seizures (convulsions)
- severe injury
- an unusual or allergic reaction to fluvastatin, other medicines, foods, dyes, or preservatives
- pregnant or trying to get pregnant
- breast-feeding

How should I take this medicine?

Take fluvastatin capsules or tablets by mouth. Follow the directions on the prescription label. Swallow the capsules with a drink of water. The capsules can be take with the evening meal or at bedtime. Take your doses at regular intervals. Do not take your medicine more often than directed. Contact your pediatrician or health care professional regarding the use of this medicine in children. Special care may be needed.

What if I miss a dose?

If you miss a dose, take it as soon as you can. If it is almost time for your next dose, take only that dose. Do not take double or extra doses.

What may interact with fluvastatin?

- alcohol
- cimetidine
- clopidogrel
- digoxin
- herbal medicines such as went yeast (Cholestin™)
- irbesartan

- medicines for treating fungal infections (fluconazole, voriconazole)
- medicines for treating HIV infections (delavirdine, efavirenz)
- medicines that suppress your immune response (cyclosporine)
- medicines to lower cholesterol or triglycerides (examples: cholestyramine, fenofibrate, gemfibrozil, niacin)
- omeprazole
- ranitidine
- rifampin, rifabutin, or rifapentine
- warfarin

Tell your prescriber or health care professional about all other medicines you are taking, including non-prescription medicines, nutritional supplements, or herbal products. Also tell your prescriber or health care professional if you are a frequent user of drinks with caffeine or alcohol, if you smoke, or if you use illegal drugs. These may affect the way your medicine works. Check with your health care professional before stopping or starting any of your medicines.

What should I watch for while taking fluvastatin?

Visit your prescriber or health care professional for regular checks on your progress. You will need to have regular tests to make sure your liver is working properly. Tell your prescriber or health care professional as soon as you can if you get any unexplained muscle pain, tenderness, or weakness, especially if you also have a fever and tiredness. Fluvastatin is only part of a total cholesterol-lowering program. Your physician or dietician can suggest a low-cholesterol and low-fat diet that will reduce your risk of getting heart and blood vessel disease. Avoid alcohol and smoking, and keep a proper exercise schedule. If you are going to have surgery tell your prescriber or health care professional that you are taking fluvastatin.

What side effects may I notice from taking fluvastatin?

Side effects that you should report to your prescriber or health care professional as soon as possible:
Rare or uncommon:
- dark yellow or brown urine
- decreased urination, difficulty passing urine
- fever
- muscle pain, tenderness, cramps, or weakness
- redness, blistering, peeling or loosening of the skin, including inside the mouth
- skin rash, itching

F

- unusual tiredness or weakness
- yellowing of the skin or eyes

Side effects that usually do not require medical attention (report to your prescriber or health care professional if they continue or are bothersome):

- diarrhea
- difficulty sleeping
- headache
- joint pain

- muscle soreness after exercise
- nausea, vomiting
- stomach upset or pain

Where can I keep my medicine?

Keep out of the reach of children in a container that small children cannot open. Store at room temperature below 30 degrees C (86 degrees F). Keep container tightly closed. Protect from light. Throw away any unused medicine after the expiration date.

Fluvoxamine tablets

FLUVOXAMINE;
50 mg; Tablet
Apotex Corp

FLUVOXAMINE;
100 mg; Tablet
Eon Labs Inc

What are fluvoxamine tablets?

FLUVOXAMINE (Luvox®) helps people with an obsessive-compulsive disorder. It relieves the anxiety and unpleasant thoughts that make a person repeat everyday tasks (like hand-washing). Fluvoxamine is also used as an antidepressant, and may be used to treat other conditions such as panic disorder, premenstrual syndrome, or traumatic stress. Generic fluvoxamine tablets are available.

What should my health care professional know before I take fluvoxamine?

They need to know if you have any of these conditions:

- heart disease
- history of manic illness
- liver disease
- seizures (convulsions)
- suicidal thoughts
- tobacco smoker
- an unusual or allergic reaction to fluvoxamine, other medicines, foods, dyes, or preservatives
- pregnant or trying to get pregnant
- breast-feeding

How should I take this medicine?

Take fluvoxamine tablets by mouth. Follow the directions on the prescription label. Swallow the tablets with a drink of water. You may take fluvoxamine with or without food. Take your doses at regular intervals. Do not take your medicine more often than directed. Do not stop taking except on your prescriber's advice.

What if I miss a dose?

If you miss a dose, take it as soon as you can. If it is almost time for your next dose, skip the missed dose and go back to your regular dosing schedule. Do not take double or extra doses.

What may interact with fluvoxamine?

Fluvoxamine has the potential to interact with a variety of medications, check with your healthcare professional. The following list contains some of these interactions.

Do not take fluvoxamine with any of the following medications:

- astemizole (Hismanal®)
- cisapride (Propulsid®)
- pimozide (Orap®)
- terfenadine (Seldane®)
- thioridazine (Mellaril®)
- medicines called MAO inhibitors—phenelzine (Nardil®), tranylcypromine (Parnate®), isocarboxazid (Marplan®), selegiline (Eldepryl®)

Fluvoxamine may also interact with the following medications:

- alcohol
- amphetamine
- caffeine
- carbamazepine
- certain diet drugs (dexfenfluramine, fenfluramine, phentermine, sibutramine)
- cimetidine
- dextroamphetamine
- dextromethorphan
- diltiazem
- dofetilide
- ergonovine
- grapefruit juice
- kava kava
- linezolid
- medications for the treatment of HIV infection or AIDS
- melatonin
- migraine headache medicines (almotriptan, eletriptan, frovatriptan, naratriptan, rizatriptan, sumatriptan, zolmitriptan, dihydroergotamine, ergotamine, methysergide)
- medications for anxiety or sleep problems; examples include alprazolam or diazepam
- methylergonovine
- metoprolol
- other medicines used for mental problems like depression or psychosis
- propranolol
- sildenafil
- some medicines for the treatment of pain
- St. John's wort, Hypericum perforatum

- theophylline
- tizanidine
- valerian
- verapamil
- voriconazole
- warfarin

Tell your prescriber or health care professional about all other medicines you are taking, including non-prescription medicines, nutritional supplements, and herbal products. Also tell your prescriber or health care professional if you are a frequent user of drinks with caffeine or alcohol, if you smoke, or if you use illegal drugs. These may affect the way your medicine works. Check with your health care professional before stopping or starting any of your medicines.

What should I watch for while taking fluvoxamine?

Visit your prescriber or health care professional for regular checks on your progress. Continue to take your tablets even if you do not immediately feel better. It can take several weeks before you feel the full effect of fluvoxamine. If you get suicidal thoughts, extreme agitation, or inability to sleep or sit still, call your prescriber or health care professional at once. If you have been taking fluvoxamine regularly for some time, do not suddenly stop taking it. You must gradually reduce the dose or your symptoms may get worse. Ask your prescriber or health care professional for advice. You may get drowsy or dizzy. Do not drive, use machinery, or do anything that needs mental alertness until you know how fluvoxamine affects you. Do not stand or sit up quickly, especially if you are an older patient. This reduces the risk of dizzy or fainting spells. Alcohol can make you more drowsy and dizzy. Avoid alcoholic drinks. Do not treat yourself for coughs, colds or allergies without asking your prescriber or health care professional for advice. Some ingredients can increase possible side effects. In general, do not drink grapefruit juice if you are taking fluvoxamine. If you have been drinking grapefruit juice with fluvoxamine that was previously prescribed, discuss this with your health care provider. If you stop drinking grapefruit juice, your dose of fluvoxamine may need to be adjusted. Your mouth may get dry. Chewing sugarless gum or sucking hard candy, and drinking plenty of water will help. If you are going to have surgery, tell your prescriber or health care professional that you are taking fluvoxamine.

What side effects may I notice from taking fluvoxamine?

Side effects that you should report to your prescriber or health care professional as soon as possible:
- fast talking and excited feelings or actions that are out of control
- irregular heartbeat (palpitations)
- muscle spasms or weakness
- seizures (convulsions)
- skin rash
- unusual tiredness or weakness
- vomiting

Side effects that usually do not require medical attention (report to your prescriber or health care professional if they continue or are bothersome):
- agitation or restlessness
- anxiety or nervousness
- daytime drowsiness
- diarrhea or constipation
- difficulty sleeping
- dry mouth
- headache
- increased sweating
- indigestion
- loss of appetite
- sexual difficulties (decreased sexual desire or ability)
- tremor (shaking)

Where can I keep my medicine?

Keep out of the reach of children in a container that small children cannot open. Store at room temperature between 15 and 30 degrees C (59 and 86 degrees F). Throw away any unused medicine after the expiration date.

Fosamprenavir tablets

LEXIVA™;
700 mg; Tablet
Glaxo Wellcome

What are fosamprenavir tablets?

FOSAMPRENAVIR (Lexiva™) is an antiviral drug called a protease inhibitor. Fosamprenavir is used to treat human immunodeficiency virus (HIV) infection. Fosamprenavir may reduce the amount of HIV in the blood and increase the number of CD4 cells (T-cells) in the blood. Fosamprenavir is used in combination with other drugs to treat the HIV virus. Fosamprenavir will not cure or prevent HIV infection or AIDS. You may still develop other infections or conditions associated with HIV. Generic fosamprenavir tablets are not yet available.

What should my health care professional know before I take fosamprenavir?

They need to know if you have any of these conditions:
- diabetes or high blood sugar
- hemophilia A or B
- high cholesterol or triglycerides

- liver disease
- vitamin K deficiency
- an unusual or allergic reaction to fosamprenavir, amprenavir, sulfa drugs, other medicines, foods, dyes, or preservatives
- pregnant or trying to get pregnant
- breast-feeding

How should this medicine be taken?

Take fosamprenavir tablets by mouth. Follow the directions on the prescription label. Swallow the tablet with a drink of water. Fosamprenavir can be taken with or without food. Do not take fosamprenavir with antacids. Take your doses at regular intervals. Do not take your medicine more often than directed. To help to make sure that your anti-HIV therapy works as well as possible, be very careful to take all of your medicine exactly as prescribed. Do not stop taking except on your prescriber's advice. Contact your pediatrician or health care professional regarding the use of this medicine in children. Special care may be needed.

What if I miss a dose?

If you miss a dose, take it as soon as you can. If it is almost time for your next dose, take only that dose. Do not take double or extra doses.

What may interact with fosamprenavir?

Many medicines may interact with fosamprenavir. If you have a question concerning other medicines you may be taking, talk with your pharmacist, prescriber or other health care professional.

Do not take fosamprenavir with any of these medicines:

- astemizole
- bepridil
- birth control pills or other hormonal birth control medicines (like the patch, ring, or injections)
- cisapride
- dihydroergotamine
- ergotamine
- lovastatin
- methadone
- methylergonovine
- methysergide
- midazolam
- rifampin
- sildenafil
- simvastatin
- St. John's wort
- triazolam
- vitamin E supplements
- warfarin
- went yeast (Cholestin™)

Other medicines that may interact with amprenavir:

- amiodarone
- antacids
- bosentan
- certain medicines for anxiety or difficulty sleeping

- certain medicines for high cholesterol (atorvastatin)
- certain medicines for depression (e.g., amitriptyline, imipramine)
- didanosine, ddI
- dofetilide
- lidocaine
- medicines for diabetes
- medicines for seizures
- medicines to lower your cholesterol (e.g., atorvastatin or cerivastatin)
- other medicines for HIV
- quinidine
- rifabutin

Tell your prescriber or health care professional about all other medicines you are taking, including non-prescription medicines, nutritional supplements, or herbal products. Also tell your prescriber or health care professional if you are a frequent user of drinks with caffeine or alcohol, if you smoke, or if you use illegal drugs. These may affect the way your medicine works. Check with your health care professional before stopping or starting any of your medicines.

What should I watch for while taking fosamprenavir?

Visit your prescriber or health care professional for regular checks on your progress. Discuss any new symptoms with your prescriber or health care professional. Fosamprenavir will not cure HIV and you can still get other illnesses or complications associated with your disease. Taking fosamprenavir does not reduce the risk of passing HIV infection to others through sexual or blood contact. It is best to avoid sexual contact so that you do not spread the disease to others. For any sexual contact, use a condom. Be careful about cuts, abrasions and other possible sources of blood contact. Never share a needle or syringe with anyone. If you are a women of childbearing age and are using hormone contraceptives, then you should use another form of birth control while taking fosamprenavir. Fosamprenavir may decrease the effectiveness of hormone birth control agents, including birth control pills and injections. Do not take antacids or didanosine, ddI within 1 hour of taking fosamprenavir. Antacids may decrease the amount of fosamprenavir you absorb.

What side effects may I notice from taking fosamprenavir?

Side effects that you should report to your prescriber or health care professional as soon as possible:

- changes in body appearance (such as weight gain or loss around the waist and/or face)
- skin rash or itchy skin
- increased hunger or thirst
- increased urination
- redness, blistering, peeling or loosening of the skin, including inside the mouth
- unusual tiredness or weakness

Side effects that usually do not require medical attention (report to your prescriber or health care professional if they continue or are bothersome):

- diarrhea
- headache
- nausea and vomiting
- stomach pain
- tingling around the mouth

Where can I keep my medicine?

Keep out of the reach of children in a container that small children cannot open. Store at room temperature between 15 and 30 degrees C (59 and 86 degrees F). Keep container tightly closed. Throw away any unused medicine after the expiration date.

Fosinopril tablets

MONOPRIL®;
20 mg; Tablet
Bristol Myers Squibb
Co

MONOPRIL®;
10 mg; Tablet
Bristol Myers Squibb
Co

What are fosinopril tablets?

FOSINOPRIL (Monopril®) is an antihypertensive (blood pressure lowering agent) known as an ACE inhibitor. Fosinopril controls high blood pressure (hypertension) by relaxing blood vessels; it is not a cure. High blood pressure levels can damage your kidneys, and may lead to a stroke or heart failure. Generic fosinopril tablets are available.

What should my health care professional know before I take fosinopril?

They need to know if you have any of these conditions:
- autoimmune disease (such as lupus), or suppressed immune function
- previous swelling of the tongue, face, or lips with difficulty breathing, difficulty swallowing, hoarseness, or tightening of the throat (angioedema)
- bone marrow disease
- heart or blood vessel disease
- liver disease
- low blood pressure
- kidney disease
- if you are on a special diet, such as a low-salt diet
- an unusual or allergic reaction to fosinopril, other ACE inhibitors, foods, dyes, or preservatives
- pregnant or trying to get pregnant
- breast-feeding

How should I take this medicine?

Take fosinopril tablets by mouth. Follow the directions on the prescription label. Swallow the tablets with a drink of water. It is best to take fosinopril on an empty stomach, at least 1 hour before or 2 hours after meals. Take your doses at regular intervals. Do not take your medicine more often than directed. Do not stop taking fosinopril except on your prescriber's advice. Contact your pediatrician or health care professional regarding the use of this medicine in children. Special care may be needed.

What if I miss a dose?

If you miss a dose, take it as soon as you can. If it is almost time for your next dose, take only that dose. Do not take double or extra doses. If you take only one dose a day and forget to take it that day, do not take a double dose the next day.

What may interact with fosinopril?

- anti-inflammatory drugs (NSAIDs, such as ibuprofen)
- hawthorn
- heparin
- lithium
- medicines for high blood pressure
- potassium salts
- water pills

Tell your prescriber or health care professional about all other medicines you are taking, including non-prescription medicines, nutritional supplements, or herbal products. Also tell your prescriber or health care professional if you are a frequent user of drinks with caffeine or alcohol, if you smoke, or if you use illegal drugs. These may affect the way your medicine works. Check with your health care professional before stopping or starting any of your medicines.

What should I watch for while taking fosinopril?

Visit your prescriber or health care professional for regular checks on your progress. Check your blood pressure regularly while you are taking fosinopril. Ask your prescriber or health care professional what your blood pressure should be and when you should contact him or her. Call your prescriber or health care professional if you notice an uneven or fast heart beat. Do not treat yourself for a fever or sore throat; check with your prescriber or health care professional as these may be the result of a fosinopril side effect. Check with your prescriber or health care professional if you get an attack of severe diarrhea, nausea and vomiting, or if you sweat a lot. The loss of body fluid can make it dangerous to take fosinopril. You may get dizzy. Do not drive, use machinery, or do anything that needs mental alertness until you know how fosinopril affects you. To avoid dizzy or fainting spells, do not stand or sit up quickly, especially if you are an older person. Alcohol can make you more dizzy. Avoid alcoholic drinks. If you are going to have surgery, tell your prescriber or health care professional that you are using fosinopril. Avoid salt substitutes or other foods or substances high in potassium salts. Do not treat yourself for coughs, colds, or pain while you are using fosinopril without asking your prescriber or health care professional for advice.

F

What side effects may I notice from taking fosinopril?

Side effects that you should report to your prescriber or health care professional as soon as possible:
- decreased amount of urine passed
- difficulty breathing, or difficulty swallowing
- dizziness, lightheadedness or fainting spells
- fast or uneven heart beat, palpitations, or chest pain
- fever or chills
- numbness or tingling in your fingers or toes
- skin rash, itching
- swelling of your face, lips, or tongue

Side effects that usually do not require medical attention (report to your prescriber or health care professional if they continue or are bothersome):
- change in taste
- cough
- headache
- tiredness

Where can I keep my medicine?

Keep out of the reach of children in a container that small children cannot open. Store at room temperature between 15 and 30 degrees C (59 and 86 degrees F). Protect from moisture. Keep container tightly closed. Throw away any unused medicine after the expiration date.

Fosinopril; Hydrochlorothiazide, HCTZ tablets

MONOPRIL-HCT®;
10 mg/12.5 mg;
Tablet
Bristol Myers Squibb
Co

MONOPRIL-HCT®;
20 mg/12.5 mg;
Tablet
Bristol Myers Squibb
Co

What are fosinopril; hydrochlorothiazide, HCTZ tablets?

FOSINOPRIL; HYDROCHLOROTHIAZIDE (Monopril-HCT®) is a combination of two drugs used to lower blood pressure. Fosinopril is an ACE inhibitor that controls high blood pressure (hypertension) by relaxing blood vessels. Hydrochlorothiazide is a diuretic. High blood pressure can damage the blood vessels of the brain, heart, and kidneys, resulting in a stroke, heart failure, or kidney failure. By lowering blood pressure, fosinopril-hydrochlorothiazide can help reduce your risk of having damage to your kidneys, heart, or other organs. This medicine does not cure high blood pressure. Generic fosinopril-hydrochlorothiazide tablets are available.

What should my health care professional know before I take fosinopril; hydrochlorothiazide?

They need to know if you have any of these conditions:
- autoimmune disease (e.g., lupus), or suppressed immune function
- previous swelling of the tongue, face, or lips with difficulty breathing, difficulty swallowing, hoarseness, or tightening of the throat (angioedema)
- bone marrow disease
- diabetes mellitus
- gout
- heart or blood vessel disease
- liver disease
- recent heart attack or stroke
- kidney disease, (e.g. renal failure or renal artery stenosis)
- pancreatitis
- electrolyte imbalance (e.g. low or high levels of potassium in the blood)
- if you are on a special diet, such as a low-salt diet (e.g. using salt substitutes)
- sulfonamide (sulfa) or thiazide allergy
- an unusual or allergic reaction to fosinopril, hydrochlorothiazide, other medicines, foods, dyes, or preservatives
- pregnant or trying to get pregnant
- breast-feeding

How should I take this medicine?

Take fosinopril-hydrochlorothiazide tablets by mouth with or without food. Follow the directions on the prescription label. Swallow the tablets with a drink of water. Take your doses at regular intervals. Do not take your medicine more often than directed. Do not stop taking this medicine except on your prescriber's advice. Many patients with high blood pressure will not notice any signs of the problem. Therefore, it is very important that you take this medicine exactly as directed and that you keep your appointments with your prescriber or health care professional even if you feel well. Contact your pediatrician or health care professional regarding the use of this medicine in children. Special care may be needed.

What if I miss a dose?

If you miss a dose, take it as soon as you can. If it is almost time for your next dose, take only that dose. Do not take double or extra doses.

What may interact with fosinopril-hydrochlorothiazide?

- allopurinol
- aminolevulinic acid
- antacids
- anti-inflammatory drugs (NSAIDs such as ibuprofen)
- aspirin
- azathioprine
- blood pressure medications
- cholesterol-lowering medications (e.g. cholestyramine or colestipol)
- diabetic medications
- dofetilide

- hawthorn
- lithium
- methoxsalen
- porfimer
- potassium salts or potassium supplements
- tetracycline
- vitamin A (retinol) creams or pills such as tretinoin Retin-A®, Renova®, Solage®, Atragen®, and others
- water pills (especially potassium-sparing diuretics such as triamterene or amiloride)

Tell your prescriber or health care professional about all other medicines you are taking, including non-prescription medicines, nutritional supplements, or herbal products. Also tell your prescriber or health care professional if you are a frequent user of drinks with caffeine or alcohol, if you smoke, or if you use illegal drugs. These may affect the way your medicine works. Check with your health care professional before stopping or starting any of your medicines.

What should I watch for while taking fosinopril-hydrochlorothiazide?

Check your blood pressure regularly while you are taking fosinopril-hydrochlorothiazide. Ask your prescriber or health care professional what your blood pressure should be and when you should contact him or her. When you check your blood pressure, write down the measurements to show your prescriber or health care professional. You must not get dehydrated, ask your prescriber or health care professional how much fluid you need to drink a day. If you are taking this medicine for a long time you must visit your prescriber or health care professional for regular checks on your progress. Make sure you schedule appointments on a regular basis. Check with your prescriber or health care professional if you get severe diarrhea, nausea and vomiting, or if you sweat a lot. The loss of too much body fluid can make it dangerous for you to take fosinopril-hydrochlorothiazide. You may get dizzy. Do not drive, use machinery, or do anything that requires mental alertness until you know how fosinopril-hydrochlorothiazide affects you. To avoid dizzy or fainting spells, do not stand or sit up quickly. Alcohol may increase the possibility of dizziness. Avoid alcoholic drinks until you have discussed their use with your prescriber or health care professional. If you are going to have surgery tell your prescriber or health care professional that you are taking fosinopril-hydrochlorothiazide. Fosinopril-hydrochlorothiazide may affect your blood sugar level.

If you have diabetes, check with your prescriber or health care professional before changing the dose of your diabetic medicine. Avoid salt substitutes unless you are told otherwise by your prescriber or health care professional. Do not take medicines for appetite control, asthma, colds, cough, hay fever, or sinus problems without asking your prescriber or health care professional for advice. Do not treat yourself for a fever or sore throat; check with your prescriber or health care professional first.

What side effects may I notice from taking fosinopril-hydrochlorothiazide?

Side effects that you should report to your prescriber or health care professional as soon as possible:

Rare or uncommon:
- difficulty breathing, difficulty swallowing, hoarseness, or tightening of the throat
- redness, blistering, peeling or loosening of the skin, including inside the mouth
- swelling of your face, lips, tongue, hands, or feet
- unusual rash, bleeding or bruising
- decreased sexual function

Other:
- confusion, dizziness, lightheadedness or fainting spells
- decreased amount of urine passed
- fast or uneven heart beat, palpitations, or chest pain
- fever or chills
- irregular heartbeat
- muscle cramps
- stomach pain
- vomiting
- unusual tiredness or weakness
- worsened gout pain
- yellowing of the eyes or skin

Side effects that usually do not require medical attention (report to your prescriber or health care professional if they continue or are bothersome):
- cough
- diarrhea or constipation
- increased sensitivity to the sun
- nausea
- tiredness or fatigue

Where can I keep my medicine?

Keep out of the reach of children. Store at room temperature between 15 and 30 degrees C (59 and 86 degrees F). Protect from moisture. Keep container tightly closed. Throw away any unused medicine after the expiration date.

F

Frovatriptan tablets

FROVA™;
2.5 mg; Tablet
Endo Pharmaceuticals, Inc

What are frovatriptan tablets?

FROVATRIPTAN (Frova™) helps to relieve a migraine attack that starts with or without aura (an unusual feeling or change in vision that warns you of an attack). Generic frovatriptan tablets are not available.

What should my health care professional know before I take frovatriptan?

They need to know if you have any of these conditions:
- bowel disease or colitis
- diabetes
- family history of heart disease
- fast or irregular heartbeat
- headaches that are different from your usual migraine
- heart or blood vessel disease, angina (chest pain), or previous heart attack
- high blood pressure
- high cholesterol
- history of stroke, transient ischemic attacks (TIAs or "mini-strokes"), or intracranial bleeding
- overweight
- poor circulation
- postmenopausal or surgical removal of uterus and ovaries
- Raynaud's syndrome
- seizure disorder
- tobacco smoker
- an unusual or allergic reaction to frovatriptan, other medicines, foods, dyes, or preservatives
- pregnant or trying to get pregnant
- breast-feeding

How should I take this medicine?

Take frovatriptan tablets by mouth. Follow the directions on the prescription label. Frovatriptan is taken after the migraine attack starts; it is not for everyday use. Swallow the tablet whole, with a glass of water. If your migraine headache returns after one dose, you can take another dose as directed. You must allow at least 2 hours between doses, and do not take more than 3 tablets (7.5 mg) in 24 hours. If there is no improvement at all after the first dose, do not take a second dose without talking to your prescriber or health care professional. Do not take your medicine more often than directed. Contact your pediatrician or health care professional regarding the use of this medicine in children. Special care may be needed.

What if I miss a dose?

This does not apply, frovatriptan is not for regular use.

What may interact with frovatriptan?

Do not take frovatriptan with any of the following medicines:

- amphetamine or cocaine
- dihydroergotamine, ergotamine, ergoloid mesylates, methysergide, or ergot-type medication—do not take within 24 hours of taking frovatriptan
- almotriptan, eletriptan, naratriptan, rizatriptan, sumatriptan, zolmitriptan—do not take within 24 hours of taking frovatriptan
- medicines for weight loss such as dexfenfluramine, dextroamphetamine, fenfluramine, or sibutramine
- monoamine oxidase inhibitors (MAOIs) such as phenelzine (Nardil®), tranylcypromine (Parnate®), isocarboxazid (Marplan®), and selegiline (Carbex®, Eldepryl®)—do not take frovatriptan within 2 weeks of stopping MAOI therapy.

Check with your doctor or pharmacist if you take any of these medications:

- cough syrup or other products containing dextromethorphan
- feverfew
- lithium
- medicines for mental depression, anxiety or mood problems such as buspirone, citalopram, fluoxetine, fluvoxamine, mirtazapine, nefazodone, paroxetine, sertraline, trazodone, tricyclic antidepressants, or venlafaxine
- meperidine
- St. John's wort
- tryptophan

Tell your physician or health care provider: about all other medicines you are taking, including non-prescription medicines and herbal medicines; if you are a frequent user of drinks with caffeine or alcohol; if you smoke; or if you use illegal drugs. These may affect the way your medicine works. Check with your health care professional before stopping or starting any of your medicines.

What should I watch for while taking frovatriptan?

Only take frovatriptan tablets for a migraine headache. Take it if you get warning symptoms or at the start of a migraine attack. Frovatriptan is not for regular use to prevent migraine attacks. Do not take this drug if your headache symptoms are different than your usual attacks; consult your doctor first. Do not take migraine products that contain ergotamine while you are taking frovatriptan; this combination can affect your heart. You may get drowsy or dizzy. Do not drive, use machinery, or do anything that needs mental alertness until you know how frovatriptan affects you. To reduce dizzy or fainting spells, do not sit or stand up quickly, especially if you are an older patient. Alcohol can increase drowsiness, dizziness and flushing. Avoid alcoholic drinks. Smoking cigarettes may increase the risk of heart-related side effects from using frovatriptan.

F

What side effects may I notice from taking frovatriptan?

Side effects that you should report to your prescriber as soon as possible:

- chest, neck, or throat pain or tightness
- dizziness or faintness
- fast or irregular heart beat, palpitations
- feeling of chest heaviness or pressure
- increased blood pressure
- severe stomach pain and cramping, bloody diarrhea
- shortness of breath, wheezing, or difficulty breathing
- tingling, pain, or numbness in the face, hands or feet
- unusual reaction or swelling of the skin, eyelids, face, or lips

Stop using frovatriptan and call your prescriber as soon as you can if you get any of these side effects.

Side effects that usually do not require medical attention (report to your prescriber or health care professional if they continue or are bothersome):

- drowsiness
- dry mouth
- feeling hot or cold
- feeling warm, flushing, or redness of the face
- headache, other than migraine headache
- heartburn or indigestion
- nausea, vomiting, or stomach upset
- pain in the bones or joints
- tiredness or weakness.

Where can I keep my medicine?

Keep out of the reach of children in a container that small children cannot open. Store at room temperature between 20 and 25 degrees C (68 and 77 degrees F). Protect from light and moisture. Throw away any unused medicine after the expiration date.

Furosemide tablets

LASIX®;
40 mg; Tablet
Hoechst Roussel
Pharmaceuticals Div

LASIX®;
80 mg; Tablet
Hoechst Roussel
Pharmaceuticals Div

What are furosemide tablets?

FUROSEMIDE (Lasix®) is a diuretic. Diuretics increase the amount of urine passed, which causes the body to lose water and salt. Furosemide helps to treat high blood pressure (hypertension). It is not a cure. It also reduces the swelling and water retention caused by various medical conditions, such as heart, liver, or kidney disease. Generic furosemide tablets are available.

What should my health care professional know before I take furosemide?

They need to know if you have any of these conditions:

- diabetes
- diarrhea
- gout
- hearing problems
- heart disease, or previous heart attack
- kidney disease, small amounts of urine, or difficulty passing urine
- liver disease
- low blood levels of calcium, potassium, chloride, sodium or magnesium
- pancreatitis
- premature birth (newborns)
- systemic lupus erythematosus (SLE)
- an unusual or allergic reaction to furosemide, sulfa drugs, other medicines, foods, dyes, or preservatives
- pregnant or trying to get pregnant
- breast-feeding

How should I take this medicine?

Take furosemide tablets by mouth. Follow the directions on the prescription label. Swallow the tablets with a drink of water. If furosemide upsets your stomach, take it with food or milk. Take your doses at regular intervals. Do not take your medicine more often than directed. Remember that you will need to pass urine frequently after taking furosemide. Do not take your doses at a time of day that will cause you problems. Do not take at bedtime.

What if I miss a dose?

If you miss a dose, take it as soon as you can. If it is almost time for your next dose, take only that dose. Do not take double or extra doses.

What may interact with furosemide?

- alcohol
- anti-inflammatory drugs (NSAIDs, such as ibuprofen)
- certain antibiotics given by injection
- cholestyramine
- cisplatin
- clofibrate
- colestipol
- dofetilide
- heart medicines such as digoxin
- hormones such as cortisone, fludrocortisone, or hydrocortisone
- lithium
- medicine for high blood pressure
- medicines that relax muscles for surgery
- nitroglycerin
- phenytoin
- water pills

Tell your prescriber or health care professional about all other medicines you are taking, including non-prescription medicines, nutritional supplements, or herbal products. Also tell your prescriber or health care professional if you are a frequent user of drinks with caffeine or alcohol, if you smoke, or if you use illegal drugs. These may affect the way your medicine works. Check

F

with your health care professional before stopping or starting any of your medicines.

What should I watch for while taking furosemide?

Visit your prescriber or health care professional for regular checks on your progress. Check your blood pressure regularly. Ask your prescriber or health care professional what your blood pressure should be, and when you should contact him or her. You must not get dehydrated, ask your prescriber or health care professional how much fluid you need to drink a day. Do not stop taking furosemide except on your prescriber's advice. Watch your diet while you are taking furosemide. Ask your prescriber or health care professional about both potassium and sodium intake. Furosemide can make your body lose potassium and you may need an extra supply. Some foods have a high potassium content such as bananas, coconuts, dates, figs, prunes, apricots, peaches, grapefruit juice, tomato juice, and orange juice. You may get dizzy or lightheaded. Do not drive, use machinery, or do anything that needs mental alertness until you know how furosemide affects you. To reduce the risk of dizzy or fainting spells, do not sit or stand up quickly, especially if you are an older patient. Alcohol can make you lightheaded, dizzy and increase confusion. Avoid or limit intake of alcoholic drinks. Furosemide can make your skin more sensitive to sun or ultraviolet light. Keep out of the sun, or wear protective clothing outdoors and use a sunscreen (at least SPF 15). Do not use sun lamps or sun tanning beds or booths. If you are going to have surgery, tell your prescriber or health care professional that you are taking furosemide. Furosemide can increase the amount of sugar in blood or urine. If you are a diabetic keep a close check on blood and urine sugar.

What side effects may I notice from taking furosemide?

Side effects that you should report to your prescriber or health care professional as soon as possible:

- blood in urine or stools
- diarrhea
- dry mouth
- fever or chills, sore throat
- hearing loss or ringing in the ears
- increased thirst
- irregular heartbeat
- lower back or side pain
- mood changes
- muscle pain or weakness, cramps
- nausea, vomiting
- severe stomach pain
- skin rash
- tingling or numbness in the hands or feet
- unusual bleeding or bruising
- unusual tiredness or weakness
- yellowing of the eyes or skin

Side effects that usually do not require medical attention (report to your prescriber or health care professional if they continue or are bothersome):

- dizziness or lightheadedness
- headache
- increased sensitivity to the sun
- loss of appetite
- stomach upset, pain, or cramps

Where can I keep my medicine?

Keep out of the reach of children in a container that small children cannot open. Store at room temperature between 15 and 30 degrees C (59 and 86 degrees F). Protect from light. Throw away any unused medicine after the expiration date.

F

Gabapentin
capsules or tablets

NEURONTIN®;
300 mg; Capsule
Parke Davis Division
of Pfizer Co.

NEURONTIN®;
600 mg; Tablet
Parke Davis Division
of Pfizer Co.

What are gabapentin capsules or tablets?

GABAPENTIN (Neurontin®) is effective in helping to control partial seizures (convulsions) in adults with epilepsy. Gabapentin is also used to help relieve certain types of nerve pain, and may be prescribed for other nervous system disorders. Generic gabapentin capsules and tablets are available.

What should my health care professional know before I take gabapentin?

They need to know if you have any of these conditions:
- kidney disease
- an unusual or allergic reaction to gabapentin, other medicines, foods, dyes, or preservatives
- pregnant or trying to get pregnant
- breast-feeding

How should I take this medicine?

Take gabapentin capsules or tablets by mouth. Follow the directions on the prescription label. Swallow the capsules or tablets with a drink of water. If gabapentin upsets your stomach, take it with food or milk. Take your doses at regular intervals. Do not take your medicine more often than directed. If your prescriber directs you to break the 600 or 800 mg tablets in half as part of your dose, the extra half tablet should be used for the next dose. If you have not used the extra half tablet within 3 days, it should be thrown away. Contact your pediatrician or health care professional regarding the use of this medicine in children. Special care may be needed.

What if I miss a dose?

If you miss a dose, take it as soon as you can. If it is almost time for your next dose, take only that dose. Do not take double or extra doses.

What may interact with gabapentin?

- antacids
- cimetidine

Tell your prescriber or health care professional about all other medicines you are taking, including non-prescription medicines, nutritional supplements, or herbal products. Also tell your prescriber or health care professional if you are a frequent user of drinks with caffeine or alcohol, if you smoke, or if you use illegal drugs. These may affect the way your medicine works. Check with your health care professional before stopping or starting any of your medicines.

What should I watch for while taking gabapentin?

Visit your prescriber or health care professional for a regular check on your progress. You may want to keep a personal record at home of how you feel your condition is responding to gabapentin treatment. You may want to share this information with your prescriber or health care professional at each visit. Wear a Medic Alert bracelet or necklace if you are taking gabapentin for seizures. Carry an identification card with information about your condition, medications, and prescriber or health care professional. You should contact your prescriber or health care professional if your seizures get worse or if you have any new types of seizures. Do not stop taking gabapentin or any of your seizure medicines unless instructed by your prescriber or health care professional. Stopping your medicine suddenly can increase your seizures or their severity. You may get drowsy, dizzy, or have blurred vision. Do not drive, use machinery, or do anything that needs mental alertness until you know how gabapentin affects you. To reduce dizzy or fainting spells, do not sit or stand up quickly, especially if you are an older patient. Alcohol can increase drowsiness and dizziness. Avoid alcoholic drinks. If you are going to have surgery, tell your prescriber or health care professional that you are taking gabapentin.

What side effects may I notice from taking gabapentin?

Side effects that you should report to your prescriber or health care professional as soon as possible:
Rare or uncommon:
- difficulty breathing or tightening of the throat
- swelling of lips or tongue
- rash

May occur in children:
- fever
- hyperactivity
- hostile or aggressive behavior
- mood changes or changes in behavior
- difficulty concentrating

Side effects that usually do not require medical attention (report to your prescriber or health care professional if they continue or are bothersome):
- constipation
- difficulty walking or controlling muscle movements
- dizziness, drowsiness
- dry mouth
- back pain, joint aches and pains
- indigestion, gas or heartburn
- loss of appetite
- nausea
- pain, burning or tingling in the hands or feet
- restlessness
- sexual difficulty (impotence)
- skin itching
- slurred speech
- sore gums
- tremor
- weight gain

G

Where can I keep my medicine?

Keep out of reach of children in a container that small children cannot open. Store at room temperature between 15 and 30 degrees C (59 and 86 degrees F). Throw away any unused medicine after the expiration date.

Galantamine tablets

RAZADYNE®;
8 mg; Tablet
Janssen
Pharmaceutica

RAZADYNE®;
12 mg; Tablet
Janssen
Pharmaceutica

What are galantamine tablets?

GALANTAMINE (Razadyne®) helps treat the symptoms associated with Alzheimer's disease. It is not a cure for Alzheimer's disease but offers improvement in memory, attention, reason, language, and the ability to perform tasks. Benefits are greater in the early stages of the disease. Generic galantamine tablets are not yet available.

What should my health care professional know before I take galantamine?

They need to know if you have any of these conditions:
- asthma or other lung disease
- difficulty passing urine
- head injury
- heart disease, or irregular or slow heartbeat
- kidney disease
- liver disease
- low blood pressure
- Parkinson's disease
- seizures (convulsions)
- stomach or intestinal disease, ulcers, or stomach bleeding
- an unusual or allergic reaction to galantamine, other medicines, foods, dyes, or preservatives
- pregnant or trying to get pregnant
- breast-feeding

How should I take this medicine?

Take galantamine tablets by mouth. Follow the directions on the prescription label. Swallow the tablets with a drink of water. Galantamine is usually administered twice daily with food, and is recommended to be taken with the morning and evening meals. Taking the medication with food and plenty of liquid may help lessen side effects such as upset stomach. Take your doses at regular intervals. Do not take your medicine more often than directed. Continue to take your medicine even if you feel better. Do not stop taking except on your prescriber's advice. Dose increases should not occur more often than every 4 weeks; follow your prescriber's dose recommendations. If therapy has been stopped for several days or more, your prescriber will restart your therapy at a lower dose. Following your prescriber's dosing and administration directions may help avoid the most common adverse effects. Contact your pediatrician or health care professional regarding the use of this medicine in children. Special care may be needed.

What if I miss a dose?

If you miss a dose, take it as soon as you can. If it is almost time for your next dose, take only that dose. Do not take double or extra doses.

What may interact with galantamine?

- amantadine
- atropine
- benztropine
- bosentan
- carbamazepine
- clarithromycin
- cimetidine
- dicyclomine
- digoxin
- donepezil
- erythromycin
- glycopyrrolate
- hyoscyamine
- medications for fungal infections (fluconazole, itraconazole, ketoconazole, terbinafine)
- medications for motion sickness (examples: dimenhydrinate, meclizine, scopolamine)
- medications for Parkinson's disease
- medicines that relax your muscles for surgery
- non-steroidal anti-inflammatory drugs (examples: ibuprofen, naproxen)
- oxybutynin
- phenobarbital
- phenytoin
- propantheline
- rifampin, rifabutin, or rifapentine
- rivastigmine
- some medications for depression, anxiety or mood disorders
- some medications for heart disease or high blood pressure
- some medications for HIV infection
- St. John's wort
- tacrine
- tolterodine
- troglitazone

Tell your prescriber or health care professional about all other medicines you are taking, including non-prescription medicines, nutritional supplements, or herbal products. Also tell your prescriber or health care professional if you are a frequent user of drinks with caffeine or alcohol, if you smoke, or if you use illegal drugs. These may affect the way your medicine works. Check

with your health care professional before stopping or starting any of your medicines.

What should I watch for while taking galantamine?

Visit your prescriber or health care professional for regular checks on your progress. Check with your prescriber or health care professional if there is no improvement in your symptoms or if they get worse. You may get dizzy or feel faint. Do not drive, use machinery, or do anything that needs mental alertness until you know how galantamine affects you. If you are going to have surgery tell your prescriber or health care professional that you are taking galantamine.

What side effects may I notice from taking galantamine?

Side effects that you should report to your prescriber or health care professional as soon as possible:
- changes in vision or balance
- diarrhea, if it is severe or does not stop
- difficulty breathing
- difficulty or pain when urinating
- dizziness, fainting spells, or falls
- nervousness, agitation, or increased confusion

- skin rash or hives
- slow heartbeat, or palpitations
- stomach pain
- uncontrollable movements
- vomiting
- weight loss

Side effects that usually do not require medical attention (report to your prescriber or health care professional if they continue or are bothersome):
- mild diarrhea, especially when starting treatment
- drowsiness
- headache
- indigestion or heartburn
- loss of appetite
- nausea
- tiredness
- trembling
- trouble sleeping

Where can I keep my medicine?

Keep out of reach of children in a container that small children cannot open. Store at room temperature between 15 and 30 degrees C (59 and 86 degrees F). Throw away any unused medicine after the expiration date. Keep container tightly closed.

Ganciclovir capsules

CYTOVENE®;
250 mg; Capsule
Hoffmann La Roche
Inc

CYTOVENE®;
500 mg; Capsule
Hoffmann La Roche
Inc

What are ganciclovir capsules?

GANCICLOVIR (Cytovene®) is used to treat viral infections caused by cytomegalovirus (CMV), including CMV retinitis (viral eye infection) and to prevent CMV infections in patients with compromised immune systems. Generic ganciclovir capsules are available.

What should my health care professional know before I take ganciclovir capsules?

They need to know if you have any of these conditions:
- decreased bone marrow function
- kidney disease or decreased kidney function
- undergoing radiation therapy
- an unusual or allergic reaction to ganciclovir, acyclovir, famciclovir, valacyclovir, valganciclovir, other medicines, foods, dyes, or preservatives
- pregnant or trying to get pregnant
- breast-feeding

How should I take this medicine?

Take ganciclovir capsules by mouth with food. Follow the directions on the prescription label. Swallow capsules with a drink of water; do not crush or open the capsules. Take your doses at regular intervals. Do not take your medicine more often than directed. Finish the full course prescribed by your health care professional even if you think your condition is better. Do not

stop taking except on your prescriber's advice. Contact your pediatrician or health care professional regarding the use of this medicine in children. Special care may be needed.

What if I miss a dose?

If you miss a dose, take it as soon as you can. If it is almost time for your next dose, take only that dose. Do not take double or extra doses.

What may interact with ganciclovir?

- didanosine, ddI
- mycophenolate
- probenecid
- zidovudine, ZDV

Tell your prescriber or health care professional about all other medicines you are taking, including non-prescription medicines, nutritional supplements, or herbal products. Also tell your prescriber or health care professional if you are a frequent user of drinks with caffeine or alcohol, if you smoke, or if you use illegal drugs. These may affect the way your medicine works. Check with your health care professional before stopping or starting any of your medicines.

What should I watch for while taking ganciclovir capsules?

Visit your prescriber or health care professional for regular checks on your progress. You will need regular blood checks. Ganciclovir is not a cure, and repeat courses of the medication are commonly needed to prevent or treat reactivation of the virus. Long-term drug use may be necessary. If you have CMV retinitis have your ophthalmologist check your eyes regularly (about every 4 to 6 weeks). Ganciclovir may increase your risk for other infections or to bruise or bleed. Call your prescriber or health care professional if you have a fever, chills, sore throat or other symptoms of a cold or flu. Do not treat these symptoms yourself. Try to avoid being around people who are sick. Call your prescriber or health care professional if you notice any unusual bleeding. Be careful not to cut, bruise or injure yourself because you may get an infection and bleed more than usual. While you are receiving ganciclovir you must take plenty of fluids. Drink several glasses of water throughout the day. You may need to have an intravenous infusion of fluids to prevent dehydration. Ganciclovir may harm your unborn baby or, in men, decrease sperm production. You should contact your prescriber as soon as possible if you believe or suspect you or your partner has become pregnant while you are taking ganciclovir. Both men and women must use effective birth control continuously while taking ganciclovir. Men should continue to use a condom for at least 90 days after stopping ganciclovir therapy. Do not nurse your baby while you take ganciclovir. Until you know how ganciclovir makes you feel, do not drive, operate machinery or do any other tasks that require you to be alert.

What side effects may I notice from taking ganciclovir?

Side effects that you should report to your prescriber or health care professional as soon as possible:

- low blood counts: ganciclovir may decrease the number of white blood cells, red blood cells and platelets. You may be at increased risk for infections and bleeding.
- signs of infection: fever or chills, cough, sore throat, pain or difficulty passing urine
- signs of decreased platelets or bleeding: bruising, pinpoint red spots on the skin, black, tarry stools, blood in the urine
- signs of decreased red blood cells: unusual weakness or tiredness, fainting spells, lightheadedness
- mouth sores
- seizures (convulsions)
- skin rash, itching
- tingling or pain in hands or feet

Side effects that usually do not require medical attention (report to your prescriber or health care professional if they continue or are bothersome):

- confusion
- diarrhea
- dizziness
- heartburn
- nausea, vomiting
- sedation
- stomach pain
- unstable while walking

Where can I keep my medicine?

Keep out of the reach of children. Store at room temperature between 15 and 30 degrees C (59 and 86 degrees F). Throw away any unused medicine after the expiration date.

Gatifloxacin tablets

TEQUIN®; 400 mg; Tablet Mead Johnson and Co Sub Bristol Myers Co		TEQUIN®; 200 mg; Tablet Mead Johnson and Co Sub Bristol Myers Co	

What are gatifloxacin tablets?

GATIFLOXACIN (Tequin™) is an antibiotic. This drug is discontinued in the United States. It kills certain bacteria or stops their growth. It is used to treat bronchitis, kidney and other urinary tract infections, pneumonia, sinusitis, and certain sexually transmitted diseases. Generic gatifloxacin tablets are not yet available.

What should my health care professional know before I take gatifloxacin?

They need to know if you have any of these conditions:
- diabetes or problems with high or low blood sugar
- heart disease or heart rhythm disturbances
- kidney disease
- liver disease
- long exposure to sunlight (working outdoors)
- seizures (convulsions)
- stomach problems (especially colitis)
- stroke
- taking diuretics (water pills) such as furosemide or hydrochlorothiazide (HCTZ)
- tendon or joint pain
- other chronic conditions
- an unusual or allergic reaction to gatifloxacin, other fluoroquinolone antibiotics, or other medicines, foods, dyes, or preservatives
- pregnant or trying to get pregnant
- breast-feeding

How should I take this medicine?

Take gatifloxacin tablets by mouth with or without food. Follow the directions on the prescription label. Swallow tablets whole with a full glass of water. Take your doses at regular intervals. Do not take your medicine more often than directed. Do not take with magnesium/aluminum antacids, sucralfate, Videx® (didanosine) chewable/buffered tablets or pediatric powder, or with other products containing iron, magnesium, or zinc. Gatifloxacin may be taken 4 hours before taking these products. Finish the full course prescribed by your prescriber or health care professional even if you think your condition is better. Do not stop taking except on your prescriber's advice. This medicine is not for use in children.

What if I miss a dose?

If you miss a dose, take it as soon as you remember. If it is almost time for your next dose, take only that dose. Do not take double or extra doses.

What may interact with gatifloxacin?

- aluminum salts
- antacids
- arsenic trioxide
- astemizole
- bepridil
- calcium salts
- certain heart medications for irregular rhythm (e.g., amiodarone, disopyramide, dofetilide, ibutilide, quinidine, procainamide, sotalol)
- certain medicines for depression or mental problems (e.g., amoxapine, haloperidol, maprotiline, phenothiazines, risperidone, sertindole, ziprasidone)
- cisapride
- clarithromycin
- cyclosporine
- didanosine (ddI)
- digoxin
- dolasetron
- doxercalciferol
- droperidol
- erythromycin
- levomethadyl
- iron (ferrous sulfate) preparations
- magnesium salicylate
- magnesium salts
- manganese
- medicines for diabetes
- multivitamins containing calcium, iron, manganese, or zinc
- NSAIDs such as Advil®, Aleve®, ibuprofen, Motrin®, naproxen
- pentamidine
- probenecid
- probucol
- quinapril
- retinoid products such as tretinoin (Retin-A®, Renova®) or isotretinoin (Accutane®)
- sevelamer
- sucralfate
- terfenadine
- troleandomycin
- warfarin
- zinc salts

Tell your prescriber or health care professional about all other medicines you are taking, including non-prescription medicines, nutritional supplements, or herbal products. Also tell your prescriber or health care professional if you are a frequent user of drinks with caffeine or alcohol, if you smoke, or if you use illegal drugs. These may affect the way your medicine works. Check with your health care professional before stopping or starting any of your medicines.

What should I watch for while taking gatifloxacin?

Tell your prescriber or health care professional if your symptoms do not improve in 2 to 3 days. If you get an unusual reaction stop taking gatifloxacin and call your prescriber or health care professional for advice. If you have diabetes, you should not take gatifloxacin. Gatifloxacin may cause alterations in blood sugar that may be particularly harmful to patients with diabetes. Certain other patients at risk for blood sugar problems, high or low blood sugar, may need to have their blood sugar carefully monitored while taking this drug. If you notice symptoms such as pain, burning, tingling, numbness and/or weakness, stop taking gatifloxacin and contact your healthcare provider immediately. You may get drowsy or dizzy. Do not drive, use machinery, or do anything that needs mental alertness until you know how gatifloxacin affects you. To reduce the risk of dizzy or fainting spells, do not sit or stand up quickly, especially if you are an older patient. Many antacids and multivitamins can interfere with absorption of gatifloxacin. This may stop gatifloxacin from working. Make sure it has been at least 4 hours since you last took gatifloxacin before taking any of these products. Keep out of the sun, or wear protective clothing outdoors and use a sunscreen. Do not use sun lamps or sun tanning beds or booths. If you notice pain or swelling of a tendon or around a joint, stop taking gatifloxacin. Rest the affected area and call your healthcare provider. Do not exercise or resume taking gatifloxacin until your healthcare provider tells you to do so. If you are going to have surgery, tell your prescriber or health care professional that you are taking gatifloxacin.

What side effects may I notice from taking gatifloxacin?

Side effects that you should report to your prescriber or health care professional as soon as possible:
Rare or uncommon:
- confusion
- difficulty breathing
- irregular heartbeat, palpitations or chest pain
- joint, muscle or tendon pain
- redness, blistering, peeling or loosening of the skin, including inside the mouth
- seizures
- severe or watery diarrhea
- skin rash, itching
- swelling of the face or neck
- tingling in hands or feet
- tremor or restlessness
- unusual tiredness or weakness
- vision changes
- vomiting

Side effects that usually do not require medical attention (report to your prescriber or health care professional if they continue or are bothersome):

G

- constipation or diarrhea
- difficulty sleeping
- dizziness or drowsiness
- headache
- nausea or stomach upset

Where can I keep my medicine?
Keep out of the reach of children in a container that small children cannot open. Store at room temperature in a tightly closed container. Throw away any unused medicine after the expiration date.

Gefitinib tablets

IRESSA®;
250 mg; Tablet
AstraZeneca Pharmaceuticals
LP

What are gefitinib tablets?
GEFITINIB (Iressa®) targets a specific protein within cancer cells and stops the cancer cells from growing. Gefitinib is used to treat certain cancers including non-small cell lung cancer. This drug might be used to treat other cancers as well. Generic gefitinib tablets are not available.

What should my health care professional know before I take Gefitinib?
They need to know if you have any of these conditions:
- liver disease
- lung fibrosis
- previous chemotherapy or radiation therapy
- an unusual reaction to gefitinib, other medicines, foods, dyes, or preservatives
- pregnant or trying to get pregnant
- breast-feeding

How should this medicine be used?
Gefitinib tablets are taken by mouth. You may take it with or without food. Follow the directions on the prescription label. Do not take your medicine more often than directed. Contact your pediatrician or health care professional regarding the use of this medicine in children. Special care may be needed.

What if I miss a dose?
Take your missed dose as soon as you remember. If it is almost time for your next dose, take only that one, and skip your missed dose. Do not take extra or double doses.

What may interact with gefitinib?
- amiodarone
- carbamazepine
- antiviral medicines for the treatment of HIV or AIDS
- bosentan
- certain medicines for fungal infections (such as fluconazole, itraconazole, ketoconazole, or voriconazole)
- certain medicines for high blood pressure
- clarithromycin
- dextromethorphan
- erythromycin
- grapefruit juice
- medicines for depression
- phenobarbital
- phenytoin
- propafenone
- rifabutin
- rifampin
- risperidone
- St. John's wort or any herbal products containing St. John's wort
- warfarin

Tell your prescriber or health care professional about all other medicines you are taking, including non-prescription medicines, nutritional supplements, or herbal products. Also tell your prescriber or health care professional if you are a frequent user of drinks with caffeine or alcohol, if you smoke, or if you use illegal drugs. These may affect the way your medicine works. Check with your health care professional before stopping or starting any of your medicines.

What should I watch for while taking gefitinib?
Visit your prescriber or health care professional for checks on your progress. You will need to have regular blood checks. The side effects of gefitinib may continue after you finish your treatment; report side effects promptly. If you experience severe or continuing diarrhea, nausea, decreased appetite, or vomiting, contact your health care provider. Gefitinib has been associated with severe lung adverse reactions. Contact your health care provider if your breathing gets worse and/or you develop any new symptoms such as a cough. There is a risk of birth defects if gefitinib is given during pregnancy. Women should not become pregnant while being treated with gefitinib. Consult with your health care provider regarding appropriate options for birth control while taking gefitinib.

What side effects may I notice from taking Gefitinib?
Side effects that you should report to your prescriber or health care professional as soon as possible:
- eye irritation
- eye pain
- fever
- mouth sores
- problems related to breathing including shortness of breath or cough
- severe or persistent diarrhea, nausea, vomiting, or loss of appetite

Side effects that usually do not require medical attention (report to your prescriber or health care professional if they continue or are bothersome):

- decreased appetite
- diarrhea
- dry skin
- itching
- nausea, vomiting
- skin rash, including acne
- weakness
- weight loss

Where can I keep my medicine?

Keep out of the reach of children in a container that small children cannot open. Store tablets at room temperature between 15 and 30 degrees C (59 and 86 degrees F). Throw away any unused medicine after the expiration date on the label.

Gemfibrozil tablets

LOPID®;
600 mg; Tablet
Parke Davis Division
of Pfizer Co.

GEMFIBROZIL;
600 mg; Tablet
Teva
Pharmaceuticals
USA Inc

What are gemfibrozil tablets?

GEMFIBROZIL (Lopid®) can help prevent cholesterol clogging blood vessels. It lowers blood fats and cholesterol for patients who are at risk of getting heart disease or a stroke. It is only for patients whose cholesterol level is not controlled by diet. It is not a cure. Generic gemfibrozil tablets are available.

What should my health care professional know before I take gemfibrozil?

They need to know if you have any of these conditions:
- gallbladder disease
- kidney disease
- liver disease
- an unusual or allergic reaction to gemfibrozil, other medicines, foods, dyes, or preservatives
- pregnant or trying to get pregnant
- breast-feeding

How should I take this medicine?

Take gemfibrozil tablets by mouth. Follow the directions on the prescription label. Swallow the tablets with a drink of water. Take your doses twice a day, 30 minutes before the morning and evening meal unless otherwise directed. Take your doses at regular intervals. Do not take your medicine more often than directed. Contact your pediatrician or health care professional regarding the use of this medicine in children. Special care may be needed.

What if I miss a dose?

If you miss a dose, take it as soon as you can. If it is almost time for your next dose, take only that dose. Do not take double or extra doses.

What may interact with gemfibrozil?

- bexarotene
- other medications used to lower cholesterol, like colestipol, and the "statin" drugs like atorvastatin, cerivastatin, fluvastatin, lovastatin, pravastatin or simvastatin
- ursodiol
- warfarin
- went yeast

Tell your prescriber or health care professional about all other medicines you are taking, including non-prescription medicines, nutritional supplements, or herbal products. Also tell your prescriber or health care professional if you are a frequent user of drinks with caffeine or alcohol, if you smoke, or if you use illegal drugs. These may affect the way your medicine works. Check with your health care professional before stopping or starting any of your medicines.

What should I watch for while taking gemfibrozil?

Gemfibrozil will not cure your condition, but taken regularly it will help keep down your cholesterol level. Visit your prescriber or health care professional for regular checks on your progress. Do not stop taking gemfibrozil, except on your prescriber's advice. Gemfibrozil is only part of a total cholesterol-lowering program. Your physician or dietician can suggest a low-cholesterol and low-fat diet that will reduce your risk of getting heart and blood vessel disease. Avoid alcohol and smoking, and keep a proper exercise schedule. If you are going to have surgery tell your prescriber or health care professional that you are taking gemfibrozil. If you are diabetic, the dose of your antidiabetic medicine may need to be changed. Gemfibrozil can increase your blood sugar levels. Check with your prescriber or health care professional before you change the dose of your diabetic medicine. You may get drowsy or have blurred vision; until you know how gemfibrozil affects you, do not drive, use machinery, or do anything that needs mental alertness.

What side effects may I notice from taking gemfibrozil?

Side effects that you should report to your prescriber or health care professional as soon as possible:
- cough or hoarseness
- dark yellow or brown urine
- fever or chills
- lower back or side pain
- stomach pain with nausea and vomiting
- muscle pain
- pain or difficulty passing urine
- unusual tiredness
- yellowing of the eyes or skin

G

Side effects that usually do not require medical attention (report to your prescriber or health care professional if they continue or are bothersome):

- blurred vision
- drowsiness, dizziness
- headache
- sexual dysfunction (loss of sexual desire)
- stomach gas, heartburn

Where can I keep my medicine?

Keep out of the reach of children in a container that small children cannot open. Store at room temperature below 30 degrees C (86 degrees F). Keep container tightly closed. Throw away any unused medicine after the expiration date.

Gemifloxacin tablets

FACTIVE®;
320 mg; Tablet
Oscient
Pharmaceuticals

What are gemifloxacin tablets?

GEMIFLOXACIN (Factive®) is an antibacterial agent. It kills certain bacteria or stops their growth. It is used to treat bronchitis and pneumonia. Generic gemifloxacin tablets are not yet available.

What should my health care professional know before I take gemifloxacin?

They need to know if you have any of these conditions:
- diabetes
- heart disease, slow heart beat, recent heart attack
- liver or kidney disease
- long exposure to sunlight (working outdoors)
- low potassium or magnesium levels
- seizures (convulsions)
- stomach problems (especially colitis)
- stroke
- other chronic conditions
- an unusual reaction to gemifloxacin, other fluoroquinolone antibiotics, medicines, foods, dyes, or preservatives
- pregnant or trying to get pregnant
- breast-feeding

How should this medicine be taken?

Take gemifloxacin tablets by mouth with or without food. Follow the directions on the prescription label. Swallow tablets whole with a full glass of water. Take your doses at regular intervals. Do not take your medicine more often than directed. Finish the full course prescribed by your prescriber or health care professional even if you think your condition is better. Do not stop taking except on your prescriber's advice. Contact your pediatrician or health care professional regarding the use of this medicine in children. Special care may be needed.

What if I miss a dose?

If you miss a dose, take it as soon as you remember. If it is almost time for your next dose, take only that dose. Do not take double or extra doses.

What may interact with gemifloxacin?

- aluminum salts
- antacids
- arsenic trioxide
- astemizole
- bepridil
- certain medicines to control the heart rhythm (e.g., amiodarone, disopyramide, dofetilide, flecainide, ibutilide, quinidine, procainamide, propafenone, sotalol)
- certain medicines for depression or mental problems (e.g., amoxapine, haloperidol, maprotiline, phenothiazines, risperidone, sertindole, ziprasidone)
- cisapride
- clarithromycin
- cyclobenzaprine
- didanosine (ddI)
- dolasetron
- droperidol
- erythromycin
- levomethadyl
- iron (ferrous sulfate) preparations
- magnesium salicylate
- magnesium salts
- manganese
- multivitamins containing iron, manganese, or zinc
- NSAIDs such as Advil®, Aleve®, ibuprofen, Motrin®, naproxen
- pentamidine
- probenecid
- probucol
- quinapril
- retinoid products such as tretinoin (Retin-A®, Renova®) or isotretinoin (Accutane®)
- sevelamer
- sucralfate
- terfenadine
- troleandomycin
- zinc salts

Tell your prescriber or health care professional about all other medicines you are taking, including non-prescription medicines, nutritional supplements, or herbal products. Also tell your prescriber or health care professional if you are a frequent user of drinks with caffeine or alcohol, if you smoke, or if you use illegal drugs. These may affect the way your medicine works. Check with your health care professional before stopping or starting any of your medicines.

What should I watch for while taking gemifloxacin?

Tell your prescriber or health care professional if your symptoms do not improve in 2 to 3 days. If you get an unusual reaction stop taking gemifloxacin and call your prescriber or health care professional for advice. If you are a diabetic, monitor your blood glucose carefully while on this medicine. Contact your healthcare professional immediately if there are significant changes in your blood sugar. You may get drowsy or dizzy. Do not drive, use machinery, or do anything that needs mental alertness until you know how gemifloxacin affects you. To reduce the risk of dizzy or fainting spells, do not sit or stand up quickly, especially if you are an older patient. Many antacids and multivitamins can interfere with absorption of gemifloxacin. This may stop gemifloxacin from working. Make sure it has been at least 3 hours since you last took gemifloxacin before taking any of these products. Keep out of the sun, or wear protective clothing outdoors and use a sunscreen. Do not use sun lamps or sun tanning beds or booths. If you notice pain or swelling of a tendon or around a joint, stop taking gemifloxacin. Rest the affected area and call your healthcare provider. Do not exercise or resume taking gemifloxacin until your healthcare provider tells you to do so. If you are going to have surgery, tell your prescriber or health care professional that you are taking gemifloxacin.

What side effects may I notice from taking gemifloxacin?

Side effects that you should report to your prescriber or health care professional as soon as possible:

Rare or uncommon:
- confusion
- difficulty breathing
- irregular heartbeat, palpitations or chest pain
- joint, muscle or tendon pain
- numbness or tingling in hands or feet
- redness, blistering, peeling or loosening of the skin, including inside the mouth
- seizures
- severe or watery diarrhea
- skin rash, itching
- swelling of the face or neck
- tremor or restlessness
- unusual tiredness or weakness
- vomiting

Side effects that usually do not require medical attention (report to your prescriber or health care professional if they continue or are bothersome):
- mild diarrhea
- dizziness
- headache
- nausea or stomach upset
- taste disturbance

Where can I keep my medicine?

Keep out of the reach of children in a container that small children cannot open. Store at room temperature in a tightly closed container. Protect from light. Throw away any unused medicine after the expiration date.

Glimepiride tablets

AMARYL®;
2 mg; Tablet
Aventis
Pharmaceuticals Inc

AMARYL®;
1 mg; Tablet
Aventis
Pharmaceuticals Inc

What are glimepiride tablets?

GLIMEPIRIDE (Amaryl®) helps to treat type 2 diabetes mellitus. Treatment is combined with a suitable diet and balanced exercise. Glimepiride increases the amount of insulin released from the pancreas and helps your body to use insulin more efficiently. Generic glimepiride tablets are available.

What should my health care professional know before I take glimepiride?

They need to know if you have any of these conditions:
- diabetic ketoacidosis
- kidney disease
- liver disease
- major surgery
- severe infection or injury
- thyroid disease
- an unusual or allergic reaction to glimepiride, sulfonamides, other medicines, foods, dyes, or preservatives
- pregnancy or recent attempts to get pregnant
- breast-feeding

How should I take this medicine?

Take glimepiride tablets by mouth. Follow the directions on the prescription label. Swallow the tablets with a drink of water. Take your dose at the same time each day, with breakfast or your first large meal; do not take more often than directed. Contact your pediatrician or health care professional regarding the use of this medicine in children. Special care may be needed. Elderly patients over 65 years old can have a stronger reaction and need a smaller dose.

What if I miss a dose?

If you miss a dose, take it as soon as you can. If it is almost time for your next dose, take only that dose. Do not take double or extra doses.

What may interact with glimepiride?

- bosentan
- medicines for fungal or yeast infections (examples: fluconazole, itraconazole, voriconazole)
- rifampin
- warfarin

Many medications may cause changes (increase or decrease) in blood sugar, these include:
- alcohol-containing beverages
- aspirin and aspirin-like drugs

- beta-blockers, often used for high blood pressure or heart problems (examples include atenolol, metoprolol, propranolol)
- chromium
- female hormones, such as estrogens or progestins, birth control pills
- isoniazid
- male hormones or anabolic steroids
- medications for weight loss
- medicines for allergies, asthma, cold, or cough
- niacin
- pentamidine
- phenytoin
- quinolone antibiotics (examples: ciprofloxacin, levofloxacin, ofloxacin)
- some herbal dietary supplements
- steroid medicines such as prednisone or cortisone
- thyroid hormones
- water pills (diuretics)

Tell your prescriber or health care professional: about all other medicines you are taking including non-prescription medicines; if you are a frequent user of drinks with caffeine or alcohol; if you smoke; or if you use illegal drugs. These can affect the way your medicine works. Check with your health care professional before stopping or starting any of your medicines.

What should I watch for while taking glimepiride?

Visit your prescriber or health care professional for regular checks on your progress. Learn how to monitor regularly blood or urine sugar and urine ketones. Check with your prescriber or health care professional if your blood sugar is high; you might need to change the dose of glimepiride. Do not skip meals. If you are exercising much more than usual, you might need extra snacks to avoid side effects caused by low blood sugar. Alcohol can increase possible side effects of glimepiride. Ask your prescriber or health care professional if you should avoid alcohol. If you have mild symptoms of low blood sugar, eat or drink something containing sugar at once and contact your prescriber or health care professional. It is wise to check your blood sugar to confirm that it is low. It is important to recognize your own symptoms of low blood sugar so that you can treat them quickly. Make sure family members know that you can choke

if you eat and drink when you have serious symptoms of low blood sugar such as seizures or unconsciousness. They must get medical help at once. Glimepiride can increase the sensitivity of your skin to the sun. Keep out of the sun, or wear protective clothing outdoors and use a sunscreen. Do not use sun lamps or sun tanning beds or booths. If you are going to have surgery, tell your prescriber or health care professional that you are taking glimepiride. Wear a medical identification bracelet or chain to say you have diabetes, and carry a card that lists all your medications.

What side effects might I notice from taking glimepiride?

Side effects that you should report to your prescriber or health care professional as soon as possible:
- anxiety or nervousness, confusion, difficulty concentrating
- blurred vision
- breathing difficulties or excessive phlegm
- cold sweats, increased sweating
- cool, pale skin
- coughing up blood
- dark yellow or brown urine
- dizziness, drowsiness
- excessive hunger
- fast heartbeat, palpitations, chest pain
- fever, chills, sore throat
- seizures (convulsions)
- tremor or shakiness
- unusual bleeding or bruising
- unusual tiredness or weakness

Side effects that usually do not require medical attention (report to your prescriber or health care professional if they continue or are bothersome):
- diarrhea
- headache
- heartburn, stomach discomfort
- increased sensitivity to the sun
- nausea, vomiting
- skin rash, redness, swelling, or itching

Where can I keep my medicine?

Keep out of the reach of children in a container that small children cannot open. Store at room temperature below 30 degrees C (86 degrees F). Throw away any unused medicine after the expiration date.

Glipizide tablets and extended-release tablets

GLUCOTROL®; 5 mg; Tablet Roerig Division of Pfizer

GLUCOTROL® XL; 10 mg; Tablet, Extended Release Roerig Division of Pfizer

What are glipizide tablets?

GLIPIZIDE (Glucotrol®, Glucotrol® XL) helps to treat type 2 diabetes mellitus. Treatment is combined with diet and exercise. Glipizide increases the amount of insulin in the blood. Glipizide helps your body to use insulin more efficiently. Generic glipizide tablets and extended-release tablets are available.

What should my health care professional know before I take glipizide?

They need to know if you have any of these conditions:
- kidney disease
- liver disease
- major surgery
- severe infection or injury
- thyroid disease
- an unusual or allergic reaction to glipizide or other sulfonylureas, other medicines, foods, dyes, or preservatives
- pregnant or trying to get pregnant
- breast-feeding

How should I take this medicine?

Take glipizide tablets by mouth. Follow the directions on the prescription label. Swallow the tablets with a drink of water. If you take glipizide once a day, take it 30 minutes before breakfast. Do not take with food. Take your doses at the same time each day; do not take more often than directed. Contact your pediatrician or health care professional regarding the use of this medicine in children. Special care may be needed. Elderly patients over 65 years old may have a stronger reaction and need a smaller dose.

What if I miss a dose?

If you miss a dose, take it as soon as you can. If it is almost time for your next dose, take only that dose. Do not take double or extra doses.

What may interact with glipizide?

- alcohol
- beta-blockers (used for high blood pressure or heart conditions)
- bosentan
- cisapride
- clofibrate
- diazoxide
- medicines for fungal or yeast infections (examples: fluconazole, itraconazole, miconazole, voriconazole)
- metoclopramide
- rifampin
- warfarin (a blood thinner)

Many medications may cause changes (increase or decrease) in blood sugar, these include:

- alcohol-containing beverages
- aspirin and aspirin-like drugs
- beta-blockers, often used for high blood pressure or heart problems (examples include atenolol, metoprolol, propranolol)
- chromium
- female hormones, such as estrogens or progestins, birth control pills
- isoniazid
- male hormones or anabolic steroids
- medications for weight loss
- medicines for allergies, asthma, cold, or cough
- niacin
- pentamidine

- phenytoin
- quinolone antibiotics (examples: ciprofloxacin, levofloxacin, ofloxacin)
- some herbal dietary supplements
- steroid medicines such as prednisone or cortisone
- thyroid hormones
- water pills (diuretics)

Tell your prescriber or health care professional about all other medicines you are taking, including non-prescription medicines, nutritional supplements, or herbal products. Also tell your prescriber or health care professional if you are a frequent user of drinks with caffeine or alcohol, if you smoke, or if you use illegal drugs. These may affect the way your medicine works. Check with your health care professional before stopping or starting any of your medicines.

What should I watch for while taking glipizide?

Visit your prescriber or health care professional for regular checks on your progress. Learn how to monitor blood or urine sugar and urine ketones regularly. Check with your prescriber or health care professional if your blood sugar is high, you may need a change of dose of glipizide. Do not skip meals. If you are exercising much more than usual you may need extra snacks to avoid side effects caused by low blood sugar. Alcohol can increase possible side effects of glipizide. Ask your prescriber or health care professional if you should avoid alcohol. If you have mild symptoms of low blood sugar, eat or drink something containing sugar at once and contact your prescriber or health care professional. It is wise to check your blood sugar to confirm that it is low. It is important to recognize your own symptoms of low blood sugar so that you can treat them quickly. Make sure family members know that you can choke if you eat or drink when you have serious symptoms of low blood sugar, such as seizures or unconsciousness. They must get medical help at once. Glipizide can increase the sensitivity of your skin to the sun. Keep out of the sun, or wear protective clothing outdoors and use a sunscreen. Do not use sun lamps or sun tanning beds or booths. If you are going to have surgery, tell your prescriber or health care professional that you are taking glipizide. Wear a medical identification bracelet or chain to say you have diabetes, and carry a card that lists all your medications.

What side effects may I notice from taking glipizide?

Side effects that you should report to your prescriber or health care professional as soon as possible:
- hypoglycemia (low blood glucose) which can cause symptoms such as anxiety or nervousness, confusion, difficulty concentrating, hunger, pale skin, nausea, fatigue, perspiration, headache, palpitations, numbness of the mouth, tingling in the fingers, tremors, muscle weakness, blurred vision, cold sensations, uncontrolled yawning, irritability, rapid heartbeat, shallow breathing, and loss of consciousness
- breathing difficulties, severe skin reactions or exces-

G

sive phlegm, which may indicate that you are having an allergic reaction to the drug
- dark yellow or brown urine, or yellowing of the eyes or skin, indicating that the drug is affecting your liver
- fever, chills, sore throat; which means the drug may be affecting your immune system
- skin rash, redness, swelling or itching
- unusual bleeding or bruising; which occurs when the drug is affecting your blood clotting system

Side effects that usually do not require medical attention (report to your prescriber or health care professional if they continue or are bothersome):

- diarrhea
- headache
- heartburn, stomach discomfort
- increased sensitivity of the skin to the sun
- nausea, vomiting

Where can I keep my medicine?

Keep out of the reach of children in a container that small children cannot open. Store at room temperature below 30 degrees C (86 degrees F). Throw away any unused medicine after the expiration date.

Glipizide; Metformin tablets

METAGLIP™;
2.5 mg/250 mg;
Tablet
Bristol Myers Squibb Co

METAGLIP™;
2.5 mg/500 mg;
Tablet
Bristol Myers Squibb Co

What are glipizide; metformin tablets?

GLIPIZIDE; METFORMIN (Metaglip™) helps to treat type 2 diabetes mellitus. Treatment is combined with a balanced diet and exercise. This medicine lowers blood sugar and helps your body to use insulin more efficiently. Generic glipizide; metformin tablets are available.

What should my health care professional know before I take glipizide; metformin?

They need to know if you have any of these conditions:
- frequently drink alcohol or alcohol-containing beverages
- become easily dehydrated
- heart attack
- heart failure
- hormone changes or problems
- kidney disease
- liver disease
- polycystic ovaries
- serious infection or injury
- stroke
- thyroid disease
- undergoing surgery or certain x-ray procedures with injectable contrast agents
- an unusual or allergic reaction to glipizide, sulfonamides, metformin, other medicines, foods, dyes, or preservatives
- pregnant or trying to get pregnant
- breast-feeding

How should this medicine be used?

Take glipizide; metformin tablets by mouth with meals. Follow the directions on the prescription label. Swallow the tablets with a drink of water. Take your doses at the same time each day; do not take more often than directed. Contact your pediatrician or health care professional regarding the use of this medicine in children. Special care may be needed. Patients over 65 years old may need a smaller dose than younger adults.

What if I miss a dose?

If you miss a dose, take it as soon as you can. If it is almost time for your next dose, take only that dose. Do not take double or extra doses.

What may interact with glipizide; metformin?

- alcohol
- antifungal medicines like fluconazole, itraconazole or miconazole
- asparaginase
- cephalexin
- chloramphenicol
- cimetidine
- cisapride
- cyclosporine
- digoxin
- dofetilide
- entecavir
- guanethidine
- lithium
- metoclopramide
- morphine
- niacin
- nifedipine
- octreotide
- other medicines for diabetes
- procainamide
- propantheline
- quinine
- quinidine
- ranitidine
- trimethoprim
- vancomycin
- warfarin
- water pills (diuretics like amiloride, furosemide, triamterene)

Many medications may cause changes (increase or decrease) in blood sugar, these include:
- alcohol-containing beverages
- aspirin and aspirin-like drugs

- beta-blockers, often used for high blood pressure or heart problems (examples include atenolol, metoprolol, propranolol)
- chromium
- female hormones, such as estrogens or progestins, birth control pills
- isoniazid
- male hormones or anabolic steroids
- medications for weight loss
- medicines for allergies, asthma, cold or cough
- niacin
- pentamidine
- phenytoin
- quinolone antibiotics (examples: ciprofloxacin, levofloxacin, ofloxacin)
- some herbal dietary supplements
- steroid medicines such as prednisone or cortisone
- thyroid hormones
- water pills (diuretics like amiloride, furosemide, triamterene)

Tell your prescriber or health care professional about all other medicines you are taking, including non-prescription medicines, nutritional supplements, or herbal products. Also tell your prescriber or health care professional if you are a frequent user of drinks with caffeine or alcohol, if you smoke, or if you use illegal drugs. These may affect the way your medicine works. Check with your health care professional before stopping or starting any of your medicines.

What should I watch for while taking glipizide; metformin?

Visit your prescriber or health care professional for regular checks on your progress. Your prescriber will check your blood sugar, kidney function, and other tests from time to time. Learn how to monitor your blood sugar. Learn what to do if you have high or low blood sugar. Do not skip meals. If you are exercising much more than usual you may need extra snacks to avoid side effects caused by low blood sugar. Do not change your medication dose without talking to your prescriber. Alcohol can increase possible side effects of this medicine. You should avoid excessive or regular alcohol use. Ask your prescriber if you should avoid alcohol. If you have mild symptoms of low blood sugar, eat or drink something containing sugar at once and contact your health care professional. It is wise to check your blood sugar to confirm that it is low. It is important to recognize your own symptoms of low blood sugar so that you can treat them quickly. Make sure family members know that you can choke if you eat or drink when you develop serious symptoms of low blood sugar, such as seizures or unconsciousness. They must get medical help at once. If you develop a severe diarrhea or vomiting, or are unable to maintain proper fluid intake, you should contact your prescriber. "Sick-days" may require adjustments to your dosage or your illness may need to be evaluated. Ask your prescriber what you should do if you become ill. This medicine can increase the sensitivity of your skin to the sun; wear protective clothing outdoors and use a sunscreen. Do not use sun lamps or sun tanning beds or booths. If you are going to have surgery or will need an x-ray procedure that uses contrast agents, tell your prescriber or health care professional that you are taking this medicine. Wear a medical identification bracelet or chain to say you have diabetes, and carry a card that lists all your medications.

What side effects may I notice from taking glipizide; metformin?

Side effects that you should report to your prescriber or health care professional as soon as possible:

- breathing difficulties or shortness of breath
- dark yellow or brown urine
- dizziness
- fever, chills, or frequent sore throats
- muscle pain
- passing out or fainting
- severe vomiting or diarrhea
- skin rash, redness, swelling, or itching
- slow or irregular heartbeat
- unusual weakness, fatigue or discomfort
- unusual stomach pain or discomfort
- yellowing of the eyes or skin

Symptoms of low blood sugar (hypoglycemia). Know the symptoms of low blood sugar, so that you can quickly treat them; which may include:

- anxiety or nervousness, confusion, difficulty concentrating, hunger, pale skin, nausea, fatigue, sweating, headache, palpitations, numbness of the mouth, tingling in the fingers, tremors, muscle weakness, blurred vision, cold sensations, uncontrolled yawning, irritability, rapid heartbeat, shallow breathing, and loss of consciousness. Hypoglycemia may cause you to not be aware of your actions or surroundings if it is severe, so you should let others know what to do if you cannot help yourself in a severe reaction.

Symptoms of high blood sugar (hyperglycemia) include:

- dizziness, dry mouth, flushed dry-skin, loss of appetite, nausea, stomach cramping, unusual thirst, frequent passing of urine

Side effects that usually do not require medical attention (report to your prescriber or health care professional if they continue or are bothersome):

- decreased appetite
- diarrhea
- gas
- headache
- heartburn
- increased sensitivity to the sun
- metallic taste in the mouth
- mild stomachache
- nausea
- weight loss

Where can I keep my medicine?

Keep out of the reach of children in a container that small children cannot open. Store at room temperature between 15 and 25 degrees C (59 and 77 degrees F). Keep container tightly closed and protect from light. Throw away any unused medicine after the expiration date.

G

Glucagon injection

GLUCAGON®;
1 mg; Injection
Eli Lilly and Co

What is glucagon injection?

GLUCAGON occurs naturally in the body. It is produced in the pancreas and increases blood sugar. Extra glucagon sometimes has to be given as an emergency treatment for severely low blood sugar (hypoglycemia) in diabetic patients, especially if they are not able to take sugar by mouth. Glucagon is also used as a diagnostic aid in x-ray examinations of the stomach and other digestive organs. Generic glucagon injections are available.

What should my health care professional know before I receive glucagon?

They need to know if you have any of these conditions:
- adrenal gland dysfunction
- blood vessel disease
- malnutrition
- pancreatic tumors
- pheochromocytoma
- an unusual or allergic reaction to glucagon, other medicines, foods, dyes, or preservatives

How should I use this medicine?

Glucagon can be an emergency treatment for a life-threatening situation. It is extremely important that someone in your household knows how and when to use this medicine. Use exactly as directed. Do not use higher doses or more often than recommended. Give glucagon as soon as possible after discovering that the diabetic patient is unconscious. After the injection, turn the patient on his/her side to prevent choking if they vomit. If the patient does not respond in 15 to 20 minutes, give a second injection and get the patient to an emergency room. Glucagon is for injection into a muscle. Glucagon injection has to be prepared from a separate powder and liquid that must be mixed before the injection can be given. Instructions for mixing and giving the injection are included in the package. Before an emergency arises, you and the person(s) most likely to give you a glucagon injection should read these instructions carefully. Check with your prescriber, pharmacist, or health care professional, if there is something you do not understand. Make sure that your emergency kit contains an appropriately sized sterile syringe and needle. Contact your pediatrician or health care professional regarding the use of this medicine in children. Special care may be needed.

What if I miss a dose?

This does not apply.

What may interact with glucagon?

- beta-blockers, often used for high blood pressure or heart problems
- phenytoin
- warfarin

Tell your prescriber or health care professional about all other medicines you are taking, including non-prescription medicines, nutritional supplements, or herbal products. Also tell your prescriber or health care professional if you are a frequent user of drinks with caffeine or alcohol, if you smoke, or if you use illegal drugs. These may affect the way your medicine works. Check with your health care professional before stopping or starting any of your medicines.

What should I watch for while taking glucagon?

If you often have periods of low blood sugar, keep a glucagon kit with you at all times. Wear a Medic Alert bracelet or necklace or carry an identification card with details of your name, your condition, medicines, and the name of your prescriber or health care professional. Show your family members and others where you keep this kit and how to use it. They need to know how to use it before you need it. They can practice by giving you your normal insulin shots. It is important that they practice. A person who has never given you a shot will probably not be able to do it in an emergency. Symptoms of low blood sugar vary from person to person. Learn to recognize your own; they can include: confusion; cool, pale skin or cold sweats; drowsiness; extreme hunger; fast heartbeat; headache; nausea, vomiting; nervousness or anxiety; shakiness or unsteadiness; tiredness; weakness; or visual changes. Eat or drink something sweet (fruit juice, honey, soft drinks, sugar or sugar water, or syrup) if you get these symptoms. If you do not feel better, ask someone to help you get to a prescriber or health care professional or emergency room right away. Do not attempt to drive yourself. Also, remind the person that he/she may need to give you a glucagon injection before medical treatment is available. After a response to an injection of glucagon, you should eat or drink some carbohydrates to prevent secondary hypoglycemia.

What side effects may I notice from taking glucagon?

Side effects that you should report to your prescriber or health care professional as soon as possible:
- chest pain or fast, irregular heartbeat (palpitations)
- dizziness or lightheadedness
- difficulty breathing
- muscle cramps
- unusual weakness

Side effects that usually do not require medical attention (report to your prescriber or health care professional if they continue or are bothersome):

- nausea, vomiting
- rash, itching

Glucosamine tablets and capsules

500 mg; Capsule
Walgreens Health Initiatives

What is glucosamine?

GLUCOSAMINE is a non-prescription dietary supplement that is being promoted for its ability to ease osteoarthritis symptoms, which may occur with aging as our joints undergo "wear-and-tear." Glucosamine is a substance found naturally in our bodies that helps maintain healthy joint cartilage. There is some proof that supplementing this substance may help reduce symptoms associated with osteoarthritis. Glucosamine supplementation has not been shown to help rheumatoid arthritis, a different arthritic condition than osteoarthritis. Glucosamine is not officially endorsed by the FDA.

What should my health care professional know before I take glucosamine?

It is important for you to tell your prescriber or other health care professional that you are using glucosamine. You should discuss this supplement with your health care professional BEFORE taking it if you have any of these conditions:

- diabetes mellitus
- kidney disease
- liver disease
- stomach or intestinal problems
- an unusual or allergic reaction to glucosamine, other medicines, foods, dyes, or preservatives
- pregnant or trying to get pregnant
- breast-feeding

How should I take this medicine?

Glucosamine tablets and capsules should be taken orally (i.e., swallowed). Follow the directions on the product label or consult your health care professional for advice. The effects of glucosamine take several weeks to appear so it should be taken daily for several weeks for best results. Take your doses at regular intervals. Do not take this supplement more often than directed. Contact your pediatrician or health care professional regarding the use of this medicine in children. Special care may be needed.

What if I miss a dose?

Missing a dose is probably not harmful. If you miss a dose, simply resume taking it on your previous schedule. Do not take double or extra doses.

Where can I keep my medicine?

Keep out of the reach of children. After mixing the injection solution, use within 48 hours if stored in a refrigerator between 2 and 8 degrees C (36 and 46 degrees F). Throw away any unused portion.

What may interact with glucosamine?

- warfarin

For many dietary supplements, interactions with other medications are unknown. That is why you should always be careful when mixing them with traditional medications. If you take any other medications, consult with your health care professional prior to taking glucosamine. Tell your prescriber or health care professional about all other medicines you are taking, including non-prescription medicines, nutritional supplements, or herbal products. Also tell your prescriber or health care professional if you are a frequent user of drinks with caffeine or alcohol, if you smoke, or if you use illegal drugs. These may affect the way your medicine works. Check with your health care professional before stopping or starting any of your medicines.

What should I watch for while taking glucosamine?

If you notice any changes in your physical health while taking glucosamine, you should contact your health care provider. Also, different brands of glucosamine might contain different amounts of active ingredient so try to use the same brand. It is unclear if glucosamine may increase blood sugar if you have diabetes, some studies indicate that no significant change in blood sugar is expected. If you are diabetic, you may wish to monitor your blood sugar more frequently when you first start this supplement. Discuss any changes in your blood sugar control with your prescriber.

What side effects may I notice from taking glucosamine?

Side effects that you should report to your prescriber or health care professional as soon as possible:

- constipation or diarrhea
- headache
- loss of appetite
- swelling of the face, feet or ankles
- skin rash or itching
- stomach pain

Side effects that usually do not require medical attention (report to your prescriber or health care professional if they continue or are bothersome):

- gas
- nausea
- upset stomach

Where can I keep my medicine?

Keep out of the reach of children. Store at room temperature between 8 and 25 degrees C (46 and 77 degrees F); do not freeze. Throw away any unused medicine after the expiration date. GENERAL INFORMATION REGARDING DIETARY SUPPLEMENTS: Dietary supplements include amino acids, vitamins, minerals, herbs, and other plant-derived substances, and extracts of these substances. Products are easy to identify as they must state "Dietary Supplement" on the label. A "Supplement Facts" panel is provided on the label for most products. Supplements are not drugs and are not regulated like pharmaceuticals. You should note that rigid quality control standards are not required for dietary supplements. Differences in the potency and purity of these products can occur. Scientific data to support the use of a dietary supplement for a certain condition may not be available. This product is not intended to diagnose, treat, cure or prevent any disease. The Food and Drug Administration suggests the following to help consumers protect themselves:

- Always read product labels and follow directions.
- Look for products containing ingredients with the "USP" notation. This indicates the manufacturer followed the standards of the US Pharmacopoeia.
- "Natural" doesn't mean a product is safe for humans to consume.
- Supplements produced or distributed by a nationally known food or drug company are more likely to be made under tight controls as these companies have standards in place for their other products. You can write to the company or manufacturer for more information about the conditions under which the products are made.

Glyburide tablets

DIABETA®;
5 mg; Tablet
Hoechst Roussel
Pharmaceuticals Div

MICRONASE®;
5 mg; Tablet
Pharmacia and
Upjohn Div Pfizer

What are glyburide tablets?

GLYBURIDE (DiaBeta®, Glynase™, Micronase®) helps to treat type 2 diabetes mellitus. Treatment is combined with a suitable diet and balanced exercise. Glyburide increases the amount of insulin released from the pancreas and helps your body to use insulin more efficiently. Generic glyburide tablets are available.

What should my health care professional know before I take glyburide?

They need to know if you have any of these conditions:
- kidney disease
- liver disease
- major surgery
- severe infection or injury
- thyroid disease
- an unusual or allergic reaction to glyburide, sulfonamides, other medicines, foods, dyes, or preservatives
- pregnant or trying to get pregnant
- breast-feeding

How should I take this medicine?

Take glyburide tablets by mouth. Follow the directions on the prescription label. Swallow the tablets with a drink of water. If you take glyburide once a day, take it with breakfast or the first main meal of the day. Take your doses at the same time each day; do not take more often than directed. Contact your pediatrician or health care professional regarding the use of this medicine in children. Special care may be needed. Elderly patients over 65 years old may have a stronger reaction and need a smaller dose.

What if I miss a dose?

If you miss a dose, take it as soon as you can. If it is almost time for your next dose, take only that dose. Do not take double or extra doses.

What may interact with glyburide?

- alcohol
- beta-blockers (used for high blood pressure or heart conditions)
- bosentan (bosentan should not be taken with glyburide, contact your prescriber)
- cisapride
- clofibrate
- diazoxide
- medicines for fungal or yeast infections (examples: fluconazole, itraconazole, miconazole, voriconazole)
- metoclopramide
- rifampin
- warfarin (a blood thinner)

Many medications may cause changes (increase or decrease) in blood sugar, these include:

- alcohol-containing beverages
- aspirin and aspirin-like drugs
- beta-blockers, often used for high blood pressure or heart problems (examples include atenolol, metoprolol, propranolol)
- chromium
- female hormones, such as estrogens or progestins, birth control pills
- isoniazid
- male hormones or anabolic steroids
- medications for weight loss
- medicines for allergies, asthma, cold, or cough
- niacin
- pentamidine
- phenytoin
- quinolone antibiotics (examples: ciprofloxacin, levofloxacin, ofloxacin)
- some herbal dietary supplements
- steroid medicines such as prednisone or cortisone

- thyroid hormones
- water pills (diuretics)

Tell your prescriber or health care professional about all other medicines you are taking, including non-prescription medicines, nutritional supplements, or herbal products. Also tell your prescriber or health care professional if you are a frequent user of drinks with caffeine or alcohol, if you smoke, or if you use illegal drugs. These may affect the way your medicine works. Check with your health care professional before stopping or starting any of your medicines.

What should I watch for while taking glyburide?

Visit your prescriber or health care professional for regular checks on your progress. Learn how to monitor blood or urine sugar and urine ketones regularly. Check with your prescriber or health care professional if your blood sugar is high, you may need a change of dose of glyburide. Do not skip meals. If you are exercising much more than usual you may need extra snacks to avoid side effects caused by low blood sugar. Alcohol can increase possible side effects of glyburide. Ask your prescriber or health care professional if you should avoid alcohol. If you have mild symptoms of low blood sugar, eat or drink something containing sugar at once and contact your prescriber or health care professional. It is wise to check your blood sugar to confirm that it is low. It is important to recognize your own symptoms of low blood sugar so that you can treat them quickly. Make sure family members know that you can choke if you eat or drink when you develop serious symptoms of low blood sugar, such as seizures or unconsciousness. They must get medical help at once. Glyburide can increase the sensitivity of your skin to the sun. Keep out of the sun, or wear protective clothing outdoors and use a sunscreen. Do not use sun lamps or sun tanning beds or booths. If you are going to have surgery, tell your prescriber or health care professional that you are taking glyburide. Wear a medical identification bracelet or chain to say you have diabetes, and carry a card that lists all your medications.

What side effects may I notice from taking glyburide?

Side effects that you should report to your prescriber or health care professional as soon as possible:
- hypoglycemia (low blood glucose), which can cause symptoms such as anxiety or nervousness, confusion, difficulty concentrating, hunger, pale skin, nausea, fatigue, perspiration, headache, palpitations, numbness of the mouth, tingling in the fingers, tremors, muscle weakness, blurred vision, cold sensations, uncontrolled yawning, irritability, rapid heartbeat, shallow breathing, and loss of consciousness
- breathing difficulties, severe skin reactions or excessive phlegm, which may indicate that you are having an allergic reaction to the drug
- dark yellow or brown urine, or yellowing of the eyes or skin, indicating that the drug is affecting your liver
- fever, chills, sore throat; which means the drug may be affecting your immune system
- unusual bleeding or bruising; which occurs when the drug is affecting your blood clotting system

Side effects that usually do not require medical attention (report to your prescriber or health care professional if they continue or are bothersome):
- headache
- heartburn, stomach discomfort
- increased sensitivity to the sun
- nausea, vomiting
- skin rash, redness, swelling or itching

Where can I keep my medicine?

Keep out of the reach of children in a container that small children cannot open. Store at room temperature between 15 and 30 degrees C (59 and 86 degrees F). Keep container tightly closed. Throw away any unused medicine after the expiration date.

Glyburide; Metformin tablets

| GLUCOVANCE®; 2.5 mg/500 mg; Tablet Bristol Myers Squibb Co | | GLUCOVANCE®; 5 mg/500 mg; Tablet Bristol Myers Squibb Co | |

What are glyburide; metformin tablets?

GLYBURIDE; METFORMIN (Glucovance®) helps to treat type 2 diabetes mellitus. Treatment is combined with a balanced diet and exercise. This medicine lowers blood sugar and helps your body to use insulin more efficiently. Generic glyburide; metformin tablets are available.

What should my health care professional know before I take glyburide; metformin?

They need to know if you have any of these conditions:
- frequently drink alcohol or alcohol-containing beverages
- become easily dehydrated
- heart attack
- heart failure
- hormone changes or problems
- kidney disease
- liver disease
- polycystic ovaries
- serious infection or injury
- stroke
- thyroid disease
- undergoing surgery or certain x-ray procedures with injectable contrast agents
- an unusual or allergic reaction to glyburide, sulfon-

amides, metformin, other medicines, foods, dyes, or preservatives
- pregnant or trying to get pregnant
- breast-feeding

How should I take this medicine?

Take glyburide; metformin tablets by mouth with meals. Follow the directions on the prescription label. Swallow the tablets with a drink of water. Take your doses at the same time each day; do not take more often than directed. Contact your pediatrician or health care professional regarding the use of this medicine in children. Special care may be needed. Patients over 65 years old may need a smaller dose than younger adults.

What if I miss a dose?

If you miss a dose, take it as soon as you can. If it is almost time for your next dose, take only that dose. Do not take double or extra doses.

What may interact with glyburide; metformin?

- alcohol
- antifungal medicines like miconazole
- asparaginase
- bosentan (bosentan should not be taken with glyburide, contact your prescriber)
- cephalexin
- chloramphenicol
- cimetidine
- cisapride
- cyclosporine
- digoxin
- dofetilide
- entecavir
- fluconazole
- guanethidine
- lithium
- metoclopramide
- morphine
- niacin
- nifedipine
- octreotide
- other medicines for diabetes
- procainamide
- propantheline
- quinine
- quinidine
- ranitidine
- trimethoprim
- vancomycin
- warfarin
- water pills (diuretics like amiloride, furosemide, triamterene)

Many medications may cause changes (increase or decrease) in blood sugar, these include:

- alcohol-containing beverages
- aspirin and aspirin-like drugs
- beta-blockers, often used for high blood pressure or heart problems (examples include atenolol, metoprolol, propranolol)
- chromium
- female hormones, such as estrogens or progestins, birth control pills
- isoniazid
- male hormones or anabolic steroids
- medications for weight loss
- medicines for allergies, asthma, cold, or cough
- niacin
- pentamidine
- phenytoin
- quinolone antibiotics (examples: ciprofloxacin, levofloxacin, ofloxacin)
- some herbal dietary supplements
- steroid medicines such as prednisone or cortisone
- thyroid hormones
- water pills (diuretics)

Tell your prescriber or health care professional about all other medicines you are taking, including non-prescription medicines, nutritional supplements, or herbal products. Also tell your prescriber or health care professional if you are a frequent user of drinks with caffeine or alcohol, if you smoke, or if you use illegal drugs. These may affect the way your medicine works. Check with your health care professional before stopping or starting any of your medicines.

What should I watch for while taking glyburide; metformin?

Visit your prescriber or health care professional for regular checks on your progress. Your prescriber will check your blood sugar, kidney function, and other tests from time to time. Learn how to monitor your blood sugar. Learn what to do if you have high or low blood sugar. Do not skip meals. If you are exercising much more than usual you may need extra snacks to avoid side effects caused by low blood sugar. Do not change your medication dose without talking to your prescriber. Alcohol can increase possible side effects of this medicine. You should avoid excessive or regular alcohol use. Ask your prescriber if you should avoid alcohol. If you have mild symptoms of low blood sugar, eat or drink something containing sugar at once and contact your health care professional. It is wise to check your blood sugar to confirm that it is low. It is important to recognize your own symptoms of low blood sugar so that you can treat them quickly. Make sure family members know that you can choke if you eat or drink when you develop serious symptoms of low blood sugar, such as seizures or unconsciousness. They must get medical help at once. If you develop a severe diarrhea or vomiting, or are unable to maintain proper fluid intake, you should contact your prescriber. "Sick-days" may require adjustments to your dosage or your illness may need to be evaluated. Ask your prescriber what you should do if you become ill. This medicine can increase the sensitivity of your skin to the sun; wear protective clothing outdoors and use a sunscreen. Do not use sun lamps or sun tanning beds or booths. If you are going to have surgery or will need an x-ray procedure that uses contrast agents, tell your prescriber or health care professional that you are taking this medicine. Wear a medical identification bracelet or chain to say you have diabetes, and carry a card that lists all your medications.

What side effects may I notice from taking glyburide; metformin?

Side effects that you should report to your prescriber or health care professional as soon as possible:
- breathing difficulties or shortness of breath
- dark yellow or brown urine
- dizziness
- fever, chills, or frequent sore throats
- muscle pain
- passing out or fainting
- severe vomiting or diarrhea
- skin rash
- slow or irregular heartbeat
- unusual weakness, fatigue or discomfort
- unusual stomach pain or discomfort
- yellowing of the eyes or skin

Symptoms of low blood sugar (hypoglycemia). Know the symptoms of low blood sugar, so that you can quickly treat them; which may include:
- anxiety or nervousness, confusion, difficulty concentrating, hunger, pale skin, nausea, fatigue, sweating, headache, palpitations, numbness of the mouth, tingling in the fingers, tremors, muscle weakness, blurred vision, cold sensations, uncontrolled yawning, irritability, rapid heartbeat, shallow breathing, and loss of consciousness. Hypoglycemia may cause you to not be aware of your actions or surroundings if it is severe, so you should let others know what to do if you cannot help yourself in a severe reaction.

Symptoms of high blood sugar (hyperglycemia) include:
- dizziness, dry mouth, flushed dry-skin, loss of appetite, nausea, stomach cramping, unusual thirst, frequent passing of urine

Side effects that usually do not require medical attention (report to your prescriber or health care professional if they continue or are bothersome):
- decreased appetite
- gas
- heartburn
- increased sensitivity to the sun
- metallic taste in the mouth
- mild stomachache
- nausea
- weight loss

Where can I keep my medicine?

Keep out of the reach of children in a container that small children cannot open. Store at room temperature between 15 and 25 degrees C (59 and 77 degrees F). Keep container tightly closed and protect from light. Throw away any unused medicine after the expiration date.

Granisetron tablets

KYTRIL®;
1 mg; Tablet
Hoffmann La Roche Inc

What are granisetron tablets?

GRANISETRON (Kytril®) helps to relieve nausea and vomiting, especially when associated with the treatment of cancer (chemotherapy). Generic granisetron tablets are not yet available.

What should my health care professional know before I take granisetron?

They need to know if you have any of these conditions:
- liver disease
- an unusual or allergic reaction to granisetron, ondansetron, other medicines, foods, dyes, or preservatives
- pregnant or trying to get pregnant
- breast-feeding

How should I take this medicine?

Take granisetron tablets by mouth. Swallow the tablets with a drink of water. Granisetron is given within 60 minutes before chemotherapy. In some cases, a second dose is given about 12 hours after the first dose. Contact your pediatrician or health care professional regarding the use of this medicine in children. Special care may be needed.

What if I miss a dose?

This does not apply. Granisetron is only given on the day(s) chemotherapy is given.

What may interact with granisetron?

- ketoconazole

Tell your prescriber or health care professional about all other medicines you are taking, including non-prescription medicines. Also tell your prescriber or health care professional if you are a frequent user of drinks with caffeine or alcohol, if you smoke, or if you use illegal drugs. These may affect the way your medicine works. Check with your health care professional before stopping or starting any of your medicines.

What should I watch for while taking granisetron?

Your condition will be monitored after taking granisetron.

What side effects may I notice from taking granisetron?

Side effects that you should report to your prescriber or health care professional as soon as possible:

Rare or uncommon:
- difficulty breathing, wheezing, shortness of breath
- fast or irregular heartbeat
- tightness in the chest
- swelling of the face, tongue, throat, hands and feet

Side effects that usually do not require medical attention (report to your prescriber or health care professional if they continue or are bothersome):
- constipation or diarrhea
- difficulty sleeping
- dizziness
- drowsiness
- fainting or lightheadedness

- fever
- headache
- nervousness
- skin rash, itching
- stomach pain
- tiredness

Where can I keep my medicine?

Keep out of the reach of children in a container that small children cannot open. Store at room temperature between 15 and 30 degrees C (56 and 86 degrees F). Protect from light. Throw away any unused medicine after the expiration date.

Griseofulvin tablets or capsules

GRIS-PEG®; 250 mg; Tablet Pedinol Pharmacal Inc

GRIS-PEG®; 125 mg; Tablet Pedinol Pharmacal Inc

What are griseofulvin tablets or capsules?

GRISEOFULVIN (Grifulvin®V, Grisactin®, Gris-PEG®) is an antifungal type of antibiotic. It treats fungus infections, caused by tinea organisms, of the skin, hair, and nails. Griseofulvin is used for infections that do not go away when treated with antifungal skin products. Generic griseofulvin tablets and capsules are available.

What should my health care professional know before I take griseofulvin?

They need to know if you have any of these conditions:
- liver disease
- on a low-fat diet
- other chronic illness
- porphyria
- systemic lupus erythematosus (SLE)
- an unusual or allergic reaction to griseofulvin, penicillin, other foods, dyes or preservatives
- pregnant or trying to get pregnant
- breast-feeding

How should I take this medicine?

Take griseofulvin capsules or tablets by mouth. Follow the directions on the prescription label. Griseofulvin works best if you take it with high-fat food or milk. Take griseofulvin at regular intervals through the day and night. For example two doses a day means one dose every 12 hours; three doses a day means one dose every 8 hours. Do not take your medicine more often than directed. Finish the full course prescribed by your prescriber or health care professional even if you feel better. Do not stop taking except on your prescriber's advice. Contact your pediatrician or health care professional regarding the use of this medicine in children. Special care may be needed.

What if I miss a dose?

If you miss a dose, take it as soon as you can. If it is almost time for your next dose, take only that dose. Do not take double or extra doses.

What may interact with griseofulvin?

- alcohol
- barbiturate medicines for inducing sleep or treating seizures (convulsions)
- cyclosporine
- female hormones, including contraceptive or birth control pills
- primidone
- warfarin

Tell your prescriber or health care professional about all other medicines you are taking, including non-prescription medicines, nutritional supplements, or herbal products. Also tell your prescriber or health care professional if you are a frequent user of drinks with caffeine or alcohol, if you smoke, or if you use illegal drugs. These may affect the way your medicine works. Check with your health care professional before stopping or starting any of your medicines.

What should I watch for while taking griseofulvin?

Tell your prescriber or health care professional if your symptoms do not begin to improve in 1 to 2 weeks. Some fungal infections need many weeks or months of treatment to cure. Use your medicine regularly for as long as your prescriber or health care professional tells you to. Oral contraceptives that contain estrogen may not work properly while you take griseofulvin. Use an additional method of birth control while you take griseofulvin and for one month afterwards. You may get drowsy or dizzy; until you know how griseofulvin affects you, do not drive, use machinery, or do anything that needs mental alertness. Alcohol may make you more drowsy, and increase flushing and a rapid heartbeat. Avoid alcoholic drinks. Keep out of the sun, or wear protective clothing and use a sunscreen. Do not use sun lamps or sun tanning beds or booths. To help prevent reinfection, wear freshly washed cotton, not synthetic, clothing.

After bathing make sure your skin is quite dry. Fungal infections like moist conditions. Do not walk about barefoot. You can use an antifungal powder once or twice a day.

What side effects may I notice from taking griseofulvin?

Side effects that you should report to your prescriber or health care professional as soon as possible:
- dark yellow or brown urine
- confusion
- increased sensitivity to the sun or ultraviolet light
- loss of appetite
- mouth sores
- skin rash, redness, blistering, or peeling of skin
- sore throat, fever

- tingling or numbness in the hands or feet
- unusual weakness or tiredness
- yellowing of the eyes or skin

Side effects that usually do not require medical attention (report to your prescriber or health care professional if they continue or are bothersome):
- difficulty sleeping
- dizziness
- flatulence (gas), heartburn
- headache
- nausea, vomiting
- stomach pain

Where can I keep my medicine?

Keep out of the reach of children in a container that small children cannot open. Store at room temperature between 15 and 30 degrees C (59 and 86 degrees F). Keep container tightly closed. Throw away any unused medicine after the expiration date.

Guaifenesin oral dosage forms

MUCINEX®; 600 mg; Tablet, Extended Release Adams Laboratories

BIDEX™; 400 mg; Tablet Stewart-Jackson Pharmacal Inc

What is guaifenesin?

GUAIFENESIN (Humibid®, Mucinex™, Muco-Fen®, Robitussin®, Bidex™ and others) helps treat coughs caused by colds or the flu. It loosens phlegm or mucus in the lungs. It is not intended to treat chronic cough caused by smoking, asthma, emphysema, heart failure, or problems in which there is a large amount of phlegm. Generic guaifenesin is available as prescription or non-prescription capsules, extended-release capsules, tablets, extended-release tablets, and oral liquids. Generic Mucinex™ tablets are not available.

What should my health care professional know before I take guaifenesin?

They need to know if you have any of these conditions:
- asthma
- chronic bronchitis
- emphysema
- fever
- heart problems (such as heart failure)
- smoker
- an unusual or allergic reaction to guaifenesin, other medicines, foods, dyes, or preservatives
- pregnant or trying to get pregnant
- breast-feeding

How should I take this medicine?

Take guaifenesin by mouth. Follow the directions on the prescription label. Swallow the medicine with a full glass of water. Do not cut, crush, bite, or chew the delayed-release tablets or capsules. Use a specially marked spoon or container to measure the liquid medicine. Ask your pharmacist if you do not have one; household spoons are not always accurate. Take your doses at regular intervals. Do not take your medicine more often than directed.

What if I miss a dose?

If you are taking guaifenesin on a regular schedule and miss a dose, take it as soon as you can. If it is almost time for your next dose, take only that dose. Do not take double or extra doses.

What may interact with guaifenesin?

No interactions between guaifenesin and other medicines have been recorded.

Some medications can cause a cough such as ACE inhibitors (captopril, enalapril, and others) which are used to treat high blood pressure or heart failure. Tell your doctor about all the prescription medications you are taking. Tell your prescriber or health care professional about all other medicines you are taking, including non-prescription medicines, nutritional supplements, or herbal products. Also tell your prescriber or health care professional if you are a frequent user of drinks with caffeine or alcohol, if you smoke, or if you use illegal drugs. These may affect the way your medicine works. Check with your health care professional before stopping or starting any of your medicines.

What should I watch for while taking guaifenesin?

Do not treat yourself for a cough for more than 1 week without consulting your prescriber or health care professional. If you also have a high fever, skin rash, continuing headache, or sore throat, ask your prescriber or health care professional for advice. You may feel drowsy or dizzy. Do not drive, use machinery, or do anything that needs mental alertness until you know

G

how guaifenesin affects you. Alcohol can make you more drowsy or dizzy; avoid alcoholic drinks. Drink plenty of water while you are taking guaifenesin; this will help loosen the mucus.

What side effects may I notice from taking guaifenesin?

Side effects that you should report to your prescriber or health care professional as soon as possible:
Rare (more likely with excessive doses of guaifenesin):
- side pain or back pain that extends to the groin (signs of kidney stones)

Side effects that usually do not require medical attention (report to your prescriber or health care professional if they continue or are bothersome):

Uncommon:
- diarrhea
- drowsiness or dizziness
- headache
- nausea or vomiting
- stomach pain
- rash

Where can I keep my medicine?

Keep out of the reach of children in a container that small children cannot open. Store at room temperature between 15 and 30 degrees C (59 and 86 degrees F). Do not freeze liquid products. Keep container tightly closed. Throw away any unused medicine after the expiration date.

Guaifenesin; Hydrocodone tablets

What are guaifenesin; hydrocodone tablets?

GUAIFENESIN; HYDROCODONE (Pneumotussin® Tablets) helps to stop or reduce coughing due to the common cold or inhaled irritants. Federal law prohibits the transfer of hydrocodone to any person other than the patient for whom it was prescribed. Do not share this medicine with anyone else. Generic guaifenesin; hydrocodone tablets are not available.

What should my health care professional know before I take guaifenesin; hydrocodone?

They need to know if you have any of these conditions:
- asthma or difficulties breathing
- chronic bronchitis
- constipation or diarrhea
- emphysema or other lung disease
- glaucoma
- heart disease
- intestinal or stomach problems
- kidney disease or a history of kidney stones
- liver disease
- other chronic illness
- pain or difficulty passing urine
- recent head trauma
- smoker
- an allergic or unusual reaction to codeine, hydromorphone, hydrocodone, oxycodone, morphine, guaifenesin, other medicines, foods, dyes, or preservatives
- pregnant or trying to get pregnant
- breast-feeding

How should I take this medicine?

Take guaifenesin; hydrocodone tablets by mouth. Follow the directions on the prescription label. Swallow the tablets whole with a full glass of water. Take guaifenesin; hydrocodone with food or milk if it upsets your stomach. Take your doses at regular intervals. Do not take your medicine more often than directed. Contact your pediatrician or health care professional regarding the use of this medicine in children. Special care may be needed. The tablets may not be swallowed easily by younger children. It is important that doses are only given at the time intervals recommended by your health care professional. Do not share this medicine with anyone.

What if I miss a dose?

If it is almost time for your next dose, take only that dose. Do not take double doses. Each dose of this cough medicine should be taken at least 4 hours apart from the previous dose. Do not take more frequently than how it was prescribed by your health care professional.

What may interact with guaifenesin; hydrocodone?

- alcohol and alcohol-containing medicines
- chloroquine
- certain medicines used for pain
- certain medicines used for Parkinson's disease
- certain medicines used to control the heart's rhythm
- cimetidine
- medicines for diarrhea
- medicines used for psychosis
- medicines used for sleep, anxiety or depression
- quinacrine
- rifabutin
- rifampin
- ritonavir
- seizure medications
- some antihistamines

Tell your prescriber or health care professional about all other medicines you are taking, including non-prescription medicines, nutritional supplements, or herbal products. Also tell your prescriber or health care professional if you are a frequent user of drinks with caffeine or alcohol, if you smoke, or if you use illegal drugs. These may affect the way your medicine works. Check

with your health care professional before stopping or starting any of your medicines.

What should I watch for while taking guaifenesin; hydrocodone?

Tell your prescriber or health care professional if your cough does not improve in 7 days. If you have a high fever, skin rash, or persistent headache as well as a cough, see your prescriber or health care professional. Use exactly as directed by your prescriber or health care professional. If you are taking guaifenesin; hydrocodone on a regular basis, do not suddenly stop taking it. Your prescriber may want to slowly lower your dose. You may get drowsy or dizzy when you first start taking this medicine. Be careful taking other medications that may also make you tired. Do not drive, use machinery, or do anything that needs mental alertness until you know how this medicine affects you. Stand or sit up slowly to reduce the risk of dizzy or fainting spells. The drowsiness should decrease after taking this medicine for a couple of days. Alcohol can increase the possible drowsiness, dizziness or confusion from this medicine. Do not drink alcoholic beverages while taking this medicine. Your mouth may get dry. Drinking plenty of water, chewing sugarless gum or sucking on hard candy may help to relieve dry mouth symptoms. Also, this medicine may cause dry eyes and blurred vision. If you wear contact lenses you may feel some discomfort. Lubricating drops may help. See your ophthalmologist if the problem does not go away or is severe. This cough medicine may cause constipation. You may need to take a laxative and/or a stool softener. Try to have a bowel movement at least every 2 to 3 days. If you do not have a bowel movement for 3 days or more call your prescriber or health care professional. They may recommend using an enema or suppository to help you move your bowels. If you are going to have surgery, tell your prescriber or health care professional that you are taking this medicine.

What side effects may I notice from taking guaifenesin; hydrocodone?

Side effects that you should report to your prescriber or health care professional as soon as possible:
Rare or uncommon:
- side or back pain that extends to the groin (signs of kidney stones)
- confusion
- difficulty breathing
- decreased ability to pass urine
- feeling faint
- slow or fast heartbeat

Side effects that usually do not require medical attention (report to your prescriber or health care professional if they continue or are bothersome):
More common:
- blurred vision
- constipation or diarrhea
- drowsiness, dizziness
- dry mouth
- headache
- itching
- stomach upset, nausea

Where can I keep my medicine?

Keep out of the reach of children in a container that small children cannot open. Avoid accidental swallowing of guaifenesin; hydrocodone by someone (especially children) other than the person for whom it was prescribed as this may result in severe effects and possibly death. Store at room temperature between 15 and 30 degrees C (59 and 86 degrees F). Protect from light. Throw away any unused medicine after the expiration date.

Guaifenesin; Hydrocodone; Pseudoephedrine tablets

What are guaifenesin; hydrocodone; pseudoephedrine tablets?

GUAIFENESIN; HYDROCODONE; PSEUDO-EPHEDRINE (Deconamine CX®, Entuss-D® and others) helps to stop or reduce coughing and nasal congestion (stuffiness) due to the common cold or respiratory infections. Federal law prohibits the use of hydrocodone in any person other than the patient for whom it was prescribed. Do not share this medicine with anyone else. Generic guaifenesin; hydrocodone; pseudoephedrine oral tablets are available.

What should my health care professional know before I take guaifenesin; hydrocodone; pseudoephedrine?

They need to know if you have any of these conditions:
- asthma or breathing problems
- blood vessel disease
- chronic bronchitis
- constipation or diarrhea
- diabetes
- emphysema or other lung disease
- fever
- glaucoma
- heart disease or heart rhythm problems
- high blood pressure
- intestinal or stomach problems
- kidney disease
- liver disease
- other chronic illness
- overactive thyroid
- pain or difficulty passing urine
- peripheral vascular disease
- prostate trouble

- recent head trauma
- smoker
- an allergic or unusual reaction to codeine, hydrocodone, hydromorphone, oxycodone, morphine, guaifenesin, pseudoephedrine, other medicines, foods, dyes, or preservatives
- pregnant or trying to get pregnant
- breast-feeding

How should this medicine be taken?

Take guaifenesin; hydrocodone; pseudoephedrine tablets by mouth. Follow the directions on the prescription label. Take this medicine with food or milk if it upsets your stomach. Take your doses at regular intervals. Do not take your medicine more often than directed. Do not share this medicine with anyone. Take this medicine with a full glass of water to help loosen and clear mucus from your throat. Elderly patients over 60 years old may have a stronger reaction to this medicine. Contact your pediatrician or health care professional regarding the use of this medicine in children. Special care may be needed.

What if I miss a dose?

If it is almost time for your next dose (less than 2 hours), take only that dose. Do not take double doses. Each dose of this cough medicine should be taken at least 4 hours apart. Do not take more frequently than how it was prescribed by your health care professional.

What may interact with guaifenesin; hydrocodone; pseudoephedrine?

- alcohol and alcohol-containing medicines
- amphetamine or other stimulant drugs
- bicarbonate, citrate, or acetate products (such as sodium bicarbonate, sodium acetate, sodium citrate, sodium lactate, and potassium citrate)
- caffeine
- chloroquine
- certain medicines used for pain
- certain medicines used for Parkinson's disease
- cimetidine
- furazolidone
- linezolid
- medicines for diabetes
- medicines for diarrhea
- medicines known as MAO inhibitors, such as phenelzine (Nardil®), tranylcypromine (Parnate®), isocarboxazid (Marplan®), and selegiline (Carbex®, Eldepryl®)
- medicines used for depression or psychosis
- medicines used for sleep or anxiety
- procarbazine
- quinacrine
- rifabutin
- rifampin
- ritonavir
- seizure medications
- some antihistamines
- some medicines for chest pain, heart disease, high blood pressure or heart rhythm problems

- some medicines for weight loss (including some herbal products, ephedrine, dextroamphetamine)
- St. John's wort
- theophylline
- thyroid hormones

Tell your prescriber or health care professional about all other medicines you are taking, including non-prescription medicines, nutritional supplements, or herbal products. Also tell your prescriber or health care professional if you are a frequent user of drinks with caffeine or alcohol, if you smoke, or if you use illegal drugs. These may affect the way your medicine works. Check with your health care professional before stopping or starting any of your medicines.

What should I watch for while taking guaifenesin; hydrocodone; pseudoephedrine?

Tell your prescriber or health care professional if your cough does not improve in 7 days. If you have a high fever, skin rash, or persistent headache as well as a cough, see your prescriber or health care professional. Use exactly as directed by your prescriber or health care professional. If you are taking guaifenesin; hydrocodone; pseudoephedrine on a regular basis, do not suddenly stop taking it. Your prescriber may want to slowly lower your dose. You may get drowsy or dizzy when you first start taking this medicine. Be careful taking other medications that may also make you tired. Do not drive, use machinery, or do anything that needs mental alertness until you know how this medicine affects you. Stand or sit up slowly to reduce the risk of dizzy or fainting spells. The drowsiness should decrease after taking this medicine for a couple of days. Alcohol can increase the possible drowsiness, dizziness or confusion from this medicine. Do not drink alcoholic beverages while taking this medicine. Your mouth may get dry. Drinking plenty of water, chewing sugarless gum, or sucking on hard candy may help to relieve dry mouth symptoms. Also, this medicine may cause dry eyes and blurred vision. If you wear contact lenses you may feel some discomfort. Lubricating drops may help. See your ophthalmologist if the problem does not go away or is severe. This cough medicine may cause constipation. You may need to take a laxative and/or a stool softener. Try to have a bowel movement at least every 2 to 3 days. If you do not have a bowel movement for 3 days or more call your prescriber or health care professional. They may recommend using an enema or suppository to help you move your bowels. If this medicine makes it difficult for you to sleep at night; take your last dose at least 2 hours before bedtime. If nervousness, dizziness, or sleeplessness occur, stop using this medicine and consult your health care provider. If you are going to have surgery, tell your prescriber or health care professional that you are taking this medicine.

What side effects may I notice from taking guaifenesin; hydrocodone; pseudoephedrine?

Side effects that you should report to your prescriber or health care professional as soon as possible:

Rare or uncommon:
- chest pain, palpitations
- confusion
- decreased ability to pass urine
- difficulty breathing
- fainting spells, or dizziness which does not go away
- numbness or tingling in the hands or feet
- skin rash or itching
- severe, persistent, or worsening headache

More common:
- anxiety or nervousness
- blurred vision
- fast, slow, or irregular heartbeat
- increased blood pressure
- excessive sweating
- sleeplessness (insomnia)
- tremor or muscle contractions

- vomiting

Side effects that usually do not require medical attention (report to your prescriber or health care professional if they continue or are bothersome):
- constipation
- drowsiness
- dry mouth
- headache (mild)
- stomach upset, nausea

Where can I keep my medicine?

Keep out of the reach of children in a container that small children cannot open. Store at room temperature, between 15 and 30 degrees C (59 and 86 degrees F); do not freeze. Keep the container tightly closed. Throw away any unused medicine after the expiration date.

Guaifenesin; Phenylephrine extended-release capsules and tablets

DECONSAL II;
20 mg; 375 mg;
Capsule Carolina
Pharmaceuticals

ENTEX LA;
30 mg; 600 mg;
Tablet Andrx
Pharmaceuticals

What are guaifenesin; phenylephrine extended-release capsules and tablets?

GUAIFENESIN; PHENYLEPHRINE (Deconsal®, Entex® ER, Entex® LA, Guaifed®, Guaifed-PD®, Guaitex® LA, PhenaVent™, Prolex® PD, Respa® PE, and others) is a combination product used to decrease congestion and help with cough symptoms. Phenylephrine is a decongestant that decreases nasal or sinus congestion (stuffiness). Guaifenesin is an expectorant that loosens phlegm or mucus. This product is not intended to treat chronic cough caused by smoking, asthma, emphysema, heart failure. Extended-release guaifenesin; phenylephrine capsules can give relief for up to 12 hours. Generic extended-release capsules and tablets are available.

What should my health care professional know before I take guaifenesin; phenylephrine?

They need to know if you have any of these conditions:
- asthma
- blood vessel disease
- chronic bronchitis
- diabetes
- difficulty urinating (urinary retention)
- emphysema
- fever
- glaucoma
- heart disease or heart rhythm problems
- high blood pressure
- kidney disease
- liver disease
- overactive thyroid
- peripheral vascular disease
- prostate trouble

- an unusual reaction to guaifenesin; phenylephrine, other medicines, foods, dyes, or preservatives
- pregnant or trying to get pregnant
- breast-feeding

How should this medicine be used?

Take guaifenesin; phenylephrine extended-release capsules or tablets by mouth. Follow the directions on the prescription label. Swallow whole with a drink of water; do not bite, crush or chew. Take your doses at regular intervals. Do not take your medicine more often than directed. Contact your pediatrician or health care professional regarding the use of this medicine in children. Special care may be needed. Elderly patients over 60 years old may have a stronger reaction to this medicine.

What if I miss a dose?

If you miss a dose, and you are taking it on a regular schedule, take it as soon as you can. If it is almost time for your next dose (less than 12 hours), take only that dose. Do not take double or extra doses.

What may interact with guaifenesin; phenylephrine?

- amphetamine or other stimulant drugs
- bromocriptine
- cocaine
- furazolidone
- linezolid
- medicines for colds and breathing difficulties
- medicines for diabetes
- medicines known as MAO inhibitors, such as phenelzine (Nardil®), tranylcypromine (Parnate®), isocar-

boxazid (Marplan®), and selegiline (Carbex®, Elde-pryl®)
- medicines for mental depression
- medicines for migraine
- procarbazine
- some medicines for chest pain, heart disease, high blood pressure or heart rhythm problems
- some medicines for weight loss (including some herbal products, ephedrine, dextroamphetamine)
- St. John's wort
- theophylline
- thyroid hormones

Some medications can cause a cough such as ACE inhibitors (captopril, enalapril, and others) which are used to treat high blood pressure or heart failure. Tell your doctor about all the prescription medications you are taking. Tell your prescriber or health care professional about all other medicines you are taking, including non-prescription medicines, nutritional supplements, or herbal products. Also tell your prescriber or health care professional if you are a frequent user of drinks with caffeine or alcohol, if you smoke, or if you use illegal drugs. These may affect the way your medicine works. Check with your health care professional before stopping or starting any of your medicines.

What should I watch for while taking guaifenesin; phenylephrine?

Check with your prescriber or health care professional if your congestion has not improved within 7 days, or if you have a high fever, skin rash, continuing headache, or sore throat with your cough. These signs may mean that you have other medical problems. If guaifenesin; phenylephrine extended-release products make it difficult for you to sleep at night; take your last dose at least 12 hours before bedtime. If nervousness, dizziness, or sleeplessness occur, stop using this drug and consult a physician. Drink plenty of fluids while you are taking this drug; this will help loosen the mucus. If you are going to have surgery, tell your prescriber you are taking guaifenesin; phenylephrine.

What side effects may I notice from taking guaifenesin; phenylephrine?

Side effects that you should report to your prescriber or health care professional as soon as possible:

Rare (more likely with excessive doses):
- pain in the side or back pain that extends to the groin (signs of kidney stones)
- persistent or unusual rash

Uncommon:
- bloody diarrhea and abdominal pain
- chest pain
- confusion
- dizziness or fainting spells
- numbness or tingling in the hands or feet
- pain or difficulty passing urine
- rapid or troubled breathing
- severe, persistent, or worsening headache

More common:
- anxiety or nervousness
- fast or irregular heartbeat, palpitations
- increased blood pressure
- increased sweating
- sleeplessness (insomnia)
- tremor or muscle contractions
- vomiting

Side effects that usually do not require medical attention (report to your prescriber or health care professional if they continue or are bothersome):
- diarrhea
- difficulty sleeping
- headache (mild)
- increased sensitivity to sunlight
- loss of appetite
- stomach upset, nausea
- restlessness

Where can I keep my medicine?

Keep out of the reach of children in a container that small children cannot open. Store at room temperature, between 15 and 30 degrees C (59 and 86 degrees F), unless otherwise specified on the product label. Protect from heat and moisture. Throw away any unused medicine after the expiration date.

Guaifenesin; Potassium Guaiacolsulfonate extended-release tablets

HUMIBID® LA;
600 mg/300 mg; Tablet, Carolina
Pharmaceuticals

What is guaifenesin; potassium guaiacolsulfonate?

GUAIFENESIN; POTASSIUM GUAIACOLSULFONATE (Humibid® LA) helps treat cough caused by colds or the flu. It loosens phlegm or mucus in the lungs. It is not intended to treat chronic cough caused by smoking, asthma, emphysema, heart failure, or problems in which there is a large amount of phlegm. Generic guaifenesin; potassium guaiacolsulfonate extended-release tablets are not available.

What should my health care professional know before I take guaifenesin; potassium guaiacolsulfonate?

They need to know if you have any of these conditions:
- asthma
- chronic bronchitis
- emphysema
- fever
- heart problems
- smoker

- an unusual reaction to guaifenesin; potassium guaiacolsulfonate, medicines, foods, dyes, or preservatives
- pregnant or trying to get pregnant
- breast-feeding

How should this medicine be taken?

Take guaifenesin; potassium guaiacolsulfonate tablets by mouth. Follow the directions on the prescription label. Swallow tablets with only small amounts of water. Do not crush, bite, or chew the tablets. Take your doses at regular intervals. Do not take your medicine more often than directed. Guaifenesin; potassium guaiacolsulfonate should not be given to children less than 12 years of age.

What if I miss a dose?

If you are taking guaifenesin; potassium guaiacolsulfonate on a regular schedule and miss a dose, take it as soon as you can. If it is almost time for your next dose, take only that dose. Do not take double or extra doses.

What may interact with guaifenesin; potassium guaiacolsulfonate?

No interactions between guaifenesin; potassium guaiacolsulfonate and other medicines have been recorded. Some medications can cause a cough such as ACE inhibitors (captopril, enalapril, and others) which are used to treat high blood pressure or heart failure. Tell your doctor about all the prescription medications you are taking. Tell your prescriber or health care professional about all other medicines you are taking, including non-prescription medicines, nutritional supplements, or herbal products. Also tell your prescriber or health care professional if you are a frequent user of drinks with caffeine or alcohol, if you smoke, or if you use illegal drugs. These may affect the way your medicine works. Check with your health care professional before stopping or starting any of your medicines.

What should I watch for while taking guaifenesin; potassium guaiacolsulfonate?

Do not treat yourself for a cough for more than 1 week without consulting your prescriber or health care professional. If you also have a high fever, skin rash, continuing headache, or sore throat, ask your prescriber or health care professional for advice. You may feel drowsy or dizzy. Do not drive, use machinery, or do anything that needs mental alertness until you know how this medicine affects you. Alcohol can make you more drowsy or dizzy; avoid alcoholic drinks. Drink plenty of water while you are taking guaifenesin; this will help loosen the mucus.

What side effects may I notice from taking guaifenesin; potassium guaiacolsulfonate?

Side effects that you should report to your prescriber or health care professional as soon as possible:
Rare (more likely with excessive doses of guaifenesin):
- side pain or back pain that extends to the groin (signs of kidney stones)

Side effects that usually do not require medical attention (report to your prescriber or health care professional if they continue or are bothersome):
Uncommon:
- diarrhea
- drowsiness or dizziness
- headache
- nausea or vomiting
- stomach pain
- rash

Where can I keep my medicine?

Keep out of the reach of children in a container that small children cannot open. Store at room temperature between 20 and 25 degrees C (68 and 77 degrees F) in a dry location. Keep container tightly closed. Throw away any unused medicine after the expiration date.

G

Guaifenesin; Pseudoephedrine regular and extended-release tablets or capsules

NASABID™ SR; 600 mg/90 mg; Tablet, Extended Release Anabolic Inc		SUDAFED® NON-DRYING SINUS; 200 mg/30 mg; Capsule Pfizer Consumer Healthcare

What are guaifenesin; pseudoephedrine regular or extended-release tablets or capsules?

GUAIFENESIN; PSEUDOEPHEDRINE (Duratuss™, Nasabid™ SR, Sudafed® Non-Drying Sinus, Ru-Tuss® DE, Nalex®, Mucinex® D, Sudafed®, Zephrex®, and others) is a combination product which is a decongestant and cough expectorant. It contains pseudoephedrine which can decrease nasal or sinus congestion (stuffiness) due to colds, the flu, or allergies. It also contains guaifenesin which loosens phlegm or mucus in the lungs, but is not intended to treat chronic cough caused by smoking, asthma, emphysema, heart failure, or problems in which there is a large amount of phlegm. Extended-release guaifenesin; pseudoephedrine tablets can give relief for up to 12 hours. Generic guaifenesin; pseudoephedrine regular and extended-release tablets or capsules are available.

What should my health care professional know before I take guaifenesin; pseudoephedrine?

They need to know if you have any of the following conditions:
- asthma
- blood vessel disease

- chronic bronchitis
- diabetes
- difficulty urinating (urinary retention)
- emphysema
- fever
- glaucoma
- heart disease or heart rhythm problems
- high blood pressure
- kidney disease
- overactive thyroid
- peripheral vascular disease
- prostate trouble
- an unusual or allergic reaction to guaifenesin, pseudo-ephedrine, other medicines, foods, dyes, or preservatives
- pregnant or trying to get pregnant
- breast-feeding

How should I take this medicine?

Take guaifenesin; pseudoephedrine extended-release tablets or capsules by mouth. Follow the directions on the prescription label. Swallow whole with a drink of water; do not bite, crush or chew. If the tablet has a groove in it, the tablet may be divided in half for a smaller dose by breaking the tablet along the groove. The tablet piece (one-half tablet) should be swallowed whole (do not bite or chew). Take your doses at regular intervals. Do not take your medicine more often than directed. Contact your pediatrician or health care professional regarding the use of this medicine in children. Elderly patients over 60 years old may have a stronger reaction to this medicine. Do not use extended-release products until you know how you react to guaifenesin; pseudoephedrine.

What if I miss a dose?

If you miss a dose, and you are taking it on a regular schedule, take it as soon as you can. If it is almost time for your next dose (less than 12 hours), take only that dose. Do not take double or extra doses.

What may interact with guaifenesin; pseudoephedrine?

- ammonium chloride
- amphetamine or other stimulant drugs
- bicarbonate, citrate, or acetate products (such as sodium bicarbonate, sodium acetate, sodium citrate, sodium lactate, and potassium citrate)
- bromocriptine
- cocaine
- furazolidone
- linezolid
- medicines for colds and breathing difficulties
- medicines for diabetes
- medicines known as MAO inhibitors, such as phenelzine (Nardil®), tranylcypromine (Parnate®), isocarboxazid (Marplan®), and selegiline (Carbex®, Eldepryl®)
- medicines for mental depression
- medicines for migraine
- procarbazine
- some medicines for chest pain, heart disease, high blood pressure or heart rhythm problems
- some medicines for weight loss (including some herbal products, ephedrine, dextroamphetamine)
- St. John's wort
- theophylline
- thyroid hormones

Some medications can cause a cough such as ACE inhibitors (captopril, enalapril, and others) which are used to treat high blood pressure or heart failure. Tell your doctor about all the prescription medications you are taking. Tell your prescriber or health care professional about all other medicines you are taking, including non-prescription medicines, nutritional supplements, or herbal products. Also tell your prescriber or health care professional if you are a frequent user of drinks with caffeine or alcohol, if you smoke, or if you use illegal drugs. These may affect the way your medicine works. Check before starting or stopping any of your medicines.

What should I watch for while taking guaifenesin; pseudoephedrine?

Check with your prescriber or health care professional if your congestion has not improved within 7 days, or if you have a high fever, skin rash, continuing headache, or sore throat with your cough. These signs may mean that you have other medical problems. If guaifenesin; pseudoephedrine extended-release products make it difficult for you to sleep at night; take your last dose at least 12 hours before bedtime. If nervousness, dizziness, or sleeplessness occur, stop using guaifenesin-pseudoephedrine and consult a physician. Drink plenty of water while you are taking guaifenesin; pseudoephedrine; this will help loosen the mucus. If you are going to have surgery, tell your prescriber you are taking guaifenesin; pseudoephedrine.

What side effects may I notice from taking guaifenesin; pseudoephedrine?

Side effects that you should report to your prescriber or health care professional as soon as possible:

Rare (more likely with excessive doses of guaifenesin; pseudoephedrine):
- pain in the side or back pain that extends to the groin (signs of kidney stones)
- persistent or unusual rash

Uncommon:
- bloody diarrhea and abdominal pain
- chest pain
- confusion
- dizziness or fainting spells
- numbness or tingling in the hands or feet
- pain or difficulty passing urine
- rapid or troubled breathing
- severe, persistent, or worsening headache

More common:
- anxiety or nervousness
- fast or irregular heartbeat, palpitations
- increased blood pressure
- increased sweating

- sleeplessness (insomnia)
- tremor or muscle contractions
- vomiting

Side effects that usually do not require medical attention (report to your prescriber or health care professional if they continue or are bothersome):

- diarrhea
- difficulty sleeping
- drowsiness
- headache (mild)
- increased sensitivity to sunlight

- loss of appetite
- stomach upset, nausea
- reddening of the skin (mild or temporary skin rash)
- restlessness

Where can I keep my medicine?

Keep out of the reach of children in a container that small children cannot open. Store at room temperature, between 15 and 30 degrees C (59 and 86 degrees F), unless otherwise specified on the product label. Protect from heat and moisture. Throw away any unused medicine after the expiration date.

Guanabenz tablets

GUANABENZ; 4 mg; Tablet Ivax Pharmaceuticals Inc	
GUANABENZ; 8 mg; Tablet Ivax Pharmaceuticals Inc	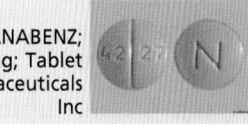

What are guanabenz tablets?

GUANABENZ (Wytensin®) is an antihypertensive. Guanabenz relaxes blood vessels, relieving high blood pressure (hypertension). It is not a cure and has to be used regularly. Untreated high blood pressure can cause a stroke, heart failure, or damage to your kidneys. Generic guanabenz tablets are available.

What should my health care professional know before I take guanabenz?

They need to know if you have any of these conditions:

- heart or blood vessel disease
- kidney disease
- liver disease
- recent heart attack or stroke
- an unusual or allergic reaction to guanabenz, other medicines, foods, dyes, or preservatives
- pregnant or trying to get pregnant
- breast-feeding

How should I take this medicine?

Take guanabenz tablets by mouth. Follow the directions on the prescription label. Swallow the tablets with a drink of water. Take your doses at regular intervals. Do not take your medicine more often than directed. Do not stop taking except on your prescriber's advice. Contact your pediatrician or health care professional regarding the use of this medicine in children. Special care may be needed.

What if I miss a dose?

If you miss a dose, take it as soon as you can. If it is almost time for your next dose, take only that dose. Do not take double or extra doses.

What may interact with guanabenz?

- hawthorn
- medicine for mental depression

Tell your prescriber or health care professional about all other medicines you are taking, including non-prescription medicines, nutritional supplements, or herbal products. Also tell your prescriber or health care professional if you are a frequent user of drinks with caffeine or alcohol, if you smoke, or if you use illegal drugs. These may affect the way your medicine works. Check with your health care professional before stopping or starting any of your medicines.

What should I watch for while taking guanabenz?

Visit your prescriber or health care professional for regular checks on your progress. Check your heart rate and blood pressure regularly while you are taking guanabenz. Ask your prescriber or health care professional what your heart rate should be and when you should contact him or her. Do not suddenly stop taking guanabenz. You must gradually reduce the dose or you may get a dangerous increase in blood pressure. Ask your prescriber or health care professional for advice. You may get drowsy or dizzy. Do not drive, use machinery, or do anything that needs mental alertness until you know how guanabenz affects you. To avoid dizzy or fainting spells, do not stand or sit up quickly, especially if you are an older person. Alcohol can make you more drowsy and dizzy. Avoid alcoholic drinks. Your mouth may get dry. Chewing sugarless gum or sucking hard candy, and drinking plenty of water will help. Do not treat yourself for coughs, colds or allergies without asking your prescriber or health care professional for advice. Some ingredients can affect your blood pressure control. If you are going to have surgery tell your prescriber or health care professional that you are taking guanabenz.

What side effects may I notice from taking guanabenz?

Stopping taking guanabenz can produce some of these side effects. Ask your prescriber or health care professional before you reduce your dose, or stop taking guanabenz.

Side effects that you should report to your prescriber or health care professional as soon as possible:

- difficulty breathing
- dizziness

- increased sweating
- increase in the amount of urine passed
- irregular heartbeat or palpitations, chest pain
- muscle weakness or pain
- nausea, vomiting
- ringing in the ears
- stomach pain
- swelling of feet or legs
- trembling, shakiness

Side effects that usually do not require medical attention (report to your prescriber or health care professional if they continue or are bothersome):

- blurred vision
- breast tenderness in men or women

- depression
- drowsiness
- dry mouth
- headache
- nasal congestion
- sexual difficulties (reduced sexual desire or ability)
- skin rash, itching
- weakness or tiredness

Where can I keep my medicine?

Keep out of the reach of children in a container that small children cannot open. Store at room temperature, approximately 25 degrees C (77 degrees F). Protect from light. Keep container tightly closed. Throw away any unused medicine after the expiration date.

Guanfacine tablets

TENEX®;
2 mg; Tablet
ESP Pharma Inc

TENEX®;
1 mg; Tablet
ESP Pharma Inc

What are guanfacine tablets?

GUANFACINE (Tenex®) is an antihypertensive. Guanfacine relaxes blood vessels, relieving high blood pressure (hypertension). It is not a cure and must be taken regularly to prevent complications of uncontrolled blood pressure. Untreated high blood pressure can cause a stroke, heart failure, or damage to your kidneys. Generic guanfacine tablets are available.

What should my health care professional know before I take guanfacine?

They need to know if you have any of these conditions:

- an unusual or allergic reaction to guanfacine, other medicines, foods, dyes, or preservatives
- breast-feeding
- depression
- heart or blood vessel disease
- kidney disease
- liver disease
- pregnant or trying to get pregnant
- recent heart attack or stroke

How should I take this medicine?

Take guanfacine tablets by mouth. Follow the directions on the prescription label. Swallow the tablets with a drink of water. Take your doses at regular intervals. Do not take your medicine more often than directed. Do not stop taking except on your prescriber's advice. Contact your pediatrician or health care professional regarding the use of this medicine in children. Special care may be needed. Older patients (over 65 years old) may have a stronger reaction to this medicine and need smaller doses.

What if I miss a dose?

If you miss a dose, take it as soon as you can. If it is almost time for your next dose, take only that dose. Do not take double or extra doses. It is important not to miss a dose of guanfacine. Even one or two missed

doses can cause serious side effects. If you do miss more than one or two doses, check with your prescriber or health care professional.

What may interact with guanfacine?

- alcohol
- barbiturate medicines for inducing sleep or treating seizures (convulsions)
- beta blockers, often used for high blood pressure or heart problems
- diet pills
- hawthorn
- medicines for anxiety such as benzodiazepines
- medicines for colds and breathing difficulties
- medicines for high blood pressure
- medicine for mental depression
- medicine for pain or inflammation
- phenytoin, often used for treating seizures (convulsions)
- water pills or diuretics

Tell your prescriber or health care professional about all other medicines you are taking, including non-prescription medicines, nutritional supplements, or herbal products. Also tell your prescriber or health care professional if you are a frequent user of drinks with caffeine or alcohol, if you smoke, or if you use illegal drugs. These may affect the way your medicine works. Check with your health care professional before stopping or starting any of your medicines.

What should I watch for while taking guanfacine?

Visit your prescriber or health care professional for regular checks on your progress. Check your heart rate and blood pressure regularly while you are taking guanfacine. Ask your prescriber or health care professional what your heart rate should be and when you should contact him or her. Do not suddenly stop taking guanfacine. You must gradually reduce the dose or you may get a dangerous increase in blood pressure. Ask your prescriber or health care professional for advice. You may get drowsy or dizzy. Do not drive, use machinery, or do anything that needs mental alertness until you know how guanfacine affects you. To avoid dizzy or fainting spells, do not stand or sit up quickly, especially if you are an older person. Alcohol can make you more drowsy and dizzy. Avoid alcoholic drinks. Your mouth may get dry. Chewing sugarless gum or sucking hard candy, and drinking plenty of water will help. Do not treat yourself for coughs, colds or allergies without asking your prescriber or health care professional for advice. Some ingredients can affect your blood pressure control. If you are going to have surgery tell your prescriber or health care professional that you are taking guanfacine.

What side effects may I notice from taking guanfacine?

Stopping taking guanfacine can produce some of these side effects. Ask your prescriber or health care professional before you reduce your dose, or stop taking guanfacine.

Side effects that you should report to your prescriber or health care professional as soon as possible:

- agitation, anxiety, trembling, or shakiness
- confusion or excessive drowsiness
- difficulty breathing
- dizziness or faintness
- increased sweating
- increased urine passed
- irregular, fast or slow heartbeat
- muscle weakness or pain
- nausea, vomiting
- palpitations or chest pain
- significant sexual dysfunction
- stomach pain
- unusual skin rash or reaction

Side effects that usually do not require medical attention (report to your prescriber or health care professional if they continue or are bothersome):

- blurred vision
- constipation
- depression
- difficulty sleeping
- drowsiness
- dry mouth
- headache
- minor sexual difficulties (reduced sexual desire or abilities)
- skin rash, itching
- sweating
- weakness or tiredness

Where can I keep my medicine?

Keep out of the reach of children in a container that small children cannot open. Store at room temperature, approximately 20 and 25 degrees C (68 and 77 degrees F). Protect from light. Keep container tightly closed. Throw away any unused medicine after the expiration date.

G

Haloperidol tablets

HALOPERIDOL;
5 mg; Tablet
Sandoz
Pharmaceuticals

HALOPERIDOL;
1 mg; Tablet
Mylan
Pharmaceuticals Inc

What are haloperidol tablets?

HALOPERIDOL (Haldol®) helps to treat schizophrenia. Haloperidol can help you to keep in touch with reality and reduce your mental problems. Haloperidol can help to control tics and vocal outbursts in patients with Tourette's syndrome and treat behavioral problems in children with severe conduct disorders (hyperactivity, mood swings, aggressive behavior, or difficulty maintaining attention). Generic haloperidol tablets are available.

What should my health care professional know before I take haloperidol?

They need to know if you have any of these conditions:
- blood disease
- breast cancer
- difficulty passing urine
- glaucoma
- head injury
- heart disease
- low blood calcium
- lung disease
- overactive thyroid
- Parkinson's disease
- prostate trouble
- seizures (convulsions)
- tobacco smoker
- an unusual or allergic reaction to haloperidol, tartrazine, other medicines, foods, dyes, or preservatives
- pregnant or trying to get pregnant
- breast-feeding

How should I take this medicine?

Take haloperidol tablets by mouth. Follow the directions on the prescription label. Swallow the tablets with a drink of water. If haloperidol upsets your stomach you can take it with food. Take your doses at regular intervals. Do not take your medicine more often than directed. Do not stop taking except on your prescriber's advice. Contact your pediatrician or health care professional regarding the use of this medicine in children. Special care may be needed. Elderly patients over age 65 years may have a stronger reaction to this medicine and need smaller doses.

What if I miss a dose?

If you miss a dose, take it as soon as you can. If it is almost time for your next dose, take only that dose and space remaining doses through the rest of the day. Do not take double or extra doses.

What may interact with haloperidol?

- alcohol
- atropine
- barbiturate medicines for inducing sleep or treating seizures (convulsions)
- benztropine
- cabergoline
- carbamazepine
- dicyclomine
- dopamine
- epinephrine
- levodopa or other medicines for Parkinson's disease
- lithium
- medicines for hay fever and other allergies
- medicines for fungal infections
- medicines for high blood pressure
- medicines for pain
- medicines to control heart rate
- other medicines for mental problems, like mental depression
- rifampin
- water pills

Tell your prescriber or health care professional about all other medicines you are taking, including non-prescription medicines, nutritional supplements, or herbal products. Also tell your prescriber or health care professional if you are a frequent user of drinks with caffeine or alcohol, if you smoke, or if you use illegal drugs. These may affect the way your medicine works. Check with your health care professional before stopping or starting any of your medicines.

What should I watch for while taking haloperidol?

Visit your prescriber or health care professional for regular checks on your progress. It may be several weeks before you see the full effects of haloperidol. Do not suddenly stop taking haloperidol. You may need to gradually reduce the dose. Only stop taking haloperidol on your prescriber's advice. You may get dizzy or drowsy. Do not drive, use machinery, or do anything that needs mental alertness until you know how haloperidol affects you. Do not stand or sit up quickly, especially if you are an older patient. This reduces the risk of dizzy or fainting spells. Alcohol can increase dizziness and drowsiness. Avoid alcoholic drinks. You can get a hangover effect the morning after a bedtime dose. Do not treat yourself for colds, diarrhea or allergies. Ask your prescriber or health care professional for advice, as some nonprescription medicines may increase possible side effects. Your mouth may get dry. Chewing sugarless gum or sucking hard candy, and drinking plenty of water will help. Be careful when brushing and flossing your teeth to avoid mouth infections or damage to your gums. See your dentist regularly. If you are going to have surgery tell your prescriber or health care professional that you are taking haloperidol. Avoid extreme

H

heat or cold. Haloperidol can stop your sweating and increase your body temperature. It can also make your body unable to stand extreme cold. Avoid hot baths and saunas. Be careful about exercising especially in hot weather. Dress warmly in cold weather and do not stay out long in the cold. Haloperidol may make you more sensitive to sun or ultraviolet light. Keep out of the sun, or wear protective clothing outdoors and use a sunscreen (at least SPF 15). Do not use sun lamps, or sun tanning beds or booths. To protect your eyes wear sunglasses even on cloudy days.

What side effects may I notice from taking haloperidol?

Side effects that you should report to your prescriber or health care professional as soon as possible:
- confusion
- difficulty breathing
- difficulty in speaking or swallowing
- difficulty passing urine, or sudden loss of bladder control
- dizziness or lightheadedness
- fast or irregular heartbeat (palpitations)
- fever, chills, or sore throat
- hot, dry skin or lack of sweating
- loss of balance or difficulty walking
- seizures (convulsions)
- stiffness, spasms, trembling
- uncontrollable tongue or chewing movements, smacking lips or puffing cheeks
- uncontrollable muscle spasms, in the face hands, arms, or legs, twisting body movements
- unusual weakness or tiredness

Side effects that usually do not require medical attention (report to your prescriber or health care professional if they continue or are bothersome):
- anxiety or agitation
- blurred vision
- breast pain or swelling
- constipation
- decreased sexual ability
- drowsiness
- dry mouth
- increased sensitivity to the sun (severe sunburn)
- menstrual changes
- nausea or vomiting
- skin rash
- unusual production of breast milk
- weight gain

Where can I keep my medicine?

Keep out of the reach of children in a container that small children cannot open. Store at room temperature between 15 and 30 degrees C (59 and 86 degrees F). Protect from light. Keep container tightly closed. Throw away any unused medicine after the expiration date.

Hydralazine tablets

HYDRALAZINE;
50 mg; Tablet
Par Pharmaceutical
Inc

HYDRALAZINE;
50 mg; Tablet
Pliva Inc

What are hydralazine tablets?

HYDRALAZINE (Apresoline®) is a vasodilator that relaxes blood vessels. It reduces blood pressure, increases the blood and oxygen supply to the heart, and decreases the workload on the heart. It helps to treat high blood pressure, high blood pressure emergencies (hypertensive crisis), and congestive heart failure. It is not a cure and must be taken regularly to control blood pressure. Generic hydralazine tablets are available.

What should my health care professional know before I take hydralazine?

They need to know if you have any of these conditions:
- blood vessel disease
- heart disease including angina or history of heart attack
- kidney disease
- rheumatic heart disease
- systemic lupus erythematosus (SLE)
- an unusual or allergic reaction to hydralazine, tartrazine dye, other medicines, foods, dyes, or preservatives
- pregnant or trying to get pregnant
- breast-feeding

How should I take this medicine?

Take hydralazine tablets by mouth. Follow the directions on the prescription label. Swallow the tablets with a drink of water. If hydralazine upsets your stomach you can take it with food. It is best to take your tablets at the same time each day. Take your doses at regular intervals. Do not take your medicine more often than directed.

What if I miss a dose?

If you miss a dose, take it as soon as you can. If it is almost time for your next dose, take only that dose. Do not take double or extra doses.

What may interact with hydralazine?

- anti-inflammatory drugs (NSAIDs, such as ibuprofen)
- female hormones, including contraceptive or birth control pills
- medicines for colds and breathing difficulties
- medicines for high blood pressure
- medicines for mental depression
- water pills

Tell your prescriber or health care professional about all other medicines you are taking, including non-pre-

scription medicines, nutritional supplements, or herbal products. Also tell your prescriber or health care professional if you are a frequent user of drinks with caffeine or alcohol, if you smoke, or if you use illegal drugs. These may affect the way your medicine works. Check with your health care professional before stopping or starting any of your medicines.

What should I watch for while taking hydralazine?

Visit your prescriber or health care professional for regular checks on your progress. Check your blood pressure and pulse rate regularly; this is important while you are taking hydralazine. Ask your prescriber or health care professional what your blood pressure and pulse rate should be and when you should contact him or her. You may get drowsy or dizzy. Do not drive, use machinery, or do anything that needs mental alertness until you know how hydralazine affects you. To reduce the risk of dizzy or fainting spells, do not sit or stand up quickly, especially if you are an older patient. Alcohol can make you more dizzy, increase flushing and rapid heartbeats; avoid alcoholic drinks. Do not treat yourself for coughs, colds, headache or pain while you are taking hydralazine, without asking your prescriber or health care professional for advice. If you are going to have surgery tell your prescriber or health care professional that you are taking hydralazine. You may need to follow a special low-sodium diet while taking hydralazine. Check with your prescriber or health care professional.

What side effects may I notice from taking hydralazine?

Side effects that you should report to your prescriber or health care professional as soon as possible:
- chest pain, or fast or irregular heartbeat (palpitations)
- fever, chills, or sore throat
- numbness or tingling in the hands or feet
- shortness of breath
- skin rash, redness, blisters or itching
- stiff or swollen joints
- sudden weight gain
- swelling of the feet or legs
- swollen lymph glands
- unusual weakness

Side effects that usually do not require medical attention (report to your prescriber or health care professional if they continue or are bothersome):
- diarrhea, or constipation
- dizziness or lightheadedness
- headache
- loss of appetite
- nausea, vomiting

Where can I keep my medicine?

Keep out of the reach of children in a container that small children cannot open. Store below 30 degrees C (86 degrees F). Protect from light. Keep container tightly closed. Throw away any unused medicine after the expiration date.

Hydralazine; Hydrochlorothiazide, HCTZ capsules

HYDRAZIDE®; 25 mg/25 mg; Capsule Par Pharmaceutical Inc

HYDRAZIDE®; 50 mg/50 mg; Capsule Par Pharmaceutical Inc

what are hydralazine; hydrochlorothiazide, HCTZ capsules?

HYDRALAZINE; HYDROCHLOROTHIAZIDE, HCTZ (Apresazide®, Hydra-Zide®) is a combination of two drugs used to treat hypertension. Hydralazine controls high blood pressure (hypertension) by relaxing blood vessels. Hydrochlorothiazide is a diuretic. High blood pressure can damage the blood vessels of the brain, heart, and kidneys, resulting in a stroke, heart failure, or kidney failure. By lowering blood pressure, hydralazine; hydrochlorothiazide can help reduce your risk of having damage to your kidneys, heart, or other organs. This medicine does not cure high blood pressure. Generic hydralazine; hydrochlorothiazide capsules are available.

What should my health care professional know before I take hydralazine; hydrochlorothiazide, HCTZ?

They need to know if you have any of these conditions:
- blood vessel disease
- diabetes
- gout
- heart disease including angina or history of heart attack
- kidney disease, small amounts of urine, or difficulty passing urine
- liver disease
- pancreatitis
- rheumatic heart disease
- systemic lupus erythematosus (SLE)
- an unusual or allergic reaction to hydralazine, hydrochlorothiazide, sulfa drugs, carbonic anhydrase inhibitors like acetazolamide, other medicines, foods, dyes, or preservatives
- pregnant or trying to get pregnant
- breast-feeding

How should this medicine be used?

Take hydralazine; hydrochlorothiazide capsules by mouth. Follow the directions on the prescription label. Swallow the capsules with a drink of water. If hydralazine; hydrochlorothiazide upsets your stomach you can take it with food. It is best to take your doses at the same time each day. Take your doses at regular intervals. Do not take your medicine more often than directed. Contact your pediatrician or health care professional regarding the use of this medicine in children. Special care may be needed.

what if I miss a dose?

If you miss a dose, take it as soon as you can. If it is almost time for your next dose, take only that dose. Do not take double or extra doses.

what may interact with hydralazine; hydrochlorothiazide, HCTZ?

- amantadine
- amphotericin B
- anti-inflammatory drugs (NSAIDs, such as ibuprofen)
- cholestyramine
- colestipol
- diazoxide
- digoxin
- dofetilide
- female hormones, including contraceptive or birth control pills
- hormones such as cortisone, hydrocortisone, prednisone
- lithium
- medicines for colds and breathing difficulties
- medicines for diabetes that are taken by mouth
- medicines for high blood pressure, heart disease, or to control the heart rhythm
- medicines for mental depression
- water pills

Tell your prescriber or health care professional about all other medicines you are taking, including non-prescription medicines, nutritional supplements, or herbal products. Also tell your prescriber or health care professional if you are a frequent user of drinks with caffeine or alcohol, if you smoke, or if you use illegal drugs. These may affect the way your medicine works. Check with your health care professional before stopping or starting any of your medicines.

what should I watch for while taking hydralazine; hydrochlorothiazide, HCTZ?

Visit your prescriber or health care professional for regular checks on your progress. Check your blood pressure regularly. Ask your prescriber or health care professional what your blood pressure should be, and when you should contact him or her. You must not get dehydrated, ask your prescriber or health care professional how much fluid you need to drink a day. Do not stop taking this medicine except on your prescriber's advice. You may get drowsy, dizzy or lightheaded. Do not drive, use machinery, or do anything that needs mental alertness until you know how this medicine affects you. To reduce the risk of dizzy or fainting spells, do not sit or stand up quickly, especially if you are an older patient. Alcohol can make you more dizzy, increase flushing and rapid heartbeats; avoid alcoholic drinks. Do not treat yourself for coughs, colds, headache or pain while you taking this medicine without asking your health care professional for advice. Watch your diet while you are taking this hydralazine; hydrochlorothiazide. Ask your prescriber or health care professional about both potassium and sodium intake. This medicine contains a diuretic which can make your body lose potassium and you may need an extra supply. Too high or too low potassium can cause problems. Some foods have a high potassium content such as bananas, coconuts, dates, figs, prunes, apricots, peaches, grapefruit juice, tomato juice, and orange juice. This medicine can make your skin more sensitive to sun or ultraviolet light. Keep out of the sun, or wear protective clothing outdoors and use a sunscreen (at least SPF 15). Do not use sun lamps or sun tanning beds or booths. If you are going to have surgery, tell your prescriber or health care professional that you are taking hydralazine; hydrochlorothiazide. Hydralazine; hydrochlorothiazide can increase the amount of sugar in blood or urine. If you are a diabetic keep a close check on blood and urine sugar.

what side effects may I notice from taking hydralazine; hydrochlorothiazide, HCTZ?

Side effects that you should report to your prescriber or health care professional as soon as possible:

- blood in urine or stools
- chest pain, or fast or irregular heartbeat (palpitations)
- diarrhea
- dry mouth
- fever or chills, sore throat
- increased thirst
- lower back or side pain
- mood changes
- muscle pain or weakness, cramps
- nausea, vomiting
- redness, blistering, peeling or loosening of the skin, including inside the mouth
- severe stomach pain
- shortness of breath
- skin rash, redness, blisters or itching
- stiff or swollen joints
- sudden weight gain
- swelling of the feet or legs
- swollen lymph glands
- tingling or numbness in the hands or feet
- unusual bleeding or bruising
- unusual tiredness or weakness
- yellowing of the eyes or skin

Side effects that usually do not require medical attention (report to your prescriber or health care professional if they continue or are bothersome):

- diarrhea or constipation
- dizziness or lightheadedness
- headache
- increased sensitivity to the sun
- loss of appetite
- stomach upset, pain, or cramps

Where can I keep my medicine?

Keep out of the reach of children in a container that small children cannot open. Store between 15 and 30 degrees C (59 and 86 degrees F). Protect from light and moisture. Keep container tightly closed. Throw away any unused medicine after the expiration date.

H

Hydrochlorothiazide, HCTZ capsules or tablets

HYDROCHLOROTHIAZIDE, HCTZ;
25 mg; Tablet
Qualitest
Pharmaceuticals Inc

MICROZIDE®;
12.5 mg; Capsule
Watson Pharmaceuticals Inc

What are hydrochlorothiazide capsules or tablets?

HYDROCHLOROTHIAZIDE (HydroDIURIL®, Esidrix®, Microzide®, Oretic®) is a diuretic. Diuretics increase the amount of urine passed, which causes the body to lose water and salt. Hydrochlorothiazide helps to treat high blood pressure (hypertension). It is not a cure. It also reduces the swelling and water retention caused by various medical conditions, such as heart, liver, or kidney disease. Generic hydrochlorothiazide capsules or tablets are available.

What should my health care professional know before I take hydrochlorothiazide?

They need to know if you have any of these conditions:
- diabetes
- gout
- kidney disease, small amounts of urine, or difficulty passing urine
- liver disease
- pancreatitis
- systemic lupus erythematosus (SLE)
- an unusual or allergic reaction to hydrochlorothiazide, sulfa drugs, carbonic anhydrase inhibitors like acetazolamide, other medicines, foods, dyes, or preservatives
- pregnant or trying to get pregnant
- breast-feeding

How should I take this medicine?

Take hydrochlorothiazide capsules or tablets by mouth. Follow the directions on the prescription label. Swallow the tablets with a drink of water. Take your doses at regular intervals. Do not take your medicine more often than directed. Remember that you will need to pass urine frequently after taking hydrochlorothiazide. Do not take your doses at a time of day that will cause you problems. Do not take at bedtime.

What if I miss a dose?

If you miss a dose, take it as soon as you can. If it is almost time for your next dose, take only that dose. Do not take double or extra doses.

What may interact with hydrochlorothiazide?

- amantadine
- amphotericin B
- anti-inflammatory drugs (NSAIDs, such as ibuprofen)
- cholestyramine
- colestipol
- diazoxide
- digoxin
- dofetilide
- hormones such as cortisone, hydrocortisone, prednisone
- lithium
- medicines for diabetes
- medicines for high blood pressure, heart disease, or to control the heart rhythm
- water pills

Tell your prescriber or health care professional about all other medicines you are taking, including non-prescription medicines, nutritional supplements, or herbal products. Also tell your prescriber or health care professional if you are a frequent user of drinks with caffeine or alcohol, if you smoke, or if you use illegal drugs. These may affect the way your medicine works. Check with your health care professional before stopping or starting any of your medicines.

What should I watch for while taking hydrochlorothiazide?

Visit your prescriber or health care professional for regular checks on your progress. Check your blood pressure regularly. Ask your prescriber or health care professional what your blood pressure should be, and when you should contact him or her. You must not get dehydrated, ask your prescriber or health care professional how much fluid you need to drink a day. Do not stop taking hydrochlorothiazide except on your prescriber's advice. Watch your diet while you are taking hydrochlorothiazide. Ask your prescriber or health care professional about both potassium and sodium intake. Hydrochlorothiazide can make your body lose potassium and you may need an extra supply. Too high or too low potassium can cause problems. Some foods have a high potassium content such as bananas, coconuts, dates, figs, prunes, apricots, peaches, grapefruit juice, tomato juice, and orange juice. You may get dizzy or lightheaded. Do not drive, use machinery, or do anything that needs mental alertness until you know how hydrochlorothiazide affects you. To reduce the risk of dizzy or fainting spells, do not sit or stand up quickly, especially if you are an older patient. Alcohol can make you lightheaded, dizzy and increase confusion. Avoid or limit intake of alcoholic drinks. Hydrochlorothiazide can make your skin more sensitive to sun or ultraviolet light. Keep out of the sun, or wear protective clothing outdoors and use a sunscreen (at least SPF 15). Do not use sun lamps or sun tanning beds or booths. If you are going to have surgery, tell your prescriber or health care professional that you are taking hydrochlorothiazide. Hydrochlorothiazide can increase the amount of sugar in blood or urine. If you are a diabetic keep a close check on blood and urine sugar.

What side effects may I notice from taking hydrochlorothiazide?

Side effects that you should report to your prescriber or health care professional as soon as possible:

- blood in urine or stools
- diarrhea
- dry mouth
- fever or chills, sore throat
- increased thirst
- irregular heartbeat
- lower back or side pain
- mood changes
- muscle pain or weakness, cramps
- nausea, vomiting
- redness, blistering, peeling or loosening of the skin, including inside the mouth
- severe stomach pain
- skin rash, itching

- tingling or numbness in the hands or feet
- unusual bleeding or bruising
- unusual tiredness or weakness
- yellowing of the eyes or skin

Side effects that usually do not require medical attention (report to your prescriber or health care professional if they continue or are bothersome):

- constipation
- dizziness or lightheadedness
- headache
- increased sensitivity to the sun
- loss of appetite
- stomach upset, pain, or cramps

Where can I keep my medicine?

Keep out of the reach of children in a container that small children cannot open. Store at room temperature between 15 and 30 degrees C (59 and 86 degrees F). Protect from light and moisture. Keep container tightly closed. Throw away any unused medicine after the expiration date.

Hydrochlorothiazide, HCTZ; Irbesartan tablets

AVALIDE®;
150 mg; 12.5 mg;
Tablet Bristol-Myers
Squibb

AVALIDE®;
300 mg; 12.5 mg;
Tablet Bristol-Myers
Squibb

What are irbesartan-hydrochlorothiazide tablets?

IRBESARTAN-HYDROCHLOROTHIAZIDE (Avalide®) is a combination of two drugs used to lower blood pressure. Irbesartan controls high blood pressure (hypertension) by relaxing blood vessels. Hydrochlorothiazide is a diuretic. High blood pressure can damage the blood vessels of the brain, heart, and kidneys, resulting in a stroke, heart failure, or kidney failure. This medicine does not cure high blood pressure. By lowering blood pressure, irbesartan-hydrochlorothiazide can help reduce your risk of having damage to your kidneys, heart, or other organs. Generic irbesartan-hydrochlorothiazide tablets are not yet available.

What should my health care professional know before I take irbesartan-hydrochlorothiazide?

They need to know if you have any of these conditions:

- autoimmune disease (e.g., lupus) or suppressed immune function
- diabetes mellitus
- gout
- heart or blood vessel disease (e.g. heart failure)
- liver disease
- recent heart attack or stroke
- kidney disease, (e.g. renal failure or renal artery stenosis)
- pancreatitis
- electrolyte imbalance (e.g. low or high levels of potassium in the blood)
- if you are on a special diet, such as a low-salt diet (e.g. using potassium substitutes)

- sulfonamide (sulfa) or thiazide allergy
- an unusual or allergic reaction to irbesartan, hydrochlorothiazide, other medicines, foods, dyes, or preservatives
- pregnant or trying to get pregnant
- breast-feeding

How should I take this medicine?

Take irbesartan-hydrochlorothiazide tablets by mouth. Follow the directions on the prescription label. Swallow the tablets with a drink of water. Irbesartan-hydrochlorothiazide can be taken with or without food. Take your doses at regular intervals. Do not take your medicine more often than directed.

What if I miss a dose?

If you miss a dose, take it as soon as you can. If it is almost time for your next dose, take only that dose. Do not take double or extra doses.

What may interact with irbesartan-hydrochlorothiazide?

- allopurinol
- anti-inflammatory drugs (NSAIDs, such as ibuprofen)
- blood pressure medications
- bosentan
- delavirdine
- diabetic medications
- dofetilide
- fluconazole
- griseofulvin
- hawthorn or horse chestnut
- imatinib

H

- lithium
- potassium salts or potassium supplements
- prochlorperazine
- rifampin
- some antibiotics that increase sensitivity to sunlight (sulfonamides, tetracyclines)
- some cholesterol-lowering medications (e.g. cholestyramine or colestipol)
- some medicines for mental disorders (phenothiazines)
- vitamin A (retinol) creams or pills such as tretinoin Retin-A®, Renova®, Solage®, Atragen®, and others
- voriconazole
- water pills (especially potassium-sparing diuretics such as triamterene or amiloride)

Tell your prescriber or health care professional about all other medicines you are taking, including non-prescription medicines, nutritional supplements, or herbal products. Also tell your prescriber or health care professional if you are a frequent user of drinks with caffeine or alcohol, if you smoke, or if you use illegal drugs. These may affect the way your medicine works. Check with your health care professional before stopping or starting any of your medicines.

What should I watch for while taking irbesartan-hydrochlorothiazide?

Check your blood pressure regularly while you are taking irbesartan-hydrochlorothiazide. Ask your prescriber or health care professional what your blood pressure should be and when you should contact him or her. When you check your blood pressure, write down the measurements to show your prescriber or health care professional. You must not get dehydrated. Ask your prescriber or health care professional how much fluid you need to drink a day. If you are taking this medicine for a long time you must visit your prescriber or health care professional for regular checks on your progress. Make sure you schedule appointments on a regular basis. Check with your prescriber or health care professional if you get an attack of severe diarrhea, nausea and vomiting, or if you sweat a lot. The loss of too much body fluid can make it dangerous for you to take irbesartan-hydrochlorothiazide. You may get dizzy. Do not drive, use machinery, or do anything that requires mental alertness until you know how irbesartan-hydrochlorothiazide affects you. To avoid dizzy or fainting spells, do not stand or sit up quickly. Alcohol may increase the possibility of dizziness. Avoid alcoholic drinks until you have discussed their use with your prescriber or health care professional. If you are going to have surgery tell your prescriber or health care professional that you are taking irbesartan-hydrochlorothia-

zide. Irbesartan-hydrochlorothiazide may affect your blood sugar level. If you have diabetes, check with your prescriber or health care professional before changing the dose of your diabetic medicine. Avoid salt substitutes unless you are told otherwise by your prescriber or health care professional. Do not take medicines for appetite control, asthma, colds, cough, hay fever, or sinus problems without asking your prescriber or health care professional for advice. Do not treat yourself for a fever or sore throat; check with your prescriber or health care professional first.

What side effects may I notice from taking irbesartan-hydrochlorothiazide?

Side effects that you should report to your prescriber or health care professional as soon as possible:
Rare or uncommon:
- difficulty breathing, difficulty swallowing, hoarseness, or tightening of the throat
- redness, blistering, peeling or loosening of the skin, including inside the mouth
- swelling of your face, lips, tongue, hands, or feet
- unusual rash, bleeding or bruising, or pinpoint red spots on the skin

Other:
- confusion, dizziness, lightheadedness or fainting spells
- decreased amount of urine passed
- decreased sexual function
- fast or uneven heart beat, palpitations, or chest pain
- fever or chills
- irregular heartbeat
- muscle cramps
- stomach pain
- vomiting
- unusual tiredness or weakness
- worsened gout pain
- yellowing of the eyes or skin

Side effects that usually do not require medical attention (report to your prescriber or health care professional if they continue or are bothersome):
- cough
- diarrhea
- headache
- increased sensitivity to the sun
- nausea
- tiredness or fatigue

Where can I keep my medicine?

Keep out of the reach of children in a container that small children cannot open. Store at room temperature between 15 and 30 degrees C (59 and 86 degrees F). Protect from light. Keep container tightly closed. Throw away any unused medicine after the expiration date.

Hydrochlorothiazide, HCTZ; Lisinopril tablets

PRINZIDE®;
25 mg/20 mg; Tablet
Merck and Co Inc

ZESTORETIC®;
25 mg/20 mg; Tablet
AstraZeneca
Pharmaceuticals LP

What are lisinopril; hydrochlorothiazide tablets?

LISINOPRIL; HYDROCHLOROTHIAZIDE (Prinzide® or Zestoretic®) is a combination of two drugs used to lower blood pressure. Lisinopril is an ACE inhibitor that controls high blood pressure (hypertension) by relaxing blood vessels. Hydrochlorothiazide is a diuretic. High blood pressure can damage the blood vessels of the brain, heart, and kidneys, resulting in a stroke, heart failure, or kidney failure. By lowering blood pressure, lisinopril-hydrochlorothiazide can help reduce your risk of having damage to your kidneys, heart, or other organs. This medicine does not cure high blood pressure. Generic lisinopril-hydrochlorothiazide tablets are available.

What should my health care professional know before I take lisinopril-hydrochlorothiazide?

They need to know if you have any of these conditions:

- autoimmune disease (e.g. lupus) or suppressed immune function
- previous swelling of the tongue, face, or lips with difficulty breathing, difficulty swallowing, hoarseness, or tightening of the throat (angioedema)
- bone marrow disease
- diabetes mellitus
- gout
- heart or blood vessel disease
- liver disease
- recent heart attack or stroke
- kidney disease, (e.g. renal failure or renal artery stenosis)
- pancreatitis
- electrolyte imbalance (e.g. low or high levels of potassium in the blood)
- if you are on a special diet, such as a low-salt diet (e.g. using potassium substitutes)
- sulfonamide (sulfa) or thiazide allergy
- an unusual or allergic reaction to lisinopril, hydrochlorothiazide, other medicines, foods, dyes, or preservatives
- pregnant or trying to get pregnant
- breast-feeding

How should I take this medicine?

Take lisinopril-hydrochlorothiazide tablets by mouth. Follow the directions on the prescription label. You may take lisinopril-hydrochlorothiazide with or without food. Swallow the tablets with a drink of water. Take your doses at regular intervals. Do not take your medicine more often than directed. Do not stop taking this medicine except on your prescriber's advice. Many patients with high blood pressure will not notice any signs of the problem. Therefore, it is very important that you take this medicine exactly as directed and that you keep your appointments with your prescriber or health care professional even if you feel well. Contact your pediatrician or health care professional regarding the use of this medicine in children. Special care may be needed.

What if I miss a dose?

If you miss a dose, take it as soon as you can. If it is almost time for your next dose, take only that dose. Do not take double or extra doses.

What may interact with lisinopril-hydrochlorothiazide?

- anti-inflammatory drugs (NSAIDs, such as ibuprofen)
- cholestyramine
- colestipol
- dofetilide
- hawthorn
- lithium
- medicines for diabetes
- medicines for high blood pressure
- potassium salts or potassium supplements
- potassium-sparing diuretics (e.g. amiloride, triamterene)

Tell your prescriber or health care professional about all other medicines you are taking, including nonprescription medicines, nutritional supplements, or herbal products. Also tell your prescriber or health care professional if you are a frequent user of drinks with caffeine or alcohol, if you smoke, or if you use illegal drugs. These may affect the way your medicine works. Check with your health care professional before stopping or starting any of your medicines.

What should I watch for while taking lisinopril-hydrochlorothiazide?

Check your blood pressure regularly while you are taking lisinopril-hydrochlorothiazide. Ask your prescriber or health care professional what your blood pressure should be and when you should contact him or her. When you check your blood pressure, write down the measurements to show your prescriber or health care professional. You must not get dehydrated, ask your prescriber or health care professional how much fluid you need to drink a day. If you are taking this medicine for a long time you must visit your prescriber or health care professional for regular checks on your progress. Make sure you schedule appointments on a regular basis. Check with your prescriber or health care professional if you get an attack of severe diarrhea, nausea and vomiting, or if you sweat a lot. The loss of too much body fluid can make it dangerous for you to take lisinopril-hydrochlorothiazide. You may get dizzy. Do

H

not drive, use machinery, or do anything that requires mental alertness until you know how lisinopril-hydrochlorothiazide affects you. To avoid dizzy or fainting spells, do not stand or sit up quickly. Alcohol may increase the possibility of dizziness. Avoid alcoholic drinks until you have discussed their use with your prescriber or health care professional. If you are going to have surgery, tell your prescriber or health care professional that you are taking lisinopril-hydrochlorothiazide. Avoid salt substitutes unless you are told otherwise by your prescriber or health care professional. Do not take medicines for appetite control, asthma, colds, cough, hay fever, or sinus problems without asking your prescriber or health care professional for advice. Do not treat yourself for a fever or sore throat; check with your prescriber or health care professional first. Lisinopril-hydrochlorothiazide may affect your blood sugar level. If you have diabetes, check with your prescriber or health care professional before changing the dose of your diabetic medicine.

What side effects may I notice from taking lisinopril-hydrochlorothiazide?

Side effects that you should report to your prescriber or health care professional as soon as possible:
Rare or uncommon:
- difficulty breathing, difficulty swallowing, hoarseness, or tightening of the throat
- redness, blistering, peeling or loosening of the skin, including inside the mouth
- swelling of your face, lips, tongue, hands, or feet
- unusual rash, bleeding or bruising, or pinpoint red spots on the skin

Other:
- confusion, dizziness, lightheadedness or fainting spells
- decreased amount of urine passed
- decreased sexual function
- fast or uneven heart beat, palpitations, or chest pain
- fever or chills
- irregular heartbeat
- muscle cramps
- stomach pain
- vomiting
- unusual tiredness or weakness
- worsened gout pain
- yellowing of the eyes or skin

Side effects that usually do not require medical attention (report to your prescriber or health care professional if they continue or are bothersome):
- cough
- diarrhea
- headache
- increased sensitivity to the sun
- nausea
- tiredness or fatigue

Where can I keep my medicine?

Keep out of the reach of children. Store at room temperature below 15 and 30 degrees C (59 and 86 degrees F). Protect from moisture and excessive light. Keep container tightly closed. Throw away any unused medicine after the expiration date.

Hydrochlorothiazide, HCTZ; Losartan tablets

HYZAAR®;
25 mg/100 mg;
Tablet
Merck and Co Inc

HYZAAR®;
12.5 mg/50 mg;
Tablet
Merck and Co Inc

What are losartan-hydrochlorothiazide tablets?

LOSARTAN-HYDROCHLOROTHIAZIDE (Hyzaar®) is a combination of two drugs used to lower blood pressure. Losartan controls high blood pressure (hypertension) by relaxing blood vessels. Hydrochlorothiazide is a diuretic. High blood pressure can damage the blood vessels of the brain, heart, and kidneys, resulting in a stroke, heart failure, or kidney failure. By lowering blood pressure, losartan-hydrochlorothiazide can help reduce your risk of having damage to your kidneys, heart, or other organs. This medicine does not cure high blood pressure. Generic losartan-hydrochlorothiazide tablets are not yet available.

What should my health care professional know before I take losartan-hydrochlorothiazide?

They need to know if you have any of these conditions:
- autoimmune disease (e.g. lupus) or suppressed immune function
- diabetes mellitus
- gout
- heart or blood vessel disease (e.g. heart failure)
- liver disease
- recent heart attack or stroke
- kidney disease, (e.g. renal failure or renal artery stenosis)
- pancreatitis
- electrolyte imbalance (e.g. low or high levels of potassium in the blood)
- if you are on a special diet, such as a low-salt diet (e.g. using potassium substitutes)
- sulfonamide (sulfa) or thiazide allergy
- an unusual or allergic reaction to losartan, hydrochlorothiazide, other medicines, foods, dyes, or preservatives
- pregnant or trying to get pregnant
- breast-feeding

How should I take this medicine?

Take losartan-hydrochlorothiazide tablets by mouth. Follow the directions on the prescription label. Swallow the tablets with a drink of water. Losartan-hydrochlorothiazide can be taken with or without food. Take your doses at regular intervals. Do not take your medicine more often than directed.

What if I miss a dose?

If you miss a dose, take it as soon as you can. If it is almost time for your next dose, take only that dose. Do not take double or extra doses.

What may interact with losartan-hydrochlorothiazide?

- allopurinol
- anti-inflammatory drugs (NSAIDs, such as ibuprofen)
- blood pressure medicines
- bosentan
- delavirdine
- diabetic medications
- dofetilide
- fluconazole
- griseofulvin
- hawthorn or horse chestnut
- lithium
- potassium salts or potassium supplements
- prochlorperazine
- rifampin
- some antibiotics which increase sensitivity to sunlight (sulfonamides, tetracyclines)
- some cholesterol-lowering medications (e.g. cholestyramine or colestipol)
- some medicines for mental disorders (phenothiazines)
- vitamin A (retinol) creams or pills such as tretinoin Retin-A®, Renova®, Solage®, Atragen®, and others
- voriconazole
- water pills (especially potassium-sparing diuretics such as triamterene or amiloride)

Tell your prescriber or health care professional about all other medicines you are taking, including non-prescription medicines, nutritional supplements, or herbal products. Also tell your prescriber or health care professional if you are a frequent user of drinks with caffeine or alcohol, if you smoke, or if you use illegal drugs. These may affect the way your medicine works. Check with your health care professional before stopping or starting any of your medicines.

What should I watch for while taking losartan-hydrochlorothiazide?

Check your blood pressure regularly while you are taking losartan-hydrochlorothiazide. Ask your prescriber or health care professional what your blood pressure should be and when you should contact him or her. When you check your blood pressure, write down the measurements to show your prescriber or health care professional. You must not get dehydrated. Ask your prescriber or health care professional how much fluid you need to drink a day. If you are taking this medicine for a long time, you must visit your health care professional for regular checks on your progress. Make sure you schedule appointments on a regular basis. Check with your prescriber or health care professional if you get an attack of severe diarrhea, nausea and vomiting, or if you sweat a lot. The loss of too much body fluid can make it dangerous for you to take losartan-hydrochlorothiazide. You may get dizzy. Do not drive, use machinery, or do anything that requires mental alert-ness until you know how losartan-hydrochlorothiazide affects you. To avoid dizzy or fainting spells, do not stand or sit up quickly. Alcohol may increase the possibility of dizziness. Avoid alcoholic drinks until you have discussed their use with your prescriber or health care professional. If you are going to have surgery tell your prescriber or health care professional that you are taking losartan-hydrochlorothiazide. Losartan-hydrochlorothiazide may affect your blood sugar level. If you have diabetes, check with your prescriber or health care professional before changing the dose of your diabetic medicine. Avoid salt substitutes unless you are told otherwise by your prescriber or health care professional. Do not take medicines for appetite control, asthma, colds, cough, hay fever, or sinus problems without asking your prescriber or health care professional for advice. Do not treat yourself for a fever or sore throat; check with your prescriber or health care professional first.

What side effects may I notice from taking losartan-hydrochlorothiazide?

Side effects that you should report to your prescriber or health care professional as soon as possible:
Rare or uncommon:
- difficulty breathing, difficulty swallowing, hoarseness, or tightening of the throat
- redness, blistering, peeling or loosening of the skin, including inside the mouth
- swelling of your face, lips, tongue, hands, or feet
- unusual rash, bleeding or bruising, or pinpoint red spots on the skin

Other:
- confusion, dizziness, lightheadedness or fainting spells
- decreased amount of urine passed
- decreased sexual function
- fast or uneven heart beat, palpitations, or chest pain
- fever or chills
- irregular heartbeat
- muscle cramps
- stomach pain
- vomiting
- unusual tiredness or weakness
- worsened gout pain
- yellowing of the eyes or skin

Side effects that usually do not require medical attention (report to your prescriber or health care professional if they continue or are bothersome):
- cough
- diarrhea
- headache
- increased sensitivity to the sun
- nausea
- tiredness or fatigue

Where can I keep my medicine?

Keep out of the reach of children in a container that small children cannot open. Store at room temperature between 15 and 30 degrees C (59 and 86 degrees F). Protect from light. Keep container tightly closed. Throw away any unused medicine after the expiration date.

Hydrochlorothiazide, HCTZ; Metoprolol tablets

LOPRESSOR® HCT;
25 mg/50 mg;
Tablet
Novartis
Pharmaceuticals

LOPRESSOR® HCT;
25 mg/100 mg;
Tablet
Novartis
Pharmaceuticals

What are metoprolol; hydrochlorothiazide tablets?

METOPROLOL; HYDROCHLOROTHIAZIDE (Lopressor HCT®) is a combination of two drugs used to lower blood pressure. Metoprolol is a beta-blocker and hydrochlorothiazide is a diuretic ("water pill"). Metoprolol; hydrochlorothiazide is used to control, but not cure, high blood pressure (hypertension). Generic metoprolol; hydrochlorothiazide tablets are available.

What should my health care professional know before I take metoprolol; hydrochlorothiazide?

They need to know if you have any of these conditions:
- asthma, bronchitis or bronchospasm
- autoimmune disease such as lupus (SLE)
- bradycardia (unusually slow heartbeat)
- chest pain (angina)
- circulation problems, or blood vessel disease (such as Raynaud's disease)
- depression
- diabetes
- electrolyte imbalance (such as low or high levels of potassium in the blood)
- emphysema, COPD, or other lung disease
- gout
- heart disease (such as heart failure or a history of heart attack)
- kidney disease
- liver disease
- muscle weakness or myasthenia gravis
- pancreatitis
- pheochromocytoma
- post-sympathectomy
- psoriasis
- thyroid disease
- an unusual or allergic reaction to hydrochlorothiazide, metoprolol, other beta-blockers, diuretics, sulfonamides, or other medicines, foods, dyes, or preservatives
- if you are on a special diet, such as a low-salt diet (using potassium substitutes)
- pregnant or trying to get pregnant
- breast-feeding

How should I take this medicine?

Take metoprolol; hydrochlorothiazide tablets by mouth with food or after a meal. Follow the directions on the prescription label. Swallow the tablets with a drink of water. Take your doses at regular intervals. Do not take your medicine more often than directed. Do not stop taking except on your prescriber's advice. Contact your pediatrician or health care professional regarding the use of this medicine in children. Special care may be needed. Elderly patients over 65 years old may have a stronger reaction to this medicine and need smaller doses.

What if I miss a dose?

If you miss a dose, take it as soon as you can. If it is almost time for your next dose, take only that dose. Do not take double or extra doses.

What may interact with metoprolol; hydrochlorothiazide?

- allopurinol
- anti-inflammatory drugs (NSAIDs, such as ibuprofen)
- cevimeline
- cimetidine
- clonidine
- cocaine or amphetamine
- fluvoxamine or fluoxetine (Prozac®)
- ginger, Zingiber officinale
- griseofulvin
- hawthorn
- lithium
- liothyronine
- mefloquine
- medicines for chest pain or angina
- medicines for colds and breathing difficulties
- medicines for diabetes
- medicines for high blood pressure or heart failure
- medicines known as MAO inhibitors, such as phenelzine (Nardil®), tranylcypromine (Parnate®), isocarboxazid (Marplan®), and selegiline (Carbex®, Eldepryl®)
- medicines to control heart rhythm (including amiodarone, digoxin, disopyramide, dofetilide, flecainide, propafenone, quinidine, and sotalol)
- porfimer
- prochlorperazine (Compazine®)
- rifampin
- some antibiotics which increase sensitivity to sunlight (sulfonamides, tetracyclines)
- some medicines for lowering cholesterol (colestipol or cholestyramine)
- some medicines for weight loss (including some herbal products, ephedrine, dextroamphetamine)
- vitamin A (retinol) creams or pills such as tretinoin Retin-A®, Renova®, Solage®, Atragen®, and others
- water pills (diuretics)

Tell your prescriber or health care professional about all other medicines you are taking, including nonprescription medicines, nutritional supplements, or herbal products. Also tell your prescriber or health care professional if you are a frequent user of drinks with caffeine or alcohol, if you smoke, or if you use illegal drugs. These may affect the way your medicine works. Check with your health care professional before stopping or starting any of your medicines.

What should I watch for while taking metoprolol; hydrochlorothiazide?

Check your heart rate and blood pressure regularly while you are taking metoprolol; hydrochlorothiazide. Ask your prescriber or health care professional what your blood pressure should be and when you should contact him or her. When you check your blood pressure, write down the measurements to show your prescriber or health care professional. If you are taking this medicine for a long time you must visit your prescriber or health care professional for regular checks on your progress. Make sure you schedule appointments on a regular basis. Do not stop taking this medicine suddenly. This could lead to serious heart-related effects. You may get drowsy or dizzy. Do not drive, use machinery, or do anything that requires mental alertness until you know how metoprolol; hydrochlorothiazide affects you. To reduce the risk of dizzy or fainting spells, do not sit or stand up quickly. Alcohol can make you more drowsy, and increase the risk of flushing and rapid heartbeats. Therefore, it is best to avoid alcoholic drinks. Check with your health care professional if you get an attack of severe diarrhea, nausea and vomiting, or sweat a lot. Ask your health care professional how much fluid you need to drink each day. The loss of too much body fluid while you are taking a diuretic can cause dehydration and lower the blood pressure below normal. Metoprolol; hydrochlorothiazide can affect blood sugar levels. If you have diabetes, check with your prescriber or health care professional before you change your diet or the dose of your diabetic medicine. Do not take medicines for appetite control, asthma, colds, cough, hay fever, or sinus problems without asking your prescriber or health care professional for advice. Do not treat yourself for a fever or sore throat; check with your prescriber or health care professional first. Avoid exposure to excessive sunlight (such as sunlamps, sunbathing) while taking this medicine. If you are going to have surgery, tell your prescriber or health care professional that you are taking metoprolol; hydrochlorothiazide.

What side effects may I notice from taking metoprolol; hydrochlorothiazide?

Side effects that you should report to your prescriber or health care professional as soon as possible:

- changes in vision (e.g. blurred vision)
- cold, tingling, or numb hands or feet
- confusion, dizziness, lightheadedness or fainting spells
- difficulty breathing, wheezing
- fever or chills
- increased thirst or sweating
- increase or decrease in the amount of urine passed
- fast or uneven heart beat, palpitations, or chest pain
- slow heart rate
- muscle cramps
- redness, blistering, peeling or loosening of the skin, including inside the mouth
- stomach pain
- swollen legs or ankles
- tremor, shakes
- unusual skin rash or bruising
- unusual tiredness or weakness
- vomiting
- worsened gout pain
- yellowing of the eyes or skin

Side effects that usually do not require medical attention (report to your prescriber or health care professional if they continue or are bothersome):

- depression, nightmares
- diarrhea, heartburn, or constipation
- dry eyes or dry mouth
- headache
- increased sensitivity to the sun
- nausea
- sexual difficulties, impotence
- tiredness or fatigue

Where can I keep my medicine?

Keep out of the reach of children in a container that small children cannot open. Store at room temperature at 15 to 30 degrees C (59 to 86 degrees F). Protect from light and moisture. Throw away any unused medicine after the expiration date.

Hydrochlorothiazide, HCTZ; Moexipril tablets

UNIRETIC®;
25 mg/15 mg; Tablet
Schwarz Pharma Inc

UNIRETIC®;
12.5 mg/15 mg;
Tablet
Schwarz Pharma Inc

What are moexipril; hydrochlorothiazide tablets?
MOEXIPRIL; HYDROCHLOROTHIAZIDE (Uniretic®) is a combination of two drugs used to lower blood pressure. Moexipril is an ACE inhibitor that controls high blood pressure (hypertension) by relaxing blood vessels. Hydrochlorothiazide is a diuretic. High blood pressure can damage the blood vessels of the brain, heart, and kidneys, resulting in a stroke, heart failure, or kidney failure. By lowering blood pressure, moexipril; hydrochlorothiazide can help reduce your risk of having damage to your kidneys, heart, or other organs. This medicine does not cure high blood pressure. Generic moexipril; hydrochlorothiazide tablets are not yet available.

What should my health care professional know before I take moexipril; hydrochlorothiazide?

They need to know if you have any of these conditions:
- autoimmune disease (e.g. lupus) or suppressed immune function
- previous swelling of the tongue, face, or lips with difficulty breathing, difficulty swallowing, hoarseness, or tightening of the throat (angioedema)
- bone marrow disease
- diabetes mellitus
- gout
- heart or blood vessel disease
- liver disease
- recent heart attack or stroke
- kidney disease, (e.g. renal failure or renal artery stenosis)
- pancreatitis
- electrolyte imbalance (e.g. low or high levels of potassium in the blood)
- if you are on a special diet, such as a low-salt diet (e.g. using potassium substitutes)
- sulfonamide (sulfa) or thiazide allergy
- an unusual or allergic reaction to moexipril, hydrochlorothiazide, other medicines, foods, dyes, or preservatives
- pregnant or trying to get pregnant
- breast-feeding

How should I take this medicine?

Take moexipril; hydrochlorothiazide tablets by mouth. Follow the directions on the prescription label. You should take moexipril; hydrochlorothiazide on an empty stomach (one hour before a meal). Swallow the tablets with a drink of water. Take your doses at regular intervals. Do not take your medicine more often than directed. Do not stop taking this medicine except on your prescriber's advice. Many patients with high blood pressure will not notice any signs of the problem. Therefore, it is very important that you take this medicine exactly as directed and that you keep your appointments with your prescriber or health care professional even if you feel well. Contact your pediatrician or health care professional regarding the use of this medicine in children. Special care may be needed.

What if I miss a dose?

If you miss a dose, take it as soon as you can. If it is almost time for your next dose, take only that dose. Do not take double or extra doses.

What may interact with moexipril; hydrochlorothiazide?

- anti-inflammatory drugs (NSAIDs, such as ibuprofen)
- blood pressure medications
- cholesterol-lowering medications (e.g. cholestyramine or colestipol)
- dofetilide
- hawthorn
- diabetic medications
- lithium
- potassium salts or potassium supplements
- water pills (especially potassium-sparing diuretics such as triamterene or amiloride)

Tell your prescriber or health care professional about all other medicines you are taking, including non-prescription medicines, nutritional supplements, or herbal products. Also tell your prescriber or health care professional if you are a frequent user of drinks with caffeine or alcohol, if you smoke, or if you use illegal drugs. These may affect the way your medicine works. Check with your health care professional before stopping or starting any of your medicines.

What should I watch for while taking moexipril; hydrochlorothiazide?

Check your blood pressure regularly while you are taking moexipril; hydrochlorothiazide. Ask your prescriber or health care professional what your blood pressure should be and when you should contact him or her. When you check your blood pressure, write down the measurements to show your prescriber or health care professional. You must not get dehydrated, ask your prescriber or health care professional how much fluid you need to drink a day. If you are taking this medicine for a long time you must visit your prescriber or health care professional for regular checks on your progress. Make sure you schedule appointments on a regular basis. Check with your prescriber or health care professional if you get an attack of severe diarrhea, nausea and vomiting, or if you sweat a lot. The loss of too much body fluid can make it dangerous for you to take moexipril; hydrochlorothiazide. You may get dizzy. Do not drive, use machinery, or do anything that requires mental alertness until you know how moexipril; hydrochlorothiazide affects you. To avoid dizzy or fainting spells, do not stand or sit up quickly. Alcohol may increase the possibility of dizziness. Avoid alcoholic drinks until you have discussed their use with your prescriber or health care professional. If you are going to have surgery tell your prescriber or health care professional that you are taking moexipril; hydrochlorothiazide. Moexipril; hydrochlorothiazide may affect your blood sugar level. If you have diabetes, check with your prescriber or health care professional before changing the dose of your diabetic medicine. Avoid salt substitutes unless you are told otherwise by your prescriber or health care professional. Do not take medicines for appetite control, asthma, colds, cough, hay fever, or sinus problems without asking your prescriber or health care professional for advice. Do not treat yourself for a fever or sore throat; check with your prescriber or health care professional first.

What side effects may I notice from taking moexipril; hydrochlorothiazide?

Side effects that you should report to your prescriber or health care professional as soon as possible:
Rare or uncommon:
- difficulty breathing, difficulty swallowing, hoarseness, or tightening of the throat

- redness, blistering, peeling or loosening of the skin, including inside the mouth
- swelling of your face, lips, tongue, hands, or feet
- unusual rash, bleeding or bruising, or pinpoint red spots on the skin
- decreased sexual function

Other:
- confusion, dizziness, lightheadedness or fainting spells
- decreased amount of urine passed
- fast or uneven heart beat, palpitations, or chest pain
- fever or chills
- irregular heartbeat
- muscle cramps
- stomach pain
- vomiting
- unusual tiredness or weakness
- worsened gout pain

- yellowing of the eyes or skin

Side effects that usually do not require medical attention (report to your prescriber or health care professional if they continue or are bothersome):
- cough
- diarrhea
- headache
- increased sensitivity to the sun
- nausea
- tiredness or fatigue

Where can I keep my medicine?

Keep out of the reach of children. Store at room temperature below 20 to 25 degrees C (68 to 77 degrees F). Protect from moisture and light. Keep container tightly closed. Throw away any unused medicine after the expiration date.

Hydrochlorothiazide, HCTZ; Olmesartan Tablets

BENICAR HCT™;
40 mg/12.5 mg;
Tablet
Sankyo Pharma Inc

BENICAR HCT™;
20 mg/12.5 mg;
Tablet
Sankyo Pharma Inc

What are hydrochlorothiazide, HCTZ; olmesartan tablets?

HYDROCHLOROTHIAZIDE, HCTZ; OLMESARTAN (Benicar HCT™) is a combination of two drugs used to lower blood pressure. Olmesartan controls high blood pressure (hypertension) by relaxing blood vessels. Hydrochlorothiazide is a diuretic. High blood pressure can damage the blood vessels of the brain, heart, and kidneys, resulting in a stroke, heart failure, or kidney failure. This medicine does not cure high blood pressure. By lowering blood pressure, olmesartan; hydrochlorothiazide can help reduce your risk of having damage to your kidneys, heart, or other organs. Generic tablets are not yet available.

What should my health care professional know before I take hydrochlorothiazide, HCTZ; olmesartan?

They need to know if you have any of these conditions:
- autoimmune disease (like lupus), or suppressed immune function
- diabetes mellitus
- gout
- heart or blood vessel disease (such as heart failure)
- liver disease
- recent heart attack or stroke
- kidney disease (such as renal failure or renal artery stenosis)
- pancreatitis
- electrolyte imbalance (such as low or high levels of potassium in the blood)
- if you are on a special diet, such as a low-salt diet (such as using potassium substitutes)
- an unusual reaction to hydrochlorothiazide, HCTZ,

olmesartan, sulfonamides (sulfa), thiazide diuretics, other medicines, foods, dyes, or preservatives
- pregnant or trying to get pregnant
- breast-feeding

How should this medicine be taken?

Take hydrochlorothiazide, HCTZ; olmesartan tablets by mouth. Follow the directions on the prescription label. Swallow the tablets with a drink of water. This medicine can be taken with or without food. Take your doses at regular intervals. Do not take your medicine more often than directed. Contact your pediatrician or health care professional regarding the use of this medicine in children. Special care may be needed. Elderly patients over 65 years old may have a stronger reaction to this medicine and need smaller doses.

What if I miss a dose?

If you miss a dose, take it as soon as you can. If it is almost time for your next dose, take only that dose. Do not take double or extra doses.

What may interact with hydrochlorothiazide, HCTZ; olmesartan?

- allopurinol
- anti-inflammatory drugs (NSAIDs, such as ibuprofen)
- blood pressure medications
- dofetilide
- drospirenone; ethinyl estradiol
- griseofulvin
- hawthorn or horse chestnut
- lithium
- medicines for diabetes
- potassium salts or potassium supplements
- prochlorperazine

H

- some antibiotics which increase sensitivity to sunlight (sulfa antibiotics, tetracyclines)
- some cholesterol-lowering medications (examples, cholestyramine or colestipol)
- some medicines for mental disorders which increase sensitivity to sunlight
- vitamin A-related (retinol) creams, pills, or supplements
- water pills (especially potassium-sparing diuretics such as spironolactone, triamterene or amiloride)

Tell your prescriber or health care professional about all other medicines you are taking, including non-prescription medicines, nutritional supplements, or herbal products. Also tell your prescriber or health care professional if you are a frequent user of drinks with caffeine or alcohol, if you smoke, or if you use illegal drugs. These may affect the way your medicine works. Check with your health care professional before stopping or starting any of your medicines.

What should I watch for while taking hydrochlorothiazide, HCTZ; olmesartan?

Check your blood pressure regularly while you are taking this medicine. Ask your prescriber or health care professional what your blood pressure should be and when you should contact him or her. When you check your blood pressure, write down the measurements to show your prescriber or health care professional. Visit your prescriber or health care professional for regular checks on your progress. Check with your prescriber or health care professional if you get an attack of severe diarrhea, nausea and vomiting, or if you sweat a lot. You must not get dehydrated. Ask your prescriber or health care professional how much fluid you need to drink a day. The loss of too much body fluid can make it dangerous for you to take this medicine. You may get dizzy. Do not drive, use machinery, or do anything that requires mental alertness until you know how this medicine affects you. To avoid dizzy or fainting spells, do not stand or sit up quickly. Alcohol may increase the possibility of dizziness. Avoid alcoholic drinks until you have discussed their use with your prescriber or health care professional. This medicine may affect your blood sugar level if you have diabetes. Check with your prescriber or health care professional before changing the dose of your diabetic medicine. Avoid salt substitutes unless you are told otherwise by your prescriber or health care professional. Do not treat yourself for a fever or sore throat; check with your prescriber or health care professional first. If you are going to have surgery tell your prescriber or health care professional that you are taking hydrochlorothiazide; olmesartan.

What side effects may I notice from taking hydrochlorothiazide, HCTZ; olmesartan?

Side effects that you should report to your prescriber or health care professional as soon as possible:
Rare or uncommon:
- difficulty breathing, difficulty swallowing, hoarseness, or tightening of the throat
- redness, blistering, peeling or loosening of the skin, including inside the mouth
- swelling of your face, lips, tongue, hands, or feet
- unusual rash, bleeding or bruising, or pinpoint red spots on the skin

Other:
- confusion, dizziness, lightheadedness, or fainting spells
- decreased amount of urine passed
- decreased sexual function
- fast or uneven (irregular) heart beat, palpitations, or chest pain
- fever or chills
- muscle cramps or pain
- stomach pain
- unusual tiredness or weakness
- vomiting
- worsened gout pain
- yellowing of the eyes or skin

Side effects that usually do not require medical attention (report to your prescriber or health care professional if they continue or are bothersome):
- cough
- diarrhea
- headache
- increased sensitivity to the sun

Where can I keep my medicine?

Keep out of the reach of children in a container that small children cannot open. Store your medicine at room temperature between 20 and 25 degrees C (68 and 77 degrees F). Throw away any unused medication after the expiration date on the label.

Hydrochlorothiazide, HCTZ; Quinapril tablets

ACCURETIC®;
12.5 mg/20 mg;
Tablet
Parke Davis Division
of Pfizer Co.

ACCURETIC®;
12.5 mg/10 mg;
Tablet
Parke Davis Division
of Pfizer Co.

What are quinapril-hydrochlorothiazide tablets?

QUINAPRIL-HYDROCHLOROTHIAZIDE (Accuretic®, Quinaretic™) is a combination of two drugs used to lower blood pressure. Quinapril is an ACE inhibitor that controls high blood pressure (hypertension) by relaxing blood vessels. Hydrochlorothiazide is a diuretic. High blood pressure can damage the blood vessels of the brain, heart, and kidneys, resulting in a stroke, heart failure, or kidney failure. By lowering blood pressure, quinapril-hydrochlorothiazide can help reduce your risk of having damage to your kidneys, heart, or other organs. This medicine does not cure high blood pressure. Generic quinapril-hydrochlorothiazide tablets are available.

What should my health care professional know before I take quinapril-hydrochlorothiazide?

They need to know if you have any of these conditions:
- autoimmune disease (e.g. lupus) or suppressed immune function
- previous swelling of the tongue, face, or lips with difficulty breathing, difficulty swallowing, hoarseness, or tightening of the throat (angioedema)
- bone marrow disease
- diabetes mellitus
- gout
- heart or blood vessel disease
- liver disease
- recent heart attack or stroke
- kidney disease, (e.g. renal failure or renal artery stenosis)
- pancreatitis
- electrolyte imbalance (e.g. low or high levels of potassium in the blood)
- if you are on a special diet, such as a low-salt diet (e.g. using potassium substitutes)
- sulfonamide (sulfa) or thiazide allergy
- an unusual or allergic reaction to quinapril, hydrochlorothiazide, other medicines, foods, dyes, or preservatives
- pregnant or trying to get pregnant
- breast-feeding

How should I take this medicine?

Take quinapril-hydrochlorothiazide tablets by mouth with or without food. Follow the directions on the prescription label. Swallow the tablets with a drink of water. Take your doses at regular intervals. Do not take your medicine more often than directed. Do not stop taking this medicine except on your prescriber's advice. Many patients with high blood pressure will not notice any signs of the problem. Therefore, it is very important that you take this medicine exactly as directed and that you keep your appointments with your prescriber or health care professional even if you feel well. Contact your pediatrician or health care professional regarding the use of this medicine in children. Special care may be needed.

What if I miss a dose?

If you miss a dose, take it as soon as you can. If it is almost time for your next dose, take only that dose. Do not take double or extra doses.

What may interact with quinapril-hydrochlorothiazide?

- allopurinol
- aminolevulinic acid
- anti-inflammatory drugs (NSAIDs such as ibuprofen)
- aspirin
- azathioprine
- blood pressure medications
- cholesterol-lowering medications (e.g. cholestyramine or colestipol)
- diabetic medications
- dofetilide
- hawthorn
- lithium
- methoxsalen
- porfimer
- potassium salts or potassium supplements
- tetracycline
- water pills (especially potassium-sparing diuretics such as triamterene or amiloride)

Tell your prescriber or health care professional about all other medicines you are taking, including non-prescription medicines, nutritional supplements, or herbal products. Also tell your prescriber or health care professional if you are a frequent user of drinks with caffeine or alcohol, if you smoke, or if you use illegal drugs. These may affect the way your medicine works. Check with your health care professional before stopping or starting any of your medicines.

What should I watch for while taking quinapril-hydrochlorothiazide?

Check your blood pressure regularly while you are taking quinapril-hydrochlorothiazide. Ask your prescriber or health care professional what your blood pressure should be and when you should contact him or her. When you check your blood pressure, write down the measurements to show your prescriber or health care professional. You must not get dehydrated, ask your prescriber or health care professional how much fluid you need to drink a day. If you are taking this medicine for a long time you must visit your prescriber or health care professional for regular checks on your progress. Make sure you schedule appointments on a regular

H

basis. Check with your prescriber or health care professional if you get an attack of severe diarrhea, nausea and vomiting, or if you sweat a lot. The loss of too much body fluid can make it dangerous for you to take quinapril-hydrochlorothiazide. You may get dizzy. Do not drive, use machinery, or do anything that requires mental alertness until you know how quinapril-hydrochlorothiazide affects you. To avoid dizzy or fainting spells, do not stand or sit up quickly. Alcohol may increase the possibility of dizziness. Avoid alcoholic drinks until you have discussed their use with your prescriber or health care professional. If you are going to have surgery tell your prescriber or health care professional that you are taking quinapril-hydrochlorothiazide. Quinapril-hydrochlorothiazide may affect your blood sugar level. If you have diabetes, check with your prescriber or health care professional before changing the dose of your diabetic medicine. Avoid salt substitutes unless you are told otherwise by your prescriber or health care professional. Do not take medicines for appetite control, asthma, colds, cough, hay fever, or sinus problems without asking your prescriber or health care professional for advice. Do not treat yourself for a fever or sore throat; check with your prescriber or health care professional first.

What side effects may I notice from taking quinapril-hydrochlorothiazide?

Side effects that you should report to your prescriber or health care professional as soon as possible:
Rare or uncommon:
- difficulty breathing, difficulty swallowing, hoarseness, or tightening of the throat
- redness, blistering, peeling or loosening of the skin, including inside the mouth
- swelling of your face, lips, tongue, hands, or feet
- unusual rash, bleeding or bruising, or pinpoint red spots on the skin
- decreased sexual function

Other:
- confusion, dizziness, lightheadedness, or fainting spells
- decreased amount of urine passed
- fast or uneven heart beat, palpitations, or chest pain
- fever or chills
- irregular heartbeat
- muscle cramps
- stomach pain
- vomiting
- unusual tiredness or weakness
- worsened gout pain
- yellowing of the eyes or skin

Side effects that usually do not require medical attention (report to your prescriber or health care professional if they continue or are bothersome):
- cough
- diarrhea
- increased sensitivity to the sun
- nausea
- tiredness or fatigue

Where can I keep my medicine?

Keep out of the reach of children. Store at room temperature below 20 to 25 degrees C (68 to 77 degrees F). Keep container tightly closed. Throw away any unused medicine after the expiration date.

Hydrochlorothiazide, HCTZ; Telmisartan tablets

MICARDIS® HCT;
12.5 mg/40 mg; Tablet
Boehringer Ingelheim
Pharmaceuticals Inc

What are telmisartan-hydrochlorothiazide tablets?

TELMISARTAN-HYDROCHLOROTHIAZIDE (Micardis® HCT) is a combination of two drugs used to lower blood pressure. Telmisartan controls high blood pressure (hypertension) by relaxing blood vessels. Hydrochlorothiazide is a diuretic. High blood pressure can damage the blood vessels of the brain, heart, and kidneys, resulting in a stroke, heart failure, or kidney failure. This medicine does not cure high blood pressure. By lowering blood pressure, telmisartan-hydrochlorothiazide can help reduce your risk of having damage to your kidneys, heart, or other organs. Generic telmisartan-hydrochlorothiazide tablets are not yet available.

What should my health care professional know before I take telmisartan-hydrochlorothiazide?

They need to know if you have any of these conditions:
- autoimmune disease (like lupus) or suppressed immune function
- diabetes mellitus
- gout
- heart or blood vessel disease (such as heart failure)
- liver disease
- recent heart attack or stroke
- kidney disease (such as renal failure or renal artery stenosis)
- pancreatitis
- electrolyte imbalance (e.g. low or high levels of potassium in the blood)
- if you are on a special diet, such as a low-salt diet (e.g. using potassium substitutes)
- sulfonamide (sulfa) or thiazide allergy
- an unusual or allergic reaction to telmisartan, hydrochlorothiazide, other medicines, foods, dyes, or preservatives
- pregnant or trying to get pregnant
- breast-feeding

How should I take this medicine?

Take telmisartan-hydrochlorothiazide tablets by mouth. Follow the directions on the prescription label.

Swallow the tablets with a drink of water. This medicine can be taken with or without food. Take your doses at regular intervals. Do not take your medicine more often than directed. Contact your pediatrician or health care professional regarding the use of this medicine in children. Special care may be needed. Elderly patients over 65 years old may have a stronger reaction to this medicine and need smaller doses.

What if I miss a dose?

If you miss a dose, take it as soon as you can. If it is almost time for your next dose, take only that dose. Do not take double or extra doses.

What may interact with telmisartan-hydrochlorothiazide?

- allopurinol
- anti-inflammatory drugs (NSAIDs, such as ibuprofen)
- blood pressure medications
- diabetic medications
- dofetilide
- griseofulvin
- hawthorn or horse chestnut
- lithium
- potassium salts or potassium supplements
- prochlorperazine
- some antibiotics which increase sensitivity to sunlight (sulfonamides, tetracyclines)
- some cholesterol-lowering medications (e.g. cholestyramine or colestipol)
- some medicines for mental disorders (phenothiazines)
- vitamin A (retinol) creams or pills such as tretinoin Retin-A®, Renova®, Solage®, Atragen®, and others
- water pills (especially potassium-sparing diuretics such as triamterene or amiloride)

Tell your prescriber or health care professional about all other medicines you are taking, including nonprescription medicines, nutritional supplements, or herbal products. Also tell your prescriber or health care professional if you are a frequent user of drinks with caffeine or alcohol, if you smoke, or if you use illegal drugs. These may affect the way your medicine works. Check with your health care professional before stopping or starting any of your medicines.

What should I watch for while taking telmisartan-hydrochlorothiazide?

Check your blood pressure regularly while you are taking this medicine. Ask your prescriber or health care professional what your blood pressure should be and when you should contact him or her. When you check your blood pressure, write down the measurements to show your prescriber or health care professional. If you are taking this medicine for a long time you must visit your prescriber or health care professional for regular checks on your progress. Make sure you schedule appointments on a regular basis. Check with your prescriber or health care professional if you get an attack of severe diarrhea, nausea and vomiting, or if you sweat a lot. You must not get dehydrated. Ask your prescriber

or health care professional how much fluid you need to drink a day. The loss of too much body fluid can make it dangerous for you to take this medicine. You may get dizzy. Do not drive, use machinery, or do anything that requires mental alertness until you know how telmisartan-hydrochlorothiazide affects you. To avoid dizzy or fainting spells, do not stand or sit up quickly. Alcohol may increase the possibility of dizziness. Avoid alcoholic drinks until you have discussed their use with your prescriber or health care professional. If you are going to have surgery tell your prescriber or health care professional that you are taking telmisartan-hydrochlorothiazide. Telmisartan-hydrochlorothiazide may affect your blood sugar level. If you have diabetes, check with your prescriber or health care professional before changing the dose of your diabetic medicine. Avoid salt substitutes unless you are told otherwise by your prescriber or health care professional. Do not treat yourself for a fever or sore throat; check with your prescriber or health care professional first.

What side effects may I notice from taking telmisartan-hydrochlorothiazide?

Side effects that you should report to your prescriber or health care professional as soon as possible:
Rare or uncommon:
- difficulty breathing, difficulty swallowing, hoarseness, or tightening of the throat
- redness, blistering, peeling or loosening of the skin, including inside the mouth
- swelling of your face, lips, tongue, hands, or feet
- unusual rash, bleeding or bruising, or pinpoint red spots on the skin

Other:
- confusion, dizziness, lightheadedness or fainting spells
- decreased amount of urine passed
- decreased sexual function
- fast or uneven (irregular) heart beat, palpitations, or chest pain
- fever or chills
- muscle cramps or pain
- stomach pain
- unusual tiredness or weakness
- vomiting
- worsened gout pain
- yellowing of the eyes or skin

Side effects that usually do not require medical attention (report to your prescriber or health care professional if they continue or are bothersome):
- cough
- diarrhea
- increased sensitivity to the sun

Where can I keep my medicine?

Keep out of the reach of children in a container that small children cannot open. Store your medicine at room temperature between 15 and 30 degrees C (59 and 86 degrees F). Tablets should not be removed from the blisters until right before use. Throw away any unused medicine after the expiration date.

H

Hydrochlorothiazide, HCTZ; Triamterene tablets or capsules

DYAZIDE®;
25 mg/37.5 mg;
Capsule
SmithKline Beecham
Pharmaceuticals Div
SmithKline Beecham
Co

MAXZIDE®;
50 mg/75 mg; Tablet
Mylan Bertek
Pharmaceuticals Inc

What are hydrochlorothiazide; triamterene tablets or capsules?

HYDROCHLOROTHIAZIDE; HCTZ TRIAMTERENE (MAXIDE® or DYAZIDE®) is a diuretic (water or fluid pill). Diuretics increase the amount of urine passed, which causes the body to lose water and salt. Dyazide® or Maxzide® are used to treat water retention and swelling caused by conditions such as heart, kidney, and liver disease. Triamterene is combined with hydrochlorothiazide to treat high blood pressure. Triamterene does not cause your body to lose potassium the way that many diuretics do. Generic hydrochlorothiazide; triamterene is available.

What should my health care professional know before I take hydrochlorothiazide; triamterene?

They need to know if you have any of these conditions:
- an unusual or allergic reaction to sulfonamide drugs, triamterene, hydrochlorothiazide, other diuretics, medicines, foods, dyes, or preservatives
- breast-feeding
- diabetes mellitus
- difficulty breathing or chronic lung disease
- gout or high blood levels of uric acid
- high blood levels of potassium
- kidney disease or kidney stones
- liver disease or jaundice
- low blood levels of sodium
- pancreatitis
- pregnant or trying to get pregnant
- small amount of urine, or difficulty passing urine
- systemic lupus erythematosus (SLE)

How should I take this medicine?

Take hydrochlorothiazide; triamterene by mouth. Follow the directions on the prescription label. Swallow the capsules or tablets with a drink of water. Take this medication with food or milk. Take your doses at regular intervals. Do not take your medicine more often than directed. Remember that you will need to pass urine frequently after taking hydrochlorothiazide; triamterene. Do not take your doses at a time of day that will cause you problems. Do not take at bedtime. Contact your pediatrician or health care professional regarding the use of this medicine in children. Special care may be needed.

What if I miss a dose?

If you miss a dose, take it as soon as you can. If it is almost time for your next dose, take only that dose. Do not take double or extra doses.

What may interact with hydrochlorothiazide, triamterene?

- alcohol
- allopurinol
- amantadine
- amphotericin B
- anti-inflammatory drugs including NSAIDs (e.g. ibuprofen), aspirin, or salicylates
- arsenic trioxide
- barbiturate medicines for inducing sleep or treating seizures (convulsions)
- bepridil
- cisplatin
- corticosteroids
- cyclosporine
- dofetilide
- drospirenone; ethinyl estradiol
- griseofulvin
- hawthorn
- heparin
- hormones such as cortisone, hydrocortisone, prednisone
- horse chestnut
- levomethadyl
- lithium
- medicines for asthma such as bronchodilators (inhalers such as Alupent®, Serevent®)
- medicines for diabetes
- medicines for high blood pressure or heart failure (ACE inhibitors, digoxin, angiotensin II antagonists, and others)
- methazolamide
- neuromuscular blockers used during anesthesia
- some antibiotics which increase sensitivity to sunlight (sulfonamides, tetracyclines)
- some medicines for mental disorders (phenothiazines)
- vitamin A (retinol) creams or pills such as tretinoin Retin-A®, Renova®, Solage®, Atragen®, and others
- some cholesterol-lowering medications (e.g. cholestyramine or colestipol)
- some medications for pain (e.g. codeine, Darvocet®, morphine, Percocet®)
- potassium salts
- sotalol
- tacrolimus
- water pills or diuretics

Tell your prescriber or health care professional about all other medicines you are taking, including non-prescription medicines, nutritional supplements, or herbal products. Also tell your prescriber or health care professional if you are a frequent user of drinks with caffeine or alcohol, if you smoke, or if you use illegal drugs.

These may affect the way your medicine works. Check with your health care professional before stopping or starting any of your medicines.

What should I watch for while taking hydrochlorothiazide; triamterene?

Visit your prescriber or health care professional for regular checks on your progress. Check your blood pressure regularly. Ask your prescriber or health care professional what your blood pressure should be, and when you should contact him or her. You must not get dehydrated, ask your prescriber or health care professional how much fluid you need to drink a day. Older patients may be more sensitive to the dehydrating effects of diuretics. Hydrochlorothiazide; triamterene will increase the amount of urine you pass. Do not stop taking this medication except on your prescriber's advice. Check with your prescriber or health care professional if you get severe nausea, vomiting or diarrhea. Watch your diet while you are taking hydrochlorothiazide; triamterene. Ask your prescriber or health care professional about diet and your potassium and sodium intake. Too much potassium can be harmful in some patients. Elderly patients, the severely ill, diabetics, or patients with kidney problems are more likely to suffer from the effects of too much potassium. Avoid salt-substitutes and nutritional supplements which contain potassium, unless your prescriber or health care professional tells you otherwise. You may get dizzy or lightheaded. Do not drive, use machinery, or do anything that needs mental alertness until you know how hydrochlorothiazide; triamterene affects you. To reduce the risk of dizzy or fainting spells, do not sit or stand up quickly, especially if you are an older patient. Alcohol can make you lightheaded, dizzy and increase confusion. Avoid or limit intake of alcoholic drinks. Hydrochlorothiazide; triamterene may increase your blood sugar levels. If you are diabetic, keep a close check on blood and urine sugar. Check with your prescriber or health care professional before you change the dose of your diabetic medicine. Hydrochlorothiazide; triamterene may make your skin more sensitive to sun or ultraviolet light. Keep out of the sun, or wear protective clothing and use a sunscreen. Do not use sun lamps or sun tanning beds or booths. If you are going to have surgery, tell your prescriber or health care professional that you are taking hydrochlorothiazide; triamterene.

What side effects may I notice from taking hydrochlorothiazide; triamterene?

Side effects that you should report to your prescriber or health care professional as soon as possible:
- abdominal pain
- black, tarry stools
- blood in urine
- bright red tongue, burning feeling in tongue, dry mouth, cracked corners of mouth
- confusion
- cough, hoarseness
- fast or irregular heartbeat, palpitations, chest pain
- fever, chills
- faintness or moderate dizziness
- lower back, abdominal or side pain
- muscle pain or cramps
- numbness or tingling in hands, feet, or lips
- pain or difficulty passing urine, reduced amount of urine passed
- redness, blistering, peeling or loosening of the skin, including inside the mouth
- skin rash, itching
- unusual bleeding or bruising, pinpoint red spots on the skin
- unusual tiredness or weakness
- yellowing of the eyes or skin
- blurred vision
- worsened gout pain
- decreased sexual function

Side effects that usually do not require medical attention (report to your prescriber or health care professional if they continue or are bothersome):
- constipation
- diarrhea
- mild dizziness
- dry mouth
- fatigue or weakness
- decreased appetite
- headache
- increased sensitivity to the sun
- increased frequency of urination
- nausea, vomiting

Where can I keep my medicine?

Keep out of the reach of children in a container that small children cannot open. Store at room temperature between 20 and 25 degrees C (68 and 77 degrees F). Protect from light. Throw away any unused medicine after the expiration date.

H

Hydrochlorothiazide, HCTZ; Valsartan tablets

DIOVAN HCT®;
12.5 mg/160 mg; Tablet
Novartis
Pharmaceuticals

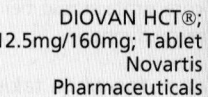

DIOVAN HCT®;
12.5mg/160mg; Tablet
Novartis
Pharmaceuticals

What are valsartan-hydrochlorothiazide tablets?

VALSARTAN-HYDROCHLOROTHIAZIDE (Diovan HCT®) is a combination of two drugs used to lower blood pressure. Valsartan controls high blood pressure (hypertension) by relaxing blood vessels. Hydrochlorothiazide is a diuretic. High blood pressure can damage the blood vessels of the brain, heart, and kidneys, resulting in a stroke, heart failure, or kidney failure. By lowering blood pressure, valsartan-hydrochlorothiazide can help reduce your risk of having damage to your kidneys, heart, or other organs. This medicine does not cure high blood pressure. Generic valsartan-hydrochlorothiazide tablets are not yet available.

What should my health care professional know before I take valsartan-hydrochlorothiazide?

They need to know if you have any of these conditions:

- autoimmune disease (e.g. lupus) or suppressed immune function
- diabetes mellitus
- gout
- heart or blood vessel disease (e.g. heart failure)
- liver disease
- recent heart attack or stroke
- kidney disease, (e.g. renal failure or renal artery stenosis)
- pancreatitis
- electrolyte imbalance (e.g. low or high levels of potassium in the blood)
- if you are on a special diet, such as a low-salt diet (e.g. using potassium substitutes)
- sulfonamide (sulfa) or thiazide allergy
- an unusual or allergic reaction to valsartan, hydrochlorothiazide, other medicines, foods, dyes, or preservatives
- pregnant or trying to get pregnant
- breast-feeding

How should I take this medicine?

Take valsartan-hydrochlorothiazide tablets by mouth. Follow the directions on the prescription label. Swallow the tablets with a drink of water. Valsartan-hydrochlorothiazide can be taken with or without food. Take your doses at regular intervals. Do not take your medicine more often than directed.

What if I miss a dose?

If you miss a dose, take it as soon as you can. If it is almost time for your next dose, take only that dose. Do not take double or extra doses.

What may interact with valsartan-hydrochlorothiazide?

- allopurinol
- anti-inflammatory drugs (NSAIDs, such as ibuprofen)
- diabetic medications
- blood pressure medications
- dofetilide
- griseofulvin
- hawthorn or horse chestnut
- lithium
- potassium salts or potassium supplements
- prochlorperazine
- some antibiotics which increase sensitivity to sunlight (sulfonamides, tetracyclines)
- some cholesterol-lowering medications (e.g. cholestyramine or colestipol)
- some medicines for mental disorders (phenothiazines)
- vitamin A (retinol) creams or pills such as tretinoin Retin-A®, Renova®, Solage®, Atragen®, and others
- water pills (especially potassium-sparing diuretics such as triamterene or amiloride

Tell your prescriber or health care professional about all other medicines you are taking, including non-prescription medicines, nutritional supplements, or herbal products. Also tell your prescriber or health care professional if you are a frequent user of drinks with caffeine or alcohol, if you smoke, or if you use illegal drugs. These may affect the way your medicine works. Check with your health care professional before stopping or starting any of your medicines.

What should I watch for while taking valsartan-hydrochlorothiazide?

Check your blood pressure regularly while you are taking valsartan-hydrochlorothiazide. Ask your prescriber or health care professional what your blood pressure should be and when you should contact him or her. When you check your blood pressure, write down the measurements to show your prescriber or health care professional. You must not get dehydrated. Ask your prescriber or health care professional how much fluid you need to drink a day. If you are taking this medicine for a long time, you must visit your health care professional for regular checks on your progress. Make sure you schedule appointments on a regular basis. Check with your prescriber or health care professional if you get an attack of severe diarrhea, nausea and vomiting, or if you sweat a lot. The loss of too much body fluid can make it dangerous for you to take valsartan-hydrochlorothiazide. You may get dizzy. Do not drive, use machinery, or do anything that requires mental alertness until you know how valsartan-hydrochlorothiazide affects you. To avoid dizzy or fainting spells, do not stand or sit up quickly. Alcohol may increase the possibility of dizziness. Avoid alcoholic drinks until you have discussed their use with your prescriber or health care professional. If you are going to have surgery tell

H

your prescriber or health care professional that you are taking valsartan-hydrochlorothiazide. Valsartan-hydrochlorothiazide may affect your blood sugar level. If you have diabetes, check with your prescriber or health care professional before changing the dose of your diabetic medicine. Avoid salt substitutes unless you are told otherwise by your prescriber or health care professional. Do not take medicines for appetite control, asthma, colds, cough, hay fever, or sinus problems without asking your prescriber or health care professional for advice. Do not treat yourself for a fever or sore throat; check with your prescriber or health care professional first.

What side effects may I notice from taking valsartan-hydrochlorothiazide?

Side effects that you should report to your prescriber or health care professional as soon as possible:
Rare or uncommon:
- difficulty breathing or swallowing, hoarseness, or tightening of the throat
- redness, blistering, peeling or loosening of the skin, including inside the mouth
- swelling of your face, lips, tongue, hands, or feet
- unusual rash, bleeding or bruising, or pinpoint red spots on the skin

Other:
- confusion, dizziness, lightheadedness or fainting spells
- decreased amount of urine passed
- decreased sexual function
- fast or uneven heart beat, palpitations, or chest pain
- fever or chills
- irregular heartbeat
- muscle cramps
- stomach pain
- unusual tiredness or weakness
- vomiting
- worsened gout pain
- yellowing of the eyes or skin

Side effects that usually do not require medical attention (report to your prescriber or health care professional if they continue or are bothersome):
- cough
- diarrhea
- headache
- increased sensitivity to the sun
- nausea
- tiredness or fatigue

Where can I keep my medicine?

Keep out of the reach of children and in a container that small children cannot open. Store your medicine at room temperature below 30 degrees C (86 degrees F). Protect from moisture. Keep your medicine container tightly closed and protect it from light. Throw away any unused medicine after the expiration date.

Hydrochlorothiazide; Spironolactone tablets

ALDACTAZIDE®; 25 mg/25 mg; Tablet GD Searle LLC a Subsidiary of Pharmacia Company Pfizer

ALDACTAZIDE®; 50 mg/50 mg; Tablet GD Searle LLC a Subsidiary of Pharmacia Company Pfizer

What do hydrochlorothiazide; spironolactone tablets do?

HYDROCHLOROTHIAZIDE; SPIRONOLACTONE (Aldactazide®) is a diuretic combination, which is also known as a water pill. Diuretics increase the amount of urine passed, which causes the body to lose water and salt. This drug is used to treat high blood pressure or water retention and swelling caused by conditions such as heart, kidney, and liver disease. Spironolactone does not cause your body to lose potassium the way that many diuretics do. Generic hydrochlorothiazide; spironolactone tablets are available.

What should my health care professional know before I take hydrochlorothiazide; spironolactone?

They need to know if you have any of these conditions:
- diabetes mellitus
- difficulty breathing or asthma
- drink a lot of water
- gout or high blood levels of uric acid
- heart disease
- high blood levels of cholesterol
- high blood levels of potassium
- hyperparathyroidism or high blood levels of calcium
- kidney disease
- liver disease or jaundice
- low blood levels of sodium
- menstrual irregularity
- pancreatitis
- small amount of urine, or difficulty passing urine
- systemic lupus erythematosus (SLE)
- an unusual reaction to hydrochlorothiazide, spironolactone, other diuretics, sulfonamide drugs, carbonic anhydrase inhibitors like acetazolamide, other medicines, foods, dyes, or preservatives
- breast-feeding
- pregnant or trying to get pregnant

How should I take this medicine?

Take hydrochlorothiazide; spironolactone tablets by mouth. Follow the directions on the prescription label. Swallow the tablets with a drink of water. Take this medication with food. Take your doses at regular intervals. Do not take your medicine more often than directed. Remember that you will need to pass urine frequently after taking hydrochlorothiazide; spironolactone. Do not take your doses at a time of day that will cause you problems. Do not take at bedtime. Contact your pediatrician or health care professional regarding the use of this medicine in children. Special care may be needed.

What if I miss a dose?

If you miss a dose, take it as soon as you can. If it is almost time for your next dose, take only that dose. Do not take double or extra doses.

What other medicines can interact with hydrochlorothiazide; spironolactone?

- alcohol
- allopurinol
- amantadine
- amphotericin B
- anti-inflammatory drugs including NSAIDs (e.g. ibuprofen), aspirin, or salicylates
- arsenic trioxide
- barbiturate medicines for inducing sleep or treating seizures (convulsions)
- bepridil
- caffeine; ergotamine
- cisplatin
- cyclosporine
- diazoxide
- digoxin
- dofetilide
- drospirenone; ethinyl estradiol
- ephedra, Ma huang
- eplerenone
- griseofulvin
- hawthorn
- heparin
- hormones such as cortisone, hydrocortisone, prednisone
- horse chestnut
- levomethadyl
- lithium
- medicines for asthma such as bronchodilators (inhalers such as Alupent®, Serevent®)
- medicines for diabetes
- medicines for high blood pressure or heart failure (ACE inhibitors, digoxin, angiotensin II antagonists, beta-blockers, and others)
- methazolamide
- neuromuscular blockers used during anesthesia
- potassium salts
- quinidine
- some antibiotics which increase sensitivity to sunlight (sulfonamides, tetracyclines)
- some cholesterol-lowering medications (e.g. cholestyramine or colestipol)
- some medicines for mental disorders (phenothiazines)
- some medicines for pain (e.g. codeine, Darvocet®, morphine, Percocet®)
- sotalol
- tacrolimus
- vitamin A (retinol) creams or pills such as tretinoin Retin-A®, Renova®, Solage®, and others
- warfarin
- water pills or diuretics

Tell your prescriber or health care professional about all other medicines you are taking, including non-prescription medicines, nutritional supplements, or herbal products. Also tell your prescriber or health care professional if you are a frequent user of drinks with caffeine or alcohol, if you smoke, or if you use illegal drugs. These may affect the way your medicine works. Check with your health care professional before stopping or starting any of your medicines.

What do I need to watch for while I take hydrochlorothiazide; spironolactone?

Visit your prescriber or health care professional for regular checks on your progress. Check your blood pressure regularly. Ask your prescriber or health care professional what your blood pressure should be and when you should contact him or her. You must not get dehydrated, ask your prescriber or health care professional how much fluid you need to drink a day. Older patients may be more sensitive to the dehydrating effects of diuretics. This drug will increase the amount of urine you pass. Do not stop taking this medication except on your prescriber's advice. Check with your prescriber or health care professional if you get severe nausea, vomiting or diarrhea. Watch your diet while you are taking this medication. Ask your prescriber or health care professional about diet and your potassium and sodium intake. Spironolactone can make your body hold onto potassium. Too much potassium can be very harmful. Elderly patients, the severely ill, patients with diabetes, or patients with kidney problems are more likely to suffer from the effects of too much potassium. Avoid salt-substitutes and nutritional supplements that contain potassium, unless your prescriber or health care professional tells you otherwise. You may need to avoid foods that are high in potassium, such as bananas, coconuts, dates, figs, prunes, apricots, peaches, grapefruit juice, tomato juice, and orange juice. You may get dizzy or lightheaded. Do not drive, use machinery, or do anything that needs mental alertness until you know how this drug affects you. To reduce the risk of dizzy or fainting spells, do not sit or stand up quickly, especially if you are an older patient. Alcohol can make you lightheaded, dizzy and increase confusion. Avoid or limit intake of alcoholic drinks. Hydrochlorothiazide; spironolactone may increase your blood sugar levels. If you have diabetes, keep a close check on your blood and urine sugar. Check with your prescriber or health care professional before you change the dose of your medicine(s) for diabetes. Hydrochlorothiazide; spironolactone may make your skin more sensitive to sun or ultraviolet light. Keep out of the sun, or wear protective clothing outdoors and use a sunscreen (at least SPF 15). Do not use sun lamps or sun tanning beds or booths. If you are going to have surgery, tell your prescriber or health care professional that you are taking hydrochlorothiazide; spironolactone.

What side effects may I notice from taking hydrochlorothiazide; spironolactone?

Side effects that you should report to your prescriber or health care professional as soon as possible:
- blood in urine
- blurred vision, change in vision
- confusion
- diarrhea
- difficulty breathing
- fainting spells
- fast or irregular heartbeat, palpitations, chest pain
- fever or chills, sore throat, cough
- muscle pain or weakness, cramps
- nausea, vomiting
- nervousness
- numbness or tingling in hands, feet, or lips
- pain or difficulty passing urine, reduced amount of urine passed
- redness, blistering, peeling or loosening of the skin, including inside the mouth
- severe stomach pain
- skin rash, itching
- unusual bleeding or bruising, pinpoint red spots on the skin
- unusual or severe tiredness or weakness
- yellowing of the eyes or skin
- worsened gout pain

Side effects that usually do not require medical attention (report to your prescriber or health care professional if they continue or are bothersome):
- breast tenderness in females
- constipation
- decreased appetite
- dizziness or lightheadedness
- drowsiness
- dry mouth
- enlarged breasts in males
- fatigue or weakness
- headache
- increased frequency of urination
- increased sensitivity to the sun
- increased thirst
- irregular menstrual periods
- sexual difficulty, inability to have an erection
- stomach upset, pain, or cramps, indigestion

Where can I keep my medicine?

Keep out of the reach of children in a container that small children cannot open. Store below 25 degrees C (77 degrees F). Throw away any unused medicine after the expiration date.

Hydrocodone tablets and capsules

HYCODAN®;
1.5 mg/5 mg; Tablet
Eckerd Drug Co

What are hydrocodone tablets and capsules?

HYDROCODONE (Hycodan®) is used to relieve cough due to colds or minor upper respiratory infections. Federal law prohibits the transfer of hydrocodone to any person other than the patient for whom it was prescribed. Do not share this medicine with anyone else. Generic hydrocodone combination capsules or tablets are available.

What should my health care professional know before I take hydrocodone?

They need to know if you have any of these conditions:
- diarrhea
- head injury
- heart disease
- kidney disease
- liver disease
- lung disease or breathing difficulties
- seizures
- an allergic or unusual reaction to hydrocodone, codeine, morphine, other medicines, foods, dyes, or preservatives
- pregnant or trying to get pregnant
- breast-feeding

How should I take this medicine?

Take hydrocodone tablets or capsules by mouth. Follow the directions on the prescription label. If hydrocodone upsets your stomach, take it with food or milk. Do not take your medicine more often than directed. Contact your pediatrician or health care professional regarding the use of this medicine in children. Special care may be needed. Do not share this medicine with anyone.

What if I miss a dose?

If you miss a dose, take it as soon as you can. If it is almost time for your next dose, take only that dose. Do not take double or extra doses.

What may interact with hydrocodone?

- medicines for diarrhea
- medicines for high blood pressure
- medicines for seizures
- rifampin
- ritonavir

Because hydrocodone can cause drowsiness, other medicines that also cause drowsiness may increase this effect of hydrocodone. Some medicines that cause drowsiness are:

- alcohol and alcohol-containing medicines
- barbiturates such as phenobarbital
- certain antidepressants or tranquilizers
- certain antihistamines used in cold medicines

Tell your prescriber or health care professional about all other medicines you are taking, including non-pre-

scription medicines, nutritional supplements, or herbal products. Also tell your prescriber or health care professional if you are a frequent user of drinks with caffeine or alcohol, if you smoke, or if you use illegal drugs. These may affect the way your medicine works. Check with your health care professional before stopping or starting any of your medicines.

What should I watch for while taking hydrocodone?

Tell your prescriber or health care professional if your symptoms do not improve or get worse. Use exactly as directed by your prescriber or health care professional. You may get drowsy or dizzy when you first start taking hydrocodone or change doses. Do not drive, use machinery, or do anything that needs mental alertness until you know how hydrocodone affects you. Stand or sit up slowly, this reduces the risk of dizzy or fainting spells. These effects may be worse if you are an older patient. The drowsiness should decrease after taking hydrocodone for a couple of days. Be careful taking other medicines which may also make you tired. This effect may be worse when taking these medicines with hydrocodone. Alcohol can increase possible drowsiness, dizziness, confusion and affect your breathing. Avoid alcohol while taking hydrocodone. Hydrocodone may cause constipation. You may need to take a laxative and/or a stool softener while taking hydrocodone. Try to have a bowel movement every 2 to 3 days, at least. If you do not have a bowel movement for 3 days or more call your prescriber or health care professional. Your mouth may get dry. Drinking plenty of water, chewing sugarless gum or sucking on hard candy may help to relieve dry mouth symptoms. Have regular dental checks. If you are going to have surgery, tell your prescriber or health care professional that you are taking hydrocodone.

What side effects may I notice from taking hydrocodone?

Side effects that you should report to your prescriber or health care professional as soon as possible:

Rare or uncommon:
- cold, clammy skin
- decreased ability to pass urine
- difficulty breathing, wheezing
- severe rash
- seizures
- slow or fast heart beat

More common:
- confusion
- lightheadedness or fainting spells
- nervousness or restlessness

Side effects that usually do not require medical attention (report to your prescriber or health care professional if they continue or are bothersome):
- blurred vision
- constipation
- dizziness or drowsiness
- dry mouth
- headache
- nausea, vomiting
- pinpoint pupils
- sweating

Where can I keep my medicine?

Keep out of the reach of children in a container that small children cannot open. Do not share or give this medicine to anyone else. Avoid accidental swallowing of hydrocodone by someone (especially children) other than the person for whom it was prescribed as this may result in severe effects and possibly death. Store at room temperature between 15 and 30 degrees C (5 and 86 degrees F). Protect from light. Throw away any unused medicine after the expiration date.

Hydrocodone; Ibuprofen tablets

VICOPROFEN®; 7.5 mg/200 mg; Tablet Abbott Pharmaceutical Product Division

HYDROCODONE; IBUPROFEN; 7.5 mg/ 200 mg; Tablet Teva Pharmaceuticals USA Inc

What are hydrocodone; ibuprofen tablets?

HYDROCODONE; IBUPROFEN (Vicoprofen®, Reprexain™) is a combination of two different types of pain medicine. Hydrocodone; ibuprofen is used to treat moderate to severe pain. Federal law prohibits the transfer of this product to any person other than the patient for whom it was prescribed. Generic hydrocodone; ibuprofen tablets are available.

What should my health care professional know before I take hydrocodone; ibuprofen?

They need to know if you have any of these conditions:
- anemia
- asthma
- bleeding problems
- cigarette smoker
- dental disease
- diabetes
- diarrhea
- drink more than 3 alcohol-containing beverages a day
- head injury
- heart or circulation problems
- kidney disease
- liver disease
- lung disease or breathing difficulties
- nasal polyps
- seizures

- stomach or duodenal ulcers
- systemic lupus erythematosus
- ulcerative colitis
- an unusual or allergic reaction to hydrocodone, ibuprofen, other pain medicines, foods, dyes or preservatives
- pregnant or trying to get pregnant
- breast-feeding

How should I take this medicine?

Take hydrocodone; ibuprofen tablets by mouth. Follow the directions on the prescription label. Swallow tablets whole with a full glass of water; take tablets in an upright or sitting position. Taking a sip of water first, before taking the tablets, may help you swallow them. If possible take bedtime doses at least 10 minutes before lying down. You can take this medicine with food to prevent stomach upset. Do not take your medicine more often than directed. This medicine is not for use in children. Do not share this medicine with anyone.

What if I miss a dose?

If you miss a dose, take it as soon as you can. If it is almost time for your next dose, take only that dose. Do not take double or extra doses.

What may interact with hydrocodone; ibuprofen?

- anti-inflammatory drugs (other NSAIDs)
- aspirin and aspirin-like medicines
- cyclosporine
- entecavir
- herbal products that contain feverfew, garlic, ginger, or ginkgo biloba
- hormones such as prednisone or cortisone
- lithium
- medicines for diabetes that are taken by mouth
- medicines for high blood pressure
- medicines that affect platelets
- medicines that treat or prevent blood clots such as warfarin and other "blood thinners"
- medicines for seizures
- methotrexate
- pemetrexed
- water pills (diuretics)

Because hydrocodone can cause drowsiness, other medicines that also cause drowsiness may increase this effect of hydrocodone; ibuprofen. Some other medicines that cause drowsiness are:

- alcohol-containing medicines
- barbiturates such as phenobarbital
- certain antidepressants or tranquilizers
- muscle relaxants
- certain antihistamines used in cold medicines

Tell your prescriber or health care professional about all other medicines you are taking, including non-prescription medicines, nutritional supplements, or herbal products. Also tell your prescriber or health care professional if you are a frequent user of drinks with caffeine or alcohol, if you smoke, or if you use illegal drugs. These may affect the way your medicine works. Check with your health care professional before stopping or starting any of your medicines.

What should I watch for while taking hydrocodone; ibuprofen?

Tell your prescriber or health care professional if your pain does not go away, if it gets worse, or if you have new or different type of pain. Do not take other pain medicines with hydrocodone; ibuprofen without advice. Many non-prescription pain medicines contain ibuprofen as an ingredient. Always read the labels carefully to avoid taking too much ibuprofen. Use exactly as directed by your prescriber or health care professional. Do not take more than the recommended dose. If you are receiving cancer chemotherapy or other immunosuppression medicine, do not take hydrocodone; ibuprofen without checking with your prescriber or health care professional. These products may hide the signs of an infection such as fever or pain. To reduce unpleasant effects on your throat and stomach, take hydrocodone; ibuprofen with a full glass of water and never just before lying down. You may also take it with food or milk. Hydrocodone; ibuprofen may make you drowsy when you first start taking it or change doses. Do not drive, use machinery, or do anything that needs mental alertness until you know how this medicine affects you. Do not sit or stand up quickly. This reduces the risk of dizzy or fainting spells. These effects may be worse if you are an older patient. The drowsiness should decrease after taking the medicine for a couple of days. If you have not slept because of your pain, you may sleep more the first few days your pain is controlled to catch-up on missed sleep. Be careful taking other medicines that may also make you tired. This effect may be worse when taking these medicines with hydrocodone; ibuprofen. Alcohol can increase drowsiness, dizziness, confusion and affect your breathing. Avoid alcohol while taking hydrocodone; ibuprofen. Do not smoke cigarettes or drink alcohol; these may increase the irritation to your stomach when taking this medicine. If you get black, tarry stools or vomit up what looks like coffee grounds, call your prescriber or health care professional at once. Hydrocodone; ibuprofen can cause constipation. Make sure to take a laxative and/or a stool softener. Try to have a bowel movement at least every 2 to 3 days. If you do not have a bowel movement for 3 days or more call your prescriber or health care professional. They may recommend using an enema or suppository to help you move your bowels. It is especially important not to use hydrocodone; ibuprofen during the last 3 months of pregnancy unless specifically directed to do so by your health care provider. Hydrocodone; ibuprofen might cause problems in the unborn child or complications during delivery. If you are going to have surgery, tell your prescriber or health care professional that you are taking hydrocodone; ibuprofen. Hydrocodone; ibuprofen can cause you to bleed more easily. Problems can arise if you need dental work, and in the day to day care of your teeth. Try to avoid damage to your teeth and gums when you brush or floss your teeth.

What side effects may I notice from taking hydrocodone; ibuprofen?

Elderly patients are more likely to get side effects. Side effects that you should report to your prescriber or health care professional as soon as possible:

- signs of bleeding—bruising, pinpoint red spots on the skin, black, tarry stools, blood in the urine, unusual tiredness or weakness
- signs of an allergic reaction—difficulty breathing, wheezing, skin rash, redness, blistering, peeling or itching, swelling of eyelids, throat, lips or feet
- change in the amount of urine passed
- chest pain
- cold, clammy skin
- confusion
- fast heartbeat
- fever, chills, muscle aches and pains
- lightheadedness or fainting spells
- nervousness or restlessness

- pain or difficulty passing urine
- seizures
- slow or fast heart beat
- stomach pain or cramps

Side effects that usually do not require medical attention (report to your prescriber or health care professional if they continue or are bothersome):

- confusion
- constipation
- diarrhea
- dizziness, drowsiness
- flushing
- gas or heartburn
- headache
- itching
- nausea, vomiting

Where can I keep my medicine?

Keep out of the reach of children in a container that small children cannot open. Do not share or give this medicine to anyone else. Avoid accidental swallowing of hydrocodone; ibuprofen by someone (especially children) other than for whom it was prescribed as this may result in severe side effects and possibly death. Store at 25 degrees C (77 degrees F). Keep container tightly closed. Protect from light. Throw away any unused medicine after the expiration date.

Hydrocortisone tablets

CORTEF®; 5 mg; Tablet Pharmacia and Upjohn Div Pfizer

CORTEF®; 10 mg; Tablet Pharmacia and Upjohn Div Pfizer

What are hydrocortisone tablets?

HYDROCORTISONE (Cortef®, Hydrocortone®) is a corticosteroid. It helps to reduce swelling, redness, itching, and allergic reactions. Hydrocortisone is similar to natural steroid hormone produced by the adrenal gland. Hydrocortisone treats severe allergies, skin problems, asthma, arthritis, or many other conditions. Generic hydrocortisone tablets are available.

What should my health care professional know before I take hydrocortisone?

They need to know if you have any of these conditions:

- blood clotting disorder
- Cushing's syndrome
- diabetes
- high blood pressure
- infection, including chicken-pox, herpes, measles, or tuberculosis
- liver disease
- myasthenia gravis
- osteoporosis
- previous heart attack
- psychosis
- seizures (convulsions)
- stomach or intestinal disease
- underactive thyroid

- an unusual or allergic reaction to hydrocortisone, corticosteroids, other medicines, foods, dyes, or preservatives
- pregnant or trying to get pregnant
- breast-feeding

How should I take this medicine?

Take hydrocortisone tablets by mouth. Follow the directions on the prescription label. Swallow the tablets with a drink of water. Take with milk or food to avoid stomach upset. If you are only taking hydrocortisone once a day, take it in the morning, which is the time your body normally secretes cortisol. Take your doses at regular intervals. Do not take your medicine more often than directed. Do not stop taking hydrocortisone except on your prescriber's advice. Contact your pediatrician or health care professional regarding the use of this medicine in children. Special care may be needed.

What if I miss a dose?

If you miss a dose, take it as soon as you can. If it is almost time for your next dose, consult your prescriber or health care professional. You may need to miss a dose or take a double dose, depending on your condition and treatment. Do not take double or extra doses without advice.

What may interact with hydrocortisone?

- anti-inflammatory drugs (NSAIDs, such as ibuprofen)
- aspirin
- barbiturate medicines for inducing sleep or treating seizures (convulsions)
- bosentan
- carbamazepine
- female hormones, including contraceptive or birth control pills
- heart medicines
- medicines for diabetes
- medicines that improve muscle strength or tone for conditions like myasthenia gravis
- phenytoin
- rifampin
- toxoids and vaccines
- water pills

Tell your prescriber or health care professional about all other medicines you are taking, including non-prescription medicines, nutritional supplements, or herbal products. Also tell your prescriber or health care professional if you are a frequent user of drinks with caffeine or alcohol, if you smoke, or if you use illegal drugs. These may affect the way your medicine works. Check with your health care professional before stopping or starting any of your medicines.

What should I watch for while taking hydrocortisone?

Visit your prescriber or health care professional for regular checks on your progress. If you are taking corticosteroids for a long time, carry an identification card with your name, the type and dose of corticosteroid, and your prescriber's name and address. Do not suddenly stop taking hydrocortisone. You may need to gradually reduce the dose, so that your body can adjust. Follow the advice of your prescriber or health care professional. If you take corticosteroids for a long time, avoid contact with people who have an infection. You may be at an increased risk from infection while taking hydrocortisone. Tell your prescriber or health care professional if you are exposed to anyone with measles or chickenpox, or if you develop sores or blisters that do not heal properly. People who are taking certain dosages of hydrocortisone may need to avoid immunization with certain vaccines or may need to have changes in their vaccination schedules to ensure adequate protection from certain diseases. Make sure to tell your prescriber or health care professional that you are taking hydrocortisone before receiving any vaccine. If you are diabetic, hydrocortisone can affect your blood sugar. Check with your prescriber or health care professional if you need help adjusting the dose of your diabetic medicine. If you take hydrocortisone tablets every day, you may need to watch your diet. Your body can also lose potassium while you take this medicine. Ask your prescriber or health care professional about your diet, especially about your salt intake. If you are going

to have surgery tell your prescriber or health care professional that you are taking hydrocortisone, or have taken it within the last 12 months. Alcohol can increase the risk of getting serious side effects while you are taking hydrocortisone. Avoid alcoholic drinks. Elderly patients have an increased risk of side effects from hydrocortisone. Hydrocortisone can interfere with certain lab tests and can cause false skin test results.

What side effects may I notice from taking hydrocortisone?

Some side effects can be reduced by taking single daily doses in the morning. Check with your prescriber or health care professional to determine the best schedule for your condition.

Side effects that you should report to your prescriber or health care professional as soon as possible:
- bloody or black, tarry stools
- confusion, excitement, restlessness, a false sense of well-being
- eye pain, decreased or blurred vision, or bulging eyes
- fever, sore throat, sneezing, cough, or other signs of infection
- frequent passing of urine
- hallucinations (seeing and hearing things that are not really there)
- increased thirst
- irregular heartbeat
- menstrual problems
- mental depression, mood swings, mistaken feelings of self-importance, mistaken feelings of being mistreated
- muscle cramps or muscle weakness
- nausea, vomiting
- pain in hips, back, ribs, arms, shoulders, or legs
- rounding out of face
- skin problems, acne
- stomach pain
- swelling of feet or lower legs
- unusual bruising or red pinpoint spots on the skin
- unusual tiredness or weakness
- weight gain or weight loss
- wounds that will not heal

Side effects that usually do not require medical attention (report to your prescriber or health care professional if they continue or are bothersome):
- diarrhea or constipation
- change in taste
- headache
- increased appetite or loss of appetite
- increased sweating
- nervousness, restlessness, or difficulty sleeping
- unusual increased growth of hair on the face or body
- upset stomach

Where can I keep my medicine?

Keep out of the reach of children in a container that small children cannot open. Store at room temperature between 15 and 30 degrees C (59 and 86 degrees F). Throw away any unused medicine after the expiration date.

This drug requires an FDA medication guide. See page xxxvii.

Hydromorphone tablets

DILAUDID®;
4 mg; Tablet
Abbott
Pharmaceutical
Product Division

DILAUDID®;
2 mg; Tablet
Abbott
Pharmaceutical
Product Division

What are hydromorphone tablets?

HYDROMORPHONE (Dilaudid®) relieves moderate to severe pain. Hydromorphone may be used to control pain following surgery, child birth, and other procedures. Hydromorphone may also be used to treat pain associated with cancer, heart attacks, sickle cell disease and other medical conditions. Federal law prohibits the transfer of hydromorphone to any person other than the patient for whom it was prescribed. Do not share this medicine with anyone else. Generic hydromorphone tablets are available.

What should my health care professional know before I take hydromorphone?

They need to know if you have any of these conditions:
- diarrhea
- head injury
- heart disease
- intestinal disease
- liver disease
- lung disease, asthma or breathing problems
- prostate trouble
- seizures
- an allergic or unusual reaction to hydromorphone, codeine, morphine, other medicines, sulfites, foods, dyes, or preservatives
- pregnant or trying to get pregnant
- breast-feeding

How should I take this medicine?

Take hydromorphone tablets by mouth. Follow the directions on the prescription label. Swallow the tablets with a drink of water. If hydromorphone upsets your stomach, you can take it with food or milk. Do not share this medicine with any one. Contact your pediatrician or health care professional regarding the use of this medicine in children. Special care may be needed.

What if I miss a dose?

If you miss a dose, take it as soon as you can. If it is almost time for your next dose, take only that dose. Do not take double or extra doses.

What may interact with hydromorphone?

- medicines for high blood pressure
- medicines for seizures

Because hydromorphone causes drowsiness, other medicines that also cause drowsiness may increase this effect of hydromorphone. Some medicines that cause drowsiness are:

- alcohol and alcohol-containing medicines
- barbiturates such as phenobarbital
- certain antidepressants and tranquilizers
- muscle relaxants
- certain antihistamines used in cold medicines

Tell your prescriber or health care professional about all other medicines you are taking, including non-prescription medicines, nutritional supplements, or herbal products. Also tell your prescriber or health care professional if you are a frequent user of drinks with caffeine or alcohol, if you smoke, or if you use illegal drugs. These may affect the way your medicine works. Check with your health care professional before stopping or starting any of your medicines.

What should I watch for while taking hydromorphone?

Tell your prescriber or health care professional if your pain does not go away, if it gets worse or it you have a new or different type of pain. Use exactly as directed by your prescriber or health care professional. If you are taking hydromorphone on a regular basis, do not suddenly stop taking it. Your body becomes used to the hydromorphone and when you suddenly stop taking it, you may develop a severe reaction. This DOES NOT mean you are "addicted" to hydromorphone. Addiction is a behavior related to getting and using a drug for a non-medical reason. If you have pain, you have a medical reason to take pain medicine such as hydromorphone to control your pain. You may get drowsy or dizzy when you first start taking hydromorphone or change doses. Do not drive, use machinery, or do anything that needs mental alertness until you know how hydromorphone affects you. Stand or sit up slowly, this reduces the risk of dizzy or fainting spells. These effects may be worse if you are an older patient. The drowsiness should decrease after taking hydromorphone for a couple of days. If you have not slept because of your pain, you may sleep more the first few days your pain is controlled to catch-up on missed sleep. Be careful taking other medicines which may also make you tired. This effect may be worse when taking these medicines with hydromorphone. Alcohol can increase possible drowsiness, dizziness, confusion and affect your breathing. Avoid alcohol while taking hydromorphone. Hydromorphone will cause constipation. Make sure to take a laxative and/or a stool softener while taking hydromorphone. Try to have a bowel movement every 2 to 3 days, at least. If you do not have a bowel movement for 3 days or more call your prescriber or health care professional. They may recommend using an enema or suppository to help you move your bowels. Your mouth may get dry. Drinking plenty of water, chewing sugarless gum or sucking on hard candy may help to relieve dry mouth symptoms. Have regular dental checks. If you are going to have surgery, tell your prescriber or health care professional that you are taking hydromorphone. Rarely, hydromorphone may cause you to have hallucinations (to see things that are not really there) or cause your legs or arms to "jerk" or have spasms. If you experience these effects, call your prescriber or health care professional.

What side effects may I notice from taking hydromorphone?

Side effects that you should report to your prescriber or health care professional as soon as possible.
Rare or uncommon:
- cold, clammy skin
- difficulty breathing, wheezing
- irregular heartbeat, palpitations
- seizures
- severe rash
- unusual weakness

More common:
- confusion
- lightheadedness or fainting spells
- nervousness or restlessness
- difficulty passing urine

Side effects that usually do not require medical attention (report to your prescriber or health care professional if they continue or are bothersome):
- blurred vision
- constipation
- drowsiness, dizziness
- flushing
- dry mouth
- headache
- nausea, vomiting
- pinpoint pupils

Where can I keep my medicine?

Keep out of the reach of children in a container that small children cannot open. Do not share or give this medicine to anyone else. Avoid accidental swallowing of hydromorphone by someone (especially children) other than the person for whom it was prescribed as this may result in severe effects and possibly death. Store at room temperature between 15 and 30 degrees C (59 and 86 degrees F). Protect from light. Throw away any unused medicine after the expiration date.

Hydroxychloroquine tablets

PLAQUENIL®;
200 mg; Tablet
Sanofi-Synthelabo Inc

HYDROXYCHLOROQUINE,
200 mg; Tablet
Teva Pharmaceuticals
USA Inc

What are hydroxychloroquine tablets?

HYDROXYCHLOROQUINE (Plaquenil®) helps to relieve swelling, stiffness and joint pain associated with rheumatoid arthritis. It is effective in controlling the symptoms of systemic lupus erythematosus. Hydroxychloroquine is also sometimes used to suppress and treat acute attacks of malaria. Generic hydroxychloroquine tablets are available.

What should my health care professional know before I take hydroxychloroquine?

They need to know if you have any of these conditions:
- an alcohol problem
- blood disorders
- dental disease
- eye disease
- glucose-6-phosphate dehydrogenase (G6PD) deficiency
- liver disease
- nerve or brain disease
- porphyria
- psoriasis
- seizures (convulsions)
- stomach or intestinal disease
- an unusual or allergic reaction to chloroquine, hydroxychloroquine, other medicines, foods, dyes, or preservatives
- pregnant or trying to get pregnant
- breast-feeding

How should I take this medicine?

Take hydroxychloroquine tablets by mouth. Follow the directions on the prescription label. Swallow tablets with a drink of water. If hydroxychloroquine upsets your stomach take it with food or milk. If you are taking hydroxychloroquine to treat arthritis or lupus erythematosus you will need to take daily doses for several weeks. If you are taking hydroxychloroquine to prevent malaria, you should start taking it two weeks before entering the endemic area, and continue for 8 weeks after leaving. If you are treating an acute attack of malaria you will need treatment for several days. Take your doses at regular intervals. Do not take your medicine more often than directed.

What if I miss a dose?

If you miss a daily dose, take it as soon as you can. If it is almost time for your next dose, take only that dose. If you forget a once-a-week dose, take it as soon as you can. Do not take double or extra doses.

What may interact with hydroxychloroquine?

- antacids
- botulinum toxins
- digoxin
- kaolin
- magnesium trisilicate
- metoprolol
- penicillamine

H

Tell your prescriber or health care professional about all other medicines you are taking, including non-prescription medicines, nutritional supplements, or herbal products. Also tell your prescriber or health care professional if you are a frequent user of drinks with caffeine or alcohol, if you smoke, or if you use illegal drugs. These may affect the way your medicine works. Check with your health care professional before stopping or starting any of your medicines.

What should I watch for while taking hydroxychloroquine?

If you are being treated for arthritis it may take several weeks of treatment before you notice an improvement in your symptoms. If you are taking hydroxychloroquine for a long time, visit your prescriber or health care professional for regular checks. If you notice any changes in your vision see your ophthalmologist for an eye exam. If you are being treated for malaria tell your prescriber or health care professional if your malarial symptoms do not improve in 2 to 3 days. Check with your pharmacist before you visit a new area where there are malaria-carrying mosquitoes. You may need to take a different antimalarial medicine. You may get drowsy. Do not drive, use machinery, or do anything that needs mental alertness until you know how hydroxychloroquine affects you. Hydroxychloroquine can cause blood problems. This can mean slow healing and a risk of infection. Try to avoid cutting or injuring yourself. Problems can arise if you need dental work, and in the day to day care of your teeth. Try to avoid damage to your teeth and gums when you brush or floss your teeth. Antacid can stop hydroxychloroquine working. If you get an upset stomach and want to take an antacid, make sure there is an interval of at least 2 hours since you last took hydroxychloroquine, or 4 hours before your next dose.

What side effects may I notice from taking hydroxychloroquine?

Serious side effects are more likely to occur with long-term use for rheumatoid arthritis rather than in the short-term use for acute malarial attacks.

Side effects that you should report to your prescriber or health care professional as soon as possible:

- blurred vision, or change in vision
- fainting spells
- fever or chills, sore throat
- hearing loss
- headaches, confusion, or other mental changes
- muscle weakness
- ringing in the ears
- seizures (convulsions)
- skin rash, itching
- tingling or numbness in the hands or feet
- unusual bleeding or bruising
- unusual tiredness or weakness

Side effects that usually do not require medical attention (report to your prescriber or health care professional if they continue or are bothersome):

- bleaching of body hair (with prolonged use)
- blue-black coloration of the skin, nails and hair
- diarrhea
- drowsiness
- hair loss
- loss of appetite
- nausea, vomiting

Where can I keep my medicine?

Keep out of the reach of children in a container that small children cannot open. It is important to keep hydroxychloroquine out of reach of children; overdose is very dangerous. Store at room temperature between 15 and 30 degrees C (59 and 86 degrees F). Throw away any unused medicine after the expiration date.

Hydroxyurea capsules

HYDREA®; 500 mg; Capsule ER Squibb and Sons Inc	DROXIA®; 200 mg; Capsule ER Squibb and Sons Inc

What are hydroxyurea capsules?

HYDROXYUREA (Droxia®, Hydrea®) is used to treat sickle cell disease or certain types of cancer. Hydroxyurea is used for treating cancers of the blood, skin, ovary and head and neck. Hydroxyurea is also used to decrease the painful episodes associated with sickle cell disease. Hydroxyurea does not cure sickle cell disease, but may help to control the symptoms when used on a regular basis. Generic hydroxyurea capsules are available.

What should my health care professional know before I take hydroxyurea?

They need to know if you have any of these conditions:
- bleeding problems
- blood disorders
- dental disease
- having intramuscular injections
- infection (especially virus infection such as chickenpox or herpes)
- kidney disease
- an unusual or allergic reaction to hydroxyurea, other chemotherapy, other medicines, foods, dyes, or preservatives
- pregnant or trying to get pregnant
- breast-feeding

How should I take this medicine?

Take hydroxyurea capsules by mouth. Follow the directions on the prescription label. Swallow the capsules with a drink of water. Do not take your medicine more often than directed. Finish the full course prescribed by your doctor or health care professional, even if the capsules make you feel unwell. Do not stop taking except on your prescriber's advice. If you have difficulty swallowing the capsule, carefully open it and empty the contents into a glass of water. Drink at once, some ingredients may not dissolve, but float on the surface; this does not matter. Make sure to drink all of the water to get the entire dose. Rinse and wash the glass thoroughly after using. Hydroxyurea is a medicine that must be handled with care. People who are not taking hydroxyurea should not be exposed to the powder in the open capsules. If the powder from the capsule is spilled, it should be wiped up immediately with a damp towel. The towel should then be put in a closed container such as a plastic bag and thrown away.

What if I miss a dose?

If you miss a dose, skip that dose unless you remember within a few hours, or your prescriber or health care professional tells you otherwise. Do not take double or extra doses. If you vomit after taking a dose, call your prescriber or health care professional for advice.

What may interact with hydroxyurea?

- didanosine, ddI
- medicines that affect your blood such as cilostazol or warfarin
- other chemotherapy agents may increase the side effects seen with hydroxyurea
- stavudine, d4T
- vaccines

Talk to your prescriber or health care professional before taking any of these medicines:

- aspirin
- acetaminophen
- ibuprofen
- naproxen
- ketoprofen

Tell your prescriber or other health care professional about all other medicines you are taking including nonprescription medicines, nutritional supplements, or herbal products. Also, tell your prescriber or health care professional if you are a frequent user of drinks with caffeine or alcohol, if you smoke or if you use illegal drugs. These may affect the way your medicine works. Check before stopping or starting any of your medications.

What should I watch for while taking hydroxyurea?

Visit your prescriber or health care professional for checks on your progress. You will need to have regular blood checks. The side effects of hydroxyurea can continue after you finish your treatment; report side effects promptly. Hydroxyurea may make you feel generally unwell. Report any side effects as above, but continue your course of medicine even though you feel ill, unless your prescriber or health care professional tells you to stop. When given alone or with other chemotherapy agents, hydroxyurea may decrease your body's ability to fight infections or increase your risk to bruise or

bleed. Call your prescriber or health care professional if you have a fever, chills, sore throat or other symptoms of a cold or flu. Do not treat these symptoms yourself. Try to avoid being around people who are sick. Call your prescriber or health care professional if you notice any unusual bleeding. Be careful not to cut, bruise or injure yourself because you may get an infection and bleed more than usual. Hydroxyurea may harm your unborn baby. You should contact your prescriber immediately if you believe or suspect you or your partner has become pregnant while you are taking hydroxyurea. Both men and women must use effective birth control continuously while taking hydroxyurea. It is recommended that you use 2 reliable forms of contraception together. Avoid taking aspirin, acetaminophen (Tylenol®), ibuprofen (Advil®), naproxen (Aleve®), or ketoprofen (Orudis® KT) products as these may hide a fever, unless instructed to by your prescriber or health care professional. Be careful brushing and flossing your teeth or using a toothpick while receiving hydroxyurea because you may get an infection or bleed more easily. If you have any dental work done, tell your dentist you are receiving hydroxyurea. Drink several glasses of water a day. This will help to reduce possible kidney problems. If you are going to have surgery, tell your prescriber or health care professional that you are taking hydroxyurea.

What side effects may I notice from taking hydroxyurea?

Side effects that you should report to your prescriber or health care professional as soon as possible:

- low blood counts—hydroxyurea may decrease the number of white blood cells, red blood cells and platelets. You may be at increased risk for infections and bleeding.
- signs of infection—fever or chills, cough, sore throat, pain or difficulty passing urine
- signs of decreased platelets or bleeding—bruising, pinpoint red spots on the skin, black, tarry stools, blood in the urine
- signs of decreased red blood cells—unusual weakness or tiredness, fainting spells, lightheadedness
- burning, redness or pain at the site of radiation therapy
- lower back pain
- sore mouth or lips (ulcers)
- vomiting

Side effects that usually do not require medical attention (report to your prescriber or health care professional if they continue or are bothersome):

- constipation or diarrhea
- loss of appetite
- nausea
- red face
- skin rash, itching

Where can I keep my medicine?

Keep out of the reach of children in a container that small children cannot open. Store at room temperature, approximately 25 degrees C (77 degrees F). Throw away any unused medicine after the expiration date.

Hydroxyzine tablets or capsules

ATARAX®;
50 mg; Tablet
Roerig Division of
Pfizer

VISTARIL®;
50 mg; Capsule
Pfizer Laboratories
Div Pfizer Inc

What are hydroxyzine tablets or capsules?

HYDROXYZINE (Atarax®, Vistaril®) is an antihistamine. This drug relieves itching and allergic skin reactions; may relieve emotional conditions that result in anxiety and tension; reduces nausea and vomiting; helps make you sleep before surgery or at bedtime, and may help with pain relief after surgery. Generic hydroxyzine tablets or capsules are available.

What should my health care professional know before I take hydroxyzine?

They need to know if you have any of these conditions:
- asthma or chronic obstructive lung disease (COPD)
- glaucoma
- heart disease
- kidney disease
- liver disease
- pain or difficulty passing urine
- prostate trouble
- other chronic illness
- ulcers or other stomach problems
- an unusual or allergic reaction to hydroxyzine, cetirizine, other medicines, foods, dyes, or preservatives
- pregnant or trying to get pregnant
- breast-feeding

How should I take this medicine?

Take hydroxyzine tablets or capsules by mouth. Follow the directions on the prescription label. Take hydroxyzine with food or milk if it upsets your stomach. Take your doses at regular intervals. Do not take your medicine more often than directed. Contact your pediatrician or health care professional regarding the use of this medicine in children. Special care may be needed.

What if I miss a dose?

If you miss a dose, take it as soon as you can. If it is almost time for your next dose, take only that dose. Do not take double or extra doses.

What may interact with hydroxyzine?

Because hydroxyzine can cause drowsiness and other effects, other medicines may increase these effects. Some medicines that may interact include:

- alcohol
- barbiturate medicines for inducing sleep or treating seizures (convulsions), like phenobarbital
- medicines for colds, hay fever or other allergies
- medicines for mental depression, anxiety, or emotional disturbances
- medicines for pain
- medicines for sleep
- muscle relaxants

Tell your prescriber or health care professional about all other medicines you are taking, including non-prescription medicines, nutritional supplements, or herbal products. Also tell your prescriber or health care professional if you are a frequent user of drinks with caffeine or alcohol, if you smoke, or if you use illegal drugs. These may affect the way your medicine works. Check with your health care professional before stopping or starting any of your medicines.

What should I watch for while taking hydroxyzine?

Tell your prescriber or health care professional if your symptoms do not improve within a few days. If you are taking hydroxyzine on a regular schedule, visit your prescriber or health care professional for regular checks on your progress. You may get drowsy or dizzy. Do not drive, use machinery, or do anything that needs mental alertness until you know how this drug affects you. To reduce the risk of dizzy or fainting spells, do not stand or sit up quickly, especially if you are an older patient. Alcohol may increase dizziness and drowsiness. Avoid alcoholic drinks. Your mouth may get dry. Chewing sugarless gum or sucking hard candy, and drinking plenty of water will help. This drug may cause dry eyes and blurred vision. If you wear contact lenses you may feel some discomfort. Lubricating drops may help. See your ophthalmologist if the problem does not go away or is severe. If you are receiving skin tests for allergies, tell your physician you are using hydroxyzine. If you are going to have surgery, including dental surgery, tell your dentist or surgeon you are using hydroxyzine.

What side effects may I notice from taking hydroxyzine?

Side effects that you should report to your prescriber or health care professional as soon as possible:
- agitation, nervousness, excitability, not able to sleep (these are more likely in children)
- dilated pupils or blurred vision
- fast or irregular heartbeat or palpitations
- muscle or facial twitches
- pain or difficulty passing urine
- seizures (convulsions)
- slurred speech or confusion
- tremor
- unusual weakness

Side effects that usually do not require medical attention (report to your prescriber or health care professional if they continue or are bothersome):
- constipation
- drowsiness, dizziness or fatigue
- dry mouth
- headache
- mild stomach upset

Where can I keep my medicine?

Keep out of the reach of children in a container that small children cannot open. Store at room tempera- ture, between 15 and 30 degrees C (59 and 86 degrees F). Keep container tightly closed. Throw away any un- used medicine after the expiration date.

Hyoscyamine oral disintegrating tablets

HYOSCYAMINE;
0.125 mg; Tablet,
Orally
Disintegrating
Ethex Corporation

NULEV®;
0.125 mg; Tablet,
Orally
Disintegrating
Schwarz Pharma Inc

What are hyoscyamine oral disintegrating tablets?

HYOSCYAMINE (NuLev®) treats different bowel problems including irritable bowel syndrome. This drug relaxes the muscles of the intestines and slows down their movement, which helps ease pain of cramps and spasms. Generic hyoscyamine oral disintegrating tab- lets are not available.

What should my health care professional know before I take hyoscyamine?

They need to know if you have any of these conditions:

- closed-angle glaucoma
- diarrhea
- difficulty passing urine
- heart disease, or previous heart attack
- hiatal hernia
- myasthenia gravis
- prostate trouble
- stomach infection
- stomach obstruction
- ulcerative colitis
- an unusual reaction to hyoscyamine, medicines, foods, dyes, or preservatives
- pregnant or trying to get pregnant
- breast-feeding

How should this medicine be used?

Take hyoscyamine oral disintegrating tablets by mouth. Follow the directions on the prescription label. These tablets are made to dissolve in the mouth. Place the tablet in the mouth and allow it to dissolve, then swal- low. While you may take these tablets with water, it is not necessary to do so. Take before meals to help prevent discomfort related to food. Do not take more than 12 tablets within 24 hours. Contact your pediatri- cian or health care professional regarding the use of this medicine in children. Special care may be needed. Children up to 12 years of age should not take more than 6 tablets within 24 hours.

What if I miss a dose?

If you miss a dose, take it as soon as you can. If it is almost time for your next dose, take only that dose. Do not take double or extra doses.

What may interact with hyoscyamine?

- amantadine
- benztropine
- cisapride
- digoxin
- donepezil
- galantamine
- medicines for heart problems
- medicines for hay fever and other allergies
- medicines for mental problems or psychotic distur- bances
- opiate prescription pain medications such as codeine, hydromorphone, and morphine
- potassium salts
- quinidine
- rivastigmine
- tacrine
- tegaserod

Tell your prescriber or health care professional about all other medicines you are taking, including non-pre- scription medicines, nutritional supplements, or herbal products. Also tell your prescriber or health care profes- sional if you are a frequent user of drinks with caffeine or alcohol, if you smoke, or if you use illegal drugs. These may affect the way your medicine works. Check with your health care professional before stopping or starting any of your medicines.

What should I watch for while taking hyoscyamine?

You may get dizzy or have blurred vision. Do not drive, use machinery, or do anything that needs mental alert- ness until you know how hyoscyamine affects you. To reduce the risk of dizzy or fainting spells, do not sit or stand up quickly, especially if you are an older patient. Alcohol can make you more dizzy, avoid alcoholic drinks. Stay out of bright light and wear sunglasses if hyoscyamine makes your eyes more sensitive to light. Your mouth may get dry. Chewing sugarless gum or sucking hard candy, and drinking plenty of water will help. Hyoscyamine may cause dry eyes and blurred vi- sion. If you wear contact lenses, you may feel some discomfort. Lubricating drops may help. See your ophthalmologist if the problem does not go away or is severe. Avoid extreme heat (e.g., hot tubs, saunas). Hyoscyamine can cause you to sweat less than normal. Your body temperature could increase to dangerous lev- els, which may lead to heat stroke.

What side effects may I notice from taking hyoscyamine?

Side effects that you should report to your prescriber or health care professional as soon as possible:

H

- anxiety, nervousness
- blurred vision or other eye problems
- confusion
- dizziness or fainting spells
- fast heartbeat
- fever
- pain or difficulty passing urine
- unusual weakness or tiredness
- vomiting

Side effects that usually do not require medical attention (report to your prescriber or health care professional if they continue or are bothersome):

- altered taste
- constipation
- drowsiness
- dry mouth
- headache
- increased sensitivity of the eyes to sun or ultraviolet light
- nausea

Where can I keep my medicine?

Keep out of the reach of children in a container that small children cannot open. Store at room temperature between 15 and 30 degrees C (59 and 86 degrees F). Throw away any unused medicine after the expiration date.

Hyoscyamine tablets or extended-release capsules or tablets

ANASPAZ®; 0.125 mg; Tablet BF Ascher and Co Inc

CYSTOSPAZ-M®; 0.375 mg; Capsule, Extended Release Polymedica Pharmaceuticals USA Inc

What are hyoscyamine tablets or extended-release tablets and capsules?

HYOSCYAMINE (Anaspaz®, Cystospaz®, Cytospaz-M®, Gastrosed®, Levbid®, Levsin®, Levsin/SL®, Levsinex®) treats different bowel problems including irritable bowel syndrome. Generic hyoscyamine regular-release tablets and extended-release capsules and tablets are available.

What should my health care professional know before I take hyoscyamine?

They need to know if you have any of these conditions:
- closed-angle glaucoma
- diarrhea
- difficulty passing urine
- heart disease, or previous heart attack
- hiatal hernia
- myasthenia gravis
- prostate trouble
- stomach infection
- stomach obstruction
- ulcerative colitis
- an unusual or allergic reaction to hyoscyamine, other medicines, foods, dyes, or preservatives
- pregnant or trying to get pregnant
- breast-feeding

How should I take this medicine?

Take hyoscyamine tablets by mouth. Follow the directions on the prescription label. Swallow the regular tablets with a drink of water. Take the tablets 30 to 60 minutes before food. Swallow extended-release tablets whole; do not crush or chew. Do not take your medicine more often than directed. Contact your pediatrician or health care professional regarding the use of this medicine in children. Special care may be needed.

What if I miss a dose?

If you miss a dose, take it as soon as you can. If it is almost time for your next dose, take only that dose. Do not take double or extra doses.

What may interact with hyoscyamine?

- amantadine
- benztropine
- cisapride
- digoxin
- donepezil
- galantamine
- medicines for heart problems
- medicines for hay fever and other allergies
- medicines for mental problems or psychotic disturbances
- opiate prescription pain medications such as codeine, hydromorphone, and morphine
- potassium salts
- quinidine
- rivastigmine
- tacrine
- tegaserod

Tell your prescriber or health care professional about all other medicines you are taking, including nonprescription medicines, nutritional supplements, or herbal products. Also tell your prescriber or health care professional if you are a frequent user of drinks with caffeine or alcohol, if you smoke, or if you use illegal drugs. These may affect the way your medicine works. Check with your health care professional before stopping or starting any of your medicines.

What should I watch for while taking hyoscyamine?

You may get dizzy or have blurred vision. Do not drive, use machinery, or do anything that needs mental alert-

H

ness until you know how hyoscyamine affects you. To reduce the risk of dizzy or fainting spells, do not sit or stand up quickly, especially if you are an older patient. Alcohol can make you more dizzy, avoid alcoholic drinks. Stay out of bright light and wear sunglasses if hyoscyamine makes your eyes more sensitive to light. Your mouth may get dry. Chewing sugarless gum or sucking hard candy, and drinking plenty of water will help. Hyoscyamine may cause dry eyes and blurred vision. If you wear contact lenses, you may feel some discomfort. Lubricating drops may help. See your ophthalmologist if the problem does not go away or is severe. Avoid extreme heat (e.g., hot tubs, saunas). Hyoscyamine can cause you to sweat less than normal. Your body temperature could increase to dangerous levels, which may lead to heat stroke.

What side effects may I notice from taking hyoscyamine?

Side effects that you should report to your prescriber or health care professional as soon as possible:

- anxiety, nervousness
- blurred vision or other eye problems
- confusion
- dizziness or fainting spells
- fast heartbeat
- fever
- pain or difficulty passing urine
- unusual weakness or tiredness
- vomiting

Side effects that usually do not require medical attention (report to your prescriber or health care professional if they continue or are bothersome):

- altered taste
- constipation
- drowsiness
- dry mouth
- increased sensitivity of the eyes to sun or ultraviolet light
- nausea

Where can I keep my medicine?

Keep out of the reach of children in a container that small children cannot open. Store at room temperature between 15 and 30 degrees C (59 and 86 degrees F). Throw away any unused medicine after the expiration date.

H

Ibandronate tablets

What are ibandronate tablets?

IBANDRONATE (Boniva™) reduces calcium loss from bones. It helps prevent bone loss and increases production of normal healthy bone in patients with osteoporosis and other conditions which place someone at risk for bone loss, including after menopause in females. Generic ibandronate tablets are not yet available.

What should my health care professional know before I take ibandronate?

They need to know if you have any of these conditions:
- dental disease
- kidney disease
- low level of blood calcium
- problems swallowing
- stomach, intestinal, or esophageal problems, like acid-reflux or GERD
- vitamin D deficiency
- an unusual or allergic reaction to ibandronate, other medicines, foods, dyes, or preservatives
- pregnant or trying to get pregnant
- breast-feeding

How should this medicine be taken?

Follow the directions on the prescription label. Take ibandronate tablets by mouth in the morning, after you have risen for the day. Swallow the tablets with a full glass (6 to 8 fluid ounces) of plain water first thing in the morning. Do not take the tablets with any other type of liquid except plain water. Do not take with mineral water, orange juice, coffee, or other fluids as these may decrease the absorption of ibandronate. Do not chew or suck on the tablets; this may cause mouth ulcers (sores). Do not eat or drink anything before you take your tablets and do not eat breakfast, drink, or take any other medicines for at least 1 hour after taking ibandronate. If you can wait for 2 hours before eating, your body will absorb even more of the medicine. After taking this medicine, remain sitting or standing upright (do not lie down) for at least 1 hour to avoid irritation of your throat and esophagus (tube connecting mouth to stomach). Do not take this medicine at the same time as antacids, calcium, magnesium or iron supplements, or vitamins with minerals; if you take these medications, take them later in the day. Do not take your medicine more often than directed. Contact your pediatrician or health care professional regarding the use of this medicine in children. Special care may be needed.

What if I miss a dose?

If you take a daily dose of ibandronate: If you miss a dose, do not take it later in the day. Continue your normal schedule starting the next morning, before you have eaten. Do not take double or extra doses. If you take a once-monthly dose of ibandronate: If you miss a dose of ibandronate 150-mg once a month and your next scheduled ibandronate administration day is more than 7 days away, take the dose on the morning after you remember. Then return to taking your dose just once a month, as originally scheduled on your regular chosen day of the month. NEVER take 2 tablets in the same week. If your next scheduled ibandronate day is only 1 to 7 days away, wait until your scheduled day to take your tablet. Then return to taking one ibandronate 150-mg tablet every month in the morning of your chosen day, according to your original schedule. Do not take double or extra doses.

What may interact with ibandronate?

- aluminum hydroxide
- antacids
- anti-inflammatory drugs like ibuprofen, naproxen, and others
- aspirin
- calcium supplements
- iron supplements
- magnesium supplements
- parathyroid hormone
- teriparatide
- vitamins with minerals

Tell your prescriber or health care professional about all other medicines you are taking, including non-prescription medicines, nutritional supplements, or herbal products. Also tell your prescriber or health care professional if you are a frequent user of drinks with caffeine or alcohol, if you smoke, or if you use illegal drugs. These may affect the way your medicine works. Check with your health care professional before stopping or starting any of your medicines.

What should I watch for while taking ibandronate?

Visit your prescriber or health care professional for regular checks on your progress. Do not stop taking ibandronate except on your prescriber's advice. Low blood levels of phosphorus and calcium can occur but usually do not cause serious problems. Your prescriber or health care professional may order regular blood tests to check for these problems. It is very important to take ibandronate with a full glass of plain water (6 to 8 ounces). Do not take with mineral water, orange juice, coffee, or other fluids as these may decrease the absorption of ibandronate. Do not take ibandronate with food. Wait at least 1 hour or longer after taking ibandronate before you eat, drink, or take other medicines. Because ibandronate may irritate your throat, remain sitting or standing upright for at least 1 hour after taking ibandronate; do not lie down. If you begin to have pain when swallowing, difficulty swallowing, heartburn or stomach pain, call your prescriber or health care professional right away. You should make sure you get enough calcium and vitamin D in your diet while you are taking ibandronate, unless directed otherwise by your health care provider. Discuss your dietary needs with your health care professional or nutritionist. If you get bone pain, or a worsening of bone pain, check with your doctor. However, many patients have improvement in their bone pain during and after treatment with ibandronate. If you are taking an antacid, a mineral supplement like calcium or iron, or a vitamin with minerals, make sure that you wait at least 1 hour, and preferably 2 hours before or after taking ibandronate. Do not take them at the same time.

What side effects may I notice from taking ibandronate?

Side effects that you should report to your prescriber or health care professional as soon as possible:
More common:
- stomach pain
- heartburn
- pain or difficulty swallowing

Rare or uncommon:
- black or tarry stools
- constant jaw pain, especially burning or cramping
- eye inflammation, pain or change in vision
- skin rash, itching (hives)
- swelling of the lips, arms, legs, face, tongue, or throat
- vomiting
- allergic reactions such as hives, swelling of the face, lips or tongue

Side effects that usually do not require medical attention (report to your prescriber or health care professional if they continue or are bothersome):
- diarrhea or constipation
- headache
- nausea
- bone, muscle or joint pain
- rash

Where can I keep my medicine?

Keep out of the reach of children in a container that small children cannot open. Store at room temperature between 15 and 30 degrees C (59 and 86 degrees F). Throw away any unused medicine after the expiration date.

Ibuprofen chewable tablets

MOTRIN® JUNIOR STRENGTH; 100 mg; Tablet, Chewable
McNeil Consumer Healthcare
Div McNeil Ppc Inc

This drug requires an FDA medication guide. See page xxxvii.

What do ibuprofen chewable tablets do?

IBUPROFEN (Children's Motrin®, Junior Strength Motrin®, Children's Advil®, Junior Strength Advil®) is an anti-inflammatory drug. Ibuprofen reduces inflammation and helps ease mild to moderate pain. It relieves the symptoms of minor aches and pains, headaches, or toothaches. Ibuprofen chewable tablets also reduce fever, but these products are intended only for children who are 2 to 11 years of age. Generic ibuprofen chewable tablets are available.

What should my health care professional know before I take ibuprofen?

Ibuprofen chewable tablets are intended for use in children; however, some of the following conditions may only apply to adults. They need to know if you have any of these conditions:
- anemia
- asthma, especially aspirin sensitive asthma
- bleeding problems or taking medicines that make you bleed easily such as anticoagulants ("blood thinners")
- cigarette smoker
- diabetes
- drink more than 3 alcohol-containing beverages a day
- heart failure
- high blood pressure

- kidney disease
- liver disease
- lost a lot of fluid due to continued vomiting or diarrhea
- stomach ulcers or pain
- systemic lupus erythematosus
- ulcerative colitis
- an unusual or allergic reaction to aspirin, other salicylates, other NSAIDs, other medicines, foods, dyes or preservatives
- pregnant or trying to get pregnant
- breast-feeding

How should I take this medicine?

Chew ibuprofen chewable tablets thoroughly. Follow the directions on the label. Use the weight of your child to determine the dose if possible, otherwise use age. Do not give more than directed and doses should not be given more than 4 times a day. If ibuprofen causes stomach upset, it may be given with food. Contact your pediatrician or health care professional regarding the use of ibuprofen chewable tablets in children under 2 years of age. Special care may be needed.

What if I miss a dose?

If you miss a dose, take it as soon as you can. If it is almost time for your next dose, take only that dose. Do not take double or extra doses.

What other medicines can interact with ibuprofen?

- alcohol
- anti-inflammatory drugs (other NSAIDs, prednisone)
- aspirin and aspirin-like medicines
- cidofovir
- cyclosporine
- entecavir
- herbal products that contain feverfew, garlic, ginger, or ginkgo biloba
- lithium
- medicines for high blood pressure
- medicines that affect platelets
- medicines that treat or prevent blood clots such as warfarin and other "blood thinners"
- methotrexate
- pemetrexed
- water pills (diuretics)

Tell your prescriber or health care professional about all other medicines you are taking, including non-prescription medicines, nutritional supplements, or herbal products. Also tell your prescriber or health care professional if you are a frequent user of drinks with caffeine or alcohol, if you smoke, or if you use illegal drugs. These may affect the way your medicine works. Check with your health care professional before stopping or starting any of your medicines.

What do I need to watch for while I take ibuprofen?

Let your prescriber or health care professional know if your pain continues. Do not take with other pain medicines or fever medicine without advice. In children, if the fever or pain gets worse, lasts for more than 3 days, or there is no relief of symptoms within the first day (24 hours), contact your health care provider. You may be covering up a more serious illness. If stomach pain or upset gets worse or continues, if redness or swelling occur in the painful area, or if new symptoms appear, contact your health care provider. Severe or persistent sore throat or sore throat accompanied by high fever, nausea, and vomiting may be serious. Consult your health care provider promptly if your child has these symptoms. Do not use for more than 2 days or give to children under 3 years of age with these symptoms unless directed by your health care provider. Discuss the use of this medicine with your health care provider if your child has not been drinking fluids, has lost a lot of fluid due to continued vomiting or diarrhea, has stomach pain, or has problems or serious side effects from taking fever reducers or pain medicine. To reduce unpleasant effects on your throat and stomach, take ibuprofen with a full glass of water and never just before lying down. If you notice black, tarry stools or experience severe stomach pain and/or vomit blood or what looks like coffee grounds, notify your health care pre-

scriber immediately. You may get drowsy. Do not drive, use machinery, or do anything that needs mental alertness until you know how ibuprofen affects you. Do not sit or stand up quickly, especially if you are an older patient. This reduces the risk of dizzy or fainting spells. Do not smoke cigarettes or drink alcohol; these increase irritation to your stomach and can make it more susceptible to damage from ibuprofen. If you are taking medicines that affect the clotting of your blood, such as aspirin or blood thinners such as Coumadin®, talk to your health care provider or prescriber before taking this medicine. If you are going to have surgery, tell your prescriber or health care professional that you are taking ibuprofen. Problems can arise if you need dental work, and in the day to day care of your teeth. Try to avoid damage to your teeth and gums when you brush or floss your teeth. It is especially important not to use ibuprofen during the last 3 months of pregnancy unless specifically directed to do so by your health care provider. Ibuprofen may cause problems in the unborn child or complications during delivery.

What side effects may I notice from taking ibuprofen?

Side effects that you should report to your prescriber or health care professional as soon as possible:

- signs of bleeding—pinpoint red spots on the skin, black tarry stools, blood in the urine, unusual tiredness or weakness, vomiting blood or vomit that looks like coffee grounds
- signs of an allergic reaction—difficulty breathing, wheezing, skin rash, redness, blistering or peeling skin, hives, or itching, swelling of eyelids, throat, lips
- blurred vision
- change in the amount of urine passed
- difficulty swallowing, severe heartburn or burning, pain in throat
- pain or difficulty passing urine
- stomach pain or cramps
- swelling of feet or ankles
- yellowing of eyes or skin

Side effects that usually do not require medical attention (report to your prescriber or health care professional if they continue or are bothersome):

- bruising
- diarrhea
- dizziness, drowsiness
- gas or heartburn
- headache
- nausea, vomiting

Where can I keep my medicine?

Keep out of the reach of children in a container that small children cannot open. Store at room temperature between 20 and 25 degrees C (68 and 77 degrees F). Keep container tightly closed. Throw away any unused medicine after the expiration date.

Ibuprofen tablets or capsules

MOTRIN®;
400 mg; Tablet
Pharmacia and
Upjohn Div Pfizer

ADVIL® LIQUI-
GELS®;
200 mg; Capsule
Whitehall-Robins

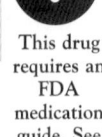

This drug
requires an
FDA
medication
guide. See
page
xxxvii.

What are ibuprofen tablets or capsules?

IBUPROFEN (Motrin®, Advil®, Rufen®, Nuprin®) is an anti-inflammatory drug. Ibuprofen reduces inflammation and eases mild to moderate pain. It reduces fever and relieves the symptoms of rheumatoid arthritis (rheumatism), osteoarthritis, menstrual cramps or premenstrual pain and swelling. Generic ibuprofen tablets and capsules are available.

What should my health care professional know before I take ibuprofen?

They need to know if you have any of these conditions:
- anemia
- asthma, especially aspirin sensitive asthma
- bleeding problems or taking medicines that make you bleed easily such as anticoagulants ("blood thinners")
- cigarette smoker
- diabetes
- drink more than 3 alcohol-containing beverages a day
- heart failure
- high blood pressure
- kidney disease
- liver disease
- stomach or duodenal ulcers
- systemic lupus erythematosus
- ulcerative colitis
- an unusual or allergic reaction to aspirin, other salicylates, other NSAIDs, other medicines, foods, dyes or preservatives
- pregnant or trying to get pregnant
- breast-feeding

How should I take this medicine?

Take ibuprofen tablets or capsules by mouth. Follow the directions on the label. Swallow tablets whole with a full glass of water; take tablets in an upright or sitting position. Taking a sip of water first, before taking the tablets, may help you swallow them. If possible take bedtime doses at least 10 minutes before lying down. Ibuprofen may be taken with food if it upsets your stomach. Take your doses at regular intervals. Do not take your medicine more often than directed. Contact your pediatrician or health care professional regarding the use of this medicine in children. Special care may be needed.

What if I miss a dose?

If you miss a dose, take it as soon as you can. If it is almost time for your next dose, take only that dose. Do not take double or extra doses.

What may interact with ibuprofen?

- alcohol
- anti-inflammatory drugs (other NSAIDs, prednisone)
- aspirin and aspirin-like medicines
- cidofovir
- cyclosporine
- entecavir
- herbal products that contain feverfew, garlic, ginger, or ginkgo biloba
- lithium
- medicines for high blood pressure
- medicines that affect platelets
- medicines that treat or prevent blood clots such as warfarin and other "blood thinners"
- methotrexate
- pemetrexed
- water pills (diuretics)

Tell your prescriber or health care professional about all other medicines you are taking, including non-prescription medicines. Also tell your prescriber or health care professional if you are a frequent user of drinks with caffeine or alcohol, if you smoke, or if you use illegal drugs. These may affect the way your medicine works. Check with your health care professional before stopping or starting any of your medicines.

What should I watch for while taking ibuprofen?

Let your prescriber or health care professional know if your pain continues. Do not take with other pain-killers without advice. Do not treat yourself for a fever with ibuprofen for more than 3 days, or for pain for more than 10 days without asking your prescriber or health care professional for advice. You may be covering up a more serious illness. To reduce unpleasant effects on your throat and stomach, take ibuprofen with a full glass of water and never just before lying down. If you notice black, tarry stools or experience severe stomach pain and vomit blood or what looks like coffee grounds, notify your health care prescriber immediately. If you are taking medicines that affect the clotting of your blood, such as aspirin or blood thinners such as Coumadin®, talk to your health care provider or prescriber before taking this medicine. You may get dizzy. Do not drive, use machinery, or do anything that needs mental alertness until you know how ibuprofen affects you. Do not sit or stand up quickly, especially if you are an older patient. This reduces the risk of dizzy or fainting spells. Do not smoke cigarettes or drink alcohol; these may increase the irritation to your stomach when taking this medicine. It is especially important not to use ibuprofen during the last 3 months of pregnancy unless specifically directed to do so by your health care provider. Ibuprofen may cause problems in the unborn child or complications during delivery. If you are going to have surgery, tell your prescriber or health care professional that you are taking ibuprofen.

Problems can arise if you need dental work, and in the day to day care of your teeth. Try to avoid damage to your teeth and gums when you brush or floss your teeth.

What side effects may I notice from taking ibuprofen?

Elderly patients are at increased risk for developing side effects.

Side effects that you should report to your prescriber or health care professional as soon as possible:

- signs of bleeding—bruising, pinpoint red spots on the skin, black tarry stools, blood in the urine, unusual tiredness or weakness
- signs of an allergic reaction—difficulty breathing or wheezing, skin rash, redness, blistering or peeling skin, hives, or itching, swelling of eyelids, throat, lips
- blurred vision
- change in the amount of urine passed
- difficulty swallowing, severe heartburn or burning, pain in throat
- pain or difficulty passing urine
- stomach pain or cramps
- swelling of feet or ankles
- vomiting blood or vomit that looks like coffee grounds

Side effects that usually do not require medical attention (report to your prescriber or health care professional if they continue or are bothersome):

- diarrhea
- dizziness, drowsiness
- gas or heartburn
- headache
- nausea, vomiting

Where can I keep my medicine?

Keep out of the reach of children in a container that small children cannot open. Store at room temperature between 15 and 30 degrees C (59 and 86 degrees F). Keep container tightly closed. Throw away any unused medicine after the expiration date.

Ibuprofen; Oxycodone tablets

COMBUNOX℗;
400 mg/5 mg; Tablet
Forest Pharmaceuticals, Inc

What are ibuprofen; oxycodone tablets?

IBUPROFEN; OXYCODONE (Combunox℗) is a combination of two different types of pain medicine and is used to treat moderate to severe pain. Federal law prohibits the transfer of this product to any person other than the patient for whom it was prescribed. Generic ibuprofen; oxycodone tablets are not available.

What should my health care professional know before I take ibuprofen; oxycodone?

They need to know if you have any of these conditions:

- anemia
- asthma
- bleeding problems
- dental disease
- diabetes
- diarrhea
- drink more than 3 alcohol-containing beverages a day
- head injury
- heart or circulation problems
- kidney disease
- liver disease
- lung disease or breathing difficulties
- nasal polyps
- seizures
- stomach or duodenal ulcers
- systemic lupus erythematosus
- ulcerative colitis
- an unusual or allergic reaction to oxycodone, ibuprofen, other medicines, foods, dyes or preservatives
- pregnant or trying to get pregnant
- breast-feeding

How should this medicine be taken?

Take ibuprofen; oxycodone combination tablets by mouth. Follow the directions on the prescription label. Swallow tablets whole with a full glass of water; take tablets in an upright or sitting position. Taking a sip of water first, before taking the tablets, may help you swallow them. If possible take bedtime doses at least 10 minutes before lying down. You can take this medicine with food to prevent stomach upset. Do not take your medicine more often than directed. Contact your pediatrician or health care professional regarding the use of this medicine in children under 14 years of age. Special care may be needed. Do not share this medicine with anyone.

What if I miss a dose?

If you miss a dose, take it as soon as you can. If it is almost time for your next dose, take only that dose. Do not take double or extra doses.

What may interact with ibuprofen; oxycodone?

- anti-inflammatory drugs (other NSAIDs)
- aspirin and aspirin-like medicines
- cyclosporine
- entecavir
- herbal products that contain feverfew, garlic, ginger, or ginkgo biloba
- hormones such as prednisone or cortisone
- lithium
- medicines for diabetes that are taken by mouth
- medicines for high blood pressure
- medicines that affect platelets

- medicines that treat or prevent blood clots such as warfarin and other "blood thinners"
- medicines for seizures
- methotrexate
- pemetrexed
- water pills (diuretics)

Because oxycodone can cause drowsiness, other medicines that also cause drowsiness may increase this effect of ibuprofen; oxycodone. Some other medicines that cause drowsiness are:

- alcohol-containing medicines
- barbiturates such as phenobarbital
- certain antidepressants or tranquilizers
- muscle relaxants
- certain antihistamines used in cold medicines

Tell your prescriber or health care professional about all other medicines you are taking, including non-prescription medicines, nutritional supplements, or herbal products. Also tell your prescriber or health care professional if you are a frequent user of drinks with caffeine or alcohol, if you smoke, or if you use illegal drugs. These may affect the way your medicine works. Check with your health care professional before stopping or starting any of your medicines.

What should I watch for while taking ibuprofen; oxycodone?

Tell your prescriber or health care professional if your pain does not go away, if it gets worse, or if you have new or different type of pain. Do not take other pain medicines with ibuprofen; oxycodone without advice. Many non-prescription pain medicines contain ibuprofen as an ingredient. Always read the labels carefully to avoid taking too much ibuprofen. Use exactly as directed by your prescriber or health care professional. Do not take more than the recommended dose. If you are receiving cancer chemotherapy or other immuno-suppression medicine, do not take ibuprofen; oxycodone without checking with your prescriber or health care professional. These products may hide the signs of an infection such as fever or pain. To reduce unpleasant effects on your throat and stomach, take ibuprofen; oxycodone with a full glass of water and never just before lying down. You may also take it with food or milk. Ibuprofen; oxycodone may make you drowsy when you first start taking it or change doses. Do not drive, use machinery, or do anything that needs mental alertness until you know how this medicine affects you. Do not sit or stand up quickly. This reduces the risk of dizzy or fainting spells. These effects may be worse if you are an older patient. The drowsiness should decrease after taking the medicine for a couple of days. If you have not slept because of your pain, you may sleep more the first few days your pain is controlled to catch-up on missed sleep. Be careful taking other medicines that may also make you tired. This effect

may be worse when taking these medicines with ibuprofen; oxycodone. Alcohol can increase drowsiness, dizziness, confusion and affect your breathing. Avoid alcohol while taking ibuprofen; oxycodone. Do not smoke cigarettes or drink alcohol; these may increase the irritation to your stomach when taking this medicine. If you get black, tarry stools or vomit up what looks like coffee grounds, call your prescriber or health care professional at once. Ibuprofen; oxycodone can cause constipation. Make sure to take a laxative and/or a stool softener. Try to have a bowel movement at least every 2 to 3 days. If you do not have a bowel movement for 3 days or more call your prescriber or health care professional. They may recommend using an enema or suppository to help you move your bowels. It is especially important not to use ibuprofen; oxycodone during the last 3 months of pregnancy unless specifically directed to do so by your health care provider. Ibuprofen; oxycodone might cause problems in the unborn child or complications during delivery. If you are going to have surgery, tell your prescriber or health care professional that you are taking ibuprofen; oxycodone. Ibuprofen; oxicodone can cause you to bleed more easily. Problems can arise if you need dental work, and in the day to day care of your teeth. Try to avoid damage to your teeth and gums when you brush or floss your teeth.

What side effects may I notice from taking ibuprofen; oxycodone?

Side effects that you should report to your prescriber or health care professional as soon as possible:

- signs of bleeding—bruising, pinpoint red spots on the skin, black, tarry stools, blood in the urine, unusual tiredness or weakness
- signs of an allergic reaction—difficulty breathing, wheezing, skin rash, redness, blistering, peeling or itching, swelling of eyelids, throat, lips or feet
- change in the amount of urine passed
- chest pain
- cold, clammy skin
- confusion
- fast heartbeat
- fever, chills, muscle aches and pains
- lightheadedness or fainting spells
- nervousness or restlessness
- pain or difficulty passing urine
- seizures
- slow or fast heart beat
- stomach pain or cramps

Side effects that usually do not require medical attention (report to your prescriber or health care professional if they continue or are bothersome):

- confusion
- constipation
- diarrhea
- dizziness, drowsiness
- flushing
- gas or heartburn

- headache
- itching
- nausea, vomiting

Where can I keep my medicine?

Keep out of the reach of children in a container that small children cannot open. Do not share or give this medicine to anyone else. Avoid accidental swallowing of ibuprofen; oxycodone by someone (especially children) other than for whom it was prescribed as this may result in severe side effects and possibly death. Store at 25 degrees C (77 degrees F). Keep container tightly closed. Protect from light. Throw away any unused medicine after the expiration date.

Ibuprofen; Pseudoephedrine tablets or caplets

What are ibuprofen; pseudoephedrine tablets or caplets?

IBUPROFEN; PSEUDOEPHEDRINE (Advil Cold & Sinus®, Dimetapp® Sinus, Dristan® Sinus, Motrin® IB Sinus, Sine-Aid® IB, Vicks DayQuil® Sinus Pressure & Pain Relief with Ibuprofen) is a decongestant, fever-reducer and pain-reliever. It can help relieve nasal or sinus congestion (stuffiness), fever, body aches or mild pain, sore throat, and headache associated with the common cold, flu, or sinusitis. Generic ibuprofen; pseudoephedrine tablets are available.

What should my health care professional know before I take ibuprofen; pseudoephedrine?

They need to know if you have any of the following conditions:
- anemia
- asthma
- cigarette smoker
- dental disease
- diabetes
- difficulty urinating (urinary retention)
- drink more than 3 alcohol-containing beverages a day
- glaucoma
- heart disease or circulation problems (e.g., heart failure, heart rhythm problems)
- high blood pressure
- immunosuppression (suppressed immune function)
- kidney disease
- liver disease
- nasal polyps
- overactive thyroid
- prostate trouble
- stomach bleeding or ulcers
- taking blood thinners
- taking hormones such as prednisone (steroids)
- ulcerative colitis
- an unusual or allergic reaction to ibuprofen, pseudoephedrine, other medicines, foods, dyes, or preservatives
- pregnant or trying to get pregnant
- breast-feeding

How should I take this medicine?

Take ibuprofen; pseudoephedrine tablets or caplets by mouth. Swallow tablets whole with a full glass of water; take tablets in an upright or sitting position. Taking a sip of water first, before taking the tablets, may help you swallow them. If possible take bedtime doses at least 10 minutes before lying down. Ibuprofen products may be taken with food if it upsets your stomach. Follow the directions on the prescription label. Take your doses at regular intervals. Do not take your medicine more often than directed. Contact your pediatrician or health care professional regarding the use of this medicine in children. Special care may be needed. Elderly patients over 60 years old may have a stronger reaction to this medicine and need smaller doses.

What if I miss a dose?

If you miss a dose, and you are taking it on a regular schedule, take it as soon as you can. If it is almost time for your next dose (less than 2 hours), take only that dose. Do not take double or extra doses.

What may interact with ibuprofen; pseudoephedrine?

- alcohol
- ammonium chloride
- amphetamine or other stimulant drugs
- anti-inflammatory drugs such as naproxen (Aleve® or prednisone)
- bicarbonate, citrate, or acetate products (such as sodium bicarbonate, sodium acetate, sodium citrate, sodium lactate, and potassium citrate)
- bromocriptine
- caffeine
- cidofovir
- cocaine
- cyclosporine
- entecavir
- furazolidone
- linezolid
- lithium
- medicines for colds and breathing difficulties
- medicines for diabetes
- medicines known as MAO inhibitors, such as phenelzine (Nardil®), tranylcypromine (Parnate®), isocarboxazid (Marplan®), and selegiline (Carbex®, Eldepryl®)
- medicines for mental depression
- medicines for migraine
- medicines that affect platelets

- medicines that treat or prevent blood clots such as warfarin and other "blood thinners"
- methotrexate
- pemetrexed
- procarbazine
- some medicines for chest pain, heart disease, high blood pressure or heart rhythm problems
- some medicines for weight loss (including some herbal products, ephedrine, dextroamphetamine)
- St. John's wort
- theophylline
- thyroid hormones
- water pills (diuretics)

Tell your prescriber or health care professional about all other medicines you are taking, including non-prescription medicines, nutritional supplements, or herbal products. Also tell your prescriber or health care professional if you are a frequent user of drinks with caffeine or alcohol, if you smoke, or if you use illegal drugs. These may affect the way your medicine works. Check before starting or stopping any of your medicines.

What should I watch for while taking ibuprofen; pseudoephedrine?

Check with your prescriber or health care professional if your symptoms have not improved within 7 days, or if you have a high fever. Do not treat yourself for a fever with ibuprofen for more than 3 days, or for pain for more than 10 days without asking your prescriber or health care professional for advice. You may be covering up a more serious illness. If ibuprofen; pseudoephedrine makes it difficult for you to sleep at night; take your last dose at least a few hours before bedtime. If nervousness, dizziness, or sleeplessness occur, stop using this product and consult a health care professional. If you are going to have surgery, tell your prescriber or health care professional that you are taking ibuprofen; pseudoephedrine. Problems can arise if you need dental work, and in the day to day care of your teeth. Try to avoid damage to your teeth and gums when you brush or floss your teeth. To reduce unpleasant effects on your throat and stomach, take ibuprofen products with a full glass of water and never just before lying down. Do not smoke cigarettes or drink alcohol; these may increase the irritation to your stomach when taking this medicine. You may get dizzy. Do not drive, use machinery, or do anything that needs mental alertness until you know how ibuprofen; pseudoephedrine affects you. Do not sit or stand up quickly, especially if you are an older patient. This reduces the risk of dizzy or fainting spells. It is especially important not to use ibuprofen products during the last 3 months of pregnancy unless specifically directed to do so by your health care provider. Ibuprofen may cause problems in the unborn child or complications during delivery.

What side effects may I notice from taking ibuprofen; pseudoephedrine?

Side effects that you should report to your prescriber or health care professional as soon as possible:
Rare or uncommon:
- blurred vision or visual changes
- chest pain
- confusion
- dizziness or fainting spells
- neck stiffness
- numbness or tingling in the hands or feet
- rapid or troubled breathing
- ringing in the ears
- seizures
- severe, persistent, or worsening headache
- signs of decreased platelets or bleeding—bruising, pinpoint red spots on the skin, black, tarry stools, blood in the urine or stools, unusual tiredness or weakness
- signs of an allergic reaction—difficulty breathing, wheezing, skin rash, redness, blistering, peeling or itching, swelling of eyelids, throat, lips or feet
- yellowing of the skin or eyes

More common:
- anxiety or nervousness
- cold, clammy skin
- difficulty swallowing
- fever, chills, muscle aches and pains
- high blood pressure
- increased sweating
- irregular heartbeat (fast or slow heartbeat), palpitations
- pain or difficulty passing urine
- stomach pain, tenderness, bleeding, or cramps
- sleeplessness (insomnia)
- swelling of eyelids, throat, lips, legs, ankles, or feet
- tremor or muscle contractions
- unexplained weight gain or fluid retention
- vomiting

Side effects that usually do not require medical attention (report to your prescriber or health care professional if they continue or are bothersome):
- constipation or diarrhea
- difficulty sleeping
- drowsiness
- gas or heartburn
- increased sensitivity to sunlight
- loss of appetite
- minor upset stomach, nausea
- restlessness

Where can I keep my medicine?

Keep out of the reach of children in a container that small children cannot open. Store at room temperature, between 20 and 25 degrees C (68 and 77 degrees F), unless otherwise specified on the product label. Protect from heat and moisture. Throw away any unused medicine after the expiration date.

Imatinib, STI-571 capsules or tablets

GLEEVEC®;
100 mg; Tablet
Novartis
Pharmaceuticals
Corp Dba Sandoz
Pharmaceuticals
Corp

GLEEVEC®;
400 mg; Tablet
Novartis
Pharmaceuticals
Corp Dba Sandoz
Pharmaceuticals
Corp

What are imatinib tablets?

IMATINIB (Gleevec®) targets specific proteins within distinct cancer cells and stops the cancer cells from growing. Imatinib is used to treat certain cancers including chronic myelogenous leukemia (CML) and specific sarcomas called GISTs. This drug might be used to treat other cancers as well. Generic imatinib tablets are not available.

What should my health care professional know before I receive imatinib?

They need to know if you have any of these conditions:
- bleeding problems
- dental disease
- infection (especially cold sores or shingles)
- heart disease (such as heart failure)
- jaundice
- kidney disease
- liver disease
- an unusual or allergic reaction to imatinib, other medicines, foods, dyes, or preservatives
- pregnant or trying to get pregnant
- breast-feeding

How should I use this medicine?

Imatinib is taken by mouth. You should take imatinib with food and a full glass of water to decrease the chance of it upsetting your stomach. Follow the directions on the prescription label. Do not take your medicine more often than directed. Contact your pediatrician or health care professional regarding the use of this medicine in children. Special care may be needed.

What if I miss a dose?

Take your missed dose as soon as you remember. If it is almost time for your next dose, take only that one, and skip your missed dose. Do not take extra or double doses.

What may interact with imatinib?

There are many possible drug interactions with imatinib. Make sure to tell your health care professional about all the medicines you are taking.

- amiodarone
- antiviral medicines (such as protease inhibitors, delavirdine, efavirenz, or nevirapine)
- astemizole
- bepridil
- bosentan
- certain medicines for anxiety or difficulty sleeping
- certain medicines for fungal infections
- certain medicines for high blood pressure

- certain medicines for high cholesterol (such as atorvastatin, cerivastatin, lovastatin, simvastatin)
- certain pain medicines
- cisapride
- clarithromycin
- cyclosporine
- dofetilide
- doxercalciferol
- ergot medicines (such as Cafergot(R), Migranal(R), D.H.E. 45(R), and others)
- flecainide
- medicines for depression
- medicines for seizures
- paricalcitol
- pimozide
- propafenone
- quinidine
- rifabutin
- rifampin
- sildenafil
- sirolimus
- St. John's wort or any herbal products containing St. John's wort
- tacrolimus
- terfenadine
- vaccines
- warfarin

Talk to your prescriber or health care professional before taking any of these medicines:
- acetaminophen
- aspirin
- ibuprofen
- ketoprofen
- naproxen

Tell your prescriber or health care professional about all other medicines that you are taking, including nonprescription medicines, nutritional supplements, or herbal products. Also tell your prescriber or health care professional if you are a frequent user of drinks with caffeine or alcohol, if you smoke, or if you use illegal drugs. These may affect the way your medicine works. Check with your health care professional before stopping or starting any of your medicines.

What should I watch for while taking imatinib?

Visit your prescriber or health care professional for checks on your progress. You will need to have regular blood checks. The side effects of imatinib may continue after you finish your treatment; report side effects promptly. Imatinib will decrease your body's ability to fight infections. Call your prescriber or health care professional if you have a fever, chills, sore throat, or other symptoms of a cold or flu. Do not treat these symptoms yourself. Try to avoid being around people who are sick. Imatinib may increase your risk to bruise or bleed. Call your prescriber or health care professional if you notice any unusual bleeding. Be careful not to cut, bruise or injure yourself because you may get an infection and bleed more than usual. Avoid taking aspirin, acetaminophen (Tylenol®), ibuprofen (Advil®), ketoprofen (Orudis KT®), or naproxen (Aleve®) products as these may mask a fever, unless instructed to by your prescriber or health care professional. Be careful brushing and flossing your teeth or using a toothpick while taking imatinib because you may get an infection or bleed more easily. If you have any dental work done, tell your dentist you are taking imatinib. Do not have any vaccinations without your prescriber's approval and avoid anyone who has recently had the oral polio vaccine. There is a risk of birth defects if imatinib is given during pregnancy. Women should not become pregnant while being treated with imatinib. If you are going to have surgery or any other procedures, tell your doctor you are taking imatinib.

What side effects may I notice from taking imatinib?

Side effects that you should report to your prescriber or health care professional as soon as possible:
- low blood counts—imatinib may decrease the number of white blood cells, red blood cells and platelets. You may be at increased risk for infections and bleeding.

- signs of infection—fever or chills, cough, sore throat, pain or difficulty passing urine
- signs of decreased platelets or bleeding—bruising, pinpoint red spots on the skin, black, tarry stools, blood in the urine, nosebleeds
- signs of decreased red blood cells—unusual weakness or tiredness, fainting spells, lightheadedness
- difficulty breathing
- swelling around the eyes or in your legs
- sores or white patches in your mouth or throat
- sudden weight gain
- yellowing of skin or eyes, dark colored urine

Side effects that usually do not require medical attention (report to your prescriber or health care professional if they continue or are bothersome):
- anxiety
- bone or muscle pain
- constipation
- decreased appetite
- diarrhea
- difficulty sleeping
- fatigue
- headache
- heartburn
- muscle cramps
- nausea/vomiting
- night sweats
- skin rash, itching
- stomach discomfort
- weakness

Where can I keep my medicine?

Keep out of reach of children. Store capsules at room temperature between 15 and 30 degrees C (59 and 86 degrees F). Throw away any unused medicine after the expiration date on the label.

Imipramine tablets and capsules

TOFRANIL®;
50 mg; Tablet
Mallinckrodt Inc
Pharmaceuticals
Group

TOFRANIL-PM®;
100 mg; Capsule
Mallinckrodt Inc
Pharmaceuticals
Group

This drug requires an FDA medication guide. See page xxxvii.

What are imipramine tablets and capsules?

IMIPRAMINE (Tofranil®, Tofranil-PM®) is an antidepressant. Imipramine can help to lift your spirits by treating your depression. Imipramine can help children who have a nighttime bed-wetting problem. Generic imipramine tablets are available, but generic capsules are not available.

What should my health care professional know before I take imipramine?

They need to know if you have any of these conditions:
- an alcohol problem
- asthma, difficulty breathing
- blood disorders or disease
- diabetes
- difficulty passing urine, prostate trouble
- glaucoma
- having intramuscular injections

- heart disease, or recent heart attack
- liver disease
- overactive thyroid
- Parkinson's disease
- schizophrenia
- seizures (convulsions)
- stomach disease
- an unusual or allergic reaction to imipramine, other medicines, foods, dyes, or preservatives
- pregnant or trying to get pregnant
- breast-feeding

How should I take this medicine?

Take imipramine tablets and capsules by mouth. Follow the directions on the prescription label. Swallow with a drink of water. Take your doses at regular intervals. Do not take your medicine more often than directed. Do not stop taking except on your prescriber's advice.

Contact your pediatrician or health care professional regarding the use of this medicine in children. Special care may be needed. Elderly patients over 65 years old and adolescents may have a stronger reaction to this medicine and need smaller doses.

What if I miss a dose?

If you miss a dose normally taken only at bedtime, it may be better to miss that dose to avoid daytime drowsiness. Ask your health care professional for advice. If you take more than one dose per day and miss a dose, take it as soon as you can. However, if it is almost time for your next dose, take only that dose. Do not take double or extra doses.

What may interact with imipramine?

Imipramine can interact with many other medicines. Some interactions can be very important. Make sure your prescriber or health care professional knows about all other medicines you are taking. Many important interactions are listed below:

Do not take imipramine with any of the following medications:

- astemizole (Hismanal®)
- cisapride (Propulsid®)
- probucol
- terfenadine (Seldane®)
- thioridazine (Mellaril®)
- medicines called MAO inhibitors-phenelzine (Nardil®), tranylcypromine (Parnate®), isocarboxazid (Marplan®), selegiline (Eldepryl®)
- other medicines for mental depression (may be duplicate therapies or cause additive side effects)

Imipramine may also interact with any of the following medications:

- alcohol
- antacids
- atropine and related drugs like hyoscyamine, scopolamine, tolterodine and others
- barbiturate medicines for inducing sleep or treating seizures (convulsions), such as phenobarbital
- blood thinners, such as warfarin
- bromocriptine
- bupropion
- cimetidine
- clonidine
- cocaine
- delavirdine
- diphenoxylate
- disulfiram
- donepezil
- drugs for treating HIV infection
- female hormones, including contraceptive or birth control pills and estrogen
- galantamine
- herbs and dietary supplements like ephedra (Ma huang), kava kava, SAM-e, St. John's wort, valerian, or others
- imatinib, STI-571
- kaolin; pectin

- labetalol
- levodopa and other medicines for movement problems like Parkinson's disease
- lithium
- medicines for anxiety or sleeping problems
- medicines for colds, flu and breathing difficulties, like pseudoephedrine
- medicines for hay fever or allergies (antihistamines)
- medicines for weight loss or appetite control
- medicines used to regulate abnormal heartbeat or to treat other heart conditions (examples: amiodarone, bepridil, disopyramide, dofetilide, encainide, flecainide, ibutilide, mibefradil, procainamide, propafenone, quinidine, and others)
- metoclopramide
- muscle relaxants, like cyclobenzaprine
- other medicines for mental or mood problems and psychotic disturbances
- prescription pain medications like morphine, codeine, tramadol and others
- procarbazine
- seizure (convulsion) or epilepsy medicine such as carbamazepine or phenytoin
- stimulants like dexmethylphenidate or methylphenidate
- some antibiotics (examples: erythromycin, gatifloxacin, levofloxacin, linezolid, moxifloxacin, sotalol, sparfloxacin)
- tacrine
- thyroid hormones such as levothyroxine

Tell your prescriber or health care professional about all other medicines you are taking, including non-prescription medicines, nutritional supplements, or herbal products. Also tell your prescriber or health care professional if you are a frequent user of drinks with caffeine or alcohol, if you smoke, or if you use illegal drugs. These may affect the way your medicine works. Check with your health care professional before stopping or starting any of your medicines.

What should I watch for while taking imipramine?

Visit your prescriber or health care professional for regular checks on your progress. It can take several days or weeks before you feel the full effect of imipramine. If you have been taking imipramine regularly for some time, do not suddenly stop taking it. You must gradually reduce the dose or you may get severe side effects. Ask your prescriber or health care professional for advice. Even after you stop taking imipramine it can still affect your body for several days. You may get drowsy or dizzy. Do not drive, use machinery, or do anything that needs mental alertness until you know how imipramine affects you. Do not stand or sit up quickly, especially if you are an older patient. This reduces the risk of dizzy or fainting spells. Alcohol can increase dizziness and drowsiness. Avoid alcoholic drinks. Do not treat yourself for coughs, colds or allergies without asking your prescriber or health care professional for advice. Some ingredients can increase possible side effects. Your mouth may get dry. Chewing sugarless gum or sucking hard candy, and drinking plenty of water will help. Imipramine may cause dry eyes and blurred vision. If you wear contact lenses you may feel some discomfort. Lubricating drops may help. See your ophthalmologist if the problem does not go away or is severe. Imipramine may make your skin more sensitive to the sun. Keep out of the sun, or wear protective clothing outdoors and use a sunscreen. Do not use sun lamps or sun tanning beds or booths. Imipramine can affect blood glucose (sugar) levels. If you are a diabetic, check your blood sugar more often than usual, especially during the first few weeks of imipramine treatment. Call your prescriber or health care professional for advice if you notice a change in the results of blood or urine glucose tests. If you are going to have surgery or will need an x-ray procedure that uses contrast agents, tell your prescriber or health care professional that you are taking this medicine.

What side effects may I notice from taking imipramine?

Side effects that you should report to your prescriber or health care professional as soon as possible:
- abnormal production of milk in females
- blurred vision or eye pain
- breast enlargement in both males and females
- confusion, hallucinations (seeing or hearing things that are not really there)
- difficulty breathing
- fainting spells
- fever
- irregular or fast, pounding heartbeat, palpitations
- muscle stiffness, or spasms
- pain or difficulty passing urine, loss of bladder control
- seizures (convulsions)
- sexual difficulties (decreased sexual ability or desire, difficulty ejaculating)
- stomach pain
- swelling of the testicles
- tingling, pain, or numbness in the feet or hands
- tremor (shaking)
- unusual weakness or tiredness
- yellowing of the eyes or skin

Side effects that usually do not require medical attention (report to your prescriber or health care professional if they continue or are bothersome):
- anxiety
- constipation, or diarrhea
- drowsiness or dizziness
- dry mouth
- headache
- increased sensitivity of the skin to sun or ultraviolet light
- loss of appetite
- nausea, vomiting
- skin rash or itching
- weight gain or loss

Where can I keep my medicine?

Keep out of the reach of children in a container that small children cannot open. Store at room temperature between 15 and 30 degrees C (59 and 86 degrees F). Throw away any unused medicine after the expiration date.

Indapamide tablets

LOZOL®;
2.5 mg; Tablet
Aventis
Pharmaceutical
Products Inc

LOZOL®;
1.25 mg; Tablet
Aventis
Pharmaceutical
Products Inc

What are indapamide tablets?

INDAPAMIDE (Lozol®) is a diuretic. Diuretics increase the amount of urine passed, which causes the body to lose water and salt. Indapamide helps to treat high blood pressure (hypertension). It is not a cure. It also reduces the swelling and water retention caused by various medical conditions, such as heart, liver, or kidney disease. Generic indapamide tablets are available.

What should my health care professional know before I take indapamide?

They need to know if you have any of these conditions:
- diabetes
- gout
- kidney disease, small amounts of urine, or difficulty passing urine
- liver disease
- low blood levels of potassium, chloride, or sodium
- thyroid disease
- an unusual or allergic reaction to indapamide, sulfa drugs, other medicines, foods, dyes, or preservatives
- pregnant or trying to get pregnant
- breast-feeding

How should I take this medicine?

Take indapamide tablets by mouth. Follow the directions on the prescription label. Swallow the tablets with a drink of water. Take your doses at regular intervals. Do not take your medicine more often than directed. Remember that you will need to pass urine frequently after taking indapamide. Do not take your doses at a time of day that will cause you problems. Do not take at bedtime. Contact your pediatrician or health care professional regarding the use of this medicine in children. Special care may be needed.

What if I miss a dose?

If you miss a dose, take it as soon as you can. If it is almost time for your next dose, take only that dose. Do not take double or extra doses.

What may interact with indapamide?

- amiodarone
- dofetilide
- heart medicines such as digoxin
- lithium
- medicines for diabetes
- medicines for high blood pressure
- medicines that relax muscles for surgery
- medicine for colds and breathing difficulties
- water pills

Tell your prescriber or health care professional about all other medicines you are taking, including non-prescription medicines, nutritional supplements, or herbal products. Also tell your prescriber or health care professional if you are a frequent user of drinks with caffeine or alcohol, if you smoke, or if you use illegal drugs. These may affect the way your medicine works. Check with your health care professional before stopping or starting any of your medicines.

What should I watch for while taking indapamide?

Visit your prescriber or health care professional for regular checks on your progress. Check your blood pressure regularly. Ask your prescriber or health care professional what your blood pressure should be, and when you should contact him or her. You must not get dehydrated, ask your prescriber or health care professional how much fluid you need to drink a day. Do not stop taking indapamide except on your prescriber's advice. Watch your diet while you are taking indapamide. Ask your prescriber or health care professional about both potassium and sodium intake. Indapamide can make your body lose potassium and you may need an extra supply. Too high or too low potassium can cause problems. Some foods have a high potassium content such as bananas, coconuts, dates, figs, prunes, apricots, peaches, grapefruit juice, tomato juice, and orange juice. You may get dizzy or lightheaded. Do not drive, use machinery, or do anything that needs mental alertness until you know how indapamide affects you. To reduce the risk of dizzy or fainting spells, do not sit or stand up quickly, especially if you are an older patient.

Alcohol can make you lightheaded, dizzy and increase confusion. Avoid or limit intake of alcoholic drinks. Indapamide may make your skin more sensitive to sun or ultraviolet light. Keep out of the sun, or wear protective clothing outdoors and use a sunscreen (at least SPF 15). Do not use sun lamps or sun tanning beds or booths. If you are going to have surgery, tell your prescriber or health care professional that you are taking indapamide. Indapamide can increase the amount of sugar in blood or urine. If you are a diabetic keep a close check on blood and urine sugar.

What side effects may I notice from taking indapamide?

Side effects that you should report to your prescriber or health care professional as soon as possible:
- blurred vision
- change in the amount or frequency of urination
- dry mouth
- increased thirst
- irregular heartbeat (palpitations)
- mood changes
- muscle cramps or spasm
- nausea, vomiting
- seizures (convulsions)
- skin rash, itching, or hives
- unusual tiredness or weakness
- yellowing of the eyes or skin

Side effects that usually do not require medical attention (report to your prescriber or health care professional if they continue or are bothersome):
- diarrhea
- difficulty sleeping
- dizziness or lightheadedness
- headache
- increased sensitivity to the sun
- loss of appetite
- sexual difficulties (impotence)
- stomach upset

Where can I keep my medicine?

Keep out of the reach of children in a container that small children cannot open. Store at room temperature between 15 and 30 degrees C (59 and 86 degrees F). Keep container tightly closed. Throw away any unused medicine after the expiration date.

Indinavir capsules

CRIXIVAN®;
200 mg; Capsule
Merck and Co Inc

CRIXIVAN®;
400 mg; Capsule
Merck and Co Inc

What are indinavir capsules?

INDINAVIR (Crixivan®) is an antiviral drug called a protease inhibitor. Indinavir is used to treat human immunodeficiency virus (HIV) infection. Indinavir may reduce the amount of HIV in the blood and increase the number of CD4 cells (T-cells) in the blood. Indinavir is used in combination with other drugs to treat the HIV virus. Indinavir will not cure or prevent HIV infection or AIDS. You may still develop other infections or conditions associated with HIV. Generic indinavir capsules are not yet available.

What should my health care professional know before I take indinavir?

They need to know if you have any of these conditions:

- diabetes or high blood sugar
- hemophilia
- high blood cholesterol, lipids or triglycerides
- history of kidney stones
- history of pancreatitis
- liver disease
- an unusual or allergic reaction to indinavir, other medicines, foods, dyes, or preservatives
- breast-feeding
- pregnancy or trying to get pregnant

How should I take this medicine?

Take indinavir capsules by mouth. Follow the directions on the prescription label. Take the capsules at least 1 hour before or 2 hours after a meal. Take the capsules with a drink of water, skim milk, juice, coffee, or tea. You may take indinavir with a light meal, such as dry toast with jelly, juice, and coffee with skim milk and sugar; or corn flakes, skim milk, and sugar. Take your doses at regular intervals. Do not take your medicine more often than directed. To help to make sure that your anti-HIV therapy works as well as possible, be very careful to take all of your medicine exactly as prescribed. Do not stop taking except on your prescriber's advice. Contact your pediatrician or health care professional regarding the use of this medicine in children. Special care may be needed.

What if I miss a dose?

If you miss a dose, take it as soon as you can. If it is almost time for your next dose, take only that dose. Do not take double or extra doses.

What may interact with indinavir?

- amiodarone
- aripiprazole
- astemizole
- atazanavir
- birth control pills or other hormonal birth control medicines (like the patch, ring, or injections)
- carbamazepine
- certain medicines for anxiety or difficulty sleeping
- certain medicines for chest pain or high blood pressure, like calcium channel blockers (examples: amlodipine, diltiazem, felodipine, nifedipine, verapamil)
- cisapride
- citalopram
- cyclosporine
- delavirdine
- didanosine, ddI
- dihydroergotamine
- dofetilide
- efavirenz
- eplerenone
- ergotamine
- escitalopram
- ethotoin
- fluconazole
- itraconazole
- ketoconazole
- medicines for diabetes

- medicines to lower your cholesterol, such as atorvastatin, cerivastatin, lovastatin, or simvastatin
- methadone
- mifepristone, RU-486
- nelfinavir
- omeprazole
- phenytoin
- pimozide
- rifabutin
- rifampin
- rifapentine
- ritonavir
- sildenafil
- sirolimus
- St. John's wort
- tacrolimus
- tadalafil
- terfenadine
- trazodone
- vardenafil
- went yeast (Cholestin™)

Tell your prescriber or health care professional about all other medicines you are taking, including nonprescription medicines, nutritional supplements, or herbal products. Also tell your prescriber or health care professional if you are a frequent user of drinks with caffeine or alcohol, if you smoke, or if you use illegal drugs. These may affect the way your medicine works. Check with your health care professional before stopping or starting any of your medicines.

What should I watch for while taking indinavir?

Visit your prescriber or health care professional for regular checks on your progress. Discuss any new symptoms with your prescriber or health care professional. Indinavir will not cure HIV and you can still get other illnesses or complications associated with your disease. Taking indinavir does not reduce the risk of passing HIV infection to others through sexual or blood contact. It is best to avoid sexual contact so that you do not spread the disease to others. For any sexual contact, use a condom. Be careful about cuts, abrasions and other possible sources of blood contact. Never share a needle or syringe with anyone. Make sure to drink plenty of fluids while taking indinavir. Try to drink at least 6 glasses of water a day (48 ounces). If you notice pain or difficulty passing urine, call your health care provider immediately. Do not take antacids or didanosine, ddI, within 1 hour of taking indinavir. Antacids may decrease the amount of indinavir you absorb.

What side effects might I notice from taking indinavir?

Side effects that you should report to your prescriber or health care professional as soon as possible:
- blood in the urine
- difficulty or pain passing urine
- pain in the back or kidney

- redness, blistering, peeling or loosening of the skin, including inside the mouth
- severe dizziness
- skin rash
- unusual tiredness or weakness
- yellowing of skin or eyes

Side effects that usually do not require medical attention (report to your prescriber or health care professional if they continue or are bothersome):
- acid reflux
- back pain
- changes in taste
- dizziness
- drowsiness

- dry skin
- headache
- loss of appetite
- nausea, vomiting
- stomach pain
- tiredness or weakness

Where can I keep my medicine?

Keep out of the reach of children in a container that small children cannot open. Store at room temperature between 15 and 30 degrees C (59 and 86 degrees F). Keep container tightly closed. Indinavir capsules are sensitive to moisture and should remain in the original container. Throw away any unused medicine after the expiration date.

Indomethacin capsules

INDOCIN®;
50 mg; Capsule
Merck and Co Inc

INDOCIN®;
25 mg; Capsule
Merck and Co Inc

This drug requires an FDA medication guide. See page xxxvii.

What are indomethacin capsules?

INDOMETHACIN (Indocin®) is a nonsteroidal anti-inflammatory drug (NSAID). Indomethacin relieves the inflammation and pain associated with rheumatoid arthritis, osteoarthritis, ankylosing spondylitis, and gout. Generic indomethacin capsules and sustained-release capsules are available.

What should my health care professional know before I take indomethacin?

They need to know if you have any of these conditions:
- asthma, especially aspirin sensitive asthma
- bleeding problems or taking medicines that make you bleed more easily such as anticoagulants ("blood thinners")
- cigarette smoker
- dental disease
- depression
- diabetes
- drink more than 3 alcohol-containing beverages a day
- heart or circulation problems such as heart failure or leg edema (fluid retention)
- high blood pressure
- kidney disease
- liver disease
- Parkinson's disease
- seizures (convulsions)
- stomach or duodenal ulcers
- systemic lupus erythematosus
- ulcerative colitis
- an unusual or allergic reaction to aspirin, other salicylates, other NSAIDs, foods, dyes or preservatives
- pregnant or trying to get pregnant
- breast-feeding

How should I take this medicine?

Take indomethacin capsules by mouth. Follow the directions on the prescription label. Swallow capsules whole with a full glass of water; take capsules in an upright or sitting position. Taking a sip of water first, before taking the capsules, may help you swallow them. If possible, take bedtime doses at least 10 minutes before lying down. Do not crush or chew the sustained-release capsules. It is better to take indomethacin with food to prevent stomach upset. Take your doses at regular intervals. Do not take your medicine more often than directed. Contact your pediatrician or health care professional regarding the use of this medicine in children. Special care may be needed.

What if I miss a dose?

If you miss a dose, take it as soon as you can. If it is almost time for your next dose, take only that dose. Do not take double or extra doses.

What may interact with indomethacin?

- alcohol
- alendronate
- aspirin and aspirin-like medicines
- cidofovir
- cyclosporine
- drospirenone; ethinyl estradiol (Yasmin®)
- entecavir
- herbal products that contain feverfew, garlic, ginger, or ginkgo biloba
- lithium
- medicines for high blood pressure
- medicines that affect platelets
- medicines that treat or prevent blood clots such as warfarin and other "blood thinners"
- methotrexate
- other anti-inflammatory drugs (such as ibuprofen or prednisone)
- pemetrexed
- water pills (diuretics)

Tell your prescriber or health care professional about all other medicines you are taking, including non-

prescription medicines, nutritional supplements, or herbal products. Also tell your prescriber or health care professional if you are a frequent user of drinks with caffeine or alcohol, if you smoke, or if you use illegal drugs. These may affect the way your medicine works. Check with your health care professional before stopping or starting any of your medicines.

What should I watch for while taking indomethacin?

Let your prescriber or health care professional know if your pain continues, do not take with other pain-killers without advice. If you get flu-like symptoms (fever, chills, muscle aches and pains), call your prescriber or health care professional; do not treat yourself. To reduce unpleasant effects on your throat and stomach, take indomethacin with a full glass of water and never just before lying down. If you notice black, tarry stools or experience severe stomach pain and vomit blood or what looks like coffee grounds, notify your health care prescriber immediately. If you are taking medicines that affect the clotting of your blood, such as aspirin or blood thinners such as Coumadin®, talk to your health care provider or prescriber before taking this medicine. You may get dizzy. Do not drive, use machinery, or do anything that needs mental alertness until you know how indomethacin affects you. Do not sit or stand up quickly, especially if you are an older patient. This reduces the risk of dizzy or fainting spells. Do not smoke cigarettes or drink alcohol; these increase irritation to your stomach and can make it more susceptible to damage from indomethacin. If you are going to have surgery, tell your prescriber or health care professional that you are taking indomethacin. Problems can arise if you need dental work, and in the day to day care of your teeth. Try to avoid damage to your teeth and gums when you brush or floss your teeth. It is especially important not to use indomethacin during the last 3 months of pregnancy unless specifically directed to do so by your health care provider. Indomethacin may cause problems in the unborn child or complications during delivery.

What side effects may I notice from taking indomethacin?

Elderly patients are at increased risk for developing side effects.

Side effects that you should report to your prescriber or health care professional as soon as possible:

- signs of bleeding from the stomach—black tarry stools, blood in the urine, unusual tiredness or weakness, vomiting blood or vomit that looks like coffee grounds
- signs of an allergic reaction—difficulty breathing or wheezing, skin rash, redness, blistering or peeling skin, hives, or itching, swelling of eyelids, throat, lips
- blurred vision
- change in the amount of urine passed
- difficulty swallowing, severe heartburn or burning, pain in throat
- pain or difficulty passing urine
- stomach pain or cramps
- swelling of feet or ankles

Side effects that usually do not require medical attention (report to your prescriber or health care professional if they continue or are bothersome):

- diarrhea or constipation
- dizziness, drowsiness
- gas or heartburn
- headache
- nausea, vomiting

Where can I keep my medicine?

Keep out of the reach of children in a container that small children cannot open. Store at room temperature below 30 degrees C (86 degrees F). Keep container tightly closed. Throw away any unused medicine after the expiration date.

Insulin injection

What is insulin injection?

INSULIN (Iletin II®, Humulin®, Humalog®, Lantus®, Novolin®, NovoLog™, etc.) is a hormone produced naturally by the pancreas. Insulin regulates the amount of sugar in your blood and prevents or reduces long-term complications including damage to the blood vessels, eyes, kidneys, or nerves. There are different types of insulin available. Each type has a different onset of action and a different duration of action in the body. You should learn which types you take and how you should administer them, and how each type acts in your body. Insulin is labeled with a large, black letter (example: R for regular, L for lente) to help you easily identify the type, or with the name of the type you take (examples: Humalog®, NovoLog™, Humalog®Mix™, Lantus®, Novolog™Mix™). Only certain types of insulin may be used in insulin pumps. Insulin is obtained from beef, pork or human sources. Beef insulin is no longer being produced in the US due to concerns of transmission of certain infections through cow tissues. Talk to your prescriber if you take beef insulin currently. Once you are stabilized, do not change the type of insulin you use unless directed to do so by your health care professional. If you must switch the type of insulin you use, you should realize that you may need to monitor your blood sugar more frequently and that dosage adjustments may be needed before you are stabilized on the new type. Take care to learn and recognize the symptoms of hypoglycemia (low blood sugar) and know how you should treat these reactions. Insulin is available from several manufacturers. Some types of insulin can only be obtained by prescription; your prescriber or health care professional will probably write one. A prescription to obtain insulin syringes may or may not be required in the state where you live.

What does my health care professional need to know before I receive insulin?

They need to know if you have any of these conditions:
- adrenal or pituitary gland problems
- diarrhea
- fever or infection
- injury or trauma
- kidney disease
- nausea, vomiting
- recent surgery
- thyroid disease
- an unusual or allergic reaction to insulin, beef or pork products, other medicines, foods, dyes, or preservatives

How should I use this medicine?

Insulin is for injection under the skin. Use daily exactly as directed. Do not use more insulin than prescribed. Do not use more or less often than prescribed. To prepare a dose: Clean the rubber stopper of the vial with an alcohol wipe. Roll the bottle gently between the palms of your hands to mix and warm the solution (not necessary for regular insulin, insulin aspart, or insulin lispro). Be sure to mix the solution well, but do not shake vigorously. Pull back the plunger of a disposable syringe to fill the syringe with an amount of air equal to your dose of insulin (if your dose is 30 units, pull the plunger to the 30 unit mark). Insert the needle into the rubber stopper of the vial, and inject the air into the vial (this will make the insulin easier to remove). Turn the vial upside down, and pull back on the plunger to fill the syringe with prescribed number of units of insulin. Remove any air bubbles trapped in the syringe. If you are mixing two types of insulin in the syringe, measure the regular, aspart, or lispro insulin first. To inject a dose: Select an injection site on the stomach, arm, buttocks, or thigh, and clean with an alcohol wipe. Pinch the skin up with your fingers about three inches apart, and insert the needle at an angle of 45 to 90 degrees. Pull back on the plunger to make sure the needle is not in a blood vessel before injecting the insulin. If blood appears, remove the needle, reinsert it in a different (nearby) location, and repeat the process. If no blood appears, press the plunger to deliver the insulin. Remove the needle from the skin and press gently on the injection site for a moment (but do not rub

or massage). Rotate your injection site such that each site is not used more than once every 1 to 2 months. If you utilize a insulin injector device, you will be taught how to use it and how to refill the device with the insulin cartridges. Depending on the type of insulin and the type of injector device you use, you should gently roll the injector device between your hands or gently tip it up-side down then right-side up, until the insulin appears uniformly white and cloudy. You will be taught how to administer doses for meals or adjust doses for activities. Your health care prescriber and diabetic educators will teach you. If you utilize an insulin pump, you will be taught how to program the pump; refill the pump cartridges; and how to administer doses for meals or adjust doses for activities. Your health care prescriber and diabetic educators will teach you.

What if I miss a dose?

It is important not to miss a dose. If you do miss a dose, use it as soon as you can. If it is almost time for your next dose, use only that dose, do not take double doses. Know the signs of low and high blood sugar and make sure a close family contact or friend can also recognize these signs. Contact your prescriber or health care professional at once if you have any problems.

What may interact with insulin?

- diazoxide
- epinephrine
- glucagon
- guanethidine
- other medicines for diabetes

Many medications may cause changes (increase or decrease) in blood sugar, these include:
- alcohol-containing beverages
- aspirin and aspirin-like drugs
- beta-blockers, often used for high blood pressure or heart problems (examples include atenolol, metoprolol, propranolol)
- chromium
- female hormones, such as estrogens, progestins, or contraceptive pills
- isoniazid
- male hormones or anabolic steroids
- medications to suppress appetite or for weight loss
- medicines for allergies, asthma, cold, or cough
- niacin
- pentamidine
- phenytoin
- some herbal dietary supplements
- steroid medicines such as prednisone or cortisone
- thyroid hormones
- water pills (diuretics)

Tell your prescriber or health care professional about all other medicines you are taking, including non-prescription medicines, nutritional supplements, or herbal products. Also tell your prescriber or health care professional if you are a frequent user of drinks with caffeine

or alcohol, if you smoke, or if you use illegal drugs. These may affect the way your medicine works. Check with your health care professional before stopping or starting any of your medicines.

What should I watch for while taking insulin?

Visit your prescriber or health care professional for regular checks on your progress. To control your diabetes properly you must use insulin regularly, follow a regular diet and exercise schedule. Diabetes cannot be cured. Careful, daily control of blood sugar can postpone or prevent many of the long-term complications of diabetes. Dangerously high or low blood sugar can occur when meals and insulin are not spaced properly. Checking and recording your blood glucose and urine ketone levels regularly is important. It is sometimes hard to tell the difference between low and high blood sugar on the basis of symptoms (see side effects). Use a glucometer (blood glucose or sugar measuring device), whenever possible, before treating a suspected increase or decrease in blood sugar. Make sure that you have the right kind of syringe for the type of insulin you use. Try not to change the brand and type of insulin syringe unless told to switch by your prescriber. Use a syringe only once and throw away syringe and needle in a closed container to prevent accidental needle sticks. Do not switch brands or types of insulin without consulting your prescriber or health care professional; this can result in dangerously high or low blood sugar. Wear a Medic Alert bracelet or necklace and/or carry an identification card with your name and address, condition, medication, and prescriber's name and address. If you develop a cold, diarrhea, vomiting or other acute infection or illness, you should contact your health care prescriber. "Sick-days" may require adjustments to your insulin dosage or your illness may need to be evaluated. Ask your prescriber what you should do if you become ill. Do not stop taking your insulin; check with your prescriber for advice. If you are a long time smoker and suddenly stop, you may need a change in insulin dose. Talk to your prescriber or health care professional first. Many nonprescription cough and cold products contain sugar or alcohol. These can affect diabetes control or can alter the results of tests used to monitor blood sugar control. Avoid alcohol and products that contain alcohol or sugar. If you are going to have surgery, make sure you tell the health care professionals that you take insulin.

What side effects may I notice from receiving insulin?

Learn how and when you should monitor your blood sugar, and what you should do if high or low blood sugar occurs. Side effects that you should report to your prescriber or health care professional as soon as possible:

Symptoms of hypoglycemia (low blood glucose). Contact your health care professional if you experience symptoms of low blood sugar, which may include:

- anxiety or nervousness, confusion, difficulty concentrating, hunger, pale skin, nausea, fatigue, sweating, headache, palpitations, numbness of the mouth, tingling in the fingers, tremors, muscle weakness, blurred vision, cold sensations, uncontrolled yawning, irritability, rapid heartbeat, shallow breathing, and loss of consciousness. Hypoglycemia may cause you to not be aware of your actions or surroundings if it is severe, so you should let others know what to do if you cannot help yourself in a severe reaction.

Symptoms of high blood sugar (hyperglycemia) include:

- dizziness, dry mouth, flushed dry skin, fruit-like breath odor, loss of appetite, nausea, stomachache, unusual thirst, frequent passing of urine

Insulin also can cause rare but serious allergic reactions in some patients, including:

- severe skin rash and itching (hives)
- difficulty breathing

Side effects that usually do not require medical attention (report to your prescriber or health care professional if they continue or are bothersome):

- increase or decrease in fatty tissue under the skin, through overuse of a particular injection site
- itching, burning, swelling, or rash at the injection site

Where can I keep my medicine?

Keep out of the reach of children. Store unopened insulin vials or pen-injector cartridges in a refrigerator between 2 and 8 degrees C (36 and 46 degrees F). Do not freeze. Return to room temperature before use. Opened vials (vials currently in use) may be safely stored at room temperature, at approximately 25 degrees C (77 degrees F) or cooler for up to 28 days. Pen-injector cartridges in use may be kept at room temperature, approximately 25 degrees C (77 degrees F or cooler) for up to 10 days. Protect from light and excessive heat. Throw away any unused medicine after the expiration date or after the specified time for room temperature storage has passed.

Interferon Alfa-2a injection

ROFERON® A;
3 million unit/0.5 ml; Injection
Hoffmann La Roche Inc

This drug requires an FDA medication guide. See page xxxvii.

What is interferon alfa-2a injection?

INTERFERON ALFA-2a (Roferon-A®) is a man-made protein. Natural interferons are produced to help the immune system fight viral infections and certain cancer growths. Interferon alfa-2a has similar actions to natural interferons and is used to treat AIDS-related Kaposi's sarcoma, certain types of hepatitis, and leukemia or other cancers. Generic interferon alfa-2a injections are not available.

What should my health care professional know before I receive interferon alfa-2a?

They need to know if you have any of these conditions:
- autoimmune disease
- blood or bleeding disorders
- depression or mental disorders
- diabetes
- heart or lung disease
- kidney disease
- liver disease
- psoriasis
- seizures
- thyroid disease
- undergoing radiation therapy
- an unusual or allergic reaction to interferons, other medicines, foods, dyes, or preservatives
- pregnant or trying to get pregnant
- breast-feeding

How should I use this medicine?

Interferon alfa-2a is for injection into a muscle or under the skin. Injections of interferon alfa-2a can be given in the hospital or clinic, or by a home health-care nurse. If you are giving yourself the injections, make sure you follow the directions carefully. You can inject your dose at bedtime if you experience flu-like effects. Do not reuse syringes or needles. Dispose of needles and syringes in a puncture-resistant container. Contact your pediatrician or health care professional regarding the use of this medicine in children. Special care may be needed.

What if I miss a dose?

If you miss a dose, use it as soon as you can. If it is almost time for your next dose, use only that dose. Do not use double or extra doses.

What may interact with interferon alfa-2a?

- theophylline
- zidovudine, AZT

Tell your prescriber or health care professional about all other medicines that you are taking, including non-prescription medicines. Also tell your prescriber or health care professional if you are a frequent user of drinks with caffeine or alcohol, if you smoke, or if you use illegal drugs. These may affect the way your medicine works. Check with your health care professional before stopping or starting any of your medicines.

What should I watch for while taking interferon alfa-2a?

Visit your prescriber or health care professional for regular checks on your progress. You will need regular blood checks. Do not change brands without consulting your prescriber or health care professional. Different brands of interferon can act differently in your body. Check with your pharmacist if your refills do not look like your original product. You may get drowsy or dizzy. Do not drive, use machinery, or do anything that needs mental alertness until you know how interferon alfa-2a affects you. Alcohol can make you more drowsy or dizzy, increase confusion and lightheadedness. Avoid alcoholic drinks. Interferon alfa-2a can cause flu-like symptoms and make you feel generally unwell. If you get a fever or sore throat that does not go away after the first few weeks of treatment, do not treat yourself. Other signs of infection include cough, lower back or side pain, pain or difficulty passing urine. Report any side effects, but continue your medicine even though you feel ill, unless your prescriber or health care professional tells you to stop. Call your prescriber or health care professional as soon as you can if you think you have an infection. Females who are able to have children should use effective birth control methods while receiving interferon alfa-2a. Interferon alfa-2a can cause blood problems and may decrease your body's ability to fight certain types of infections or increase your risk to bruise or bleed. This may be more of a concern if you are receiving high doses or other chemotherapy agents with your interferon treatment. Call your prescriber or health care professional if you have symptoms of a cold or flu that do not get better. Do not treat these symptoms yourself. Call your prescriber or health care professional if you notice any unusual bleeding. Be careful not to cut, bruise, or injure yourself because you may get an infection and bleed more than usual. Be careful brushing and flossing your teeth or using a toothpick while receiving interferon alfa-2a because you may get an infection or bleed more easily. If you have any dental work done, tell your dentist you are receiving interferon alfa-2a. Your mouth may get dry. Chewing sugarless gum or sucking hard candy, and drinking plenty of water will help. Make sure to drink plenty of water while you are taking interferon alfa-2a. Use disposable syringes only once. Place used syringes and needles in a closed container to prevent accidental needle sticks.

What side effects may I notice from receiving interferon alfa-2a?

The side effects you may experience with interferon alfa-2a therapy depend upon the dose, other types of medicine given at the same time, and the disease being treated. Not all of these effects occur in all patients. Discuss any concerns or questions with your prescriber or health care professional.

Side effects that you should report to your prescriber or health care professional as soon as possible:

Uncommon:

- low blood counts—interferon alfa-2a may decrease the number of white blood cells, red blood cells and platelets. You may be at increased risk for infections and bleeding.
- signs of infection—fever or chills, cough, sore throat, pain or difficulty passing urine
- signs of decreased platelets or bleeding—bruising, pinpoint red spots on the skin, black, tarry stools, blood in the urine
- signs of decreased red blood cells—unusual weakness or tiredness, fainting spells, lightheadedness

Common:

- confusion
- depression
- difficulty breathing
- difficulty sleeping
- difficulty thinking or concentrating

- irregular heartbeat, palpitations or chest pain
- menstrual changes
- nervousness
- numbness or tingling in the fingers and toes

Side effects that usually do not require medical attention (report to your prescriber or health care professional if they continue or are bothersome):

- blurred vision
- changes in taste (metallic taste)
- cough
- diarrhea
- dry or sore mouth
- fever, chills
- hair loss
- headaches
- joint, leg, or back pain
- loss of appetite
- muscle aches
- nasal congestion
- nausea, vomiting
- sexual difficulties
- skin rash, itching
- tiredness

Where can I keep my medicine?

Keep out of the reach of children. Store in a refrigerator between 2 and 8 degrees C (36 and 46 degrees F). Do not freeze. Throw away any unused vials or syringes after the expiration date.

Interferon Alfa-2b injection

INTRON® A
MULTIDOSE PEN;
3 million IU/0.2ml;
Injection
Schering Corp

INTRON® A;
10 million IU/ml;
Injection
Schering Corp

What is interferon alfa-2b injection?

INTERFERON ALFA-2b (Intron® A) is a man-made protein. Natural interferons are produced to help the immune system fight viral infections and certain cancer growths. Interferon alfa-2b has similar actions to natural interferons and is used to treat AIDS-related Kaposi's sarcoma, certain types of hepatitis, and leukemia or other cancers. Generic interferon alfa-2b injections are not yet available.

What should my health care professional know before I receive interferon alfa-2b?

They need to know if you have any of these conditions:

- autoimmune disease
- blood or bleeding disorders
- depression or other mental disorders
- diabetes
- heart or lung disease
- liver disease
- psoriasis
- thyroid disease
- undergoing radiation therapy

- an unusual or allergic reaction to interferons, other medicines, foods, dyes, or preservatives
- pregnant or trying to get pregnant
- breast-feeding

How should I use this medicine?

Interferon alfa-2b is for injection into a muscle or under the skin or may be given as an infusion into your veins. Injections of interferon alfa-2b can be given in the hospital or clinic, or by a home health care nurse. If you are giving yourself the injections, make sure you follow the directions carefully. You can inject your dose at bedtime if you experience flu-like effects. Do not reuse syringes or needles. Dispose of needles and syringes in a puncture-resistant container. Contact your pediatrician or health care professional regarding the use of this medicine in children. Special care may be needed.

What if I miss a dose?

If you miss a dose, use it as soon as you can. If it is almost time for your next dose, contact your health care provider for instructions and if you need to change your schedule. Do not use double or extra doses.

What may interact with interferon alfa-2b?

- theophylline
- zidovudine, AZT

Tell your prescriber or health care professional about all other medicines that you are taking, including non-prescription medicines. Also tell your prescriber or health care professional if you are a frequent user of drinks with caffeine or alcohol, if you smoke, or if you use illegal drugs. These may affect the way your medicine works. Check with your health care professional before stopping or starting any of your medicines.

What should I watch for while taking interferon alfa-2b?

Visit your prescriber or health care professional for regular checks on your progress. You will need regular blood checks. Do not change brands without consulting your prescriber or health care professional. Different brands of interferon can act differently in your body. Check with your pharmacist if your refills do not look like your original product. You may get drowsy or dizzy. Do not drive, use machinery, or do anything that needs mental alertness until you know how interferon alfa-2b affects you. Alcohol can make you more drowsy or dizzy, increase confusion and lightheadedness. Avoid alcoholic drinks. Interferon alfa-2b can cause flu-like symptoms and make you feel generally unwell. If you get a fever or sore throat that do not go away after the first few weeks of treatment, do not treat yourself. Report any side effects as above, but continue your course of medicine even though you feel ill, unless your prescriber or health care professional tells you to stop. Call your prescriber or health care professional as soon as you can if you think you have an infection. Other signs of infection include cough, lower back or side pain, pain or difficulty passing urine. Females who are able to have children should use effective birth control methods while receiving interferon alfa-2b. Interferon alfa-2b can cause blood problems and may decrease your body's ability to fight certain types of infections or increase your risk to bruise or bleed. This may be more of a concern if you are receiving high doses or other chemotherapy agents with your interferon treatment. Call your prescriber or health care professional if you have symptoms of a cold or flu that do not get better. Do not treat these symptoms yourself. Call your prescriber or health care professional if you notice any unusual bleeding. Be careful not to cut, bruise, or injure yourself because you may get an infection and bleed more than usual. Be careful brushing and flossing your teeth or using a toothpick while receiving interferon alfa-2b because you may get an infection or bleed more easily. If you have any dental work done, tell your dentist you are receiving interferon alfa-2b. Your mouth may get dry. Chewing sugarless gum or sucking hard candy, and drinking plenty of water will help. Make sure to drink plenty of fluids while you are taking interferon alfa-2b. Use disposable syringes only once. Place used syringes and needles in a closed container to prevent accidental needle sticks.

What side effects may I notice from receiving interferon alfa-2b?

The side effects you may experience with interferon alfa-2b therapy depend upon the dose, other types of medicine given at the same time, and the disease being treated. Not all of these effects occur in all patients. Discuss any concerns or questions with your prescriber or health care professional.

Side effects that you should report to your prescriber or health care professional as soon as possible:
Uncommon:
- low blood counts—interferon alfa-2b may decrease the number of white blood cells, red blood cells and platelets. You may be at increased risk for infections and bleeding.
- signs of infection—fever or chills, cough, sore throat, pain or difficulty passing urine
- signs of decreased platelets or bleeding—bruising, pinpoint red spots on the skin, black, tarry stools, blood in the urine
- signs of decreased red blood cells—unusual weakness or tiredness, fainting spells, lightheadedness

Common:
- confusion
- depression
- difficulty breathing
- difficulty sleeping
- difficulty thinking or concentrating
- irregular heartbeat, palpitations or chest pain
- nervousness
- numbness or tingling in the fingers and toes

Side effects that usually do not require medical attention (report to your prescriber or health care professional if they continue or are bothersome):
- blurred vision
- changes in taste (metallic taste)
- cough
- diarrhea
- dry or sore mouth
- fever, chills
- hair loss
- headaches
- joint, leg, or back pain
- loss of appetite
- muscle aches
- nasal congestion
- nausea, vomiting
- skin rash, itching
- tiredness

Where can I keep my medicine?

Keep out of the reach of children. Store in a refrigerator between 2 and 8 degrees C (36 and 46 degrees F). Do not freeze. Throw away any unused vials or syringes after the expiration date.

Interferon Alfa-2b; Ribavirin kit

REBETRON™;
3 million IU/0.2 ml/200 mg;
Injection
Schering Corp

What is the interferon alfa-2b; ribavirin kit?
The **REBETRON**™ kit contains **RIBAVIRIN** (Rebetol®) capsules and **INTERFERON ALFA-2b** (Intron® A) injection. Ribavirin and interferon-alfa are used together to treat chronic hepatitis C infections. Ribavirin is an antiviral agent. It is not for the treatment of simple viral infections or other types of hepatitis infections. Interferon alfa-2b is a synthetic (man-made) protein produced by genetic engineering. Natural interferons are produced to help the immune system fight viral infections. Interferon alfa-2b, which has similar actions to natural interferons, has protective activity against viruses. Generic ribavirin capsules and interferon alfa injections are not yet available.

What should my health care professional know before I take interferon alfa-2b ribavirin?
They need to know if you have any of these conditions:
- anemia
- autoimmune disease
- bone marrow suppression (low white blood cell, red blood cells, or platelets)
- breathing problems
- depression or other mental illness
- diabetes
- heart disease such as angina or history of a heart attack
- high blood pressure
- human immunodeficiency virus (HIV) infection
- kidney disease
- liver disease (other than hepatitis C)
- pancreatitis
- past interferon treatment for hepatitis C that did not work
- prior organ transplant
- psoriasis
- recent radiation therapy (within 4 weeks)
- sickle cell disease
- thalassemia
- thyroid problems
- an unusual or allergic reaction to ribavirin, interferons, other medicines, foods, dyes, or preservatives
- pregnant or trying to get pregnant
- breast-feeding

How should I take this medicine?
Finish the full course prescribed by your prescriber or health care professional even if you think your condition is better. Do not stop taking except on your prescriber's advice. Ribavirin capsules are taken by mouth in the morning and the evening. Swallow capsules with a drink of water. You can take ribavirin capsules with or without food, but you should take it the same way every day. The exact dose will be determined by your prescriber or health care professional. Follow the directions on your prescription package. Take your doses at regular intervals. Do not take your medicine more often than directed Interferon alfa is for injection into a muscle or under the skin. Injections of interferon alfa can be given in the hospital or clinic, or by a home health care nurse. If you are giving yourself the injections, make sure you follow the directions carefully. Give interferon injections in the evening or at bedtime to decrease the degree of side effects. Do NOT share this medicine with anyone else. Contact your pediatrician or health care professional regarding the use of this medicine in children. Special care may be needed.

What if I miss a dose?
If you miss a dose, take it as soon as you can. If it is almost time for your next dose, take only that dose. Do not take double or extra doses.

What may interact with interferon alfa-2b; ribavirin?
- zidovudine, ZDV (AZT)
- theophylline
- oral contraceptives

Tell your prescriber or other health care professional about all other medicines you are taking including non-prescription medicines, nutritional supplements, or herbal products. Also, tell your prescriber or health care professional if you are a frequent user of drinks with caffeine or alcohol, if you smoke or if you use illegal drugs. These may affect the way your medicine works. Check before stopping or starting any of your medications.

What should I watch for while taking interferon alfa-2b; ribavirin?
Treatment with interferon alfa-2b; ribavirin may last for 24 to 48 weeks. It is important not to stop treatment even if you are feeling better. You may need to have blood tests done during therapy to evaluate your progress. Ribavirin may cause severe birth defects or death to the unborn child if taken during pregnancy; therefore if you are pregnant, you must not take ribavirin. Women who can still have children must have a negative pregnancy test before starting treatment then monthly pregnancy tests until 6 months after stopping ribavirin. Female patients and female partners of men taking ribavirin must use 2 forms of effective birth control methods during treatment with ribavirin and for 6 months after stopping ribavirin therapy. If you think you may have become pregnant and are taking ribavirin, contact your prescriber or health care professional right away. There is no information regarding whether treatment with interferon alfa-2b; ribavirin will prevent the spreading hepatitis C to other people. Also, it is not known if interferon alfa-2b; ribavirin can cure

hepatitis C or prevent other complications of hepatitis C infection such as cirrhosis, liver failure, or liver cancer. Many patients may experience flu-like symptoms after receiving interferon alfa injections. These symptoms may include headache, fatigue, fever, and muscle aches. You may be able to decrease these effects by giving the interferon injection at bedtime. Some patients may be able to take acetaminophen (Tylenol®) before the interferon injection. Check with your prescriber or health care professional before taking any products containing acetaminophen as these may worsen your liver disease. Interferon alfa-2b; ribavirin therapy may cause anemia (low red blood counts). You will need to have frequent blood checks during the first month of treatment with interferon alfa-2b; ribavirin to follow your counts. Make sure to drink plenty of fluids while taking interferon alfa-2b; ribavirin, especially during the first part of treatment. If you will be administering interferon alfa to yourself at home, your prescriber or health care professional should provide you with a puncture-resistant container for the proper disposal of syringes and needles. Never reuse syringes or needles.

What side effects may I notice from using interferon alfa-2b; ribavirin?

Side effects that you should report to your prescriber or health care professional as soon as possible:

- changes in your heart rate
- depression
- dizziness or light-headedness
- increased fatigue
- increased weakness, fatigue or tiredness
- missed menstrual cycle

Side effects that usually do not require medical attention (report to your prescriber or health care professional if they continue or are bothersome):

- flu-like symptoms
- hair thinning
- headache
- heartburn
- itching
- nausea
- skin rash
- vomiting

Where can I keep my medicine?

Keep out of the reach of children. NEVER share this medicine with anyone. Ribavirin capsules may be kept in the refrigerator between 2 and 8 degrees C (36 and 46 degrees F) or at room temperature, 25 degrees C (77 degrees F). Interferon vials or multidose pens should be kept in the refrigerator between 2 and 8 degrees C (36 and 46 degrees F).

This drug requires an FDA medication guide. See page xxxvii.

Interferon Alfacon-1 injection

INFERGEN®;
9 mcg/0.3 ml;
Injection
Intermune Inc

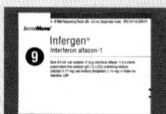

INFERGEN®;
15 mcg/0.5 ml;
Injection
Intermune Inc

What is interferon alfacon-1 injection?

INTERFERON ALFACON-1 (Infergen®) is a man-made substance similar to natural interferon made by your body. Natural interferons help your immune system work better. Interferon alfacon-1 has similar actions to natural interferons. It is used to treat hepatitis C. Interferon alfacon-1 may also be used to treat other types of viral infections or certain types of cancer. Generic interferon alfacon-1 injections are not yet available.

What should my health care professional know before I receive interferon alfacon-1?

They need to know if you have any of these conditions:

- autoimmune disease
- blood or bleeding disorders
- depression or mental disorders
- diabetes
- heart or lung disease
- thyroid disease
- an unusual or allergic reaction to interferons, other medicines, foods, dyes, or preservatives
- pregnant or trying to get pregnant
- breast-feeding

How should I use this medicine?

Interferon alfacon-1 is for injection under the skin. Injections of interferon alfacon-1 can be given in the hospital or clinic, or by a home health care nurse. If you are giving yourself the injections, make sure you follow the directions carefully. If you give interferon alfacon-1 at bedtime, you may be able to decrease some of the side effects. Do not reuse syringes or needles. Dispose of needles and syringes in a puncture-resistant container. Contact your pediatrician or health care professional regarding the use of this medicine in children. Special care may be needed.

What if I miss a dose?

If you miss a dose, use it as soon as you can. Wait at least 48 hours before taking your next dose.

What may interact with interferon alfacon-1?

- zidovudine (AZT)

Tell your prescriber or health care professional about all other medicines that you are taking, including non-prescription medicines. Also tell your prescriber or health care professional if you are a frequent user of drinks with caffeine or alcohol, if you smoke, or if you use illegal drugs. These may affect the way your medicine works. Check with your health care professional before stopping or starting any of your medicines.

What should I watch for while taking interferon alfacon-1?

Visit your prescriber or health care professional for regular checks on your progress. You will need regular blood checks. Do not change brands without consulting your prescriber or health care professional. Different brands of interferon can act differently in your body. Check with your pharmacist if your refills do not look like your original product. Use disposable syringes only once. Place used syringes and needles in a closed container to prevent accidental needle sticks. Interferon alfacon-1 can cause flu-like symptoms especially during the first few weeks of treatment. These symptoms may include fever, chills, fatigue, muscle aches, nausea, and decreased appetite. If you get a fever or sore throat after the first few weeks of treatment, do not treat yourself. Call your prescriber or health care professional as soon as you can if you think you have an infection. Your mouth may get dry. Chewing sugarless gum or sucking hard candy, and drinking plenty of water will help. Females who are able to have children should use effective birth control methods while receiving interferon alfacon-1.

What side effects may I notice from receiving interferon alfacon-1?

Side effects that you should report to your prescriber or health care professional as soon as possible:
- confusion

- depression
- difficulty breathing
- dizziness
- irregular heartbeat, palpitations, or chest pain
- numbness or tingling in the fingers and toes

Side effects that usually do not require medical attention (report to your prescriber or health care professional if they continue or are bothersome):
- blurred vision or eye pain
- changes in taste (metallic taste)
- cough
- diarrhea
- difficulty sleeping
- difficulty thinking or concentrating
- dry or sore mouth
- fever, chills during the first 2 weeks of treatment
- hair loss
- headaches
- indigestion
- joint, leg, or back pain
- loss of appetite
- menstrual changes
- muscle aches
- nasal congestion
- nervousness
- nausea or stomach upset
- skin rash, itching
- tiredness, especially during the first 1 to 2 weeks of treatment

Where can I keep my medicine?

Keep out of the reach of children. Store in a refrigerator between 2 and 8 degrees C (36 and 46 degrees F). Do not freeze. Throw away any unused vials or syringes after the expiration date.

Interferon Alfa-n3 injection

ALFERON® N;
5,000,000 unit/ml; Injection
Interferon Sciences Inc

What is interferon alfa-n3 injection?

INTERFERON ALFA-n3 (Alferon N®) is made of many different subtypes of natural interferon alpha. Interferon alpha is made by your body to attack viral infections and certain types of cancer. Interferon alfa-n3 is used to treat genital warts, which are caused by a viral infection. This drug is only occasionally used to treat hepatitis C. Generic interferon alfa-n3 injections are not yet available.

What should my health care professional know before I receive interferon alfa-n3?

They need to know if you have any of these conditions:
- diabetes
- heart or lung disease
- psoriasis
- seizures
- an unusual or allergic reaction to interferons, neomycin, mouse or egg proteins, other medicines, foods, dyes, or preservatives

- pregnant or trying to get pregnant
- breast-feeding

How should I use this medicine?

Interferon alfa-n3 is injected directly into the lesions by a trained health care professional.

What if I miss a dose?

If you miss an appointment, reschedule it as soon as you can.

What may interact with interferon alfa-n3?

There are no reported drug interactions with interferon alfa-n3 when it is given to treat genital warts.

Tell your prescriber or health care professional about all other medicines that you are taking, including nonprescription medicines. Also tell your prescriber or health care professional if you are a frequent user of drinks with caffeine or alcohol, if you smoke, or if you use illegal drugs. These may affect the way your medicine works. Check with your health care professional before stopping or starting any of your medicines.

What should I watch for while taking interferon alfa-n3?

Visit your prescriber or health care professional for regular checks on your progress. You will need regular blood checks. Do not change brands without consulting your prescriber or health care professional. Different brands of interferon can act differently in your body. Check with your pharmacist if your refills do not look like your original product. You may get drowsy or dizzy. Do not drive, use machinery, or do anything that needs mental alertness until you know how interferon alfa-n3 affects you. Alcohol can make you more drowsy or dizzy, increase confusion and lightheadedness. Avoid alcoholic drinks. Females who are able to have children should use effective birth control methods while receiving interferon alfa-n3.

What side effects may I notice from receiving interferon alfa-n3?

Side effects that you should report to your prescriber or health care professional as soon as possible:
- signs of allergic reactions including hives, tightness of chest, wheezing, difficulty breathing

Side effects that usually do not require medical attention (report to your prescriber or health care professional if they continue or are bothersome):
- fever, chills
- headaches
- joint, leg, or back pain
- muscle aches
- nausea, vomiting
- skin rash, itching
- tiredness

Where can I keep my medicine?

You will receive this medicine in a clinic or office setting; you will not keep this medicine at home.

This drug requires an FDA medication guide. See page xxxvii.

Interferon Beta-1a injection

AVONEX®; 30 mcg/ml; Injection Biogen Inc

AVONEX®; 30 mcg/0.5 ml; Injection Biogen Inc

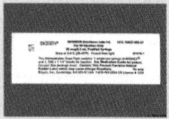

What is interferon beta-1a injection?

INTERFERON BETA-1a (Avonex®) is a drug that acts like a protein in your body called interferon beta. Interferon beta helps to control your immune system. Interferon beta-1a is used in the treatment of multiple sclerosis to decrease the number and severity of attacks. Beta interferons are occasionally used to treat other diseases. Generic interferon beta-1a injections are not yet available.

What should my health care professional know before I receive interferon beta-1a?

They need to know if you have any of these conditions:
- depression or other mental health disorder
- heart disease or irregular heart beats/rhythm
- liver disease
- low blood counts
- previous heart attack
- seizure disorder
- thyroid disease
- an unusual or allergic reaction to interferon, albumin, hamster proteins, latex, other medicines, foods, dyes, or preservatives
- pregnant or trying to get pregnant
- breast-feeding

How should I use this medicine?

Interferon beta-1a is for injection into a muscle. It may be given by a health care professional in a hospital or clinic setting. Your health care professional may teach you how to give these injections at home. Make sure you understand how to give the injections and are comfortable with it before you give them yourself. Before preparing an injection always wash your hands well

with soap and water. Do not shake the solution before measuring or injecting a dose. Do not use more than the prescribed dose. Using larger or more frequent doses increases the risk of getting serious side effects. The manufacturer of Avonex® offers free information to patients and their health care partners. Contact MS ActiveSource for more information (1-800-456-2255). Avonex® prefilled syringes should be allowed to warm to room temperature before using. This usually takes about 30 minutes. Do not reuse needles or syringes. Discard needles and syringes in a puncture-resistant container provided to you by your health care professional. Contact your pediatrician or health care professional regarding the use of this medicine in children. Special care may be needed.

What if I miss a dose?

If you miss a dose or an appointment for a dose, take it as soon as possible or reschedule your appointment as soon as possible. You may continue your regular schedule but do not give 2 injections within 2 days of each other.

What may interact with interferon beta-1a?

- zidovudine

Tell your prescriber or health care professional about all other medicines that you are taking, including non-prescription medicines, nutritional supplements, or herbal products. Also tell your prescriber or health care professional if you are a frequent user of drinks with caffeine or alcohol, if you smoke, or if you use illegal drugs. These may affect the way your medicine works.

Check with your health care professional before stopping or starting any of your medicines.

What should I watch for while taking interferon beta-1a?

Visit your prescriber or health care professional for regular checks on your progress. Tell your prescriber or health care professional if you are feeling depressed. Females of childbearing age should use a reliable method of birth control. If you do become pregnant, stop using interferon beta-1a at once and contact your prescriber or health care professional. Reactions at the site of injection may occur. Ask your prescriber or health care professional to suggest a series of injection sites, so that you do not have to use the same site repeatedly. Flu-like symptoms are common with interferon beta-1a therapy. Using this medicine at night can reduce these symptoms. Your prescriber or health care professional may suggest taking acetaminophen (Tylenol®) or ibuprofen (Motrin®, Advil®, etc.) before your dose and for 24 hours after you receive your injection. Use disposable syringes only once, and throw away syringes and needles in a closed, puncture-resistant container to prevent accidental needle sticks.

What side effects may I notice from receiving interferon beta-1a?

Side effects that you should report to your prescriber or health care professional as soon as possible:
- confusion
- depression
- difficulty breathing, swelling of face or throat, rash, hives, or other signs of a severe allergic reaction
- fainting

- mood changes, anxiety
- seizures
- unusual weakness or tiredness

Side effects that usually do not require medical attention (report to your prescriber or health care professional if they continue or are bothersome):
- diarrhea
- dizziness
- fever, chills, or flu-like symptoms
- headache
- muscle aches
- nausea, vomiting
- pain, redness, swelling, and irritation at the injection site
- stomach pain
- weakness

Where can I keep my medicine?

Keep out of the reach of children. Except as listed, this medicine must be kept cold. Store in a refrigerator between 2 and 8 degrees C (36 and 46 degrees F); do not freeze. Do not use beyond the expiration date on the syringe or vial.

- *Avonex® vials:* If a refrigerator is not available, the vials may be kept at room temperature at or below 25 degrees C (77 degrees F) for up to 30 days. Use as soon as possible after preparing the solution. If necessary, the prepared solution may be kept in a refrigerator for up to 6 hours. Throw away any unused solution.
- *Avonex® pre-filled syringes:* Once removed from the refrigerator, the pre-filled syringes should be used within 12 hours. Do not expose to high temperatures. Protect from light.

Interferon Beta-1a injection

REBIF®;
22 mcg/0.5 ml;
Injection
Serono Inc

REBIF®;
44 mcg/0.5 ml;
Injection
Serono Inc

What is interferon beta-1a injection?

INTERFERON BETA-1a (Rebif®) is a drug that acts like a protein in your body called interferon beta. Interferon beta helps to control your immune system. Interferon beta-1a is used in the treatment of multiple sclerosis to decrease the number and severity of attacks. Beta interferons are occasionally used to treat other diseases. Generic interferon beta-1a injections are not yet available.

What should my health care professional know before I take interferon beta-1a?

They need to know if you have any of these conditions:
- frequently or regularly drink alcohol-containing beverages
- depression or other mental health disorder
- heart disease or irregular heart beats/rhythm
- liver disease
- low blood counts

- previous heart attack
- seizure disorder
- thyroid disease
- an unusual or allergic reaction to interferon, albumin, hamster proteins, other medicines, foods, dyes, or preservatives
- pregnant or trying to get pregnant
- breast-feeding

How should I use this medicine?

Interferon beta-1a is for injection under the skin, three days a week (preferably late in the afternoon or evening) on the same days of the week at least 48 hours apart. It may be given by a health care professional in a hospital or clinic setting. Your health care professional may teach you how to give these injections at home. Before you try to use this injection, carefully read the instructions provided. Make sure you are comfortable and understand how to prepare, inject, and

This drug requires an FDA medication guide. See page xxxvii.

store interferon beta-1a. Before giving an injection always wash your hands well with soap and water. Do not use more than the prescribed dose. Using larger or more frequent doses increases the risk of getting serious side effects. The manufacturer offers complimentary services including injection training and reimbursement support. Contact MS LifeLines at 1-877-44-REBIF. Do not reuse needles or syringes. Discard needles and syringes in a puncture-resistant container provided to you by your health care professional. Contact your pediatrician or health care professional regarding the use of this medicine in children. Special care may be needed.

What if I miss a dose?

If you miss a dose or an appointment for a dose, take it as soon as possible or reschedule your appointment as soon as possible. If a dose is missed, administer the dose as soon as possible then skip the following day. Do not give on two consecutive days. Return to the regular schedule the following week.

What may interact with interferon beta-1a?

- zidovudine

Tell your prescriber or health care professional about all other medicines that you are taking, including nonprescription medicines, nutritional supplements, or herbal products. Also tell your prescriber or health care professional if you are a frequent user of drinks with caffeine or alcohol, if you smoke, or if you use illegal drugs. These may affect the way your medicine works. Check with your health care professional before stopping or starting any of your medicines.

What should I watch for while taking interferon beta-1a?

Visit your prescriber or health care professional for regular checks on your progress. Tell your prescriber or health care professional if you are feeling depressed. Females of childbearing age should use a reliable method of birth control. If you do become pregnant, stop using interferon beta-1a at once and contact your prescriber or health care professional. Reactions at the site of injection may occur. Ask your prescriber or

health care professional to suggest a series of injection sites, so that you do not have to use the same site repeatedly. Flu-like symptoms are common with interferon beta-1a therapy. Using this medicine at night can reduce these symptoms. Your prescriber or health care professional may suggest taking acetaminophen (Tylenol®) or ibuprofen (Motrin®, Advil®, etc.) before your dose and for 24 hours after you receive your injection. Use disposable syringes only once, and throw away syringes and needles in a closed, puncture-resistant container to prevent accidental needle sticks.

What side effects may I notice from receiving interferon beta-1a?

Side effects that you should report to your prescriber or health care professional as soon as possible:

- confusion
- depression
- difficulty breathing, swelling of face or throat, rash, hives, or other signs of a severe allergic reaction
- fainting
- mood changes, anxiety
- seizures
- unusual weakness or tiredness
- yellow coloring of skin or eyes

Side effects that usually do not require medical attention (report to your prescriber or health care professional if they continue or are bothersome):

- diarrhea
- dizziness
- fever, chills, or flu-like symptoms
- headache
- muscle aches
- nausea, vomiting
- pain, redness, swelling, and irritation at the injection site
- stomach pain
- weakness

Where can I keep my medicine?

Keep out of the reach of children. This medicine must be kept cold. Store in a refrigerator between 2 and 8 degrees C (36 and 46 degrees F); do not freeze. If a refrigerator is temporarily not available, Rebif® should be kept cool below 25 degrees C (77 degrees F) and away from heat and light. Throw away any unused solution.

Interferon Beta-1b injection

BETASERON;
0.3 mg; Injection
Berlex Laboratories Inc

What is interferon beta-1b injection?

INTERFERON BETA-1b (Betaseron®) is a manmade drug that acts like a substance in your body called interferon beta. Interferon beta helps to control your immune system. Interferon beta-1b helps to decrease the number and severity of attacks in multiple sclerosis. Interferon betas are occasionally used to treat other

diseases. Generic interferon beta-1b injections are not yet available.

What should my health care professional know before I receive interferon beta-1b?

- depression
- heart disease or irregular heart beats
- low blood counts

- previous heart attack
- an unusual or allergic reaction to interferon, albumin, proteins, other medicines, foods, dyes, or preservatives
- pregnant or trying to get pregnant
- breast-feeding

How should I use this medicine?

Interferon beta-1b is for injection under the skin. Before you try to use this injection, carefully read the instructions provided. Make sure you understand how to prepare, inject, and store interferon beta-1b. Before preparing an injection always wash your hands well with soap and water. Do not shake the solution before measuring or injecting a dose. Do not use more than the prescribed dose. Using larger or more frequent doses increases the risk of getting serious side effects. Do not reuse needles or syringes. Discard needles and syringes in a puncture-resistant container provided to you by your health care professional.

What if I miss a dose?

If you miss a dose, use it as soon as you can. Reschedule your next dose about 48 hours later. Contact your prescriber or health care professional if you have questions about adjusting your schedule.

What may interact with interferon beta-1b?

- zidovudine, AZT

Tell your prescriber or health care professional about all other medicines that you are taking, including non-prescription medicines, nutritional supplements, or herbal products. Also tell your prescriber or health care professional if you are a frequent user of drinks with caffeine or alcohol, if you smoke, or if you use illegal drugs. These may affect the way your medicine works. Check with your health care professional before stopping or starting any of your medicines.

What should I watch for while taking interferon beta-1b?

Visit your prescriber or health care professional for regular checks on your progress. Tell your prescriber or health care professional if you are feeling depressed. Females of child-bearing age should use a reliable method of birth control. If you do get pregnant, stop using interferon beta-1b at once and contact your prescriber or health care professional. Reactions at the site of injection are common. Ask your prescriber or health care professional to suggest a series of injection sites, so that you do not have to use the same site repeatedly. You can use an injection site again after one week, providing the skin is not tender, red, or hard. Serious reactions at the injection site may occur in a small number of patients. Contact your prescriber or health care professional immediately if an injection site becomes black-blue, swells, or starts to drain fluid. Flu-like symptoms are common with interferon beta-1b therapy. Using this medicine at night can reduce the impact of these symptoms. Your prescriber or health care professional may suggest taking acetaminophen (Tylenol®) or ibuprofen (Motrin®, Advil®, etc) before your dose and for 24 hours after you receive your injection. Use disposable syringes only once, and throw away syringes and needles in a closed container to prevent accidental needle sticks.

What side effects may I notice from receiving interferon beta-1b?

Side effects that you should report to your prescriber or health care professional as soon as possible:

- a skin sore with a black-blue color, swelling, or drainage
- confusion
- depression or nervousness
- irregular heartbeat (palpitations)
- mood changes, anxiety
- unusual bruising or bleeding

Side effects that usually do not require medical attention (report to your prescriber or health care professional if they continue or are bothersome):

- constipation or diarrhea
- drowsiness, dizziness
- fever, chills, or flu-like symptoms
- headache
- increased sweating
- menstrual changes
- muscle aches
- nausea, vomiting
- pain, redness, swelling, and irritation at the injection site
- unusual weakness or tiredness

Where can I keep my medicine?

Keep out of the reach of children. Store at room temperature between 15 and 30 degrees C (59 and 86 degrees F). After mixing, if not used immediately, the product should be refrigerated and used within 3 hours. Avoid freezing. Throw away any unused diluted injection.

Interferon Gamma-1b injection

ACTIMMUNE®;
100 mcg (2 million IU)/0.5 ml;
Injection
Intermune Inc

What is interferon gamma-1b injection?

INTERFERON Gamma-1b (Actimmune®) is a man-made drug that acts like a substance in your body called interferon gamma. Interferon gamma helps your immune system work better. In patients with chronic granulomatous disease, interferon gamma helps to fight infections. In children with osteopetrosis, interferon gamma helps to slow the progression of the disease. Interferon gamma is also being studied in the treatment of other infections and diseases. Generic interferon gamma-1b injections are not available.

What should my health care professional know before I receive interferon gamma-1b?

They need to know if you have any of these conditions:
- blood disorders
- heart disease, especially heart failure or an irregular heart beat
- seizure disorder
- an unusual or allergic reaction to interferon, proteins, other medicines, foods, dyes, or preservatives
- pregnant or trying to get pregnant
- breast-feeding

How should I use this medicine?

Interferon gamma-1b is for injection under the skin. A health care professional can give it, or you may be able to give yourself the injections. Before you try to use this injection, carefully read the instructions provided. Make sure you understand how to prepare, inject, and store interferon gamma-1b. Before preparing an injection always wash your hands well with soap and water. Do not shake the solution before measuring or injecting a dose. Do not use more than the prescribed dose. Using larger or more frequent doses increases the risk of getting serious side effects. If you will be giving interferon gamma-1b at home, make sure you receive a puncture resistant container for the disposal of used syringes and needles. Do not reuse needles or syringes.

What if I miss a dose?

If you miss a dose, use it as soon as you can. Reschedule your next dose about 48 hours later. Contact your prescriber or health care professional if you have questions about adjusting your schedule.

What may interact with interferon gamma-1b?

- phenytoin
- theophylline
- warfarin

Tell your prescriber or health care professional about all other medicines that you are taking, including non-prescription medicines, nutritional supplements, or herbal products. Also tell your prescriber or health care professional if you are a frequent user of drinks with caffeine or alcohol, if you smoke, or if you use illegal drugs. These may affect the way your medicine works. Check with your health care professional before stopping or starting any of your medicines.

What should I watch for while taking interferon gamma-1b?

Visit your prescriber or health care professional for regular checks on your progress. Females of child-bearing age should use a reliable method of birth control. If you do get pregnant, stop using interferon gamma-1b at once and contact your prescriber or health care professional. Reactions at the site of injection may occur. Ask your prescriber or health care professional to suggest a series of injection sites, so that you do not have to use the same site repeatedly. You can use an injection site again after one week, providing the skin is not tender, red, or hard. Flu-like symptoms are common with interferon gamma-1b therapy. Using this medicine at night can reduce the impact of these symptoms. After checking with your prescriber or health care professional and getting their approval, you may also take acetaminophen (Tylenol®) or ibuprofen (Advil®, Motrin®) before your injection to help lessen any fever or headache. Use disposable syringes only once, and throw away syringes and needles in a closed container to prevent accidental needle sticks.

What side effects may I notice from receiving interferon gamma-1b?

Side effects that you should report to your prescriber or health care professional as soon as possible:
- skin rash, itching
- unusual weakness or tiredness

Side effects that usually do not require medical attention (report to your prescriber or health care professional if they continue or are bothersome):
- fever, chills, or flu-like symptoms
- headache
- increased sweating
- muscle aches
- nausea, vomiting
- redness, swelling, tenderness, and irritation at the injection site

Where can I keep my medicine?

Keep out of the reach of children. Store in a refrigerator between 2 and 8 degrees C (36 and 46 degrees F); do not freeze. Use within 12 hours of taking out of the refrigerator. Throw away any unused vials if they have been out of the refrigerator longer than 12 hours. Do not use any vials after the expiration date.

Iodoquinol tablets

YODOXIN®;
650 mg; Tablet
Glenwood Llc

What are iodoquinol tablets?

IODOQUINOL (Yodoxin®) is an amebicide antimicrobial agent. This medicine is used to treat infections caused by amebas (a type of parasite) when these parasites are present in the gut (intestines). Generic iodoquinol tablets are available.

What should my health care professional know before I take iodoquinol?

They need to know if you have any of these conditions:
- eye disorders
- kidney disease
- liver disease
- nerve disease
- thyroid disease
- zinc deficiency
- an unusual reaction to Iodoquinol, iodine, chloroxine, pamaquine, pentaquine, primaquine, other medicines, foods, dyes, or preservatives
- pregnant or trying to get pregnant
- breast-feeding

How should this medicine be used?

Take iodoquinol tablets by mouth. Follow the directions on the prescription label. Iodoquinol causes less stomach side effects if taken with food. You can chew the tablets if needed or swallow them whole or crush and mix with food (such as applesauce). Do not take this medication more often than prescribed. Finish the full course of medicine even if you feel better. Space your doses evenly through the day and night and take at the same time each day. Parasite (ameba) death can be slow. To remove all parasites from the intestines can take several days. Contact your pediatrician or health care professional regarding the use of this medicine in children. Special care may be needed.

What if I miss a dose?

If you miss a dose, take it as soon as you can. If it is almost time for your next dose, take only that dose. Do not take double or extra doses. You must leave a suitable interval between doses. If you are taking three doses per day, make sure at least 3 to 4 hours pass between each dose.

What may interact with iodoquinol?

- medications for thyroid problems

Tell your prescriber or health care professional about all other medicines you are taking, including non-prescription medicines, nutritional supplements, or herbal products. Also tell your prescriber or health care professional if you are a frequent user of drinks with caffeine or alcohol, if you smoke, or if you use illegal drugs. These may affect the way your medicine works. Check with your health care professional before stopping or starting any of your medicines.

What should I watch for while taking iodoquinol?

Visit you prescriber or health care professional to check that your infection has gone. If you still have an infection after 20 days of therapy, you may need a second course of tablets. Follow up as indicated by your prescriber or health care professional. You may need a simple blood test to check for changes in thyroid and liver function. Wash your hands; scrub your fingernails and shower often. Every day, change and launder bedclothes, linens and undergarments. This will help other family members from getting infected.

What side effects may I notice from taking iodoquinol?

Side effects that you should report to your prescriber or health care professional as soon as possible:
- blurred vision, loss of vision, or color blindness
- swelling of the throat
- fever, chills
- numbness or pain in feet or hands

Side effects that usually do not require medical attention (report to your prescriber or health care professional if they continue or are bothersome):
- diarrhea
- dizziness
- headache
- nausea, vomiting
- stomach pain
- skin discoloration
- skin irritation

Where can I keep my medicine?

Keep out of the reach of children in a container that small children cannot open. Store at room temperature between 15 and 30 degrees C (59 and 86 degrees F). Throw away any unused medicine after the expiration date.

Irbesartan tablets

AVAPRO®;
150 mg; Tablet
Bristol Myers Squibb
Co

AVAPRO®;
300 mg; Tablet
Bristol Myers Squibb
Co

What are irbesartan tablets?

IRBESARTAN (Avapro®) helps lower blood pressure to normal levels. It controls high blood pressure, but it is not a cure. High blood pressure can damage your kidneys, and may lead to a stroke or heart failure. Irbesartan helps prevent these things from happening. Generic irbesartan tablets are not yet available.

What should my health care professional know before I take irbesartan?

They need to know if you have any of these conditions:
- heart failure
- kidney disease
- liver disease
- electrolyte imbalance (e.g. low or high levels of potassium in the blood)
- if you are on a special diet, such as a low-salt diet (e.g. using potassium substitutes)
- an unusual or allergic reaction to irbesartan, other medicines, foods, dyes, or preservatives
- pregnant or trying to get pregnant
- breast-feeding

How should I take this medicine?

Take irbesartan tablets by mouth. Follow the directions on the prescription label. Swallow the tablets with a drink of water. Irbesartan can be taken with or without food. Take your doses at regular intervals. Do not take your medicine more often than directed.

What if I miss a dose?

If you miss a dose, take it as soon as you can. If it is almost time for your next dose, take only that dose. Do not take double or extra doses.

What may interact with irbesartan?

- anti-inflammatory pain medicines such as ibuprofen (Motrin®)
- blood pressure medications
- bosentan
- delavirdine
- imatinib
- fluconazole
- hawthorn
- lithium
- rifampin
- potassium salts or potassium supplements
- voriconazole
- water pills (especially potassium-sparing diuretics such as triamterene or amiloride)

Tell your prescriber or health care professional about all other medicines you are taking, including non-prescription medicines, nutritional supplements, or herbal products. Also tell your prescriber or health care professional if you are a frequent user of drinks with caffeine or alcohol, if you smoke, or if you use illegal drugs. These may affect the way your medicine works. Check with your health care professional before stopping or starting any of your medicines.

What should I watch for while taking irbesartan?

Check your blood pressure regularly while you are taking irbesartan. Ask your prescriber or health care professional what your blood pressure should be and when you should contact him or her. When you check your blood pressure, write down the measurements to show your prescriber or health care professional. If you are taking this medicine for a long time you must visit your prescriber or health care professional for regular checks on your progress. Make sure you schedule appointments on a regular basis. You may experience dizziness. Do not drive, use machinery, or do anything that requires mental alertness until you know how irbesartan affects you. To avoid dizziness, do not stand or sit up quickly. Avoid salt substitutes unless you are told otherwise by your prescriber or health care professional. If you are going to have surgery tell your prescriber or health care professional that you are taking irbesartan.

What side effects may I notice from taking irbesartan?

Side effects that you should report to your prescriber or health care professional as soon as possible:
Rare or uncommon:
- difficulty breathing or swallowing, hoarseness, or tightening of the throat
- swelling of your face, lips, tongue, hands, or feet
- unusual rash or hives
- decreased sexual function

Other:
- confusion, dizziness, lightheadedness or fainting spells
- decreased amount of urine passed
- fast or uneven heart beat or palpitations

Side effects that usually do not require medical attention (report to your prescriber or health care professional if they continue or are bothersome):
- cough
- diarrhea
- fatigue or tiredness
- nasal congestion or stuffiness
- sore or cramping muscles
- upset stomach

Where can I keep my medicine?

Keep out of the reach of children in a container that small children cannot open. Store at room temperature between 15 and 30 degrees C (59 and 86 degrees F). Protect from light. Keep container tightly closed. Throw away any unused medicine after the expiration date.

Iron Salts tablets or capsules

FERROUS SULFATE;
325 mg; Tablet
Mutual/United
Research
Laboratories

FERROUS
GLUCONATE;
300 mg; Tablet
Upsher-Smith
Laboratories Inc

What are iron salts tablets?

IRON SALTS (e.g. ferrous sulfate, ferrous gluconate, ferrous fumarate, carbonyl iron) are iron supplements. Iron is a mineral needed by your body to make new red blood cells. Iron also helps red blood cells function. Red blood cells carry oxygen to all of your body tissues. There are many different kinds of iron supplements. However, extra iron should only be taken under the advice of a health care professional. Adults or kids with anemia due to low iron levels or a low red blood cell count may be prescribed iron. Pregnant women in their last 3 to 6 months of pregnancy may need to take extra iron, but should only take iron if their doctor tells them to. Do not treat yourself with iron if you are feeling tired or fatigued. Most healthy people get adequate iron in their diets, particularly if they eat fortified cereals, meat, poultry, and fish. Generic iron tablets are available.

What should my health care professional know before I take iron salts?

They need to know if you have any of these conditions:
- an alcohol problem
- blood transfusions
- bowel disease
- hemolytic anemia
- iron overload (hemochromatosis, hemosiderosis)
- liver disease
- peptic ulcer
- an unusual or allergic reaction to iron, other medicines, foods, dyes, or preservatives
- pregnant or trying to get pregnant
- breast-feeding

How should I take this medicine?

Take the tablets or capsules by mouth. Follow the directions on the prescription label. Swallow the tablets or capsules whole with a glass of water or fruit juice. If you are taking enteric-coated or extended-release tablets or capsules, swallow them whole; do not crush or chew. It is best to take iron on an empty stomach. Take at least 1 hour before or 2 hours after food. Take tablets or capsules in an upright or sitting position. Taking a sip of water first, before taking the tablets or capsules, may help you swallow them. If possible take bedtime doses at least 10 minutes before lying down. If the iron causes your stomach to be upset, you may take it with food. Take your doses at regular intervals. Do not take your medicine more often than directed.

What if I miss a dose?

If you miss a dose, and are taking iron salts as a dietary supplement, skip the missed dose. If you are being treated for anemia and you miss a dose, take it as soon as you can. If it is almost time for your next dose, take only that dose. Do not take double or extra doses.

What may interact with iron salts?

If you are taking this iron product, you should not take iron in any other medicine or dietary supplement. *Other medications that may interact with iron:*

- alendronate
- antacids
- ascorbic acid (vitamin C)
- calcium carbonate
- cefdinir
- chloramphenicol
- cholestyramine
- deferoxamine
- dimercaprol
- etidronate
- levodopa or combination drugs containing levodopa
- medicines for stomach ulcers or other stomach problems
- methyldopa
- pancreatic enzyme supplements
- penicillamine
- quinolone antibiotics (examples: Cipro®, Floxin®, Tequin® and others)
- risedronate
- tetracycline antibiotics (examples: doxycycline, tetracycline, minocycline, and others)
- thyroid hormones
- zinc supplements

Tell your prescriber or health care professional about all other medicines you are taking, including non-prescription medicines. Also tell your prescriber or health care professional if you are a frequent user of drinks with caffeine or alcohol, if you smoke, or if you use illegal drugs. These may affect the way your medicine works. Check with your health care professional before stopping or starting any of your medicines.

What should I watch for while taking iron salts?

You should only use iron supplements under the supervision of your health care professional. If you are told by your health care provider that you need iron supplements, you should visit your health care professional for regular blood checks. Do not use iron longer than prescribed, and do not take a higher dose than recommended. Long-term use may cause excess iron to build-up in the body. Once the cause of a low red blood cell count is treated by your prescriber, it usually takes 3 to 6 months of iron therapy to reverse the problem. Pregnant women should follow the dose and length of iron treatment as directed by their doctors. Do not take iron with dairy products or antacids. If you need to take an antacid, take it 2 hours after a dose of iron. Alcohol can reduce the amount of iron taken in from your diet; avoid large amounts of alcohol.

What side effects may I notice from taking iron salts?

Side effects that you should report to your prescriber or health care professional as soon as possible:
- blue lips, nails, or palms
- dark colored stools (this may be due to discoloration from the iron, but can indicate a more serious condition)
- drowsiness
- pain on swallowing
- pale or clammy skin
- seizures (convulsions)
- stomach pain

- unusual tiredness
- vomiting
- weak, fast, or irregular heartbeat

Side effects that usually do not require medical attention (report to your prescriber or health care professional if they continue or are bothersome):
- constipation
- indigestion
- nausea or stomach upset

Where can I keep my medicine?

Keep out of the reach of children in a container that small children cannot open. Even small amounts of iron-containing products can be poisonous to a child. Store at room temperature between 15 and 30 degrees C (59 and 86 degrees F). Keep container tightly closed. Throw away any unused medicine after the expiration date.

This drug requires an FDA medication guide. See page xxxvii.

Isocarboxazid tablets

MARPLAN®;
10 mg; Tablet
Oxford Pharmaceutical
Services Inc

What are isocarboxazid tablets?

ISOCARBOXAZID (Marplan®) belongs to a class of drugs called monoamine oxidase inhibitors (MAOIs). Isocarboxazid increases the level of certain chemicals in the brain that help fight depression and other mood problems, including certain anxiety disorders. Isocarboxazid can interact with certain foods and other medicines to cause unpleasant side effects. You must know what foods and medicines to avoid (see below). Generic isocarboxazid tablets are not yet available.

What should my health care professional know before I take isocarboxazid?

They need to know if you have any of these conditions:
- frequently drink alcohol-containing beverages
- asthma or bronchitis
- attempted suicide
- bipolar disorder or mania
- diabetes
- headaches or migraine
- heart or blood vessel disease, or irregular heart beats
- high blood pressure
- kidney disease
- liver disease
- overactive thyroid
- Parkinson's disease
- pheochromocytoma
- recent head trauma
- seizures or convulsions
- schizophrenia or psychosis
- stroke or other cerebrovascular disease
- an unusual or allergic reaction to isocarboxazid, other medicines, foods, dyes, or preservatives
- pregnant or trying to get pregnant
- breast-feeding

How should I take this medicine?

Take isocarboxazid tablets by mouth. Follow the directions on the prescription label. Swallow the tablets with a drink of water. Take your doses at regular intervals. Do not take your medicine more often than directed. Do not stop taking the tablets except on your prescriber's advice. Contact your pediatrician or health care professional regarding the use of this medicine in children. Special care may be needed. Elderly patients over age 65 years may have a stronger reaction to this medicine and should use this medicine with caution.

What if I miss a dose?

If you miss a dose, take it as soon as you can. If it is less than 2 hours to your next dose, take only that dose and skip the missed dose. Do not take double or extra doses.

What may interact with isocarboxazid?

- alcohol
- barbiturates such as phenobarbital
- bupropion
- buspirone
- caffeine
- carbamazepine
- certain medicines for blood pressure (especially beta-blockers, methyldopa, reserpine, guanadrel, and guanethidine)
- cocaine
- dextromethorphan
- diet pills or stimulants, like amphetamines or ephedra
- furazolidone
- ginseng
- guarana
- kava kava

- levodopa
- linezolid
- local anesthetics
- medicines for allergies, colds, flu symptoms, sinus congestion, and breathing difficulties
- medicines for diabetes
- medicines for migraine headaches
- medicines for movement abnormalities as in Parkinson's disease (examples: entacapone, levodopa, selegiline, tolcapone)
- muscle relaxants
- other medicines for mental depression, anxiety, or mood or mental problems
- meperidine
- procarbazine
- SAM-e
- seizure (convulsion) or epilepsy medicine
- St. John's wort
- tramadol
- tryptophan
- tyramine—see below for foods that contain tyramine
- valerian
- water pills (diuretics)
- yohimbine

Tell your prescriber or health care professional about all other medicines you are taking, including non-prescription medicines, nutritional supplements, or herbal products. Also tell your prescriber or health care professional if you are a frequent user of drinks with caffeine or alcohol, if you smoke, or if you use illegal drugs. These may affect the way your medicine works. Check with your health care professional before stopping or starting any of your medicines.

What should I watch for while taking isocarboxazid?

Visit your prescriber or health care professional for regular checks on your progress. It can take up to 3 to 6 weeks to see the full effects of isocarboxazid. Do not suddenly stop taking your medicine; this may make your condition worse or give you withdrawal symptoms. Ask your prescriber or health care professional for advice about gradually reducing your dosage. Even after you stop taking isocarboxazid the effects can last for at least two weeks. Continue to take all precautions and avoid all food and medicine that interact with isocarboxazid. Isocarboxazid can interact with certain foods that contain tyramine to produce severe headaches, a rise in blood pressure, or irregular heart beat. Foods that contain significant amounts of tyramine include aged cheeses; meats and fish (especially aged, smoked, pickled, or processed such as bologna, pepperoni, salami, summer sausage); beer and ale; alcohol-free beer; wine (especially red); sherry; hard liquor; liqueurs; avocados; bananas; figs; raisins; soy sauce; miso soup; yeast/protein extracts; bean curd; fava or broad bean pods; or any over-ripe fruit. Ask your prescriber or health

care professional, pharmacist, or nutritionist for a complete listing of tyramine-containing foods. Also, avoid drinks containing caffeine, such as tea, coffee, chocolate, or cola. Call your prescriber or health care professional as soon as you can if you get frequent headaches or have palpitations. You may get drowsy, dizzy or have blurred vision. Do not drive, use machinery, or do anything that needs mental alertness until you know how isocarboxazid affects you. Do not stand or sit up quickly, especially if you are an older patient. This reduces the risk of dizzy or fainting spells. Alcohol may increase dizziness or drowsiness; avoid alcoholic drinks. Isocarboxazid can make your mouth dry. Chewing sugarless gum, sucking hard candy and drinking plenty of water will help. Do not treat yourself for coughs, colds, flu or allergies without asking your prescriber or health care professional for advice. Do not take any medications for weight loss without advice either. Some ingredients in these products may increase possible side effects. If you are diabetic there is a possibility that isocarboxazid may affect your blood sugar. Ask your prescriber or health care professional for advice if there is any change in your blood or urine sugar tests. Notify your health care professional if you are scheduled to have any surgery, procedure or medical testing (including myelography). You should usually stop taking this drug at least 10 days before elective surgery; tell your prescriber or health care professional that you have been taking isocarboxazid.

What side effects may I notice from taking isocarboxazid?

Side effects that you should report to your prescriber or health care professional as soon as possible:

- agitation, excitability, restlessness, or nervousness
- chest pain
- confusion or changes in mental state
- convulsions or seizures (uncommon)
- difficulty breathing
- difficulty passing urine
- enlarged pupils, sensitivity of the eyes to light
- fever, clammy skin, increased sweating
- headache or increased blood pressure
- lightheadedness or fainting spells
- muscle or neck stiffness or spasm
- sexual dysfunction
- slow, fast, or irregular heartbeat (palpitations)
- sore throat and fever
- yellowing of the skin or eyes

Side effects that usually do not require medical attention (report to your prescriber or health care professional if they continue or are bothersome):

- blurred vision or change in vision
- constipation or diarrhea
- difficulty sleeping
- drowsiness or dizziness
- dry mouth

- increased appetite; weight increase
- increased sensitivity to sunlight
- muscle aches or pains, trembling
- nausea or vomiting
- sexual dysfunction
- swelling of the feet or legs
- tiredness or weakness

Where can I keep my medicine?

Keep out of the reach of children in a container that small children cannot open. Store at room temperature between 15 and 30 degrees C (59 and 86 degrees F). Keep container tightly closed. Throw away any unused medicine after the expiration date.

Isoniazid, INH tablets

ISONIAZID, INH℠; 300 mg; Tablet Eon Labs Inc

ISONIAZID, INH℠; 100 mg; Tablet Barr Laboratories Inc

What are isoniazid tablets?

ISONIAZID (INH℠) is used to treat or prevent tuberculosis. For treatment of tuberculosis, other medicines may be used in together with isoniazid. For prevention of tuberculosis, isoniazid may be given alone. Generic isoniazid tablets are available.

What should my health care professional know before I take isoniazid?

They need to know if you have any of these conditions:
- acne
- diabetes mellitus
- kidney disease
- if you frequently drink alcohol-containing beverages
- liver disease
- malnutrition
- seizures (convulsions)
- tingling of the fingers or toes, or other nerve disorder
- an unusual or allergic reaction to isoniazid, other medicines, foods, dyes or preservatives
- pregnant or trying to get pregnant
- breast-feeding

How should I take this medicine?

Take isoniazid tablets by mouth. Follow the directions on the prescription label. Swallow tablets whole with a full glass of water. Take isoniazid on an empty stomach; 1 to 2 hours before food, or at least 2 hours after food. Take your doses at regular intervals and try not to miss any doses. Do not take your medicine more often than directed. Finish the full course prescribed by your prescriber or health care professional even if you think your condition is better. Do not stop taking except on your prescriber's advice.

What if I miss a dose?

If you miss a dose, take it as soon as you can. If you do not remember until the next day, take only that dose. Do not take double or extra doses.

What may interact with isoniazid?

- alcohol
- carbamazepine
- chlorzoxazone
- cycloserine
- diazepam
- disulfiram
- furazolidone
- histamine-containing foods (examples: aged cheeses and fish such as tuna, skipjack, sardinella and especially raw fish or spoiled fish)
- hormones such as prednisone or cortisone
- itraconazole
- linezolid
- medicines called MAO inhibitors-phenelzine (Nardil®), tranylcypromine (Parnate®), isocarboxazid (Marplan®), selegiline (Eldepryl®)
- medicines for diabetes
- phenytoin
- procarbazine
- rifampin
- some medications for Parkinson's disease, such as entacapone, levodopa or tolcapone
- tyramine-containing foods (such as cheeses; meats and fish, especially those that are aged, smoked, pickled, or processed; beer and ale; wine; avocados; bananas; figs; raisins; soy sauce; miso soup; yeast extract; and bean curd)
- valproic acid
- voriconazole
- warfarin

Tell your prescriber or health care professional about all other medicines you are taking, including non-prescription medicines, nutritional supplements, or herbal products. Also tell your prescriber or health care professional if you are a frequent user of drinks with caffeine or alcohol, if you smoke, or if you use illegal drugs. These may affect the way your medicine works. Check with your health care professional before stopping or starting any of your medicines.

What should I watch for while taking isoniazid?

Keep taking your isoniazid even if you feel better. You may need to take this medicine for a long time. Visit your prescriber or health care professional for regular checks; tell him of any change in your vision. Report any other side effects promptly. Ask your prescriber or health care professional if you need to take pyridoxine, vitamin B_6. Isoniazid can make your body short of this vitamin. Avoid alcoholic drinks while you are taking isoniazid. Alcohol can increase the damage to your liver from isoniazid. An interaction between isoniazid and certain foods can make you feel ill (see interactions list). If you get red or itching skin, fast heartbeat, sweat, get chills or feel clammy, feel lightheaded and have a headache, do not treat yourself. Call your prescriber or health care professional as soon as you can and avoid these foods. Antacids can prevent isoniazid from working correctly. If you get an upset stomach and want to take an antacid, make sure there is an interval of at least 2 hours since you last took isoniazid, or at least 4 hours before your next dose. If you are diabetic, you may get a false-positive result for sugar in your urine. Check with your prescriber or health care professional before you change your diet or the dose of your diabetic medicine.

What side effects may I notice from taking isoniazid?

Elderly patients are more likely to get side effects. Side effects that you should report to your prescriber or health care professional as soon as possible:
- blood in urine
- blurred vision, eye pain
- changes in how you see color (especially seeing the difference between red and green)
- clumsiness, unsteadiness
- dark yellow or brown urine
- difficulty breathing
- fever or chills, sore throat
- headache
- loss of appetite
- nausea, vomiting
- reduced amount of urine passed
- seizures (convulsions)
- skin rash, itching
- stomach pain
- tingling, pain, or numbness in the hands or feet
- unusual bleeding or bruising
- unusual tiredness or weakness
- yellowing of the eyes or skin

Side effects that usually do not require medical attention (report to your prescriber or health care professional if they continue or are bothersome):
- diarrhea
- upset stomach

Where can I keep my medicine?

Keep out of the reach of children in a container that small children cannot open. Store at room temperature between 15 and 30 degrees C (59 and 86 degrees F). Protect from light. Keep container tightly closed. Throw away any unused medicine after the expiration date.

Isosorbide Dinitrate, ISDN sublingual or chewable tablets

SORBITRATE® CHEWABLE;
5 mg; Tablet, Chewable
AstraZeneca Pharmaceuticals
LP

What are isosorbide dinitrate sublingual or chewable tablets?

ISOSORBIDE DINITRATE (Isordil®, Sorbitrate® Chewable) is a type of vasodilator. It relaxes blood vessels, increasing the blood and oxygen supply to your heart. It relieves the pain you can get with angina. There are several different types of tablets and capsules. Each type has a special design, to give the most effective action. Sublingual (under the tongue) or chewable tablets can also provide prompt relief as soon as chest pain indicates the start of an angina attack. Isosorbide dinitrate can also help to prevent pain before activities that can cause an attack (such as climbing stairs, exercise, going outdoors in cold weather, or having sex). Isosorbide dinitrate is available as chewable tablets, or sublingual (under the tongue) tablets. Generic sublingual tablets are available, but not generic chewable tablets.

What should my health care professional know before I take isosorbide dinitrate?

They need to know if you have any of these conditions:
- anemia
- glaucoma
- head injury, recent stroke, or bleeding in the brain
- liver disease
- low blood pressure
- previous heart attack
- overactive thyroid
- stomach or intestinal disease
- an unusual or allergic reaction to isosorbide dinitrate, other medicines, foods, dyes, or preservatives
- pregnant or trying to get pregnant
- breast-feeding

How should I take this medicine?

Sublingual and chewable tablets can be taken on an as needed basis. Follow the directions on the prescription label. Let the sublingual tablets dissolve under the tongue. Chew the chewable tablets well, to allow the medicine to be absorbed through the mouth. Make sure your mouth is not dry, saliva (fluid) around the tablet will help it to dissolve more quickly. Do not swallow whole. If you are treating an acute attack your symptoms should improve in 5 to 10 minutes. You can repeat the dose every 10 to 15 minutes for up to 3 doses. If you are no better after 3 doses and 20 to 30 minutes, contact your prescriber or health care professional or have someone take you straight to an emergency room. Do not eat, drink, smoke, or chew tobacco while a tablet is dissolving. Do not take your medicine more often than directed.

What if I miss a dose?

This only applies if you are taking tablets for prevention of angina on a regular basis. If you miss a dose, take it as soon as you can. If it is almost time for your next dose, take only that dose. Do not take double or extra doses.

What may interact with isosorbide dinitrate?

- acetylcholine
- alcohol
- aspirin
- beta-blockers, often used for high blood pressure or heart problems
- histamine
- medicines for colds and breathing difficulties
- medicines for high blood pressure
- medicines for mental problems or psychotic disturbances
- medicines for pain
- sildenafil (Viagra®)
- tadalafil (Cialis)
- vardenafil (Levitra®)
- water pills

Viagra® (sildenafil), Cialis (tadalafil), or Levitra® (vardenafil) should not be taken with this medication to avoid severe side effects including very low blood pressure and other complications. Tell your prescriber or health care professional about all other medicines you are taking, including non-prescription medicines, nutritional supplements, or herbal products. Also tell your prescriber or health care professional if you are a frequent user of drinks with caffeine or alcohol, if you smoke, or if you use illegal drugs. These may affect the way your medicine works. Check with your health care professional before stopping or starting any of your medicines.

What should I watch for while taking isosorbide dinitrate?

Check your heart rate and blood pressure regularly while you are taking isosorbide dinitrate. Ask your prescriber or health care professional what your heart rate and blood pressure should be and when you should contact him or her. Tell your prescriber or health care professional if you feel your medicine is no longer hav-

ing any effect. You may get dizzy. Do not drive, use machinery, or do anything that needs mental alertness until you know how isosorbide dinitrate affects you. To reduce the risk of dizzy or fainting spells, do not sit or stand up quickly, especially if you are an older patient. Alcohol can make you more dizzy, and increase flushing and rapid heartbeats. Avoid alcoholic drinks. Try to remain calm; this will help you to feel better faster. If you feel dizzy, take several deep breaths and lie down with your feet propped up, or bend forward with your head resting between your knees. If you are taking isosorbide dinitrate on a regular schedule, do not stop taking it suddenly or your symptoms may get worse. Ask your prescriber or health care professional how to gradually reduce the dose.

What side effects may I notice from taking isosorbide dinitrate?

Side effects that you should report to your prescriber or health care professional as soon as possible:
- bluish discoloration of lips, fingernails, or palms of hands
- dizziness or fainting
- dry mouth
- irregular heartbeat, palpitations
- low blood pressure
- skin rash
- sweating
- the feeling of extreme pressure in the head
- unusual tiredness or weakness

Side effects that usually do not require medical attention (report to your prescriber or health care professional if they continue or are bothersome):
- flushing of the face or neck
- headache
- nausea, vomiting

Where can I keep my medicine?

Keep out of the reach of children. Store at room temperature, approximately 25 degrees C (77 degrees F). Protect from light. Keep container tightly closed. Throw away any unused medicine after the expiration date.

Isosorbide Dinitrate, ISDN tablets or extended-release tablets or capsules

ISORDIL® TITRADOSE®;
5 mg; Tablet Biovail
Pharmaceuticals Inc

DILATRATE®-SR;
40 mg; Capsule,
Extended Release
Schwarz Pharma Inc

What are isosorbide dinitrate tablets or extended-release tablets or capsules?

ISOSORBIDE DINITRATE (Isordil®, Isordil® Titradose®, Dilatrate®-SR, Sorbitrate®, Sorbitrate® SA) is a type of vasodilator. It relaxes blood vessels, increasing the blood and oxygen supply to your heart. It relieves the pain you can get with angina. There are several different types of tablets and capsules. Each type has

a special design, to give the most effective action. Taken on a regular schedule, isosorbide dinitrate tablets, capsules, or sustained-release tablets or capsules, can help prevent attacks of angina. It is effective in the long-term treatment of angina associated with coronary artery disease. Isosorbide dinitrate is available as tablets, capsules, sustained-release tablets, and sustained-release capsules. Some of these are available as generics.

What should my health care professional know before I take isosorbide dinitrate?

They need to know if you have any of these conditions:

- anemia
- glaucoma
- head injury, recent stroke, or bleeding in the brain
- liver disease
- low blood pressure
- previous heart attack
- overactive thyroid
- stomach or intestinal disease
- an unusual or allergic reaction to isosorbide dinitrate, other medicines, foods, dyes, or preservatives
- pregnant or trying to get pregnant
- breast-feeding

How should I take this medicine?

Take isosorbide tablets or capsules by mouth. Follow the directions on the prescription label. The way you take this medicine depends on what type of tablet or capsule you are using. Swallow regular tablets or capsules with a drink of water. Swallow sustained-release tablets or capsules whole; do not crush or chew. Take isosorbide dinitrate on an empty stomach, 1 hour before or 2 hours after food. Take at regular intervals. Try to take your doses at the same time each day, and continue to take them even if you feel better. Do not stop taking except on your prescriber's advice. Do not take your medicine more often than directed. Contact your pediatrician or health care professional regarding the use of this medicine in children. Special care may be needed.

What if I miss a dose?

If you miss a dose, take it as soon as you can. If it is almost time for your next dose, take only that dose (less than 2 hours for regular tablets, or 6 hours for extended-release preparations). Do not take double or extra doses.

What may interact with isosorbide dinitrate?

- acetylcholine
- alcohol
- aspirin
- beta-blockers, often used for high blood pressure or heart problems
- histamine
- medicines for colds and breathing difficulties
- medicines for high blood pressure
- medicines for mental problems or psychotic disturbances
- medicines for pain
- sildenafil (Viagra®)
- tadalafil (Cialis)
- vardenafil (Levitra®)
- water pills

Viagra® (sildenafil), Cialis (tadalafil), or Levitra® (vardenafil) should not be taken with this medication to avoid severe side effects including very low blood pressure and other complications. Tell your prescriber or health care professional about all other medicines you are taking, including non-prescription medicines, nutritional supplements, or herbal products. Also tell your prescriber or health care professional if you are a frequent user of drinks with caffeine or alcohol, if you smoke, or if you use illegal drugs. These may affect the way your medicine works. Check with your health care professional before stopping or starting any of your medicines.

What should I watch for while taking isosorbide dinitrate?

Check your heart rate and blood pressure regularly while you are taking isosorbide dinitrate. Ask your prescriber or health care professional what your heart rate and blood pressure should be and when you should contact him or her. Tell your prescriber or health care professional if you feel your medicine is no longer having any effect. You may get dizzy. Do not drive, use machinery, or do anything that needs mental alertness until you know how isosorbide dinitrate affects you. To reduce the risk of dizzy or fainting spells, do not sit or stand up quickly, especially if you are an older patient. Alcohol can make you more dizzy, and increase flushing and rapid heartbeats. Avoid alcoholic drinks. Try to remain calm; this will help you to feel better faster. If you feel dizzy, take several deep breaths and lie down with your feet propped up, or bend forward with your head resting between your knees. If you are taking isosorbide dinitrate on a regular schedule, do not stop taking it suddenly or your symptoms may get worse. Ask your prescriber or health care professional how to gradually reduce the dose.

What side effects may I notice from taking isosorbide dinitrate?

Side effects that you should report to your prescriber or health care professional as soon as possible:

- bluish discoloration of lips, fingernails, or palms of hands
- dizziness or fainting
- dry mouth
- irregular heartbeat, palpitations
- low blood pressure
- skin rash
- sweating
- the feeling of extreme pressure in the head
- unusual tiredness or weakness

Side effects that usually do not require medical attention (report to your prescriber or health care professional if they continue or are bothersome):

- flushing of the face or neck
- headache
- nausea, vomiting

Where can I keep my medicine?

Keep out of the reach of children in a container that small children cannot open. Store at room temperature, approximately 25 degrees C (77 degrees F). Protect from light. Keep container tightly closed. Throw away any unused medicine after the expiration date.

Isosorbide Mononitrate tablets or extended-release tablets

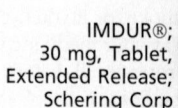

IMDUR®;
30 mg, Tablet,
Extended Release;
Schering Corp

ISMO®;
20 mg, Tablet; ESP
Pharma Inc

What are isosorbide mononitrate tablets or extended-release tablets?

ISOSORBIDE MONONITRATE (Ismo®, Imdur®, Monoket®) is a type of vasodilator. It relaxes blood vessels, increasing the blood and oxygen supply to your heart. It is effective in the long-term treatment of angina associated with coronary artery disease. Generic isosorbide mononitrate is available.

What should my health care professional know before I take isosorbide mononitrate?

They need to know if you have any of these conditions:
- anemia
- dizziness or fainting spells when rising from a sitting position
- glaucoma
- head injury, recent stroke, or bleeding in the brain
- low blood pressure, or low blood volume
- previous heart attack
- overactive thyroid
- stomach or intestinal disease
- an unusual or allergic reaction to isosorbide dinitrate, other medicines, foods, dyes, or preservatives
- pregnant or trying to get pregnant
- breast-feeding

How should I take this medicine?

Take isosorbide tablets by mouth. Follow the directions on the prescription label. Unless your prescriber or health care professional tells you otherwise for the regular tablets (Ismo®), take the first dose when you get up in the morning and the second dose about 7 hours later. Swallow regular tablets with a drink of water. Unless your prescriber or health care professional tells you otherwise for the sustained-release tablets (Imdur®), take once a day when you get up in the morning. Swallow sustained-release tablets whole; do not crush or chew. Take isosorbide mononitrate on an empty stomach, 1 hour before or 2 hours after food. Take at regular intervals. Try to take your doses at the same time each day, and continue to take them even if you feel better. It can take several weeks or longer to see the full effects of this medicine. Do not stop taking except on your prescriber's advice. Do not take your medicine more often than directed. Contact your pediatrician or health care professional regarding the use of this medicine in children. Special care may be needed.

What if I miss a dose?

If you miss a dose, take it as soon as you can. If it is almost time for your next dose (less than 6 hours for regular tablets or 12 hours for sustained-release tablets), take only that dose. Do not take double or extra doses.

What may interact with isosorbide mononitrate?

- acetylcholine
- alcohol
- beta-blockers, often used for high blood pressure or heart problems
- histamine
- norepinephrine
- medicines for angina or high blood pressure
- medicines for colds and breathing difficulties
- medicines for high blood pressure
- medicines for pain
- tadalafil (Cialis)
- sildenafil (Viagra®)
- vardenafil (Levitra®)
- water pills

Viagra® (sildenafil), Cialis (tadalafil), or Levitra® (vardenafil) should not be taken with this medication to avoid severe side effects including very low blood pressure and other complications. Tell your prescriber or health care professional about all other medicines you are taking, including non-prescription medicines, nutritional supplements, or herbal products. Also tell your prescriber or health care professional if you are a frequent user of drinks with caffeine or alcohol, if you smoke, or if you use illegal drugs. These may affect the way your medicine works. Check with your health care professional before stopping or starting any of your medicines.

What should I watch for while taking isosorbide mononitrate?

Check your heart rate and blood pressure regularly while you are taking isosorbide mononitrate. Ask your prescriber or health care professional what your heart rate and blood pressure should be and when you should contact him or her. Tell your prescriber or health care professional if you feel your medicine is no longer having any effect. You may get dizzy. Do not drive, use machinery, or do anything that needs mental alertness until you know how isosorbide mononitrate affects you. To reduce the risk of dizzy or fainting spells, do not sit or stand up quickly, especially if you are an older patient. Alcohol can make you more dizzy, and increase flushing and rapid heartbeats. Avoid alcoholic drinks. Do not stop taking isosorbide mononitrate suddenly or your symptoms may get worse. Ask your prescriber or health care professional how to gradually reduce the dose.

What side effects may I notice from taking isosorbide mononitrate?

Side effects that you should report to your prescriber or health care professional as soon as possible:

- bluish discoloration of lips, fingernails, or palms of hands
- dizziness or fainting
- dry mouth
- irregular heartbeat, palpitations
- low blood pressure
- skin rash
- sweating
- the feeling of extreme pressure in the head

- unusual tiredness or weakness

Side effects that usually do not require medical attention (report to your prescriber or health care professional if they continue or are bothersome):

- flushing of the face or neck
- headache
- nausea, vomiting

Where can I keep my medicine?

Keep out of the reach of children. Store between 15 and 30 degrees C (59 and 86 degrees F). Keep container tightly closed. Throw away any unused medicine after the expiration date.

Isotretinoin capsules

| ACCUTANE®; 20 mg; Capsule Hoffmann La Roche Inc | | ACCUTANE®; 40 mg; Capsule Hoffmann La Roche Inc | |

This drug requires an FDA medication guide. See page xxxvii.

What are isotretinoin capsules?

ISOTRETINOIN (Accutane®, Claravis™) treats severe cystic acne (also called nodular acne) that has not responded to other therapy such as antibiotics. It can produce complete and prolonged remission of the disease. Isotretinoin may also be used to treat other skin conditions besides acne. Starting March 1, 2006, to receive isotretinoin, you, your physician and your pharmacy must be registered in the iPLEDGE program. You may only receive up to a 30-day supply of isotretinoin at one time, and you will need a new prescription for each refill. Your prescription must be filled within 7 days of your doctor's office visit. Make sure you receive and read the Medication Guide every time you get a prescription or refill for isotretinoin. Get a new Medication Guide with every refill. It is important that you read all of the information. Generic isotretinoin capsules are available.

What should my health care professional know before I take isotretinoin?

They need to know if you have any of these conditions:

- anorexia nervosa or an eating disorder
- back pain
- diabetes
- high blood cholesterol or triglycerides
- hearing problems
- if you frequently drink alcohol-containing beverages
- inflammatory bowel disease
- liver disease
- low white blood cell count
- mental problems, such as depression, psychosis, attempted suicide, or a family history of mental problems
- osteoporosis, osteomalacia, or other bone disorders
- pancreatitis
- participate in sports or activities where you are more likely to break a bone, such as football or rugby

- weight problem
- an unusual or allergic reaction to isotretinoin, vitamin A or related drugs, parabens, other medicines, foods, dyes, or preservatives
- pregnant or trying to get pregnant
- breast-feeding

How should I take this medicine?

Take isotretinoin capsules by mouth. Follow the directions on the prescription label. This medicine is usually taken 2 times a day with a meal, unless your prescriber tells you otherwise. Swallow the capsules with a full glass of water to help prevent throat irritation. Do not chew or suck on the capsules. Do not take your medicine more often than directed. Make sure you receive and read the isotretinoin Medication Guide every time you get a prescription or refill for isotretinoin. Get a new Medication Guide with every refill. It is important that you read and understand all of this information. Do not share this medicine with anyone else due to the risk of birth defects and other serious side effects. Contact your pediatrician or health care professional regarding the use of this medicine in children. Special care may be needed.

What if I miss a dose?

If you miss a dose, take it as soon as you can. If it is almost time for your next dose, take only that dose. Do not take double or extra doses.

What may interact with isotretinoin?

- alcohol
- benzoyl peroxide, salicylic acid, or other drying medicines used for acne
- corticosteroids (example: prednisone)
- medicines for seizures
- orlistat
- other drugs that make you more sensitive to the sun such as sulfa drugs

- progestin-only birth control hormones (examples: 'Minipills' like Aygestin®, Micronor®, Nor-QD® or injectable/implantable products such as Depo-Provera® or Norplant®)
- tetracycline antibiotics (examples: doxycycline, tetracycline)
- vitamins and other supplements containing vitamin A
- warfarin

Tell your prescriber or health care professional about all other medicines you are taking, including non-prescription medicines, nutritional supplements, or herbal products. Also tell your prescriber or health care professional if you are a frequent user of drinks with caffeine or alcohol, if you smoke, or if you use illegal drugs. These may affect the way your medicine works. Check with your health care professional before stopping or starting any of your medicines.

What should I watch for while taking isotretinoin?

You may experience a flare of acne during the initial treatment period. You will need to see your prescriber or health care professional monthly to get a new prescription and to check on your progress and for side effects. Your pharmacist cannot fill a prescription for isotretinoin without a written prescription that has a qualification sticker. Phoned-in prescriptions or refills will not be filled. If your prescription for isotretinoin does not have a yellow sticker on it, contact your prescriber. Isotretinoin can cause birth defects; do not get pregnant while taking this drug. *All females who may be able to have children:* You will receive information concerning the risks of isotretinoin therapy. It is very important for you to read and understand all of the information provided to you. You must complete 2 consent forms and review materials that describe the precautions you must take. If you do not understand any part of the consent forms, do not sign them, and do not take any isotretinoin until all of your questions have been answered. If you do not have the Medications Guide, a video, and a booklet about pregnancy prevention, do not start taking isotretinoin. Call your prescriber. You will need to have 2 negative pregnancy tests before starting isotretinoin and then monthly pregnancy tests during treatment, even if you are not sexually active. You cannot get monthly refills for isotretinoin unless there is proof of the negative pregnancy test. Use 2 reliable forms of birth control together for 1 month prior to, during, and for 1 month after stopping isotretinoin therapy. Avoid using birth control pills that do not contain estrogen; they may not work while you are taking isotretinoin. If you become pregnant, miss a menstrual cycle, or stop using birth control, you must immediately stop taking isotretinoin. Severe birth defects may occur even if just one dose of isotretinoin is taken. Do not breast-feed your infant while taking isotretinoin or for 1 month after stopping treatment. *All Males:* You will also receive information concerning the risks of isotretinoin therapy. In addition, you should read the Medication guide and review all other information

supplied. You will need to sign a consent form that indicates you understand the information and instructions. Do not donate blood while taking isotretinoin and for 30 days after completion of treatment to avoid exposing pregnant women to isotretinoin through the donated blood. Do not share your isotretinoin prescription with anyone else due to the risk of birth defects and other serious adverse effects. Some patients have become depressed or developed serious mental problems while taking isotretinoin or soon after stopping isotretinoin. Some patients have had thoughts about ending their life, have tried to end their life (attempted suicide), or have ended their own life (committed suicide). There have been reports of patients receiving isotretinoin becoming aggressive or violent. No one knows if isotretinoin caused people to act this way or if it would have happened even if the person did not take isotretinoin. Stop taking isotretinoin if you start feeling depressed or have thoughts of violence or suicide. Isotretinoin can increase cholesterol and triglyceride levels and decrease HDL (the 'good' cholesterol) levels. Your health care provider will monitor these levels and recommend appropriate therapy, including dietary changes or prescription drugs, if necessary. Alcohol can increase the risk of developing high cholesterol or high blood lipids. Avoid alcoholic drinks while you are taking isotretinoin. If you wear contact lenses, they may feel uncomfortable. If your eyes get dry, check with your eye doctor. Isotretinoin may decrease your night vision; this effect may occur suddenly. Be careful driving or operating machinery especially at night. Isotretinoin may cause other vision changes. If you experience any change in vision, stop taking isotretinoin and see an eye doctor. Your mouth may get dry. Chewing sugarless gum or sucking hard candy, and drinking plenty of water will help. Avoid multivitamins or nutritional supplements that contain vitamin A. Isotretinoin can increase sensitivity of the skin to sun or UV light. Keep out of the sun, or wear protective clothing outdoors and use a sunscreen (SPF 15 or higher). Do not use sun lamps or sun tanning beds or booths. Cosmetic procedures to smooth your skin including waxing, dermabrasion, or laser therapy should be avoided during isotretinoin therapy and for at least 6 months after you stop due to the possibility of scarring. Check with your health care provider for advice about when you can have cosmetic procedures. Isotretinoin may affect your blood sugar levels. If you are diabetic check with your prescriber or health care professional if you notice any change in your blood sugar tests. Isotretinoin may affect bones, muscles, and ligaments and cause pain in your joints or muscles. Tell your prescriber if you plan vigorous physical activity during your treatment with isotretinoin. Tell your health care provider if you develop pain, particularly back pain or joint pain. It is not known if taking isotretinoin for acne will affect your bones. Muscle weakness with or without pain can be a sign of a serious problem. If this happens, stop taking isotretinoin and call your prescriber right away.

What side effects may I notice from taking isotretinoin?

Stop taking isotretinoin and notify your prescriber at once if you have any of these symptoms:
- difficulty concentrating
- feel like you have no energy
- feel unusually sad or have crying spells
- feelings of worthlessness or inappropriate guilt
- increased irritability, anger, aggression or thoughts of violence
- loss of interest in usual activities
- sleep too much or have trouble sleeping
- start to have thoughts about hurting yourself
- withdraw from family or friends

Side effects that you should report to your prescriber or health care professional as soon as possible:
- chest pain
- changes in menstrual cycle
- changes in vision, like blurred or double vision or decreased night vision
- difficulty breathing or shortness of breath
- dizziness
- fainting
- hearing loss or ringing in the ears
- hives, skin rash
- increased urination and/or thirst or dark urine
- irregular heartbeat

- muscle or joint pain
- muscle weakness with or without pain
- nausea and vomiting
- severe headache
- slurred speech
- stomach pain
- swelling of face or mouth
- trouble swallowing
- unusual bruising or bleeding
- yellowing of the eyes or skin

Side effects that usually do not require medical attention (report to your prescriber or health care professional if they continue or are bothersome):
- chapped lips
- dry eyes
- dry mouth
- dry nose that may lead to nosebleeds
- dry skin
- flushing
- hair loss, increased fragility of hair
- headache (mild)
- increased sensitivity of skin to the sun

Where can I keep my medicine?

Keep out of the reach of children in a container that small children cannot open. Store at room temperature between 15–30 degrees C (59–86 degrees F). Throw away any unused medicine after the expiration date.

Isradipine capsules

DYNACIRC®;
5 mg; Capsule
Reliant
Pharmaceuticals Llc

DYNACIRC®;
2.5 mg; Capsule
Reliant
Pharmaceuticals Llc

What are isradipine capsules?

ISRADIPINE (DynaCirc®) is a calcium-channel blocker. It affects the amount of calcium found in your heart and muscle cells. This results in relaxation of blood vessels, which can reduce the amount of work the heart has to do. Isradipine reduces high blood pressure (hypertension). It is not a cure. Generic isradipine capsules are available.

What should my health care professional know before I take isradipine?

They need to know if you have any of these conditions:
- heart problems, low blood pressure, irregular heartbeat
- liver disease
- previous heart attack
- over 65 years old
- an unusual or allergic reaction to isradipine, other medicines, foods, dyes, or preservatives
- pregnant or trying to get pregnant
- breast-feeding

How should I take this medicine?

Take isradipine capsules by mouth. Follow the directions on the prescription label. Swallow the capsules whole with a drink of water, do not crush or chew.

This medicine may be taken with or without food. Do not significantly increase grapefruit juice intake while taking this drug, or avoid grapefruit juice if possible. Take your doses at regular intervals. Do not take your medicine more often then directed. Do not stop taking except on your prescriber's advice. Contact your pediatrician or health care professional regarding the use of this medicine in children. Special care may be needed. Elderly patients over 65 years old may have a stronger reaction to this medicine and need smaller doses.

What if I miss a dose?

If you miss a dose, take it as soon as you can. If it is almost time for your next dose, take only that dose. Do not take double or extra doses.

What may interact with isradipine?

Do not take isradipine with any of the following:

- grapefruit juice

Isradipine may also interact with the following medications:

- alcohol
- anti-inflammatory drugs (NSAIDs, such as ibuprofen)
- barbiturates such as phenobarbital
- bosentan
- cimetidine

- female hormones, including contraceptive or birth control pills
- herbal or dietary supplements such as ginger, gingko biloba, ginseng, hawthorn, *Ma huang* (ephedra), melatonin, St. John's wort, went yeast
- imatinib, STI-571
- local anesthetics or general anesthetics
- lovastatin
- medicines for fungal infections (fluconazole, itraconazole, ketoconazole, voriconazole)
- medicines for high blood pressure
- medicines for HIV infection or AIDS
- medicines for prostate problems
- medicines for seizures (carbamazepine, phenobarbital, phenytoin, primidone)
- rifampin, rifapentine, or rifabutin
- some antibiotics (clarithromycin, erythromycin, telithromycin, troleandomycin)
- some medicines for heart-rhythm problems (amiodarone, diltiazem, disopyramide, flecainide, quinidine, verapamil)
- some medicines for depression or mental problems (fluoxetine, fluvoxamine, nefazodone)
- water pills (diuretics)
- yohimbine
- zafirlukast
- zileuton

Tell your prescriber or health care professional about all other medicines you are taking, including non-prescription medicines, nutritional supplements, or herbal products. Also tell your prescriber or health care professional if you are a frequent user of drinks with caffeine or alcohol, if you smoke, or if you use illegal drugs. These may affect the way your medicine works. Check with your health care professional before stopping or starting any of your medicines.

What should I watch for while taking isradipine?

Check your blood pressure and pulse rate regularly; this is important while you are taking isradipine. Ask your prescriber or health care professional what your blood pressure and pulse rate should be and when you should contact him or her. You may feel dizzy or lightheaded. Do not drive, use machinery, or do anything that needs mental alertness until you know how isradipine affects you. To reduce the risk of dizzy or fainting spells, do not sit or stand up quickly, especially if you are an older patient. Avoid alcoholic drinks; they can make you more dizzy, increase flushing and rapid heartbeats. If you are going to have surgery, tell your prescriber or health care professional that you are taking isradipine. Do not suddenly stop taking isradipine. Ask your prescriber or health care professional how to gradually reduce the dose.

What side effects may I notice from taking isradipine?

Side effects that you should report to your prescriber or health care professional as soon as possible:
- fast heartbeat, palpitations, irregular heartbeat, chest pain
- difficulty breathing
- dizziness or drowsiness
- fainting spells, lightheadedness
- swelling of the legs and ankles

Side effects that usually do not require medical attention (report to your prescriber or health care professional if they continue or are bothersome):
- facial flushing
- headache
- weakness or tiredness

Where can I keep my medicine?

Keep out of the reach of children in a container that small children cannot open. Store at room temperature below 30 degrees C (86 degrees F). Protect from light. Keep container tightly closed. Throw away any unused medicine after the expiration date.

Isradipine extended-release tablets	DYNACIRC® CR; 5 mg; Tablet, Extended Release Reliant Pharmaceuticals Llc		DYNACIRC® CR; 10 mg; Tablet, Extended Release Reliant Pharmaceuticals Llc	

What are isradipine extended-release tablets?

ISRADIPINE (DynaCirc® CR) is a calcium-channel blocker. It affects the amount of calcium found in your heart and muscle cells. This results in relaxation of blood vessels, which can reduce the amount of work the heart has to do. Isradipine reduces high blood pressure (hypertension). It is not a cure. Generic isradipine extended-release tablets are not yet available.

What should my health care professional know before I take isradipine?

They need to know if you have any of these conditions:
- heart problems, low blood pressure, irregular heartbeat
- liver disease
- previous heart attack
- over 65 years old
- an unusual or allergic reaction to isradipine, other medicines, foods, dyes, or preservatives
- pregnant or trying to get pregnant
- breast-feeding

How should I take this medicine?

Take isradipine tablets by mouth. Follow the directions on the prescription label. Swallow the tablets whole with a drink of water, do not crush, break, or chew. This medicine may be taken with or without food. Do not significantly increase grapefruit juice intake while taking this drug, or avoid grapefruit juice if possible. Take your doses at regular intervals. Do not take your medicine more often then directed. Do not stop taking except on your prescriber's advice. Contact your pediatrician or health care professional regarding the use of this medicine in children. Special care may be needed. Elderly patients over 65 years old may have a stronger reaction to this medicine and need smaller doses.

What if I miss a dose?

If you miss a dose, take it as soon as you can. If it is almost time for your next dose, take only that dose. Do not take double or extra doses.

What may interact with isradipine?

Do not take isradipine with any of the following:

- grapefruit juice

Isradipine may also interact with the following medications:

- alcohol
- anti-inflammatory drugs (NSAIDs, such as ibuprofen)
- barbiturates such as phenobarbital
- bosentan
- cimetidine
- female hormones, including contraceptive or birth control pills
- herbal or dietary supplements such as gingko biloba, ginseng, hawthorn, *Ma huang* (ephedra), melatonin, St. John's wort, went yeast
- imatinib, STI-571
- local anesthetics or general anesthetics
- lovastatin
- medicines for fungal infections (fluconazole, itraconazole, ketoconazole, voriconazole)
- medicines for high blood pressure
- medicines for HIV infection or AIDS
- medicines for prostate problems
- medicines for seizures (carbamazepine, phenobarbital, phenytoin, primidone)
- rifampin, rifapentine, or rifabutin
- some antibiotics (clarithromycin, erythromycin, telithromycin, troleandomycin)
- some medicines for heart-rhythm problems (amiodarone, diltiazem, disopyramide, flecainide, quinidine, verapamil)
- some medicines for depression or mental problems (fluoxetine, fluvoxamine, nefazodone)
- water pills (diuretics)
- yohimbine
- zafirlukast
- zileuton

Tell your prescriber or health care professional about all other medicines you are taking, including non-prescription medicines, nutritional supplements, or herbal products. Also tell your prescriber or health care professional if you are a frequent user of drinks with caffeine or alcohol, if you smoke, or if you use illegal drugs. These may affect the way your medicine works. Check with your health care professional before stopping or starting any of your medicines.

What should I watch for while taking isradipine?

Check your blood pressure and pulse rate regularly; this is important while you are taking isradipine. Ask your prescriber or health care professional what your blood pressure and pulse rate should be and when you should contact him or her. You may feel dizzy or lightheaded. Do not drive, use machinery, or do anything that needs mental alertness until you know how isradipine affects you. To reduce the risk of dizzy or fainting spells, do not sit or stand up quickly, especially if you are an older patient. Avoid alcoholic drinks; they can make you more dizzy, increase flushing and rapid heartbeats. If you are going to have surgery, tell your prescriber or health care professional that you are taking isradipine. Do not suddenly stop taking isradipine. Ask your prescriber or health care professional how to gradually reduce the dose.

What side effects may I notice from taking isradipine?

Side effects that you should report to your prescriber or health care professional as soon as possible:

- fast heartbeat, palpitations, irregular heartbeat, chest pain
- difficulty breathing
- dizziness or drowsiness
- fainting spells, lightheadedness
- swelling of the legs and ankles

Side effects that usually do not require medical attention (report to your prescriber or health care professional if they continue or are bothersome):

- facial flushing
- headache
- weakness or tiredness

Where can I keep my medicine?

Keep out of the reach of children in a container that small children cannot open. Store at room temperature below 30 degrees C (86 degrees F). Protect from light. Keep container tightly closed. Throw away any unused medicine after the expiration date.

Itraconazole capsules

SPORANOX®;
100 mg; Capsule
Janssen Pharmaceutica Inc

What are itraconazole capsules?

ITRACONAZOLE (Sporanox®) is an antifungal type of antibiotic. It treats serious fungal infections; especially those associated with the lungs. Generic itraconazole capsules are available.

What should my health care professional know before I take itraconazole capsules?

They need to know if you have any of these conditions:
- heart disease, including angina or heart failure
- liver disease
- lung disease, including COPD
- kidney disease or on dialysis
- an unusual or allergic reaction to itraconazole, or other azole medicines, foods, dyes or preservatives
- pregnant or trying to get pregnant
- breast-feeding

How should I take this medicine?

Take itraconazole capsules by mouth. Follow the directions on the prescription label. Itraconazole capsules work best if you take them with food or a cola beverage, but do not take them with oranges or orange juice. Take your doses at regular intervals. Do not take your medicine more often than directed. Finish the full course prescribed by your prescriber or health care professional even if you feel better. Do not stop taking except on your prescriber's advice. Contact your pediatrician or health care professional regarding the use of this medicine in children. Special care may be needed.

What if I miss a dose?

If you miss a dose, take it as soon as you can. If it is almost time for your next dose, take only that dose. Do not take double or extra doses.

What may interact with itraconazole capsules?

Do not take itraconazole with the following medications or foods:

- astemizole (Hismanal®)
- bosentan (Tracleer™)
- cerivastatin (Baycol®)
- cimetidine (Tagamet®)
- cisapride (Propulsid®)
- dofetilide (Tikosyn™)
- esomeprazole (Nexium®)
- famotidine (Pepcid®)
- lansoprazole (Prevacid®)
- lovastatin (Advicor®, Altocor™, Mevacor®)
- nizatidine (Axid®)
- omeprazole (Prilosec®)
- oranges or orange juice
- pantoprazole (Protonix®)
- pimozide (Orap®)

- quinidine (Cardioquin®, Quinidex®, Quinaglute®)
- rabeprazole (AcipHex™)
- ranitidine (Zantac®)
- simvastatin (Zocor®)
- terfenadine (Seldane®)
- triazolam (Halcion®)
- went yeast (Cholestin™)

Other drugs that may interact with itraconazole include:

- antacids
- atorvastatin
- cilostazol
- clarithromycin
- cyclosporine
- digoxin
- dihydroergotamine, ergotamine, or methysergide
- erythromycin
- medicines for anxiety or sleep (e.g., alprazolam, estazolam)
- medicines for diabetes that are taken by mouth
- medicines for HIV infection or AIDS
- medicines for tuberculosis including isoniazid, INH, rifabutin, rifampin, and rifapentine
- methadone
- other medicines for fungal or yeast infections
- phenytoin
- pravastatin
- rosuvastatin

Tell your prescriber or health care professional about all other medicines you are taking, including non-prescription medicines, nutritional supplements, or herbal products. Also tell your prescriber or health care professional if you are a frequent user of drinks with caffeine or alcohol, if you smoke, or if you use illegal drugs. These may affect the way your medicine works. Check with your health care professional before stopping or starting any of your medicines.

What should I watch for while taking itraconazole capsules?

If you experience unusual fatigue, loss of appetite (anorexia), nausea and/or vomiting, yellowing of skin, dark urine, or pale stools, stop taking itraconazole immediately and contact your healthcare provider. Tell your prescriber or health care professional if your symptoms do not begin to improve in 1 to 2 weeks. Some fungal infections need many weeks or months of treatment to cure. Take your medicine regularly for as long as your prescriber or health care professional tells you to. Do not take ranitidine (Zantac®), cimetidine (Tagamet®), famotidine (Pepcid®), or other agents [e.g., omeprazole (Prilosec®), lansoprazole (Prevacid®), pantoprazole (Protonix®)] that may decrease the acid in your stomach. Itraconazole needs acid in the stomach so that it can be absorbed. If you use antacids, do not take them at the same time as itraconazole. Take itraconazole 1 hour before or 4 hours after antacids.

What side effects may I notice from taking itraconazole capsules?

Side effects that you should report to your prescriber or health care professional as soon as possible:
Rare or uncommon:
- difficulty breathing or shortness of breath
- dark yellow or brown urine
- loss of appetite
- pale stools
- redness, blistering, peeling or loosening of the skin, including inside the mouth
- skin rash, itching
- stomach pain

- skin rash, itching, hives
- swelling, fluid retention
- unusual fatigue
- vomiting
- yellowing of the eyes or skin

Side effects that usually do not require medical attention (report to your prescriber or health care professional if they continue or are bothersome):
- diarrhea
- dizziness
- headache
- nausea

Where can I keep my medicine?

Keep out of the reach of children in a container that small children cannot open. Store at or below 25 degrees C (77 degrees F). Do not freeze. Throw away any unused medicine after the expiration date.

Ivermectin tablets

STROMECTOL®;
3 mg; Tablet
Merck and Co, Inc

What are ivermectin tablets?

IVERMECTIN (Stromectol®) treats parasite infections. This medicine treats worm infections like river blindness and a type of diarrhea called strongyloidiasis. It can also be used to treat other types of resistant parasitic infections, including scabies or head lice. Generic ivermectin tablets are not yet available.

What should my health care professional know before I take ivermectin?

They need to know if you have any of these conditions:
- asthma
- liver disease
- an unusual reaction to ivermectin, other medicines, foods, dyes, or preservatives
- pregnant or trying to get pregnant
- breast-feeding

How should this medicine be used?

Take ivermectin tablets by mouth with a full glass of water. Do not take ivermectin with food. Follow the directions on the prescription label. As a general rule take ivermectin tablets 1 hour before breakfast. Do not take your medicine more often than directed. Finish the full course of medicine prescribed by your prescriber or health care professional even if you feel better. Contact your pediatrician or health care professional regarding the use of this medicine in children. Special care may be needed.

What if I miss a dose?

Since ivermectin is usually given as a one time dose, it is unlikely that you will miss a dose. However, you may need a return visit to your doctor to see if you need repeat doses to cure the infection.

What may interact with ivermectin?

Ivermectin is usually given as a one time dose and thus drug interactions are thought to be uncommon. Check with your prescriber or health care professional if you will be receiving multiple doses of ivermectin and if you are taking other medications.
Tell your prescriber or health care professional about all other medicines you are taking, including non-prescription medicines, nutritional supplements, or herbal products. Also tell your prescriber or health care professional if you are a frequent user of drinks with caffeine or alcohol, if you smoke, or if you use illegal drugs. These may affect the way your medicine works. Check with your health care professional before stopping or starting any of your medicines.

What should I watch for while taking ivermectin?

Visit your prescriber or health care professional to check that your infection has gone. Your prescriber may request that you have stool samples or other tests checked for the infection. If you have a severe infection, you may need a repeat course of treatment. You may get dizzy. Until you know how ivermectin affects you, do not drive, use machinery, or do anything that needs mental alertness. Practice good hygiene to prevent infection of others. Wash your hands, scrub your fingernails and shower often. Every day change and launder linens and undergarments. Scrub toilets often and keep floors clean. Other people in your house may need treatment. Check with your prescriber or health care professional.

What side effects may I notice from taking ivermectin?

Ivermectin is usually well tolerated and serious side effects are rare.

Side effects that you should report to your prescriber or health care professional as soon as possible:

- difficulty breathing
- eye or eyelid pain, irritation, redness or swelling
- loss or change of vision
- redness, blistering, peeling or loosening of the skin, including inside the mouth
- skin rash, hives or increased itching
- yellowing of eyes or skin
- unusual weakness or tiredness

Side effects that usually do not require medical attention (report to your prescriber or health care professional if they continue or are bothersome):

- dizziness or lightheadedness

- joint or muscle pain
- tender glands in the neck, armpits, or groin
- headache
- diarrhea
- loss of appetite
- nausea, vomiting
- tremors
- swelling of the face, hands, arms, feet, or legs

Where can I keep my medicine?

Keep out of the reach of children in a container that small children cannot open. Store at room temperature below 30 degrees C (86 degrees F). Keep container tightly closed. Throw away any unused medicine after the expiration date.

Ketoconazole tablets

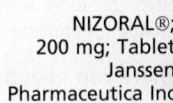

NIZORAL®;
200 mg; Tablet
Janssen
Pharmaceutica Inc

KETOCONAZOLE;
200 mg; Tablet
Mutual/United
Research
Laboratories

What are ketoconazole tablets?

KETOCONAZOLE (Nizoral®) is an antifungal type of antibiotic. It treats fungal infections such as ringworm of the body (tinea corporis), ringworm of the groin (tinea cruris or jock itch), sun fungus (tinea versicolor, pityriasis versicolor), dandruff, and other systemic (throughout the body) fungal infections. Generic ketoconazole oral tablets are available.

What should my health care professional know before I take ketoconazole?

They need to know if you have any of these conditions:
- an alcohol abuse problem
- low stomach acid production (achlorhydria or hypochlorhydria)
- liver disease
- other chronic illness
- an unusual or allergic reaction to ketoconazole, itraconazole, miconazole, other foods, dyes or preservatives
- pregnant or trying to get pregnant
- breast-feeding

How should I take this medicine?

Take ketoconazole tablets by mouth. Follow the directions on the prescription label. Take your doses at regular intervals. Ketoconazole works best if you take it with food. If you have a low production of stomach acid you may have to take your tablets dissolved in dilute hydrochloric acid. Drink this mixture through a straw to avoid contact with the teeth. Then drink a glass of water, swishing it round your teeth before you swallow. Do not take or use your medicine more often than directed. Finish the full course prescribed by your prescriber or health care professional even if you feel better. Do not stop taking except on your prescriber's advice. Contact your pediatrician or health care professional regarding the use of this medicine in children. Special care may be needed.

What if I miss a dose?

If you miss a dose, take it as soon as you can. If it is almost time for your next dose, take only that dose. Do not take double or extra doses.

What may interact with ketoconazole?

- alcohol
- antacids
- astemizole
- bosentan
- cisapride
- cyclosporine
- didanosine (ddI)
- dofetilide
- ergotamine, dihydroergotamine or methysergide
- hormones such as prednisone or cortisone
- isoniazid
- certain medicines for anxiety or difficulty sleeping
- medicines for lowering cholesterol (such as atorvastatin, lovastatin, simvastatin)
- medicines for movement abnormalities as in Parkinson's disease, or for gastrointestinal problems
- medicines for stomach ulcers and other stomach problems
- other medicines for fungal or yeast infections
- pimozide
- pioglitazone
- quinidine
- phenytoin
- rifampin
- terfenadine
- tolbutamide
- warfarin

Tell your prescriber or health care professional about all other medicines you are taking, including non-prescription medicines, nutritional supplements, or herbal products. Also tell your prescriber or health care professional if you are a frequent user of drinks with caffeine or alcohol, if you smoke, or if you use illegal drugs. These may affect the way your medicine works. Check with your health care professional before stopping or starting any of your medicines.

What should I watch for while taking ketoconazole?

Tell your prescriber or health care professional if your symptoms do not begin to improve in 1 to 2 weeks. Some fungal infections can take many weeks or months of treatment to cure. Take your medicine regularly for as long as your prescriber or health care professional tells you to. You may get dizzy; until you know how ketoconazole affects you, do not drive, use machinery, or do anything that needs mental alertness. Alcohol may make you more dizzy, feel sick and increase possible damage to your liver. Avoid alcoholic drinks while you are taking ketoconazole and for two days afterwards. Other medicines you get on prescription, or buy at the pharmacy may contain small amounts of alcohol. Do not take terfenadine (Seldane®) or astemizole (Hismanal®) with ketoconazole. This combination of medicines can produce serious effects on your heart. Ketoconazole may make your eyes more sensitive to light. Wear dark glasses in bright sun, or under any bright lights.

What side effects may I notice from taking ketoconazole?

Side effects that you should report to your prescriber or health care professional as soon as possible:
- dark yellow or brown urine
- loss of appetite

K

- redness, blistering, peeling or loosening of the skin, including inside the mouth
- skin rash, itching
- stomach pain
- yellowing of the eyes or skin

Side effects that usually do not require medical attention (report to your prescriber or health care professional if they continue or are bothersome):

- breast swelling and tenderness, or sexual difficulties (impotence) in men

- drowsiness or dizziness
- eyes get more sensitive to light
- nausea, vomiting

Where can I keep my medicine?

Keep out of the reach of children in a container that small children cannot open. Store at room temperature between 15 and 30 degrees C (59 and 86 degrees F). Keep container tightly closed. Throw away any unused medicine after the expiration date.

This drug requires an FDA medication guide. See page xxxvii.

Ketoprofen tablets or capsules

ORUVAIL®;
200 mg; Capsule,
Extended Release
Wyeth
Pharmaceuticals Inc

ORUDIS® KT;
12.5 mg; Tablet
Whitehall-Robins

What are ketoprofen tablets or capsules?

KETOPROFEN (Orudis® KT, Oruvail®) is an anti-inflammatory drug. Ketoprofen helps relieve the inflammation and pain associated with rheumatoid arthritis, osteoarthritis, menstrual cramps or premenstrual pain and swelling. Ketoprofen is available in a non-prescription strength to treat minor aches and pains associated with the common cold, backache, muscular aches, toothache and menstrual pain. Generic ketoprofen immediate- and extended-release capsules are available.

What should my health care professional know before I take ketoprofen?

They need to know if you have any of these conditions:

- asthma, especially aspirin-sensitive asthma
- bleeding problems
- cigarette smoker
- diabetes mellitus
- drink more than 3 alcohol-containing beverages a day
- heart failure
- high blood pressure
- kidney disease
- liver disease
- lost a lot of fluid due to continued vomiting or diarrhea
- stomach or duodenal ulcers
- systemic lupus erythematosus
- ulcerative colitis
- an unusual or allergic reaction to ketoprofen, aspirin, other salicylates, other NSAIDs, foods, dyes or preservatives
- pregnant or trying to get pregnant
- breast-feeding

How should I take this medicine?

Take ketoprofen tablets or capsules by mouth. Follow the directions on the label. Swallow tablets or capsules whole with a full glass of water; take tablets or capsules in an upright or sitting position. Taking a sip of water first, before taking the tablets or capsules, may help you swallow them. If possible take bedtime doses at least 10 minutes before lying down. Do not crush or chew the extended-release capsules. You can take ketoprofen with food to prevent stomach upset. Take your doses at regular intervals. Do not take your medicine more often than directed. Contact your pediatrician or health care professional regarding the use of this medicine in children. Special care may be needed.

What if I miss a dose?

If you miss a dose, take it as soon as you can. If it is almost time for your next dose, take only that dose. Do not take double or extra doses.

What other medicines can interact with ketoprofen?

- alcohol
- alendronate
- anti-inflammatory drugs (other NSAIDs, prednisone)
- aspirin and aspirin-like medicines
- cidofovir
- cyclosporine
- drospirenone; ethinyl estradiol (Yasmin®)
- entecavir
- herbal products that contain feverfew, garlic, ginger, or ginkgo biloba
- lithium
- medicines for high blood pressure
- medicines that affect platelets
- medicines that treat or prevent blood clots such as warfarin and other "blood thinners"
- methotrexate
- pemetrexed
- water pills (diuretics)

Tell your prescriber or health care professional about all other medicines you are taking, including non-prescription medicines, nutritional supplements, or herbal products. Also tell your prescriber or health care professional if you are a frequent user of drinks with caffeine or alcohol, if you smoke, or if you use illegal drugs. These may affect the way your medicine works. Check with your health care professional before stopping or starting any of your medicines.

K

What do I need to watch for while I take ketoprofen?

Let your prescriber or health care professional know if your pain continues. Do not take with other pain medicines or fever medicine without advice. If you get flu-like symptoms (fever, chills, muscle aches and pains), call your prescriber or health care professional. Do not treat yourself. To reduce unpleasant effects on your throat and stomach, take ketoprofen with a full glass of water and never just before lying down. Take ketoprofen with food or milk if stomach upset occurs. If you notice black, tarry stools or experience severe stomach pain and vomit blood or what looks like coffee grounds, notify your health care prescriber immediately. If you have stomach pain or an upset stomach that worsens or persists, redness or swelling in a painful area, or any new symptoms, call your health care professional. If you are taking medicines that affect the clotting of your blood, such as aspirin or blood thinners such as Coumadin®, talk to your health care provider or prescriber before taking this medicine. You may get dizzy. Do not drive, use machinery, or do anything that needs mental alertness until you know how ketoprofen affects you. Do not sit or stand up quickly, especially if you are an older patient. This reduces the risk of dizzy or fainting spells. Do not smoke cigarettes or drink alcohol; these increase irritation to your stomach and can make it more susceptible to damage from ketoprofen. It is especially important not to use ketoprofen during the last 3 months of pregnancy unless specifically directed to do so by your health care provider. Ketoprofen may cause problems in the unborn child or complications during delivery. If you are going to have surgery, tell your prescriber or health care professional that you are taking ketoprofen. Problems can arise if you need dental work, and in the day to day care of your teeth. Try to avoid damage to your teeth and gums when you brush or floss your teeth.

What side effects may I notice from taking ketoprofen?

Side effects that you should report to your prescriber or health care professional as soon as possible:

- signs of bleeding—black tarry stools, blood in the urine, unusual tiredness or weakness, vomiting blood or vomit that looks like coffee grounds
- signs of an allergic reaction—difficulty breathing, wheezing, skin rash, redness, blistering or peeling skin, hives, itching, swelling of eyelids, throat, lips
- blurred vision
- change in the amount of urine passed
- difficulty swallowing, severe heartburn or burning, pain in throat
- pain or difficulty passing urine
- stomach pain or cramps
- swelling of feet or ankles

Side effects that usually do not require medical attention (report to your prescriber or health care professional if they continue or are bothersome):

- diarrhea or constipation
- dizziness, drowsiness
- gas or heartburn
- headache
- nausea, vomiting

Where can I keep my medicine?

Keep out of the reach of children in a container that small children cannot open. Store at room temperature, approximately 25 degrees C (77 degrees F) away from humidity (not in the bathroom or kitchen, if possible). Keep container tightly closed. Throw away any unused medicine after the expiration date.

Ketorolac tablets

TORADOL®;
10 mg; Tablet
Hoffmann La Roche
Inc

KETOROLAC;
10 mg; Tablet
Teva
Pharmaceuticals
USA Inc

K

This drug requires an FDA medication guide. See page xxxvii.

What are ketorolac tablets?

KETOROLAC (Toradol®) is a nonsteroidal anti-inflammatory drug (NSAID). Ketorolac helps relieve mild to moderate pain in the short-term, including post-operative pain. Ketorolac should not be used for more than 5 days. Generic ketorolac tablets are available.

What should my health care professional know before I take ketorolac?

They need to know if you have any of these conditions:

- asthma, especially aspirin-sensitive asthma
- bleeding problems or taking medicines that make you bleed more easily such as anticoagulants ("blood thinners")
- cigarette smoker
- dental disease
- diabetes
- drink more than 3 alcohol-containing beverages a day
- heart failure
- high blood pressure
- kidney disease
- liver disease
- stomach or duodenal ulcers
- systemic lupus erythematosus
- ulcerative colitis
- an unusual or allergic reaction to ketorolac, aspirin,

other salicylates, other NSAIDs, foods, dyes or preservatives
- pregnant or trying to get pregnant
- breast-feeding

How should I take this medicine?

Take ketorolac tablets by mouth. Follow the directions on the prescription label. Swallow tablets whole with a full glass of water; take tablets or capsules in an upright or sitting position. Taking a sip of water first, before taking the tablets or capsules, may help you swallow them. If possible take bedtime doses at least 10 minutes before lying down. You can take ketorolac with food to prevent stomach upset. Take your doses at regular intervals. Do not take your medicine more often than directed. Do not give this medicine to any other person. Contact your pediatrician or health care professional regarding the use of this medicine in children. Special care may be needed.

What if I miss a dose?

If you miss a dose, take it as soon as you can. If it is almost time for your next dose, take only that dose. Do not take double or extra doses.

What may interact with ketorolac?

- alcohol
- alendronate
- aspirin and aspirin-like medicines
- cidofovir
- cyclosporine
- drospirenone; ethinyl estradiol (Yasmin®)
- entecavir
- herbal products that contain feverfew, garlic, ginger, or ginkgo biloba
- lithium
- medicines for high blood pressure
- medicines that affect platelets
- medicines that treat or prevent blood clots such as warfarin and other "blood thinners"
- methotrexate
- other anti-inflammatory drugs (such as ibuprofen or prednisone)
- pemetrexed
- water pills (diuretics)

Tell your prescriber or health care professional about all other medicines you are taking, including non-prescription medicines, nutritional supplements, or herbal products. Also tell your prescriber or health care professional if you are a frequent user of drinks with caffeine or alcohol, if you smoke, or if you use illegal drugs. These may affect the way your medicine works. Check with your health care professional before stopping or starting any of your medicines.

What should I watch for while taking ketorolac?

Let your prescriber or health care professional know if your pain continues after 5 days. Do not take ketorolac with other pain-killers without advice. If you get flu-like symptoms (fever, chills, muscle aches and pains), call your prescriber or health care professional; do not treat yourself. To reduce unpleasant effects on your throat and stomach, take ketorolac with a full glass of water and never just before lying down. If you notice black, tarry stools or experience severe stomach pain and vomit blood or what looks like coffee grounds, notify your health care prescriber immediately. If you are taking medicines that affect the clotting of your blood, such as aspirin or blood thinners such as Coumadin®, talk to your health care provider or prescriber before taking this medicine. You may get dizzy. Do not drive, use machinery, or do anything that needs mental alertness until you know how ketorolac affects you. Do not sit or stand up quickly, especially if you are an older patient. This reduces the risk of dizzy or fainting spells. Do not smoke cigarettes or drink alcohol; these increase irritation to your stomach and can make it more susceptible to damage from ketorolac. If you are going to have surgery or dental work, tell your prescriber or health care professional that you are taking ketorolac. Ketorolac can increase bleeding and decrease the ability for blood to clot. It is especially important not to use ketorolac during the last 3 months of pregnancy unless specifically directed to do so by your health care provider. Ketorolac may cause problems in the unborn child or complications during delivery.

What side effects may I notice from taking ketorolac?

Side effects that you should report to your prescriber—or health care professional as soon as possible:
- signs of bleeding—black tarry stools, blood in the urine, unusual tiredness or weakness, vomiting blood or vomit that looks like coffee grounds
- signs of an allergic reaction—difficulty breathing, wheezing, skin rash, redness, blistering or peeling skin, hives, or itching, swelling of eyelids, throat, lips
- blurred vision
- change in the amount of urine passed
- difficulty swallowing, severe heartburn or burning, pain in throat
- pain or difficulty passing urine
- stomach pain or cramps
- swelling of feet or ankles

Side effects that usually do not require medical attention (report to your prescriber or health care professional if they continue or are bothersome):
- diarrhea or constipation
- dizziness, drowsiness
- gas or heartburn
- headache
- nausea, vomiting

Where can I keep my medicine?

Keep out of the reach of children in a container that small children cannot open. Store at room temperature between 15 and 30 degrees C (59 and 86 degrees F). Protect from light. Throw away any unused medicine after the expiration date.

K

Labetalol tablets

TRANDATE®;
300 mg; Tablet
Prometheus
Laboratories Inc

TRANDATE®;
200 mg; Tablet
Prometheus
Laboratories Inc

What are labetalol tablets?

LABETALOL (Normodyne®, Trandate®) belongs to a group of medicines called beta-blockers. Beta-blockers reduce the workload on the heart and help it to beat more regularly. Labetalol controls, but does not cure, high blood pressure (hypertension). High blood pressure may not make you feel sick, but it can lead to serious heart problems. Generic labetalol tablets are available.

What should my health care professional know before I take labetalol?

They need to know if you have any of these conditions:
- asthma, bronchitis or bronchospasm
- circulation problems
- depression
- diabetes
- emphysema, or other lung disease
- history of heart attack or heart disease
- kidney disease
- liver disease
- muscle weakness or disease
- pheochromocytoma
- psoriasis
- thyroid disease
- an unusual or allergic reaction to labetalol, other beta-blockers, medicines, foods, dyes, or preservatives
- pregnant or trying to get pregnant
- breast-feeding

How should I take this medicine?

Take labetalol tablets by mouth. Follow the directions on the prescription label. Swallow the tablets with a drink of water. Take your doses at regular intervals. Do not take your medicine more often than directed. Do not stop taking except on your prescriber's advice. Contact your pediatrician or health care professional regarding the use of this medicine in children. Special care may be needed.

What if I miss a dose?

If you miss a dose, take it as soon as you can. If it is almost time for your next dose, take only that dose. Do not take double or extra doses. There should be at least 8 hours between doses.

What may interact with labetalol?

- cimetidine
- diltiazem
- hawthorn
- medicines for diabetes
- medicines for high blood pressure
- medicines for mental depression
- medicines for colds and breathing difficulties
- nitroglycerin
- verapamil
- water pills

Tell your prescriber or health care professional about all other medicines you are taking, including non-prescription medicines, nutritional supplements, or herbal products. Also tell your prescriber or health care professional if you are a frequent user of drinks with caffeine or alcohol, if you smoke, or if you use illegal drugs. These may affect the way your medicine works. Check with your health care professional before stopping or starting any of your medicines.

What should I watch for while taking labetalol?

Check your heart rate and blood pressure regularly while you are taking labetalol. Ask your prescriber or health care professional what your heart rate and blood pressure should be, and when you should contact him or her. Do not stop taking this medicine suddenly. This could lead to serious heart-related effects. You may get drowsy or dizzy. Do not drive, use machinery, or do anything that requires mental alertness until you know how labetalol affects you. To reduce the risk of dizzy or fainting spells, do not sit or stand up quickly. Alcohol can make you more drowsy, and increase flushing and rapid heartbeats. Therefore, it is best to avoid alcoholic drinks. Labetalol can affect blood sugar levels. If you have diabetes, check with your prescriber or health care professional before you change your diet or the dose of your diabetic medicine. If you are going to have surgery, tell your prescriber or health care professional that you are taking labetalol.

What side effects may I notice from taking labetalol?

Side effects that you should report to your prescriber or health care professional as soon as possible:
- cold hands or feet
- dark yellow or brown urine
- depression
- difficulty breathing, wheezing
- dizziness or fainting spells
- irregular heartbeat
- pain or difficulty passing urine
- skin rash
- slow heart rate (fewer than recommended by your prescriber or health care professional)
- swollen legs or ankles
- tingling of the scalp or skin
- vomiting
- yellowing of the eyes or skin

Side effects that usually do not require medical atten-

tion (report to your prescriber or health care professional if they continue or are bothersome):

- dry itching skin
- headache
- nausea
- sexual difficulties, impotence
- unusual tiredness

Where can I keep my medicine?

Keep out of the reach of children in a container that small children cannot open. Store at room temperature between 2 and 30 degrees C (36 and 86 degrees F). Protect from moisture. Throw away any unused medicine after the expiration date.

Lactase chewable tablets, tablets, caplets, or capsules

What are lactase chewable tablets, tablets, caplets, or capsules?

LACTASE (DairyEase®, Lac-Dos®, Lactaid®, Lactrase®, RiteAid® Dairy Relief™, SureLac®, Walgreen's® Dairy Digestive™) is an enzyme that aids in the digestion of lactose. Lactose is a sugar is found in dairy products such as ice cream, cheese and milk. When the lactase enzyme is not present, lactose intolerance can occur after eating dairy foods and cause symptoms like diarrhea, stomach pain, bloating and gas. Lactase supplements can break down lactose and relieve symptoms related to lactose intolerance. Lactase supplements are available without a prescription from many different manufacturers.

What should my health care professional know before I take lactase?

They need to know if you have any of these conditions:

- phenylketonuria (chewable lactase tablets may contain phenylalanine)
- an unusual or allergic reaction to lactase, other medicines, foods, dyes, or preservatives
- pregnant or trying to become pregnant
- breast-feeding

How should this medicine be taken?

Take lactase chewable tablets, tablets, caplets, or capsules by mouth with the first bite of a meal or drink that contains dairy products. Chewable tablets may be chewed prior to swallowing. You may take lactase with each dairy-containing meal or drink. Do not take lactase too early or the stomach will breakdown the enzyme and it will not be effective. It may take a trial to see what dose of lactase reduces your symptoms best. Contact your pediatrician or health care professional regarding the use of this medicine in children. Special care may be needed.

What if I miss a dose?

Missing a dose is not harmful, but you may experience lactose intolerance symptoms to some degree if the meal contains dairy foods. If you forget to take lactase with the first bite of food, you can take it during the meal.

What may interact with lactase?

- No drug interactions have been documented between lactase and other medications

Tell your prescriber or health care professional about all other medicines that you are taking, including non-prescription medicines, nutritional supplements, or herbal products. Also tell your prescriber or health care professional if you are a frequent use of drinks with caffeine or alcohol, if you smoke, or if you use illegal drugs. These may affect the way your medicine works. Check with your health care professional before stopping or starting any of your medicines.

What should I watch for while taking lactase?

Lactase should decrease symptoms of lactose intolerance such as diarrhea, stomach pain, bloating and gas. Consult your health care professional should you experience unusual symptoms.

What side effects may I notice from taking lactase?

Side effects that you should report to your prescriber or health care professional as soon as possible:

- there are no known serious side effects from taking lactase

Side effects that usually do not require medical attention (report to your prescriber or health care professional if they continue or are bothersome):

- report any perceived unusual effects

Where can I keep my medicine?

Keep out of the reach of children in a container that small children cannot open. Store at room temperature below 25 degrees C (77 degrees F). Do not refrigerate. Keep away from heat. Throw away any unused medicine after the expiration date.

Lactobacillus capsules, chewable tablets, granules, or tablets

BACID®;
Tablet
Becton Dickinson

BACID®;
Granule
Becton Dickinson

What are *Lactobacillus* capsules, chewable tablets, granules, or tablets?

LACTOBACILLUS products (Bacid®, Culturelle®, DDS®-Acidophilus, Lactinex®, MoreDophilus®, Primadophilus Reuteri™) contain a harmless bacteria that helps to reestablish the bacteria in the human colon. Products may contain one or more of the following bacteria: *Lactobacillus acidophilus*, *Lactobacillus bulgaricus*, *Lactobacillus rhamnosus* GG, or *Lactobacillus reuteri*. These products are considered dietary supplements by the FDA. They are used to treat or prevent diarrhea caused by an infection or by antibiotics. Various brand name products are available.

What should my health care professional know before I take *Lactobacillus*?

They need to know if you have any of these conditions:
- chronic disease or suppressed immune system
- prosthetic heart valve or valvular heart disease
- an unusual reaction to *Lactobacillus*, any medicines, lactose or milk, other foods, dyes, or preservatives
- pregnant or trying to get pregnant
- breast-feeding

How should this medicine be used?

Lactobacillus products are taken by mouth. Follow the directions on the label. The capsules, chewable tablets, and tablets should be taken with a small amount of milk, fruit juice, or water. The granules should be added to or taken with cereal, food, milk, fruit juice, or water. Over-the-counter (OTC) *Lactobacillus* products are not recommended for children under 3 years unless prescribed by a doctor. Contact your pediatrician or health care professional regarding the use of this medicine in children. Special care may be needed.

What if I miss a dose?

If you miss a dose, take it as soon as you can. If it is almost time for your next dose, take only that dose. Do not take double or extra doses.

What may interact with *Lactobacillus*?

There are no known interactions of *Lactobacillus* products with food, beverages, or other medications.

Tell your prescriber or health care professional about all other medicines you are taking, including non-prescription medicines, nutritional supplements, or herbal products. Also tell your prescriber or health care professional if you are a frequent user of drinks with caffeine or alcohol, if you smoke, or if you use illegal drugs. These may affect the way your medicine works. Check with your health care professional before stopping or starting any of your medicines.

What should I watch for while taking *Lactobacillus*?

If you have allergies to milk or you are sensitive to lactose, avoid using *Lactobacillus* products. Stop using immediately if you develop signs of an allergic reaction such as skin rash or difficulty breathing; contact your health care provider immediately. Do not use for more than 2 days unless directed by your doctor. Do not use if you have a high fever; see your health care provider for advice.

What side effects may I notice from taking *Lactobacillus*?

Side effects that you should report to your prescriber or health care professional as soon as possible:
- difficulty breathing or tightness in the chest or throat
- skin rash, hives, or severe itching
- severe nausea or vomiting
- unusual tiredness or weakness

Side effects that usually do not require medical attention (report to your prescriber or health care professional if they continue or are bothersome):
- constipation
- flatulence
- hiccups

Where can I keep my medicine?

Keep out of the reach of children in a container that small children cannot open. Most *Lactobacillus* products require refrigeration to maintain potency. Read the label for the specific product you are using. Do not freeze. Throw away any unused product after the expiration date.

L

Lamivudine, 3TC tablets

EPIVIR®;
150 mg; Tablet
Physicians Total Care Inc

EPIVIR-HBV®;
100 mg; Tablet
Glaxo Wellcome

What are lamivudine tablets?

LAMIVUDINE, 3TC (Epivir®, Epivir-HBV®) is an antiviral drug called a nucleoside reverse transcriptase inhibitor or NRTI. Lamivudine is used to treat infections due to hepatitis B and human immunodeficiency virus (HIV). When used for hepatitis B, lamivudine can slow the damage to your liver. When used for HIV lamivudine may reduce the amount of HIV in the blood and increase the number of CD4 cells (T-cells) in the blood. When used to treat HIV, lamivudine is used in combination with other medicines for HIV. Lamivudine will not cure or prevent hepatitis B infection, HIV infection, or AIDS. You may still develop other infections or conditions associated with your infection. Generic lamivudine tablets are not yet available.

What should my health care professional know before I take lamivudine?

They need to know if you have any of these conditions:

- if you frequently drink alcohol-containing beverages
- kidney disease
- organ transplant
- other liver disease
- pancreatitis
- tingling or numbness in the hands or feet
- an unusual or allergic reaction to lamivudine, other medicines, foods, dyes, or preservatives
- pregnant or trying to get pregnant
- breast-feeding

How should I take this medicine?

Take lamivudine tablets by mouth. Follow the directions on the prescription label. Swallow tablets with a drink of water. If lamivudine upsets your stomach, you can take it with food. If you find it difficult to swallow the tablets, ask your prescriber or health care professional if you can take lamivudine oral solution. Take your doses at regular intervals. Do not take your medicine more often than directed. To help to make sure that your anti-HIV therapy works as well as possible, be very careful to take all of your medicine exactly as prescribed. Do not stop taking except on your prescriber's advice. Contact your pediatrician or health care professional regarding the use of this medicine in children. Special care may be needed.

What if I miss a dose?

If you miss a dose, take it as soon as you can. If it is almost time for your next dose, take only that dose. Do not take double or extra doses.

What may interact with lamivudine?

- amiloride
- dofetilide
- entecavir
- indinavir
- metformin
- memantine
- procainamide
- ribavirin
- sulfamethoxazole; trimethoprim, SMX-TMP (Bactrim®, Septra®)
- trimethoprim
- zalcitabine, ddC

Epivir-HBV® tablets contain a lower dose of the same drug (lamivudine) as Epivir® Oral solution and tablets, Combivir®, and Trizivir®; therefore, Epivir-HBV® tablets should not be taken with any of these products. Discuss any changes in your treatment with your health care provider.

Tell your prescriber or health care professional about all other medicines you are taking, including non-prescription medicines, nutritional supplements, or herbal products. Also tell your prescriber or health care professional if you are a frequent user of drinks with caffeine or alcohol, if you smoke, or if you use illegal drugs. These may affect the way your medicine works. Check with your health care professional before stopping or starting any of your medicines.

What should I watch for while taking lamivudine?

Visit your prescriber or health care professional for regular checks on your progress. Discuss any new symptoms with your prescriber or health care professional. Lamivudine will not cure HIV or hepatitis B infection and you can still get other illnesses or complications associated with your disease. Taking lamivudine does not reduce the risk of passing HIV or hepatitis B infection to others through sexual or blood contact. It is best to avoid sexual contact so that you do not spread the disease to others. For any sexual contact, use a condom. Be careful about cuts, abrasions and other possible sources of blood contact. Never share a needle or syringe with anyone. The doses of lamivudine are different depending upon the disease for which you are being treated. If you are receiving lamivudine for hepatitis B infection only, you should be tested for HIV prior to starting and during treatment to avoid inappropriate therapy for HIV. Patients with both HIV and hepatitis B who are planning to change their HIV treatment regimen to a regimen that does not contain lamivudine should discuss continued therapy for hepatitis B with their prescriber or health care professional. Some people have worsening of hepatitis after stopping lamivudine therapy. Tell your prescriber or health care professional if you get tingling, pain or numbness in your hands or feet. Tell your prescriber or health care professional at once, especially for children less than

12 years of age, if you have nausea and vomiting accompanied by severe stomach pain.

What side effects may I notice from taking lamivudine?

Side effects that you should report to your prescriber or health care professional as soon as possible:
- breathing difficulties or shortness of breath
- changes in body appearance (weight gain around waist and/or face)
- dizziness
- muscle aches, pains, or weakness
- pain, tingling, or numbness in the hands or feet
- passing out or fainting
- severe vomiting or diarrhea
- slow or irregular heartbeat
- symptoms of high blood sugar: dizziness, dry mouth, flushed dry skin, fruit-like breath odor, loss of appetite, nausea, stomachache, unusual thirst, frequent passing of urine
- unusual stomach pain or discomfort
- unusual weakness, fatigue or discomfort
- worsening jaundice or other signs of hepatitis

Side effects that usually do not require medical attention (report to your prescriber or health care professional if they continue or are bothersome):
- cough
- diarrhea
- nausea, vomiting
- difficulty sleeping
- hair loss
- headache
- runny or stuffy nose
- skin rash

Where can I keep my medicine?

Keep out of the reach of children in a container that small children cannot open. Store between 2 and 30 degrees C (36 and 86 degrees F). Keep the container tightly closed. Throw away any unused medicine after the expiration date.

Lamivudine, 3TC; Zidovudine, ZDV tablets

COMBIVIR®;
150 mg / 300 mg ; Tablet
Glaxo Wellcome Division

What are Lamivudine; Zidovudine tablets?

LAMIVUDINE, 3TC; ZIDOVUDINE, ZDV TABLETS (Combivir®) is a combination of two antiviral drugs in one tablet. Combivir® can slow down the damage caused by the human immunodeficiency virus (HIV), the virus that causes acquired immune deficiency syndrome (AIDS). The amount of HIV virus in the blood is called "viral load." Lamivudine; Zidovudine can reduce the viral load, especially when combined with another anti-HIV drug. Lamivudine; Zidovudine will not cure or prevent HIV infection or AIDS. Generic lamivudine/zidovudine combination tablets are not yet available.

What should my health care professional know before I take Lamivudine; Zidovudine?

They need to know if you have any of these conditions:
- dental problems
- kidney disease
- liver disease
- pancreatitis
- tingling or numbness in the hands or feet
- an unusual or allergic reaction to lamivudine, zidovudine, other medicines, foods, dyes, or preservatives
- pregnant or trying to get pregnant
- breast-feeding

How should I take this medicine?

Take Combivir® tablets by mouth. Follow the directions on the prescription label. Swallow the tablets with a drink of water. You can take Combivir® with or without food. Take your doses at regular intervals.

Do not take your medicine more often than directed. It is very important that you take this medicine exactly as instructed by your prescriber or health care professional. Try not to miss any doses of Combivir®. Also, do not stop taking this medicine unless you are told to stop by your prescriber or health care professional. Contact your pediatrician or health care professional regarding the use of this medicine in children. Special care may be needed.

What if I miss a dose?

If you miss a dose, take it as soon as you can. If it is almost time for your next dose, take only that dose. Do not take double or extra doses.

What may interact with Lamivudine; Zidovudine?

- atovaquone
- fluconazole
- interferon
- probenecid
- valproic acid
- zalcitabine, ddC

Tell your prescriber or health care professional about all other medicines you are taking, including nonprescription medicines, nutritional supplements, or herbal products. Also tell your prescriber or health care professional if you are a frequent user of drinks with caffeine or alcohol, if you smoke, or if you use illegal drugs. These may affect the way your medicine works.

L

Check with your health care professional before stopping or starting any of your medicines.

What should I watch for while taking Lamivudine; Zidovudine?

You must visit your prescriber or health care professional for regular checks on your progress. Combivir® will not cure HIV infection and you can still get other illnesses associated with HIV. Tell your prescriber or health care professional if you get tingling, pain or numbness in your hands or feet. Tell your prescriber or health care professional at once if you have nausea and vomiting accompanied by severe stomach pain. Combivir® can cause blood problems. This can mean slow healing and a risk of infection. Try to avoid cutting or injuring yourself. Problems can arise if you need dental work, and in the day to day care of your teeth. Try to avoid damage to your teeth and gums when you brush or floss your teeth. Your prescriber or health care professional will check your blood counts while you are receiving Combivir®. It is very important that you keep any appointments that are scheduled by your prescriber or health care professional. Taking Combivir® does not reduce the risk of passing HIV infection to others through sexual or blood contact. It is best to avoid sexual contact so that you do not spread the disease to others. For any sexual contact, use a condom. Be careful about cuts, abrasions and other possible sources of blood contact. Never share a needle or syringe with anyone.

What side effects may I notice from taking Combivir®?

Side effects that you should report to your prescriber or health care professional as soon as possible:
- depression
- dizziness
- fever or chills, sore throat
- loss of appetite
- muscle pain or weakness
- nausea, vomiting
- pain, tingling, or numbness in the hands or feet
- shortness of breath
- unusual bleeding or bruising
- unusual tiredness or weakness

Side effects that usually do not require medical attention (report to your prescriber or health care professional if they continue or are bothersome):
- change in nail color
- cough
- diarrhea
- difficulty sleeping
- headache
- runny or stuffy nose
- skin rash
- tiredness
- upset stomach

Where can I keep my medicine?

Keep out of the reach of children in a container that small children cannot open. Store between 2 and 30 degrees C (36 and 86 degrees F). Keep the container tightly closed. Throw away any unused medicine after the expiration date.

Lamotrigine tablets or chewable tablets

LAMICTAL®;
200 mg; Tablet
Glaxo Wellcome
Division

LAMICTAL®;
100 mg; Tablet
Glaxo Wellcome
Division

What are lamotrigine tablets or chewable tablets?

LAMOTRIGINE (Lamictal®) is effective in helping to control partial seizures (convulsions) in adults and children with epilepsy. Lamotrigine is also used in adults and children who have generalized (major) seizures (convulsions) due to a special condition named Lennox-Gastaut syndrome. Lamotrigine is usually prescribed with other medications that also help to control the convulsions, although sometimes lamotrigine may be used by itself. Generic lamotrigine tablets are not yet available.

What should my health care professional know before I take lamotrigine?

They need to know if you have any of these conditions:
- folate deficiency
- kidney disease
- liver disease
- an unusual or allergic reaction (including rash) to lamotrigine, other medicines, foods, dyes, or preservatives

- pregnant or trying to get pregnant
- breast-feeding

How should I take this medicine?

If you take regular Lamictal® tablets: Take lamotrigine tablets by mouth. Follow the directions on the prescription label. Swallow the tablets with a drink of water. Do not chew these tablets—they have a bitter taste. If lamotrigine upsets your stomach, take it with food or milk. Take your doses at regular intervals. Do not take your medicine more often than directed.
If you take Lamictal® chewable dispersible tablets: Take these lamotrigine tablets by mouth. These tablets may be swallowed whole, chewed, mixed in water, or in diluted fruit juice to aid swallowing. To mix the tablets in water or juice, add the tablets to a small amount of liquid (enough to cover the medication) in a glass or spoon. The tablets will dissolve in about 1 minute. Once dissolved, mix or swirl the liquid and take the entire solution immediately. It is important that you swallow all of the liquid used to prepare the

dose, so that the full prescribed dose is given. Take your doses at regular intervals. Do not take your medicine more often than directed.

Contact your pediatrician or health care professional regarding the use of this medication in children. Special care may be needed.

What if I miss a dose?

If you miss a dose, take it as soon as you can. If it is almost time for your next dose, take only that dose. Do not take double or extra doses.

What may interact with lamotrigine?

- acetaminophen (e.g. Tylenol®)
- bosentan
- carbamazepine
- medicines used to treat HIV or AIDS infection (examples: indinavir, ritonavir)
- methotrexate
- phenobarbital
- phenytoin
- primidone
- pyrimethamine
- rifampin
- trimethoprim
- valproic acid

Tell your prescriber or health care professional about all other medicines you are taking, including non-prescription medicines, nutritional supplements, or herbal products. Also tell your prescriber or health care professional if you are a frequent user of drinks with caffeine or alcohol, if you smoke, or if you use illegal drugs. These may affect the way your medicine works. Check with your health care professional before stopping or starting any of your medicines.

What should I watch for while taking lamotrigine?

Visit your prescriber or health care professional for a regular check on your progress. Wear a Medic Alert bracelet or necklace. Carry an identification card with information about your condition, medications, and prescriber or health care professional. It is important to take lamotrigine exactly as instructed by your health care professional. When first starting lamotrigine treatment, you prescriber will have to adjust your dosage slowly, and it may take weeks or months before your dose is stable. You should contact your prescriber or health care professional if your seizures get worse or if you have any new types of seizures. Do not stop taking lamotrigine or any of your seizure medicines unless instructed by your prescriber or health care professional. Stopping your medicine suddenly can increase your seizures or their severity. You may get drowsy, dizzy (more common in women than in men), or have blurred vision. Do not drive, use machinery, or do anything that needs mental alertness until you know how lamotrigine affects you. To reduce dizzy or fainting spells, do not sit or stand up quickly, especially if you are an older

patient. Alcohol can increase drowsiness and dizziness. Avoid alcoholic drinks or medicines containing alcohol. If you are going to have surgery, tell your prescriber or health care professional that you are taking lamotrigine.

What side effects may I notice from taking lamotrigine?

Most people who take lamotrigine tolerate it well. The most common side effects are dizziness, drowsiness, headache, blurred vision, nausea, and rash. If a skin rash occurs at any time while taking lamotrigine, contact your prescriber immediately. Rashes may be very severe and sometimes requires being treatment in the hospital. Deaths from rashes have occurred. Serious rashes occur more often in children than adults taking lamotrigine. It is more common for these serious rashes to occur during the first 2 months of treatment, but a rash can occur at any time.

Side effects that you should report to your prescriber or health care professional immediately:
- fever
- painful sores in the mouth, eyes, or nose
- redness, blistering, peeling or loosening of the skin, including inside the mouth
- skin rash of any type, itching
- swelling of the face, lips or tongue
- swollen lymph glands

Side effects you should report to your prescriber or health care professional as soon as possible:
- blurred, or double vision
- changes in seizure type or frequency
- depression, or mood changes
- difficulty walking or controlling muscle movements
- uncontrollable eye movements
- unusual weakness or tiredness

Side effects that usually do not require medical attention (report to your prescriber or health care professional if they continue or are bothersome):
- back pain, joint aches and pains
- diarrhea, or constipation
- difficulty sleeping
- dizziness, drowsiness
- dry mouth
- headache
- hot flashes
- loss of appetite
- menstrual disorder
- nausea, vomiting
- slurred speech
- stomach upset, indigestion
- stuffy, runny nose
- tremor

Where can I keep my medicine?

Keep out of reach of children in a container that small children cannot open. Store at room temperature between 15 and 30 degrees C (59 and 86 degrees F). Throw away any unused medicine after the expiration date.

L

Lansoprazole capsules and disintegrating tablets

PREVACID®;
30 mg; Capsule,
Delayed Release
Tap Pharmaceuticals
Inc

PREVACID®
SOLUTAB™;
30 mg; Tablet,
Orally
Disintegrating
Tap Pharmaceuticals
Inc

What are lansoprazole capsules or disintegrating tablets?

LANSOPRAZOLE (Prevacid®, Prevacid® Solutab™) prevents the production of acid in the stomach. It reduces symptoms and prevents injury to the esophagus or stomach in patients with gastroesophageal reflux disease (GERD) or ulcers. Lansoprazole is also useful in conditions that produce too much stomach acid such as Zollinger-Ellison syndrome. Generic lansoprazole capsules or disintegrating tablets are not yet available.

What should my health care professional know before I take lansoprazole?

They need to know if you have any of these conditions:
- liver disease
- an unusual or allergic reaction to lansoprazole, other medicines, foods, dyes, or preservatives
- pregnant or trying to get pregnant
- breast-feeding

How should I take this medicine?

Capsules

Take lansoprazole capsules by mouth. Follow the directions on the prescription label. Swallow the capsules whole with a drink of water; do not crush or chew. Lansoprazole works best if taken on an empty stomach. It is best to take the capsules 30 to 60 minutes before food. Take your doses at regular intervals. Do not take your medicine more often than directed. If you have difficulty swallowing the capsules, you may open the Prevacid® capsule and sprinkle the contents on a tablespoon of any of the following foods: applesauce, pudding, cottage cheese, yogurt, or a spoonful of Ensure® drink. Do not crush the contents of the capsule into the food. Swallow the dose immediately after preparing it; do not chew. Follow with a drink of water. Contact your pediatrician or health care professional regarding the use of this medicine in children. Special care may be needed.

Disintegrating Tablets

Take lansoprazole disintegrating tablets by mouth. Follow the directions on the prescription label. Place the tablet on your tongue and allow it to dissolve in your mouth. The tablet will dissolve rapidly, usually in less than one minute. Swallow the medicine once completely dissolved. Do not swallow the tablets whole or chew them. Take your doses at regular intervals. Do not take your medicine more often than directed. Contact your pediatrician or health care professional re-

garding use of this medicine in children. Special care may be needed.

What if I miss a dose?

If you miss a dose, take it as soon as you can. If it is almost time for your next dose, take only that dose. Do not take double or extra doses.

What may interact with lansoprazole?

- ampicillin
- bisacodyl
- delavirdine
- digoxin
- fluvoxamine
- iron salts
- itraconazole
- ketoconazole
- sucralfate
- theophylline
- voriconazole

Tell your prescriber or health care professional about all other medicines you are taking, including non-prescription medicines, nutritional supplements, or herbal products. Also tell your prescriber or health care professional if you are a frequent user of drinks with caffeine or alcohol, if you smoke, or if you use illegal drugs. These may affect the way your medicine works. Check with your health care professional before stopping or starting any of your medicines.

What should I watch for while taking lansoprazole?

It can take several days of therapy with lansoprazole before your stomach pains improve. Check with your prescriber or health care professional if your condition does not improve, or if it gets worse. You can take antacids for the occasional relief of pain unless your prescriber or health care professional tells you otherwise.

What side effects may I notice from taking lansoprazole?

Side effects that you should report to your prescriber or health care professional as soon as possible.
Rare or uncommon:
- dark yellow or brown urine
- fever or sore throat
- unusual skin rash, blistering, or peeling
- unusual bleeding or bruising
- yellowing of the eyes or skin
- vomiting

Side effects that usually do not require medical attention (report to your prescriber or health care professional if they continue or are bothersome):

- abdominal pain
- diarrhea or constipation
- headache
- nausea

Lansoprazole; Naproxen tablets and capsules

PREVACID® NAPRAPAC™ 500;
15 mg/500 mg;
Tap Pharmaceuticals Inc

What are lansoprazole; naproxen tablets and capsules?

NAPROXEN; LANSOPRAZOLE (Prevacid® NapraPAC™) is a combination of medications used to treat pain associated with osteoarthritis, rheumatoid arthritis, or ankylosing spondylitis. The Prevacid® NapraPAC™ "kit" contains Naprosyn® (naproxen tablets), and Prevacid® (lansoprazole capsules) packaged together. Generic Prevacid® NapraPAC™ therapy kits are not available.

What should my health care professional know before I take lansoprazole; naproxen?

They need to know if you have any of these conditions:

- anemia
- asthma, especially aspirin sensitive asthma
- bleeding problems or taking medicines that make you bleed easily such as anticoagulants ("blood thinners")
- cigarette smoker
- diabetes
- drink more than 3 alcohol-containing beverages a day
- heart failure
- high blood pressure
- kidney disease
- liver disease
- stomach or duodenal ulcers
- systemic lupus erythematosus
- ulcerative colitis
- an unusual or allergic reaction to naprosyn, aspirin or other NSAIDs, lansoprazole or other proton pump inhibitors, other medicines, foods, dyes, or preservatives
- pregnant or trying to get pregnant
- breast-feeding

How should this medicine be used?

Each daily "dose" of Prevacid® NapraPAC™ contains three pills: one pink and green capsule (Prevacid®) and two pink tablets (Naprosyn® 375) or two yellow tablets (Naprosyn® 500). One tablet should be taken in the morning before breakfast along with the capsule. The other tablet should be taken in the early evening. Follow the directions on the prescription label. Swallow capsules and tablets whole with a drink of water; do not crush or chew. Take your doses at regular intervals. Do not take your medicine more often than directed. Contact your pediatrician or health care profes-

sional regarding the use of this medicine in children. Special care may be needed.

What if I miss a dose?

If you miss a dose, take it as soon as you can. If it is almost time for your next dose, take only that dose. Do not take double or extra doses.

What may interact with lansoprazole; naproxen?

- alcohol
- alendronate
- ampicillin
- aspirin and aspirin-like medicines
- cidofovir
- cyclosporine
- delavirdine
- digoxin
- entecavir
- fluvoxamine
- gefitinib
- herbal products that contain feverfew, garlic, ginger, or ginkgo biloba
- iron salts
- itraconazole
- ketoconazole
- lithium
- medicines for high blood pressure
- medicines that affect platelets
- medicines that treat or prevent blood clots such as warfarin and other "blood thinners"
- methotrexate
- other anti-inflammatory drugs (such as ibuprofen, naproxen or prednisone)
- pemetrexed
- sucralfate
- theophylline
- voriconazole
- water pills (diuretics)

Tell your prescriber or health care professional about all other medicines you are taking, including non-prescription medicines, nutritional supplements, or herbal products. Also tell your prescriber or health care professional if you are a frequent user of drinks with caffeine or alcohol, if you smoke, or if you use illegal drugs. These may affect the way your medicine works. Check

Where can I keep my medicine?

Keep out of the reach of children in a container that small children cannot open. Store at room temperature between 15 and 30 degrees C (59 and 86 degrees F). Protect from moisture. Throw away any unused medicine after the expiration date.

L

with your health care professional before stopping or starting any of your medicines.

What should I watch for while taking lansoprazole; naproxen?

Do not smoke cigarettes or drink alcohol; these increase irritation of your stomach and can make your stomach more susceptible to damage from naproxen. Let your prescriber or health care professional know if you develop stomach or throat pain. Do not take lansoprazole; naproxen with other pain-killers without advice. Naproxen is available over-the-counter without a prescription. Do not take any prescription or over-the-counter product without talking to your health care professional. To reduce unpleasant effects on your throat and stomach, do not take lansoprazole; naproxen just before lying down. If you notice black, tarry stools or experience severe stomach pain and vomit blood or what looks like coffee grounds, notify your health care prescriber immediately. If you are taking medicines that affect the clotting of your blood, such as aspirin or blood thinners such as Coumadin®, talk to your health care provider or prescriber before taking this medicine. You may get dizzy or sleepy. Do not drive, use machinery, or do anything that needs mental alertness until you know how lansoprazole; naproxen affects you. Stand or sit up slowly, this reduces the risk of dizzy or fainting spells. These effects may be worse if you are an older patient. It is especially important not to use lansoprazole; naproxen during the last 3 months of pregnancy unless specifically directed to do so by your health care provider. Problems in the unborn child or complications during delivery could occur. If you are going to have surgery or dental work, tell your prescriber or health care professional that you are taking lansoprazole; naproxen. Brush and floss your teeth and gums gently.

What side effects may I notice from taking lansoprazole; naproxen?

Side effects that you should report to your prescriber or health care professional as soon as possible:

- signs of bleeding—bruising, pinpoint red spots on the skin, black tarry stools, blood in the urine, unusual tiredness or weakness, vomiting blood or vomit that looks like coffee grounds
- signs of an allergic reaction—difficulty breathing or wheezing, skin rash, redness, blistering or peeling skin, hives, or itching, swelling of eyelids, throat, lips
- blurred vision
- change in the amount of urine passed
- difficulty swallowing, severe heartburn or burning, pain in throat
- fever
- pain or difficulty passing urine
- stomach pain, cramps, or vomiting
- ringing sound in your ears or hearing loss
- swelling of feet or ankles
- yellowing of eyes or skin

Side effects that usually do not require medical attention (report to your prescriber or health care professional if they continue or are bothersome):

- diarrhea or constipation
- dizziness
- drowsiness
- headache
- nausea

Where can I keep my medicine?

Keep out of the reach of children in the original container. Store at room temperature between 15 and 30 degrees C (59 and 86 degrees F). Protect from light and moisture. Throw away any unused medicine after the expiration date.

Lanthanum Carbonate chewable tablets

FOSRENOL®;
500 mg; Tablet
Shire Biologics, Div Shire
Biochem Inc

What are lanthanum carbonate chewable tablets?

LANTHANUM CARBONATE (Fosrenol®) helps decrease the amount of phosphate in your blood that may build up due to kidney disease. Generic lanthanum carbonate chewable tablets are not available.

What should my health care professional know before I take lanthanum carbonate?

They need to know if you have any of these conditions:

- stomach or intestinal problems (such as stomach or intestinal obstruction, Crohn's disease, ulcerative colitis, or peptic ulcer disease)
- an unusual reaction to lanthanum carbonate, other medicines, foods, dyes, or preservatives
- pregnant or trying to get pregnant
- breast-feeding

How should this medicine be used?

Chew the lanthanum carbonate chewable tablets completely, then swallow. The chewable tablets should never be swallowed whole. Take this medicine with meals. Follow the directions on the prescription label. Take your doses at regular intervals. Do not take your medicine more often than directed. Contact your pediatrician or health care professional regarding the use of this medicine in children. Special care may be needed.

What if I miss a dose?

If you miss a dose, take it as soon as you can. If it is almost time for your next dose, take only that dose. Do not take double or extra doses.

What may interact with lanthanum carbonate?

Tell your prescriber or health care professional about all other medicines you are taking, including non-prescription medicines, nutritional supplements, or herbal products. Also tell your prescriber or health care professional if you are a frequent user of drinks with caffeine or alcohol, if you smoke, or if you use illegal drugs. These may affect the way your medicine works. Check with your health care professional before stopping or starting any of your medicines.

What should I watch for while taking lanthanum carbonate?

Visit your prescriber or health care professional for regular checks on your progress. If you have bothersome stomach problems, feel unusually tired or weak, become confused or irritable, or develop a headache that does not get better. Make sure to take this medicine with or immediately after meals. Adhering to the diet prescribed by your physician will help with the phosphate-lowering benefits of this medicine.

What side effects may I notice from taking lanthanum carbonate?

Side effects that you should report to your prescriber or health care professional as soon as possible:

- drowsiness, dizziness, or fainting spells
- confusion or irritability
- nausea, vomiting
- loss of appetite
- headache

Side effects that usually do not require medical attention (report to your prescriber or health care professional if they continue or are bothersome):

- abdominal pain
- constipation
- diarrhea
- runny nose

Where can I keep my medicine?

Keep out of the reach of children in a container that small children cannot open. Store at room temperature of 20 to 25 degrees C (68 to 77 degrees F). Throw away any unused medicine after the expiration date.

Latanoprost; Timolol eye solution

XALATAN®; 0.005%; Solution Pharmacia and Upjohn Div Pfizer

XALATAN®; 0.005%; Solution Pharmacia and Upjohn Div Pfizer

What is latanoprost; timolol eye solution?

LATANOPROST; TIMOLOL (Xalatan®, Xalcom™) helps to reduce pressure inside the eye when it is elevated (ocular hypertension) or for patients with a certain type of glaucoma (open-angle glaucoma). Timolol belongs to a group of medicines called beta-blockers, while latanoprost is a prostaglandin. Generic latanoprost; timolol eye solution is not yet available.

What should my health care professional know before I use latanoprost; timolol?

They need to know if you have, or have had any of these conditions:

- angina (chest pain)
- asthma, bronchitis or bronchospasm, emphysema, COPD, or other lung disease
- closed-angle glaucoma
- contact lenses
- depression
- diabetes
- eye infection, irritation, or damage (such as corneal abrasion, iritis, keratitis)
- heart disease including heart failure, heart rhythm problems, or blood vessel disease (Raynaud's disease)
- kidney disease
- liver disease
- low blood pressure
- muscle weakness or disease (such as myasthenia gravis)
- pheochromocytoma
- stroke, cerebrovascular disease, or history of TIA (transient ischemic attack)
- thyroid disease
- an unusual or allergic reaction to latanoprost, timolol, or other medicines, foods, dyes, or preservatives
- pregnant or trying to get pregnant
- breast-feeding

How should I use this medicine?

Contact lenses should be removed prior to using latanoprost; timolol eye solution. Ask your health care professional regarding when you can reinsert your contact lenses after applying latanoprost; timolol eye drops. Latanoprost; timolol eye solution is only for use in the eye. Do not take by mouth. Follow the directions on the prescription label. Wash hands before and after use. Tilt the head back slightly and pull down the lower lid with your index finger to form a pouch. Try not to touch the tip of the dropper to your eye, fingertips, or any other surface. Squeeze the prescribed number of drops into the pouch. Close the eye for a few moments to spread the drops and apply gentle finger pressure to the inner corner of the eye (tear duct) for 1 to 2 minutes. Use your doses at regular intervals. Do not use your medicine more often than directed. Do not stop using except on your prescriber's advice. Contact your pediatrician or health care professional regarding the use of this medicine in children. Special care may be needed.

L

What if I miss a dose?

If you miss a dose, use it as soon as you can. If it is almost time for your next dose, use only that dose. Do not use double or extra doses.

What may interact with latanoprost; timolol?

Eye drops containing thimerosal can interact with latanoprost eye solution when given at the same time. Eye drops containing latanoprost should be given at least 5 minutes apart from eye drops containing thimerosal.

- atropine
- beta-blockers or calcium-channel blockers, often used for high blood pressure or heart problems
- cimetidine
- cevimeline
- clonidine
- diet drugs or stimulant drugs (such as ephedrine or amphetamine)
- medicines for high blood pressure
- medicines for colds, sinus problems, or breathing difficulties
- medicines for diabetes
- medicines for mental depression
- medicines for mental problems and psychotic disturbances
- medicines to control heart rhythm (such as amiodarone, digoxin, quinidine, and others)
- mefloquine
- thimerosal

If you are using another eye preparation for your eye condition, ask your health care professional regarding how long to wait before applying each product to the eyes after using the latanoprost; timolol eye drops. Do not use any other eye products with latanoprost; timolol without asking your prescriber or health care professional.

Tell your prescriber or health care professional about all other medicines you are taking, including non-prescription medicines, nutritional supplements, or herbal products. Also tell your prescriber or health care professional if you are a frequent user of drinks with caffeine or alcohol, if you smoke, or if you use illegal drugs. These may affect the way your medicine works. Check with your health care professional before stopping or starting any of your medicines.

What should I watch for while taking latanoprost; timolol?

Visit your prescriber or health care professional for regular eye pressure exams. Report any serious side effects promptly. Ask your prescriber or health care professional if you should continue to use latanoprost; timolol if you injure your eyes, get an eye infection, or need eye surgery. You may get drowsy or dizzy. Do not drive, use machinery, or do anything that requires mental alertness until you know how latanoprost; timolol affects you. To reduce the risk of dizzy or fainting spells, do not sit or stand up quickly. This medicine may cause your eye, eyelashes, and eyelids to change color (darkening or brown coloring). Tell your prescriber or health care professional if this occurs. These changes may be permanent. If you wear soft contact lenses, you should not put latanoprost; timolol eye drops in your eyes while wearing the lenses. Ask your prescriber or health care professional about how long you should wait before inserting your contact lenses after placing the latanoprost; timolol eye drops into the eye. Certain chemicals in the solution can be absorbed by contact lenses. Be careful not to touch the tip of the dispensing container onto the eye, or any other surface. Serious eye infections can result from contamination of eye solutions. If your eyes are more sensitive to light, stay out of bright light and wear dark sunglasses. If you are going to have surgery, tell your prescriber or health care professional that you are taking latanoprost; timolol.

What side effects may I notice from using latanoprost; timolol?

Side effects that you should report to your prescriber or health care professional as soon as possible:
- blurred vision or other changes in vision
- changes in the color of the eye (increase in brown color), or darkening of the eyelashes or eyelid
- confusion, hallucinations (seeing and hearing things that are not really there)
- difficulty breathing, shortness of breath, or wheezing
- difficulty sleeping, nightmares
- dizziness or fainting spells
- hives
- inflamed or infected eyes or eyelids
- irregular or slow heartbeat, fast heartbeat or palpitations, chest pain
- skin rash, peeling, blistering or loosening of skin
- swelling of the legs or ankles
- unusual weakness or tiredness

Side effects that usually do not require medical attention (report to your prescriber or health care professional if they continue or are bothersome):
- burning, stinging, itching or discomfort of the eyes or eyelids
- dry eyes, or the feeling of something in the eye
- headache
- increased flow of tears
- increased sensitivity of the eyes to light

Where can I keep my medicine?

Keep out of the reach of children in a container that small children cannot open. Ask your pharmacist regarding proper storage information of latanoprost; timolol.

Leflunomide tablets

ARAVA®;
20 mg; Tablet
Aventis
Pharmaceuticals Inc

ARAVA®;
10 mg; Tablet
Aventis
Pharmaceuticals Inc

What are leflunomide tablets?

LEFLUNOMIDE (Arava®) is a medication that reduces inflammation and swelling due to rheumatoid arthritis. The response of the immune system may contribute to rheumatoid arthritis. Leflunomide affects this system and is able to slow down the progression of the disease, especially in the affected joints. Leflunomide helps to treat all stages of adult rheumatoid arthritis. Leflunomide can be used with some of the other medications that are used to treat the inflammation and pain of this condition (for example, aspirin, other salicylates, or nonsteroidal anti-inflammatory drugs like ibuprofen). Generic leflunomide tablets are not yet available.

What should my health care professional know before I take leflunomide?

They need to know if you have, or have ever had, any of these conditions:
- an alcohol problem
- anemia or other blood disorders
- cancer or cancer treatments (radiation therapy)
- an immune deficiency (natural or due to cancer, cancer chemotherapy, infection with the HIV virus or AIDS, radiation, or steroid therapy)
- fever or infection
- high blood pressure
- kidney disease
- liver disease
- lung disease or breathing problems
- an unusual or allergic reaction to leflunomide, other medicines, foods, dyes, or preservatives
- pregnant or trying to get pregnant
- breast-feeding

How should I take this medicine?

Take leflunomide tablets by mouth. Follow the directions on the prescription label. Swallow the tablets with a drink of water. You can take leflunomide with food or milk. Take your doses at the same time every day. Do not take your medicine more often than directed. Continue to take your medicine even if you feel better. Do not stop taking your medicine unless your prescriber or health care professional tells you to discontinue taking it. Contact your pediatrician or health care professional regarding the use of this medicine in children. Special care may be needed.

What if I miss a dose?

If you miss a dose, take it as soon as you can. If it is almost time for your next dose, take only that dose. Do not take double or extra doses.

What may interact with leflunomide?

- some anti-inflammatory medicines
- azathioprine
- charcoal
- cholestyramine
- cyclosporine
- fos phenytoin
- isoniazid
- itraconazole
- ketoconazole
- methotrexate
- phenytoin
- rifampin
- some vaccines
- sulfasalazine
- tacrine
- troglitazone, and some other medicines for diabetes
- warfarin

Tell your prescriber or health care professional about all other medicines you are taking, including non-prescription medicines, nutritional supplements, or herbal products. Also tell your prescriber or health care professional if you are a frequent user of drinks with caffeine or alcohol, if you smoke, or if you use illegal drugs. These may affect the way your medicine works. Check with your health care professional before stopping or starting any of your medicines.

What should I watch for while taking leflunomide?

Visit your prescriber or health care professional for checks on your progress. A few side effects occur commonly with leflunomide. They include diarrhea, abdominal pain or nausea, rash, changes in hair texture or growth. In some persons, liver function can be altered. Sometimes the side effects can be more serious. Your prescriber or health care professional will be observing you closely and will monitor blood tests related to your medicine. You will need to have regular tests to see if your liver is working properly. The side effects of leflunomide can continue after you finish your treatment; report side effects promptly. If you are a woman who has the potential to become pregnant, it is important that you discuss birth control options with your prescriber or health care professional prior to taking leflunomide. You must not be pregnant and must be using a reliable form of birth control to prevent pregnancy. Leflunomide has the potential to harm an unborn baby. If you think that you might be pregnant at any time during your treatment with leflunomide, you should see your health care provider at once. While you are taking medications for rheumatoid arthritis you might be more susceptible to infection. Try to avoid people with colds, flu, and bronchitis. Do not have any vaccinations without your doctor's approval. Call your health care professional for advice if you get a fever, chills or sore throat, do not treat yourself. If you are

L

going to have surgery tell your doctor or dentist that you are taking leflunomide. Alcoholic drinks can make you more dizzy and increase possible damage to your liver. Avoid alcoholic drinks while taking leflunomide.

What side effects may I notice from taking leflunomide?

Side effects you should report to your prescriber or health care professional as soon as possible:

- dark yellow or brown urine
- diarrhea, especially if severe or does not stop
- difficulty breathing or shortness of breath
- dizziness
- fever or chills, cough or sore throat
- increases in blood pressure, especially if you are being treated for high blood pressure
- numbness, pain, or tingling in an arm, hand, leg, or foot
- pain in the stomach or abdomen
- skin rash or hives
- ulcers of the mouth or difficulty or pain on swallowing
- unusual bleeding or bruising, pinpoint red spots on the skin, nose bleeds or bleeding gums

- unusual tiredness or weakness
- vomiting
- yellowing of eyes or skin

Side effects that do usually do not require medical attention (report to your prescriber or health care professional if they continue or are bothersome):

- change in the taste of foods or drinks
- changes in the appearance of the fingernails or toenails
- hair loss (reversible)
- headache
- itching of the skin
- loss of appetite
- nausea, indigestion, or vomiting
- weight loss
- worsening of joint pain

Where can I keep my medicine?

Keep out of the reach of children in a container that small children cannot open. Store at room temperature between 15 and 30 degrees C (59 and 86 degrees F). Protect from moisture and light. Throw away any unused medicine after the expiration date.

Letrozole tablets

FEMARA®;
2.5 mg; Tablet
Novartis Pharmaceuticals

What are letrozole tablets?

LETROZOLE (Femara®) blocks the formation of the hormone estrogen. Some types of breast cancer need estrogen, and letrozole stops tumor growth by decreasing estrogen levels. Letrozole is for the treatment of breast cancer in postmenopausal women only. Generic letrozole tablets are not yet available.

What should my health care professional know before I take letrozole?

They need to know if you have any of these conditions:

- liver disease
- osteoporosis
- an unusual or allergic reaction to letrozole, other medicines, foods, dyes, or preservatives
- pregnant or trying to get pregnant
- breast-feeding

How should I take this medicine?

Take letrozole tablets by mouth at the same time each day. Follow the directions on the prescription label. Swallow the tablets with a drink of water. Do not take your medicine more often than directed. Do not stop taking except on your prescriber's advice. Contact your pediatrician or health care professional regarding the use of this medicine in children. Special care may be needed.

What if I miss a dose?

If you miss a dose, take it as soon as you can. If it is almost time for your next dose, take only that dose.

Do not take double or extra doses. If you vomit after taking a dose, call your prescriber or health care professional for advice.

What may interact with letrozole?

- androstenedione
- any medicine containing estrogens (this may include some herbal products and some birth control pills)
- DHEA

Tell your prescriber or health care professional about all other medicines you are taking, including non-prescription medicines, nutritional supplements, or herbal products. Also tell your prescriber or health care professional if you are a frequent user of drinks with caffeine or alcohol, if you smoke, or if you use illegal drugs. These may affect the way your medicine works. Check with your health care professional before stopping or starting any of your medicines.

What should I watch for while taking letrozole?

Visit your prescriber or health care professional for regular checks on your progress. Let your prescriber or health care professional know about any unusual vaginal bleeding. Do not treat yourself for diarrhea, nausea, vomiting or other side effects. Ask your prescriber or health care professional for advice.

What side effects may I notice from taking letrozole?

Side effects that you should report to your prescriber or health care professional as soon as possible:

- difficulty breathing
- chest pain
- leg pain or swelling
- skin rash

Side effects that usually do not require medical attention (report to your prescriber or health care professional if they continue or are bothersome):

- back or bone pain
- cough, or throat infection
- diarrhea or constipation
- dizziness
- headache
- hair loss

- hot flashes
- loss of appetite
- nausea, vomiting
- stomach pain or upset stomach
- sweating
- weakness or tiredness
- weight gain

Where can I keep my medicine?

Keep out of the reach of children in a container that small children cannot open. Store between 15 and 30 degrees C (59 and 86 degrees F). Throw away any unused medicine after the expiration date.

Leucovorin tablets

LEUCOVORIN;
5 mg; Tablet
Barr Laboratories
Inc

LEUCOVORIN;
5 mg; Tablet
Roxane Laboratories
Inc

What are leucovorin tablets?

LEUCOVORIN (Wellcovorin®) helps to prevent or treat some of the harmful effects of certain medicines, including methotrexate. Leucovorin can also treat certain kinds of anemia (low blood counts). Generic leucovorin tablets are available.

What should my health care professional know before I take leucovorin?

They need to know if you have any of these conditions:

- diarrhea
- mouth sores (stomatitis or mucositis)
- pernicious anemia or any other type of anemia
- vitamin B_{12} deficiency
- vomiting
- an unusual or allergic reaction to leucovorin, folic acid, other medicines, foods, dyes, or preservatives
- pregnant or trying to get pregnant
- breast-feeding

How should I take this medicine?

Take leucovorin tablets by mouth. Follow the directions on the prescription label. Swallow the tablets with a drink of water. Take your doses at regular intervals. Do not take your medicine more often than directed. It is very important to take this medicine exactly how it is prescribed. Do not stop taking except on your prescriber's advice even if you feel better.

What if I miss a dose?

Try not to miss any doses. If you do forget to take a dose or if you vomit after taking a dose, call your prescriber or health care professional for advice as soon as you can. Do not take double or extra doses unless your prescriber or health care professional tells you to.

What may interact with leucovorin?

- barbiturate medicines for inducing sleep or treating seizures
- phenytoin

Tell your prescriber or health care professional about all other medicines that you are taking, including non-prescription medicines, nutritional supplements, or herbal products. Also tell your prescriber or health care professional if you are a frequent user of drinks with caffeine or alcohol, if you smoke, or if you use illegal drugs. These may affect the way your medicine works. Check with your health care professional before stopping or starting any of your medicines.

What should I watch for while taking leucovorin?

Visit your prescriber or health care professional for regular checks on your progress. If you have nausea and vomit regularly talk to your prescriber or health care professional about the possibility of having injections of leucovorin instead of tablets. Do not stop taking leucovorin without your prescriber's advice.

What side effects may I notice from taking leucovorin?

Leucovorin has few side effects; they include:

- difficulty breathing
- skin rash, or itching

Where can I keep my medicine?

Keep out of the reach of children in a container that small children cannot open. Store at room temperature between 15 and 25 degrees C (59 and 77 degrees F). Protect from light and moisture. Throw away any unused medicine after the expiration date.

L

Levetiracetam tablets

KEPPRA®;
500 mg; Tablet
UCB Pharma Inc

KEPPRA®;
250 mg; Tablet
UCB Pharma Inc

What are levetiracetam tablets?

LEVETIRACETAM (Keppra®) is effective in helping to control partial seizures (convulsions). Levetiracetam is prescribed with other medications that also help to control the convulsions. Levetiracetam may occasionally be prescribed to help control other types of seizures. Generic levetiracetam tablets are not yet available.

What should my health care professional know before I take levetiracetam?

They need to know if you have any of these conditions:
- kidney disease
- an unusual or allergic reaction to levetiracetam, other medicines, foods, dyes, or preservatives
- pregnant or trying to get pregnant
- breast-feeding

How should I take this medicine?

Take levetiracetam tablets by mouth. Follow the directions on the prescription label. Swallow the tablets with a drink of water. You may take this medicine with food. The tablets may be crushed if they are difficult to swallow, but they will have a bitter taste. Take your doses at regular intervals. Do not take your medicine more often than directed. Contact your pediatrician or health care professional regarding the use of this medication in children. Special care may be needed.

What if I miss a dose?

If you miss a dose, take it as soon as you can. If it is almost time for your next dose, take only that dose. Do not take double or extra doses.

What may interact with levetiracetam?

Levetiracetam is unlikely to interact with other prescribed medications.

Tell your prescriber or health care professional about all other medicines you are taking, including non-prescription medicines, nutritional supplements, or herbal products. Also tell your prescriber or health care professional if you are a frequent user of drinks with caffeine or alcohol, if you smoke, or if you use illegal drugs. These may affect the way your medicine works. Check with your health care professional before stopping or starting any of your medicines.

What should I watch for while taking levetiracetam?

Visit your prescriber or health care professional for a regular check on your progress. Wear a Medic Alert bracelet or necklace. Carry an identification card with information about your condition, medications, and prescriber or health care professional. It is important to take levetiracetam exactly as instructed by your health care professional. When first starting levetiracetam treatment, you prescriber may have to adjust your dosage. It may take weeks or months before your dose is stable. You should contact your prescriber or health care professional if your seizures get worse or if you have any new types of seizures. Do not stop taking levetiracetam or any of your seizure medicines unless instructed by your prescriber or health care professional. Stopping your medicine suddenly can increase your seizures or their severity. You may get drowsy or dizzy. Do not drive, use machinery, or do anything that needs mental alertness until you know how levetiracetam affects you. To reduce dizzy spells, do not sit or stand up quickly, especially if you are an older patient. Alcohol can increase drowsiness and dizziness. Avoid alcoholic drinks or medicines containing alcohol. If you are going to have surgery, tell your prescriber or health care professional that you are taking levetiracetam.

What side effects may I notice from taking levetiracetam?

Side effects that you should report to your prescriber or health care professional immediately:
- difficulty breathing or tightening of the throat
- rash
- swelling of lips or tongue

Side effects you should report to your prescriber or health care professional as soon as possible:
- agitation, restlessness, irritability, or other changes in mood
- changes in seizure type or frequency
- difficulty walking or controlling muscle movements
- unusual weakness or tiredness

Side effects that usually do not require medical attention (report to your prescriber or health care professional if they continue or are bothersome):
- dizziness, drowsiness

Where can I keep my medicine?

Keep out of reach of children in a container that small children cannot open. Store at room temperature between 15 and 30 degrees C (59 and 86 degrees F). Throw away any unused medicine after the expiration date.

L

Levocarnitine tablets, capsules, and oral solution

CARNITOR®;
330 mg; Tablet
Sigma Tau Pharmaceuticals
Inc

What are levocarnitine tablets, capsules, and oral solution?

LEVOCARNITINE (Carnitor®) is a prescription nutritional supplement used to treat conditions of carnitine deficiency and various other conditions. Generic levocarnitine oral solution and tablets are available.

What should my health care professional know before I use levocarnitine?

They need to know if you have any of these conditions:
- history of seizures, or receiving any medications for the treatment of seizures.
- pregnant or trying to get pregnant
- breast-feeding
- heart disease
- liver disease
- kidney disease
- swollen ankles or problems with fluid retention
- history of headaches

How should I use this medicine?

Take levocarnitine capsules, tablets, and oral solution by mouth. Follow the directions on the prescription label. Swallow the capsules and tablets with a drink of water. Do not chew or open the capsules or tablets. Take the capsules, tablets or oral solution with food to lessen the risk of nausea/vomiting, diarrhea and upset stomach. The oral solution may be mixed with soft drink or juice. Take your doses at regular intervals. Levocarnitine is usually taken in 3 or 4 divided daily doses. Do not take your medicine more often than directed. Do not stop taking except on your prescriber's advice.

What if I miss a dose?

If you miss a dose, take a dose as soon as you can. If it is almost time for your next dose, use only that dose. Do not use double or extra doses without advice.

What may interact with levocarnitine?

- Prescription levocarnitine should not be taken with carnitine that is available at most health food stores.

Tell your prescriber or health care professional about all other medicines you are taking, including non-prescription medicines, nutritional supplements, or herbal products. Also tell your prescriber or health care professional if you are a frequent user of drinks with caffeine or alcohol, if you smoke, or if you use illegal drugs. These may affect the way your medicine works. Check with your health care professional before stopping or starting any of your medicines.

What should I watch for while taking levocarnitine?

Visit your prescriber or health care professional for checks on your progress. You will need to have regular blood checks. If you have kidney disease and are receiving levocarnitine injections, you should not try to treat your condition with levocarnitine capsules, tablets or solutions. These other formulations of levocarnitine may be harmful when you have kidney problems. Talk to your health care professional if you have questions.

What side effects may I notice from using levocarnitine?

Side effects that you should report to your prescriber or health care professional as soon as possible:
- diarrhea
- dizziness
- fast heart rate
- fever
- increased blood pressure
- seizures
- swollen ankles or problems with fluid retention
- tingling in the hands or feet

Side effects that usually do not require medical attention (report to your prescriber or health care professional if they continue or are bothersome):
- body odor
- nausea/vomiting
- upset stomach

Where can I keep my medicine?

Store at room temperature between 15 and 30 degrees C (59 and 86 degrees F). Avoid excessive heat above 40 degrees C (104 degrees F); do not freeze. Throw away any unused medicine after the expiration date. Keep out of the reach of children.

L

Levofloxacin tablets

LEVAQUIN®;
500 mg; Tablet
OMP Div, Ortho-
McNeil
Pharmaceuticals

LEVAQUIN®;
750 mg; Tablet
OMP Div, Ortho-
McNeil
Pharmaceuticals

What are levofloxacin tablets?

LEVOFLOXACIN (Levaquin®) is an antibiotic. Levofloxacin kills certain bacteria or stops their growth. It is used to treat urinary tract, prostate, skin, sinus and lung infections, as well as other infections. Generic levofloxacin tablets are not yet available.

What should my health care professional know before I take levofloxacin?

They need to know if you have any of these conditions:
- dehydration
- kidney disease
- seizures (convulsions)
- stomach problems (especially colitis)
- stroke
- an unusual or allergic reaction to fluoroquinolone antibiotics, foods, dyes, or preservatives
- pregnant or trying to get pregnant
- breast-feeding

How should I take this medicine?

Take levofloxacin tablets by mouth with or without food. Follow the directions on the prescription label. Swallow tablets whole with a full glass of water. Take your doses at regular intervals. Do not take your medicine more often than directed. Finish the full course prescribed by your prescriber or health care professional even if you think your condition is better. Do not stop taking except on your prescriber's advice. Contact your pediatrician or health care professional regarding the use of this medicine in children. Special care may be needed.

What if I miss a dose?

If you miss a dose, take it as soon as you remember. If it is almost time for your next dose, take only that dose. Do not take double or extra doses.

What may interact with levofloxacin?

- aluminum salts
- antacids
- arsenic trioxide
- astemizole
- bepridil
- calcium salts
- caffeine
- certain heart medications for irregular rhythm (e.g., amiodarone, disopyramide, dofetilide, ibutilide, quinidine, procainamide, sotalol)
- certain medicines for depression or mental problems (e.g., amoxapine, haloperidol, maprotiline, phenothiazines, risperidone, sertindole, ziprasidone)
- cimetidine
- cisapride
- clarithromycin
- cyclobenzaprine
- cyclosporine
- dairy products
- didanosine (ddI)
- dolasetron
- droperidol
- erythromycin
- levomethadyl
- iron (ferrous sulfate) preparations
- magnesium salicylate
- magnesium salts
- manganese
- medicines for diabetes
- multivitamins containing calcium, iron, manganese, or zinc
- NSAIDs such as Advil®, Aleve®, ibuprofen, Motrin®, naproxen
- pentamidine
- probucol
- retinoid products such as tretinoin (Retin-A®, Renova®) or isotretinoin (Accutane®)
- sevelamer
- sucralfate
- terfenadine
- theophylline
- troleandomycin
- warfarin
- zinc salts

Tell your prescriber or health care professional about all other medicines you are taking, including non-prescription medicines. Also tell your prescriber or health care professional if you are a frequent user of drinks with caffeine or alcohol, if you smoke, or if you use illegal drugs. These may affect the way your medicine works. Check with your health care professional before stopping or starting any of your medicines.

What should I watch for while taking levofloxacin?

Tell your prescriber or health care professional if your symptoms do not improve in 2 to 3 days. If you are a diabetic monitor your blood glucose carefully. If you get an unusual reaction stop taking levofloxacin and call your prescriber or health care professional for advice. You may get drowsy or dizzy. Do not drive, use machinery, or do anything that needs mental alertness until you know how levofloxacin affects you. To reduce the risk of dizzy or fainting spells, do not sit or stand up quickly, especially if you are an older patient. Drink several glasses of water a day. Cut down on drinks that contain caffeine. Antacids can stop levofloxacin from working. If you get an upset stomach and want to take an antacid, make sure it has been at least 2 hours since you last took levofloxacin, or at least 2 to 4 hours before your next dose. Calcium, iron, and zinc preparations can also stop levofloxacin from working properly. Take calcium tablets, iron tablets, zinc tablets, or vitamins that contain calcium, iron, or zinc at least 2 hours before or two hours after levofloxacin. Keep out of the sun, or wear protective clothing outdoors and use a sunscreen. Do not use sun lamps or sun tanning beds or booths. If you notice symptoms such as pain, burning, tingling, numbness and/or weakness, stop taking levofloxacin and contact your healthcare provider immediately. If you notice pain or swelling of a tendon or around a joint, stop taking levofloxacin. Call your healthcare provider. Rest the affected area. Do not exercise or take levofloxacin until your healthcare provider tells you to do so. If you are going to have surgery, tell your prescriber or health care professional that you are taking levofloxacin.

What side effects may I notice from taking levofloxacin?

Side effects that you should report to your prescriber or health care professional as soon as possible:
Rare or uncommon:
- confusion
- difficulty breathing
- irregular heartbeat, palpitations or chest pain
- joint, muscle or tendon pain

- nightmares
- changes in your thought process
- redness, blistering, peeling or loosening of the skin, including inside the mouth
- seizures
- severe or watery diarrhea
- skin rash, itching
- swelling of the face or neck
- tremor or restlessness
- vision changes
- vomiting

Side effects that usually do not require medical attention (report to your prescriber or health care professional if they continue or are bothersome):
- constipation or diarrhea
- difficulty sleeping
- dizziness or drowsiness
- headache
- intestinal gas or bloating
- nausea or stomach upset

Where can I keep my medicine?

Keep out of the reach of children in a container that small children cannot open. Store at room temperature between 25 and 30 degrees C (59 to 85 degrees F) and keep in a tightly closed container. Throw away any unused medicine after the expiration date.

Levothyroxine tablets

SYNTHROID®;
150 mg; Tablet
Abbott
Pharmaceutical
Product Division

LEVOXYL®;
0.1 mg; Tablet
Jones Pharma Inc
Sub King
Pharmaceuticals Inc

What are levothyroxine tablets?

LEVOTHYROXINE (Levothroid®, Levoxyl®, Levo-T®, Synthroid®, Unithroid®, and others) acts as a replacement for people whose thyroid gland does not produce enough thyroid hormone. Levothyroxine can improve symptoms of thyroid deficiency such as slow speech, lack of energy, weight gain, hair loss, dry thick skin and unusual sensitivity to cold. Levothyroxine also helps to treat a condition called goiter, which is an enlarged thyroid gland. Generic levothyroxine tablets are available.

What should my health care professional know before I take levothyroxine?

They need to know if you have any of these conditions:
- angina
- diabetes mellitus
- heart disease
- high blood pressure
- low levels of pituitary hormone
- dieting or on a weight loss program
- previous heart attack
- an unusual or allergic reaction to levothyroxine, other thyroid hormones, medicines, foods, dyes, or preservatives
- pregnant or trying to get pregnant

How should I take this medicine?

Take levothyroxine tablets by mouth 30 to 60 minutes before a meal (on an empty stomach) with a full glass of water. The doses should be taken at regular intervals as indicated on the medication label. Do not take your medication more often than directed. Contact your pediatrician or health care professional regarding the use of this medicine in children. Special care may be needed.

What if I miss a dose?

If you miss a dose, take it as soon as you can. If it is almost time for your next dose, take only that dose. Do not take double or extra doses.

What may interact with levothyroxine?

- amiodarone
- antacids
- calcium supplements, like Tums® and many others
- carbamazepine
- cholestyramine
- colestipol
- digoxin
- female hormones, including contraceptive or birth control pills
- ketamine
- medicines for colds and breathing difficulties

L

- medicines for diabetes
- medicines for mental depression
- medicines or herbals used to decrease weight or appetite
- phenobarbital or other barbiturate medications
- phenytoin
- prednisone or other corticosteroids
- rifabutin
- rifampin
- soy isoflavones
- sucralfate
- theophylline
- warfarin

Tell your prescriber or health care professional about all other medicines you are taking, including non-prescription medicines, nutritional supplements, or herbal products. Also tell your prescriber or health care professional if you are a frequent user of drinks with caffeine or alcohol, if you smoke, or if you use illegal drugs. These may affect the way your medicine works. Check with your health care professional before stopping or starting any of your medicines.

What should I watch for while taking levothyroxine?

If you are taking levothyroxine for an underactive thyroid, it may be several weeks before you notice an improvement. Check with your prescriber or health care professional if your symptoms do not improve or if you develop any of the above side effects. It may be necessary for you to take this medicine for the rest of your life; do not stop taking except on your prescriber's advice. Do not switch brands of levothyroxine unless your prescriber agrees with the change. Ask your prescriber or health care professional for advice if you are uncertain. Thyroid hormones can affect blood sugar levels. If you also have diabetes, you may need to adjust the dose of your diabetic medicine once you are stabilized on levothyroxine. You may lose some of your hair while using levothyroxine. With time, this usually corrects itself. If you are going to have surgery, tell your prescriber or health care professional that you are taking levothyroxine. Be sure to take your levothyroxine tablets with a full glass of water. Certain brands of levothyroxine tablets may rapidly swell and disintegrate, which causes choking, gagging, the tablet getting stuck in your throat, or difficulty swallowing. Most of these problems disappear when the tablets are taken with water.

What side effects may I notice from taking levothyroxine?

Side effects that you should report to your prescriber or health care professional as soon as possible:
- difficulty breathing, wheezing, or shortness of breath
- chest pain
- excessive sweating or intolerance to heat
- fast or irregular heartbeat or pulse rate
- nervousness
- skin rash or hives
- swelling of ankles, feet or legs

Side effects that usually do not require medical attention (report to your prescriber or health care professional if they continue or are bothersome):
- changes in appetite
- changes in menstrual periods
- diarrhea
- fever
- hair loss
- headache
- irritability
- leg cramps
- nausea, vomiting
- tremors
- trouble sleeping
- weight loss

Where can I keep my medicine?

Keep out of the reach of children in a container that small children cannot open. Store at room temperature between 15 and 30 degrees C (59 and 86 degrees F). Protect from light and moisture. Keep container tightly closed. Throw away any unused medicine after the expiration date.

L

Linezolid tablets

ZYVOX®;
600 mg; Tablet
Pharmacia and Upjohn Div
Pfizer

What are linezolid tablets?

LINEZOLID (Zyvox®) is an antibiotic. Linezolid kills or stops the growth of certain bacteria that cause certain infections. Linezolid is used to treat infections of the skin, bone, blood, lung and respiratory tract, and other tissues. Generic linezolid tablets are not yet available.

What should my health care professional know before I take linezolid?

They need to know if you have any of these conditions:
- frequently drink alcoholic beverages, including wine or beer
- anxiety disorder

- asthma or bronchitis
- diabetes
- headaches or migraine
- heart or blood vessel disease, or irregular heart beats
- high blood pressure
- kidney disease
- liver disease
- overactive thyroid
- Parkinson's disease
- pheochromocytoma
- recent head trauma
- seizures or convulsions
- schizophrenia, psychosis or mania
- stroke or other cerebrovascular disease
- an unusual or allergic reaction to linezolid, other antibiotics or other medicines, foods, dyes, or preservatives
- pregnant or trying to get pregnant
- breast-feeding

How should I take this medicine?

Take linezolid tablets by mouth. Follow the directions on the prescription label. You can take this medicine with food. Take your doses at regular intervals. Do not take your medicine more often than directed. Finish the full course prescribed by your prescriber or health care professional even if you think your condition is better. Do not stop using except on your prescriber's advice. Ask your prescriber or health care professional if you have any questions. Contact your pediatrician or health care professional regarding the use of this medicine in children. Special care may be needed.

What if I miss a dose?

If you miss a dose, use it as soon as you can. If it is almost time for your next dose, use only that dose. Do not use double or extra doses.

What may interact with linezolid?

- alcohol
- bupropion
- caffeine
- cocaine
- cyclobenzaprine
- dextromethorphan
- diet pills, stimulants or amphetamine-like drugs
- furazolidone
- guarana
- medicines for allergies, colds, hayfever, sinus, and breathing difficulties
- medicines for headaches or migraine (such as naratriptan, rizatriptan, sumatriptan, zolmitriptan or Midrin®)
- medicines for high blood pressure and heart medicines
- medicines called MAO inhibitors—examples: phenelzine (Nardil®), tranylcypromine (Parnate®), isocarboxazid (Marplan®)
- medicines for mental depression, anxiety, psychotic disturbances or other mental problems
- meperidine
- procarbazine

- some medications for Parkinson's disease, such as entacapone, levodopa or tolcapone
- St. John's wort, Hypericum perforatum
- tramadol
- tryptophan
- tyramine—see below for foods that contain tyramine

Tell your prescriber or health care professional about all other medicines you are taking, including non-prescription medicines, nutritional supplements, or herbal products. Also tell your prescriber or health care professional if you are a frequent user of drinks with caffeine or alcohol, if you smoke, or if you use illegal drugs. These may affect the way your medicine works. Check with your health care professional before stopping or starting any of your medicines.

What should I watch for while taking linezolid?

Tell your prescriber or health care professional if your symptoms do not begin to improve in a few days. If you get severe or watery diarrhea, do not treat yourself. Call your prescriber or health care professional for advice. Because linezolid may interact with many over-the-counter medications, you must check with your prescriber before taking any non-prescription medicines while on this antibiotic. Do not treat yourself for coughs, colds, or allergies. Do not take any medications for weight loss. Some ingredients in these products may increase possible side effects. Linezolid can interact with certain foods that contain tyramine to produce severe headaches, a rise in blood pressure, or irregular heart beat. Foods that contain significant amounts of tyramine include aged cheeses; meats and fish (especially aged, smoked, pickled, or processed such as bologna, pepperoni, salami, summer sausage); beer and ale; alcohol-free beer; wine (especially red); sherry; hard liquor; liqueurs; avocados; bananas; figs; raisins; soy sauce; miso soup; yeast/protein extracts; bean curd; fava or broad bean pods; or any over-ripe fruit. Ask your prescriber or health care professional, pharmacist, or nutritionist for a complete listing of tyramine-containing foods. Also, avoid drinks containing caffeine, such as tea, coffee, chocolate, or cola. Call your prescriber or health care professional as soon as you can if you get frequent or severe headaches or have palpitations. You may get drowsy, dizzy or have blurred vision. Do not drive, use machinery, or do anything that needs mental alertness until you know how this medicine affects you. Do not stand or sit up quickly, especially if you are an older patient. This reduces the risk of dizzy or fainting spells. Avoid alcoholic drinks. Notify your health care professional if you are scheduled to have any surgery, procedure or medical testing (including myelography); tell your prescriber or health care professional that you have been taking linezolid.

What side effects may I notice from taking linezolid?

Side effects that you should report to your prescriber or health care professional as soon as possible:

L

Rare or uncommon:
- increased blood pressure
- irregular heart beat or palpitations
- severe or watery diarrhea
- skin bruising
- tremor
- unusual weakness or tiredness
- blurred vision or other changes in vision

More common:
- skin rash, itching

Side effects that usually do not require medical attention (report to your prescriber or health care professional if they continue or are bothersome):
- change in taste

- headache
- mild diarrhea
- dizziness
- mild stomach upset
- nausea, vomiting
- temporary tongue discoloration

Where can I keep my medicine?

Keep this medicine out of reach of children. Store the linezolid tablets at room temperature 15 to 30 degrees C (59 to 86 degrees F), away from direct heat and light. Do not freeze. Keep the prescription bottle tightly closed. Throw away any unused tablets after the expiration date.

Liothyronine tablets

CYTOMEL®;
5 mcg; Tablet
Jones Pharma Inc
Sub King
Pharmaceuticals Inc

CYTOMEL®;
25 mcg; Tablet
Jones Pharma Inc
Sub King
Pharmaceuticals Inc

What are liothyronine tablets?

LIOTHYRONINE (Cytomel®) is for people whose thyroid gland does not produce enough thyroid hormone. Replacing thyroid hormone can improve symptoms of thyroid deficiency such as slow speech, lack of energy, weight gain, hair loss, dry thick skin and unusual sensitivity to cold. Liothyronine also helps to treat a condition called goiter, which is an enlarged thyroid gland. Liothyronine tablets may also be used as a diagnostic agent. Generic liothyronine tablets are not available.

What should my health care professional know before I take liothyronine?

They need to know if you have any of these conditions:
- angina
- diabetes mellitus or insipidus
- heart disease
- high blood pressure
- low levels of pituitary hormone
- dieting or on a weight loss program
- previous heart attack
- an unusual or allergic reaction to liothyronine, other thyroid hormones, medicines, foods, dyes, or preservatives
- pregnant or trying to get pregnant

How should I take this medicine?

Take liothyronine tablets by mouth 30 to 60 minutes before a meal (on an empty stomach) with a full glass of water. The doses should be taken at regular intervals as indicated on the medication label. Do not take your medication more often than directed. Contact your pediatrician or health care professional regarding the use of this medicine in children. Special care may be needed.

What if I miss a dose?

If you miss a dose, take it as soon as you can. If it is almost time for your next dose, take only that dose. Do not take double or extra doses.

What may interact with liothyronine?

- amiodarone
- antacids
- calcium supplements, like Tums® and many others
- carbamazepine
- cholestyramine
- colestipol
- digoxin
- female hormones, including contraceptive or birth control pills
- ketamine
- medicines for colds and breathing difficulties
- medicines for diabetes
- medicines for mental depression
- medicines or herbals used to decrease weight or appetite
- phenobarbital or other barbiturate medications
- phenytoin
- prednisone or other corticosteroids
- rifabutin
- rifampin
- soy isoflavones
- sucralfate
- theophylline
- warfarin

Tell your prescriber or health care professional about all other medicines you are taking, including non-prescription medicines, nutritional supplements, or herbal products. Also tell your prescriber or health care professional if you are a frequent user of drinks with caffeine or alcohol, if you smoke, or if you use illegal drugs. These may affect the way your medicine works. Check with your health care professional before stopping or starting any of your medicines.

What should I watch for while taking liothyronine?

If you are taking liothyronine for an underactive thyroid, it may be several weeks before you notice an improvement. Check with your prescriber or health care professional if your symptoms do not improve or if you develop any of the above side effects. It may be necessary for you to take this medicine for the rest of your life; do not stop taking except on your prescriber's advice. Thyroid hormones can affect blood sugar levels. If you also have diabetes, you may need to adjust the dose of your diabetic medicine once you are stabilized on liothyronine. Careful monitoring of blood glucose is often necessary. You may lose some hair during the first few months while using liothyronine. With time, this usually corrects itself. If you are going to have surgery, tell your prescriber or health care professional that you are taking liothyronine.

What side effects may I notice from taking liothyronine?

Side effects that you should report to your prescriber or health care professional as soon as possible:
- difficulty breathing, wheezing, or shortness of breath
- chest pain
- excessive sweating or intolerance to heat
- fast or irregular heartbeat or pulse rate
- nervousness
- skin rash or hives
- swelling of ankles, feet or legs

Side effects that usually do not require medical attention (report to your prescriber or health care professional if they continue or are bothersome):
- changes in appetite
- changes in menstrual periods
- diarrhea
- fever
- hair loss
- headache
- irritability
- leg cramps
- nausea, vomiting
- tremors
- trouble sleeping
- weight loss

Where can I keep my medicine?

Keep out of the reach of children in a container that small children cannot open. Store tablets at room temperature between 15 and 30 degrees C (59 and 86 degrees F). Protect from light. Keep container tightly closed. Throw away any unused medicine after the expiration date.

Liotrix tablets

THYROLAR®;
0.15 mg/37.5 mcg;
Tablet
Forest
Pharmaceuticals Inc

THYROLAR®;
0.1 mg/25 mcg;
Tablet
Forest
Pharmaceuticals Inc

What are liotrix tablets?

LIOTRIX (Thyrolar® and others) acts as a replacement for people whose thyroid gland does not produce enough thyroid hormone. Liotrix can improve symptoms of thyroid deficiency such as slow speech, lack of energy, weight gain, hair loss, dry thick skin and unusual sensitivity to cold. Liotrix also helps to treat a condition called goiter, which is an enlarged thyroid gland. Generic liotrix tablets are not available.

What should my health care professional know before I take liotrix?

They need to know if you have any of these conditions:
- angina
- diabetes mellitus
- heart disease
- high blood pressure
- low levels of pituitary hormone
- dieting or on a weight loss program
- previous heart attack
- an unusual or allergic reaction to liotrix, other thyroid hormones, medicines, foods, dyes, or preservatives
- pregnant or trying to get pregnant

How should I take this medicine?

Take liotrix tablets by mouth 30 to 60 minutes before a meal (on an empty stomach) with a full glass of water. The doses should be taken at regular intervals as indicated on the medication label. Do not take your medi-

cation more often than directed. Contact your pediatrician or health care professional regarding the use of this medicine in children. Special care may be needed.

What if I miss a dose?

If you miss a dose, take it as soon as you can. If it is almost time for your next dose, take only that dose. Do not take double or extra doses.

What may interact with liotrix?

- amiodarone
- antacids
- calcium supplements, like Tums® and many others
- carbamazepine
- cholestyramine
- colestipol
- digoxin
- female hormones, including contraceptive or birth control pills
- ketamine
- medicines for colds and breathing difficulties
- medicines for diabetes
- medicines for mental depression
- medicines or herbals used to decrease weight or appetite
- phenobarbital or other barbiturate medications
- phenytoin
- prednisone or other corticosteroids
- rifabutin
- rifampin

L

- soy isoflavones
- sucralfate
- theophylline
- warfarin

Tell your prescriber or health care professional about all other medicines you are taking, including non-prescription medicines, nutritional supplements, or herbal products. Also tell your prescriber or health care professional if you are a frequent user of drinks with caffeine or alcohol, if you smoke, or if you use illegal drugs. These may affect the way your medicine works. Check with your health care professional before stopping or starting any of your medicines.

What should I watch for while taking liotrix?

If you are taking liotrix for an underactive thyroid, it may be several weeks before you notice an improvement. Check with your prescriber or health care professional if your symptoms do not improve or if you develop any of the above side effects. It may be necessary for you to take this medicine for the rest of your life; do not stop taking except on your prescriber's advice. Do not switch brands of liotrix unless your prescriber agrees with the change; not all brands contain equivalent amounts of hormones. Ask your prescriber or health care professional for advice if you are uncertain. Thyroid hormones can affect blood sugar levels. If you also have diabetes, you may need to adjust the dose of your diabetic medicine once you are stabilized on liotrix. Careful monitoring of blood glucose is often necessary. You may lose some of your hair during the first few months while using liotrix. With time, this condition usually corrects itself. If you are going to have surgery,

tell your prescriber or health care professional that you are taking liotrix.

What side effects may I notice from taking liotrix?

Side effects that you should report to your prescriber or health care professional as soon as possible:
- difficulty breathing, wheezing, or shortness of breath
- chest pain
- excessive sweating or intolerance to heat
- fast or irregular heartbeat or pulse rate
- nervousness
- skin rash or hives
- swelling of ankles, feet or legs

Side effects that usually do not require medical attention (report to your prescriber or health care professional if they continue or are bothersome):
- changes in appetite
- changes in menstrual periods
- diarrhea
- fever
- hair loss
- headache
- irritability
- leg cramps
- nausea, vomiting
- tremors
- trouble sleeping
- weight loss

Where can I keep my medicine?

Keep out of the reach of children in a container that small children cannot open. Store tablets in the refrigerator between 2 and 8 degrees C (36 and 46 degrees F) in a tightly closed container. Protect from light and moisture. Throw away any unused medicine after the expiration date.

Lisinopril tablets

ZESTRIL®;
5 mg; Tablet
AstraZeneca
Pharmaceuticals LP

PRINIVIL®;
5 mg; Tablet
Merck and Co Inc

What are lisinopril tablets?

LISINOPRIL (Prinivil®, Zestril®) is an antihypertensive (blood pressure lowering agent) known as an ACE inhibitor. Lisinopril controls high blood pressure (hypertension) by relaxing blood vessels; it is not a cure. High blood pressure levels can damage your kidneys, and may lead to a stroke or heart failure. Lisinopril also helps to treat patients with heart failure (heart does not pump strongly enough). Generic lisinopril tablets are available.

What should my health care professional know before I take lisinopril?

They need to know if you have any of these conditions:
- autoimmune disease (such as lupus), or suppressed immune function
- previous swelling of the tongue, face, or lips with diffi-

culty breathing, difficulty swallowing, hoarseness, or tightening of the throat (angioedema)
- bone marrow disease
- heart or blood vessel disease
- low blood pressure
- kidney disease
- if you are on a special diet, such as a low-salt diet
- an unusual or allergic reaction to lisinopril, other ACE inhibitors, foods, dyes, or preservatives
- pregnant or trying to get pregnant
- breast-feeding

How should I take this medicine?

Take lisinopril tablets by mouth. Follow the directions on the prescription label. Swallow the tablets with a drink of water. Take your doses at regular intervals. Do not take your medicine more often than directed. Do not stop taking lisinopril except on your prescriber's advice. Contact your pediatrician or health care professional regarding the use of this medicine in children. Special care may be needed.

What if I miss a dose?

If you miss a dose, take it as soon as you can. If it is almost time for your next dose, take only that dose. Do not take double or extra doses. If you take only one dose a day and forget to take it that day, do not take a double dose the next day.

What may interact with lisinopril?

- anti-inflammatory drugs (NSAIDs, such as ibuprofen)
- hawthorn
- heparin
- lithium
- medicines for high blood pressure
- potassium salts
- water pills

Tell your prescriber or health care professional about all other medicines you are taking, including non-prescription medicines, nutritional supplements, or herbal products. Also tell your prescriber or health care professional if you are a frequent user of drinks with caffeine or alcohol, if you smoke, or if you use illegal drugs. These may affect the way your medicine works. Check with your health care professional before stopping or starting any of your medicines.

What should I watch for while taking lisinopril?

Visit your prescriber or health care professional for regular checks on your progress. Check your blood pressure regularly while you are taking lisinopril. Ask your prescriber or health care professional what your blood pressure should be and when you should contact him or her. Call your prescriber or health care professional if you notice an uneven or fast heart beat. Do not treat yourself for a fever or sore throat; check with your prescriber or health care professional as these may be the result of a lisinopril side effect. Check with your prescriber or health care professional if you get an attack of severe diarrhea, nausea and vomiting, or if you sweat

a lot. The loss of body fluid can make it dangerous to take lisinopril. You may get dizzy. Do not drive, use machinery, or do anything that needs mental alertness until you know how lisinopril affects you. To avoid dizzy or fainting spells, do not stand or sit up quickly, especially if you are an older person. Alcohol can make you more dizzy. Avoid alcoholic drinks. If you are going to have surgery, tell your prescriber or health care professional that you are using lisinopril. Avoid salt substitutes or other foods or substances high in potassium salts. Do not treat yourself for coughs, colds, or pain while you are using lisinopril without asking your prescriber or health care professional for advice.

What side effects may I notice from taking lisinopril?

Side effects that you should report to your prescriber or health care professional as soon as possible:
- decreased amount of urine passed
- difficulty breathing, or difficulty swallowing
- dizziness, lightheadedness or fainting spells
- fast or uneven heart beat, palpitations, or chest pain
- fever or chills
- numbness or tingling in your fingers or toes
- skin rash, itching
- swelling of your face, lips, or tongue

Side effects that usually do not require medical attention (report to your prescriber or health care professional if they continue or are bothersome):
- change in taste
- cough
- headache
- tiredness

Where can I keep my medicine?

Keep out of the reach of children in a container that small children cannot open. Store at room temperature between 15 and 30 degrees C (59 and 86 degrees F). Protect from moisture, Keep container tightly closed. Do not freeze. Throw away any unused medicine after the expiration date.

Lithium extended-release tablets

LITHOBID®;
300 mg; Tablet,
Extended Release
Solvay
Pharmaceuticals Inc

ESKALITH CR®;
450 mg; Tablet,
Extended Release
SmithKline Beecham
Pharmaceuticals Div
SmithKline Beecham
Co

What are lithium extended-release tablets?

LITHIUM (Eskalith CR®, Lithobid®) helps to control extreme mood swings in manic-depressive illness. Lithium helps you to maintain a more balanced state, without swinging from a highly elated, over-excited state to that of being very sad and depressed. Lithium can prevent or reduce these episodes. Generic lithium extended-release tablets are available.

What should my health care professional know before I take lithium?

They need to know if you have any of these conditions:
- dehydration (diarrhea or sweating)
- heart or blood vessel disease
- kidney disease
- leukemia
- low level of salt in the blood, or low-salt diet

- Parkinson's disease
- psoriasis
- seizures (convulsions)
- underactive thyroid, or thyroid disease
- an unusual or allergic reaction to lithium, other medicines, foods, dyes, or preservatives
- pregnant or trying to get pregnant
- breast-feeding

How should I take this medicine?

Take lithium extended-release tablets by mouth. Follow the directions on the prescription label. Swallow the tablets whole with a drink of water; do not break, crush or chew. Take after a meal or snack to avoid stomach upset. Take your doses at regular intervals. Do not take your medicine more often than directed. Do not stop taking except on your prescriber's advice. Contact your pediatrician or health care professional regarding the use of this medicine in children. Special care may be needed. Elderly patients over age 65 years may have a stronger reaction to this medicine and need smaller doses.

What if I miss a dose?

If you miss a dose, take it as soon as you can. If it is almost time for your next dose (less than 4 hours), take only that dose. Do not take double or extra doses.

What may interact with lithium?

- anti-inflammatory drugs (NSAIDs, such as ibuprofen, or COX-2 inhibitors, such as celecoxib)
- caffeine
- calcium iodide
- carbamazepine
- guarana
- medicines for diabetes
- medicines for high blood pressure
- medicines for mental problems and psychotic disturbances
- metronidazole
- potassium iodide, KI
- sodium bicarbonate
- sodium chloride
- verapamil
- water pills

Tell your prescriber or health care professional about all other medicines you are taking, including non-prescription medicines, nutritional supplements, or herbal products. Also tell your prescriber or health care professional if you are a frequent user of drinks with caffeine or alcohol, if you smoke, or if you use illegal drugs. These may affect the way your medicine works. Check with your health care professional before stopping or starting any of your medicines.

What should I watch for while taking lithium?

Visit your prescriber or health care professional for regular checks on your progress. It can take several weeks of treatment to get improvement in your condition.

You must continue to take lithium at regular intervals even when your symptoms are better. Do not stop taking lithium except on your prescriber's advice. The amount of lithium you take is very important. Taking more than the prescribed dose can cause serious side effects. You are taking a slow-release form of lithium. Do not change with any other brand without your prescriber's advice. The amount of salt (sodium) in your body influences the effects of lithium, and lithium can increase salt loss from the body. Eat a normal diet that includes salt. Do not change to salt substitutes. Avoid changes involving diet, or medications that include large amounts of sodium (such as sodium bicarbonate). Ask your prescriber or health care professional for advice if you are not sure. Drink plenty of fluids while you are taking lithium. Avoid drinks that contain caffeine, such as coffee, tea and colas. You will need extra fluids if you have diarrhea or sweat a lot. This will help prevent toxic effects from lithium. Be careful not to get overheated during exercise, saunas, hot baths, and hot weather. Consult your prescriber or health care professional if you have a high fever or persistent diarrhea. You may get dizzy, drowsy, or have blurred vision. Do not drive, use machinery, or do anything that needs mental alertness until you know how lithium affects you. Make sure that family members or friends know of early signs of lithium toxicity (see side effects above). If you are going to have surgery, tell your prescriber or health care professional that you are taking lithium.

What side effects may I notice from taking lithium?

Side effects that you should report to your prescriber or health care professional as soon as possible:
More common:
- diarrhea
- drowsiness
- loss of appetite
- muscle weakness
- nausea, vomiting
- slurred speech

These symptoms can progress to:
- blurred vision
- clumsiness or loss of balance
- confusion
- dizziness
- seizures
- trembling

Rare or uncommon:
- difficulty speaking or swallowing
- fainting
- hair loss
- hoarseness
- slow, fast, or irregular heartbeat (palpitations)
- pain, coldness, or blue coloration of fingers or toes
- rough, dry skin
- sensitivity to cold
- swelling in the neck
- unusual tiredness or weakness
- unusual weight gain

L

Side effects that usually do not require medical attention (report to your prescriber or health care professional if they continue or are bothersome):

- increased thirst
- increased frequency and urgency to pass urine
- muscle twitches
- nausea
- skin rash
- stomach bloating, full feeling

- trembling of the hands

Where can I keep my medicine?

Keep out of the reach of children in a container that small children cannot open. Store at room temperature between 15 and 30 degrees C (59 and 86 degrees F). Keep container tightly closed. Protect from light. Throw away any unused medicine after the expiration date.

Lithium tablets or capsules

ESKALITH®;
300 mg; Capsule
SmithKline Beecham
Pharmaceuticals Div
SmithKline Beecham
Co

LITHIUM;
300 mg; Tablet
Roxane Laboratories
Inc

What are lithium tablets or capsules?

LITHIUM (Eskalith®, Lithonate®, Lithane®, Lithotabs®) helps to control extreme mood swings in manic-depressive illness. Lithium helps you to maintain a more balanced state, without swinging from a highly elated, over-excited state to that of being very sad and depressed. Lithium can prevent or reduce these episodes. Generic lithium tablets or capsules are available.

What should my health care professional know before I take lithium?

They need to know if you have any of these conditions:

- dehydration (diarrhea or sweating)
- heart or blood vessel disease
- kidney disease
- leukemia
- low level of salt in the blood, or low-salt diet
- Parkinson's disease
- psoriasis
- seizures (convulsions)
- underactive thyroid, or thyroid disease
- an unusual or allergic reaction to lithium, other medicines, foods, dyes, or preservatives
- pregnant or trying to get pregnant
- breast-feeding

How should I take this medicine?

Take lithium tablets or capsules by mouth. Follow the directions on the prescription label. Swallow the tablets or capsules with a drink of water. Take after a meal or snack to avoid stomach upset. Take your doses at regular intervals. Do not take your medicine more often than directed. Do not stop taking except on your prescriber's advice. Contact your pediatrician or health care professional regarding the use of this medicine in children. Special care may be needed. Elderly patients over age 65 years may have a stronger reaction to this medicine and need smaller doses.

What if I miss a dose?

If you miss a dose, take it as soon as you can. If it is almost time for your next dose (less than 2 hours), take only that dose. Do not take double or extra doses.

What may interact with lithium?

- anti-inflammatory drugs (NSAIDs, such as ibuprofen, or COX-2 inhibitors, such as celecoxib)
- caffeine
- calcium iodide
- carbamazepine
- guarana
- medicines for diabetes
- medicines for high blood pressure
- medicines for mental problems and psychotic disturbances
- metronidazole
- potassium iodide, KI
- sodium bicarbonate
- sodium chloride
- verapamil
- water pills

Tell your prescriber or health care professional about all other medicines you are taking, including non-prescription medicines, nutritional supplements, or herbal products. Also tell your prescriber or health care professional if you are a frequent user of drinks with caffeine or alcohol, if you smoke, or if you use illegal drugs. These may affect the way your medicine works. Check with your health care professional before stopping or starting any of your medicines.

What should I watch for while taking lithium?

Visit your prescriber or health care professional for regular checks on your progress. It can take several weeks of treatment to get improvement in your condition. You must continue to take lithium at regular intervals even when your symptoms are better. Do not stop taking lithium except on your prescriber's advice. The amount of lithium you take is very important. Taking more than the prescribed dose can cause serious side effects. The amount of salt (sodium) in your body influences the effects of lithium, and lithium can increase salt loss from the body. Eat a normal diet that includes salt. Do not change to salt substitutes. Avoid changes involving diet, or medications that include large amounts of sodium (such as sodium bicarbonate). Ask

L

your prescriber or health care professional for advice if you are not sure. Drink plenty of fluids while you are taking lithium. Avoid drinks that contain caffeine, such as coffee, tea and colas. You will need extra fluids if you have diarrhea or sweat a lot. This will help prevent toxic effects from lithium. Be careful not to get overheated during exercise, saunas, hot baths, and hot weather. Consult your prescriber or health care professional if you have a high fever or persistent diarrhea. You may get dizzy, drowsy, or have blurred vision. Do not drive, use machinery, or do anything that needs mental alertness until you know how lithium affects you. Make sure that family members or friends know of early signs of lithium toxicity (see side effects above). If you are going to have surgery, tell your prescriber or health care professional that you are taking lithium.

What side effects may I notice from taking lithium?

Side effects that you should report to your prescriber or health care professional as soon as possible:
More common:
- diarrhea
- drowsiness
- loss of appetite
- muscle weakness
- nausea, vomiting
- slurred speech

These symptoms can progress to:
- blurred vision
- clumsiness or loss of balance
- confusion
- dizziness
- seizures
- trembling

Rare or uncommon:
- difficulty speaking or swallowing
- fainting
- hair loss
- hoarseness
- slow, fast, or irregular heartbeat (palpitations)
- pain, coldness, or blue coloration of fingers or toes
- rough, dry skin
- sensitivity to cold
- swelling in the neck
- unusual tiredness or weakness
- unusual weight gain

Side effects that usually do not require medical attention (report to your prescriber or health care professional if they continue or are bothersome):
- increased thirst
- increased frequency and urgency to pass urine
- muscle twitches
- nausea
- skin rash
- stomach bloating, full feeling
- trembling of the hands

Where can I keep my medicine?

Keep out of the reach of children in a container that small children cannot open. Store at room temperature between 15 and 30 degrees C (59 and 86 degrees F). Keep container tightly closed. Protect from light. Throw away any unused medicine after the expiration date.

Lomefloxacin tablets

MAXAQUIN®;
400 mg; Tablet
Pharmacia and Upjohn Div
Pfizer

What are lomefloxacin tablets?

LOMEFLOXACIN (Maxaquin®) is a fluoroquinolone antibiotic. Lomefloxacin kills certain bacteria or stops their growth. It treats respiratory and urinary tract infections, or prevents infection during surgery on the urinary tract. Generic lomefloxacin tablets are not yet available.

What should my health care professional know before I take lomefloxacin?

They need to know if you have any of these conditions:
- arteriosclerosis
- dehydration
- kidney disease
- long exposure to sunlight (working outdoors)
- seizures (convulsions)
- stomach problems (especially colitis)
- stroke
- other chronic illness
- an unusual or allergic reaction to fluoroquinolone antibiotics, foods, dyes, or preservatives
- pregnant or trying to get pregnant
- breast-feeding

How should I take this medicine?

Take lomefloxacin tablets by mouth. Follow the directions on the prescription label. Swallow tablets whole with a full glass of water. It is best to take lomefloxacin on an empty stomach. If it upsets your stomach, lomefloxacin can be taken with food, but avoid any dairy products, iron-containing products or antacids. Take your doses at regular intervals. Do not take your medicine more often than directed. Finish the full course prescribed by your prescriber or health care professional even if you think your condition is better. Do not stop taking except on your prescriber's advice. Contact your pediatrician or health care professional regarding the use of this medicine in children. Special care may be needed.

What if I miss a dose?

If you miss a dose, take it as soon as you can. If it is almost time for your next dose, take only that dose.

Do not take double or extra doses. There should be an interval of at least 10 to 12 hours between doses.

What may interact with lomefloxacin?

- aluminum salts
- antacids
- calcium salts
- certain heart medications for irregular rhythm (e.g., amiodarone, disopyramide, dofetilide, flecainide, ibutilide, quinidine, procainamide, sotalol)
- cyclobenzaprine
- didanosine (Videx® tablets or oral solution)
- iron supplements
- magnesium salts
- manganese
- multivitamins containing iron, calcium, zinc, or manganese
- NSAIDs such as Advil®, Aleve®, ibuprofen, Motrin®, naproxen
- sucralfate
- warfarin
- zinc salts

Tell your prescriber or health care professional about all other medicines you are taking, including non-prescription medicines, nutritional supplements, or herbal products. Also tell your prescriber or health care professional if you are a frequent user of drinks with caffeine or alcohol, if you smoke, or if you use illegal drugs. These may affect the way your medicine works. Check with your health care professional before stopping or starting any of your medicines.

What should I watch for while taking lomefloxacin?

Tell your prescriber or health care professional if your symptoms do not improve in 2 to 3 days. Keep out of the sun, or wear protective clothing outdoors and use a sunscreen. Do not use sun lamps or sun tanning beds or booths. If you get a sunburn reaction, with skin burning, redness, swelling, blisters, rash, itching, or dermatitis, stop taking your tablets at once and call your prescriber or health care professional for advice. You may get drowsy or dizzy. Do not drive, use machinery, or do anything that needs mental alertness until you know how lomefloxacin affects you. To reduce the risk of dizzy or fainting spells, do not sit or stand up quickly, especially if you are an older patient. Drink several glasses of water a day. Cut down on drinks that contain caffeine. Antacids can stop lomefloxacin from working.

If you get an upset stomach and want to take an antacid, make sure there is an interval of at least 2 hours since you last took lomefloxacin, or 6 hours before your next dose. Calcium, iron, and zinc preparations can also stop lomefloxacin from working properly. Take calcium tablets, iron tablets, zinc tablets, or vitamins that contain calcium, iron, or zinc at least 6 hours before your dose of lomefloxacin or at least 2 hours after your dose of lomefloxacin. If you notice pain or swelling of a tendon or around a joint, stop taking lomefloxacin. Call your healthcare provider. Rest the affected area. Do not exercise or take lomefloxacin until your healthcare provider tells you to do so. If you notice pain, burning, tingling, numbness and/or weakness of the hands or feet, discontinue lomefloxacin and call your healthcare professional immediately. If you are going to have surgery, tell your prescriber or health care professional that you are taking lomefloxacin.

What side effects may I notice from taking lomefloxacin?

Side effects that you should report to your prescriber or health care professional as soon as possible:
- difficulty breathing
- increased sensitivity to the sun or ultraviolet light
- irregular heartbeat, palpitations or chest pain
- joint, muscle or tendon pain
- nervousness, excitability, restlessness
- severe or watery diarrhea
- skin rash, itching
- seizures (convulsions)
- swelling of the face or neck
- vomiting

Side effects that usually do not require medical attention (report to your prescriber or health care professional if they continue or are bothersome):
- diarrhea
- difficulty sleeping
- dizziness, drowsiness
- gas or heartburn
- headache
- nausea
- stomach pain

Where can I keep my medicine?

Keep out of the reach of children in a container that small children cannot open. Store at room temperature between 15 and 30 degrees C (59 and 86 degrees F). Throw away any unused medicine after the expiration date.

L

Lomustine, CCNU capsules

CEENU®;
100 mg; Capsule
Mead Johnson and
Co Sub Bristol Myers
Co

CEENU®;
40 mg; Capsule
Mead Johnson and
Co Sub Bristol Myers
Co

What are lomustine capsules?

LOMUSTINE (CeeNU®) is a type of chemotherapy for treating cancer. Lomustine belongs to a group of medicines known as alkylating agents. Lomustine interferes with cell growth and is used to treat brain tumors and certain cancers of the blood (Hodgkin's disease). Generic lomustine capsules are not yet available.

What should my health care professional know before I take lomustine?

They need to know if you have any of these conditions:
- bleeding problems
- blood disorders
- dental disease
- infection (especially virus infection such as chickenpox or herpes)
- kidney disease
- lung disease
- an unusual or allergic reaction to lomustine, other chemotherapy, other medicines, foods, dyes, or preservatives
- pregnant or trying to get pregnant
- breast-feeding

How should I take this medicine?

Take lomustine capsules by mouth. To provide the correct dose of lomustine for you, there may be capsules of different types and colors to take as a single dose, dispensed by your pharmacist. Follow the directions on the prescription label. Swallow the capsules with a drink of water. Do not take the capsules with food. Lomustine is usually taken as a single dose once every 6 weeks. Do not take your medicine more often than directed. Finish the full course prescribed by your doctor or health care professional even if the capsules make you feel unwell. Do not stop taking except on your prescriber's advice. Contact your pediatrician or health care professional regarding the use of this medicine in children. Special care may be needed.

What if I miss a dose?

It is important not to miss a dose. You will only take one dose every 6 weeks. If you vomit after taking a dose, call your prescriber or health care professional for advice.

What may interact with lomustine?

- cimetidine
- vaccines

Talk to your prescriber or health care professional before taking any of these medicines:
- acetaminophen
- aspirin
- ibuprofen
- ketoprofen
- naproxen

Tell your prescriber or health care professional about all other medicines you are taking, including non-prescription medicines, nutritional supplements, or herbal products. Also tell your prescriber or health care professional if you are a frequent user of drinks with caffeine or alcohol, if you smoke, or if you use illegal drugs. These may affect the way your medicine works. Check with your health care professional before stopping or starting any of your medicines.

What should I watch for while taking lomustine?

Visit your prescriber or health care professional for checks on your progress. You will need to have regular blood checks. The side effects of lomustine can continue after you finish your treatment; report side effects promptly. Lomustine may make you feel generally unwell. This is not uncommon because lomustine affects good cells as well as cancer cells. Report any side effects as above, but continue your course of medicine even though you feel ill, unless your prescriber or health care professional tells you to stop. Lomustine may decrease your body's ability to fight infections. Call your prescriber or health care professional if you have a fever, chills, sore throat or other symptoms of a cold or flu. Do not treat these symptoms yourself. Try to avoid being around people who are sick. Lomustine may increase your risk to bruise or bleed. Call your prescriber or health care professional if you notice any unusual bleeding. Be careful not to cut, bruise or injure yourself because you may get an infection and bleed more than usual. Avoid taking aspirin, acetaminophen (Tylenol®), ibuprofen (Advil®), naproxen (Aleve®), or ketoprofen (Orudis® KT) products as these may hide a fever, unless instructed to by your prescriber or health care professional. Be careful brushing and flossing your teeth or using a toothpick while receiving lomustine because you may get an infection or bleed more easily. If you have any dental work done, tell your dentist you are received lomustine. Do not have any vaccinations without your prescriber's approval and avoid anyone who has recently had the oral polio vaccine. Women of childbearing age should use effective birth control methods during lomustine treatment. There is a risk of birth defects if lomustine is given during pregnancy. Women should not become pregnant while being treated with lomustine. If you are going to have surgery, tell your prescriber or health care professional that you are taking lomustine.

What side effects may I notice from taking lomustine?

The side effects you may experience with lomustine therapy depend upon the dose, other types of chemotherapy or radiation therapy given, and the disease being treated. Not all of these effects occur in all patients. Discuss any concerns or questions with your prescriber or health care professional.

Side effects that you should report to your prescriber or health care professional as soon as possible:

- difficulty breathing, wheezing or shortness of breath
- low blood counts—lomustine may decrease the number of white blood cells, red blood cells and platelets. You may be at increased risk for infections and bleeding.
- signs of infection—fever or chills, cough, sore throat, pain or difficulty passing urine
- signs of decreased platelets or bleeding—bruising, pin-point red spots on the skin, black, tarry stools, blood in the urine
- signs of decreased red blood cells—unusual weakness or tiredness, fainting spells, lightheadedness
- yellowing of skin or eyes

Side effects that usually do not require medical attention (report to your prescriber or health care professional if they continue or are bothersome):

- confusion
- hair loss
- loss of appetite (this may last for several days)
- mouth sores
- nausea, vomiting

Where can I keep my medicine?

Keep out of the reach of children in a container that small children cannot open. Store at room temperature below 40 degrees C (104 degrees F). Keep container tightly closed. Throw away any unused medicine after the expiration date.

Loperamide tablets or capsules

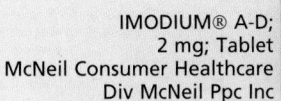 IMODIUM® A-D;
2 mg; Tablet
McNeil Consumer Healthcare
Div McNeil Ppc Inc

What are loperamide tablets or capsules?

LOPERAMIDE (Imodium®, Imodium® A-D) helps to control and relieve the symptoms of diarrhea including traveler's diarrhea and the diarrhea associated with inflammatory bowel diseases. Generic loperamide capsules are available.

What should my health care professional know before I take loperamide?

They need to know if you have any of these conditions:

- a black or bloody stool
- bacterial food poisoning
- colitis or mucus in your stool
- currently taking an antibiotic medication for an infection
- diarrhea for more than 2 days
- fever
- liver disease
- severe abdominal pain, swelling or bulging
- an unusual or allergic reaction to loperamide, other medicines, foods, dyes, or preservatives
- pregnant or trying to get pregnant
- breast-feeding

How should I take this medicine?

Take loperamide tablets or capsules by mouth. Follow the directions on the prescription label. Swallow the tablets or capsules with a drink of water. Take your doses at regular intervals. Do not take your medicine more often than directed. Contact your pediatrician or health care professional regarding the use of this medicine in children. Special care may be needed. Elderly patients may have a more variable response to the effects of loperamide, and are more susceptible to the effects of dehydration.

What if I miss a dose?

This does not apply. Once your diarrhea has been brought under control you should only take a dose after a loose bowel movement.

What may interact with loperamide?

- alosetron
- cholestyramine
- cisapride
- erythromycin
- metoclopramide
- quinidine

Tell your prescriber or health care professional about all other medicines you are taking, including non-prescription medicines, nutritional supplements, or herbal products. Also tell your prescriber or health care professional if you are a frequent user of drinks with caffeine or alcohol, if you smoke, or if you use illegal drugs. These may affect the way your medicine works. Check with your health care professional before stopping or starting any of your medicines.

What should I watch for while taking loperamide?

Do not take loperamide for more than 1 week without consulting your prescriber or health care professional. If your symptoms do not improve after taking loperamide for two days, you may have a problem that needs further evaluation. Check with your prescriber or health care professional at once if you develop a fever, severe abdominal pain, swelling or bulging, or if you

L

have bloody/black diarrhea or stools. You may get drowsy or dizzy. Do not drive, use machinery, or do anything that needs mental alertness until you know how loperamide affects you. Alcohol can increase possible drowsiness and dizziness; avoid alcoholic drinks. Your mouth may get dry. Sucking hard candy or chewing sugarless gum and drinking plenty of water can help. Drinking plenty of water can also help prevent dehydration that can occur with diarrhea.

What side effects may I notice from taking loperamide?

Side effects that you should report to your prescriber or health care professional as soon as possible:
- black or bloody stools
- bloated, swollen feeling in your abdomen
- blurred vision
- loss of appetite
- skin rash
- stomach pain

Side effects that usually do not require medical attention (report to your prescriber or health care professional if they continue or are bothersome):
- drowsiness or dizziness
- dry mouth
- constipation
- nausea, vomiting
- tiredness

Where can I keep my medicine?

Keep out of the reach of children in a container that small children cannot open. Store at room temperature between 15 and 30 degrees C (59 and 86 degrees F). Keep container tightly closed. Throw away any unused medicine after the expiration date.

Lopinavir; Ritonavir capsules

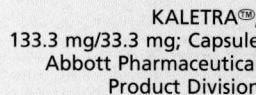 KALETRA™;
133.3 mg/33.3 mg; Capsule
Abbott Pharmaceutical
Product Division

What are lopinavir; ritonavir capsules?

LOPINAVIR; RITONAVIR (Kaletra™) are antiviral drugs called protease inhibitors. Lopinavir; ritonavir is used to treat human immunodeficiency virus (HIV) infection. Lopinavir; ritonavir may reduce the amount of HIV in the blood and increase the number of CD4 cells (T-cells) in the blood. Lopinavir; ritonavir is used in combination with other drugs used to treat the HIV virus. Lopinavir; ritonavir will not cure or prevent HIV infection or AIDS. You may still develop other infections or conditions associated with HIV. Generic lopinavir; ritonavir capsules are not available.

What should my health care professional know before I take lopinavir; ritonavir?

They need to know if you have any of these conditions:
- diabetes mellitus or high blood sugar
- hemophilia
- high cholesterol levels
- high triglyceride levels
- liver disease, including hepatitis
- an unusual or allergic reaction to lopinavir, ritonavir, castor oil, other medicines, foods, dyes, or preservatives
- breast-feeding
- pregnancy or recent attempts to get pregnant

How should I take this medicine?

Take lopinavir; ritonavir capsules by mouth. Follow the directions on the prescription label exactly. Take the capsules with meals or food. Take your doses at regular intervals. Do not take your medicine more often than directed. To help to make sure that your therapy works as well as possible, be very careful to take all of your medicine exactly as prescribed. Do not stop taking except on your prescriber's advice. Contact your pedia-

trician or health care professional regarding the use of this medicine in children. Special care may be needed. Lopinavir; ritonavir may be given to children and infants greater than 6 months of age.

What if I miss a dose?

If you miss a dose, take it as soon as you can. If it is almost time for your next dose, take only that dose. Do not take double or extra doses.

What may interact with lopinavir; ritonavir?

Many medicines may interact with lopinavir; ritonavir, if you have a question concerning other medicines you may be taking, talk with your pharmacist, prescriber or other health care professional.
Do not take lopinavir; ritonavir with any of these medicines:

- alfuzosin (Uroxatral®)
- amiodarone (Cordarone®)
- astemizole (Hismanal®)
- bepridil (Vascor®)
- cisapride (Propulsid®)
- dofetilide (Tylosin®)
- ergotamine medicines (Cafergot®, Migranal®, D.H.E. 45®, and others)
- lovastatin (Mevacor®)
- midazolam (Versed®)
- pimozide (Orap®)
- quinidine (Quinaglute®, Cardioquin®, Quinidex®, and others)
- simvastatin (Zocor®)
- St. John's wort or products containing St. John's wort
- terfenadine (Seldane®)
- triazolam (Halcion®)
- went yeast (Cholestin™)
- zolpidem (Ambien®)

L

Other medicines that may interact with lopinavir; ritonavir:

- atovaquone
- birth control pills or other hormonal birth control medicines (like the patch, ring, or injections)
- bosentan
- certain medicines for anxiety or difficulty sleeping
- certain medicines for fungal infections
- certain medicines for high cholesterol (e.g., atorvastatin or cerivastatin)
- certain medicines for high blood pressure
- certain pain medicines
- medicines for seizures
- medicines for depression
- medicines for diabetes
- other antiviral medicines such as didanosine, ddI, saquinavir, or zidovudine
- clarithromycin
- cyclosporine
- erythromycin
- imatinib, STI-571
- rifabutin
- rifampin
- rifapentine
- theophylline
- sildenafil
- warfarin

Tell your prescriber or health care professional about all other medicines you are taking, including non-prescription medicines, nutritional supplements, or herbal products. Also tell your prescriber or health care professional if you are a frequent user of drinks with caffeine or alcohol, if you smoke, or if you use illegal drugs. These may affect the way your medicine works. Check with your health care professional before stopping or starting any of your medicines.

What should I watch for while taking lopinavir; ritonavir?

You must visit your prescriber or health care professional for regular checks on your progress. Lopinavir; ritonavir will not cure HIV infection, and you can still get other illnesses associated with HIV. Lopinavir; ritonavir may cause abnormal liver function tests, changes in your cholesterol or triglyceride levels, and may increase the level of your blood sugar. Visit your health care professional or prescriber regularly to check for any of these side effects. Some of these effects may become serious. Taking lopinavir; ritonavir does not reduce the risk of passing HIV infection to others through sexual or blood contact. It is best to avoid sexual contact so that you do not spread the disease to others. For any sexual contact, use a condom. Be careful about cuts, abrasions, and other possible sources of blood contact. Never share a needle or syringe with anyone. If you are a woman of childbearing age and are using hormone contraceptives, then you should use another form of birth control while taking lopinavir; ritonavir. Lopinavir; ritonavir may decrease the effectiveness of hormone birth control agents, including birth control pills and injections. Do not breast-feed your infant if you have HIV.

What side effects might I notice from taking lopinavir; ritonavir?

Side effects that you should report to your prescriber or health care professional as soon as possible:
- abdominal pain
- increases in your blood sugar
- redness, blistering, peeling or loosening of the skin, including inside the mouth
- signs of a severe allergic reaction including difficulty breathing, tightness in throat, or swelling of your tongue
- skin rash, hives
- unusual tiredness or weakness

Side effects that usually do not require medical attention (report to your prescriber or health care professional if they continue or are bothersome):
- abnormal bowel movements
- changes in taste
- changes in body fat
- diarrhea
- difficulty sleeping
- dizziness
- headache
- heartburn
- loss of appetite
- nausea, vomiting
- tingling or numbness in the hands or feet or around the mouth
- tiredness or weakness

Where can I keep my medicine?

Keep out of the reach of children in a container that small children cannot open. Store the capsules in the refrigerator. You do not need to keep them in the refrigerator if you use them all within 2 months and keep them below 77 degrees F. Do not expose the capsules to very hot or cold temperatures. Keep the container tightly closed. Throw away any unused medicine after the expiration date.

L

Loracarbef capsules

LORABID®;
400 mg; Capsule
Monarch
Pharmaceuticals Inc

LORABID®;
200 mg; Capsule
Monarch
Pharmaceuticals Inc

What are loracarbef capsules?

LORACARBEF (Lorabid®) is an antibiotic very similar to the cephalosporins. It treats many kinds of infections including those of the skin (impetigo), respiratory tract (bronchitis, tonsillitis or pneumonia), sinuses (sinusitis), and ear (otitis media). Generic loracarbef capsules are not yet available.

What should my health care professional know before I take loracarbef?

They need to know if you have any of these conditions:
- kidney disease
- stomach or intestinal problems (especially colitis)
- other chronic illness
- an unusual or allergic reaction to loracarbef, cephalosporin antibiotics, penicillins, other foods, dyes or preservatives.
- pregnant or trying to get pregnant
- breast-feeding

How should I take this medicine?

Take loracarbef capsules by mouth. Follow the directions on the prescription label. Swallow the capsules with a drink of water. Take loracarbef 1 to 2 hours before or at least 2 hours after eating; taking it with food can make it less effective. Do not take your medicine more often than directed. Finish the full course prescribed by your prescriber or health care professional even if you think your condition is better. Do not stop taking except on your prescriber's advice. Contact your pediatrician or health care professional regarding the use of this medicine in children. Special care may be needed. Loracarbef is regularly prescribed to children 6 months and older.

What if I miss a dose?

If you miss a dose, take it as soon as you can. If it is almost time for your next dose, take only that dose. Do not take double or extra doses. There should be an interval of at least 10 to 12 hours between doses.

What may interact with loracarbef?

- medicines used to treat or prevent blood clots
- probenecid

Tell your prescriber or health care professional about all other medicines you are taking, including non-prescription medicines, nutritional supplements, or herbal products. Also tell your prescriber or health care professional if you are a frequent user of drinks with caffeine or alcohol, if you smoke, or if you use illegal drugs. These may affect the way your medicine works. Check with your health care professional before stopping or starting any of your medicines.

What should I watch for while taking loracarbef?

Tell your prescriber or health care professional if symptoms do not begin to improve in a few days. If you get severe or watery diarrhea, do not treat yourself. Call your prescriber or health care professional for advice.

What side effects may I notice from using loracarbef?

Side effects that you should report to your prescriber or health care professional as soon as possible:
- fever or chills, sore throat
- dizziness
- headache
- severe or watery diarrhea
- redness, blistering, peeling or loosening of the skin, including inside the mouth
- skin rash, itching
- swollen joints
- unusual bleeding or bruising
- unusual weakness or tiredness

Side effects that usually do not require medical attention (report to your prescriber or health care professional if they continue or are bothersome):
- diarrhea
- difficulty sleeping
- loss of appetite
- nausea, vomiting
- stomach pain
- vaginal itching

Where can I keep my medicine?

Keep out if the reach of children in a container that small children cannot open. Store the capsules at room temperature, 15 to 30 degrees C (59 to 86 degrees F). Protect from heat. Keep container tightly closed. Throw away any unused medicine after the expiration date.

L

Loratadine tablets

CLARITIN®;
10 mg; Tablet
Schering Corp

LORATADINE;
10 mg; Tablet
Sandoz
Pharmaceuticals

What are loratadine tablets?

LORATADINE (Alavert™, Claritins, Claritin® Reditabs, Claritin® Hives Relief) is an antihistamine. It relieves the symptoms of hay fever (sneezing, runny nose, and itchy, watery eyes), and can also treat hives and associated itching of the skin. Generic loratadine tablets are available.

What should my health care professional know before I take loratadine?

They need to know if you have any of these conditions:
- asthma
- kidney disease
- liver disease
- an unusual or allergic reaction to loratadine, other medicines, foods, dyes, or preservatives
- pregnant or trying to get pregnant
- breast-feeding

How should I take this medicine?

Take loratadine tablets by mouth. Follow the directions on the prescription label. Take your doses at regular intervals. You may take this medicine with food. Do not take your medicine more often than directed. If you are taking Claritin® Reditabs or Alavert™: Place the tablet on your tongue, allow to dissolve completely and then swallow. You can take the Claritin® Reditabs or Alavert™ tablets with or without water. Contact your pediatrician or health care professional regarding the use of this medicine in children. Special care may be needed. This medicine may be used in children as young as 6 years old; younger children can receive the syrup form of this medicine.

What if I miss a dose?

If you miss a dose, take it as soon as you can. If it is almost time for your next dose, take only that dose. Do not take double doses.

What may interact with loratadine?

- certain antibiotics (clarithromycin, erythromycin)
- medicines for fungal infections (fluconazole, itraconazole, ketoconazole, voriconazole)
- medicines for HIV infection or AIDS

In addition, the following medicines can make you feel drowsy:

- alcohol
- barbiturate medicines for inducing sleep or treating seizures (convulsions)

- medicines for anxiety or sleeping problems, such as alprazolam, diazepam, or temazepam
- medicines for hay fever and other allergies such as antihistamines
- medicines for mental problems, including anxiety, depression and psychotic disturbances
- medicines for pain

Tell your prescriber or health care professional about all other medicines you are taking, including non-prescription medicines, nutritional supplements, or herbal products. Also tell your prescriber or health care professional if you are a frequent user of drinks with caffeine or alcohol, if you smoke, or if you use illegal drugs. These may affect the way your medicine works. Check with your health care professional before stopping or starting any of your medicines.

What should I watch for while taking loratadine?

Tell your prescriber or health care professional if your symptoms do not improve in 1 to 2 days. Do not drive, use machinery, or do anything that needs mental alertness until you know how loratadine affects you. To reduce the risk of dizzy or fainting spells, do not stand or sit up quickly, especially if you are an older patient. Alcohol may increase dizziness and drowsiness. Avoid alcoholic drinks. Your mouth may get dry. Chewing sugarless gum or sucking hard candy, and drinking plenty of water will help.

What side effects may I notice from taking loratadine?

Side effects that you should report to your prescriber or health care professional as soon as possible:
- unusual restlessness or nervousness in children

Side effects that usually do not require medical attention (report to your prescriber or health care professional if they continue or are bothersome):
- dry mouth
- headache
- tiredness or drowsiness

Where can I keep my medicine?

Keep out of the reach of children in a container that small children cannot open. Store at room temperature or between 2 and 25 degrees C (36 and 77 degrees F). Keep the Claritin® Reditabs in the foil pouch until ready to use. Protect from moisture. Throw away any unused medicine after the expiration date.

L

Loratadine; Pseudoephedrine tablets

CLARITIN-D® 12 HOUR; 5 mg/120 mg; Tablet, Extended Release Schering Corp

CLARITIN-D®; 10 mg/240 mg; Tablet, Extended Release Schering-Plough HealthCare Products Inc

What are loratadine; pseudoephedrine tablets?

LORATADINE; PSEUDOEPHEDRINE (Claritin-D® 12 Hour, Claritin-D® 24 Hour) is an antihistamine and decongestant. It relieves the symptoms of hay fever (seasonal rhinitis) and the common cold, including nasal and sinus congestion. Generic loratadine; pseudoephedrine tablets are available.

What should my health care professional know before I take loratadine; pseudoephedrine?

They need to know if you have any of these conditions:
- blood vessel disease
- diabetes
- difficulty swallowing
- glaucoma
- heart disease
- high blood pressure
- kidney disease
- liver disease
- overactive thyroid
- stomach ulcer
- urinary tract or prostate trouble
- an unusual or allergic reaction to acrivastine; pseudoephedrine, other medicines, foods, dyes, or preservatives
- pregnant or trying to get pregnant
- breast-feeding

How should I take this medicine?

Take loratadine; pseudoephedrine tablets by mouth. Follow the directions on the prescription label. Swallow the tablets whole with water. Do not cut, crush or chew the tablets. Take your doses at regular intervals. Do not take your medicine more often than directed. Contact your pediatrician or health care professional regarding the use of this medicine in children. Special care may be needed. Older patients may have a stronger reaction to this medicine.

What if I miss a dose?

If you miss a dose, take it as soon as you can. If it is almost time for your next dose, take only that dose. Do not take double doses.

What may interact with loratadine; pseudoephedrine?

- alcohol or illicit drugs such as cocaine
- bromocriptine
- caffeine
- certain antibiotics (clarithromycin, erythromycin)
- cimetidine

- barbiturate medicines for inducing sleep or treating seizures (convulsions), like phenobarbital
- erythromycin
- furazolidone
- linezolid
- MAO inhibitors (examples: Eldepryl®, Marplan®, Nardil® and Parnate®)
- mecamylamine
- medicines for anxiety or sleeping problems, such as alprazolam, diazepam or temazepam
- medicines for colds, breathing difficulties or weight loss, such as ephedra
- medicines for fungal infections (fluconazole, itraconazole, ketoconazole, voriconazole)
- medicines for hay fever and other allergies such as antihistamines
- medicines for heart disease such as digoxin or beta-blockers
- medicines for HIV infection or AIDS
- medicines for mental problems, including anxiety, depression and psychotic disturbances
- medicines for migraine headaches such as dihydroergotamine or ergotamine
- medicines for nasal congestion, such as more pseudoephedrine
- medicines for pain such as codeine or morphine
- methyldopa
- procarbazine
- reserpine
- sodium bicarbonate

Tell your prescriber or health care professional about all other medicines you are taking, including non-prescription medicines, nutritional supplements, or herbal products. Also tell your prescriber or health care professional if you are a frequent user of drinks with caffeine or alcohol, if you smoke, or if you use illegal drugs. These may affect the way your medicine works. Check with your health care professional before stopping or starting any of your medicines.

What should I watch for while taking loratadine; pseudoephedrine?

Tell your prescriber or health care professional if your symptoms do not improve in 1 to 2 days or if you have a high fever. Do not drive, use machinery, or do anything that needs mental alertness until you know how loratadine affects you. To reduce the risk of dizzy or fainting spells, do not stand or sit up quickly, especially if you are an older patient. Alcohol may increase dizziness and drowsiness. Avoid alcoholic drinks. Your mouth may get dry. Chewing sugarless gum or sucking hard candy, and drinking plenty of water will help.

L

What side effects may I notice from taking loratadine; pseudoephedrine?

Side effects that you should report to your prescriber or health care professional as soon as possible:
- abdominal pain or rectal bleeding
- chest pain
- confusion
- convulsions (seizures)
- difficulty breathing or wheezing
- difficulty swallowing or enlarged tongue
- difficulty urinating
- dizziness or fainting spells
- fast or irregular heartbeat, palpitations
- high blood pressure
- numbness or tingling in the hands or feet
- rash
- severe, persistent, or worsening headache
- tremor or muscle contractions
- visual changes
- vomiting

Side effects that usually do not require medical attention (report to your prescriber or health care professional if they continue or are bothersome):
- cough
- dry mouth
- headache (mild)
- loss of appetite or nausea
- nervousness or difficulty sleeping

Where can I keep my medicine?

Keep out of the reach of children in a container that small children cannot open. Store at room temperature or between 2 and 25 degrees C (36 and 77 degrees F). Protect from moisture. Throw away any unused medicine after the expiration date.

Lorazepam tablets

ATIVAN®;
1 mg; Tablet
Biovail
Pharmaceuticals Inc

LORAZEPAM;
1 mg; Tablet
UDL Laboratories
Inc

What are lorazepam tablets?

LORAZEPAM (Ativan®) is a benzodiazepine. Benzodiazepines belong to a group of medicines that slow down the central nervous system. Lorazepam relieves anxiety and nervousness. Federal law prohibits the transfer of lorazepam to any person other than the patient for whom it was prescribed. Do not share this medicine with anyone else. Generic lorazepam tablets are available.

What should my health care professional know before I take lorazepam?

They need to know if you have any of these conditions:
- an alcohol or drug abuse problem
- bipolar disorder, depression, psychosis or other mental health condition
- glaucoma
- kidney disease
- liver disease
- lung disease, such as chronic obstructive pulmonary disease (COPD), sleep apnea or other breathing difficulties
- myasthenia gravis
- Parkinson's disease
- seizures or a history of seizures
- shortness of breath
- snoring
- suicidal thoughts
- an unusual or allergic reaction to lorazepam, other benzodiazepines, foods, dyes, or preservatives
- pregnant or trying to get pregnant
- breast-feeding

How should I take this medicine?

Take lorazepam tablets by mouth. Follow the directions on the prescription label. Swallow the tablets with a drink of water. If lorazepam upsets your stomach, take it with food or milk. Take your doses at regular intervals. Do not take your medicine more often than directed. Do not stop taking except on your prescriber's advice. Contact your pediatrician or health care professional regarding the use of this medicine in children. Special care may be needed.

What if I miss a dose?

If you miss a dose and remember within an hour, take it as soon as you can. If it is more than an hour since you missed a dose, skip that dose and go back to your regular schedule. Do not take double or extra doses.

What may interact with lorazepam?

- alcohol
- barbiturate medicines for inducing sleep or treating seizures (convulsions), like phenobarbital
- caffeine
- female hormones, including contraceptive or birth control pills
- herbal or dietary supplements such as kava kava, melatonin, or valerian
- levodopa
- medicines for anxiety or sleeping problems, such as alprazolam, diazepam or triazolam
- medicines for depression, mental problems or psychiatric disturbances
- phenytoin
- prescription pain medicines
- probenecid
- some medicines for colds, hay fever or other allergies
- theophylline
- valproic acid

L

Tell your prescriber or health care professional about all other medicines you are taking, including non-prescription medicines, nutritional supplements, or herbal products. Also tell your prescriber or health care professional if you are a frequent user of drinks with caffeine or alcohol, if you smoke, or if you use illegal drugs. These may affect the way your medicine works. Check with your health care professional before stopping or starting any of your medicines.

What should I watch for while taking lorazepam?

Visit your prescriber or health care professional for regular checks on your progress. Your body may become dependent on lorazepam; ask your prescriber or health care professional if you still need to take it. However, if you have been taking lorazepam regularly for some time, do not suddenly stop taking it. You must gradually reduce the dose or you may get severe side effects. Ask your prescriber or health care professional for advice before increasing or decreasing the dose. Even after you stop taking lorazepam it can still affect your body for several days. You may get drowsy or dizzy. Do not drive, use machinery, or do anything that needs mental alertness until you know how lorazepam affects you. To reduce the risk of dizzy and fainting spells, do not stand or sit up quickly, especially if you are an older patient. Alcohol may increase dizziness and drowsiness. Avoid alcoholic drinks. Do not treat yourself for coughs, colds or allergies without asking your prescriber or health care professional for advice. Some ingredients can increase possible side effects. If you are going to have surgery, tell your prescriber or health care professional that you are taking lorazepam.

What side effects may I notice from taking lorazepam?

Side effects that you should report to your prescriber or health care professional as soon as possible:
- confusion
- depression
- double vision or abnormal eye movements
- hallucinations (seeing and hearing things that are not really there)
- lightheadedness or fainting spells
- mood changes, excitability or aggressive behavior
- movement difficulty, staggering or jerky movements
- muscle cramps
- restlessness
- tremors
- weakness or tiredness

Side effects that usually do not require medical attention (report to your prescriber or health care professional if they continue or are bothersome):
- constipation or diarrhea
- difficulty sleeping, nightmares
- dizziness, drowsiness, clumsiness, or unsteadiness; a "hangover" effect
- headache
- loss of memory
- nausea, vomiting

Where can I keep my medicine?

Keep out of the reach of children in a container that small children cannot open. Store at room temperature, approximately 25 degrees C (77 degrees F). Protect from light. Keep container tightly closed. Throw away any unused medicine after the expiration date.

Losartan tablets

COZAAR®;
50 mg; Tablet
Merck and Co Inc

COZAAR®;
25 mg; Tablet
Merck and Co Inc

What are losartan tablets?

LOSARTAN (Cozaar®) helps lower blood pressure to normal levels. It controls high blood pressure, but it is not a cure. High blood pressure can damage your kidneys, and may lead to a stroke or heart failure. Losartan helps prevent these things from happening. Losartan is also used to improve symptoms in patients with heart failure. Generic losartan tablets are not yet available.

What should my health care professional know before I take losartan?

They need to know if you have any of these conditions:
- heart failure
- kidney disease
- liver disease
- electrolyte imbalance (e.g. low or high levels of potassium in the blood)
- if you are on a special diet, such as a low-salt diet (e.g. using potassium substitutes)
- an unusual or allergic reaction to losartan, other medicines, foods, dyes, or preservatives
- pregnant or trying to get pregnant
- breast-feeding

How should I take this medicine?

Take losartan tablets by mouth. Follow the directions on the prescription label. Swallow the tablets with a drink of water. Losartan can be taken with or without food. Take your doses at regular intervals. Do not take your medicine more often than directed.

What if I miss a dose?

If you miss a dose, take it as soon as you can. If it is almost time for your next dose, take only that dose. Do not take double or extra doses.

What may interact with losartan?

- anti-inflammatory pain medicines such as ibuprofen (Motrin®)
- blood pressure medications
- bosentan
- cimetidine
- delavirdine
- fluconazole
- hawthorn
- lithium
- phenobarbital
- potassium salts or potassium supplements
- rifampin
- voriconazole
- water pills (especially potassium-sparing diuretics such as triamterene or amiloride)

Tell your prescriber or health care professional about all other medicines you are taking, including non-prescription medicines, nutritional supplements, or herbal products. Also tell your prescriber or health care professional if you are a frequent user of drinks with caffeine or alcohol, if you smoke, or if you use illegal drugs. These may affect the way your medicine works. Check with your health care professional before stopping or starting any of your medicines.

What should I watch for while taking losartan?

Check your blood pressure regularly while you are taking losartan. Ask your prescriber or health care professional what your blood pressure should be and when you should contact him or her. When you check your blood pressure, write down the measurements to show your prescriber or health care professional. If you are taking this medicine for a long time you must visit your prescriber or health care professional for regular checks on your progress. Make sure you schedule appointments on a regular basis. You may experience dizziness. Do not drive, use machinery, or do anything that requires mental alertness until you know how losartan affects you. To avoid dizziness, do not stand or sit up quickly. Avoid salt substitutes unless you are told otherwise by your prescriber or health care professional. If you are going to have surgery tell your prescriber or health care professional that you are taking losartan.

What side effects may I notice from taking losartan?

Side effects that you should report to your prescriber or health care professional as soon as possible:
Rare or uncommon:
- difficulty breathing or swallowing, hoarseness, or tightening of the throat
- swelling of your face, lips, tongue, hands, or feet
- unusual rash

Other:
- confusion, dizziness, lightheadedness or fainting spells
- decreased amount of urine passed
- decreased sexual function
- fast or uneven heart beat, palpitations, or chest pain

Side effects that usually do not require medical attention (report to your prescriber or health care professional if they continue or are bothersome):
- cough
- diarrhea
- fatigue or tiredness
- headache
- inability to sleep
- nausea or stomach pain
- nasal congestion or stuffiness
- sore or cramping muscles
- upset stomach

Where can I keep my medicine?

Keep out of the reach of children in a container that small children cannot open. Store at room temperature between 15 and 30 degrees C (59 and 86 degrees F). Protect from light. Keep container tightly closed. Throw away any unused medicine after the expiration date.

Lovastatin extended-release tablets

ALTOPREV™; 20 mg; Tablet, Extended Release Andrx Laboratories Inc

ALTOPREV™; 40 mg; Tablet, Extended Release Andrx Laboratories Inc

What are lovastatin extended-release tablets?

LOVASTATIN (Altoprev™) extended-release tablets block the body's ability to make cholesterol. Lovastatin can help lower blood cholesterol for patients who are at risk of getting heart disease or a stroke. It is only for patients whose cholesterol level is not controlled by diet. It is not a cure. Generic lovastatin extended-release tablets are not yet available.

What should my health care professional know before I take lovastatin?

They need to know if you have any of these conditions:

- an alcohol problem
- any hormone disorder (such as diabetes, underactive thyroid)
- blood salt imbalance
- infection
- kidney disease
- liver disease
- low blood pressure
- muscle disorder or condition
- recent surgery
- seizures (convulsions)
- severe injury

L

- an unusual or allergic reaction to lovastatin, other medicines, foods, dyes, or preservatives
- pregnant or trying to get pregnant
- breast-feeding

How should this medicine be taken?

Take lovastatin extended-release tablets by mouth in the evening, at bedtime. Follow the directions on the prescription label. Swallow the tablets whole with a drink of water. Do not crush or chew these tablets. It is best to take this medicine on an empty stomach without food. Do not take lovastatin with grapefruit juice. Take your doses at regular intervals. Do not take your medicine more often than directed. Contact your pediatrician or health care professional regarding the use of this medicine in children. Special care may be needed.

What if I miss a dose?

If you miss a dose, take it as soon as you can. If it is almost time for your next dose, take only that dose. Do not take double or extra doses.

What may interact with lovastatin?

Do not take lovastatin with any of the following:

- amprenavir
- atazanavir
- clarithromycin
- delavirdine
- erythromycin
- grapefruit juice
- indinavir
- itraconazole
- ketoconazole
- lopinavir; ritonavir
- mibefradil
- nefazodone
- nelfinavir
- ritonavir
- saquinavir
- troleandomycin
- went yeast (dietary supplement)

Lovastatin may also interact with the following medications:

- alcohol
- amiodarone
- barbiturates (examples: phenobarbital, butalbital, primidone)
- bosentan
- carbamazepine
- cilostazol
- cyclosporine
- danazol
- diltiazem
- efavirenz
- imatinib, STI-571
- isradipine
- fluconazole
- medicines to lower cholesterol or triglycerides (examples: clofibrate, fenofibrate, gemfibrozil, niacin)
- medicine used to stop early pregnancy (mifepristone, RU-486)
- nicardipine

- oxcarbazepine
- phenytoin
- rifampin, rifabutin, or rifapentine
- St. John's wort
- telithromycin
- verapamil
- voriconazole
- warfarin

Tell your prescriber or health care professional about all other medicines you are taking, including non-prescription medicines, nutritional supplements, or herbal products. Also tell your prescriber or health care professional if you are a frequent user of drinks with caffeine or alcohol, if you smoke, or if you use illegal drugs. These may affect the way your medicine works. Check with your health care professional before stopping or starting any of your medicines.

What should I watch for while taking lovastatin?

Visit your prescriber or health care professional for regular checks on your progress. You may need to have blood tests drawn to make sure your liver is working properly. Tell your prescriber or health care professional as soon as you can if you get any unexplained muscle pain, tenderness, or weakness, especially if you also have a fever and tiredness. Some medicines increase the risk of muscle side effects while taking lovastatin. Discuss your drug regimen with your health care provider if you are prescribed certain antibiotics or antifungals which are not recommended with lovastatin (examples: clarithromycin, erythromycin, itraconazole, ketoconazole). Your prescriber may decide to temporarily stop the lovastatin treatment while you are taking a short course of the antibiotic or antifungal therapy. Alternatively, your health care provider may prescribe another antibiotic or antifungal medicine for your condition. Lovastatin is only part of a total cholesterol-lowering program. Your physician or dietician can suggest a low-cholesterol and low-fat diet that will reduce your risk of getting heart and blood vessel disease. Avoid alcohol and smoking, and keep a proper exercise schedule. If you are going to have surgery, tell your prescriber or health care professional that you are taking lovastatin.

What side effects may I notice from taking lovastatin?

Side effects that you should report to your prescriber or health care professional as soon as possible:
Rare or uncommon:

- blurred vision, or vision changes
- dark yellow or brown urine
- decreased urination, difficulty passing urine
- fever
- muscle pain, tenderness, cramps, or weakness
- redness, blistering, peeling or loosening of the skin, including inside the mouth
- skin rash, itching

- unusual tiredness or weakness
- yellowing of the skin or eyes

Side effects that usually do not require medical attention (report to your prescriber or health care professional if they continue or are bothersome):
- constipation or diarrhea
- difficulty sleeping
- dizziness
- headache

- nausea, vomiting
- stomach pain or indigestion

Where can I keep my medicine?

Keep out of the reach of children in a container that small children cannot open. Store at room temperature between 20 and 25 degrees C (68 and 77 degrees F). Avoid exposure to heat and moisture. Throw away any unused medicine after the expiration date.

Lovastatin tablets

MEVACOR®;
20 mg; Tablet
Merck and Co Inc

MEVACOR®;
10 mg; Tablet
Merck and Co Inc

What are lovastatin tablets?

LOVASTATIN (Mevacor®) blocks the body's ability to make cholesterol. Lovastatin can help lower blood cholesterol for patients who are at risk of getting heart disease or a stroke. It is only for patients whose cholesterol level is not controlled by diet. It is not a cure. Generic lovastatin tablets are available.

What should my health care professional know before I take lovastatin?

They need to know if you have any of these conditions:
- an alcohol problem
- any hormone disorder (such as diabetes, underactive thyroid)
- blood salt imbalance
- infection
- kidney disease
- liver disease
- low blood pressure
- muscle disorder or condition
- recent surgery
- seizures (convulsions)
- severe injury
- an unusual or allergic reaction to lovastatin, other medicines, foods, dyes, or preservatives
- pregnant or trying to get pregnant
- breast-feeding

How should I take this medicine?

Take lovastatin tablets by mouth. Follow the directions on the prescription label. Take lovastatin tablets with food. If you take lovastatin once a day, take the dose with the evening meal. Swallow the tablets with a drink of water. Do not take lovastatin with grapefruit juice; orange juice may be used instead. Take your doses at regular intervals. Do not take your medicine more often than directed. Contact your pediatrician or health care professional regarding the use of this medicine in children. Special care may be needed.

What if I miss a dose?

If you miss a dose, take it as soon as you can. If it is almost time for your next dose, take only that dose. Do not take double or extra doses.

What may interact with lovastatin?

Do not take lovastatin with any of the following:
- amprenavir
- atazanavir
- clarithromycin
- delavirdine
- erythromycin
- grapefruit juice
- indinavir
- itraconazole
- ketoconazole
- lopinavir; ritonavir
- mibefradil
- nefazodone
- nelfinavir
- ritonavir
- saquinavir
- troleandomycin
- went yeast (dietary supplement)

Lovastatin may also interact with the following medications:
- alcohol
- amiodarone
- barbiturates (examples: phenobarbital, butalbital, primidone)
- bosentan
- carbamazepine
- cilostazol
- cyclosporine
- danazol
- diltiazem
- efavirenz
- imatinib, STI-571
- isradipine
- fluconazole
- medicines to lower cholesterol or triglycerides (examples: clofibrate, fenofibrate, gemfibrozil, niacin)
- medicine used to stop early pregnancy (mifepristone, RU-486)
- nicardipine
- oxcarbazepine
- phenytoin
- rifampin, rifabutin, or rifapentine
- St. John's wort
- telithromycin
- verapamil

L

- voriconazole
- warfarin

Tell your prescriber or health care professional about all other medicines you are taking, including non-prescription medicines, nutritional supplements, or herbal products. Also tell your prescriber or health care professional if you are a frequent user of drinks with caffeine or alcohol, if you smoke, or if you use illegal drugs. These may affect the way your medicine works. Check with your health care professional before stopping or starting any of your medicines.

What should I watch for while taking lovastatin?

Visit your prescriber or health care professional for regular checks on your progress. You may need to have blood tests drawn to make sure your liver is working properly. Tell your prescriber or health care professional as soon as you can if you get any unexplained muscle pain, tenderness, or weakness, especially if you also have a fever and tiredness. Some medicines increase the risk of muscle side effects while taking lovastatin. Discuss your drug regimen with your health care provider if you are prescribed certain antibiotics or antifungals which are not recommended with lovastatin (examples: clarithromycin, erythromycin, itraconazole, ketoconazole). Your prescriber may decide to temporarily stop the lovastatin while you are taking a short course of the antibiotic or antifungal therapy. Alternatively, your health care provider may prescribe another antibiotic or antifungal medicine for your condition. Lovastatin is only part of a total cholesterol-lowering program. Your physician or dietician can suggest a low-cholesterol and low-fat diet that will reduce your risk of getting heart and blood vessel disease.

Avoid alcohol and smoking, and keep a proper exercise schedule. If you are going to have surgery, tell your prescriber or health care professional that you are taking lovastatin.

What side effects may I notice from taking lovastatin?

Side effects that you should report to your prescriber or health care professional as soon as possible:
Rare or uncommon:
- blurred vision, or vision changes
- dark yellow or brown urine
- decreased urination, difficulty passing urine
- fever
- muscle pain, tenderness, cramps, or weakness
- redness, blistering, peeling or loosening of the skin, including inside the mouth
- skin rash, itching
- unusual tiredness or weakness
- yellowing of the skin or eyes

Side effects that usually do not require medical attention (report to your prescriber or health care professional if they continue or are bothersome):
- constipation or diarrhea
- difficulty sleeping
- dizziness
- headache
- nausea, vomiting
- stomach pain or indigestion

Where can I keep my medicine?

Keep out of the reach of children in a container that small children cannot open. Store at room temperature between 5 and 30 degrees C (41 and 86 degrees F). Protect from light. Throw away any unused medicine after the expiration date.

Lovastatin; Niacin extended-release tablets	ADVICOR™; 20 mg/1000 mg; Tablet Kos Pharmaceuticals Inc		ADVICOR™; 20 mg/750 mg; Tablet Kos Pharmaceuticals Inc	

What are lovastatin; niacin extended-release tablets?

LOVASTATIN; NIACIN (Advicor™) blocks the body's ability to make cholesterol. Advicor™ can help lower your cholesterol level. The combination of lovastatin and niacin lowers the "bad" cholesterol level (LDL) and increases the "good" cholesterol level (HDL). By improving your cholesterol levels, you may decrease your risk of having a heart attack or stroke. This medicine is only for patients whose cholesterol levels are not controlled by diet and exercise alone. Generic tablets are not available.

What should my health care professional know before I take lovastatin; niacin?

They need to know if you have any of these conditions:

- an alcohol problem
- blood salt imbalance
- diabetes or other hormone disorder
- gallbladder disease
- gout
- heart disease or a history of heart attack
- infection
- kidney disease
- liver disease
- low blood counts, low platelets, or bleeding problems
- low blood pressure or taking drugs to lower blood pressure
- muscle disorder or condition
- recent surgery or severe injury
- seizures (convulsions)
- ulcers of intestine or stomach
- an unusual or allergic reaction to lovastatin; niacin, other medicines, foods, dyes, or preservatives

- pregnant or trying to get pregnant
- breast-feeding

How should I take this medicine?

Take lovastatin; niacin tablets by mouth. Follow the directions on the prescription label. Swallow the tablet with a drink of water. Do not crush, break, or chew the tablet. The tablet should be taken in the evening with a low-fat snack. Do not take lovastatin; niacin with grapefruit juice, hot beverages, or alcohol-containing beverages. Take your doses at regular intervals. Do not take your medicine more often than directed. If skin flushing (skin warmth, redness) becomes a problem, ask your health care provider if you can take aspirin (or ibuprofen) before taking your lovastatin; niacin doses. Taking one dose of aspirin (or ibuprofen) 30 minutes before taking lovastatin; niacin can help to decrease the amount of flushing you experience. If you also take resins such as cholestyramine (Questran®) or colestipol (Colestid®) to lower your cholesterol, you should take lovastatin; niacin at least 1 hour before or 4 hours after a dose of these medications. Contact your pediatrician or health care professional regarding the use of this medicine in children. Special care may be needed.

What if I miss a dose?

If you miss a dose, take it as soon as you can. If it is almost time for your next dose, take only that dose. Do not take double or extra doses.

What may interact with lovastatin; niacin?

Do not take lovastatin; niacin with any of the following:

- alcohol-containing beverages
- amprenavir
- atazanavir
- clarithromycin
- delavirdine
- erythromycin
- grapefruit juice
- indinavir
- itraconazole
- ketoconazole
- lopinavir; ritonavir
- mibefradil
- nefazodone
- nelfinavir
- other niacin products
- ritonavir
- saquinavir
- troleandomycin
- went yeast (Cholestin™, a dietary supplement)

Lovastatin; niacin may also interact with the following medications:

- amiodarone
- barbiturates (examples: phenobarbital, butalbital, primidone)
- bosentan
- carbamazepine
- cilostazol
- cyclosporine

- danazol
- diltiazem
- efavirenz
- imatinib, STI-571
- isradipine
- fluconazole
- medicines for diabetes
- medicines for high blood pressure or heart disease
- medicine used to stop early pregnancy (mifepristone, RU-486)
- nitroglycerin or nitrates (amyl nitrate, isosorbide dinitrate, isosorbide mononitrate)
- other medicines to lower cholesterol or triglycerides (cholestyramine, colestipol, fenofibrate, gemfibrozil)
- oxcarbazepine
- phenytoin
- rifampin, rifabutin, or rifapentine
- St. John's wort
- telithromycin
- verapamil
- warfarin

Tell your prescriber or health care professional about all other medicines you are taking, including non-prescription medicines, nutritional supplements, or herbal products. Also tell your prescriber or health care professional if you are a frequent user of drinks with caffeine or alcohol, if you smoke, or if you use illegal drugs. These may affect the way your medicine works. Check with your health care professional before stopping or starting any of your medicines.

What should I watch for while taking lovastatin; niacin?

Visit your prescriber or health care professional for regular checks on your progress. Do not take more lovastatin; niacin than is prescribed. You will need to have regular tests to make sure your liver is working properly. Lovastatin; niacin is only part of a total cholesterol-lowering program. Your physician or dietician can suggest a low-cholesterol and low-fat diet that will reduce your risk of getting heart and blood vessel disease. Avoid alcohol and smoking, and keep a proper exercise schedule. Tell your prescriber or health care professional as soon as you can if you get any unexplained muscle pain, tenderness, or weakness, especially if you also have a fever and tiredness. Some medicines increase the risk of muscle side effects while taking lovastatin; niacin. Discuss your drug regimen with your health care provider if you are prescribed certain antibiotics or antifungals which are not recommended with lovastatin; niacin (examples: clarithromycin, erythromycin, itraconazole, ketoconazole). Your prescriber may decide to temporarily stop taking lovastatin; niacin while you are taking a short course of the antibiotic or antifungal therapy. Alternatively, your health care provider may prescribe another antibiotic or antifungal medicine for your condition. You may get dizzy, faint, or have blurred vision; until you know how niacin affects you, do not drive, use machinery, or do anything that needs mental alertness. To avoid dizzy or fainting spells, do not stand or sit up quickly, especially if you are an older person. Do not drink hot drinks or alcohol at the same time you take your lovastatin; niacin dose. Hot drinks and alcohol can increase the flushing caused by lovastatin; niacin, which can be uncomfortable. Alcohol also can increase possible dizziness. If you are going to have surgery tell your prescriber or health care professional that you are taking lovastatin; niacin. You may notice the empty shell of the tablet in your stool; this is no cause for concern.

What side effects may I notice from taking lovastatin; niacin?

Side effects that you should report to your prescriber or health care professional as soon as possible:
Rare or uncommon:
- blurred vision
- breathing problems
- chest pain
- dark yellow or brown urine
- decreased urination, difficulty passing urine
- fever
- sexual problems
- unexplained muscle pain, tenderness, cramps, or weakness
- unusual or severe tiredness or weakness or eyes
- yellowing of the skin or eyes

More common:
- dizziness that does not go away or fainting spells
- increased blood sugar, especially if you have diabetes
- nausea, vomiting
- palpitations
- skin rash, hives, peeling or itching of the skin
- stomach pain, loss of appetite
- swelling of the body (e.g., legs, ankles, arms)

Side effects that usually do not require medical attention (report to your prescriber or health care professional if they continue or are bothersome):
- chills
- diarrhea or constipation
- difficulty sleeping
- dizziness (mild), lightheadedness
- flushing (skin redness), warmth, and burning or tingling of the skin
- gas
- headache
- stomach upset, discomfort, or bloating
- sweating

Where can I keep my medicine?

Keep out of the reach of children in a container that small children cannot open. Store at controlled room temperature between 20 and 25 degrees C (68 and 77 degrees F). Keep container tightly closed. Throw away any unused medicine after the expiration date.

L

Magnesium Salts
capsules, tablets, or oral solution

MAG DELAY®;
64 mg; Tablet,
Extended Release
Major
Pharmaceuticals Inc

MAG-OX® 400;
400 mg; Tablet
Blaine Company Inc

What are magnesium salts?

MAGNESIUM SALTS (MAG-Delay®, MAG-OX) can be given as a dietary supplement to prevent or correct low blood magnesium caused by malnutrition or certain diseases. Magnesium salts can also be taken to relieve constipation or to cleanse the bowel before medical procedures.

What should my health care professional know before I take magnesium salts?

They need to know if you have any of these conditions:
- dehydration
- heart disease
- kidney disease
- stomach blockage

How should I take this medicine?

Directions for taking the capsules or tablets:
Magnesium capsules and tablets are taken by mouth with a full glass of water. Follow the directions on the label. Take your doses at regular intervals only if you are treating a mineral deficiency. Otherwise only take as needed. Do not take more often than prescribed.
Directions for taking the oral solution:
Add the prescribed dose to a full glass of water (at least 8 oz). Drink the solution at least 1 hour before or 2 hours after a meal. Follow the directions on the label. Take your doses at regular intervals only if you are treating a mineral deficiency. Otherwise only take as needed. Do not take more often than prescribed.

What if I miss a dose?

If you are taking magnesium salts on a regular basis and miss a dose, take it as soon as you can. If it is almost time for your next dose, take only that dose. Do not take double or extra doses.

What may interact with magnesium salts?

- barbiturate medicines for inducing sleep or treating seizures (convulsions)
- certain antibiotics
- ethanol
- medicines for anxiety or sleeping problems, such as diazepam or temazepam
- medicines for hay fever and other allergies
- medicines for heart problems
- medicines for mental depression
- medicines for mental problems or psychotic disturbances
- medicines for pain
- other magnesium-containing antacids, laxatives or supplements
- water pills

Tell your prescriber or health care professional about all other medicines you are taking, including non-prescription medicines, nutritional supplements, or herbal products. Also tell your prescriber or health care professional if you are a frequent user of drinks with caffeine or alcohol, if you smoke, or if you use illegal drugs. These may affect the way your medicine works. Check with your health care professional before stopping or starting any of your medicines.

What should I watch for while taking magnesium salts?

Do not use magnesium salts as a laxative for more than one week without consulting your prescriber or health care professional. Laxative products should only be taken as single and infrequent doses. Continued use can lead to problems with the amounts of water and salts in your blood. Continued constipation may indicate a more serious problem needing medical attention. Take magnesium salts with plenty of water to improve the laxative effect and prevent dehydration.

What side effects may I notice from taking magnesium salts?

Side effects that you should report to your prescriber or health care professional as soon as possible:
Rare:
- flushing
- lightheadedness or fainting spells
- low body temperature
- slow or difficult breathing
- slow reflexes
- sweating
- unusual tiredness or weakness

Side effects that usually do not require medical attention (report to your prescriber or health care professional if they continue or are bothersome):
- diarrhea

Where can I keep my medicine?

Keep out of the reach of children in a container that small children cannot open. Store at room temperature between 15 and 30 degrees C (59 and 86 degrees F). Keep container tightly closed. Throw away any unused medicine after the expiration date.

Recommended Dietary Allowance (RDA):

The Recommended Dietary Allowance (RDA) is the daily amount of a vitamin or mineral needed to supply adequate nutrition for healthy persons. The RDA is different for each group of people based on age, physical state (i.e. pregnancy), and sex. Your needs can be met by the foods you eat, by taking a supplement, or the

M

two of these together. Ask your health care professional if you have questions regarding these recommendations. The RDA for magnesium is:

Group

Females, pregnant or breast-feeding: 350 and 400 mg

Adult females: 310 and 320 mg
Adult males: 400 and 420 mg
Adolescents 14 to 18 years old: 360 and 410 mg
Children 9 to 13 years old: 240 mg
Children 1 to 8 years old: 80 and 130 mg

This drug requires an FDA medication guide. See page xxxvii.

Maprotiline tablets

MAPROTILINE;
50 mg; Tablet
Mylan
Pharmaceuticals Inc

MAPROTILINE;
75 mg; Tablet
Watson
Pharmaceuticals Inc

What are maprotiline tablets?

MAPROTILINE (Ludiomil®) is an antidepressant, a medicine that helps to lift mental depression. Maprotiline helps to relieve different types of depression and also helps to relieve anxiety associated with depression. Generic maprotiline tablets are available.

What should my health care professional know before I take maprotiline?

They need to know if you have any of these conditions:
- an alcohol abuse problem
- asthma
- bipolar disorder
- blood disorders
- breathing difficulties
- diabetes
- difficulty passing urine
- having intramuscular injections
- heart disease
- liver disease
- over-active thyroid
- Parkinson's disease
- previous heart attack
- prostate trouble
- schizophrenia
- seizures (convulsions)
- stomach or intestinal disease
- an unusual or allergic reaction to maprotiline, other medicines, foods, dyes, or preservatives
- pregnant or trying to get pregnant
- breast-feeding

How should I take this medicine?

Take maprotiline tablets by mouth. Follow the directions on the prescription label. Swallow the tablets with a drink of water. Take your doses at regular intervals. Do not take your medicine more often than directed. Do not stop taking the tablets except on your prescriber's advice. Contact your pediatrician or health care professional regarding the use of this medicine in children. Special care may be needed. Elderly patients over 60 years old may have a stronger reaction to this medicine and need smaller doses.

What if I miss a dose?

If you miss a dose, take it as soon as you can. If it is less than four hours to your next dose, take only that dose and skip the missed dose. If you only take a single dose at bedtime and forget, do not take it in the morning without checking with your prescriber or health care professional. Do not take double or extra doses.

What may interact with maprotiline?

Maprotiline can interact with many other medicines. An interaction can be very important or fairly insignificant. Make sure your prescriber or health care professional knows about all other medicines you are taking; the most important are listed below:
- alcohol
- barbiturate medicines for inducing sleep or treating seizures (convulsions)
- blood thinners
- cimetidine or ranitidine
- clonidine
- disulfiram
- erythromycin
- female hormones, including contraceptive or birth control pills
- labetalol
- linezolid
- medicines for anxiety or sleeping problems, such as diazepam or temazepam
- medicines for colds and breathing difficulties
- medicines for hay fever and other allergies
- medicines for high blood pressure
- medicines for mental depression
- medicines for mental problems and psychotic disturbances
- medicines for movement abnormalities as in Parkinson's disease, or for gastrointestinal problems
- medicines for over- or under-active thyroid
- seizure (convulsion) or epilepsy medicine

Tell your prescriber or health care professional about all other medicines you are taking, including non-prescription medicines, nutritional supplements, or herbal products. Also tell your prescriber or health care professional if you are a frequent user of drinks with caffeine or alcohol, if you smoke, or if you use illegal drugs. These may affect the way your medicine works. Check with your health care professional before stopping or starting any of your medicines.

What should I watch for while taking maprotiline?

Visit your prescriber or health care professional for regular checks on your progress. You may have to take

M

maprotiline for several weeks before you feel better. If you have been taking maprotiline for some time, do not suddenly stop taking it. Your prescriber or health care professional may want you to gradually reduce the dose; ask for advice. You may get drowsy, dizzy or have blurred vision. Do not drive, use machinery, or do anything that needs mental alertness until you know how maprotiline affects you. Do not stand or sit up quickly, especially if you are an older patient. This reduces the risk of dizzy or fainting spells. Alcohol may increase dizziness or drowsiness; avoid alcoholic drinks. Maprotiline can make your mouth dry. Chewing sugarless gum, sucking hard candy and drinking plenty of water will help. Maprotiline may make your skin more sensitive to sun or ultraviolet light. Keep out of the sun, or wear protective clothing outdoors and use a sunscreen (at least SPF 15). Do not use sun lamps or sun tanning beds or booths. Do not treat yourself for coughs, colds, or allergies without asking your prescriber or health care professional for advice. Some ingredients may increase possible side effects. If you are going to have surgery or will need an x-ray procedure that uses contrast agents, tell your prescriber or health care professional that you are taking this medicine.

What side effects may I notice from taking maprotiline?

Side effects that you should report to your prescriber or health care professional as soon as possible:
- difficulty breathing
- eye pain
- fainting spells
- fast or irregular heartbeat (palpitations)

- fever with increased sweating
- hallucinations (seeing or hearing things that are not really there)
- loss of bladder control, or problems passing urine
- muscle stiffness or problems with movement
- pale skin
- seizures (convulsions)
- skin rash or itching (hives)
- swelling or tenderness of breasts or testicles
- unusual and uncontrollable muscle twitches or movements of the mouth (lip-smacking, puckering, chewing)
- yellowing of the eyes or skin

Side effects that usually do not require medical attention (report to your prescriber or health care professional if they continue or are bothersome):
- blurred vision
- confusion or nervousness
- constipation or diarrhea
- drowsiness, dizziness or lightheadedness
- dry mouth
- headache
- increased appetite and weight gain
- increased sensitivity to sunlight
- nausea, vomiting
- sexual difficulties (decreased sexual ability or desire)
- trouble sleeping (insomnia)
- unusual tiredness or weakness

Where can I keep my medicine?

Keep out of the reach of children in a container that small children cannot open. Store at room temperature below 30 degrees C (86 degrees F). Keep container tightly closed. Throw away any unused medicine after the expiration date.

Mebendazole tablets

VERMOX®;
100 mg; Tablet, Chewable
McNeil Consumer and
Specialty Pharmaceuticals

What are mebendazole tablets?

MEBENDAZOLE (Vermox®) is an anthelmintic. This medicine treats parasitic (worm) infections from roundworms, hookworms, pinworms, whipworms, or infections with two or more of these worms. Generic mebendazole tablets are available.

What should my health care professional know before I take mebendazole?

They need to know if you have any of these conditions:
- Crohn's disease
- inflammatory bowel disease
- liver disease
- ulcerative colitis
- an unusual or allergic reaction to mebendazole or other substances, such as foods, preservatives or dyes
- pregnant or trying to get pregnant
- breast-feeding

How should I take this medicine?

Take mebendazole tablets by mouth. Follow the directions on the prescription label. Mebendazole works best when taken with food, especially fatty foods such as whole milk, cheese, or ice cream. You can chew the tablets, swallow them whole or crush and mix with food (such as ice cream or pudding), which is an easy way to give the tablets to children. Do not take your medicine more often than directed. Finish the full course of medicine prescribed by your prescriber or health care professional even if you feel better. Space your doses evenly through the day and night and take at the same time each day. Parasite (worm) death can be slow. To remove all parasites (worms) from the intestines can take several days. Contact your pediatrician or health care professional regarding the use of this medicine in children. Special care may be needed.

M

What if I miss a dose?

If you miss a dose, take it as soon as you can. If it is almost time for your next dose, take only that dose. Do not take double or extra doses. You must leave a suitable interval between doses. If you are taking one dose a day and have to take a missed dose, make sure there is at least 10 to 12 hours between doses. If you are taking two doses a day and have to take a missed dose, make sure there is at least 5 to 6 hours between doses.

What may interact with mebendazole?

- carbamazepine
- phenytoin

Tell your prescriber or health care professional about all other medicines you are taking, including non-prescription medicines, nutritional supplements, or herbal products. Also tell your prescriber or health care professional if you are a frequent user of drinks with caffeine or alcohol, if you smoke, or if you use illegal drugs. These may affect the way your medicine works. Check with your health care professional before stopping or starting any of your medicines.

What should I watch for while taking mebendazole?

Visit your prescriber or health care professional to check that your infection has gone. If you still have an infection after 3 weeks you may need a second course of tablets. If you have hookworms or whipworms you may be anemic. Check with your prescriber or health care professional to see if you need iron supplements. If you have pinworms other people in your house may need treatment. Pinworms are spread easily by close contact. Wash your hands, scrub your fingernails and shower often. Every day change and launder bedclothes, linens, and undergarments. This will help keep other family members from getting infected. Disinfect the toilet every day, and damp mop the floors often to reduce the number of worm eggs.

What side effects may I notice from taking mebendazole?

Side effects that you should report to your prescriber or health care professional as soon as possible:
- fever or chills, sore throat
- rash, itching
- unusual weakness or tiredness

Side effects that usually do not require medical attention (report to your prescriber or health care professional if they continue or are bothersome):
- diarrhea
- dizziness
- headache
- nausea, vomiting
- ringing in the ears
- stomach pain, which can occur when large numbers of worms are present

Where can I keep my medicine?

Keep out of the reach of children in a container that small children cannot open. Store at room temperature between 15 and 30 degrees C (59 and 86 degrees F). Throw away any unused medicine after the expiration date.

Meclizine tablets, capsules, or chewable tablets

ANTIVERT®;
25 mg; Tablet
Roerig Division of
Pfizer

ANTIVERT®;
50 mg; Tablet
Roerig Division of
Pfizer

What are meclizine tablets or capsules?

MECLIZINE (Antivert®, Bonine®) is an antihistamine. It helps to prevent nausea, vomiting, or dizziness associated with motion sickness, and to treat or prevent vertigo (extreme dizziness or a sensation that you or your surroundings are tilting or spinning around). Generic meclizine tablets and capsules are available.

What should my health care professional know before I take meclizine?

They need to know if you have any of these conditions:
- asthma
- glaucoma
- prostate trouble
- stomach problems
- urinary problems
- an unusual or allergic reaction to meclizine, other medicines, foods, dyes, or preservatives
- breast-feeding

How should I take this medicine?

Take meclizine tablets or capsules by mouth. Follow the directions on the prescription label. Swallow the tablets or capsules with a drink of water (chewable tablets can be chewed or swallowed whole). If you are using meclizine to prevent motion sickness, take the dose at least 1 hour before travel. If meclizine upsets your stomach, take it with food or milk. Take your doses at regular intervals. Do not take your medicine more often than directed. Contact your pediatrician or health care professional regarding the use of this medicine in children. Special care may be needed.

What if I miss a dose?

If you miss a dose and are taking meclizine on a regular schedule, take it as soon as you can. If it is almost time for your next dose, take only that dose. Do not take double or extra doses.

What may interact with meclizine?

- alcohol
- barbiturate medicines for inducing sleep or treating seizures (convulsions)
- certain antibiotics given by injection
- digoxin
- medicines for anxiety or sleeping problems, such as alprazolam, diazepam or temazepam
- medicines for hay fever and other allergies
- medicines for mental depression
- medicines for movement abnormalities as in Parkinson's disease, or for gastrointestinal problems
- medicines for pain
- medicines that relax skeletal muscle

Tell your prescriber or health care professional about all other medicines you are taking, including non-prescription medicines, nutritional supplements, or herbal products. Also tell your prescriber or health care professional if you are a frequent user of drinks with caffeine or alcohol, if you smoke, or if you use illegal drugs. These may affect the way your medicine works. Check with your health care professional before stopping or starting any of your medicines.

What should I watch for while taking meclizine?

If you are taking meclizine on a regular schedule, visit your prescriber or health care professional for regular checks on your progress. You may get dizzy, drowsy or have blurred vision. Do not drive, use machinery, or do anything that needs mental alertness until you know how meclizine affects you. Do not stand or sit up quickly, especially if you are an older patient. This reduces the risk of dizzy or fainting spells. Alcohol can increase possible dizziness; avoid alcoholic drinks. Meclizine may make your mouth dry. Chewing sugarless gum, sucking hard candy and drinking plenty of water may help. Visit your dentist regularly. Meclizine may cause dry eyes and blurred vision. If you wear contact lenses you may feel some discomfort. Lubricating drops may help. See your ophthalmologist if the problem does not go away or is severe.

What side effects may I notice from taking meclizine?

Side effects that you should report to your prescriber or health care professional as soon as possible:
- fainting spells
- fast or irregular heartbeat (palpitations)

Side effects that usually do not require medical attention (report to your prescriber or health care professional if they continue or are bothersome):
- blurred vision
- constipation
- difficulty passing urine
- difficulty sleeping
- drowsiness, dizziness
- dry mouth
- headache
- stomach upset

Where can I keep my medicine?

Keep out of the reach of children in a container that small children cannot open. Store at room temperature between 15 and 30 degrees C (59 and 86 degrees F). Keep container tightly closed. Throw away any unused medicine after the expiration date.

Meclofenamate, mefenamic acid capsules

PONSTEL®;
250 mg; Capsule
First Horizon
Pharmaceutical Corp

MECLOFENAMATE;
100 mg; Capsule
Mylan
Pharmaceuticals Inc

This drug requires an FDA medication guide. See page xxxvii.

What are meclofenamate or mefenamic acid capsules?

MECLOFENAMATE (meclofenamate sodium) and **MEFENAMIC ACID** (Ponstel®) are nonsteroidal anti-inflammatory drugs (NSAIDs). Meclofenamate helps relieve inflammation and pain associated with rheumatoid arthritis and osteoarthritis. Both drugs help relieve mild to moderate pain, including menstrual cramps or premenstrual discomfort. Generic meclofenamate capsules are available, but generic mefenamic acid capsules are not yet available.

What should my health care professional know before I take meclofenamate or mefenamic acid?

They need to know if you have any of these conditions:
- asthma, especially aspirin-sensitive asthma
- bleeding problems or taking medicines that make you bleed easily such as anticoagulants ("blood thinners")
- cigarette smoker
- dental disease
- diabetes mellitus
- drink more than 3 alcohol-containing beverages a day
- heart failure
- high blood pressure
- kidney disease
- liver disease
- lost a lot of fluid due to continued vomiting or diarrhea
- stomach ulcers or pain
- systemic lupus erythematosus
- ulcerative colitis
- an unusual or allergic reaction to mefenamic acid, meclofenamate, aspirin, other salicylates, other NSAIDs, foods, dyes or preservatives
- pregnant or trying to get pregnant
- breast-feeding

M

How should I take this medicine?

Take meclofenamate or mefenamic capsules by mouth. Follow the directions on the prescription label. Swallow capsules whole with a full glass of water; take capsules in an upright or sitting position. Taking a sip of water first, before taking the capsules, may help you swallow them. If possible take bedtime doses at least 10 minutes before lying down. You can take meclofenamate or mefenamic acid with food to prevent stomach upset. Take your doses at regular intervals. Do not take your medicine more often than directed. Contact your pediatrician or health care professional regarding the use of this medicine in children. Special care may be needed.

What if I miss a dose?

If you miss a dose, take it as soon as you can. If it is almost time for your next dose, take only that dose. Do not take double or extra doses.

What other medicines can interact with meclofenamate or mefenamic acid?

- alcohol
- alendronate
- anti-inflammatory drugs (other NSAIDs, prednisone)
- aspirin and aspirin-like medicines
- cidofovir
- cyclosporine
- drospirenone; ethinyl estradiol (Yasmin®)
- entecavir
- herbal products that contain feverfew, garlic, ginger, or ginkgo biloba
- lithium
- medicines for high blood pressure
- medicines that affect platelets
- medicines that treat or prevent blood clots such as warfarin and other "blood thinners"
- methotrexate
- pemetrexed
- water pills (diuretics)

Tell your prescriber or health care professional about all other medicines you are taking, including non-prescription medicines, nutritional supplements, or herbal products. Also tell your prescriber or health care professional if you are a frequent user of drinks with caffeine or alcohol, if you smoke, or if you use illegal drugs. These may affect the way your medicine works. Check with your health care professional before stopping or starting any of your medicines.

What do I need to watch for while I take meclofenamate or mefenamic acid?

Let your prescriber or health care professional know if your pain continues. Do not take your capsules with other pain killers without advice. If you get flu-like symptoms (fever, chills, muscle aches and pains), call your prescriber or health care professional; do not treat yourself. To reduce unpleasant effects on your throat and stomach, take meclofenamate or mefenamic acid with a full glass of water and never just before lying down. If you notice black, tarry stools or experience severe stomach pain and/or vomit blood or what looks like coffee grounds, notify your health care prescriber immediately. If you are taking medicines that affect the clotting of your blood, such as aspirin or blood thinners such as Coumadin®, talk to your health care provider or prescriber before taking this medicine. You may get dizzy. Do not drive, use machinery, or do anything that needs mental alertness until you know how meclofenamate or mefenamic acid affects you. Do not sit or stand up quickly, especially if you are an older patient. This reduces the risk of dizzy or fainting spells. Do not smoke cigarettes or drink alcohol; these increase irritation to your stomach and can make it more susceptible to damage from this medicine. If you are going to have surgery, tell your prescriber or health care professional that you are taking this medicine. Problems can arise if you need dental work, and in the day-to-day care of your teeth. Try to avoid damage to your teeth and gums when you brush or floss your teeth. It is especially important not to use meclofenamate or mefenamic acid during the last 3 months of pregnancy unless specifically directed to do so by your health care provider. Meclofenamate or mefenamic acid may cause problems in the unborn child or complications during delivery.

What side effects may I notice from taking meclofenamate or mefenamic acid?

Side effects that you should report to your prescriber or health care professional as soon as possible:

- signs of bleeding—black tarry stools, blood in the urine, unusual tiredness or weakness, or vomiting blood or vomit that looks like coffee grounds
- signs of an allergic reaction—difficulty breathing, wheezing, skin rash, redness, blistering or peeling skin, hives, or itching, swelling of eyelids, throat, lips
- blurred vision
- change in the amount of urine passed
- difficulty swallowing, severe heartburn or burning, pain in throat
- pain or difficulty passing urine
- stomach pain or cramps
- swelling of feet or ankles

Side effects that usually do not require medical attention (report to your prescriber or health care professional if they continue or are bothersome):

- diarrhea or constipation
- dizziness, drowsiness
- gas or heartburn
- headache
- nausea, vomiting

Where can I keep my medicine?

Keep out of the reach of children in a container that small children cannot open. Store at room temperature between 15 and 30 degrees C (59 and 86 degrees F). Keep container tightly closed. Protect meclofenamate sodium capsules from light. Throw away any unused medicine after the expiration date.

M

Medroxyprogesterone tablets

PROVERA®;
5 mg; Tablet
Pharmacia and
Upjohn Div Pfizer

PROVERA®;
2.5 mg; Tablet
Pharmacia and
Upjohn Div Pfizer

What are medroxyprogesterone tablets?

MEDROXYPROGESTERONE (Provera®) helps to treat an irregular menstrual cycle, lack of menstrual periods, or abnormal uterine bleeding caused by a hormonal imbalance. Medroxyprogesterone acts like the natural hormone progesterone. Natural progesterone is essential to normal reproductive functioning of the womb and reproductive system. Generic medroxyprogesterone tablets are available.

What should my health care professional know before I take medroxyprogesterone?

They need to know if you have any of these conditions:
- asthma
- blood vessel disease, blood clotting disorder, or suffered a stroke
- breast cancer
- heart, kidney or liver disease
- high blood lipids or cholesterol
- mental depression
- migraine
- seizures (convulsions)
- vaginal bleeding
- an unusual or allergic reaction to medroxyprogesterone, other hormones, medicines, foods, dyes, or preservatives
- pregnant or trying to get pregnant
- breast-feeding

How should I take this medicine?

Take medroxyprogesterone tablets by mouth. Follow the directions on the prescription label. Swallow the tablets with a drink of water. Take your doses at regular intervals. Do not take your medicine more often than directed. Bleeding generally begins in 3 to 7 days after completing the drug treatment. Contact your pediatrician or health care professional regarding the use of this medicine in children. Special care may be needed.

What if I miss a dose?

If you miss a dose, take it as soon as you can. If it is almost time for your next dose, take only that dose. Do not take double or extra doses.

What may interact with medroxyprogesterone?

- antibiotics or medicines for infections, especially rifampin, rifabutin, rifapentine, and griseofulvin
- barbiturate medicines such as phenobarbital, which may be used to induce sleep or to treat seizures
- bosentan
- bromocriptine
- medications for treating seizures (convulsions) such as carbamazepine, phenytoin, or primidone
- modafinil
- St. John's wort

Tell your prescriber or health care professional about all other medicines you are taking, including non-prescription medicines, nutritional supplements, or herbal products. Also tell your prescriber or health care professional if you are a frequent user of drinks with caffeine or alcohol, if you smoke, or if you use illegal drugs. These may affect the way your medicine works. Check with your health care professional before stopping or starting any of your medicines.

What should I watch for while taking medroxyprogesterone?

Visit your prescriber or health care professional for regular checks on your progress. You should have a complete check-up every 6 to 12 months. Stop taking medroxyprogesterone at once and contact your prescriber or health care professional if you think you are pregnant. The effect of medroxyprogesterone on fertility can last for a long time. If you want to get pregnant when you have stopped taking this medicine it may be some time before you can conceive. Progestins can cause swelling, tenderness, or bleeding of the gums; be careful when brushing and flossing teeth. See your dentist regularly for routine dental care.

What side effects may I notice from taking medroxyprogesterone?

Side effects that you should report to your prescriber or health care professional as soon as possible:
- breast tenderness or discharge
- numbness or pain in the arm or leg
- pain in the chest, groin or leg
- severe headache
- stomach pain
- sudden shortness of breath
- unusual weakness or tiredness
- vision or speech problems
- yellowing of skin or eyes

Side effects that usually do not require medical attention (report to your prescriber or health care professional if they continue or are bothersome):
- changes in sexual desire or ability
- changes in vaginal bleeding
- facial hair growth
- fluid retention and swelling
- headache
- increased sweating or hot flashes
- loss of appetite or increase in appetite
- mood changes, anxiety, depression, frustration, anger, or emotional outbursts
- skin rash
- stomach discomfort
- weight gain or weight loss
- vaginal yeast infection (irritation and white discharge)

M

Where can I keep my medicine?

Keep out of the reach of children in a container that small children cannot open. Store at room temperature between 15 and 30 degrees C (59 and 86 degrees F). Keep container tightly closed. Throw away any unused medicine after the expiration date.

Megestrol tablets

MEGACE®;
40 mg; Tablet
Mead Johnson

MEGACE®;
20 mg; Tablet
Mead Johnson

What are megestrol tablets?

MEGESTROL (Megace®, Pallace®) is similar to the natural female hormone called progesterone. Megestrol tablets are used for treating breast cancer and endometrial cancer. Generic megestrol tablets are available.

What should my health care professional know before I take megestrol?

They need to know if you have any of these conditions:
- a history of adrenal gland problems
- a history of blood clotting in the blood vessels of the legs, lungs or other parts of the body
- diabetes
- liver disease
- menstrual bleeding problems
- vaginal bleeding
- an unusual or allergic reaction to megestrol, other medicines, foods, dyes, or preservatives
- pregnant or trying to get pregnant
- breast-feeding

How should I take this medicine?

Take megestrol tablets by mouth, Follow the directions on the prescription label. Swallow the tablets with a drink of water. Do not take your medicine more often than directed. Finish the full course prescribed by your doctor or health care professional, even if the tablets make you feel unwell. Do not stop taking except on your prescriber's advice. Contact your pediatrician or health care professional regarding the use of this medicine in children. Special care may be needed.

What if I miss a dose?

If you miss a dose, take it as soon as you can. If it is almost time for your next dose, take only that dose. Do not take double or extra doses.

What may interact with megestrol?

- carbamazepine
- dofetilide
- fosphenytoin
- medicines used to treat diabetes
- phenobarbital
- phenytoin
- primidone
- rifampin
- rifabutin
- rifapentine
- warfarin

Tell your prescriber or health care professional about all other medicines you are taking, including non-prescription medicines, nutritional supplements, or herbal products. Also tell your prescriber or health care professional if you are a frequent user of drinks with caffeine or alcohol, if you smoke, or if you use illegal drugs. These may affect the way your medicine works. Check with your health care professional before stopping or starting any of your medicines.

What should I watch for while taking megestrol?

Visit your prescriber or health care professional for regular checks on your progress. Continue taking megestrol even if you feel better. It may take 2 months of regular use before you know if this medicine is working for your condition. Do not stop taking except on your prescriber's advice. You may have an increased appetite and put on weight. Discuss this with your prescriber if it is a problem. Discuss any unusual or unpleasant side effects with your prescriber. If you are a female of child-bearing age, use an effective method of birth control while you are taking megestrol.

What side effects may I notice from taking megestrol?

Side effects that you should report to your prescriber or health care professional as soon as possible:
- difficulty breathing
- chest pain
- fluid retention or swelling
- increased blood pressure
- leg pain or swelling
- nausea and vomiting
- unusual fatigue, weakness or dizziness

Side effects that usually do not require medical attention (report to your prescriber or health care professional if they continue or are bothersome):
More common:
- breakthrough menstrual bleeding (females)
- hot flashes or flushing
- sexual difficulties (men)
- weight gain

Less common:
- breast tenderness (men and women)
- hair loss
- increased blood sugar
- skin rash

M

Where can I keep my medicine?

Keep out of the reach of children in a container that small children cannot open. Store at controlled room temperature, 15 and 30 degrees C (59 and 86 degrees F). Protect from heat; do not expose to temperatures above 40 degrees C (104 degrees F). Throw away any unused medicine after the expiration date.

Melatonin oral dosage forms

MELATONIN;
3 mg; Tablet
Nature's Bounty

What are melatonin oral dosage forms?

MELATONIN is a hormone that the body produces. Melatonin performs many functions; some functions are not well understood. It is known that the melatonin in the body contributes to the natural regulation of sleep during night hours. Melatonin products are used to help some people who have difficulty maintaining normal sleep patterns. Although melatonin is claimed to be helpful for other problems related to hormones and aging, there is no proof at this time that melatonin is effective for such uses. Melatonin products are either chemically synthesized or are from animal sources, such as cattle. The use of melatonin products from animal sources is not recommended due to the risk of viral contamination of these products. Melatonin is available over-the-counter as a nutritional supplement from many manufacturers.

What should my health care professional know before I take melatonin?

It is important for you to tell your prescriber or other health care professional that you are using melatonin. Some hormones exert potent effects and may interact with other drugs you are taking. You should discuss melatonin with your health care professional BEFORE taking it if you have any of these conditions:

- are a frequent user of alcohol or have a history of drug abuse
- difficulty sleeping
- heart, kidney or liver disease
- history of emotional illness, such as anxiety or depression
- immunosuppression, or if you are receiving treatment for cancer
- seizure disorder (convulsions) or any other neurologic condition
- an unusual or allergic reaction to melatonin, hormones, other medicines, foods, dyes, or preservatives
- pregnant or trying to get pregnant
- breast-feeding

How should I take this medicine?

Follow the directions on the package labeling, or talk to your health care professional. Most forms of this medicine should be taken orally (i.e., swallowed). Sublingual tablets should be placed under the tongue or between the cheek and gum and allowed to dissolve. Do not chew sublingual tablets. If you are taking an extended release form of melatonin, do not crush or chew the tablets or capsules. Aerosol spray forms of this medication should not be inhaled into the lungs, but sprayed into the mouth. Self-treatment with melatonin should not continue for longer than 2 weeks without the advice of a health care professional. Contact your pediatrician or health care professional regarding the use of this hormone in children. Special care may be needed.

What if I miss a dose?

Missing a dose is probably not harmful. If you miss a dose, simply resume taking it on your previous schedule. Do not take double doses to catch up, however.

What may interact with melatonin?

- amphetamine and dextroamphetamine
- blood pressure medicines such as nifedipine
- herbal dietary supplements like kava kava or valerian
- hormonal medications
- medications for depression, anxiety, or other emotional or psychiatric problems.
- medications for treating seizures (convulsions)
- medications for sleep
- tamoxifen
- treatments for cancer or immune disorders

For many over-the-counter products sold as nutritional supplements, interactions with other medications are unknown. That is why you should always be careful when mixing these remedies with traditional medications. If you take any other medications, consult with your health care professional prior to taking melatonin. Tell your prescriber or health care professional about all other medicines you are taking, including non-prescription medicines, nutritional supplements, or herbal products. Also tell your prescriber or health care professional if you are a frequent user of drinks with caffeine or alcohol, if you smoke, or if you use illegal drugs. These may affect the way your medicine works. Check with your health care professional before stopping or starting any of your medicines.

What should I watch for while taking melatonin?

Because some melatonin products can be derived from animals, particularly cattle, allergic reactions are possible. Stop using this hormone if you develop a rash. You may want to see your health care professional, or inform them that this occurred. Melatonin may cause drowsiness. Driving or operating machinery, or performing other tasks that require mental alertness requires caution when taking melatonin. You should not participate in these activities until you determine how mela-

M

tonin affects you. Do not drink alcohol while taking melatonin. Alcohol might increase side effects. Do not use melatonin without approval from your health care professional if you are currently being treated for a mental or emotional problem such as depression or anxiety. Melatonin might interfere with your treatments. Also do not stop your prescribed treatments without talking to your prescriber or health care professional. Self treatment should continue for no longer than 2 weeks. You should contact your health care professional for advice prior to prolonged use. Different brands of melatonin might contain different amounts of active ingredient so be careful to use the same brand. It is recommended that you use a brand from a reliable manufacturer and one that has been standardized. A standardized product is more likely to contain the same amount of hormone from dose to dose. Your health care professional or pharmacist can assist you in finding a standardized product.

What side effects may I notice from taking melatonin?

Side effects that you should report to your prescriber or health care professional as soon as possible:

- confusion, forgetfulness
- depressed mood, nervousness, or other mood changes
- difficulty staying awake or alert during the day
- rash
- rapid heartbeat or "palpitations"
- shortness of breath or difficulty breathing

Side effects that usually do not require medical attention (report to your prescriber or health care professional if they continue or are bothersome):

- drowsiness, dizziness
- headache
- upset stomach

Where can I keep my medicine?

Keep out of the reach of children. Store at room temperature; do not freeze. Throw away any unused medicine after the expiration date.

GENERAL INFORMATION REGARDING DIETARY SUPPLEMENTS:

Dietary supplements include amino acids, hormones, vitamins, minerals, herbs, and other plant-derived substances, and extracts of these substances. Products are easy to identify as they must state "Dietary Supplement" on the label. A "Supplement Facts" panel is provided on the label for most products. Supplements are not drugs and are not regulated like pharmaceuticals. You should note that rigid quality control standards are not required for dietary supplements. Differences in the potency and purity of these products can occur. Scientific data to support the use of a dietary supplement for a certain condition may not be available. This product is not intended to diagnose, treat, cure or prevent any disease. The Food and Drug Administration suggests the following to help consumers protect themselves:

- Always read product labels and follow directions.
- Look for products containing ingredients with the "USP" notation. This indicates the manufacturer followed the standards of the US Pharmacopoeia.
- "Natural" doesn't mean a product is safe for humans to consume.
- Supplements produced or distributed by a nationally known food or drug company are more likely to be made under tight controls as these companies have standards in place for their other products. You can write to the company or manufacturer for more information about the conditions under which the products are made.

Meloxicam tablets

MOBIC®;
7.5 mg; Tablet
Boehringer
Ingelheim
Pharmaceuticals Inc

MOBIC®;
15 mg; Tablet
Boehringer
Ingelheim
Pharmaceuticals Inc

What are meloxicam tablets?

MELOXICAM (Mobic®) is used for osteoarthritis or rheumatoid arthritis to reduce pain and inflammation. Meloxicam has also been used to treat mild to moderate pain due to other conditions. Generic meloxicam is available.

What should my health care professional know before I take meloxicam?

They need to know if you have any of these conditions:

- asthma, especially aspirin sensitive asthma
- bleeding problems or taking medicines that make you bleed more easily such as anticoagulants ("blood thinners")
- cigarette smoker
- dental disease

- diabetes
- drink more than 3 alcohol-containing beverages a day
- heart or circulation problems such as heart failure or leg edema (fluid retention)
- high blood pressure
- kidney disease
- liver disease
- stomach or duodenal ulcers
- systemic lupus erythematosus
- ulcerative colitis
- an unusual or allergic reaction to aspirin, other salicylates, meloxicam, piroxicam, other NSAIDs, other medicines, foods, dyes or preservatives
- pregnant or trying to get pregnant
- breast-feeding

How should I take this medicine?

Take meloxicam tablets by mouth. Follow the directions on the prescription label. Swallow tablets whole with a full glass of water; take tablets in an upright or sitting position. Taking a sip of water first, before taking the tablets, may help you swallow them. If possible take bedtime doses at least 10 minutes before lying down. If meloxicam upsets your stomach, take it with food or milk. Take your doses at regular intervals. Do not take your medicine more often than directed. Contact your pediatrician or health care professional regarding the use of this medicine in children. Special care may be needed. Elderly patients over 65 years old may have a stronger reaction to this medicine and need smaller doses.

What if I miss a dose?

If you miss a dose, take it as soon as you can. If it is almost time for your next dose, take only that dose. Do not take double or extra doses.

What may interact with meloxicam?

- alcohol
- alendronate
- aspirin and aspirin-like medicines
- cidofovir
- cyclosporine
- drospirenone; ethinyl estradiol (Yasmin®)
- entecavir
- herbal products that contain feverfew, garlic, ginger, or ginkgo biloba
- lithium
- medicines for high blood pressure
- medicines that affect platelets
- medicines that treat or prevent blood clots such as warfarin and other "blood thinners"
- methotrexate
- other anti-inflammatory drugs (such as ibuprofen or prednisone)
- pemetrexed
- water pills (diuretics)

Tell your prescriber or health care professional about all other medicines you are taking, including non-prescription medicines, nutritional supplements, or herbal products. Also tell your prescriber or health care professional if you are a frequent user of drinks with caffeine or alcohol, if you smoke, or if you use illegal drugs. These may affect the way your medicine works. Check with your health care professional before stopping or starting any of your medicines.

What should I watch for while taking meloxicam?

Let your prescriber or health care professional know if your pain continues; do not take with other pain killers without advice. If you get flu-like symptoms (fever, chills, muscle aches and pains), call your prescriber or health care professional; do not treat yourself. To re-duce unpleasant effects on your stomach, take meloxicam with a full glass of water and never just before lying down. You may also take this medicine with food to decrease stomach upset. If you notice black, tarry stools or experience severe stomach pain and/or vomit blood or what looks like coffee grounds, notify your health care prescriber immediately. Meloxicam cannot take the place of aspirin for the prevention of heart attack or stroke. If you are taking medicines that affect the clotting of your blood, such as aspirin or blood thinners such as Coumadin®, talk to your health care provider or prescriber before taking this medicine. If you are currently taking aspirin for this purpose, you should not discontinue taking aspirin without checking with your prescriber or health care professional. Do not smoke cigarettes or drink alcohol; these increase irritation to your stomach and can make it more susceptible to damage from meloxicam. It is especially important not to use meloxicam during the last 3 months of pregnancy unless specifically directed to do so by your health care provider. Meloxicam may cause problems in the unborn child or complications during delivery.

What side effects may I notice from taking meloxicam?

Side effects that you should report to your prescriber or health care professional as soon as possible:

- signs of bleeding—bruising, pinpoint red spots on the skin, black tarry stools, blood in the urine, unusual tiredness or weakness, vomiting blood or vomit that looks like coffee grounds
- signs of an allergic reaction—difficulty breathing or wheezing, skin rash, redness, blistering or peeling skin, hives, or itching, swelling of eyelids, throat, lips
- blurred vision
- change in the amount of urine passed
- difficulty swallowing, severe heartburn or burning, pain in throat
- pain or difficulty passing urine
- stomach pain or cramps
- swelling of feet or ankles
- unexplained weight gain or edema
- yellowing of eyes or skin

Side effects that usually do not require medical attention (report to your prescriber or health care professional if they continue or are bothersome):

- constipation or diarrhea
- difficulty swallowing
- dizziness
- gas or heartburn
- minor upset stomach
- nausea or vomiting

Where can I keep my medicine?

Keep out of the reach of children in a container that small children cannot open. Store at room temperature 15 and 30 degrees C (59 and 86 degrees F). Protect from moisture. Keep container tightly closed. Throw away any unused medicine after the expiration date.

M

Melphalan tablets

ALKERAN®;
2 mg; Tablet
Glaxo Wellcome Division
SmithKline Beecham Corp

What are melphalan tablets?

MELPHALAN (Alkeran®) is a type of chemotherapy for treating cancer. Melphalan interferes with cell growth and treats cancers of the ovaries and bone marrow. Generic melphalan tablets are not yet available.

What should my health care professional know before I take melphalan?

They need to know if you have any of these conditions:
- bleeding problems
- blood disorders
- dental disease
- gout
- infection (especially virus infection such as chickenpox or herpes)
- kidney disease
- liver disease
- recent radiation therapy
- an unusual or allergic reaction to melphalan, other chemotherapy, other medicines, foods, dyes, or preservatives
- pregnant or trying to get pregnant
- breast-feeding

How should I take this medicine?

Take melphalan tablets by mouth. Follow the directions on the prescription label. Swallow the tablets with a drink of water. Take your doses at regular intervals. Do not take your medicine more often than directed. Finish the full course prescribed by your doctor or health care professional, even if the tablets make you feel unwell. Your dosage schedule will depend on the type of cancer being treated. Some cancers require many months of therapy. Do not stop taking except on your prescriber's advice. Contact your pediatrician or health care professional regarding the use of this medicine in children. Special care may be needed.

What if I miss a dose?

If you miss a dose, miss that dose and continue with your regular schedule. Do not double the next dose. If you vomit after taking a dose, call your prescriber or health care professional for advice.

What may interact with melphalan?

- immune globulins
- interferon alfa
- live virus vaccines and killed virus vaccines

Tell your prescriber or health care professional about all other medicines you are taking, including non-prescription medicines, nutritional supplements, or herbal products. Also tell your prescriber or health care professional if you are a frequent user of drinks with caffeine or alcohol, if you smoke, or if you use illegal drugs. These may affect the way your medicine works. Check with your health care professional before stopping or starting any of your medicines.

What should I watch for while taking melphalan?

Visit your prescriber or health care professional for checks on your progress. You will need to have regular blood checks. The side effects of melphalan can continue after you finish your treatment; report side effects promptly. Melphalan may make you feel generally unwell. This is not uncommon because melphalan affects good cells as well as cancer cells. Report any side effects as above, but continue your course of medicine even though you feel ill, unless your prescriber or health care professional tells you to stop. While you are using melphalan, you will be more susceptible to infection. Try to avoid people with colds, flu, and bronchitis. Do not have any vaccinations without your prescriber's approval and avoid anyone who has recently had oral polio vaccine. Call your prescriber or health care professional for advice if you get a fever, chills or sore throat. Do not treat yourself. Melphalan can cause blood problems. This can mean slow healing and a risk of infection. Try to avoid cutting or injuring yourself. Problems can arise if you need dental work, and in the day-to-day care of your teeth. Try to avoid damage to your teeth and gums when you brush or floss your teeth. If you are going to have surgery, tell your prescriber or health care professional that you are taking melphalan. Melphalan can change male sperm or female eggs. Talk to your prescriber or health care professional about how this medicine can affect your ability to have normal babies.

What side effects may I notice from taking melphalan?

Side effects that you should report to your prescriber or health care professional as soon as possible:
- black tarry stools
- blood in the urine
- chest pain
- difficulty breathing, wheezing
- fever or chills, cough or sore throat
- lower back pain
- pain or difficulty passing urine
- unusual bleeding or bruising, pinpoint red spots on your skin
- unusual tiredness or weakness
- vomiting

Side effects that usually do not require medical attention (report to your prescriber or health care professional if they continue or are bothersome):

M

- diarrhea
- hair loss
- missed menstrual periods
- mouth ulcers
- nausea
- skin rash, itching

Where can I keep my medicine?

Keep out of the reach of children in a container that small children cannot open. Store at room temperature between 15 and 25 degrees C (59 and 77 degrees F). Protect from light and moisture. Throw away any unused medicine after the expiration date.

Memantine tablets

NAMENDA®;
10 mg; Tablet
Forest
Pharmaceuticals Inc

NAMENDA®;
5 mg; Tablet
Forest
Pharmaceuticals Inc

What are memantine tablets?

MEMANTINE (Namenda®) helps treat the symptoms associated with Alzheimer's disease or dementia. It is not a cure for Alzheimer's disease but offers improvement in memory, attention, reason, language, and the ability to perform simple tasks. Benefits are usually greater in the later stages of the disease. Generic memantine tablets are not yet available.

What should my health care professional know before I take memantine?

They need to know if you have any of these conditions:
- kidney disease
- seizures (convulsions) or a seizure disorder
- an unusual reaction to memantine, other medicines, foods, dyes, or preservatives
- pregnant or trying to get pregnant
- breast-feeding

How should this medicine be taken?

Take memantine tablets by mouth. Follow the directions on the prescription label. Swallow the tablets with a drink of water. You may take memantine with food. Take your doses at regular intervals. Do not take your medicine more often than directed. Continue to take your medicine even if you feel better. Do not stop taking except on your prescriber's advice. Contact your pediatrician or health care professional regarding the use of this medicine in children. Special care may be needed.

What if I miss a dose?

If you miss a dose, take it as soon as you can. If it is almost time for your next dose, take only that dose. Do not take double or extra doses.

What may interact with memantine?

- amantadine
- dextromethorphan
- levodopa
- medicines for colds, flu, or hayfever and other allergies (antihistamines)
- pergolide
- pramipexole
- ropinirole
- trihexyphenidyl

Tell your prescriber or health care professional about all other medicines you are taking, including non-prescription medicines, nutritional supplements, or herbal products. Also tell your prescriber or health care professional if you are a frequent user of drinks with caffeine or alcohol, if you smoke, or if you use illegal drugs. These may affect the way your medicine works. Check with your health care professional before stopping or starting any of your medicines.

What should I watch for while taking memantine?

Visit your prescriber or health care professional for regular checks on your progress. Check with your prescriber or health care professional if there is no improvement in your symptoms or if they get worse. You may get dizzy or feel faint. Do not drive, use machinery, or do anything that needs mental alertness until you know how memantine affects you. If you are going to have surgery tell your prescriber or health care professional that you are taking memantine.

What side effects may I notice from taking memantine?

Side effects that you should report to your prescriber or health care professional as soon as possible:
- agitation or a feeling of restlessness
- confusion
- dizziness
- hallucinations (seeing or hearing things that are not really there)
- not able to hold your urine
- shortness of breath
- swelling in throat or tongue
- skin rash or redness, peeling of skin
- vomiting

Side effects that usually do not require medical attention (report to your prescriber or health care professional if they continue or are bothersome):
- constipation or diarrhea (mild)
- drowsiness or unable to sleep
- feeling of nausea, upset stomach
- headache

Where can I keep my medicine?

Keep out of the reach of children in a container that small children cannot open. Store at room temperature between 15 degrees and 30 degrees C (59 degrees and 86 degrees F). Throw away any unused medicine after the expiration date.

M

Meperidine tablets

DEMEROL®;
50 mg; Tablet
Sanofi-Synthelabo
Inc

DEMEROL®;
100 mg; Tablet
Sanofi-Synthelabo
Inc

What are meperidine tablets?

MEPERIDINE (Demerol®) relieves moderate to severe pain. Meperidine may be used to control pain following surgery, child birth, and other procedures. Meperidine may also be used to treat pain associated with cancer, heart attacks, sickle cell disease and other medical conditions. Federal law prohibits the transfer of meperidine to any person other than the patient for whom it was prescribed. Do not share this medicine with anyone else. Generic meperidine tablets are available.

What should my health care professional know before I take meperidine?

They need to know if you have any of these conditions:
- diarrhea
- glaucoma
- heart disease
- intestinal disease
- kidney disease
- liver disease
- lung disease or breathing difficulties
- pain or difficulty passing urine
- prostate problems
- seizures
- an unusual or allergic reaction to meperidine, other medicines, foods, dyes, or preservatives
- pregnant or trying to get pregnant
- breast-feeding

How should I take this medicine?

Take meperidine tablets by mouth. Follow the directions on the prescription label. Swallow the tablets with a drink of water. If meperidine upsets your stomach, you can take it with food or milk. Take your doses at regular intervals. Do not take your medicine more often than directed. Do not share this medicine with any one. Contact your pediatrician or health care professional regarding the use of this medicine in children. Special care may be needed.

What if I miss a dose?

If you miss a dose, take it as soon as you can. If it is almost time for your next dose, take only that dose. Do not take double or extra doses.

What may interact with meperidine?

- acyclovir
- furazolidone
- linezolid
- medicines for high blood pressure
- medicines called MAO inhibitors-phenelzine (Nardil®), tranylcypromine (Parnate®), isocarboxazid (Marplan®)

- medicines for seizures
- procarbazine
- other medicines for depression
- ritonavir
- selegiline
- valacyclovir

Because meperidine causes drowsiness, other medicines that also cause drowsiness may increase this effect of meperidine. Some medicines that cause drowsiness are:
- alcohol and alcohol containing medicines
- barbiturates such as phenobarbital
- certain antidepressants and tranquilizers
- certain antihistamines used in cold medicines
- muscle relaxants

Tell your prescriber or health care professional about all other medicines you are taking, including non-prescription medicines, nutritional supplements, or herbal products. Also tell your prescriber or health care professional if you are a frequent user of drinks with caffeine or alcohol, if you smoke, or if you use illegal drugs. These may affect the way your medicine works. Check with your health care professional before stopping or starting any of your medicines.

What should I watch for while taking meperidine?

Tell your prescriber or health care professional if your pain does not go away, if it gets worse or if you have a new or different type of pain. Use exactly as directed by your prescriber or health care professional. If you are taking meperidine on a regular basis, do not suddenly stop taking it. Your body becomes used to the meperidine and when you suddenly stop taking it, you may develop a severe reaction. This DOES NOT mean you are "addicted" to meperidine. Addiction is a behavior related to getting and using a drug for a non-medical reason. If you have pain, you have a medical reason to take pain medicine such as meperidine to control your pain. You may get drowsy or dizzy when you first start taking meperidine or change doses. Do not drive, use machinery, or do anything that needs mental alertness until you know how meperidine affects you. Stand or sit up slowly, as this reduces the risk of dizzy or fainting spells. These effects may be worse if you are an older patient. The drowsiness should decrease after taking meperidine for a couple of days. If you have not slept because of your pain, you may sleep more the first few days your pain is controlled to catch-up on missed sleep. Be careful taking other medicines which may also make you tired. This effect may be worse when taking these medicines with meperidine. Alcohol can increase possible drowsiness, dizziness, confusion and may affect your breathing. Avoid alcohol while taking meperidine. Meperidine will cause constipation. Make sure to take a laxative and/or a stool softener while taking meperidine. Try to have a bowel movement every 2 to 3 days, at least. If you do not have a bowel movement for 3 days or more call your prescriber or health care professional. They may recommend using an enema or suppository to help you move your bowels. Your mouth may get dry. Drinking plenty of water, chewing sugarless gum or sucking on hard candy may help to relieve dry mouth symptoms. Have regular dental checks. If you are going to have surgery, tell your prescriber or health care professional that you are taking meperidine. Rarely, meperidine may cause you to have hallucinations (to see things that are not really there) or cause your legs or arms to "jerk" or have spasms. If you experience these effects, call your prescriber or health care professional.

What side effects may I notice from taking meperidine?

Some side effects can be eased if you lie down after taking your medicine.

Rare or uncommon:

- cold, clammy skin
- difficulty breathing, wheezing
- irregular heartbeat, palpitations
- seizures
- severe rash
- unusual weakness

More common:

- confusion
- lightheadedness or fainting spells
- nervousness or restlessness
- difficulty passing urine

Side effects that usually do not require medical attention (report to your prescriber or health care professional if they continue or are bothersome):

- blurred vision
- constipation
- drowsiness, dizziness
- flushing
- dry mouth
- headache
- nausea, vomiting

Where can I keep my medicine?

Keep out of the reach of children in a container that small children cannot open. Do not share or give this medicine to anyone else. Avoid accidental swallowing of meperidine by someone (especially children) other than the person for whom it was prescribed as this may result in severe effects and possibly death. Store at room temperature between 15 and 30 degrees C (59 and 86 degrees F). Protect from light. Keep container tightly closed. Throw away any unused medicine after the expiration date.

Meprobamate tablets

MILTOWN®; 400 mg; Tablet MedPointe Pharmaceuticals	
MEPROBAMATE; 200 mg; Tablet Watson Pharmaceuticals Inc	

What are meprobamate tablets?

MEPROBAMATE (Equanil®, Miltown®, Trancot®) has a sedative action that can cause relaxation and help reduce tension or anxiety. It is recommended for short-term use only. Meprobamate is sometimes used as a sedative before surgical procedures. Federal law prohibits the transfer of meprobamate to any person other than the patient for whom it was prescribed. Generic meprobamate tablets are available.

What should my health care professional know before I take meprobamate?

They need to know if you have any of these conditions:

- frequently drink alcoholic beverages
- attempted suicide
- drug abuse
- kidney disease
- liver disease
- porphyria
- seizures (convulsions)
- an unusual or allergic reaction to meprobamate, carisoprodol, felbamate, mebutamate, carbromal, or other medicines, foods, dyes, or preservatives
- pregnant or trying to get pregnant
- breast-feeding

How should I take this medicine?

Take meprobamate by mouth. Follow the directions on the prescription label. Swallow the tablets or capsules with a drink of water. Swallow the capsules whole; do not crush or chew. Take your doses at regular intervals. Do not take your medicine more often than directed. Tablets or capsules may be taken with food or milk to reduce stomach upset. Contact your pediatrician or health care professional regarding the use of this medicine in children. Special care may be needed.

What if I miss a dose?

If you miss a dose, take it if you remember within 1 hour. If you remember after more than 1 hour, skip the missed dose and resume your schedule at the next dose. Do not take double or extra doses.

What may interact with meprobamate?

- alcohol
- dietary supplements for relaxation or sleep, like kava kava, melatonin, or valerian
- medicines for allergies, hay fever, colds or flu-like symptoms
- medicines for mood problems like anxiety, depression, or severe mental disturbances

M

- pain medications
- seizure (convulsion) or epilepsy medicine

Tell your prescriber or health care professional about all other medicines you are taking, including non-prescription medicines, nutritional supplements, or herbal products. Also tell your prescriber or health care professional if you are a frequent user of drinks with caffeine or alcohol, if you smoke, or if you use illegal drugs. These may affect the way your medicine works. Check with your health care professional before stopping or starting any of your medicines.

What should I watch for while taking meprobamate?

Visit your prescriber or health care professional for regular checks on your progress. If you have been taking meprobamate regularly for a few weeks and suddenly stop taking it, you may get unpleasant withdrawal symptoms. Your prescriber or health care professional may want to gradually reduce the dose. Do not stop taking except on your prescriber's advice. After taking meprobamate you may get a residual hangover effect that leaves you drowsy or dizzy. Until you know how meprobamate affects you, do not drive, use machinery, or do anything that needs mental alertness. To reduce dizzy or fainting spells, do not sit or stand up quickly, especially if you are an older patient. Alcohol can increase possible unpleasant effects. Avoid alcoholic drinks while taking this drug. Many medications can cause additive drowsiness or dizziness. Ask your doctor or pharmacist before taking any non-prescription medications with meprobamate. If you are going to have surgery or other procedures, tell your prescriber or health care professional that you are taking meprobamate.

What side effects may I notice from taking meprobamate?

Side effects that you should report to your prescriber or health care professional as soon as possible:
- confusion
- difficulty breathing, wheezing
- fever, chills, or sore throat
- hallucinations
- fast or irregular heartbeat (palpitations)
- fainting spells
- numbness, tingling in the hands or feet
- skin rash and itching (hives)
- slurred speech
- staggering, unable to coordinate movement
- swelling of the feet and ankles
- unusual bleeding or bruising
- unusual tiredness or weakness

Side effects that usually do not require medical attention (report to your prescriber or health care professional if they continue or are bothersome):
- blurred vision
- diarrhea
- drowsiness or dizziness, lightheadedness, "hangover effect"
- false sense of well being
- headache
- indigestion
- loss of appetite
- nausea, vomiting

Where can I keep my medicine?

Keep out of the reach of children in a container that small children cannot open. Store at room temperature between 15 and 30 degrees C (59 and 86 degrees F). Keep container tightly closed. Throw away any unused medicine after the expiration date.

Mercaptopurine, 6-MP tablets

PURINETHOL®;
50 mg; Tablet
Gate
Pharmaceuticals

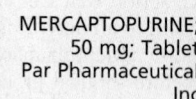

MERCAPTOPURINE;
50 mg; Tablet
Par Pharmaceutical
Inc

What are mercaptopurine tablets?

MERCAPTOPURINE, 6-MP (Purinethol®) is a type of chemotherapy for treating cancer. Mercaptopurine interferes with the growth of cancer cells. It is used for treating acute lymphocytic leukemia (ALL). Mercaptopurine may also be used to treat inflammatory bowel conditions such as ulcerative colitis or Crohn's disease. Generic mercaptopurine tablets are available.

What should my health care professional know before I take mercaptopurine?

They need to know if you have any of these conditions:
- biliary disease (cholestasis)
- bleeding problems
- blood disorders
- dental disease

- infection (especially virus infection such as chickenpox or herpes)
- kidney disease
- liver disease
- recent radiation therapy
- thiopurine methyltransferase (TPMT) deficiency
- an unusual or allergic reaction to mercaptopurine, other chemotherapy, other medicines, foods, dyes, or preservatives
- pregnant or trying to get pregnant
- breast-feeding

How should I take this medicine?

Take mercaptopurine tablets by mouth. Follow the directions on the prescription label. Swallow the tablets with a drink of water. Do not take your medicine more often than directed. Finish the full course prescribed

M

by your doctor or health care professional, even if the tablets make you feel unwell. Do not stop taking except on your prescriber's advice. Contact your pediatrician or health care professional regarding the use of this medicine in children. Special care may be needed.

What if I miss a dose?

If you miss a dose, skip that dose unless your prescriber or health care professional tells you otherwise. Do not take double or extra doses. If you vomit after taking a dose, call your prescriber or health care professional for advice.

What may interact with mercaptopurine?

- agents that treat or prevent blood clots (example: warfarin)
- allopurinol
- balsalazide
- mesalamine, 5-ASA
- olsalazine
- sulfasalazine
- vaccines

Talk to your prescriber or health care professional before taking any of these medicines:

- acetaminophen
- aspirin
- ibuprofen
- naproxen
- ketoprofen

Tell your prescriber or health care professional about all other medicines you are taking, including non-prescription medicines, nutritional supplements, or herbal products. Also tell your prescriber or health care professional if you are a frequent user of drinks with caffeine or alcohol, if you smoke, or if you use illegal drugs. These may affect the way your medicine works. Check with your health care professional before stopping or starting any of your medicines.

What should I watch for while taking mercaptopurine?

Visit your prescriber or health care professional for checks on your progress. You will need to have regular blood checks. The side effects of mercaptopurine can continue after you finish your treatment; report side effects promptly. Mercaptopurine may make you feel generally unwell. This is not uncommon because mercaptopurine affects good cells as well as cancer cells. Report any side effects as above, but continue your course of medicine even though you feel ill, unless your prescriber or health care professional tells you to stop. Mercaptopurine may decrease your body's ability to fight infections. Call your prescriber or health care professional if you have a fever, chills, sore throat, or other symptoms of a cold or flu. Do not treat these symptoms yourself. Try to avoid being around people who are sick. Mercaptopurine may increase your risk to bruise or bleed. Call your prescriber or health care

professional if you notice any unusual bleeding. Be careful not to cut, bruise or injure yourself because you may get an infection and bleed more than usual. Avoid taking aspirin, acetaminophen (Tylenol®), ibuprofen (Advil®), naproxen (Aleve®), or ketoprofen (Orudis® KT) products as these may hide a fever, unless instructed to by your prescriber or health care professional. Mercaptopurine can harm your unborn child if taken during pregnancy. Women who are able to have children should avoid becoming pregnant while taking mercaptopurine. Be careful brushing and flossing your teeth or using a toothpick while receiving mercaptopurine because you may get an infection or bleed more easily. If you have any dental work done, tell your dentist you are receiving mercaptopurine. If you are going to have surgery, tell your prescriber or health care professional that you are taking mercaptopurine.

What side effects may I notice from taking mercaptopurine?

The side effects you may experience with mercaptopurine therapy depend upon the dose, other types of chemotherapy or radiation therapy given, and the disease being treated. Not all of these effects occur in all patients. Discuss any concerns or questions with your prescriber or health care professional.

Side effects that you should report to your prescriber or health care professional as soon as possible:

- blood in the urine
- low blood counts—mercaptopurine may decrease the number of white blood cells, red blood cells and platelets. You may be at increased risk for infections and bleeding.
- signs of infection—fever or chills, cough, sore throat, pain or difficulty passing urine
- signs of decreased platelets or bleeding—bruising, pinpoint red spots on the skin, black, tarry stools, nosebleeds
- signs of decreased red blood cells—unusual weakness or tiredness, fainting spells, lightheadedness
- difficulty breathing
- mouth or lip sores
- swelling of the abdomen, lower legs or feet
- yellowing of the eyes or skin

Side effects that usually do not require medical attention (report to your prescriber or health care professional if they continue or are bothersome):

- darkening of the skin
- diarrhea
- loss of appetite
- nausea, vomiting
- rash

Where can I keep my medicine?

Keep out of the reach of children in a container that small children cannot open. Store at room temperature between 15 and 25 degrees C (59 and 77 degrees F). Protect from moisture. Keep container tightly closed. Throw away any unused medicine after the expiration date.

Mesalamine, 5-ASA extended-release tablets or capsules

PENTASA®;
250 mg; Capsule,
Extended Release
Aventis
Pharmaceuticals Inc

ASACOL®;
400 mg; Tablet,
Delayed Release
Procter and Gamble
Pharmaceuticals Inc
Sub Procter and
Gamble Co

What are mesalamine tablets or capsules?

MESALAMINE (Asacol®, Pentasa®) is an anti-inflammatory agent. It reduces inflammation inside the bowel and pain associated with ulcerative colitis and Crohn's disease. Generic mesalamine delayed-release (enteric-coated) tablets and capsules are not yet available.

What should my health care professional know before I take mesalamine?

They need to know if you have any of these conditions:
- kidney disease
- pyloric stenosis (narrowing of the tube leading out of the stomach)
- an unusual or allergic reaction to mesalamine, other medicines, sulfites, foods, dyes, or preservatives
- pregnant or trying to get pregnant
- breast-feeding

How should I take this medicine?

Take mesalamine tablets or capsules by mouth. Follow the directions on the prescription label. Swallow the tablets or capsules whole with a full glass of water; do not crush or chew. Take your doses at regular intervals. Do not take your medicine more often than directed. Contact your pediatrician or health care professional regarding the use of this medicine in children. Special care may be needed.

What if I miss a dose?

If you miss a dose, take it as soon as you can. If it is almost time for your next dose, take only that dose. Do not take double or extra doses.

What may interact with mesalamine?

- digoxin

Tell your prescriber or health care professional about all other medicines you are taking, including non-prescription medicines, nutritional supplements, or herbal products. Also tell your prescriber or health care professional if you are a frequent user of drinks with caffeine or alcohol, if you smoke, or if you use illegal drugs. These may affect the way your medicine works. Check with your health care professional before stopping or starting any of your medicines.

What should I watch for while taking mesalamine?

Tell your prescriber or health care professional if your symptoms do not start to improve after several days. There is usually an improvement in 3 to 21 days. You may need about 6 weeks of treatment to get good results. It is important that you go on taking your medicine and only stop taking it on your prescriber's advice. Do not change the brand of mesalamine that you are taking without talking to your prescriber or health care professional. All brands of mesalamine do not have the same dose. You may notice the empty shell from mesalamine tablets or capsules in your stool. This is quite normal; your body will have absorbed the contents.

What side effects may I notice from taking mesalamine?

Side effects that you should report to your prescriber or health care professional as soon as possible:
- bloody diarrhea
- chest pain
- difficulty breathing, wheezing
- fever
- pain or difficulty passing urine
- skin rash or itching
- unusual weakness or tiredness
- yellowing of the eyes or skin

Call your prescriber or health care professional for advice if you get any of these side effects.

Side effects that usually do not require medical attention (report to your prescriber or health care professional if they continue or are bothersome):
- headache
- nausea, vomiting
- stomach gas (flatulence)
- stomach pain or cramps

Where can I keep my medicine?

Keep out of the reach of children in a container that small children cannot open. Store at room temperature between 15 and 30 degrees C (59 and 86 degrees F). Throw away any unused medicine after the expiration date.

M

Mesoridazine tablets

What are mesoridazine tablets?

MESORIDAZINE (Serentil®) treats conditions such as schizophrenia that cause you to hear or see things that others do not. It may also help treat some other emotional or nervous problems. Generic mesoridazine tablets are not yet available.

What should my health care professional know before I take mesoridazine?

They need to know if you have any of these conditions:
- an alcohol abuse problem
- blood disease
- cancer
- difficulty urinating
- glaucoma
- head injury
- heart, kidney, or liver disease
- lung disease
- Parkinson's disease
- prostate trouble
- Reye's syndrome
- seizures (convulsions)
- tardive dyskinesia (uncontrollable movement disorder)
- thoughts of suicide
- vision problems
- an unusual or allergic reaction to mesoridazine, other medicines, foods, dyes, or preservatives
- pregnant or trying to get pregnant
- breast-feeding

How should I take this medicine?

Take mesoridazine tablets by mouth. Follow the directions on the prescription label. Swallow the tablets with a drink of water. If mesoridazine upsets your stomach you can take it with food. Take your doses at regular intervals. Do not take your medicine more often than directed. Do not stop taking except on your prescriber's advice. Contact your pediatrician or health care professional regarding the use of this medicine in children. Special care may be needed. Elderly patients may have a stronger reaction to this medicine and need smaller doses.

What if I miss a dose?

If you miss a dose, take it as soon as you can. If it is almost time for your next dose, take only that dose. Do not take double or extra doses.

What may interact with mesoridazine?

Do not take mesoridazine with any of the following:

- some antibiotics (clarithromycin, erythromycin, gatifloxacin, grepafloxacin, moxifloxacin, sparfloxacin)
- some antidepressants (amoxapine, maprotiline)
- arsenic trioxide
- astemizole
- bepridil
- cisapride
- daunorubicin or doxorubicin
- diltiazem
- some medicines for treating heart-rhythm problems (amiodarone, flecainide, disopyramide, dofetilide, ibutilide, procainamide, quinidine, sotalol)
- pimozide
- probucol
- terfenadine
- terodiline
- verapamil

Mesoridazine may also interact with the following:

- alcohol
- antacids
- antidiarrheal medications
- atropine
- benztropine
- bromocriptine
- cabergoline
- cocaine
- dextroamphetamine or amphetamine
- dronabinol or marijuana
- lithium
- meclizine
- medicines for anxiety
- medicines for an over-active thyroid gland
- medicines for colds and flu
- medicines for insomnia (difficulty sleeping)
- medicines for hay fever and other allergies
- medicines for mental depression
- medicines for movement abnormalities as in Parkinson's disease
- medications for treating seizures (convulsions)
- medicines for pain or for use as muscle relaxants, including tramadol
- medicines to treat urine or bladder incontinence
- metoclopramide
- other medicines for treating thought disorders such as schizophrenia
- quinine
- rifampin
- some medications for high blood pressure or heart problems
- some weight loss medications
- trihexyphenidyl
- vitamin A

Tell your prescriber or health care professional about all other medicines you are taking, including non-pre-

M

scription medicines. Also tell your prescriber or health care professional if you are a frequent user of drinks with caffeine or alcohol, if you smoke, or if you use illegal drugs. These may affect the way your medicine works. Check with your health care professional before stopping or starting any of your medicines.

What should I watch for while taking mesoridazine?

Visit your prescriber or health care professional for regular checks on your progress. It may be several weeks before you see the full effects of mesoridazine. Do not suddenly stop taking mesoridazine. Your doctor may want you to gradually reduce the dose. Only stop taking mesoridazine on your prescriber's advice. Mesoridazine may cause your skin to become more sensitive to the sun or ultraviolet light. If this reaction occurs, it can cause a severe sunburn and damage the skin. Keep out of the sun, or wear protective clothing outdoors and use a sunscreen (at least SPF 15). Do not use sun lamps or sun tanning beds or booths. Wear sunglasses to protect your eyes. Mesoridazine can change the response of your body to heat or cold. Try not to get overheated. Avoid temperature extremes, such as saunas, hot tubs, or very hot or cold baths or showers. Dress warmly in cold weather. If you experience dry mouth while taking mesoridazine, make sure to drink plenty of water. It may also be helpful to suck on sugarless hard candy or crushed ice. If your dry mouth is severe, ask your doctor about a saliva substitute. You may get dizzy or drowsy. Do not drive, use machinery, or do anything that needs mental alertness until you know how mesoridazine affects you. Alcohol can increase dizziness and drowsiness. Avoid alcoholic drinks. Do not stand or sit up quickly, especially if you are an older patient. This reduces the risk of dizzy or fainting spells. If you are going to have surgery or will need a procedure that uses contrast agents, tell your prescriber or health care professional that you are taking this medicine.

What side effects may I notice from taking mesoridazine?

Side effects that you should report to your prescriber or health care professional as soon as possible:
- breast enlargement in men or women

- breast milk in women who are not breast-feeding
- change in emotion or behavior such as feeling depressed, angry, or anxious
- change in vision
- chest pain, fast or irregular heartbeat
- confusion
- dark yellow or brown urine
- difficulty breathing
- difficulty swallowing
- fever
- inability to control muscle movements in the face, hands, arms, or legs
- increased thirst
- intolerance to heat or cold
- loss of balance or difficulty walking
- menstrual changes
- seizures
- stiff muscles or jaw
- seizures
- skin rash
- spasms of the face, tongue, or mouth
- uncontrollable tongue or mouth movements

Side effects that usually do not require medical attention (report to your prescriber or health care professional if they continue or are bothersome):

Less common or rare:
- changes in sexual desire
- excessive watering or drooling of mouth
- nausea or vomiting
- restlessness or need to keep moving
- stuffy nose
- trouble in controlling urine

More common:
- constipation
- difficulty urinating
- dizziness; especially on standing from a sitting or lying position
- drowsiness
- dry mouth
- weight gain

Where can I keep my medicine?

Keep out of the reach of children in a container that small children cannot open. Store at room temperature between 20 degrees and 25 degrees C (68 degrees and 77 degrees F). Throw away any unused medicine after the expiration date.

Metaproterenol inhalation aerosol

ALUPENT®;
0.65 mg/actuation; Aerosol;
Metered
Boehringer Ingelheim
Pharmaceuticals Inc

What is metaproterenol inhalation aerosol?

METAPROTERENOL (Alupent®) can open up air passages and make breathing easier for people with various lung problems such as asthma. Generic metaproterenol inhalation aerosol is not yet available.

What should my health care professional know before I use metaproterenol?

They need to know if you have any of the following conditions:

- diabetes
- heart disease
- high-blood pressure
- overactive thyroid
- an unusual or allergic reaction to metaproterenol, sulfites, other medicines, foods, dyes, or preservatives
- pregnant or trying to get pregnant
- breast-feeding

How should I use this medicine?

Metaproterenol aerosol is for inhalation through the mouth. Shake the canister well. Tilt your head back slightly. Breathe out fully, emptying as much air as possible from your lungs. Keep the canister upright. Keep the inhaler about 1 inch from your open mouth (or place the mouthpiece loosely between your open lips). Press down on the inhaler (one puff) while breathing in deeply and slowly. Hold your breath for at least 10 seconds and then exhale (breathe out). Wait for at least 1 to 2 minutes between puffs. Do not use more than two puffs at a time, unless your prescriber or health care professional tells you otherwise. Contact your pediatrician or health care professional regarding the use of this medicine in children. Special care may be needed.

What if I miss a dose?

If you miss a dose, use it as soon as you can. If it is almost time for your next dose, use only that dose. Do not use double or extra doses.

What may interact with metaproterenol?

- arsenic trioxide
- astemizole
- bepridil
- beta-blockers, often used for high blood pressure or heart problems
- caffeine
- certain antibiotics (such as clarithromycin, erythromycin, gatifloxacin, gemifloxacin, grepafloxacin, levofloxacin, linezolid, moxifloxacin, sparfloxacin)
- chloroquine
- cisapride
- droperidol
- halofantrine
- levomethadyl
- medicines for colds and breathing difficulties
- medicines for heart disease or high blood pressure
- medicines known as MAO inhibitors, such as phenelzine (Nardil®), tranylcypromine (Parnate®), isocarboxazid (Marplan®), and selegiline (Carbex®, Eldepryl®)
- medicines to control heart rhythm (examples: amiodarone, disopyramide, dofetilide, flecainide, procainamide, quinidine, sotalol)
- medicines for treating depression or mental illness (amoxapine, haloperidol, maprotiline, pimozide, phenothiazines, risperidone, sertindole, tricyclic antidepressants, ziprasidone)
- methadone
- pentamidine

- probucol
- some medicines for weight loss (including some herbal products, ephedra, ephedrine, dextroamphetamine)
- steroid hormones such as dexamethasone, cortisone, hydrocortisone
- terfenadine
- theophylline
- thyroid hormones
- water pills or diuretics

Tell your prescriber or health care professional about all other medicines you are taking, including nonprescription medicines, nutritional supplements, or herbal products. Also tell your prescriber or health care professional if you are a frequent user of drinks with caffeine or alcohol, if you smoke, or if you use illegal drugs. These may affect the way your medicine works. Check before starting or stopping any of your medicines.

What should I watch for while taking metaproterenol?

Check with your prescriber or health care professional if your symptoms do not improve with metaproterenol inhalation, or if they get worse. You may need a change of therapy. Make sure you are using your inhaler properly. To keep your mouth from getting dry after inhaling metaproterenol, rinse out your mouth with water. Do not get the aerosol spray in your eyes. If you also use ipratropium (Atrovent®) or an inhaled steroid (such as beclomethasone or triamcinolone), use the metaproterenol first. Wait at least 5 minutes before using the other inhaler. Do not treat yourself for coughs, colds or allergies without checking with your prescriber or health care professional. Nonprescription medicines may contain ingredients that will increase the effects of your medicine. If you are going to have surgery, tell your prescriber or health care professional that you are using metaproterenol.

What side effects may I notice from using metaproterenol?

Side effects that you should report to your prescriber or health care professional as soon as possible:

- difficulty breathing, wheezing
- dizziness, drowsiness
- flushing (reddening of the skin)
- irregular heartbeats, palpitations, chest pain
- numbness in fingers or toes
- skin rash, hives
- swelling of the lips or face
- vomiting

Side effects that usually do not require medical attention (report to your prescriber or health care professional if they continue or are bothersome):

- anxiety or nervousness
- headache
- increased sweating
- muscle cramps
- nausea
- tremor
- weakness or tiredness

M

Where can I keep my medicine?

Keep out of the reach of children. Store at room temperature between 15 and 25 degrees C (59 and 77 degrees F). Protect from light. Throw away any unused medicine after the expiration date.

Metaproterenol tablets

METAPROTERENOL;
10 mg; Tablet
Teva
Pharmaceuticals
USA Inc

METAPROTERENOL;
10 mg; Tablet
Par Pharmaceuticals
Inc

What are metaproterenol tablets?

METAPROTERENOL (Alupent®) can open up air passages and make breathing easier for people with various lung problems such as asthma. Generic metaproterenol tablets are available.

What should my health care professional know before I take metaproterenol?

They need to know if you have any of the following conditions:
- diabetes
- heart disease
- high blood pressure
- over active thyroid
- an unusual or allergic reaction to metaproterenol, sulfites, other medicines, foods, dyes, or preservatives
- pregnant or trying to get pregnant
- breast-feeding

How should I take this medicine?

Take metaproterenol tablets by mouth. Follow the directions on the prescription label. Swallow the tablets with a drink of water. If metaproterenol upsets your stomach, take with food or milk, unless your prescriber or health care professional tells you otherwise. Take your doses at regular intervals. Do not take the tablets more often than directed. Contact your pediatrician or health care professional regarding the use of this medicine in children. Special care may be needed.

What if I miss a dose?

If you miss a dose, take it as soon as you can. Do not take the missed dose if more than 1 hour has passed since it was due. Do not take double or extra doses.

What may interact with metaproterenol?

- arsenic trioxide
- astemizole
- bepridil
- beta-blockers, often used for high blood pressure or heart problems
- caffeine
- certain antibiotics (such as clarithromycin, erythromycin, gatifloxacin, gemifloxacin, grepafloxacin, levofloxacin, linezolid, moxifloxacin, sparfloxacin)
- chloroquine
- cisapride
- droperidol
- halofantrine
- levomethadyl

- medicines for colds and breathing difficulties
- medicines for heart disease or high blood pressure
- medicines known as MAO inhibitors, such as phenelzine (Nardil®), tranylcypromine (Parnate®), isocarboxazid (Marplan®), and selegiline (Carbex®, Eldepryl®)
- medicines to control heart rhythm (examples: amiodarone, disopyramide, dofetilide, flecainide, procainamide, quinidine, sotalol)
- medicines for treating depression or mental illness (amoxapine, haloperidol, maprotiline, pimozide, phenothiazines, risperidone, sertindole, tricyclic antidepressants, ziprasidone)
- methadone
- pentamidine
- probucol
- some medicines for weight loss (including some herbal products, ephedra, ephedrine, dextroamphetamine)
- steroid hormones such as dexamethasone, cortisone, hydrocortisone
- terfenadine
- theophylline
- thyroid hormones
- water pills or diuretics

Tell your prescriber or health care professional about all other medicines you are taking, including non-prescription medicines, nutritional supplements, or herbal products. Also tell your prescriber or health care professional if you are a frequent user of drinks with caffeine or alcohol, if you smoke, or if you use illegal drugs. These may affect the way your medicine works. Check before starting or stopping any of your medicines.

What should I watch for while taking metaproterenol?

Use exactly as directed by your prescriber or health care professional. Do not take more often than instructed. Check with your prescriber or health care professional if your symptoms do not improve with metaproterenol, or if they get worse. You may need a change of therapy. Do not treat yourself for coughs, colds or allergies without checking with your prescriber or health care professional. Non-prescription medicines may contain ingredients that will increase the effects of your medicine.

What side effects may I notice from taking metaproterenol?

Side effects that you should report to your prescriber or health care professional as soon as possible:

- difficulty breathing, wheezing
- dizziness, drowsiness
- flushing (reddening of the skin)
- irregular heartbeats, palpitations, chest pain
- numbness in fingers or toes
- skin rash, hives
- swelling of the lips or face
- vomiting

Side effects that usually do not require medical attention (report to your prescriber or health care professional if they continue or are bothersome):

- anxiety or nervousness
- headache

- increased sweating
- muscle cramps
- nausea
- tremor
- weakness or tiredness

Where can I keep my medicine?

Keep out of the reach of children in a container that small children cannot open. Store at room temperature between 15 and 30 degrees C (59 and 86 degrees F). Store blister packs below 25 degrees C (77 degrees F). Protect from light. Throw away any unused medicine after the expiration date.

Metaxalone tablets

SKELAXIN®;
400 mg; Tablet
King
Pharmaceuticals Inc

SKELAXIN®;
800 mg; Tablet
King
Pharmaceuticals Inc

What are metaxalone tablets?

METAXALONE (Skelaxin®) is a muscle relaxant. It helps to relieve pain and stiffness in muscles caused by strains, sprains, or other injury to your muscles. Generic metaxalone tablets are not available.

What should my health care professional know before I take metaxalone?

They need to know if you have any of these conditions:

- anemia or blood disorder
- kidney disease
- liver disease
- an unusual or allergic reaction to metaxalone, other medicines, foods, dyes, or preservatives
- pregnant or trying to get pregnant
- breast-feeding

How should I take this medicine?

Take metaxalone tablets by mouth. Swallow the tablets with a drink of water. Follow the directions on the prescription label. Take your doses at regular intervals. Do not take your medicine more often than directed. Contact your pediatrician or health care professional regarding the use of this medicine in children. Special care may be needed.

What if I miss a dose?

If you miss a dose, take it as soon as you can. If it is almost time for your next dose, take only the next dose. Do not take double or extra doses.

What may interact with metaxalone?

Because metaxalone can cause drowsiness, other medicines that also cause drowsiness may increase this effect of metaxalone. Some medicines that cause drowsiness are:

- alcohol-containing medicines
- barbiturates such as phenobarbital
- certain antidepressants or tranquilizers
- certain narcotics or pain medicines

- certain medicines used for anxiety or to help produce sleep
- certain antihistamines used in cold medicines

Ask your prescriber or health care professional about other medicines that may increase the effect of metaxalone. Tell your prescriber or health care professional about all other medicines you are taking, including non-prescription medicines, nutritional supplements, or herbal products. Also tell your prescriber or health care professional if you are a frequent user of drinks with caffeine or alcohol, if you smoke, or if you use illegal drugs. These may affect the way your medicine works. Check with your health care professional before stopping or starting any of your medicines.

What should I watch for while taking metaxalone?

Check with your prescriber or health care professional if your condition does not improve within 1 to 2 weeks. You may get drowsy or dizzy. Do not drive, use machinery, or do anything that needs mental alertness until you know how metaxalone affects you. To reduce the risk of dizzy or fainting spells, do not sit or stand up quickly, especially if you are an older patient. Alcohol can make you more drowsy; avoid alcoholic drinks.

What side effects may I notice from taking metaxalone?

Side effects that you should report to your prescriber or health care professional as soon as possible:

- skin rash
- sore throat or fever with or without chills
- unusual tiredness or weakness
- vomiting
- yellow eyes or skin

Side effects that usually do not require medical attention (report to your prescriber or health care professional if they continue or are bothersome):

M

- dizziness
- drowsiness
- headache
- irritability
- nervousness
- stomach upset

Where can I keep my medicine?

Keep out of the reach of children in a container that small children cannot open. Store at room temperature away from heat and direct light. Keep container tightly closed. Throw away any unused medicine after the expiration date.

Metformin tablets and extended-release tablets

GLUCOPHAGE®;
500 mg; Tablet
Bristol Myers Squibb
Co

GLUCOPHAGE® XR;
750 mg; Tablet,
Extended Release
Bristol Myers Squibb
Co

What are metformin tablets or extended-release tablets?

METFORMIN (Glucophage®, Glucophage® XR) is a medicine used to treat type 2 diabetes mellitus. Treatment is combined with a balanced diet and exercise. This medicine lowers blood sugar and helps your body to use insulin more efficiently. It is sometimes used with other medicines for diabetes. Generic metformin tablets and extended-release tablets are available.

What should my health care professional know before I take metformin?

They need to know if you have any of these conditions:
- frequently drink alcohol or alcohol-containing beverages
- become easily dehydrated
- heart attack
- heart failure that is treated with medications
- hormone changes or problems
- kidney disease
- liver disease
- polycystic ovaries
- serious infection or injury
- thyroid disease
- undergoing surgery or certain x-ray procedures with injectable contrast agents
- an unusual or allergic reaction to metformin, other medicines, foods, dyes, or preservatives
- pregnant or trying to get pregnant
- breast-feeding

How should I take this medicine?

Take metformin tablets by mouth, with meals. Follow the directions on the prescription label. Swallow the tablets with a drink of water. Do not crush, cut, or chew extended-release tablets. Take your doses at regular intervals. Do not take your medicine more often than directed. Glucophage® XR may be eliminated as a soft mass in your stool that may look like the original tablet; this is not harmful and will not affect the way the drug works to control your diabetes. Contact your pediatrician or health care professional regarding the use of this medicine in children. Special care may be needed.

What if I miss a dose?

If you miss a dose, take it as soon as you can. If it is almost time for your next dose, take only that dose. Do not take double or extra doses.

What may interact with metformin?

- alcohol
- cephalexin
- cimetidine
- digoxin
- dofetilide
- morphine
- nifedipine
- procainamide
- propantheline
- quinidine
- quinine
- ranitidine
- trimethoprim
- trospium
- vancomycin
- water pills (diuretics like amiloride, furosemide, triamterene)

Many medications may cause changes (increase or decrease) in blood sugar; these include:

- alcohol-containing beverages
- aspirin and aspirin-like drugs
- beta-blockers, often used for high blood pressure or heart problems (examples include atenolol, metoprolol, propranolol)
- chromium
- female hormones, such as estrogens, progestins, or contraceptive pills
- isoniazid
- male hormones or anabolic steroids
- medications for weight loss
- medicines for allergies, asthma, cold, or cough
- niacin
- pentamidine
- phenytoin
- some herbal dietary supplements
- steroid medicines such as prednisone or cortisone
- thyroid hormones
- water pills (diuretics)

M

Tell your prescriber or health care professional about all other medicines you are taking, including non-prescription medicines, nutritional supplements, or herbal products. Also tell your prescriber or health care professional if you are a frequent user of drinks with caffeine or alcohol, if you smoke, or if you use illegal drugs. These may affect the way your medicine works. Check with your health care professional before stopping or starting any of your medicines.

What should I watch for while taking metformin?

Visit your prescriber or health care professional for regular checks on your progress. Your prescriber will check your blood sugar, kidney function, and other tests from time to time. Learn how to monitor your blood sugar. Learn what to do if you have high or low blood sugar. Do not skip meals. If you are exercising much more than usual you may need extra snacks to avoid side effects caused by low blood sugar. Do not change your medication dose without talking to your prescriber. If you have mild symptoms of low blood sugar, eat or drink something containing sugar at once and contact your health care professional. It is wise to check your blood sugar to confirm that it is low. It is important to recognize your own symptoms of low blood sugar so that you can treat them quickly. Make sure family members know that you can choke if you eat or drink when you develop serious symptoms of low blood sugar, such as seizures or unconsciousness. They must get medical help at once. If you develop a severe diarrhea or vomiting, or are unable to maintain proper fluid intake, you should contact your prescriber. "Sick days" may require adjustments to your dosage or your illness may need to be evaluated. Ask your prescriber what you should do if you become ill. If you are going to have surgery or will need an x-ray procedure that uses contrast agents, tell your prescriber or health care professional that you are taking this medicine. Wear a medical identification bracelet or chain to say you have diabetes, and carry a card that lists all your medications.

What side effects may I notice from taking metformin?

Side effects that you should report to your prescriber or health care professional as soon as possible:
- breathing difficulties or shortness of breath
- dizziness
- muscle aches or pains
- passing out or fainting
- severe vomiting or diarrhea
- slow or irregular heartbeat
- unusual stomach pain or discomfort
- unusual weakness, fatigue or discomfort

In combination with other diabetic medications, (like acarbose, glyburide, glipizide, miglitol, or insulin), metformin may cause low blood sugar (hypoglycemia). Contact your health care professional if you experience symptoms of low blood sugar, which may include:
- anxiety or nervousness
- confusion
- difficulty concentrating
- hunger
- pale skin
- nausea
- fatigue
- sweating
- headache
- palpitations
- numbness of the mouth
- tingling in the fingers
- tremors
- muscle weakness
- blurred vision
- cold sensations
- uncontrolled yawning
- irritability
- rapid heartbeat
- shallow breathing
- loss of consciousness

Symptoms of high blood sugar (hyperglycemia) include:
- dizziness
- dry mouth
- flushed dry skin
- fruit-like breath odor
- loss of appetite
- nausea
- stomachache
- unusual thirst
- frequent passing of urine

Side effects that usually do not require medical attention (report to your prescriber or health care professional if they continue or are bothersome):
- decreased appetite
- gas
- heartburn
- metallic taste in the mouth
- mild stomachache
- nausea
- weight loss

Where can I keep my medicine?

Keep out of the reach of children in a container that small children cannot open. Store at room temperature between 15 and 30 degrees C (59 and 86 degrees F). Protect from moisture and light. Throw away any unused medicine after the expiration date.

M

Metformin; Rosiglitazone tablet

AVANDAMET™;
500 mg/2 mg; Tablet
SmithKline Beecham
Pharmaceuticals Div
SmithKline Beecham
Co

AVANDAMET™;
1000 mg/2 mg;
Tablet
SmithKline Beecham
Pharmaceuticals Div
SmithKline Beecham
Co

What are metformin; rosiglitazone tablets?

METFORMIN; ROSIGLITAZONE (Avandamet™) is a combination medicine used to treat type 2 diabetes mellitus. Drug therapy for diabetes should be combined with a balanced diet, weight loss, and exercise. This medicine lowers blood sugar and helps your body to use insulin more efficiently. Generic metformin; rosiglitazone tablets are not yet available.

What should my health care professional know before I take metformin; rosiglitazone?

They need to know if you have any of these conditions:
- frequently drink alcohol or alcohol-containing beverages
- become easily dehydrated
- heart attack or other heart problems
- heart failure that is treated with medications
- history of diabetic ketoacidosis (DKA)
- hormone changes or problems
- kidney disease
- liver disease
- polycystic ovaries
- serious infection or injury
- swelling of the arms, legs, or feet; water retention
- thyroid disease
- use insulin
- undergoing surgery or certain x-ray procedures with injectable contrast agents
- an unusual reaction to metformin; rosiglitazone, other medicines, foods, dyes, or preservatives
- pregnant or trying to get pregnant
- breast-feeding

How should this medicine be taken?

Take metformin; rosiglitazone tablets by mouth, with meals. Follow the directions on the prescription label. Swallow the tablets with a drink of water. Take your doses at the same time each day; do not take more often than directed. Contact your pediatrician or health care professional regarding the use of this medicine in children. Special care may be needed. Patients over 65 years old may need a smaller dose than younger adults.

What if I miss a dose?

If it is almost time for your next dose, take only that dose. Do not take double or extra doses.

What may interact with metformin; rosiglitazone?

- alcohol
- cephalexin
- cimetidine
- digoxin
- dofetilide
- entecavir
- insulin
- morphine
- nifedipine
- procainamide
- propantheline
- quinidine
- quinine
- ranitidine
- trimethoprim
- vancomycin
- water pills (diuretics like amiloride, furosemide, triamterene)

Many medications may cause changes (increase or decrease) in blood sugar; these include:

- alcohol-containing beverages
- aspirin and aspirin-like drugs
- beta-blockers, often used for high blood pressure or heart problems (examples: atenolol, metoprolol, propranolol)
- chromium
- female hormones, such as estrogens or progestins, birth control pills
- fibric acid derivatives, used to treat high cholesterol (examples: fenofibrate and gemfibrozil)
- isoniazid
- male hormones or anabolic steroids
- medications to suppress appetite or for weight loss
- medicines for allergies, asthma, cold, or cough
- niacin
- pentamidine
- phenytoin
- quinolone antibiotics (examples: ciprofloxacin, levofloxacin, ofloxacin)
- some herbal dietary supplements
- steroid medicines such as prednisone or cortisone
- thyroid hormones
- water pills (diuretics)

Tell your prescriber or health care professional about all other medicines you are taking, including non-prescription medicines, nutritional supplements, or herbal products. Also tell your prescriber or health care professional if you are a frequent user of drinks with caffeine or alcohol, if you smoke, or if you use illegal drugs. These may affect the way your medicine works. Check with your health care professional before stopping or starting any of your medicines.

M

What should I watch for while taking metformin; rosiglitazone?

Contact your health care professional if you experience symptoms of low blood sugar (hypoglycemia) or high blood sugar (hyperglycemia). Visit your prescriber or health care professional for regular checks on your progress. Your prescriber will check your blood sugar, kidney function, liver function and other tests from time to time. Learn how to monitor blood or urine sugar and urine ketones regularly. Do not skip meals. If you are exercising much more than usual you may need extra snacks to avoid side effects caused by low blood sugar. If you have mild symptoms of low blood sugar, eat or drink something containing sugar at once and contact your prescriber or health care professional. It is wise to check your blood sugar to confirm that it is low. It is important to recognize your own symptoms of low blood sugar so that you can treat them quickly. Make sure family members know that you can choke if you eat or drink when you have serious symptoms of low blood sugar, such as seizures or unconsciousness. They must get medical help at once. If you develop severe diarrhea, nausea or vomiting, or are unable to maintain proper fluid intake, you should contact your prescriber. "Sick days" may require adjustments to your dosage or your illness may need to be evaluated. Ask your prescriber what you should do if you become ill. If you are going to have surgery or will need an x-ray procedure that uses contrast agents, tell your prescriber or health care professional that you are taking this medicine. Wear a medical identification bracelet or chain that says you have diabetes, and carry a card that lists all your medications.

What side effects may I notice from taking metformin; rosiglitazone?

Side effects that you should report to your prescriber or health care professional as soon as possible:

- anxiety or nervousness, confusion, difficulty concentrating
- blurred vision
- breathing difficulties or shortness of breath
- cold sweats, increased sweating
- cool, pale skin
- dark yellow or brown urine, or yellowing of the eyes or skin
- dizziness
- muscle aches or pains
- passing out or fainting
- rapid gain in weight
- severe vomiting or prolonged diarrhea
- skin rash or hives
- slow or irregular heartbeat
- swelling of the hands, legs, and/or feet
- tremors or shakiness
- unusual stomach pain or discomfort
- unusual fatigue, tiredness or weakness

Symptoms of low blood sugar (hypoglycemia). Know the symptoms of low blood sugar, so that you can quickly treat them, which may include:

- anxiety or nervousness
- confusion
- difficulty concentrating
- hunger
- pale skin
- nausea
- fatigue
- sweating
- headache
- palpitations
- numbness of the mouth
- tingling in the fingers
- tremors
- muscle weakness
- blurred vision
- cold sensations
- uncontrolled yawning
- irritability
- rapid heartbeat
- shallow breathing
- loss of consciousness

Hypoglycemia may cause you to not be aware of your actions or surroundings if it is severe, so you should let others know what to do if you cannot help yourself in a severe reaction.

Symptoms of high blood sugar (hyperglycemia) include:

- dizziness
- dry mouth
- flushed, dry skin
- loss of appetite
- nausea
- stomach cramping
- unusual thirst
- frequent passing of urine

Side effects that usually do not require medical attention (report to your prescriber or health care professional if they continue or are bothersome):

- backache
- decreased appetite
- diarrhea
- gas
- headache
- heartburn
- metallic taste in the mouth
- slow weight gain
- weight loss

Where can I keep my medicine?

Keep out of the reach of children in a container that small children cannot open. Store at room temperature between 15 and 30 degrees C (59 and 86 degrees F). Protect from moisture and light. Throw away any unused medicine after the expiration date.

M

Methadone tablets

METHADONE;
5 mg; Tablet
Roxane Laboratories
Inc

METHADONE;
10 mg; Tablet
Roxane Laboratories
Inc

What are methadone tablets?

METHADONE (Dolophine®) is strong pain medication similar to morphine. Methadone relieves moderate to severe pain. Methadone is also used as part of detoxification and maintenance programs to help prevent withdrawal symptoms in people addicted to drugs such as heroin or other illegal street drugs. Federal law prohibits the transfer of methadone to any person other than the patient for whom it was prescribed. Do not share this medicine with anyone else. Generic methadone tablets are available.

What should my health care professional know before I take methadone?

They need to know if you have any of these conditions:
- biliary tract disease
- diarrhea
- heart disease
- intestinal disease
- kidney disease
- liver disease
- lung disease or breathing difficulties
- seizures
- an unusual or allergic reaction to methadone, propoxyphene, other medicines, foods, dyes, or preservatives
- pregnant or trying to get pregnant
- breast-feeding

How should I take this medicine?

Take methadone tablets by mouth. Follow the directions on the prescription label. Swallow the tablets with a drink of water. If methadone upsets your stomach you can take it with food or milk. Take your doses at regular intervals. Do not take your medicine more often than directed. Contact your pediatrician or health care professional regarding the use of this medicine in children. Special care may be needed.

What if I miss a dose?

If you miss a dose, take it as soon as you can. If it is almost time for your next dose, take only that dose. Do not take double or extra doses.

What may interact with methadone?

- antiviral medicines such as protease inhibitors, delavirdine, didanosine (ddI), efavirenz, nevirapine, stavudine (d4T), or zidovudine
- buprenorphine
- butorphanol
- clarithromycin
- erythromycin
- fluvoxamine
- grapefruit juice
- medicines for high blood pressure
- medicines for seizures
- nalbuphine
- naltrexone
- nefazodone
- pentazocine
- rifampin
- St. John's wort

Because methadone can cause drowsiness, other medicines that also cause drowsiness may increase this effect of methadone. Some medicines that cause drowsiness are:
- alcohol and alcohol-containing medicines
- barbiturates such as phenobarbital
- certain antidepressants or tranquilizers
- muscle relaxants
- certain antihistamines used in cold medicines
- tramadol

Ask your prescriber or health care professional about other medicines that may increase the effect of methadone. Tell your prescriber or health care professional about all other medicines you are taking, including non-prescription medicines, nutritional supplements, or herbal products. Also tell your prescriber or health care professional if you are a frequent user of drinks with caffeine or alcohol, if you smoke, or if you use illegal drugs. These may affect the way your medicine works. Check with your health care professional before stopping or starting any of your medicines.

What should I watch for while taking methadone?

Tell your prescriber or health care professional if your pain does not go away, if it gets worse or if you have a new or different type of pain. Use exactly as directed by your prescriber or health care professional. If you are taking methadone on a regular basis, do not suddenly stop taking it. Your body becomes used to methadone and when you suddenly stop taking it, you may develop a severe reaction. You may get drowsy or dizzy. Be careful taking other medicines that may also make you tired. This effect may be worse when taking these medicines with methadone. Do not drive, use machinery, or do anything that needs mental alertness until you know how methadone affects you. Do not stand or sit up quickly, especially if you are an older patient. This reduces the risk of dizzy or fainting spells. Alcohol can increase possible drowsiness, dizziness, confusion, and can affect your breathing. Avoid alcohol while taking methadone. Methadone will cause constipation. Make sure to take a laxative and/or stool softener while taking methadone. Try to have a bowel movement every 2 to 3 days, at least. If you do not have a bowel movement for 3 days or more, call your prescriber or health care professional. They may recommend using an enema or suppository to help you move your bowels. Your mouth may get dry. Chewing sugarless gum or sucking hard candy, and drinking plenty of water may help. Visit the dentist regularly. If you are going to have surgery, tell your prescriber or health care professional that you are taking methadone.

What side effects may I notice from taking methadone?

Side effects that you should report to your prescriber or health care professional as soon as possible:
- breathing difficulties
- cold, clammy skin
- confusion
- lightheadedness or fainting spells
- nervousness or restlessness
- seizures
- slow or fast heartbeat
- unusual weakness
- decrease or difficulty passing urine

Side effects that usually do not require medical attention (report to your prescriber or health care professional if they continue or are bothersome):
- blurred vision
- clumsiness, unsteadiness
- constipation
- dizziness, drowsiness
- dry mouth
- flushing
- headache
- nausea/vomiting
- pinpoint pupils
- sweating

Where can I keep my medicine?

Keep out of the reach of children in a container that small children cannot open. Do not share or give this medicine to anyone else. Avoid accidental swallowing of methadone by someone (especially children) other than the person for whom it was prescribed as this may result in severe effects and possibly death. Store at room temperature between 15 and 30 degrees C (59 and 86 degrees F). Protect from light. Store in the original carton until time of use. Throw away any unused medicine after the expiration date.

Methimazole tablets

TAPAZOLE®; 10 mg; Tablet King Pharmaceuticals Inc

TAPAZOLE®; 5 mg; Tablet King Pharmaceuticals Inc

What are methimazole tablets?

METHIMAZOLE (Tapazole®) prevents the thyroid gland from producing too much thyroid hormone. Methimazole is used to treat a condition known as hyperthyroidism (over-active thyroid). Generic methimazole tablets are available.

What should my health care professional know before I take methimazole?

They need to know if you have any of these conditions:
- liver disease
- blood disorder
- an unusual or allergic reaction to methimazole, other medicines, foods, dyes, or preservatives
- pregnant or trying to get pregnant
- breast-feeding

How should I take this medicine?

Take methimazole tablets by mouth. Follow the directions on the prescription label. Swallow the tablets with a drink of water. Food can affect the amount of methimazole absorbed into the body. You may take methimazole either on an empty stomach or with food, but always take it the same way to make sure the effects are the same. Take your doses at regular intervals. Do not take your medicine more often than directed. Do not stop taking methimazole except on your prescriber's advice.

What if I miss a dose?

If you miss a dose, take it as soon as you can and space remaining doses evenly. If you do not remember the missed dose until almost time for the next dose, take both doses together. Contact your prescriber or health care professional if you miss more than one dose. Do not take extra doses.

What may interact with methimazole?

- amiodarone
- digoxin
- potassium iodide
- sodium iodide
- theophylline
- warfarin

Tell your prescriber or health care professional about all other medicines you are taking, including non-prescription medicines, nutritional supplements, or herbal products. Also tell your prescriber or health care professional if you are a frequent user of drinks with caffeine or alcohol, if you smoke, or if you use illegal drugs. These may affect the way your medicine works. Check with your health care professional before stopping or starting any of your medicines.

What should I watch for while taking methimazole?

Visit your prescriber or health care professional for regular checks on your progress, and to make sure your

M

body is producing the right amount of thyroid hormone. If you are going to have surgery, tell your prescriber or health care professional that you are taking methimazole. Methimazole can reduce your resistance to infection. Contact your prescriber or health care professional if you have any infection or injury. Avoid people who have colds, flu, bronchitis or other infectious disease. Do not have any vaccinations without your prescriber's approval. Avoid people who have recently received oral polio vaccine.

What side effects may I notice from taking methimazole?

Side effects that you should report to your prescriber or health care professional as soon as possible:
- backache
- black, tarry stools
- fever, sore throat, hoarseness
- menstrual changes
- mouth sores
- numbness or tingling in the hands or feet

- severe redness or itching of the skin, or dry cracked skin
- stomach pain
- swelling of the feet or legs
- unusual bleeding or bruising, pinpoint red spots on the skin
- unusual or sudden weight increase
- unusual tiredness or weakness
- yellowing of skin or eyes

Side effects that usually do not require medical attention (report to your prescriber or health care professional if they continue or are bothersome):
- headache
- nausea, vomiting
- mild skin rash, itching
- muscle aches and pains

Where can I keep my medicine?

Keep out of the reach of children in a container that small children cannot open. Store at room temperature between 15 and 30 degrees C (59 and 86 degrees F). Throw away any unused medicine after the expiration date.

Methocarbamol tablets

ROBAXIN®;
500 mg; Tablet
Schwarz Pharma Inc

ROBAXIN®;
750 mg; Tablet
Schwarz Pharma Inc

What are methocarbamol tablets?

METHOCARBAMOL (Robaxin®) is a muscle relaxant. It helps to relieve pain and stiffness in muscles and can treat muscle spasms. Generic methocarbamol tablets are available.

What should my health care professional know before I take methocarbamol?

They need to know if you have any of these conditions:
- an unusual or allergic reaction to methocarbamol, other medicines, foods, dyes, or preservatives
- pregnant or trying to get pregnant
- breast-feeding

How should I take this medicine?

Take methocarbamol tablets by mouth. Follow the directions on the prescription label. Swallow the tablets with a drink of water. Take your doses at regular intervals. Do not take your medicine more often than directed. Contact your pediatrician or health care professional regarding the use of this medicine in children. Special care may be needed.

What if I miss a dose?

If you miss a dose, take it as soon as you can. If it is almost time for your next dose, take only the next dose. Do not take double or extra doses.

What may interact with methocarbamol?

Because methocarbamol can cause drowsiness, other medicines that also cause drowsiness may increase this

effect of methocarbamol. Ask your prescriber or health care professional about other medicines that may increase the effect of methocarbamol.

Tell your prescriber or health care professional about all other medicines you are taking, including non-prescription medicines, nutritional supplements, or herbal products. Also tell your prescriber or health care professional if you are a frequent user of drinks with caffeine or alcohol, if you smoke, or if you use illegal drugs. These may affect the way your medicine works. Check with your health care professional before stopping or starting any of your medicines.

What should I watch for while taking methocarbamol?

You may get drowsy or dizzy. Do not drive, use machinery, or do anything that needs mental alertness until you know how methocarbamol affects you. To reduce the risk of dizzy or fainting spells, do not sit or stand up quickly, especially if you are an older patient. Alcohol can make you more drowsy; avoid alcoholic drinks.

What side effects may I notice from taking methocarbamol?

Side effects that you should report to your prescriber or health care professional as soon as possible:
- constipation
- dark urine
- lightheadedness, fainting spells
- seizures (convulsions)
- skin itching or rash

M

- slow heartbeat
- vomiting

Side effects that usually do not require medical attention (report to your prescriber or health care professional if they continue or are bothersome):
- blurred vision
- drowsiness, dizziness
- flushing
- headache

- metallic taste
- nausea
- nervousness or confusion

Where can I keep my medicine?

Keep out of the reach of children in a container that small children cannot open. Store below 40 degrees C (104 degrees F). Keep container tightly closed. Throw away any unused medicine after the expiration date.

Methotrexate tablets

TREXALL®;
5 mg; Tablet
Barr Laboratories
Inc

METHOTREXATE;
2.5 mg; Tablet
Lederle
Pharmaceutical Div
American Cyanamid
Co

What are methotrexate tablets?

METHOTREXATE (Rheumatrex®, Trexall®) is a chemotherapy agent that is used to treat certain kinds of cancer and other diseases. Methotrexate tablets are commonly used to treat inflammatory conditions such as rheumatoid arthritis and psoriasis. Methotrexate affects cells that are rapidly growing such as cancer cells, cells of psoriasis, and cells in your mouth and stomach. Methotrexate is used in treating a number of cancers including leukemias, lymphoma, breast cancer, and others. Generic methotrexate tablets are available.

What should my health care professional know before I take methotrexate tablets?

They need to know if you have any of these conditions:
- if you are HIV-positive or have acquired immunodeficiency syndrome (AIDS)
- if you frequently drink alcohol-containing beverages
- bleeding or blood disorders
- cold sores or previous chickenpox or shingles infection
- gout
- an active infection
- kidney disease, including a history of kidney stones
- liver disease
- lung disease
- recent radiation therapy or sunburn
- stomach or intestinal disease or obstruction
- ulcerative colitis
- an unusual or allergic reaction to methotrexate, other chemotherapy, other medicines, foods, dyes, or preservatives
- pregnant or trying to get pregnant
- breast-feeding

How should I take this medicine?

Take methotrexate tablets by mouth. Follow the directions on the prescription label. Swallow the tablets with a drink of water. Do not take your medicine more often than directed. Finish the full course prescribed by your doctor or health care professional, even if the tablets make you feel unwell. Do not stop taking except on your prescriber's advice. The dose of methotrexate and how often it will be given may be different depending upon your disease and other medicines you are taking. If you have questions about the proper dose of your medicine, ask your prescriber or other health care professional.

What if I miss a dose?

If you miss a dose, skip that dose unless you remember within an hour or two, or your prescriber or health care professional tells you otherwise. Do not take double or extra doses. If you vomit after taking a dose, call your prescriber or health care professional for advice.

What may interact with methotrexate?

- anti-inflammatory drugs (NSAIDs, such as ibuprofen)
- antibiotics and other medicines for infections
- aspirin and aspirin-like medicines
- leucovorin
- vaccines
- medicines for diabetes
- phenytoin
- probenecid
- pyrimethamine

Tell your prescriber or health care professional about all other medicines that you are taking, including nonprescription medicines, nutritional supplements, or herbal products. Also tell your prescriber or health care professional if you are a frequent user of drinks with caffeine or alcohol, if you smoke, or if you use illegal drugs. These may affect the way your medicine works. Check with your health care professional before stopping or starting any of your medicines.

What should I watch for while taking methotrexate tablets?

Visit your prescriber or health care professional for checks on your progress. You will need to have regular blood checks. The side effects of methotrexate can continue after you finish your treatment; report side effects promptly. It may take several weeks before you see an improvement in your rheumatoid arthritis or psoriasis. Avoid alcohol-containing beverages while taking

M

methotrexate. Methotrexate therapy for rheumatoid arthritis and psoriasis may cause damage to your liver. Your prescriber or health care professional will closely monitor your liver function while you are taking methotrexate. You may need to have a liver sample (a biopsy) taken before you receive methotrexate and during your therapy for rheumatoid arthritis or psoriasis. Methotrexate may make you feel generally unwell. This is because methotrexate affects good cells as well as the disease cells. Report any side effects as above, but continue your course of medicine even though you feel ill, unless your prescriber or health care professional tells you to stop. Methotrexate may decrease your body's ability to fight infections. Call your prescriber or health care professional if you have a fever, chills, sore throat or other symptoms of a cold or flu. Do not treat these symptoms yourself. Try to avoid being around people who are sick. Methotrexate may harm your unborn baby. You should contact your prescriber immediately if you believe or suspect you or your partner have become pregnant while you are taking methotrexate. Both men and women must use effective birth control continuously while taking methotrexate. It is recommended that you use two reliable forms of contraception together. Men should continue to use contraception for at least 3 months after stopping methotrexate therapy. Women should continue to use contraception until after their first normal menstrual cycle after stopping methotrexate therapy. If you are going to have surgery or dental work, tell your surgeon, dentist, or health care professional that you are taking methotrexate. Methotrexate may cause you to more sensitive to the sun. Also methotrexate may cause a previous sunburn or radiation therapy reaction to reappear. Keep out of the sun, or wear protective clothing outdoors and use a sunscreen. Do not use sun lamps or sun tanning beds or booths.

What side effects may I notice from taking methotrexate tablets?

Side effects will vary depending on the condition for which you are being treated, the dose, and the length of time you are taking methotrexate. If you want more information on possible side effects, ask your prescriber or health care professional to discuss this with you.

Side effects that you should report to your prescriber or health care professional as soon as possible:

- symptoms of infection—fever or chills, cough, sore throat, pain or difficulty passing urine
- symptoms of decreased platelets or bleeding—bruising, pinpoint red spots on the skin, black, tarry stools, blood in the urine
- symptoms of decreased red blood cells (anemia)—unusual weakness or tiredness, fainting spells, lightheadedness
- diarrhea
- difficulty breathing, a non-productive cough
- mouth and throat ulcers
- redness, blistering, peeling or loosening of the skin, including inside the mouth
- skin rash, hives, or itching
- changes in vision
- vomiting
- yellow coloring of skin or eyes

Side effects that usually do not require medical attention (report to your prescriber or health care professional if they continue or are bothersome):

- hair loss
- increased sensitivity to sun and ultraviolet light
- loss of appetite
- nausea

Where can I keep my medicine?

Keep out of the reach of children in a container that small children cannot open. Store at room temperature between 15 and 30 degrees C (59 and 86 degrees F). Protect from light. Throw away any unused medicine after the expiration date.

Methscopolamine tablets

PAMINE®;
2.5 mg; Tablet
Kenwood
Therapeutics Div
Bradley
Pharmaceuticals Inc

PAMINE® FORTE;
5 mg; Tablet
Kenwood
Therapeutics Div
Bradley
Pharmaceuticals Inc

What are methscopolamine tablets?

METHSCOPOLAMINE (Pamine®) is a medicine that blocks the release of stomach acid. It is used with other medications to treat ulcers in the stomach and intestines. Generic methscopolamine tablets are not available.

What should my health care professional know before I take methscopolamine?

They need to know if you have any of these conditions:
- abnormal (fast, slow, or irregular) heart rhythm
- difficulty passing urine
- glaucoma
- heart disease
- high blood pressure
- intestinal problems such as ulcerative colitis
- kidney disease
- liver disease
- myasthenia gravis
- overactive thyroid
- stomach or bowel obstruction
- an unusual reaction to methscopolamine, other medicines, foods, dyes, or preservatives
- pregnant or trying to get pregnant
- breast-feeding

M

How should this medicine be taken?

Take methscopolamine tablets by mouth. Follow the directions on the prescription label. Take methscopolamine on an empty stomach, about 30 minutes before eating. Take your doses at regular intervals. Do not take your medicine more often than directed. Elderly patients over age 65 years may have a stronger reaction to this medicine and may need smaller doses. Contact your pediatrician or health care professional regarding the use of this medicine in children. Special care may be needed.

What if I miss a dose?

If you miss a dose, take it as soon as you can. If it is almost time for your next dose, take only that dose. Do not take double or extra doses.

What may interact with methscopolamine?

- alcohol-containing beverages
- amantadine
- antacids
- atomoxetine
- barbiturates such as phenobarbital, butalbital, primidone, or secobarbital
- benztropine
- bethanechol
- cisapride
- cyclobenzaprine
- digoxin
- donepezil
- disopyramide
- drugs for erectile dysfunction
- erythromycin
- galantamine
- itraconazole
- ketoconazole
- medicines for hay fever and other allergies
- medicines for mental depression
- medicines for mental problems and psychotic disturbances
- medicine for anxiety or sleeping problems (such as alprazolam, diazepam, or temazepam)
- meperidine
- metoclopramide
- opiate prescription pain medications such as codeine, hydromorphone, oxycodone, and morphine
- quinidine
- rivastigmine
- tacrine
- tegaserod

Tell your prescriber or health care professional about all other medicines you are taking, including non-prescription medicines, nutritional supplements, or herbal products. Also tell your prescriber or health care professional if you are a frequent user of drinks with caffeine or alcohol, if you smoke, or if you use illegal drugs. These may affect the way your medicine works. Check with your health care professional before stopping or starting any of your medicines.

What should I watch for while taking methscopolamine?

Visit your prescriber or health care professional for regular checks on your progress. Do not stop taking this medicine abruptly. Your prescriber or health care professional may want to gradually reduce the dose so that you do not get side effects or make your condition worse. Your prescriber or health care professional may want you to have an eye exam from time to time. You may get dizzy or have blurred vision. Do not drive, use machinery, or do anything that requires mental alertness until you know how methscopolamine affects you. To reduce the risk of dizzy or fainting spells, do not sit or stand up quickly, especially if you are an older patient. Alcohol can make you more dizzy, and increase flushing and rapid heartbeats. Avoid alcoholic drinks. Your mouth may get dry. Chewing sugarless gum or sucking hard candy, and drinking plenty of water, will help. Methscopolamine may cause dry eyes and blurred vision. If you wear contact lenses, you may feel some discomfort. Lubricating drops may help. See your ophthalmologist (eye doctor) if the problem does not go away or is severe. Stay out of bright light and wear sunglasses if methscopolamine makes your eyes more sensitive to light. Avoid extreme heat (e.g., hot tubs, saunas). Methscopolamine can cause you to sweat less than normal. Your body temperature could increase to dangerous levels, which can lead to heat stroke.

What side effects may I notice from taking methscopolamine?

Side effects that you should report to your prescriber or health care professional as soon as possible:

- blurred vision, or other eye problems
- confusion
- decrease in sweating
- difficulty breathing
- difficulty swallowing
- dizziness or fainting
- fast or irregular heartbeat (palpitations)
- fever
- pain or difficulty passing urine
- skin rash
- vomiting
- weakness or tiredness

Side effects that usually do not require medical attention (report to your prescriber or health care professional if they continue or are bothersome):

- anxiety, nervousness
- constipation
- difficulty sleeping
- drowsiness
- dry mouth
- headache
- itching
- loss of taste
- nausea
- sexual difficulties (decreased sexual ability or desire)

M

Where can I keep my medicine?

Keep out of the reach of children in a container that small children cannot open. Store at room temperature between 15 and 30 degrees C (59 and 86 degrees F). Throw away any unused medicine after the expiration date.

Methsuximide capsules

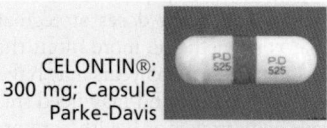

CELONTIN®;
300 mg; Capsule
Parke-Davis

What are methsuximide capsules?

METHSUXIMIDE (Celontin®) is an anticonvulsant medication. This drug can help with seizure (convulsion) control in those with absence seizures (petit mal epilepsy). Generic methsuximide capsules are not available.

What should my health care professional know before I take methsuximide?

They need to know if you have any of these conditions:
- blood disorders or disease
- depression
- kidney disease
- liver disease
- mental disorders
- systemic lupus erythematosus (SLE)
- an unusual or allergic reaction to methsuximide, other medicines, foods, dyes, or preservatives
- pregnant or trying to get pregnant
- breast-feeding

How should I take this medicine?

Take methsuximide capsules by mouth. Follow the directions on the prescription label. Swallow the capsules with a drink of water. If methsuximide upsets your stomach, take it with food or milk. Take your doses at regular intervals. Do not take your medicine more often than directed and do not stop taking it without consulting your health care provider. Stopping this medicine too quickly may cause your seizures to worsen. Contact your pediatrician or health care professional regarding the use of this medicine in children. Special care may be needed.

What if I miss a dose?

If you miss a dose, take it as soon as you can. If it is almost time for your next dose, take only that dose. Do not take double or extra doses.

What may interact with methsuximide?

- alcohol
- evening primrose oil
- lamotrigine
- phenobarbital
- phenytoin or fosphenytoin
- primidone
- valproic acid
- other seizure (convulsion) or epilepsy medicine

Tell your prescriber or health care professional about all other medicines you are taking, including non-prescription medicines, nutritional supplements, or herbal products. Also tell your prescriber or health care professional if you are a frequent user of drinks with caffeine or alcohol, if you smoke, or if you use illegal drugs. These may affect the way your medicine works. Check with your health care professional before stopping or starting any of your medicines.

What should I watch for while taking methsuximide?

Visit your prescriber or health care professional for a regular check on your progress. Do not stop taking methsuximide suddenly because this increases the risk of seizures. Wear a Medic Alert bracelet or necklace. Carry an identification card with information about your condition, medications, and prescriber or health care professional. You may get drowsy, dizzy, or have blurred vision. Do not drive, use machinery, or do anything that needs mental alertness until you know how methsuximide affects you. To reduce dizzy or fainting spells, do not sit or stand up quickly, especially if you are an older patient. Alcohol can increase drowsiness and dizziness. Avoid alcoholic drinks. Promptly report any signs of infection, including fever, sore throat, or swollen glands, to your health care professional. Also report skin rashes, or redness, blistering, peeling or loosening of the skin, including inside the mouth. If you are going to have surgery, tell your prescriber or health care professional that you are taking methsuximide.

What side effects may I notice from taking methsuximide?

Side effects that you should report to your prescriber or health care professional as soon as possible:
- blurred vision
- difficulty speaking
- fever, sore throat, swollen glands
- hallucinations (seeing or hearing things that are not really there)
- mood changes, confusion, nervousness, or hostility
- muscle or bone aches and pain
- redness, blistering, peeling or loosening of the skin, including inside the mouth
- shortness of breath, or wheezing
- skin rash and itching
- swelling or pain around eyes
- unusual bleeding or bruising
- unusual tiredness or weakness

M

Side effects that usually do not require medical attention (report to your prescriber or health care professional if they continue or are bothersome):

- bloating or gas
- clumsiness or unsteadiness
- constipation or diarrhea
- dizziness or drowsiness
- headache
- hiccups
- insomnia
- loss of appetite
- nausea, vomiting
- sensitivity to light
- stomach cramps
- weight loss

Where can I keep my medicine?

Keep out of reach of children in a container that small children cannot open. Store at room temperature below 30 degrees C (86 degrees F). Protect from light and moisture. Throw away any unused medicine after the expiration date.

Methyclothiazide tablets

ENDURON®;
5 mg; Tablet
Abbott
Pharmaceutical
Product Division

ENDURON®;
2.5 mg; Tablet
Abbott
Pharmaceutical
Product Division

What are methyclothiazide tablets?

METHYCLOTHIAZIDE (Enduron®, Aquatensen®) is a diuretic. Diuretics increase the amount of urine passed, which causes the body to lose water and salt. Methyclothiazide helps to treat high blood pressure (hypertension). It is not a cure. This drug also reduces the swelling and water retention caused by various medical conditions, such as heart, liver, or kidney disease. Generic methyclothiazide tablets are available.

What should my health care professional know before I take methyclothiazide?

They need to know if you have any of these conditions:

- diabetes mellitus
- gout
- heart disease
- kidney disease, small amounts of urine, or difficulty passing urine
- liver disease
- pancreatitis
- systemic lupus erythematosus (SLE)
- electrolyte imbalance (e.g. low or high levels of potassium in the blood) if you are on a special diet, such as a low-salt diet (e.g. using potassium substitutes)
- an unusual or allergic reaction to methyclothiazide or other thiazides, sulfonamides, or other medicines, foods, dyes, or preservatives
- pregnant or trying to get pregnant
- breast-feeding

How should I take this medicine?

Take methyclothiazide tablets by mouth. Follow the directions on the prescription label. Swallow the tablets with a drink of water. This medicine can be taken with or without food. Take your doses at regular intervals. Do not take your medicine more often than directed. Remember that you will need to pass urine frequently after taking methyclothiazide. Do not take your doses at a time of day that will cause you problems. Avoid taking this medicine at bedtime. Contact your pediatrician or health care professional regarding the use of this medicine in children. Special care may be needed. Elderly patients over 65 years old may have a stronger reaction to this medicine and may need smaller doses.

What if I miss a dose?

If you miss a dose, take it as soon as you can. If it is almost time for your next dose, take only that dose. Do not take double or extra doses.

What may interact with methyclothiazide?

- allopurinol
- amphotericin B
- anti-inflammatory drugs including NSAIDs (e.g. ibuprofen), aspirin, or salicylates
- barbiturate medicines for inducing sleep or treating seizures (convulsions)
- blood pressure medications
- diabetic medications
- digoxin
- dofetilide
- griseofulvin
- hawthorn or horse chestnut
- hormones such as cortisone, hydrocortisone, prednisone
- lithium
- potassium salts or potassium supplements
- prochlorperazine
- some antibiotics which increase sensitivity to sunlight (sulfonamides, tetracyclines)
- some cholesterol-lowering medications (e.g. cholestyramine or colestipol)
- some medicines for mental disorders (phenothiazines)
- some medications for pain (e.g. codeine, Darvocet®, morphine, Percocet®)
- water pills (especially potassium-sparing diuretics such as triamterene or amiloride)

Tell your prescriber or health care professional about all other medicines you are taking, including non-prescription medicines, nutritional supplements, or herbal products. Also tell your prescriber or health care professional if you are a frequent user of drinks with caffeine

M

or alcohol, if you smoke, or if you use illegal drugs. These may affect the way your medicine works. Check with your health care professional before stopping or starting any of your medicines.

What should I watch for while taking methyclothiazide?

Check your blood pressure regularly while you are taking this medicine. Ask your prescriber or health care professional what your blood pressure should be and when you should contact him or her. When you check your blood pressure, write down the measurements to show your prescriber or health care professional. If you are taking this medicine for a long time you must visit your prescriber or health care professional for regular checks on your progress. Make sure you schedule appointments on a regular basis. Check with your prescriber or health care professional if you get an attack of severe diarrhea, nausea and vomiting, or if you sweat a lot. You must not get dehydrated. Ask your prescriber or health care professional how much fluid you need to drink a day. The loss of too much body fluid can make it dangerous for you to take this medicine. Watch your diet while you are taking methyclothiazide. Ask your prescriber or health care professional about both potassium and sodium intake. Methyclothiazide can make your body lose potassium and you may need an extra supply. Too high or too low potassium can cause problems. Some foods have high potassium content such as bananas, coconuts, dates, figs, prunes, apricots, peaches, grapefruit juice, tomato juice, and orange juice. You may get dizzy. Do not drive, use machinery, or do anything that requires mental alertness until you know how methyclothiazide affects you. To avoid dizzy or fainting spells, do not stand or sit up quickly. Alcohol may increase the possibility of dizziness. Avoid alcoholic drinks until you have discussed their use with your prescriber or health care professional. Methyclothiazide can make your skin more sensitive to sun or ultraviolet light. Keep out of the sun, or wear protective clothing outdoors and use a sunscreen (at least SPF 15). Do not use sun lamps or sun tanning beds or booths. If you are going to have surgery, tell your prescriber or health care professional that you are taking methyclothiazide. Do not treat yourself for a fever or sore throat; check with your prescriber or health care professional first. Methyclothiazide can increase the amount of sugar in blood or urine. If you are a diabetic keep a close check on blood and urine sugar and check with your prescriber or health care professional before changing the dose of your diabetic medicine.

What side effects may I notice from taking methyclothiazide?

Side effects that you should report to your prescriber or health care professional as soon as possible:
Rare or uncommon:
- confusion
- decreased sexual function
- lower back or side pain
- nausea, vomiting
- redness, blistering, peeling or loosening of the skin, including inside the mouth
- severe stomach upset, pain, or cramps
- unusual rash, bleeding or bruising, or pinpoint red spots on the skin
- yellowing of the eyes or skin

More common:
- decreased amount of urine passed
- dizziness, lightheadedness or fainting spells
- fast or uneven heart beat, palpitations, or chest pain
- fever or chills, sore throat
- muscle pain or weakness, cramps
- tingling or numbness in the hands or feet
- unusual tiredness or weakness
- worsened gout pain

Side effects that usually do not require medical attention (report to your prescriber or health care professional if they continue or are bothersome):
- constipation or diarrhea
- headache
- increased sensitivity to the sun
- increased thirst
- loss of appetite
- stomach upset

Where can I keep my medicine?

Keep out of the reach of children in a container that small children cannot open. Store at room temperature between 15 and 30 degrees C (59 and 86 degrees F). Protect from light and moisture. Keep container tightly closed. Throw away any unused medicine after the expiration date.

M

Methyldopa tablets

METHYLDOPA;
250 mg; Tablet
UDL Laboratories
Inc

METHYLDOPA;
500 mg; Tablet
Ivax Pharmaceuticals
Inc

What are methyldopa tablets?

METHYLDOPA (Aldomet®) is an antihypertensive. Methyldopa affects nerve centers in the brain that control blood vessels. As blood vessels relax, methyldopa relieves high blood pressure (hypertension). Methyldopa is not a cure and has to be used regularly. Generic methyldopa tablets are available.

What should my health care professional know before I take methyldopa?

They need to know if you have any of these conditions:
- anemia
- depression or mental disorders
- heart or blood vessel disease
- kidney disease
- liver disease
- Parkinson's disease
- pheochromocytoma
- an unusual or allergic reaction to methyldopa, other medicines, foods, dyes, or preservatives
- pregnant or trying to get pregnant
- breast-feeding

How should I take this medicine?

Take methyldopa tablets by mouth. Follow the directions on the prescription label. Swallow the tablets with a drink of water. Take your doses at regular intervals. Do not take your medicine more often than directed. Do not stop taking except on your prescriber's advice.

What if I miss a dose?

If you miss a dose, take it as soon as you can. If it is almost time for your next dose, take only that dose. Do not take double or extra doses.

What may interact with methyldopa?

- hawthorn
- iron salts
- medicines for colds and breathing difficulties
- medicines for high blood pressure
- medicine for mental depression
- some medications for Parkinson's disease, such as entacapone, levodopa or tolcapone
- tolbutamide
- water pills

Tell your prescriber or health care professional about all other medicines you are taking, including non-prescription medicines, nutritional supplements, or herbal products. Also tell your prescriber or health care professional if you are a frequent user of drinks with caffeine or alcohol, if you smoke, or if you use illegal drugs. These may affect the way your medicine works. Check with your health care professional before stopping or starting any of your medicines.

What should I watch for while taking methyldopa?

Visit your prescriber or health care professional for regular checks on your progress. Check your heart rate and blood pressure regularly while you are taking methyldopa. Ask your prescriber or health care professional what your heart rate should be and when you should contact him or her. If you get a fever, especially in the first few months, call your prescriber or health care professional. Do not treat yourself. You may get drowsy or dizzy. Do not drive, use machinery, or do anything that needs mental alertness until you know how methyldopa affects you. To avoid dizzy or fainting spells, do not stand or sit up quickly, especially if you are an older person. Alcohol can make you more drowsy and dizzy. Avoid alcoholic drinks. Your mouth may get dry. Chewing sugarless gum or sucking hard candy, and drinking plenty of water will help. Iron can stop the absorption of methyldopa. Do not take methyldopa with iron preparations or multiple vitamins containing iron. If you have to take iron, make sure that there are at least 2 hours between iron and methyldopa doses.

What side effects may I notice from taking methyldopa?

Side effects that you should report to your prescriber or health care professional as soon as possible:
- chest pain
- black, sore tongue
- dark yellow or brown urine
- depression
- difficulty sleeping, nightmares
- fever (usually within the first 3 months of treatment)
- slow heartbeat
- stomach pain
- swelling of the feet or legs
- unusual weakness or tiredness
- yellowing of the eyes or skin

Side effects that usually do not require medical attention (report to your prescriber or health care professional if they continue or are bothersome):
- breast enlargement (men or women)
- diarrhea
- dizziness or lightheadedness
- drowsiness
- dry mouth
- headache
- menstrual irregularity

M

- nausea, vomiting
- numbness or tingling in hands or feet
- sexual difficulties (decreased sexual desire or impotence)
- skin rash
- stuffy nose
- unusual breast milk production

Where can I keep my medicine?

Keep out of the reach of children in a container that small children cannot open. Store at room temperature between 15 and 30 degrees C (59 and 86 degrees F). Keep container tightly closed. Throw away any unused medicine after the expiration date.

Methylergonovine tablets

METHERGINE®;
0.2 mg; Tablet
Novartis Pharmaceuticals

What are methylergonovine tablets?

METHYLERGONOVINE (Methergine®) belongs to a group of medicines known as ergot alkaloids. Methylergonovine is often used to stop excessive bleeding that occurs in females after childbirth or following an abortion or miscarriage. Generic methylergonovine tablets are not available.

What should my health care professional know before I take methylergonovine?

They need to know if you have any of these conditions:
- blood clots
- chest pain
- history of heart attacks
- heart or blood vessel disease
- high blood pressure
- high cholesterol
- infection
- kidney disease
- liver disease
- lung disease
- poor circulation
- stroke
- tobacco smoker
- an unusual or allergic reaction to methylergonovine, other medicines, foods, dyes, or preservatives
- pregnant or trying to get pregnant
- breast-feeding (this medicine may be used with care for up to 7 days without interfering with breast-feeding)

How should I take this medicine?

Take methylergonovine tablets by mouth. Follow the directions on the prescription label. Swallow the tablets whole with a glass of water. Do not take your medicine more often than directed. Do not stop taking except on your prescriber's advice. Contact your pediatrician or health care professional regarding the use of this medicine in children. Special care may be needed.

What if I miss a dose?

Do not take the missed dose. Take only the next dose according to your normal schedule. Do not take double or extra doses. Do not take this medicine for longer than it is prescribed.

What may interact with methylergonovine?

Do not use any of the following migraine drugs within 24 hours of this medicine:
- almotriptan
- eletriptan
- frovatriptan
- naratriptan
- rizatriptan
- sumatriptan
- zolmitriptan

Also, do not use this drug with:
- caffeine-ergotamine (example: Cafergot® or Wigraine®)
- dihydroergotamine (DHE® or Migranal®)
- ergonovine
- ergotamine (example: Ergomar®) or methysergide (Sansert®)

Methylergonovine may also interact with:
- aprepitant
- bromocriptine
- cabergoline
- clarithromycin
- cocaine
- danazol
- ergoloid mesylates (Hydergine®)
- erythromycin
- fluoxetine
- fluvoxamine
- grapefruit juice
- herbal products like feverfew
- imatinib, STI-571
- medicines for colds, flu, or breathing difficulties
- medicines for fungal infections (examples: fluconazole, itraconazole, ketoconazole, voriconazole)
- medicines or herbal products to decrease weight or appetite
- metronidazole
- nefazodone
- nicotine
- some medicines for high blood pressure or chest pain
- some medications for the treatment of HIV infection or AIDS
- troleandomycin
- zileuton

Tell your prescriber or health care professional about all other medicines you are taking, including non-prescription medicines, nutritional supplements, or herbal products. Also tell your prescriber or health care professional if you are a frequent user of drinks with caffeine or alcohol, if you smoke, or if you use illegal drugs. These may affect the way your medicine works. Check with your health care professional before stopping or starting any of your medicines.

What should I watch for while taking methylergonovine?

Follow your prescriber's instructions for how to take this medicine and what to watch for. You will need a follow-up appointment for an exam within a few days. Take it easy if you are not feeling well. If you are female, do not put anything in your vagina: no tampons, no sex, and no douching until the bleeding has stopped and your prescriber allows return to normal activities. Follow your prescriber's directions for your condition, you may need to notify them of any of the following: bleeding increases (example: using more than one pad per hour for 3 to 4 hours); fever > 100 degrees F (38 degrees C) or chills; passing tissue or large clots (save any tissue that you pass for exam by your prescriber); severe abdominal pain or cramping. Do not take any other medicines without talking to your health care professional first. If you are going to have any type of surgery, tell your prescriber or health care professional that you are taking methylergonovine.

What side effects may I notice from taking methylergonovine?

Side effects that you should report to your prescriber or health care professional as soon as possible:

Rare:

- abdominal pain or cramping
- blurred vision
- chest pain or tightness
- cold hands or feet
- confusion
- decrease in the amount of urine passed
- difficulty breathing
- fast, slow, or pounding heartbeat
- hearing or seeing things that are not really there
- itching
- leg or arm pain or cramps
- seizures
- severe, sudden headache
- swelling of hands, ankles, or feet
- tingling, pain or numbness in feet or hands
- vomiting
- weakness

Side effects that usually do not require medical attention (report to your prescriber or health care professional if they continue or are bothersome):

- change in taste
- diarrhea
- mild headache
- nausea or mild vomiting
- temporary ringing of ears

Where can I keep my medicine?

Keep out of the reach of children in a container that small children cannot open. Store tablets at room temperature, in a cool place away from exposure to heat, light or moisture. Throw away any unused medicine after the expiration date. Keep container tightly closed.

Methylphenidate extended-release tablets or capsules

RITALIN® LA; 20 mg; Capsule, Extended Release Novartis Pharmaceuticals		CONCERTA®; 36 mg; Tablet, Extended Release McNeil Consumer and Specialty Pharmaceuticals	

What are methylphenidate extended-release tablets or capsules?

METHYLPHENIDATE (Metadate® ER, Ritalin®-SR or the once-daily brands, Concerta®, Metadate® CD, Ritalin® LA) is a stimulant. It can improve attention span, concentration, and emotional control, and reduce restless or overactive behavior. This medicine treats attention-deficit hyperactivity disorder (ADHD). It can also help a condition called narcolepsy, an illness that makes it difficult to stay awake during normal daytime hours. Federal law prohibits the transfer of methylphenidate to any person other than the person for whom it was prescribed. Do not share this medicine with anyone else. Generic methylphenidate extended-release tablets or capsules may or may not be available, depending on the product you are taking.

What should my health care professional know before I take methylphenidate?

They need to know if you have any of these conditions:

- regularly drink beverages containing alcohol
- a history of drug abuse
- difficulty swallowing, problems with the esophagus (tube connecting mouth to stomach), or a history of blockage of the stomach or intestines
- glaucoma
- heart failure or other heart disease
- heart rhythm disturbance
- history of recent heart attack
- high blood pressure

M

- liver disease
- mental illness, including anxiety, bipolar disorder, depression, mania or schizophrenia
- overactive thyroid
- seizures (convulsions)
- Tourette's syndrome (speech repetition or involuntary use of obscene language)
- an unusual or allergic reaction to methylphenidate, other medicines, foods, dyes, or preservatives
- pregnant or trying to get pregnant
- breast-feeding

How should I take this medicine?

Take methylphenidate extended-release tablets or capsules by mouth. Follow the directions on the prescription label. Swallow whole with a drink of water or juice; do not crush, cut, or chew. You may take this medicine with food. Take your doses at regular intervals. Usually the last dose of the day will be taken at least 8 hours before your normal bedtime, so it will not interfere with sleep. Some brands (Concerta®, Metadate® CD, Ritalin® LA) are taken just once-daily, in the morning. Do not take your medicine more often than directed. If swallowing a Metadate® CD or Ritalin® LA capsule is difficult, this capsule may be opened and the dose gently sprinkled on a small amount (1 tablespoon) of cool applesauce. (Do not sprinkle on warm applesauce or this may result in improper dosing.) The sprinkles should not be crushed or chewed. Take the medicine immediately after sprinkling (do not store for future use). Drink some fluids (water, milk or juice) after taking the sprinkles with applesauce. Contact your pediatrician or health care professional regarding the use of this medicine in children. Special care may be needed. This medicine is commonly prescribed for children ≥ 6 years old.

What if I miss a dose?

If it is almost time for your next dose, take only that dose. Do not take double or extra doses.

What may interact with methylphenidate?

- antacids
- amphetamine or dextroamphetamine
- bretylium
- caffeine
- carbamazepine
- clonidine
- dexmethylphenidate
- furazolidone
- guarana
- linezolid
- lithium
- medicines for colds, sinus, and breathing difficulties
- medicines for high blood pressure
- medicines called MAO inhibitors- examples: phenelzine (Nardil®), tranylcypromine (Parnate®), isocarboxazid (Marplan®)
- other medicines for mental depression or anxiety
- medicines for mental problems and psychotic disturbances
- medicines to decrease appetite or cause weight loss
- modafinil
- pemoline
- procarbazine
- seizure (convulsion) or epilepsy medicine
- warfarin
- water pills

Tell your prescriber or health care professional about all other medicines you are taking, including non-prescription medicines, nutritional supplements, or herbal products. Also tell your prescriber or health care professional if you are a frequent user of drinks with caffeine or alcohol, if you smoke, or if you use illegal drugs. These may affect the way your medicine works. Check with your health care professional before stopping or starting any of your medicines.

What should I watch for while taking methylphenidate?

Visit your prescriber or health care professional for regular checks on your progress. This prescription requires that you follow special procedures with your prescriber and pharmacy; you will need to have a new written prescription from your prescriber every time you need a refill. Methylphenidate may affect your concentration, or hide signs of tiredness. Until you know how this drug affects you, do not drive, ride a bicycle, use machinery, or do anything that needs mental alertness. Tell your prescriber or health care professional if this medicine loses its effects, or if you feel you need to take more than the prescribed amount. Do not change the dosage without advice from your prescriber or health care professional. Ask your prescriber or health care professional for advice. Decreased appetite is a common side effect when starting this medicine. Eating small, frequent meals or snacks can help. Talk to your prescriber if you continue to have poor eating habits. Height and weight growth of a child taking this medication will be monitored closely. If you are going to have surgery or other medical procedures, tell your health care professional that you are taking methylphenidate. If you are taking the Concerta® tablets, you may notice the tablet shell in your stool. This is normal.

What side effects may I notice from taking methylphenidate?

Side effects that you should report to your prescriber or health care professional as soon as possible:
- anxiety or severe nervousness
- bruising
- changes in mood or behavior, including seeing or hearing things that are not really there or over-focused, staring-type behavior
- chest pain, fast or irregular heartbeat (palpitations)
- fever, or hot, dry skin
- increased blood pressure
- joint pain
- skin rash, itching

M

- uncontrollable head, mouth, neck, arm, or leg movements

Side effects that usually do not require medical attention (report to your prescriber or health care professional if they continue or are bothersome):
Less common or rare:
- a sense of well being
- blurred vision
- dizziness or lightheadedness
- stomach cramps

More common, especially in the first few weeks of treatment:

- decreased appetite or loss of appetite
- headache
- mild stomach upset
- nervousness, restlessness, or difficulty sleeping
- weight loss

Where can I keep my medicine?

Keep out of the reach of children in a container that small children cannot open. Store at room temperature below 30 degrees C (86 degrees F). Protect from light and moisture. Keep container tightly closed. Throw away any unused medicine after the expiration date.

Methylphenidate tablets

RITALIN®; 5 mg; Tablet Novartis Pharmaceuticals Corp Dba Ciba Pharmaceuticals Co

METHYLIN®; 10 mg; Tablet Mallinckrodt Inc Pharmaceuticals Group

What are methylphenidate tablets?

METHYLPHENIDATE (Methylin®, Ritalin®) is a stimulant. It can improve attention span, concentration, and emotional control, and reduce restless or overactive behavior. This medicine treats attention-deficit hyperactivity disorder (ADHD). It can also help a condition called narcolepsy, an illness that makes it difficult to stay awake during normal daytime hours. Federal law prohibits the transfer of methylphenidate to any person other than the person for whom it was prescribed. Do not share this medicine with anyone else. Generic methylphenidate tablets are available.

What should my health care professional know before I take methylphenidate?

They need to know if you have any of these conditions:
- regularly drink beverages containing alcohol
- a history of drug abuse
- glaucoma
- heart failure or other heart disease
- heart rhythm disturbance
- history of recent heart attack
- high blood pressure
- liver disease
- mental illness, including anxiety, bipolar disorder, depression, mania or schizophrenia
- overactive thyroid
- seizures (convulsions)
- Tourette's syndrome (speech repetition or involuntary use of obscene language)
- an unusual or allergic reaction to methylphenidate, other medicines, foods, dyes, or preservatives
- pregnant or trying to get pregnant
- breast-feeding

How should I take this medicine?

Take methylphenidate tablets by mouth. Follow the directions on the prescription label. Swallow the tablets with a drink of water. It is best to take methylphenidate 30 to 45 minutes before meals, unless directed otherwise by your prescriber or health care professional.

Take your doses at regular intervals. Usually the last dose of the day will be taken at least 4 to 6 hours before your normal bedtime, so it will not interfere with sleep. Do not take your medicine more often than directed. Contact your pediatrician or health care professional regarding the use of this medicine in children. Special care may be needed. This medicine is commonly prescribed for children ≥ 6 years old.

What if I miss a dose?

If you miss a dose, take it as soon as you can. If it is almost time for your next dose, take only that dose. Do not take double or extra doses.

What may interact with methylphenidate?

- amphetamine or dextroamphetamine
- bretylium
- caffeine
- carbamazepine
- clonidine
- dexmethylphenidate
- furazolidone
- guarana
- linezolid
- lithium
- medicines for colds, sinus, and breathing difficulties
- medicines for high blood pressure
- medicines called MAO inhibitors- examples: phenelzine (Nardil®), tranylcypromine (Parnate®), isocarboxazid (Marplan®)
- other medicines for mental depression or anxiety
- medicines for mental problems and psychotic disturbances
- medicines to decrease appetite or cause weight loss
- modafinil
- pemoline
- procarbazine
- seizure (convulsion) or epilepsy medicine
- warfarin
- water pills

M

Tell your prescriber or health care professional about all other medicines you are taking, including non-prescription medicines, nutritional supplements, or herbal products. Also tell your prescriber or health care professional if you are a frequent user of drinks with caffeine or alcohol, if you smoke, or if you use illegal drugs. These may affect the way your medicine works. Check with your health care professional before stopping or starting any of your medicines.

What should I watch for while taking methylphenidate?

Visit your prescriber or health care professional for regular checks on your progress. This prescription requires that you follow special procedures with your prescriber and pharmacy; you will need to have a new written prescription from your prescriber every time you need a refill. Methylphenidate may affect your concentration, or hide signs of tiredness. Until you know how this drug affects you, do not drive, ride a bicycle, use machinery, or do anything that needs mental alertness. Tell your prescriber or health care professional if this medicine loses its effects, or if you feel you need to take more than the prescribed amount. Do not change the dosage without advice from your prescriber or health care professional. Ask your prescriber or health care professional for advice. Decreased appetite is a common side effect when starting this medicine. Eating small, frequent meals or snacks can help. Talk to your prescriber if you continue to have poor eating habits. Height and weight growth of a child taking this medication will be monitored closely. If you are going to have surgery or other medical procedures, tell your health care professional that you are taking methylphenidate.

What side effects may I notice from taking methylphenidate?

Side effects that you should report to your prescriber or health care professional as soon as possible:
- anxiety or severe nervousness
- bruising
- changes in mood or behavior, including seeing or hearing things that are not really there or over-focused, staring-type behavior
- chest pain, fast or irregular heartbeat (palpitations)
- fever, or hot, dry skin
- increased blood pressure
- joint pain
- skin rash, itching
- uncontrollable head, mouth, neck, arm, or leg movements

Side effects that usually do not require medical attention (report to your prescriber or health care professional if they continue or are bothersome):
Less common or rare:
- a sense of well being
- blurred vision
- dizziness or lightheadedness
- stomach cramps

More common, especially in the first few weeks of treatment:
- decreased appetite or loss of appetite
- headache
- mild stomach upset
- nervousness, restlessness, or difficulty sleeping
- weight loss

Where can I keep my medicine?

Keep out of the reach of children in a container that small children cannot open. Store at room temperature below 30 degrees C (86 degrees F). Protect from light and moisture. Keep container tightly closed. Throw away any unused medicine after the expiration date.

Methylprednisolone tablets

METHYL-PREDNISOLONE;
4 mg; Tablet
Watson
Pharmaceuticals Inc

METHYL-PREDNISOLONE;
4 mg; Tablet
Qualitest
Pharmaceuticals Inc

What are methylprednisolone tablets?

METHYLPREDNISOLONE (Medrol®, Meprolone®) is a corticosteroid. It helps to reduce swelling, redness, itching, and allergic reactions and can be used to treat severe allergies, skin problems, asthma, arthritis and other conditions. Methylprednisolone is used in the treatment of multiple sclerosis. Generic methylprednisolone tablets are available.

What should my health care professional know before I take methylprednisolone?

They need to know if you have any of these conditions:
- cataracts or glaucoma
- Cushing's syndrome
- heart problems, or previous heart attack
- high blood pressure or blood clotting disorder
- infection, such as herpes, measles, tuberculosis or chickenpox
- myasthenia gravis
- psychosis
- osteoporosis
- recent surgery
- seizures (convulsions)
- stomach or intestinal disease, including colitis
- under-active thyroid
- an unusual or allergic reaction to methylprednisolone, other corticosteroids, medicines, foods, dyes, or preservatives

M

- pregnant or trying to get pregnant
- breast-feeding

How should I take this medicine?

Take methylprednisolone tablets by mouth. Follow the directions on the prescription label. Swallow the tablets with a drink of water. Take with food or milk to avoid stomach upset. If you are only taking methylprednisolone once a day, take it in the morning, which is the time your body normally secretes cortisol. Take your doses at regular intervals. Do not take your medicine more often than directed. Contact your pediatrician or health care professional regarding the use of this medicine in children. Special care may be needed.

What if I miss a dose?

If you miss a dose, take it a soon as you can. If it is almost time for your next dose, consult your prescriber or health care professional. You may need to miss a dose or take a double dose, depending on your condition and treatment. Do not take double or extra doses without advice.

What may interact with methylprednisolone?

- acetazolamide
- anti-inflammatory drugs (NSAIDs, such as ibuprofen)
- barbiturate medicines for inducing sleep or treating seizures
- bosentan
- certain heart medicines
- erythromycin
- female hormones, including contraceptives or birth control pills
- grapefruit juice
- itraconazole
- live virus vaccines, and other toxoids and vaccines
- medicines for diabetes
- phenytoin
- rifabutin
- rifampin
- troleandomycin
- voriconazole
- water pills
- warfarin

Tell your prescriber or health care professional about all other medicines you are taking, including non-prescription medicines, nutritional supplements, or herbal products. Also tell your prescriber or health care professional if you are a frequent user of drinks with caffeine or alcohol, if you smoke, or if you use illegal drugs. These may affect the way your medicine works. Check with your health care professional before stopping or starting any of your medicines.

What should I watch for while taking methylprednisolone?

Visit your prescriber or health care professional for regular checks on your progress. If you are taking methylprednisolone over a prolonged period, carry an identification card with your name and address, the type and dose of your medicine, and your prescriber's name and address. If you are taking methylprednisolone regularly, avoid contact with people who have an infection. You will have an increased risk from infection while taking methylprednisolone. Tell your prescriber or health care professional if you are exposed to anyone with measles or chickenpox, or if you develop sores or blisters that do not heal properly. People who are taking certain dosages of methylprednisolone may need to avoid immunization with certain vaccines or may need to have changes in their vaccination schedules to ensure adequate protection from certain diseases. Make sure to tell your prescriber or health care professional that you are taking methylprednisolone before receiving any vaccine. If you are going to have surgery, tell your prescriber or health care professional that you are taking methylprednisolone. If you receive methylprednisolone every day, you may need to watch your diet. Your body can lose potassium while you are taking this medicine. Ask your prescriber or health care professional about your diet. Methylprednisolone can affect your blood sugar. If you are diabetic check with your prescriber or health care professional if you need help adjusting the dose of your diabetic medicine. Alcohol can increase the risk of getting serious side effects while you are taking methylprednisolone. Avoid alcoholic drinks. Methylprednisolone can interfere with certain lab tests and can cause false skin test results.

What side effects may I notice from taking methylprednisolone?

Side effects that you should report to your prescriber or health care professional as soon as possible:

- bloody or black, tarry stools
- confusion, excitement, restlessness, a false sense of well-being
- eye pain, decreased or blurred vision, or bulging eyes
- fever, sore throat, sneezing, cough, or other signs of infection, wounds that will not heal
- frequent passing of urine
- increased thirst
- irregular heartbeat
- menstrual problems
- mental depression, mood swings, mistaken feelings of self-importance or of being mistreated
- muscle cramps or weakness
- nausea, vomiting
- pain in hips, back, ribs, arms, shoulders, or legs
- rounding out of face
- skin problems, acne, thin and shiny skin
- stomach pain
- swelling of feet or lower legs
- unusual bruising, pinpoint red spots on the skin
- unusual tiredness or weakness
- weight gain or weight loss

Side effects that usually do not require medical attention (report to your prescriber or health care professional if they continue or are bothersome):

- diarrhea or constipation
- headache

M

- increased or decreased appetite
- increased sweating
- nervousness, restlessness, or difficulty sleeping
- upset stomach
- unusual increased growth of hair on the face or body

Methyltestosterone tablets, capsules, or buccal tablets

ANDROID®;
10 mg; Capsule
Valeant
Pharmaceuticals

METHITEST®;
25 mg; Tablet
Global
Pharmaceuticals Div
of Impax Labs., Inc.

What are methyltestosterone tablets or capsules?

METHYLTESTOSTERONE (Android-10®, Testred®, Virilon®, Methitest®) is a synthetic (manmade) androgen or male reproductive (sex) hormone. Normal male sexual development—including the sex organs, increases in muscle mass, facial hair, and deep voice—depends on natural androgens. Methyltestosterone replaces natural hormone in men with low testosterone (androgen) production, underdeveloped testes, and/or impotence. Methyltestosterone can help to stimulate delayed puberty and help to treat certain breast cancers in women. Generic methyltestosterone tablets are available, but not generic capsules.

What should my health care professional know before I take methyltestosterone?

They need to know if you have any of these conditions:
- breast cancer
- diabetes
- heart or blood vessel disease
- high blood calcium levels
- kidney disease
- liver disease
- previous heart attack
- prostate trouble
- pregnant or trying to get pregnant
- breast-feeding
- an unusual or allergic reaction to methyltestosterone, tartrazine dye, other medicines, foods, dyes, or preservatives

How should I take this medicine?

Take methyltestosterone tablets or capsules by mouth. Follow the directions on the prescription label. Take your doses at regular intervals. Do not take your medicine more often than directed.
Tablets and capsules:
Swallow the tablets or capsules with a drink of water. It is best to take the tablets or capsules with food.
Buccal tablets:
Place a methyltestosterone buccal tablet under the upper lip against the gum, or between the cheek and the gum. Follow the directions on the prescription label. Let the tablet dissolve slowly; do not swallow whole. Try not to touch the tablet with your tongue, or drink hot liquid, as this will increase the rate at which the tablet dissolves. Do not chew tobacco while

a tablet is dissolving. Contact your pediatrician or health care professional regarding the use of this medicine in children. Special care may be needed.

Where can I keep my medicine?

Keep out of the reach of children. Store at room temperature between 15 and 30 degrees C (59 and 86 degrees F). Throw away any unused medicine after the expiration date.

What if I miss a dose?

If you miss a dose, take it as soon as you can. If it is almost time for your next dose, take only that dose. Do not take double or extra doses.

What may interact with methyltestosterone?

- blood thinners
- cyclosporine
- growth hormone
- imipramine

Tell your prescriber or health care professional about all other medicines you are taking, including non-prescription medicines, nutritional supplements, or herbal products. Also tell your prescriber or health care professional if you are a frequent user of drinks with caffeine or alcohol, if you smoke, or if you use illegal drugs. These may affect the way your medicine works. Check with your health care professional before stopping or starting any of your medicines.

What should I watch for while taking methyltestosterone?

If you are diabetic, methyltestosterone may affect your blood sugar. Check with your prescriber or health care professional before you change your diet or the dose of your diabetic medicine. Methyltestosterone is banned from use in athletes by the U.S. Olympic Committee and other athletic organizations.

What side effects may I notice from taking methyltestosterone?

Side effects that you should report to your prescriber or health care professional as soon as possible:
- anxiety, depression
- black, tarry stools or light-colored stools
- dark yellow or brown urine
- hair loss
- nausea, vomiting
- skin rash and itching (hives)
- stomach pain
- unusual bleeding
- unusual swelling
- weight gain
- yellowing of the eyes or skin

M

Additional side effects that can occur primarily in men include:

- breast tenderness or enlargement
- frequent erections
- frequent or difficult passing of urine
- groin or scrotum pain

Additional side effects that can occur primarily in women include:

- irregular vaginal bleeding/spotting
- decrease in breast size
- enlarged clitoris
- facial hair growth
- voice changes (deepening or hoarseness)

Side effects that usually do not require medical attention (report to your prescriber or health care professional if they continue or are bothersome):

- acne
- headache
- sexual difficulties; changes in sexual desire can occur in either male or female patients, and excessive doses can cause impotence in men

Where can I keep my medicine?

Keep out of the reach of children in a container that small children cannot open. Store at room temperature between 15 and 30 degrees C (59 and 86 degrees F). Keep container tightly closed.

Metoclopramide tablets

REGLAN®;
5 mg; Tablet
Richmond Div
Wyeth

REGLAN®;
10 mg; Tablet
Richmond Div
Wyeth

What are metoclopramide tablets?

METOCLOPRAMIDE (Reglan®) has a number of uses. Metoclopramide increases the movements of the stomach and intestines. It can help treat heartburn in patients who suffer from a backward flow of stomach acid into the esophagus, often called "GERD." It is also used for diabetic gastroparesis, a condition in some diabetics that causes discomfort, heartburn, nausea, and a feeling of fullness after meals. It can also be used for other purposes, like hiccups. Generic metoclopramide tablets are available.

What should my health care professional know before I take metoclopramide?

They need to know if you have any of these conditions:

- asthma
- breast cancer
- depression
- G6PD deficiency
- high blood pressure
- kidney disease
- methemoglobin reductase deficiency
- Parkinson's disease or a movement disorder
- pheochromocytoma
- seizures (convulsions)
- stomach obstruction, bleeding, or perforation
- an unusual or allergic reaction to metoclopramide, procainamide, sulfites, other medicines, foods, dyes, or preservatives
- pregnant or trying to get pregnant
- breast-feeding

How should I take this medicine?

Take metoclopramide tablets by mouth. Follow the directions on the prescription label. Swallow the tablets with a drink of water. Take metoclopramide on an empty stomach, about 30 minutes before eating. Take your doses at regular intervals. Do not take your medicine more often than directed. Contact your pediatri-

cian or health care professional regarding the use of this medicine in children. Special care may be needed.

What if I miss a dose?

If you miss a dose, take it as soon as you can. If it is almost time for your next dose, take only that dose. Do not take double or extra doses.

What may interact with metoclopramide?

- alcohol
- bromocriptine
- cyclosporine
- digoxin
- medicines for diabetes, including insulin
- medicines that treat diarrhea
- medicines for hay fever and other allergies
- medicines for mental depression
- medicines for mental problems or psychotic disturbances
- medicines for Parkinson's disease, like levodopa
- medicines for sleep or for pain

Tell your prescriber or health care professional about all other medicines you are taking, including non-prescription medicines, nutritional supplements, or herbal products. Also tell your prescriber or health care professional if you are a frequent user of drinks with caffeine or alcohol, if you smoke, or if you use illegal drugs. These may affect the way your medicine works. Check with your health care professional before stopping or starting any of your medicines.

What should I watch for while taking metoclopramide?

It may take a few weeks for your stomach condition to improve on this medicine. You may get drowsy or dizzy. Do not drive, use machinery, or do anything that needs mental alertness until you know how metoclopramide affects you. Alcohol can increase drowsiness or dizziness; avoid alcoholic drinks. If you are going to have

M

surgery, tell your prescriber or health care professional that you are taking metoclopramide.

What side effects may I notice from taking metoclopramide?

Serious or limiting side effects are uncommon, but may include:

- breast enlargement in men or women, or production of breast-milk in women who are not breast-feeding
- change in the way you walk (shuffling feet)
- difficulty moving, speaking or swallowing
- drooling, lip smacking, or rapid movements of the tongue
- involuntary or uncontrollable movements of the eyes, head, arms and legs
- irregular heartbeat or palpitations
- muscle twitches and spasms
- skin rash
- unusual tiredness or weakness

Side effects that usually do not require medical attention (report to your prescriber or health care professional if they continue or are bothersome):

- depression
- diarrhea
- difficulty sleeping
- dizziness
- drowsiness
- headache
- menstrual changes
- restlessness or nervousness
- sexual difficulties (decreased sexual desire or impotence)

Where can I keep my medicine?

Keep out of the reach of children in a container that small children cannot open. Store at room temperature between 15 and 30 degrees C (59 and 86 degrees F). Throw away any unused medicine after the expiration date.

Metolazone extended-release tablets

ZAROXOLYN®;
5 mg; Tablet
Celltech
Pharmaceuticals, Inc

ZAROXOLYN®;
10 mg; Tablet
Celltech
Pharmaceuticals, Inc

What are metolazone extended-release tablets?

METOLAZONE (Zaroxolyn®) is a diuretic. Diuretics increase the amount of urine passed, which causes the body to lose water and salt. Metolazone helps to treat high blood pressure (hypertension). It is not a cure. It also reduces the swelling and water retention caused by various medical conditions, such as heart, liver, or kidney disease. Generic metolazone tablets are available.

What should my health care professional know before I take metolazone?

They need to know if you have any of these conditions:

- diabetes
- gout
- high levels of blood calcium
- kidney disease
- liver disease
- pancreatitis
- systemic lupus erythematosus (SLE)
- an unusual or allergic reaction to metolazone, carbonic anhydrase inhibitors like acetazolamide, sulfa drugs, other medicines, foods, dyes, or preservatives
- pregnant or trying to get pregnant
- breast-feeding

How should I take this medicine?

Take metolazone extended-release tablets by mouth. Follow the directions on the prescription label. Swallow the tablets whole with a drink of water; do not crush or chew. Take your doses at regular intervals.

Do not take your medicine more often than directed. Remember that you will need to pass urine frequently after taking metolazone. Do not take your doses at a time of day that will cause you problems. Do not take at bedtime. Contact your pediatrician or health care professional regarding the use of this medicine in children. Special care may be needed.

What if I miss a dose?

If you miss a dose, take it as soon as you can. If it is almost time for your next dose, take only that dose. Do not take double or extra doses.

What may interact with metolazone?

- amphotericin B
- anti-inflammatory drugs (NSAIDs, such as ibuprofen)
- cisplatin
- dofetilide
- heart medicines such as digoxin
- hormones such as cortisone, fludrocortisone, hydrocortisone, prednisone
- lithium
- medicines for high blood pressure
- medicines for colds and breathing difficulties
- medicines for diabetes
- medicines that relax muscles for surgery
- probenecid
- water pills

Tell your prescriber or health care professional about all other medicines you are taking, including non-prescription medicines, nutritional supplements, or herbal

products. Also tell your prescriber or health care professional if you are a frequent user of drinks with caffeine or alcohol, if you smoke, or if you use illegal drugs. These may affect the way your medicine works. Check with your health care professional before stopping or starting any of your medicines.

What should I watch for while taking metolazone?

Visit your prescriber or health care professional for regular checks on your progress. Check your blood pressure regularly. Ask your prescriber or health care professional what your blood pressure should be, and when you should contact him or her. You must not get dehydrated; ask your prescriber or health care professional how much fluid you need to drink a day. Do not stop taking metolazone except on your prescriber's advice. There are different brands of metolazone. They are not the same and you must not change your regular brand without your prescriber's advice. Watch your diet while you are taking metolazone. Ask your prescriber or health care professional about both potassium and sodium intake. Metolazone can make your body lose potassium and you may need an extra supply. Too high or too low potassium can cause problems. Some foods have a high potassium content such as bananas, coconuts, dates, figs, prunes, apricots, peaches, grapefruit juice, tomato juice, and orange juice. You may get dizzy or lightheaded. Do not drive, use machinery, or do anything that needs mental alertness until you know how metolazone affects you. To reduce the risk of dizzy or fainting spells, do not sit or stand up quickly, especially if you are an older patient. Alcohol can make you lightheaded, dizzy and increase confusion. Avoid or limit intake of alcoholic drinks. Metolazone may make your skin more sensitive to sun or ultraviolet light. Keep out of the sun, or wear protective clothing outdoors and use a sunscreen (at least SPF 15). Do not use sun lamps or sun tanning beds or booths. If you are going to have surgery, tell your prescriber or health care professional that you are taking metolazone. Metolazone can increase the amount of sugar in blood or urine. If you are a diabetic keep a close check on blood and urine sugar.

What side effects may I notice from taking metolazone?

Side effects that you should report to your prescriber or health care professional as soon as possible:
Rare or uncommon:
- change in your vision (such as blurred vision)
- chest pain, irregular heartbeat (palpitations)
- lower back or side pain
- numbness or tingling in the hands or feet
- redness, blistering, peeling or loosening of the skin, including inside the mouth
- severe stomach upset, pain, or cramps
- unusual rash, bleeding or bruising, or pinpoint red spots on the skin
- unusual tiredness or weakness
- yellowing of the eyes or skin

More common:
- cough or hoarseness
- dizziness, fainting spells, or lightheadedness
- fever or chills
- increased thirst which does not go away
- joint pain, or muscle pain, cramps
- mood changes
- mouth sores
- nausea, vomiting
- pain or difficulty passing urine

Side effects that usually do not require medical attention (report to your prescriber or health care professional if they continue or are bothersome):
- constipation or diarrhea
- decreased sexual ability
- dry mouth
- increased sensitivity to the sun
- loss of appetite
- upset stomach

Where can I keep my medicine?

Keep out of the reach of children in a container that small children cannot open. Store at room temperature, between 15 and 30 degrees C (59 and 86 degrees F). Protect from light. Keep container tightly closed. Throw away any unused medicine after the expiration date.

M

Metoprolol tablets or extended-release tablets

LOPRESSOR®;
100 mg; Tablet
Novartis
Pharmaceuticals

TOPROL XL®;
100 mg; Tablet,
Extended Release
AstraZeneca LP

What are metoprolol tablets or extended-release tablets?

METOPROLOL (Lopressor®, Toprol XL®) belongs to a group of medicines called beta-blockers. Beta-blockers reduce the workload on the heart and help it to beat more regularly. Metoprolol controls, but does not cure, high blood pressure (hypertension). High blood pressure may not make you feel sick, but it can lead to serious heart problems. Metoprolol also relieves chest pain (angina) and can be helpful after a heart attack. Metoprolol is also used to improve symptoms in patients with other types of heart disease. Generic metoprolol tablets are available, but not extended-release tablets.

What should my health care professional know before I take metoprolol?

They need to know if you have any of these conditions:
- angina (chest pain)
- asthma, bronchitis or bronchospasm
- circulation problems, or blood vessel disease (such as Raynaud's disease)
- depression
- diabetes
- emphysema, or other lung disease
- history of heart attack or heart disease
- liver disease
- muscle weakness or disease
- pheochromocytoma
- psoriasis
- thyroid disease
- an unusual or allergic reaction to metoprolol, other beta-blockers, medicines, foods, dyes, or preservatives
- pregnant or trying to get pregnant
- breast-feeding

How should I take this medicine?

Take metoprolol tablets by mouth. Follow the directions on the prescription label. Swallow the tablets with a drink of water. Do not crush or chew extended-release tablets. Take tablets with or immediately after meals. Take your doses at regular intervals. Do not take your medicine more often than directed. Do not stop taking except on your prescriber's advice. Contact your pediatrician or health care professional regarding the use of this medicine in children. Special care may be needed.

What if I miss a dose?

If you miss a dose, take it as soon as you can. If it is almost time for your next dose, take only that dose. Do not take double or extra doses. There should be at least 4 hours between doses (or 8 hours if taking extended-release products).

What may interact with metoprolol?

- anti-inflammatory drugs (NSAIDs, such as ibuprofen)
- cimetidine
- cocaine
- fluoxetine
- hawthorn
- medicines for colds and breathing difficulties
- medicines for diabetes
- medicines for high blood pressure
- medicines to control heart rhythm
- medicines for malaria
- rifampin
- water pills

Tell your prescriber or health care professional about all other medicines you are taking, including non-prescription medicines, nutritional supplements, or herbal products. Also tell your prescriber or health care professional if you are a frequent user of drinks with caffeine or alcohol, if you smoke, or if you use illegal drugs. These may affect the way your medicine works. Check with your health care professional before stopping or starting any of your medicines.

What should I watch for while taking metoprolol?

Check your heart rate and blood pressure regularly while you are taking metoprolol. Ask your prescriber or health care professional what your heart rate and blood pressure should be, and when you should contact him or her. Do not stop taking this medicine suddenly. This could lead to serious heart-related effects. You may get drowsy or dizzy. Do not drive, use machinery, or do anything that requires mental alertness until you know how metoprolol affects you. To reduce the risk of dizzy or fainting spells, do not sit or stand up quickly. Alcohol can make you more drowsy, and increase flushing and rapid heartbeats. Therefore, it is best to avoid alcoholic drinks. Metoprolol can affect blood sugar levels. If you have diabetes, check with your prescriber or health care professional before you change your diet or the dose of your diabetic medicine. If you are going to have surgery, tell your prescriber or health care professional that you are taking metoprolol.

What side effects may I notice from taking metoprolol?

Side effects that you should report to your prescriber or health care professional as soon as possible:
- anxiety
- cold, tingling, or numb hands or feet
- difficulty breathing, wheezing
- dizziness or fainting spells

- increase in the amount of urine passed
- increased thirst
- irregular heartbeat
- skin rash
- slow heart rate (fewer than recommended by your prescriber or health care professional)
- sweating
- swollen legs or ankles
- tremor, shakes
- vomiting
- weight loss

Side effects that usually do not require medical attention (report to your prescriber or health care professional if they continue or are bothersome):

- diarrhea
- dry itching skin
- headache
- nausea
- sexual difficulties, impotence
- unusual tiredness

Where can I keep my medicine?

Keep out of the reach of children in a container that small children cannot open. Store at room temperature between 15 and 30 degrees C (59 and 86 degrees F). Protect from moisture. Throw away any unused medicine after the expiration date.

Metronidazole tablets, capsules, or extended-release tablets

FLAGYL®;
500 mg; Tablet
GD Searle LLC a
Subsidiary of
Pharmacia Company
Pfizer

FLAGYL®;
750 mg; Tablet,
Extended Release
GD Searle LLC a
Subsidiary of
Pharmacia Company
Pfizer

What are metronidazole tablets, capsules, or extended-release tablets?

METRONIDAZOLE (Flagyl®, Flagyl XR®) kills or prevents the growth of certain bacteria and protozoa (single cell animals). Metronidazole treats infections of the skin, central nervous system, bones and joints, respiratory tract, abdomen, gynecologic and vaginal infections (including trichomoniasis), and intestinal infections (including dysentery). Generic metronidazole tablets, capsules, and extended-release tablets are available.

What should my health care professional know before I take metronidazole?

They need to know if you have any of these conditions:
- if you drink alcoholic beverages
- anemia or other blood disorders
- liver disease
- disease of the nervous system
- seizures (convulsions)
- other chronic illness
- an unusual or allergic reaction to metronidazole, or other medicines, foods, dyes, or preservatives
- pregnant or trying to get pregnant
- breast-feeding

How should I take this medicine?

Take metronidazole tablets or capsules by mouth. Follow the directions on the prescription label.
Tablets or capsules:
Swallow tablets or capsules whole with a full glass of water. You can take this medicine with food or milk.
Extended-release tablets:
Swallow tablets whole with a full glass of water. Take this medicine on an empty stomach 1 hour before or 2 hours after meals or food. Take your doses at regular intervals. Do not take your medicine more often than directed. Finish the full course prescribed by your prescriber or health care professional even if you think your condition is better. Do not stop taking except on your prescriber's advice. Contact your pediatrician or health care professional regarding the use of this medicine in children. Special care may be needed.

What if I miss a dose?

If you miss a dose, take it as soon as you can. If it is almost time for your next dose, take only that dose. Do not take double or extra doses.

What may interact with metronidazole?

- alcohol or alcohol-containing beverages or medicines
- amprenavir
- barbiturate medicines for inducing sleep or treating seizures (convulsions)
- carbamazepine
- cimetidine
- disulfiram
- fluorouracil
- lithium
- methadone
- phenytoin
- sirolimus
- tacrolimus
- warfarin

Tell your prescriber or health care professional about all other medicines you are taking, including non-prescription medicines. Also tell your prescriber or health care professional if you are a frequent user of drinks with caffeine or alcohol, if you smoke, or if you use illegal drugs. These may affect the way your medicine works. Check with your health care professional before stopping or starting any of your medicines.

What should I watch for while taking metronidazole?

Tell your prescriber or health care professional if your symptoms do not improve in 2 or 3 days. If you are

M

taking this medicine for a long time you must visit your prescriber or health care professional for regular blood checks. Avoid alcoholic drinks while you are taking metronidazole and for 3 days afterward. Alcohol may make you dizzy, feel sick, and flushed; give you headaches and stomach pains. You may get drowsy or dizzy. Do not drive, use machinery, or do anything that needs mental alertness until you know how metronidazole affects you. To reduce the risk of dizzy or fainting spells, do not sit or stand up quickly, especially if you are an older patient. Your mouth may get dry. Chewing sugarless gum or sucking hard candy, and drinking plenty of water will help. If you are being treated for an infection of your sex organs, your sexual partner may also need treatment. You can use a condom to stop reinfection of you or your sexual partner. If you are going to have surgery, tell your prescriber or health care professional that you are using metronidazole.

What side effects may I notice from taking metronidazole?

Side effects that you should report to your prescriber or health care professional as soon as possible:
Rare or uncommon:
- clumsiness, dizziness, or unsteadiness
- fever or chills, sore throat

- numbness, tingling, pain or weakness in the hands or feet
- seizures (convulsions)
- skin rash, itching
- vomiting or severe stomach pain

More common:
- unusual tiredness or weakness
- vaginal irritation or discharge

Side effects that usually do not require medical attention (report to your prescriber or health care professional if they continue or are bothersome):
- dark brown or reddish urine
- diarrhea
- dry mouth
- food tasting unusual or like metal
- headache
- loss of appetite
- nausea
- mild stomach pain or cramps

Where can I keep my medicine?

Keep out of the reach of children in a container that small children cannot open. Store at room temperature between 15 and 30 degrees C (59 and 86 degrees F). Protect from light. Keep container tightly closed. Throw away any unused medicine after the expiration date.

Mexiletine capsules

MEXITIL®;
200 mg; Capsule
Boehringer
Ingelheim
Pharmaceuticals Inc

MEXITIL®;
250 mg; Capsule
Boehringer
Ingelheim
Pharmaceuticals Inc

What are mexiletine capsules?

MEXILETINE (Mexitil®) is an antiarrhythmic agent. Mexiletine treats irregular heart rhythm and can slow rapid heartbeats (tachycardia). Mexiletine can help your heart to return to and maintain a normal rhythm. Generic mexiletine capsules are available.

What should my health care professional know before I take mexiletine?

They need to know if you have any of these conditions:
- heart disease or problems other than rhythm and heart rate problems
- liver disease
- low blood pressure
- previous heart attack
- seizures (convulsions)
- an unusual or allergic reaction to mexiletine, other medicines, foods, dyes, or preservatives
- pregnant or trying to get pregnant
- breast-feeding

How should I take this medicine?

Take mexiletine capsules by mouth. Follow the directions on the prescription label. Swallow the capsules with a drink of water. If mexiletine upsets your stomach you can take it with food, milk or an antacid. Take

your doses at regular intervals. Do not take your medicine more often than directed. Contact your pediatrician or health care professional regarding the use of this medicine in children. Special care may be needed.

What if I miss a dose?

If you miss a dose, take it as soon as you can. If it is almost time for your next dose, take only that dose. Do not take the missed dose if it is more than 4 hours after the dose was due. Do not take double or extra doses.

What may interact with mexiletine?

- ammonium chloride
- acetazolamide
- cimetidine
- disopyramide
- medicines to control heart rhythm
- phenytoin
- sodium bicarbonate
- some antidepressants or drugs for anxiety disorders
- theophylline

Tell your prescriber or health care professional about all other medicines you are taking, including non-prescription medicines, nutritional supplements, or herbal products. Also tell your prescriber or health care professional if you are a frequent user of drinks with caffeine or alcohol, if you smoke, or if you use illegal drugs. These may affect the way your medicine works. Check with your health care professional before stopping or starting any of your medicines.

What should I watch for while taking mexiletine?

Visit your prescriber or health care professional for regular checks on your progress. Do not stop taking mexiletine suddenly; this may cause serious, heart-related side effects. Because your condition and the use of mexiletine carry some risk. it is a good idea to carry an identification card, necklace or bracelet with details of your condition, medications and prescriber or health care professional. Check your heart rate (pulse) and blood pressure regularly while you are taking mexiletine. Ask your prescriber or health care professional what your heart rate and blood pressure should be, and when you should contact him or her. Your prescriber or health care professional also may schedule regular blood tests and electrocardiograms to check your progress. You may feel dizzy or faint. Do not drive, use machinery, or do anything that needs mental alertness until you know how mexiletine affects you. To reduce the risk of dizzy or fainting spells, do not sit or stand up quickly, especially if you are an older patient. Alcohol can make you more dizzy, increase flushing and rapid heartbeats. Avoid alcoholic drinks. If you are going to have surgery, tell your prescriber or health care professional that you are taking mexiletine.

What side effects may I notice from taking mexiletine?

Side effects that you should report to your prescriber or health care professional as soon as possible:

- chest pain, continued irregular heartbeats
- difficulty breathing
- seizures (convulsions)
- redness, blistering, peeling or loosening of the skin, including inside the mouth
- skin rash
- trembling, shaking
- unusual bleeding or bruising
- unusual weakness or tiredness

Side effects that usually do not require medical attention (report to your prescriber or health care professional if they continue or are bothersome):

- blurred vision
- difficulty walking
- dizziness
- heartburn
- nausea, vomiting
- nervousness
- numbness, or tingling in the fingers or toes
- skin rash
- stomach pain

Where can I keep my medicine?

Keep out of the reach of children in a container that small children cannot open. Store at room temperature below 30 degrees C (86 degrees F). Throw away any unused medicine after the expiration date.

Midodrine tablets

PROAMATINE®;
5 mg; Tablet
Shire US Inc

PROAMATINE®;
2.5 mg Tablet
Shire US Inc

What are midodrine tablets?

MIDODRINE (ProAmatine®) is used to treat low blood pressure in someone who has symptoms such as dizziness when going from a sitting to a standing position. Generic midodrine tablets are available.

What should my health care professional know before I take midodrine?

They need to know if you have any of the following conditions:

- diabetes mellitus
- heart disease
- high blood pressure
- kidney disease
- overactive thyroid
- pheochromocytoma
- an unusual or allergic reaction to midodrine, other medicines, foods, dyes, or preservatives
- pregnant or trying to get pregnant
- problems urinating
- breast-feeding

How should I take this medicine?

Take midodrine tablets by mouth. Follow the directions on the prescription label. Swallow the tablets with a drink of water. Take your doses at the intervals prescribed by your doctor or health care professional. Your last dose for the day should be taken 3 to 4 hours before bedtime. Do not take your medicine more often than directed. If you are going to be lying down for any length of time, you should not take that dose of your medication. Contact your pediatrician or health care professional regarding the use of this medicine in children. Special care may be needed.

What if I miss a dose?

If you miss a dose, take it as soon as you can. If it is almost time for your next dose (less than 3 hours), take only that dose. There must be at least 3 hours between your doses. Do not take double or extra doses.

What may interact with midodrine?

- cimetidine
- linezolid

M

- metformin
- ranitidine
- triamterene
- medicines for correcting heart rhythm problems
- medicines for colds and breathing difficulties
- medicines for treating depression, especially monoamine oxidase inhibitors (MAOIs)
- medicines for migraine
- medicines for heart disease or high blood pressure
- medicines for weight loss

Tell your prescriber or health care professional about all other medicines you are taking, including non-prescription medicines, nutritional supplements, or herbal products. Also tell your prescriber or health care professional if you are a frequent user of drinks with caffeine or alcohol, if you smoke, or if you use illegal drugs. These may affect the way your medicine works. Check before starting or stopping any of your medicines.

What should I watch for while taking midodrine?

If you develop cold symptoms or decide to lose weight while taking midodrine, contact your prescriber or health care professional before taking any medications. Some of these medications can also increase your blood pressure.

What side effects may I notice from taking midodrine?

Side effects that you should report to your prescriber or health care professional as soon as possible:
- awareness of heart beating
- blurred vision

- difficulty breathing, wheezing
- irregular heartbeat, palpitations, or chest pain
- pounding in the ears
- skin rash, hives
- vomiting

Side effects that usually do not require medical attention (report to your prescriber or health care professional if they continue or are bothersome):
- backache
- change in heart rate
- chills
- difficulty sleeping
- dizziness
- drowsiness
- dry mouth
- dry skin
- facial flushing
- goose bumps
- headache
- heartburn
- increased need to urinate
- irritability
- itching
- leg cramps
- nausea
- restlessness
- stomach pain
- tingling in the skin or scalp

Where can I keep my medicine?

Keep out of the reach of children in a container that small children cannot open. Store at room temperature between 15 and 25 degrees C (59 and 77 degrees F). Throw away any unused medicine after the expiration date.

Miglitol tablets

 GLYSET®;
50 mg; Tablet
Pharmacia and
Upjohn Div Pfizer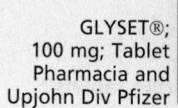

GLYSET®;
100 mg; Tablet
Pharmacia and
Upjohn Div Pfizer

What are miglitol tablets?

MIGLITOL (Glyset®) lowers blood sugar in patients with diabetes. It slows the entry of certain sugars from food in the intestine into the body. Because it acts to reduce the absorption of sugars or starches in food, it must be taken with meals. Treatment is combined with a balanced diet and exercise. Miglitol may be given with some other diabetic medications. Generic miglitol tablets are not yet available.

What should my health care professional know before I take miglitol?

They need to know if you have any of these conditions:
- hiatal hernia
- kidney disease
- stomach or bowel disease, or obstruction
- an unusual or allergic reaction to miglitol, other medicines, foods, dyes, or preservatives
- pregnant or trying to get pregnant
- breast-feeding

How should I take this medicine?

Take miglitol tablets by mouth. Follow the directions on the prescription label. Swallow the tablets at the start of a main meal, with a drink of water if necessary. Take your doses at regular intervals. Do not take your medicine more often than directed. If you develop severe vomiting or severe diarrhea that prevents you from eating meals, call your health care prescriber for advice. Contact your pediatrician or health care professional regarding the use of this medicine in children. Special care may be needed.

What if I miss a dose?

If you forgot your dose at the start of your meal and you are still eating that meal, take your dose while you are still eating. Otherwise, skip the missed dose. Miglitol is not effective if not taken during a meal. Wait for your next dose at your next main meal, and take only that dose. Do not take double or extra doses.

What may interact with miglitol?

- charcoal
- cholestyramine
- colestipol
- digoxin
- neomycin
- other medicines for diabetes
- pancrelipase, pancreatin, amylase, or other digestive enzyme supplements
- warfarin

Many medications may cause changes (increase or decrease) in blood sugar, these include:

- alcohol-containing beverages
- beta-blockers, often used for high blood pressure or heart problems (examples include atenolol, metoprolol, propranolol)
- chromium
- female hormones, such as estrogens, progestins, or contraceptive pills
- isoniazid
- male hormones or anabolic steroids
- medications to suppress appetite or for weight loss
- medicines for allergies, asthma, cold, or cough
- niacin
- pentamidine
- phenytoin
- some herbal dietary supplements
- steroid medicines such as prednisone or cortisone
- thyroid hormones
- water pills (diuretics)

Tell your prescriber or health care professional about all other medicines that you are taking, including non-prescription medicines, nutritional supplements, or herbal products. Also tell your prescriber or health care professional if you are a frequent user of drinks with caffeine or alcohol, if you smoke, or if you use illegal drugs. These may affect the way your medicine works. Check with your health care professional before stopping or starting any of your medicines.

What should I watch for while taking miglitol?

Visit your prescriber or health care professional for regular checks on your progress. Learn how to monitor your blood sugar. Miglitol does not cause symptoms of hypoglycemia (too low blood sugar) by itself, but if given with another antidiabetic medicine, it may increase their potential to lower blood sugar. If you do take miglitol in combination with other medications, you and family members must learn to recognize and how to treat symptoms of low blood sugar. *If you are taking miglitol with other diabetic medications:* Because miglitol prevents the breakdown of table sugar you must always keep a supply of glucose or dextrose tablets or solution readily available to treat low blood sugar

events if they occur. Ask your pharmacist to help you find these products at the store. Wear a medical identification bracelet or chain to say you have diabetes, and carry a card that lists all your medications.

What side effects may I notice from taking miglitol?

Side effects that you should report to your prescriber or health care professional as soon as possible:
It is rare to have serious side effects with this medicine:

- skin rash or itching
- unusual tiredness
- weight loss

In combination with other diabetic medications, like glyburide, glipizide, metformin or insulin, miglitol may cause hypoglycemia (low blood glucose). Contact your health care professional if you experience symptoms of low blood sugar that may include:

- anxiety or nervousness
- confusion
- difficulty concentrating
- hunger
- pale skin
- nausea
- fatigue
- sweating
- headache
- palpitations
- numbness of the mouth
- tingling in the fingers
- tremors
- muscle weakness
- blurred vision
- cold sensations
- uncontrolled yawning
- irritability
- rapid heartbeat
- shallow breathing
- loss of consciousness

Side effects that usually do not require medical attention (report to your prescriber or health care professional if they continue or are bothersome):
These side effects with miglitol are usually minor but very common. They include:

- bloated feeling
- diarrhea
- stomach or intestinal gas or rumbling stomach
- stomach pain or discomfort

Where can I keep my medicine?

Keep out of the reach of children in a container that small children cannot open. Store at room temperature between 15 and 30 degrees C (59 and 86 degrees F). Keep away from wet or moist areas, like the bathroom. Throw away any unused medicine after the expiration date.

M

Miglustat capsules

What are miglustat capsules?

MIGLUSTAT (Zavesca®) helps to prevent the reduction of a naturally occurring enzyme that is needed in your body to help with fat breakdown. It helps to keep normal blood levels of this enzyme, and it may help prevent your liver or spleen from getting big. Generic miglustat capsules are not yet available.

What should my health care professional know before I take miglustat?

They need to know if you have any of these conditions:
- dehydration
- diarrhea or a condition that causes diarrhea
- kidney disease
- numbness, tingling or a burning sensation in your fingers, toes or other areas
- tremors
- an unusual reaction to miglustat, other medicines, foods, dyes, or preservatives
- pregnant or trying to get pregnant
- breast-feeding

How should I take this medicine?

Take miglustat capsules by mouth. Follow the directions on the prescription label. Take your doses at regular intervals at the same times each day. You may take miglustat with or without meals. Do not take your medicine more often than directed. Contact your pediatrician or health care professional regarding the use of this medicine in children. Special care may be needed.

What if I miss a dose?

If you miss a dose of miglustat, just skip that dose. Wait until your next scheduled dose and take only that dose. Do not take double or extra doses.

What may interact with miglustat?

- imiglucerase

Tell your prescriber or health care professional about all other medicines you are taking, including non-prescription medicines, nutritional supplements, or herbal products. Also tell your prescriber or health care professional if you are a frequent user of drinks with caffeine or alcohol, if you smoke, or if you use illegal drugs. These may affect the way your medicine works. Check with your health care professional before stopping or starting any of your medicines.

What should I watch for while taking miglustat?

See your health care provider for regular checks on your progress. Your health care provider may need to monitor your kidney function while you are taking miglustat. This will usually be done by taking a blood sample. Diarrhea and tremors in your hands may be common side effects you will notice while taking miglustat. You may take other medicines to help control your diarrhea. Talk to your health care provider about which medications may be best for you. In females, this drug may cause harm to a developing baby if this drug is taken during pregnancy. It is important that you do not become pregnant while you are taking this drug. Use an effective form of birth control; talk to your health care provider regarding birth control options. Do not take this drug if you are already pregnant. Tell your health care provider if you think you may be pregnant. Men engaging in sexual intercourse should use a condom (or other form of effective birth control) while taking this drug to prevent pregnancy in their female partner, as drug-related sperm changes may lead to birth defects. Continue to use male condoms (or other forms of effective birth control) for 3 months after stopping the use of miglustat.

What side effects may I notice from taking miglustat?

Side effects that you should report to your prescriber or health care professional as soon as possible:
- a numbness, tingling or burning feeling in your hands, feet or other parts of your body
- in women, changes in your menstrual cycle (period)
- problems with your eyes or vision
- severe diarrhea
- shakiness or tremors in your hands

Side effects that usually do not require medical attention (report to your prescriber or health care professional if they continue or are bothersome):
- cramps
- dizziness
- dry mouth
- headache
- loss in appetite
- mild diarrhea
- stomach pain or upset, nausea, vomiting
- weakness
- weight loss

Where can I keep my medicine?

Keep out of the reach of children in a container that small children cannot open. Store at controlled room temperature between 20 and 25 degrees C (68 and 77 degrees F). Keep away from extreme heat, humidity or moisture. Throw away any unused medication after the expiration date.

M

Minocycline tablets or capsules

DYNACIN®;
100 mg; Capsule
Medicis
Dermatologics Inc

DYNACIN®;
100 mg; Tablet
Medicis
Dermatologics Inc

What are minocycline tablets or capsules?

MINOCYCLINE (Dynacin®, Minocin®) is a tetra-cycline-type antibiotic. Minocycline kills certain bacteria that cause infection, or stops their growth. It treats many kinds of infections of the skin, bone, stomach, respiratory tract, sinuses, ear, and urinary tract. It also treats certain sexually transmitted diseases. Generic minocycline tablets and capsules are available.

What should my health care professional know before I take minocycline?

They need to know if you have any of these conditions:
- kidney disease
- liver disease
- long exposure to sunlight (working outdoors)
- an unusual or allergic reaction to minocycline, other tetracyclines
- pregnant or trying to get pregnant
- breast-feeding

How should I take this medicine?

Take minocycline tablets or capsules by mouth. Follow the directions on the prescription label. Swallow tablets or capsules whole with a full glass of water; take tablets or capsules in an upright or sitting position. Taking a sip of water first, before taking the tablets or capsules, may help you swallow them. If possible take bedtime doses at least 10 minutes before lying down. It is best to take minocycline without food, but if it upsets your stomach take it with food. Take your doses at regular intervals. Do not take your medicine more often than directed. Finish the full course prescribed by your prescriber or health care professional even if you think your condition is better. Do not stop taking except on your prescriber's advice. Contact your pediatrician or health care professional regarding the use of this medicine in children. Special care may be needed.

What if I miss a dose?

If you miss a dose, take it as soon as you can. If it is almost time for your next dose, take only that dose. Do not take double or extra doses. There should be an interval of at least 4 to 6 hours between doses.

What may interact with minocycline?

- antacids
- calcium salts
- cholestyramine
- colestipol
- digoxin
- female hormones, including contraceptive or birth control pills
- ferrous sulfate
- magnesium salts
- other antibiotics
- phenytoin
- sodium bicarbonate
- warfarin

Tell your prescriber or health care professional about all other medicines you are taking, including non-prescription medicines, nutritional supplements, or herbal products. Also tell your prescriber or health care professional if you are a frequent user of drinks with caffeine or alcohol, if you smoke, or if you use illegal drugs. These may affect the way your medicine works. Check with your health care professional before stopping or starting any of your medicines.

What should I watch for while taking minocycline?

Tell your prescriber or health care professional if your symptoms do not improve in 3 to 5 days. Sometimes it will take longer than this before you get better. Do not take minocycline just before going to bed. It may not dissolve properly when you are lying down and can cause ulceration of your food pipe. Keep out of the sun, or wear protective clothing outdoors and use a sunscreen. Do not use sun lamps or sun tanning beds or booths. Birth control pills (contraceptive pills) may not work properly while you are taking this medicine. Use an extra method of birth control for at least one month. You may get drowsy or dizzy. Do not drive, use machinery, or do anything that needs mental alertness until you know how minocycline affects you. To reduce the risk of dizzy or fainting spells, do not sit or stand up quickly, especially if you are an older patient. If you are being treated for a sexually transmitted disease, avoid sexual contact until you have finished your treatment. Your sexual partner may also need treatment. If you are going to have surgery, tell your prescriber or health care professional that you are taking minocycline. Antacid can stop minocycline from working. If you get an upset stomach and want to take an antacid, make sure there is an interval of at least 2 hours since you last took minocycline, or 4 hours before your next dose. Never take minocycline if it is past the expiration date; it can make you seriously ill.

What side effects may I notice from taking minocycline?

Side effects that you should report to your prescriber or health care professional as soon as possible:
- dark yellow or brown urine
- difficulty breathing
- fever
- headache
- increased sensitivity to the sun or ultraviolet light
- itching in the rectal or genital area

M

- pain on swallowing
- redness, blistering, peeling or loosening of the skin, including inside the mouth
- stomach pain or cramps
- skin rash or itching
- unusual bleeding or bruising
- unusual tiredness or weakness
- yellowing of eyes or skin.

Side effects that usually do not require medical attention (report to your prescriber or health care professional if they continue or are bothersome):
- diarrhea

- discolored tongue or teeth
- drowsiness, dizziness
- loss of appetite
- nausea, vomiting
- sore mouth

Where can I keep my medicine?

Keep out of the reach of children in a container that small children cannot open. Store at room temperature between 15 and 30 degrees C (59 and 86 degrees F). Protect from light and moisture. Throw away any unused medicine after the expiration date.

Minoxidil tablets

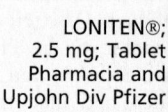

LONITEN®;
2.5 mg; Tablet
Pharmacia and
Upjohn Div Pfizer

LONITEN®;
10 mg; Tablet
Pharmacia and
Upjohn Div Pfizer

What are minoxidil tablets?

MINOXIDIL (Loniten®) is a vasodilator that relaxes blood vessels; when taken by mouth minoxidil helps to treat high blood pressure. It is not a cure and must be taken regularly to control blood pressure. Generic minoxidil tablets are available.

What should my health care professional know before I take minoxidil?

They need to know if you have any of these conditions:
- angina
- heart or blood vessel disease
- kidney disease
- lung disease
- pheochromocytoma
- previous heart attack
- an unusual or allergic reaction to minoxidil, other medicines, foods, dyes, or preservatives
- pregnant or trying to get pregnant
- breast-feeding

How should I take this medicine?

Take minoxidil tablets by mouth. Follow the directions on the prescription label. Swallow the tablets with a drink of water. Take your doses at regular intervals. Do not take your medicine more often than directed.

What if I miss a dose?

If you miss a dose, take it as soon as you can if you remember within a few hours. If it is almost time for your next dose or you do not remember until the next day, skip a dose and take only the dose for that day. Do not take double or extra doses.

What may interact with minoxidil?

- anti-inflammatory drugs (NSAIDs, such as ibuprofen)
- female hormones, including contraceptive or birth control pills
- medicines for chest pain
- medicines for colds and breathing difficulties

- medicines for high blood pressure
- water pills

Tell your prescriber or health care professional about all other medicines you are taking, including non-prescription medicines, nutritional supplements, or herbal products. Also tell your prescriber or health care professional if you are a frequent user of drinks with caffeine or alcohol, if you smoke, or if you use illegal drugs. These may affect the way your medicine works. Check with your health care professional before stopping or starting any of your medicines.

What should I watch for while taking minoxidil?

Visit your prescriber or health care professional for regular checks on your progress. Check your blood pressure and pulse rate regularly; this is important while you are taking minoxidil. Ask your prescriber or health care professional what your blood pressure and pulse rate should be and when you should contact him or her. While you are taking minoxidil, keep a check on your weight. Tell your prescriber or health care professional if you rapidly gain more then 5 pounds. You may need to follow a special low-sodium diet while taking minoxidil. Check with your prescriber or health care professional. Do not treat yourself for coughs, colds, headache or pain while you are taking minoxidil, without asking your prescriber or health care professional for advice. If you are going to have surgery tell your prescriber or health care professional that you are taking minoxidil.

What side effects may I notice from taking minoxidil?

Side effects that you should report to your prescriber or health care professional as soon as possible:
- chest pain, fast or irregular heartbeat, palpitations
- difficulty breathing
- dizziness or fainting spells
- redness, blistering, peeling or loosening of the skin, including inside the mouth

M

- skin rash or itching
- stiff or swollen joints
- sudden weight gain
- swelling of the feet or legs
- unusual weakness

Side effects that usually do not require medical attention (report to your prescriber or health care professional if they continue or are bothersome):

- headache
- unusual hair growth, on the face, arms, and back

Where can I keep my medicine?
Keep out of the reach of children in a container that small children cannot open. Store at room temperature between 20 and 25 degrees C (68 and 77 degrees F). Throw away any unused medicine after the expiration date.

Mirtazapine tablets

REMERON®;
30 mg; Tablet
Organon USA Inc

REMERON®
SOLTAB™;
30 mg; Tablet,
Orally
Disintegrating
Organon USA Inc

This drug requires an FDA medication guide. See page xxxvii.

What are mirtazapine tablets?
MIRTAZAPINE (Remeron®, Remeron® SolTab™) is an antidepressant, a medicine that helps to lift mental depression and relieve anxiety. Mirtazapine is not like other antidepressants. Mirtazapine may be used for treating some types of tremors. Generic mirtazapine tablets and a generic version of Remeron® SolTab™ (tablet that dissolves in your mouth) are available.

What should my health care professional know before I take mirtazapine?
They need to know if you have any of these conditions:
- diabetes
- heart disease or irregular heart beats
- high blood cholesterol or triglycerides
- kidney disease
- liver disease
- low blood pressure
- mania
- phenylketonuria
- receiving electroconvulsive therapy
- seizures (convulsions)
- stroke
- suicidal thoughts
- an unusual or allergic reaction to mirtazapine, other medicines, foods, dyes, or preservatives
- pregnant or trying to get pregnant
- breast-feeding

How should I take this medicine?
Take mirtazapine tablets by mouth. Follow the directions on the prescription label and for the type of product you are taking (see below). Because mirtazapine can cause drowsiness and improve sleep, it is often taken before bed. Do not take your medicine more often than directed. Do not stop taking the tablets except on your prescriber's advice.
Remeron® tablets:
Take these tablets by mouth, do not chew. Swallow the tablets with a drink of water.
Remeron® SolTab™ tablets:
These tablets are made to dissolve in the mouth without having to take them with water. Place the tablet in the mouth and allow it to dissolve, then swallow.

While you may take these tablets with water, it is not necessary to do so. Contact your pediatrician or health care professional regarding the use of this medicine in children. Special care may be needed.

What if I miss a dose?
If you miss a dose, take it as soon as you can. If it is almost time for your next dose, take only that dose. Do not take double or extra doses.

What may interact with mirtazapine?
Do not take mirtazapine with any of the following medications:

- medicines called MAO inhibitors—phenelzine (Nardil®), tranylcypromine (Parnate®), isocarboxazid (Marplan®), selegiline (Eldepryl®)

Mirtazapine may also interact with the following medications:

- alcohol
- amphetamines
- clonidine
- cocaine
- furazolidone
- herbal therapies, like St. John's wort, kava kava, tryptophan, or valerian
- linezolid
- medicines for sleep
- medicines for mental depression, anxiety, or other mood problems
- medicines for high blood pressure
- medicines for pain
- muscle relaxants
- procarbazine
- some medicines for allergies, colds, flu, or sinus trouble

Tell your prescriber or health care professional about all other medicines you are taking, including non-prescription medicines, nutritional supplements, or herbal products. Also tell your prescriber or health care professional if you are a frequent user of drinks with caffeine or alcohol, if you smoke, or if you use illegal drugs. These may affect the way your medicine works. Check with your health care professional before stopping or starting any of your medicines.

M

What should I watch for while taking mirtazapine?

Visit your prescriber or health care professional for regular checks on your progress. You may have to take mirtazapine for several weeks before you feel better. If you have suicidal thoughts, extreme agitation, or inability to sleep or sit still, call your prescriber or health care professional at once. You may get drowsy or dizzy while taking mirtazapine. Do not drive, use machinery, or do anything that needs mental alertness until you know how mirtazapine affects you. Do not stand or sit up quickly, especially if you are an older patient. This reduces the risk of dizzy or fainting spells. Alcohol may increase dizziness or drowsiness; avoid alcoholic drinks. Mirtazapine can make your mouth dry. Chewing sugarless gum, sucking hard candy and drinking plenty of water will help. Do not treat yourself for coughs, colds, or allergies without asking your prescriber or health care professional for advice. Some ingredients may increase possible side effects. If you are going to have surgery, tell your prescriber or health care professional that you are taking mirtazapine.

What side effects may I notice from taking mirtazapine?

Side effects that you should report to your prescriber or health care professional as soon as possible:
- confusion
- difficulty breathing
- difficulty passing urine
- dizziness or lightheadedness
- emotional changes or unusual thoughts
- fever, easy-bruising, sore throat, or mouth ulcers or blisters
- flu-like symptoms (fever, chills, cough, muscle or joint aches and pains)
- irregular heartbeat (palpitations)
- stomach pain with nausea and/or vomiting
- swelling of the hands or feet
- unusual tiredness or weakness
- vomiting

Side effects that usually do not require medical attention (report to your prescriber or health care professional if they continue or are bothersome):
- back pain
- dry mouth
- constipation
- drowsiness
- increased appetite
- mild nausea
- weight gain

Where can I keep my medicine?

Keep out of the reach of children in a container that small children cannot open. Store at a controlled temperature between 20 and 25 degrees C (68 and 77 degrees F) in a tight, light resistant container. Keep in a dry, cool place. Throw away any unused medicine after the expiration date.

Misoprostol tablets

CYTOTEC®;
200 mcg; Tablet
GD Searle LLC a
Subsidiary of
Pharmacia Company
Pfizer

CYTOTEC®;
100 mcg; Tablet
GD Searle LLC a
Subsidiary of
Pharmacia Company
Pfizer

What are misoprostol tablets?

MISOPROSTOL (Cytotec®) helps to prevent stomach ulcers in patients using nonsteroidal anti-inflammatory drugs (NSAIDS, drugs commonly used for arthritis, inflammation, and pain). Misoprostol reduces the amount of acid produced in the stomach and protects the stomach lining from the effects of acid. Misoprostol is also sometimes used for other purposes in females. Generic misoprostol tablets are available.

What should my health care professional know before I take misoprostol?

They need to know if you have any of these conditions:
- heart disease
- inflammatory disease of the intestine, like Crohn's disease or ulcerative colitis
- kidney disease
- ulcerative colitis
- an unusual or allergic reaction to misoprostol, prostaglandins, other medicines, foods, dyes, or preservatives
- pregnant or trying to get pregnant
- breast-feeding

How should I take this medicine?

Take misoprostol tablets by mouth. Follow the directions on the prescription label. Swallow the tablets with a drink of water. Take your doses at regular intervals; this medication is usually taken with meals and at bedtime with food. Taking this medication with food reduces the chance of diarrhea or stomach upset. Do not take your medicine more often than directed. Do not share this medication with anyone else. Before starting this medication, read the paper on your prescription provided by your pharmacist or health care professional. This paper will tell you about this drug. Make certain you understand the instructions. Contact your pediatrician or health care professional regarding the use of this medicine in children. Special care may be needed.

What if I miss a dose?

If you miss a dose, take it as soon as you can. If it is almost time for your next dose, take only that dose. Do not take double or extra doses.

M

What may interact with misoprostol?

- antacids
- cyclosporine

Tell your prescriber or health care professional about all other medicines you are taking, including non-prescription medicines, nutritional supplements, or herbal products. Also tell your prescriber or health care professional if you are a frequent user of drinks with caffeine or alcohol, if you smoke, or if you use illegal drugs. These may affect the way your medicine works. Check with your health care professional before stopping or starting any of your medicines.

What should I watch for while taking misoprostol?

It can take several days of therapy with misoprostol before your stomach pains improve. Check with your prescriber or health care professional if your condition does not improve, or if it gets worse. You can take antacids for the occasional relief of pain unless your prescriber or health care professional tells you otherwise. If you are female, you should not use this drug to prevent stomach ulcers if you are pregnant. Females should avoid pregnancy while taking this medication and for at least one month (one full menstrual cycle) after discontinuing this medication. Misoprostol can cause contractions of the uterus that may cause abortion or the medication may harm an unborn baby. You should use a reliable form of birth control while taking misoprostol; talk to your health care provider about

birth control options. If you become pregnant, think you are pregnant, or want to become pregnant during misoprostol treatment, stop taking this drug immediately and contact your health care provider for advice.

What side effects may I notice from taking misoprostol?

Side effects that you should report to your prescriber or health care professional as soon as possible:

- chest pain
- dehydration
- lightheadedness or fainting spells
- severe diarrhea
- sudden shortness of breath
- unusual vaginal bleeding, pelvic pain or cramping (females)

Side effects that usually do not require medical attention (report to your prescriber or health care professional if they continue or are bothersome):

- diarrhea (mild)
- dizziness
- headache
- menstrual irregularity, spotting, or cramps
- nausea
- stomach upset or cramps

Where can I keep my medicine?

Keep out of the reach of children in a container that small children cannot open. Store at room temperature below 25 degrees C (77 degrees F). Keep in a dry place. Protect from moisture. Throw away any unused medicine after the expiration date.

Mitotane tablets

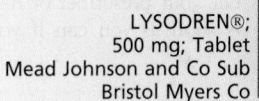 LYSODREN®;
500 mg; Tablet
Mead Johnson and Co Sub
Bristol Myers Co

What are mitotane tablets?

MITOTANE (Lysodren®) treats an overactive adrenal gland or certain cancers that affect the adrenal gland. Treatment with mitotane reduces the amount of hormones called "adrenocorticoids." Your body needs these hormones for things like growth, sexual development, and reproduction. Too much or too little of these hormones, however, can cause serious problems. Generic mitotane tablets are not yet available.

What should my health care professional know before I take mitotane?

They need to know if you have any of these conditions:

- liver disease
- infection
- nervous system disease
- serious injury
- shock
- an unusual or allergic reaction to mitotane, other medicines, foods, dyes, or preservatives
- pregnant or trying to get pregnant
- breast-feeding

How should I take this medicine?

Take mitotane tablets by mouth. Follow the directions on the prescription label. Swallow the tablets with a drink of water. Take your doses at regular intervals. Do not stop taking except on your prescriber's advice.

What if I miss a dose?

If you miss a dose, take it as soon as you can. If it is almost time for your next dose, take only that dose. Do not take double or extra doses. If you vomit after taking a dose, call your prescriber or health care professional for advice.

What may interact with mitotane?

- barbiturate medicines for inducing sleep or treating seizures (convulsions)
- cyclophosphamide
- hormones such as prednisone or cortisone
- live virus vaccines
- medicines for hay fever and other allergies
- medicines for mental depression

M

- medicines for mental problems and psychotic disturbances
- medicines for pain
- phenytoin
- spironolactone
- warfarin

Tell your prescriber or health care professional about all other medicines you are taking, including non-prescription medicines, nutritional supplements, or herbal products. Also tell your prescriber or health care professional if you are a frequent user of drinks with caffeine or alcohol, if you smoke, or if you use illegal drugs. These may affect the way your medicine works. Check with your health care professional before stopping or starting any of your medicines.

What should I watch for while taking mitotane?

Visit your prescriber or health care professional for regular checks on your progress. Many nonprescription medicines contain ingredients that increase the side effects of mitotane. Be sure to check with your prescriber or health care professional before taking any other medicines. You may get drowsy or dizzy. Do not drive, use machinery, or do anything that needs mental alertness until you know how mitotane affects you. To reduce the risk of dizzy or fainting spells, do not sit or stand up quickly, especially if you are an older patient. Alcohol can make you more drowsy and dizzy, increase confusion and lightheadedness. Avoid alcoholic drinks while you are taking mitotane. While you are taking mitotane your body will be less able to fight infection and inflammation. Let your prescriber or health care professional know as soon as you can if you get an injury, infection or any illness. Try to avoid people with colds, flu, and bronchitis. Do not have any vaccinations without your prescriber's approval and avoid anyone who has recently had oral polio vaccine. If you are going to have surgery, tell your prescriber or health care professional that you are taking mitotane.

What side effects may I notice from taking mitotane?

Side effects that you should report to your prescriber or health care professional as soon as possible:
- diarrhea
- blood in urine
- blurred vision
- dizziness or drowsiness
- fever and chills
- mental depression, confusion or irritability
- skin rash
- unusual tiredness or weakness
- vomiting

Side effects that usually do not require medical attention (report to your prescriber or health care professional if they continue or are bothersome):
- flushing of skin
- loss of appetite
- nausea
- tremor

Where can I keep my medicine?

Keep out of the reach of children in a container that small children cannot open. Store at room temperature between 15 and 30 degrees C (59 and 86 degrees F). Protect from light. Keep container tightly closed. Throw away any unused medicine after the expiration date.

Modafinil tablets

PROVIGIL®;
200 mg; Tablet
Cephalon Inc

PROVIGIL®;
100 mg; Tablet
Cephalon Inc

What are modafinil tablets?

MODAFINIL (Provigil®) is a medication that helps to promote alertness during daytime hours. Modafinil helps to improve the symptoms of a condition called narcolepsy. Narcolepsy makes people fall into a sudden deep sleep at odd times; this excessive sleepiness can interfere with the ability to participate in daytime activities. Modafinil has also been used to treat fatigue associated with other sleep disorders. Federal law prohibits giving this medication to any person other than the person for whom it was prescribed. Generic modafinil tablets are not yet available.

What should my health care professional know before I take modafinil?

They need to know if you have any of these conditions:
- if you frequently drink alcohol-containing beverages
- if you have a history of drug or alcohol abuse or rehabilitation
- heart disease (including heart valve problems, irregular heart beat, recent heart attack, or unstable chest pain)
- high blood pressure
- kidney disease
- liver disease
- mental illness
- an unusual or allergic reaction to modafinil, other medicines, foods, dyes, or preservatives
- use some method of birth control
- pregnant or trying to get pregnant
- breast-feeding

How should I take this medicine?

Take modafinil tablets by mouth. Take your daily dose in the morning hours to get the best effects during the

M

day; taking the medication in the afternoon or evening might interfere with your night-time sleep. Follow the directions on the prescription label regarding how to take this medicine. Swallow the tablets with a drink of water. Take your doses at regular intervals. Do not take your medicine more often than directed. Remember: your prescription for modafinil is only for you. You should never share or give your modafinil prescription to anyone else. Contact your pediatrician or health care professional regarding the use of this medicine in children. Special care may be needed.

What if I miss a dose?

If you miss a dose, take it as soon as you can. If it is almost time for your next dose, take only that dose. Do not take double or extra doses.

What may interact with modafinil?

Modafinil can potentially interact with a variety of medications. Doses of your other medications may need to be adjusted or you may have to be monitored more closely.

- alcohol-containing beverages
- antidepressants and other medications for the treatment of mood problems
- antifungal medications (like itraconazole or ketoconazole)
- barbiturates (like phenobarbital)
- birth control pills or other hormone-containing birth control devices or implants
- caffeine
- carbamazepine
- cimetidine
- cyclosporine
- dextroamphetamine, methylphenidate, or other stimulants
- grapefruit juice
- guarana
- linezolid
- phenytoin
- some antibiotics (like rifampin, erythromycin, clarithromycin)
- theophylline
- warfarin

Tell your prescriber or health care professional about all other medicines you are taking, including non-prescription medicines, nutritional supplements, or herbal products. Also tell your prescriber or health care professional if you are a frequent user of drinks with caffeine or alcohol, if you smoke, or if you use illegal drugs. These may affect the way your medicine works. Check with your health care professional before stopping or starting any of your medicines.

What should I watch for while taking modafinil?

The use of modafinil needs careful supervision. Patients with narcolepsy can be helped, but not cured, by modafinil treatment. Visit your prescriber or health care professional for regular checks on your progress. The full effects of modafinil may not be seen right away. Do not stop taking except on your prescriber's advice. Modafinil may affect your concentration, function, or may hide signs that you are tired. Try to maintain a regular sleeping pattern. Until you know how modafinil affects you, do not drive, use machinery, or do any activity that needs mental alertness. Because alcohol may interfere with your response to modafinil or your alertness, it is recommended that you avoid alcohol-containing beverages while on this medication. Modafinil can decrease the effectiveness of certain contraceptives including birth control pills and implantable hormonal contraceptives. If you are using this type of birth control while taking modafinil you should either: 1) use an alternate birth control method; or 2) use another effective birth control method together with your current contraceptive. You should also continue to follow this advice for 1 month after you stop treatment with modafinil. You may wish to discuss birth control options with your health care provider. Some patients with narcolepsy may experience temporary moments of limpness or loss of muscle tone as a regular problem of their condition. These episodes are called cataplexy. This problem may occur when the person laughs, gets excited, or experiences other emotions. Modafinil usually does not increase or decrease the occurrence of these episodes. It is unknown if modafinil's effects will be increased by the use of other stimulants, like caffeine. Caffeine is available in many foods, beverages, and medications. Ask your prescriber if you should limit or change your intake of caffeine-containing products while on modafinil. Do not take any non-prescription medications without the advice of your health care provider or pharmacist. If you are going to have surgery, notify your health care provider that you are on this medication.

What side effects may I notice from taking modafinil?

Side effects that you should report to your prescriber or health care professional as soon as possible:
Rare:
- chest pain
- diarrhea (severe) or vomiting
- difficulty breathing or shortness of breath
- heart palpitations, irregular heartbeat, or a fast heartbeat
- increased blood pressure, particularly if you have high blood pressure
- skin rash, itching, hives, or other allergic reactions
- sore throat, fever, or chills
- tremor or shaking movements

Side effects that usually do not require medical attention (report to your prescriber or health care professional if they continue or are bothersome):
More common:
- headache
- nausea, mild diarrhea, or stomach upset
- nervousness

M

Less common:

- decreased appetite
- depressed or elevated mood, anxiety, or other changes in your moods or emotions
- dizziness
- dry mouth or skin
- trouble sleeping at night

Where can I keep my medicine?

Keep out of the reach of children in a container that small children cannot open. Store at room temperature between 20 and 25 degrees C (68 and 77 degrees F). Keep container tightly closed. Throw away any unused medicine after the expiration date.

Moexipril tablets

UNIVASC®;
7.5 mg; Tablet
Schwarz Pharma Inc

UNIVASC®;
15 mg; Tablet
Schwarz Pharma Inc

What are moexipril tablets?

MOEXIPRIL (Univasc®) is an antihypertensive (blood pressure lowering agent) known as an ACE inhibitor. Moexipril controls high blood pressure (hypertension) by relaxing blood vessels; it is not a cure. High blood pressure levels can damage your kidneys, and may lead to a stroke or heart failure. Generic moexipril tablets are not available.

What should my health care professional know before I take moexipril?

They need to know if you have any of these conditions:

- autoimmune disease (such as lupus), or suppressed immune function
- previous swelling of the tongue, face, or lips with difficulty breathing, difficulty swallowing, hoarseness, or tightening of the throat (angioedema)
- bone marrow disease
- diabetes
- heart or blood vessel disease
- low blood pressure
- kidney disease
- if you are on a special diet, such as a low-salt diet
- an unusual or allergic reaction to moexipril, other ACE inhibitors, foods, dyes, or preservatives
- pregnant or trying to get pregnant
- breast-feeding

How should I take this medicine?

Take moexipril tablets by mouth one hour before meals. Follow the directions on the prescription label. Swallow the tablets with a drink of water. Take your doses at regular intervals. Do not take your medicine more often than directed. Do not stop taking moexipril except on your prescriber's advice. Contact your pediatrician or health care professional regarding the use of this medicine in children. Special care may be needed.

What if I miss a dose?

If you miss a dose, take it as soon as you can. If it is almost time for your next dose, take only that dose. Do not take double or extra doses. If you take only one dose a day and forget to take it that day, do not take a double dose the next day.

What may interact with moexipril?

- carbamazepine
- cerivastatin
- paclitaxel
- phenobarbital
- phenytoin
- repaglinide
- rifabutin
- rifampin
- rosiglitazone
- troglitazone

Tell your prescriber or health care professional about all other medicines you are taking, including non-prescription medicines, nutritional supplements, or herbal products. Also tell your prescriber or health care professional if you are a frequent user of drinks with caffeine or alcohol, if you smoke, or if you use illegal drugs. These may affect the way your medicine works. Check with your health care professional before stopping or starting any of your medicines.

What should I watch for while taking moexipril?

Visit your prescriber or health care professional for regular checks on your progress. Check your blood pressure regularly while you are taking moexipril. Ask your prescriber or health care professional what your blood pressure should be and when you should contact him or her. Stop taking moexipril and call your prescriber or health care professional if you have difficulty breathing, or notice any swelling of the lips, tongue or face. Check with your prescriber or health care professional if you get an attack of severe diarrhea, nausea and vomiting, or if you sweat a lot. The loss of body fluid can make it dangerous to take moexipril. You may get dizzy. Do not drive, use machinery, or do anything that needs mental alertness until you know how moexipril affects you. To avoid dizzy or fainting spells, do not stand or sit up quickly, especially if you are an older person. Alcohol can make you more dizzy. Avoid alcoholic drinks. If you are going to have surgery, tell your prescriber or health care professional that you are taking moexipril. Avoid salt substitutes or other foods or substances high in potassium salts. Do not treat yourself for cough, sore throat, colds, or pain while you are using moexipril without asking your prescriber or health care professional for advice.

What side effects may I notice from taking moexipril?

Side effects that you should report to your prescriber or health care professional as soon as possible:

- decreased amount of urine passed
- difficulty breathing, or difficulty swallowing
- dizziness, lightheadedness or fainting spells
- fast or uneven heart beat, palpitations, or chest pain
- fever or chills
- numbness or tingling in your fingers or toes
- skin rash, itching
- swelling of your face, lips, or tongue

Side effects that usually do not require medical atten-

tion (report to your prescriber or health care professional if they continue or are bothersome):

- change in taste
- cough
- flushing
- headache
- tiredness

Where can I keep my medicine?

Keep out of the reach of children in a container that small children cannot open. Store at room temperature between 15 and 30 degrees C (59 and 86 degrees F). Protect from moisture. Keep container tightly closed. Throw away any unused medicine after the expiration date.

Montelukast tablets or chewable tablets

SINGULAIR®; 10 mg; Tablet Merck and Co Inc

SINGULAIR®; 5 mg; Tablet, Chewable Merck and Co Inc

What are montelukast tablets or chewable tablets?

MONTELUKAST (Singulair®) helps to reduce asthma symptoms (coughing, wheezing, shortness of breath, or chest tightness) and control your asthma. It does not provide instant relief and cannot be used to treat a sudden asthma attack. It works only when used on a regular basis to help reduce inflammation and prevent asthma attacks. Montelukast is effective in adults and children. This drug is also helpful in improving seasonal allergies, like hay fever. Generic montelukast tablets or chewable tablets are not yet available.

What should my health care professional know before I use montelukast?

They need to know if you have any of these conditions:

- an acute asthma attack
- are on corticosteroid therapy, like prednisone or inhalers
- liver disease, like hepatitis
- phenylketonuria
- an unusual or allergic reaction to montelukast, other medicines, foods, dyes, or preservatives
- pregnant or trying to get pregnant
- breast-feeding

How should I use this medicine?

Take montelukast by mouth. You may take your tablets with food. Take montelukast every day at roughly the same time, even on days when you are not having asthma or allergy symptoms. Follow the directions on the prescription label. Do not take your medicine more often than directed. If you are taking the chewable tablets, chew them well before swallowing with water. You may take your tablets with food. Take montelukast every day at roughly the same time, even on days when you are not having asthma or allergy symptoms. Follow the directions on the prescription label. Do not take

your medicine more often than directed. Contact your pediatrician or health care professional regarding the use of this medicine in children. Special care may be needed. Montelukast chewable tablets are normally prescribed in children 2 years of age or older.

What if I miss a dose?

If you miss a dose, take it as soon as you can. If it is almost time for the next dose, skip the previous dose. Do not use double or extra doses.

What may interact with montelukast?

- carbamazepine
- phenobarbital
- phenytoin
- rifabutin
- rifampin
- troglitazone

Tell your prescriber or health care professional about all other medicines you are taking, including non-prescription medicines. Also tell your prescriber or health care professional if you are a frequent user of drinks with caffeine or alcohol, if you smoke, or if you use illegal drugs. These may affect the way your medicine works. Check with your health care professional before stopping or starting any of your medicines.

What should I watch for while taking montelukast?

Montelukast is only used to help prevent asthma attacks; it is not used as a "quick-relief" medicine to treat an asthma attack. Therefore, you should always have your "quick-relief" medicine with you to treat an asthma attack. Talk with your prescriber about what you should do if you have an acute asthma attack. Tell your prescriber or health care professional if your symptoms do not improve or if your asthma gets worse. If

M

you find that your medicines become less effective in treating your asthma, you should contact your health care professional as soon as possible. Do not to stop taking or decrease the use of your other asthma treatments, including steroids, when starting montelukast unless otherwise directed by their health care prescriber. Follow your prescriber's directions exactly. Montelukast works best if you use it regularly even when you do not have asthma symptoms. Do not stop using your medication without your prescriber's advice. If you are going to have surgery, tell your health care professional that you take montelukast.

What side effects may I notice from using montelukast?

Side effects that you should report to your prescriber or health care professional as soon as possible:
Rare or uncommon:
- a feeling of pins and needles or numbness of arms and legs
- dark brown or yellow urine
- diarrhea
- easy bruising or bleeding
- edema or swelling of the legs or ankles
- fatigue or weakness
- fever
- flu-like illness
- muscle aches or cramps
- seizure or convulsion

- skin rash and itching
- severe stomach pain
- swelling of the face, lips, tongue, and/or throat, which may cause difficulty in breathing or swallowing
- vomiting
- wheezing or continued coughing
- yellowing of the eyes or skin

Side effects that usually do not require medical attention (report to your prescriber or health care professional if they continue or are bothersome):
- cough
- difficulty sleeping
- dizziness
- drowsiness
- headache
- heartburn
- hoarseness or sore throat
- indigestion or stomach upset
- muscle aches or cramps
- nausea
- runny nose
- unusual dreams

Where can I keep my medicine?

Keep out of the reach of children. Store at room temperature, between 15 and 30 degrees C (59 and 86 degrees F); do not freeze. Protect from light and moisture. Throw away any unused medicine after the expiration date.

Morphine sustained-release tablets or capsules

MS CONTIN®; 30 mg; Tablet, Extended Release Purdue Frederick Co

KADIAN®; 60 mg; Capsule, Extended Release Alpharma USPD Inc

What are morphine sustained-release tablets or capsules?

MORPHINE (MS Contin®, Oramorph®, Kadian®) relieves moderate to severe pain. Morphine may also be used to treat pain associated with cancer, heart attacks, sickle cell disease and other medical conditions. This type of morphine is for people who need pain medicine for more than a few days. These capsules and tablets are especially designed to release morphine over a period of time. Do not share this medicine with anyone else. Federal law prohibits the transfer of morphine to any person other than the patient for whom it was prescribed. Generic morphine sustained release tablets are available and capsules are not available.

What should my health care professional know before I take morphine?

They need to know if you have any of these conditions:
- if you frequently have alcohol-containing drinks
- abnormal bladder function, difficulty urinating
- constipation
- diarrhea
- head injury
- heart disease
- intestinal disease

- kidney disease
- liver disease
- lung disease or breathing difficulties (asthma, COPD)
- seizures
- an unusual or allergic reaction to morphine, oxycodone, codeine, other medicines, foods, dyes, or preservatives
- pregnant or trying to get pregnant
- breast-feeding

How should I take this medicine?

Take morphine sustained-release tablets or capsules by mouth. Follow the directions on the prescription label. Do not take morphine sustained-release products on an "as needed" basis; morphine sustained-release products should be taken on a regular basis only for the condition for which it was prescribed. Swallow the tablets with a drink of water. Do not break, crush, or chew morphine sustained-release tablets; this will cause the release of a large amount of morphine to be absorbed into your body at once, which can be dangerous causing an overdose and serious adverse reactions. If morphine upsets your stomach, you can take it with food or milk. If you are taking the morphine sustained-release capsules and have problems swallowing them, you may open them and sprinkle the contents on some applesauce. Make sure to eat the whole portion. Do not divide up into other doses or save portions. Eat it right away. Do not chew, crush or dissolve the pellets inside the capsule. Contact your pediatrician or health care professional regarding the use of this medicine in children. Special care may be needed. Do not share this medicine with anyone.

What if I miss a dose?

If you miss a dose, take it as soon as you can. If it is almost time for your next dose, take only that dose. Do not take double or extra doses.

What may interact with morphine?

- carbamazepine
- gabapentin
- medicines for high blood pressure
- metformin
- phenytoin
- phenobarbital
- primidone
- rifampin

Because morphine can cause drowsiness, other medicines that also cause drowsiness may increase this effect of morphine. Some medicines that cause drowsiness are:

- alcohol-containing medicines
- barbiturates such as phenobarbital
- certain antidepressants or tranquilizers
- muscle relaxants
- certain antihistamines used in cold medicines

Ask your prescriber or health care professional about other medicines that may increase the effect of morphine.
Tell your prescriber or health care professional about all other medicines that you are taking, including nonprescription medicines, nutritional supplements, or herbal products. Also, tell your prescriber or health care professional if you are a frequent user of drinks with caffeine or alcohol, if you smoke, or if you use illegal drugs. These may affect the way your medicine works. Check with your health care professional before stopping or starting any of your medicines.

What should I watch for while taking morphine?

Tell your prescriber or health care professional if your pain does not go away, if it gets worse, or if you have new or different type of pain. Use exactly as directed by your prescriber or health care professional. If you are taking morphine on a regular basis, do not suddenly stop taking it. Your body becomes used to the morphine and when you suddenly stop taking it, you may develop a severe reaction. This does NOT mean you are "addicted" to morphine. Addiction is a behavior related to getting and using a drug for a non-medical reason. If you have pain, you have a medical reason to take pain medicine such as morphine to control your pain. You may get drowsy or dizzy when you first start taking

morphine or change doses. Do not drive, use machinery, or do anything that needs mental alertness until you know how morphine affects you. Stand or sit up slowly, this reduces the risk of dizzy or fainting spells. These effects may be worse if you are an older patient. The drowsiness should decrease after taking morphine for a couple of days. If you have not slept because of your pain, you may sleep more the first few days your pain is controlled to catch-up on missed sleep. Be careful taking other medicines which may also make you tired. This effect may be worse when taking these medicines with morphine. Alcohol can increase possible drowsiness, dizziness, confusion and affect your breathing. Avoid alcohol while taking morphine. Morphine will cause constipation. Make sure to take a laxative and/or a stool softener while taking morphine. Try to have a bowel movement at least every 2 to 3 days. If you do not have a bowel movement for 3 days or more call your prescriber or health care professional. They may recommend using an enema or suppository to help you move your bowels. Your mouth may get dry. Drinking plenty of water, chewing sugarless gum or sucking on hard candy may help to relieve dry mouth symptoms. Have regular dental checks. If you are going to have surgery, tell your prescriber or health care professional that you are taking morphine. Rarely, morphine may cause you to have hallucinations (to see things that are not really there) or cause your legs or arms to "jerk" or have spasms. If you experience these effects, call your prescriber or health care professional.

What side effects may I notice from taking morphine?

Side effects that you should report to your prescriber or health care professional as soon as possible:
Rare or uncommon:
- breathing difficulties, wheezing
- cold, clammy skin
- seizures
- slow or fast heartbeat
- severe rash
- unusual weakness

More common:
- confusion
- lightheadedness or fainting spells
- nervousness or restlessness

Side effects that usually do not require medical attention (report to your prescriber or health care professional if they continue or are bothersome):
- itching
- blurred vision
- clumsiness, unsteadiness
- constipation
- decrease or difficulty passing urine
- dizziness, drowsiness
- dry mouth
- flushing
- headache

M

- nausea/vomiting
- pinpoint pupils
- sweating

Where can I keep my medicine?

Keep out of the reach of children in a container that small children cannot open. Do not share or give this medicine to anyone else. Avoid accidental swallowing of morphine by someone (especially children) other than the person for whom it was prescribed as this may result in severe effects and possibly death. Store at room temperature between 15 and 30 degrees C (59 and 86 degrees F). Protect from light. Throw away any unused medicine after the expiration date.

Morphine tablets or capsules

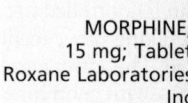

MORPHINE;
15 mg; Tablet
Roxane Laboratories
Inc

MORPHINE;
30 mg; Tablet
Ethex Corporation

What are morphine tablets or capsules?

MORPHINE (MSIR®) relieves moderate to severe pain. Morphine may be used to control the pain following surgery, child birth, and other procedures. Morphine may also be used to treat pain associated with cancer, heart attacks, sickle cell disease and other medical conditions. Do not share this medicine with anyone else. Federal law prohibits the transfer of morphine to any person other than the patient for whom it was prescribed. Generic morphine tablets are available.

What should my health care professional know before I take morphine?

They need to know if you have any of these conditions:
- if you frequently have alcohol-containing drinks
- abnormal bladder function, difficulty urinating
- constipation
- diarrhea
- head injury
- heart disease
- intestinal disease
- kidney disease
- liver disease
- lung disease or breathing difficulties (asthma, COPD)
- seizures
- an unusual or allergic reaction to morphine, oxycodone, codeine, other medicines, foods, dyes, or preservatives
- pregnant or trying to get pregnant
- breast-feeding

How should I take this medicine?

Take morphine tablets by mouth. Follow the directions on the prescription label. Swallow the tablets with a drink of water. If morphine upsets your stomach, you can take it with food or milk. If you are taking the capsules and have problems swallowing them, you may open them and sprinkle the contents on some applesauce or pudding. Make sure to eat the whole portion. Do not divide into other doses or save portions. Eat it right away. Contact your pediatrician or health care professional regarding the use of this medicine in children. Special care may be needed. Do not share this medicine with anyone.

What if I miss a dose?

If you miss a dose, take it as soon as you can. If it is almost time for your next dose, take only that dose. Do not take double or extra doses.

What may interact with morphine?

- carbamazepine
- gabapentin
- medicines for high blood pressure
- metformin
- phenytoin
- phenobarbital
- primidone
- rifampin

Because morphine can cause drowsiness, other medicines that also cause drowsiness may increase this effect of morphine. Some medicines that cause drowsiness are:

- alcohol-containing medicines
- barbiturates such as phenobarbital
- certain antidepressants or tranquilizers
- muscle relaxants
- certain antihistamines used in cold medicines

Ask your prescriber or health care professional about other medicines that may increase the effect of morphine. Tell your prescriber or health care professional about all other medicines that you are taking, including non-prescription medicines, nutritional supplements, or herbal products. Also, tell your prescriber or health care professional if you are a frequent user of drinks with caffeine or alcohol, if you smoke, or if you use illegal drugs. These may affect the way your medicine works. Check with your health care professional before stopping or starting any of your medicines.

What should I watch for while taking morphine?

Tell your prescriber or health care professional if your pain does not go away, if it gets worse, or if you have new or different type of pain. Use exactly as directed by your prescriber or health care professional. If you are taking morphine on a regular basis, do not suddenly stop taking it. Your body becomes used to the morphine and when you suddenly stop taking it, you may develop a severe reaction. This does NOT mean you are "ad-

M

dicted" to morphine. Addiction is a behavior related to getting and using a drug for a non-medical reason. If you have pain, you have a medical reason to take pain medicine such as morphine to control your pain. You may get drowsy or dizzy when you first start taking morphine or change doses. Do not drive, use machinery, or do anything that needs mental alertness until you know how morphine affects you. Stand or sit up slowly, this reduces the risk of dizzy or fainting spells. These effects may be worse if you are an older patient. The drowsiness should decrease after taking morphine for a couple of days. If you have not slept because of your pain, you may sleep more the first few days your pain is controlled to catch-up on missed sleep. Be careful taking other medicines which may also make you tired. This effect may be worse when taking these medicines with morphine. Alcohol can increase possible drowsiness, dizziness, confusion and affect your breathing. Avoid alcohol while taking morphine. Morphine will cause constipation. Make sure to take a laxative and/or a stool softener while taking morphine. Try to have a bowel movement every 2 to 3 days, at least. If you do not have a bowel movement for 3 days or more call your prescriber or health care professional. They may recommend using an enema or suppository to help you move your bowels. Your mouth may get dry. Drinking plenty of water, chewing sugarless gum or sucking on hard candy may help to relieve dry mouth symptoms. Have regular dental checks. If you are going to have surgery, tell your prescriber or health care professional that you are taking morphine. Rarely, morphine may cause you to have hallucinations (to see things that are not really there) or cause your legs or arms to "jerk" or have spasms. If you experience these effects, call your prescriber or health care professional.

What side effects may I notice from taking morphine?

Side effects that you should report to your prescriber or health care professional as soon as possible:

Rare or uncommon:
- breathing difficulties, wheezing
- cold, clammy skin
- seizures
- slow or fast heartbeat
- severe rash
- unusual weakness

More common:
- confusion
- lightheadedness or fainting spells
- nervousness or restlessness

Side effects that usually do not require medical attention (report to your prescriber or health care professional if they continue or are bothersome):
- itching
- blurred vision
- clumsiness, unsteadiness
- constipation
- decrease or difficulty passing urine
- dizziness, drowsiness
- dry mouth
- flushing
- headache
- nausea/vomiting
- pinpoint pupils
- sweating

Where can I keep my medicine?

Keep out of the reach of children in a container that small children cannot open. Do not share or give this medicine to anyone else. Avoid accidental swallowing of morphine by someone (especially children) other than the person for whom it was prescribed as this may result in severe effects and possibly death. Store at room temperature between 15 and 30 degrees C (59 and 86 degrees F). Protect from light. Throw away any unused medicine after the expiration date.

Moxifloxacin tablets

AVELOX®;
400 mg; Tablet
Schering Corp

What are moxifloxacin tablets?

MOXIFLOXACIN (Avelox®, Avelox® ABC Pack™) is an antibiotic. It kills certain bacteria or stops their growth. It is used to treat bronchitis, pneumonia, sinusitis, and certain skin infections. Generic moxifloxacin tablets are not yet available.

What should my health care professional know before I take moxifloxacin?

They need to know if you have any of these conditions:
- diabetes
- heart disease
- liver disease
- long exposure to sunlight (working outdoors)
- seizures (convulsions)
- stomach problems (especially colitis)
- stroke
- tendon or joint pain
- other chronic conditions
- an unusual or allergic reaction to fluoroquinolone antibiotics, foods, dyes, or preservatives
- pregnant or trying to get pregnant
- breast-feeding

How should I take this medicine?

Take moxifloxacin tablets by mouth with or without food. Follow the directions on the prescription label.

M

Swallow tablets whole with a full glass of water. Take your doses at regular intervals. Do not take your medicine more often than directed. Finish the full course prescribed by your prescriber or health care professional even if you think your condition is better. Do not stop taking except on your prescriber's advice. Contact your pediatrician or health care professional regarding the use of this medicine in children. Special care may be needed.

What if I miss a dose?

If you miss a dose, take it as soon as you remember. If it is almost time for your next dose, take only that dose. Do not take double or extra doses.

What may interact with moxifloxacin?

- aluminum salts
- antacids
- arsenic trioxide
- astemizole
- bepridil
- certain heart medications for irregular rhythm (e.g., amiodarone, disopyramide, dofetilide, flecainide, ibutilide, quinidine, procainamide, sotalol)
- certain medications for depression or other mental problems (e.g., tricyclic antidepressants, amoxapine, maprotiline, phenothiazines, haloperidol, pimozide, risperidone, sertindole, and ziprasidone)
- cisapride
- clarithromycin
- cyclobenzaprine
- cyclosporine
- didanosine (ddI)
- diuretics (water pills) such as furosemide or hydrochlorothiazide which can cause low potassium levels
- dolasetron
- droperidol
- erythromycin
- iron (ferrous sulfate) preparations
- levomethadyl
- magnesium salicylate
- magnesium salts
- manganese
- medicines for diabetes
- multivitamins that contain iron, magnesium, manganese, or zinc
- NSAIDs such as Advil®, Aleve®, ibuprofen, Motrin®, naproxen
- pentamidine
- probucol
- quinapril
- retinoid products such as tretinoin (Retin-A®, Renova®) or isotretinoin (Accutane®)
- sevelamer
- sucralfate
- terfenadine
- troleandomycin
- warfarin
- zinc salts
- ziprasidone

Tell your prescriber or health care professional about all other medicines you are taking, including non-prescription medicines, nutritional supplements, or herbal products. Also tell your prescriber or health care professional if you are a frequent user of drinks with caffeine or alcohol, if you smoke, or if you use illegal drugs. These may affect the way your medicine works. Check with your health care professional before stopping or starting any of your medicines.

What should I watch for while taking moxifloxacin?

Tell your prescriber or health care professional if your symptoms do not improve in 2 to 3 days. If you get an unusual reaction stop taking moxifloxacin and call your prescriber or health care professional for advice. If you are a diabetic, monitor your blood glucose carefully while on this medicine. You may get dizzy. Do not drive, use machinery, or do anything that needs mental alertness until you know how moxifloxacin affects you. To reduce the risk of dizzy or fainting spells, do not sit or stand up quickly, especially if you are an older patient. Many antacids and multivitamins can interfering with absorption of moxifloxacin. This may stop moxifloxacin from working. Take moxifloxacin either 4 hours before or 8 hours after taking any of these products. If you notice symptoms such as pain, burning, tingling, numbness and/or weakness, stop taking moxifloxacin and contact your healthcare provider immediately. If you notice pain or swelling of a tendon or around a joint, stop taking moxifloxacin. Rest the affected area and call your healthcare provider. Do not exercise or resume taking moxifloxacin until your healthcare provider tells you to do so. Keep out of the sun, or wear protective clothing outdoors and use a sunscreen. Do not use sun lamps or sun tanning beds or booths. If you are going to have surgery, tell your prescriber or health care professional that you are taking moxifloxacin.

What side effects may I notice from taking moxifloxacin?

Side effects that you should report to your prescriber or health care professional as soon as possible:
Rare or uncommon:
- confusion
- difficulty breathing
- irregular heartbeat, palpitations or chest pain
- joint, muscle or tendon pain
- seizures
- severe or watery diarrhea
- skin rash, itching
- swelling of the face or neck
- tingling in hands or feet
- tremor or restlessness
- unusual tiredness or weakness
- vision problems
- vomiting

Side effects that usually do not require medical atten-

tion (report to your prescriber or health care professional if they continue or are bothersome):

- diarrhea
- difficulty sleeping
- dizziness
- headache
- nausea or stomach upset

Mycophenolate delayed-release tablets

MYFORTIC®;
360 mg; Tablet, Delayed Release
Novartis Pharmaceuticals

What are mycophenolate delayed-release tablets?

MYCOPHENOLATE SODIUM (Myfortic®) is a medication used to decrease the immune system's response to a transplanted organ, which the body would otherwise see as foreign. Mycophenolate reduces unwanted immune responses and helps to prevent rejection in patients who receive kidney transplants. Generic mycophenolate sodium delayed-release tablets are not yet available.

What should my health care professional know before I take mycophenolate?

They need to know if you have any of these conditions:

- anemia or other blood disorder
- constipation
- diabetes mellitus
- diarrhea
- infection, bacterial or viral
- Lesch-Nyhan or Kelley-Seegmiller syndrome
- stomach ulcer
- unusual bleeding or bruising
- an unusual reaction to mycophenolate, medicines, foods, dyes, or preservatives
- pregnant or trying to get pregnant
- breast-feeding

How should I take this medicine?

Take mycophenolate sodium delayed-release tablets by mouth on an empty stomach. Follow the directions on the prescription label. Swallow the tablets with a drink of water. Take your doses at regular intervals. Do not take your medicine more often than directed. Do not cut, chew, or crush the tablets. Avoid contact with the contents of broken tablets. If contact occurs, rinse your exposed body area thoroughly with water. The mycophenolate sodium delayed-release tablets are different than the mycophenolate mofetil tablets. Do not substitute one for the other. Contact your pediatrician or health care professional regarding the use of this medicine in children. Special care may be needed.

What if I miss a dose?

If you miss a dose, take it as soon as you can. If it is almost time for your next dose, take only that dose. Do not take double or extra doses.

Where can I keep my medicine?

Keep out of the reach of children in a container that small children cannot open. Store at room temperature in a tightly closed container. Avoid high humidity. Throw away any unused medicine after the expiration date.

What may interact with mycophenolate?

- acyclovir or valacyclovir
- antacids
- cholestyramine or colestipol
- ganciclovir
- iron supplements, like ferrous sulfate
- oral contraceptives
- vaccines
- other medicines that suppress your immune system

Talk to your prescriber or health care professional before taking any of these medicines:

- aspirin
- acetaminophen
- ibuprofen
- ketoprofen
- naproxen

Tell your prescriber or health care professional about all other medicines you are taking, including non-prescription medicines, nutritional supplements, or herbal products. Also tell your prescriber or health care professional if you are a frequent user of drinks with caffeine or alcohol, if you smoke, or if you use illegal drugs. These may affect the way your medicine works. Check with your health care professional before stopping or starting any of your medicines.

What should I watch for while taking mycophenolate?

Visit your prescriber or health care professional for regular checks on your progress. You will need frequent blood checks during the first few months you are receiving mycophenolate tablets. Mycophenolate sodium can cause birth defects in animals. It is not known if it will cause birth defects in humans. Women who may have children must have a negative pregnancy test within 1 week of starting therapy. In addition, women must use two forms of effective birth control (condoms and birth control pills, for example) before, during and for 6 weeks after finishing treatment. Women who become pregnant should discuss the potential risks and options with their physician. Mycophenolate sodium will decrease your body's ability to fight infections. Call your prescriber or health care professional if you have a

M

fever, chills, sore throat or other symptoms of a cold or flu. Do not treat these symptoms yourself. Try to avoid being around people who are sick. Mycophenolate sodium may increase your risk to bruise or bleed. Call your prescriber or health care professional if you notice any unusual bruising or bleeding. After you stop taking this medication, side effects can continue. Some side effects may not occur until years after the medicine was taken. These effects can include the development of certain types of cancer. Discuss this possibility with your prescriber or health care professional. Mycophenolate sodium may increase your risk for certain types of skin cancer. To decrease your risk, wear protective clothing, including hats, and use sunscreen with a high protection factor when exposed to the sun. Avoid using tanning beds. Unless instructed otherwise by your prescriber or health care professional, avoid taking over-the-counter products that contain aspirin, acetaminophen or a nonsteroidal anti-inflammatory drug. A fever or symptoms of an infection may be masked. If you are unsure if a product contains one of these ingredients, ask your doctor or pharmacist. Your blood sugar may increase. Ask your prescriber or health care professional for advice if you have diabetes and notice a change in your blood sugar level.

What side effects may I notice from receiving mycophenolate?

Side effects that you should report to your prescriber or health care professional as soon as possible:

- back pain or general pain
- blood in urine
- chest pain, irregular heartbeats
- difficulty breathing, wheezing
- dizziness or fainting
- fever, chills or sore throat
- increased thirst
- increase in the frequency and amount of urine passed
- swelling of the feet or legs
- swollen face or tongue
- unusual bleeding or bruising
- unusual tiredness or weakness

Side effects that usually do not require medical attention (report to your prescriber or health care professional if they continue or are bothersome):

- constipation
- diarrhea or soft stools
- difficulty sleeping
- gas
- loss of appetite
- nausea, vomiting
- stomach pain or indigestion

Where can I keep my medicine?

Keep out of the reach of children in a container that small children cannot open. Store in a cool, dry place. Keep your medicine in the original container with the lid tightly closed. Throw away any unused medicine after the expiration date.

Mycophenolate mofetil tablets or capsules	CELLCEPT®; 250 mg; Capsule Hoffmann La Roche Inc		CELLCEPT®; 500 mg; Tablet Hoffmann La Roche Inc.	

What are mycophenolate mofetil tablets or capsules?

MYCOPHENOLATE MOFETIL (CellCept®) is a medication used to decrease the immune system's response to a transplanted organ, which the body would otherwise see as foreign. Mycophenolate reduces unwanted immune responses and helps to prevent rejection in patients who receive organ or bone marrow transplants. Mycophenolate mofetil also can be used to treat severe rheumatoid arthritis or psoriasis. Generic mycophenolate mofetil capsules or tablets are not yet available.

What should my health care professional know before I take mycophenolate mofetil?

They need to know if you have any of these conditions:
- anemia or other blood disorder
- diarrhea
- infection, bacterial or viral
- stomach ulcer
- unusual bleeding or bruising
- an unusual or allergic reaction to mycophenolate mofetil, other medicines, foods, dyes, or preservatives

- pregnant or trying to get pregnant
- breast-feeding

How should I take this medicine?

Take mycophenolate mofetil capsules and tablets by mouth on an empty stomach. Follow the directions on the prescription label. Swallow the capsules or tablets with a drink of water. Take your doses at regular intervals. Do not take your medicine more often than directed. Do not crush the tablets or open the capsules. Avoid contact with the contents of the capsules or broken tablets. If contact occurs, rinse thoroughly with water. Contact your pediatrician or health care professional regarding the use of this medicine in children. Special care may be needed.

What if I miss a dose?

If you miss a dose, take it as soon as you can. If it is almost time for your next dose, take only that dose. Do not take double or extra doses.

What may interact with mycophenolate mofetil?

- acyclovir or valacyclovir
- antacids

- cholestyramine or colestipol
- ganciclovir
- iron supplements, like ferrous sulfate
- oral contraceptives
- vaccines
- other medicines that suppress your immune system

Talk to your prescriber or health care professional before taking any of these medicines:

- aspirin
- acetaminophen
- ibuprofen
- ketoprofen
- naproxen

Tell your prescriber or health care professional about all other medicines you are taking, including non-prescription medicines, nutritional supplements, or herbal products. Also tell your prescriber or health care professional if you are a frequent user of drinks with caffeine or alcohol, if you smoke, or if you use illegal drugs. These may affect the way your medicine works. Check with your health care professional before stopping or starting any of your medicines.

What should I watch for while taking mycophenolate mofetil?

Visit your prescriber or health care professional for regular checks on your progress. You will need frequent blood checks during the first few months you are receiving mycophenolate capsules. Mycophenolate mofetil can cause birth defects in animals. It is not known if it will cause birth defects in humans. Women who may have children must have a negative pregnancy test within 1 week of starting therapy. In addition, women must use two forms of effective birth control (condoms and birth control pills, for example) before, during and for 6 weeks after finishing treatment. Women who become pregnant should discuss the potential risks and options with their physician. Mycophenolate mofetil will decrease your body's ability to fight infections. Call your prescriber or health care professional if you have a fever, chills, sore throat or other symptoms of a cold or flu. Do not treat these symptoms yourself. Try to avoid being around people who are sick. Mycophenolate mofetil may increase your risk to bruise or bleed. Call your prescriber or health care professional if you notice any unusual bruising or bleeding. After you stop taking this medication, side effects can continue. Some

side effects may not occur until years after the medicine was taken. These effects can include the development of certain types of cancer. Discuss this possibility with your prescriber or health care professional. Mycophenolate mofetil may increase your risk for certain types of skin cancer. To decrease your risk, were protective clothing, including hats, and use sunscreen with a high protection factor when exposed to the sun. Avoid using tanning beds. Avoid taking aspirin, acetaminophen (Tylenol®), ibuprofen (Advil®), ketoprofen (Orudis KT®), or naproxen (Aleve®) products as these may mask a fever, unless instructed to by your prescriber or health care professional. Your blood sugar may increase. Ask your prescriber or health care professional for advice if you are diabetic and notice a change in your blood sugar level.

What side effects may I notice from taking mycophenolate mofetil?

Side effects that you should report to your prescriber or health care professional as soon as possible:

- back pain or general pain
- blood in urine
- chest pain, irregular heartbeats
- difficulty breathing, wheezing
- dizziness or fainting
- fever, chills or sore throat
- increased thirst
- increase in the frequency and amount of urine passed
- swelling of the feet or legs
- swollen face or tongue
- unusual bleeding or bruising
- unusual tiredness or weakness

Side effects that usually do not require medical attention (report to your prescriber or health care professional if they continue or are bothersome):

- constipation
- diarrhea or soft stools
- difficulty sleeping
- gas
- loss of appetite
- nausea, vomiting
- stomach pain or indigestion

Where can I keep my medicine?

Keep out of the reach of children in a container that small children cannot open. Store in a cool, dry place. Throw away any unused medicine after the expiration date.

M

This drug requires an FDA medication guide. See page xxxvii.

Nabumetone tablets

RELAFEN®;
500 mg; Tablet
SmithKline Beecham
Corp

RELAFEN®;
750 mg; Tablet
SmithKline Beecham
Corp

What do nabumetone tablets do?

NABUMETONE (Relafen®) is a nonsteroidal anti-inflammatory drug (NSAID). It helps relieve pain and inflammation associated with rheumatoid arthritis and osteoarthritis. Generic nabumetone tablets are available.

What should my health care professional know before I take nabumetone?

They need to know if you have any of these conditions:
- anemia
- asthma, especially aspirin sensitive asthma
- bleeding problems or taking medicines that make you bleed more easily such as anticoagulants ("blood thinners")
- cigarette smoker
- diabetes
- drink more than three alcohol-containing beverages a day
- heart failure
- high blood pressure
- kidney disease
- liver disease
- anemia
- stomach ulcers or pain
- systemic lupus erythematosus
- ulcerative colitis
- an unusual or allergic reaction to aspirin, other salicylates, other NSAIDs, other medicines, foods, dyes or preservatives
- pregnant or trying to get pregnant
- breast-feeding

How should I take this medicine?

Take nabumetone tablets by mouth. Follow the directions on the prescription label. Swallow tablets whole with a full glass of water; take tablets in an upright or sitting position. Taking a sip of water first, before taking the tablets, may help you swallow them. If possible take bedtime doses at least 10 minutes before lying down. You can take nabumetone with food to prevent stomach upset. Take your doses at regular intervals. Do not take your medicine more often than directed. Contact your pediatrician or health care professional regarding the use of this medicine in children. Special care may be needed.

What if I miss a dose?

If you miss a dose, take it as soon as you can. If it is almost time for your next dose, take only that dose. Do not take double or extra doses.

What may interact with nabumetone?

- alcohol
- anti-inflammatory drugs (other NSAIDs, prednisone)
- aspirin and aspirin-like medicines
- cidofovir
- cyclosporine
- entecavir
- herbal products that contain feverfew, garlic, ginger, or ginkgo biloba
- lithium
- medicines for high blood pressure
- medicines that affect platelets
- medicines that treat or prevent blood clots such as warfarin and other "blood thinners"
- methotrexate
- pemetrexed
- water pills (diuretics)

Tell your prescriber or health care professional about all other medicines you are taking, including non-prescription medicines, nutritional supplements, or herbal products. Also tell your prescriber or health care professional if you are a frequent user of drinks with caffeine or alcohol, if you smoke, or if you use illegal drugs. These may affect the way your medicine works. Check with your health care professional before stopping or starting any of your medicines.

What should I watch for while taking nabumetone?

Let your prescriber or health care professional know if your pain continues. Do not take nabumetone with other pain killers without advice. If you get flu-like symptoms (fever, chills, muscle aches and pains), call your prescriber or health care professional; do not treat yourself. To reduce unpleasant effects on your throat and stomach, take nabumetone with a full glass of water and never just before lying down. If you notice black, tarry stools or experience severe stomach pain and/or vomit blood or what looks like coffee grounds, notify your health care prescriber immediately. If you are taking medicines that affect the clotting of your blood, such as aspirin or blood thinners such as Coumadin®, talk to your health care provider or prescriber before taking this medicine. You may get dizzy. Do not drive, use machinery, or do anything that needs mental alertness until you know how nabumetone affects you. Do not sit or stand up quickly, especially if you are an older patient. This reduces the risk of dizzy or fainting spells. Do not smoke cigarettes or drink alcohol; these increase irritation to your stomach and can make it more susceptible to damage from nabumetone. If you are going to have surgery, tell your prescriber or health care professional that you are taking this medicine. Problems can arise if you need dental work, and in the day-to-day care of your teeth. Try to avoid damage to your teeth and gums when you brush or floss your teeth.

N

It is especially important not to use nabumetone during the last 3 months of pregnancy unless specifically directed to do so by your health care provider. Nabumetone may cause problems in the unborn child or complications during delivery.

What side effects may I notice from taking nabumetone?

Side effects that you should report to your prescriber or health care professional as soon as possible:
- signs of bleeding—bruising, pinpoint red spots on the skin, black tarry stools, blood in the urine, unusual tiredness or weakness, vomiting blood or vomit that looks like coffee grounds
- signs of an allergic reaction—difficulty breathing or wheezing, skin rash, redness, blistering or peeling skin, hives, or itching, swelling of eyelids, throat, lips
- blurred vision
- change in the amount of urine passed
- difficulty swallowing, severe heartburn or burning, pain in throat

- pain or difficulty passing urine
- stomach pain or cramps
- swelling of feet or ankles
- yellowing of the eyes or skin

Side effects that usually do not require medical attention (report to your prescriber or health care professional if they continue or are bothersome):
- diarrhea
- dizziness
- drowsiness
- gas or heartburn
- headache
- nausea, vomiting

Where can I keep my medicine?

Keep out of the reach of children in a container that small children cannot open. Store at room temperature between 15 and 30 degrees C (59 and 86 degrees F). Protect from light. Keep container tightly closed. Throw away any unused medicine after the expiration date.

Nadolol tablets

CORGARD®;
120 mg; Tablet
Monarch
Pharmaceuticals Inc

CORGARD®;
80 mg; Tablet
Monarch
Pharmaceuticals Inc

What are nadolol tablets?

NADOLOL (Corgard®) belongs to a group of medicines called beta-blockers. Beta-blockers reduce the workload on the heart and help it to beat more regularly. Nadolol controls, but does not cure, high blood pressure (hypertension). High blood pressure may not make you feel sick, but it can lead to serious heart problems. Nadolol also relieves chest pain (angina). Nadolol is also sometimes used to help decease tremor or anxiety. Generic nadolol tablets are available.

What should my health care professional know before I take nadolol?

They need to know if you have any of these conditions:
- angina (chest pain)
- asthma, bronchitis or bronchospasm
- circulation problems, or blood vessel disease (such as Raynaud's disease)
- depression
- diabetes
- emphysema, or other lung disease
- history of heart attack or heart disease
- muscle weakness or disease
- pheochromocytoma
- psoriasis
- thyroid disease
- an unusual or allergic reaction to nadolol, other beta-blockers, medicines, foods, dyes, or preservatives
- pregnant or trying to get pregnant
- breast-feeding

How should I take this medicine?

Take nadolol tablets by mouth. Follow the directions on the prescription label. Swallow the tablets with a

drink of water. Take your doses at regular intervals. Do not take your medicine more often than directed. Do not stop taking except on your prescriber's advice. Contact your pediatrician or health care professional regarding the use of this medicine in children. Special care may be needed.

What if I miss a dose?

If you miss a dose, take it as soon as you can. If it is almost time for your next dose, take only that dose. Do not take double or extra doses.

What may interact with nadolol?

- anti-inflammatory drugs (NSAIDs, such as ibuprofen)
- atropine
- cocaine
- hawthorn
- medicines for chest pain or angina
- medicines for colds and breathing difficulties
- medicines for diabetes
- medicines for high blood pressure
- medicine for mental problems or psychotic disturbances
- medicines to control heart rhythm
- water pills

Tell your prescriber or health care professional about all other medicines you are taking, including nonprescription medicines, nutritional supplements, or herbal products. Also tell your prescriber or health care professional if you are a frequent user of drinks with caffeine or alcohol, if you smoke, or if you use illegal drugs. These may affect the way your medicine works. Check

N

with your health care professional before stopping or starting any of your medicines.

What should I watch for while taking nadolol?

Check your heart rate and blood pressure regularly while you are taking nadolol. Ask your prescriber or health care professional what your heart rate and blood pressure should be, and when you should contact him or her. Do not stop taking this medicine suddenly. This could lead to serious heart-related effects. You may get drowsy or dizzy. Do not drive, use machinery, or do anything that requires mental alertness until you know how nadolol affects you. To reduce the risk of dizzy or fainting spells, do not sit or stand up quickly. Alcohol can make you more drowsy, and increase flushing and rapid heartbeats. Therefore, it is best to avoid alcoholic drinks. Nadolol can affect blood sugar levels. If you have diabetes, check with your prescriber or health care professional before you change your diet or the dose of your diabetic medicine. If you are going to have surgery, tell your prescriber or health care professional that you are taking nadolol.

What side effects may I notice from taking nadolol?

Side effects that you should report to your prescriber or health care professional as soon as possible:

- cold, tingling, or numb hands or feet
- difficulty breathing, wheezing
- dizziness or fainting spells
- increase in the amount of urine passed
- increased thirst
- irregular heartbeat
- mental depression
- skin rash, peeling
- slow heart rate (less than 50 beats a minute)
- swelling of the legs or ankles
- weight loss

Side effects that usually do not require medical attention (report to your prescriber or health care professional if they continue or are bothersome):

- darkened skin color
- dry itching skin
- headache
- unusual tiredness

Where can I keep my medicine?

Keep out of the reach of children in a container that small children cannot open. Store at room temperature, approximately 25 degrees C (77 degrees F). Protect from light. Keep container tightly closed. Throw away any unused medicine after the expiration date.

Naltrexone tablets

DEPADE®;
100 mg; Tablet
Mallinckrodt Inc
Pharmaceuticals Group

What are naltrexone tablets?

NALTREXONE (Depade®, ReVia®) helps you to remain free of your dependence on opiate drugs (narcotics) or alcohol. Naltrexone works by blocking the "high" that these substances can give you. Naltrexone therapy is combined with counseling and support groups. You can only use naltrexone after an initial detoxification period. If you take naltrexone while you are still taking opiate drugs, you can induce withdrawal symptoms. Generic naltrexone tablets are available.

What should my health care professional know before I take naltrexone?

They need to know if you have any of these conditions:
- if you are still using opiate drugs (narcotics) or alcohol
- liver disease, including hepatitis
- kidney disease
- an unusual or allergic reaction to naltrexone, other medicines, foods, dyes, or preservatives
- pregnant or trying to get pregnant
- breast-feeding

How should I take this medicine?

Take naltrexone tablets by mouth. Follow the directions on the prescription label. Swallow the tablets with a drink of water. Take your doses at regular intervals and with food to decrease the side effects. Do not take your medicine more often than directed. Contact your pediatrician or health care professional regarding the use of this medicine in children. Special care may be needed.

What if I miss a dose?

If you miss a dose and remember on the same day, take the missed dose. If you do not remember until the next day, ask your prescriber or health care professional about rescheduling your doses. Do not take double or extra doses.

What may interact with naltrexone?

- certain medicines for mental problems and psychotic disturbances
- certain medicines for pain (for example, medicines containing codeine or propoxyphene)
- clonidine
- disulfiram

Tell your prescriber or health care professional about all other medicines you are taking, including non-prescription medicines, nutritional supplements, or herbal products. Also tell your prescriber or health care professional if you are a frequent user of drinks with caffeine

N

or alcohol, if you smoke, or if you use illegal drugs. These may affect the way your medicine works. Check with your health care professional before stopping or starting any of your medicines.

What should I watch for while taking naltrexone?

Report to your prescriber or health care professional regularly. It is important to attend any counseling or support groups that your prescriber or health care professional recommends. Attending these sessions while you are taking naltrexone will help you remain free of your dependence on opiate drugs or alcohol. Never try to overcome the effects of naltrexone by taking large amounts of narcotics because this can cause coma and death. If you are going to have surgery, tell your prescriber or health care professional that you are taking naltrexone. It is a good idea to carry a card in case of emergency to alert medical personnel that you are taking naltrexone. Do not treat yourself for coughs, colds, pain or diarrhea. Ask your prescriber or health care professional for advice. Some of the ingredients may interact with naltrexone and cause side effects. You may feel dizzy or lightheaded. Do not drive, use machinery, or do anything that needs mental alertness until you know how naltrexone affects you.

What side effects may I notice from taking naltrexone?

Naltrexone causes few side effects in patients who are not taking opiate drugs. Some of the side effects listed below can occur only if you are still taking opiate drugs. Side effects that you should report to your prescriber or health care professional as soon as possible:
- blurred vision or other eye problems
- confusion
- difficult or frequent passing of urine
- difficulty in awaking from sleep
- earache, ringing in the ears
- fast or pounding heartbeat (palpitations)
- fever

- hallucinations (seeing and hearing things that are not really there)
- mood changes
- nose bleeds
- pain, tenderness, or color changes in the legs or feet
- shortness of breath
- skin rash, itching
- slowed breathing
- swelling of the face, feet, or lower legs
- swollen glands
- weight gain
- yellow color of your eyes or skin

Side effects that usually do not require medical attention (report to your prescriber or health care professional if they continue or are bothersome):
Rare or uncommon, unless you are still taking narcotics:
- anxiety, nervousness, restlessness
- chills, sore throat
- constipation or diarrhea
- cough, hoarseness
- increased thirst
- irritability
- joint or muscle pain
- loss of appetite
- runny nose, sinus problems, sneezing
- sexual problems in males
- stomach cramps or pain

More common:
- anxiety
- difficulty sleeping
- dizziness
- headache
- increased tiredness
- nausea
- nervousness
- vomiting

Where can I keep my medicine?

Keep out of the reach of children in a container that small children cannot open. Store at room temperature between 15 and 30 degrees C (59 and 86 degrees F). Protect from light. Keep container tightly closed. Throw away any unused medicine after the expiration date.

Naproxen tablets, caplets, or delayed-release tablets

NAPROSYN®;
375 mg; Tablet,
Delayed Release
Hoffmann La Roche
Inc

ALEVE®;
220 mg; Tablet
Bayer Corp
Consumer Care Div

This drug requires an FDA medication guide. See page xxxvii.

N

What are naproxen tablets, caplets, or delayed-release tablets?

NAPROXEN (Naprosyn®, EC Naprosyn®, Naprelan®, Anaprox®, Anaprox® DS, Aleve®) is an anti-inflammatory drug. It relieves pain and inflammation associated with rheumatoid arthritis, osteoarthritis, and juvenile (childhood) arthritis. Naproxen is also effective in treating other mild to moderate pain, including menstrual pain, headache, toothache, and temporarily reduces fever. Naproxen should only be used in children who are over 12 years old. Generic naproxen tablets and delayed-release tablets are available.

What should my health care professional know before I take naproxen?

They need to know if you have any of these conditions:
- anemia
- asthma, especially aspirin sensitive asthma
- bleeding problems or taking medicines that make you bleed easily such as anticoagulants ("blood thinners")
- cigarette smoker

- diabetes
- drink more than three alcohol-containing beverages a day
- heart failure
- high blood pressure
- kidney disease
- liver disease
- stomach or duodenal ulcers
- systemic lupus erythematosus
- ulcerative colitis
- an unusual or allergic reaction to aspirin, other salicylates, other NSAIDs, other medicines, foods, dyes or preservatives
- pregnant or trying to get pregnant
- breast-feeding

How should I take this medicine?

Take naproxen tablets by mouth. Follow the directions on the prescription label. Swallow tablets whole with a full glass of water; take tablets in an upright or sitting position. Taking a sip of water first, before taking the tablets, may help you swallow them. If possible take bedtime doses at least 10 minutes before lying down. You can take naproxen with food to prevent stomach upset. If you are taking the delayed-release tablets swallow them whole; do not crush or chew. Take your doses at regular intervals. Do not take your medicine more often than directed. Contact your pediatrician or health care professional regarding the use of this medicine in children. Special care may be needed. Do not give to children less than 12 years unless directed by your health care provider.

What if I miss a dose?

If you miss a dose, take it as soon as you can. If it is almost time for your next dose, take only that dose. Do not take double or extra doses.

What other drug(s) may interact with naproxen?

- alcohol
- alendronate
- aspirin and aspirin-like medicines
- cidofovir
- cyclosporine
- entecavir
- herbal products that contain feverfew, garlic, ginger, or ginkgo biloba
- lithium
- medicines for high blood pressure
- medicines that affect platelets
- medicines that treat or prevent blood clots such as warfarin and other "blood thinners"
- methotrexate
- other anti-inflammatory drugs (such as ibuprofen or prednisone)
- pemetrexed
- water pills (diuretics)

Tell your prescriber or health care professional about all other medicines you are taking, including non-prescription medicines, nutritional supplements, or herbal products. Also tell your prescriber or health care professional if you are a frequent user of drinks with caffeine or alcohol, if you smoke, or if you use illegal drugs. These may affect the way your medicine works. Check with your health care professional before stopping or starting any of your medicines.

What should I watch for while I taking naproxen?

Let your prescriber or health care professional know if your pain continues. Do not take naproxen with other pain killers without advice. If you get flu-like symptoms (fever, chills, muscle aches and pains), call your prescriber or health care professional; do not treat yourself. Do not treat yourself for pain more than 10 days or for fever more than 3 days without consulting your health care provider. To reduce unpleasant effects on your throat and stomach, take naproxen with a full glass of water and never just before lying down. If you notice black, tarry stools or experience severe stomach pain and vomit blood or what looks like coffee grounds, notify your health care prescriber immediately. If you are taking medicines that affect the clotting of your blood, such as aspirin or blood thinners such as Coumadin®, talk to your health care provider or prescriber before taking this medicine. You may get dizzy. Do not drive, use machinery, or do anything that needs mental alertness until you know how naproxen affects you. Stand or sit up slowly, this reduces the risk of dizzy or fainting spells. These effects may be worse if you are an older patient. Do not smoke cigarettes or drink alcohol; these increase irritation to your stomach and can make it more susceptible to damage from naproxen. It is especially important not to use naproxen during the last 3 months of pregnancy unless specifically directed to do so by your health care provider. Naproxen may cause problems in the unborn child or complications during delivery. If you are going to have surgery, tell your prescriber or health care professional that you are taking naproxen. Problems can arise if you need dental work, and in the day-to-day care of your teeth. Try to avoid damage to your teeth and gums when you brush or floss your teeth.

What side effects may I notice from taking naproxen?

Side effects that you should report to your prescriber or health care professional as soon as possible:

- signs of bleeding—bruising, pinpoint red spots on the skin, black tarry stools, blood in the urine, unusual tiredness or weakness, vomiting blood or vomit that looks like coffee grounds
- signs of an allergic reaction—difficulty breathing or wheezing, skin rash, redness, blistering or peeling skin, hives, or itching, swelling of eyelids, throat, lips
- blurred vision
- change in the amount of urine passed
- difficulty swallowing, severe heartburn or burning, pain in throat

- pain or difficulty passing urine
- stomach pain or cramps
- swelling of feet or ankles
- yellowing of eyes or skin

Side effects that usually do not require medical attention (report to your prescriber or health care professional if they continue or are bothersome):
- diarrhea or constipation
- dizziness
- drowsiness

- gas or heartburn
- headache
- nausea, vomiting

Where can I keep my medicine?
Keep out of the reach of children in a container that small children cannot open. Store at room temperature between 15 and 30 degrees C (59 and 86 degrees F). Protect from light. Keep container tightly closed. Throw away any unused medicine after the expiration date.

Naratriptan tablets

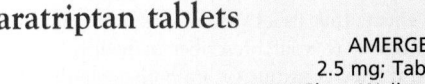

AMERGE®;
2.5 mg; Tablet
Glaxo Wellcome

AMERGE®;
1 mg; Tablet
Glaxo Wellcome

What are naratriptan tablets?
NARATRIPTAN (Amerge®) helps to relieve a migraine attack that starts with or without aura (a peculiar feeling or visual disturbance that warns you of an attack). Generic naratriptan tablets are not yet available.

What should my health care professional know before I take naratriptan?
They need to know if you have any of these conditions:
- bowel disease or colitis
- diabetes
- family history of heart disease
- fast or irregular heartbeat
- headaches that are different from your usual migraine
- heart or blood vessel disease, angina (chest pain), or previous heart attack
- high blood pressure
- high cholesterol
- history of stroke, transient ischemic attacks (TIAs or "mini-strokes"), or intracranial bleeding
- kidney disease
- liver disease
- overweight
- poor circulation
- postmenopausal or surgical removal of uterus and ovaries
- Raynaud's syndrome
- seizure disorder
- tobacco smoker
- an unusual or allergic reaction to naratriptan, other medicines, foods, dyes, or preservatives
- pregnant or trying to get pregnant
- breast-feeding

How should I take this medicine?
Take naratriptan tablets by mouth. Follow the directions on the prescription label. Naratriptan is taken after the migraine attack starts; it is not for everyday use. Swallow the tablets whole with fluids. If your migraine headache returns after one dose, you can take another dose as directed. You must allow at least 4 hours between doses, and do not take more than 5 mg in 24 hours. If there is no improvement at all after the first dose, do not take a second dose without talking to your prescriber or health care professional. Do not take your medicine more often than directed. Contact your pediatrician or health care professional regarding the use of this medicine in children. Special care may be needed.

What if I miss a dose?
This does not apply; naratriptan is not for regular use.

What may interact with naratriptan?
Do not take naratriptan with any of the following medicines:

- amphetamine or cocaine
- dihydroergotamine, ergotamine, ergoloid mesylates, methysergide, or ergot-type medication—do not take within 24 hours of taking naratriptan.
- almotriptan, eletriptan, rizatriptan, sumatriptan, zolmitriptan—do not take within 24 hours of taking naratriptan.
- medicines for weight loss such as dexfenfluramine, dextroamphetamine, fenfluramine, or sibutramine
- monoamine oxidase inhibitors (MAOIs) such as phenelzine (Nardil®), tranylcypromine (Parnate®), isocarboxazid (Marplan®), and selegiline (Carbex®, Eldepryl®)—do not take naratriptan within 2 weeks of stopping MAOI therapy.

Check with your doctor or pharmacist if you take any of these medications:

- birth control pills
- cough syrup or other products containing dextromethorphan
- feverfew
- lithium
- medicines for mental depression, anxiety or mood problems such as buspirone, citalopram, fluoxetine, fluvoxamine, mirtazapine, nefazodone, paroxetine, sertraline, trazodone, tricyclic antidepressants, or venlafaxine
- meperidine
- St. John's wort
- tryptophan

Tell your physician or health care provider about all other medicines you are taking, including non-pre-

N

scription medicines; if you are a frequent user of drinks with caffeine or alcohol; if you smoke; or if you use illegal drugs. These may affect the way your medicine works. Check with your health care professional before stopping or starting any of your medicines.

What should I watch for while taking naratriptan?

Only take naratriptan tablets for a migraine headache. Take it if you get warning symptoms or at the start of a migraine attack. Naratriptan is not for regular use to prevent migraine attacks. Do not take it if your headache symptoms are different than your usual attacks; consult your doctor first. Do not take migraine products that contain ergotamine while you are taking naratriptan; this combination can affect your heart. You may get drowsy or dizzy. Do not drive, use machinery, or do anything that needs mental alertness until you know how naratriptan affects you. To reduce dizzy or fainting spells, do not sit or stand up quickly, especially if you are an older patient. Alcohol can increase drowsiness, dizziness and flushing. Avoid alcoholic drinks. Smoking cigarettes may increase the risk of heart-related side effects from using naratriptan.

What side effects may I notice from taking naratriptan?

Side effects that you should report to your prescriber as soon as possible:

- chest, neck, or throat pain or tightness
- dizziness or faintness
- fast or irregular heart beat, palpitations
- feeling of chest heaviness or pressure
- increased blood pressure
- severe stomach pain and cramping, bloody diarrhea
- shortness of breath, wheezing, or difficulty breathing
- tingling, pain, or numbness in the face, hands or feet
- unusual reaction or swelling of the skin, eyelids, face, or lips

Stop using naratriptan and call your prescriber as soon as you can if you get any of these side effects.

Side effects that usually do not require medical attention (report to your prescriber or health care professional if they continue or are bothersome):

- drowsiness
- dry mouth
- feeling warm, flushing, or redness of the face
- nausea, vomiting, or stomach upset
- tiredness or weakness

Where can I keep my medicine?

Keep out of the reach of children in a container that small children cannot open. Store at room temperature between 20 and 25 degrees C (68 and 77 degrees F). Protect from light and moisture. Throw away any unused medicine after the expiration date.

Nateglinide tablets

STARLIX®; 120 mg; Tablet Novartis Pharmaceuticals

STARLIX®; 60 mg; Tablet Novartis Pharmaceuticals

What is nateglinide?

NATEGLINIDE (Starlix®) is a medicine used to lower blood sugar in patients with type 2 diabetes mellitus. It is sometimes used with other medicines for diabetes. Generic nateglinide tablets are not yet available.

What should my health care professional know before I use nateglinide?

They need to know if you have any of these conditions:

- diabetic ketoacidosis
- liver disease
- an unusual or allergic reaction to nateglinide, other medicines, foods, dyes, or preservatives
- pregnant or trying to get pregnant
- breast-feeding

How should I use this medicine?

Take nateglinide tablets by mouth. Follow the directions on the prescription label. Swallow the tablets with a drink of water. Do not chew the tablets. Nateglinide is usually taken three times a day with a meal. Each dose should be taken 1 to 30 minutes before each meal. If you skip a meal, do not take that dose of nateg-linide. Do not take your medicine more often than directed. Do not take nateglinide without a meal. Do not stop taking except on your prescriber's advice. Contact your pediatrician or health care professional regarding the use of this medicine in children. Special care may be needed.

What if I miss a dose?

If you miss a dose before a meal, skip that dose. If it is almost time for your next dose, take only that dose with the next scheduled meal as directed. Do not take double or extra doses.

What may interact with nateglinide?

Certain medications may interfere with the way your body maintains its blood sugar. Such medications may include:

- beta-blockers such as propranolol or nadolol
- chromium, or multivitamins with trace elements
- corticosteroids such as prednisone or cortisone
- diuretics such as hydrochlorothiazide
- estrogens
- ethanol

N

- isoniazid
- antidepressant drugs such as phenelzine
- niacin
- birth control pills
- chlorpromazine and other drugs similar to chlorpromazine
- herbal supplements such as black cohosh, ephedra, garlic, and horse chestnut
- phenytoin
- probenecid
- rifampin, rifabutin, rifapentine
- salicylates such as aspirin
- sulfonamides
- drugs used for weight loss, or decongestants such as pseudoephedrine
- thyroid hormones

Tell your prescriber or health care professional about all other medicines you are taking, including non-prescription medicines, nutritional supplements, or herbal products. Also tell your prescriber or health care professional if you are a frequent user of drinks with caffeine or alcohol, if you smoke, or if you use illegal drugs. These may affect the way your medicine works. Check with your health care professional before stopping or starting any of your medicines.

What should I watch for while taking nateglinide?

Visit your prescriber or health care professional for regular checks on your progress. Learn how to monitor blood or urine sugar and urine ketones regularly. Check with your prescriber or health care professional if your blood sugar is high, you may need a change of dose of nateglinide. Do not skip meals. If you are exercising much more than usual you may need extra snacks to avoid side effects caused by low blood sugar. Alcohol can increase possible side effects of nateglinide. Ask

your prescriber or health care professional if you should avoid alcohol. If you have mild symptoms of low blood sugar, eat or drink something containing sugar at once and contact your prescriber or health care professional. It is wise to check your blood sugar to confirm that it is low. It is important to recognize your own symptoms of low blood sugar so that you can treat them quickly. Make sure family members know that you can choke if you eat or drink when you develop serious symptoms of low blood sugar, such as seizures or unconsciousness. They must get medical help at once. If you are going to have surgery, tell your prescriber or health care professional that you are taking nateglinide. Wear a medical identification bracelet or chain to say you have diabetes, and carry a card that lists all your medications.

What side effects may I notice from using nateglinide?

Side effects that you should report to your prescriber or health care professional as soon as possible:

- dizziness
- fast heart rate
- low blood sugar
- skin rash or itchy skin
- sweating
- tremor

Side effects that usually do not require medical attention (report to your prescriber or health care professional if they continue or are bothersome):

- nausea/vomiting
- upset stomach

Where can I keep my medicine?

Keep out of the reach of children. Store at room temperature between 15 and 30 degrees C (59 and 86 degrees F). Avoid excessive exposure to heat above 40 degrees C (104 degrees F); do not freeze. Throw away any unused medicine after the expiration date.

Nefazodone tablets

| NEFAZODONE;
100 mg; Tablet
Ivax Pharmaceuticals
Inc | | NEFAZODONE;
100 mg; Tablet
Teva
Pharmaceuticals
USA Inc | |

This drug requires an FDA medication guide. See page xxxvii.

What are nefazodone tablets?

NEFAZODONE (Serzone®) is primarily used for the treatment of depression. Nefazodone may benefit patients who have unusual or limiting side effects from other antidepressants. Occasionally nefazodone is prescribed for other behavioral or emotional problems, like anxiety or traumatic stress. Generic nefazodone tablets are available.

What should my health care professional know before I take nefazodone?

They need to know if you have any of these conditions:

- angina
- bipolar disorder or mania

- heart disease or history of heart attack
- liver disease or a history of liver disease
- high blood pressure treated with medications
- low blood pressure
- previous stroke
- have had thoughts of suicide
- an unusual or allergic reaction to nefazodone, other medicines, food, dyes, or preservatives
- pregnant or trying to get pregnant
- breast-feeding

How should I take this medicine?

Take nefazodone tablets by mouth. Follow the directions on the prescription label. Swallow tablets with a drink of water. You may take nefazodone with or with-

N

out food. Take your doses at regular intervals. Do not take your medicine more often than directed. Contact your pediatrician or health care professional regarding the use of this medicine in children. Special care may be needed.

What if I miss a dose?

If you miss a dose, take it as soon as you can. If it is almost time for your next dose, take only that dose. Do not take double or extra doses. You must leave a suitable interval between doses. If you are taking two doses a day and have to take a missed dose, make sure there is at least 5 to 6 hours between doses.

What may interact with nefazodone?

Do not take nefazodone with any of the following medications:

- astemizole
- carbamazepine
- cerivastatin
- cisapride
- lovastatin
- medicines called MAO inhibitors—phenelzine (Nardil®), tranylcypromine (Parnate®), isocarboxazid (Marplan®), and selegiline (Eldepryl®)
- pimozide
- simvastatin
- terfenadine
- went yeast or Cholestin®

Other medications that can interact with nefazodone include:

- alcohol-containing beverages
- medicines for anxiety or sleeping problems, such as alprazolam, diazepam, clonazepam or triazolam
- atorvastatin
- buspirone
- cilostazol
- cyclosporine
- dextroamphetamine
- digoxin
- dofetilide
- entacapone
- furazolidone
- haloperidol
- herbal dietary supplements like kava kava, St. John's wort, and valerian
- linezolid
- loratadine
- medications used for HIV infection (examples: indinavir, nelfinavir, ritonavir)
- melatonin
- modafinil
- phenytoin
- sibutramine
- sildenafil
- some medicines for depression or anxiety (examples: citalopram, fluoxetine, fluvoxamine, paroxetine, sertraline, venlafaxine)
- tacrolimus
- tolcapone
- tolterodine
- warfarin

Tell your prescriber or health care professional about all other medicines you are taking, including non-prescription medicines, nutritional supplements, or herbal products. Also tell your prescriber or health care professional if you are a frequent user of drinks with caffeine or alcohol, if you smoke, or if you use illegal drugs. These may affect the way your medicine works. Check with your health care professional before stopping or starting any of your medicines.

What should I watch for while taking nefazodone?

If you are taking this medicine for a long time, you must visit your prescriber or health care professional for regular checks on your progress. Call your prescriber or health care professional if you feel faint or you fall. If you experience feelings or thoughts of suicide, extreme agitation, or inability to sleep or sit still, call your health care provider at once. You may get drowsy or dizzy. Do not drive, use machinery, or do anything that needs mental alertness until you know how nefazodone affects you. Do not sit up (from a lying position) or stand up quickly, especially if you are an older patient. This reduces the risk of dizzy or fainting spells. Your mouth may become dry. Chewing sugarless gum, sucking hard candy and drinking plenty of water will help. If you are going to have surgery, tell your prescriber or health care professional that you are taking nefazodone.

What side effects may I notice from taking nefazodone?

Side effects that you should report to your prescriber or health care professional as soon as possible:
Nefazodone rarely causes liver problems, but report any of the following immediately to your health care professional:
- abdominal pain
- dark yellow or brown urine
- loss of appetite for several days or more
- severe nausea or stomach pain
- yellowing of the skin or the eyes
- unusual tiredness

Other side effects you should report to your health care professional as soon as possible:
- agitation, confusion
- blurred vision, or changes in vision
- irregular heartbeat
- fainting spells, loss of balance
- flu-like symptoms (fever, chills, cough, muscle or joint aches and pains)
- pain or difficulty passing urine
- prolonged or painful erection (men, rare)
- skin rash or hives
- seizures or convulsions
- redness, blistering, peeling or loosening of the skin, including inside the mouth
- weakness

Side effects that usually do not require medical atten-

or alcohol, if you smoke, or if you use illegal drugs. These may affect the way your medicine works. Check with your health care professional before stopping or starting any of your medicines.

What should I watch for while taking naltrexone?

Report to your prescriber or health care professional regularly. It is important to attend any counseling or support groups that your prescriber or health care professional recommends. Attending these sessions while you are taking naltrexone will help you remain free of your dependence on opiate drugs or alcohol. Never try to overcome the effects of naltrexone by taking large amounts of narcotics because this can cause coma and death. If you are going to have surgery, tell your prescriber or health care professional that you are taking naltrexone. It is a good idea to carry a card in case of emergency to alert medical personnel that you are taking naltrexone. Do not treat yourself for coughs, colds, pain or diarrhea. Ask your prescriber or health care professional for advice. Some of the ingredients may interact with naltrexone and cause side effects. You may feel dizzy or lightheaded. Do not drive, use machinery, or do anything that needs mental alertness until you know how naltrexone affects you.

What side effects may I notice from taking naltrexone?

Naltrexone causes few side effects in patients who are not taking opiate drugs. Some of the side effects listed below can occur only if you are still taking opiate drugs. Side effects that you should report to your prescriber or health care professional as soon as possible:
- blurred vision or other eye problems
- confusion
- difficult or frequent passing of urine
- difficulty in awaking from sleep
- earache, ringing in the ears
- fast or pounding heartbeat (palpitations)
- fever

- hallucinations (seeing and hearing things that are not really there)
- mood changes
- nose bleeds
- pain, tenderness, or color changes in the legs or feet
- shortness of breath
- skin rash, itching
- slowed breathing
- swelling of the face, feet, or lower legs
- swollen glands
- weight gain
- yellow color of your eyes or skin

Side effects that usually do not require medical attention (report to your prescriber or health care professional if they continue or are bothersome):
Rare or uncommon, unless you are still taking narcotics:
- anxiety, nervousness, restlessness
- chills, sore throat
- constipation or diarrhea
- cough, hoarseness
- increased thirst
- irritability
- joint or muscle pain
- loss of appetite
- runny nose, sinus problems, sneezing
- sexual problems in males
- stomach cramps or pain

More common:
- anxiety
- difficulty sleeping
- dizziness
- headache
- increased tiredness
- nausea
- nervousness
- vomiting

Where can I keep my medicine?

Keep out of the reach of children in a container that small children cannot open. Store at room temperature between 15 and 30 degrees C (59 and 86 degrees F). Protect from light. Keep container tightly closed. Throw away any unused medicine after the expiration date.

Naproxen tablets, caplets, or delayed-release tablets

NAPROSYN®; 375 mg; Tablet, Delayed Release Hoffmann La Roche Inc

ALEVE®; 220 mg; Tablet Bayer Corp Consumer Care Div

This drug requires an FDA medication guide. See page xxxvii.

What are naproxen tablets, caplets, or delayed-release tablets?

NAPROXEN (Naprosyn®, EC Naprosyn®, Naprelan®, Anaprox®, Anaprox® DS, Aleve®) is an anti-inflammatory drug. It relieves pain and inflammation associated with rheumatoid arthritis, osteoarthritis, and juvenile (childhood) arthritis. Naproxen is also effective in treating other mild to moderate pain, including menstrual pain, headache, toothache, and temporarily reduces fever. Naproxen should only be used in children who are over 12 years old. Generic naproxen tablets and delayed-release tablets are available.

What should my health care professional know before I take naproxen?

They need to know if you have any of these conditions:
- anemia
- asthma, especially aspirin sensitive asthma
- bleeding problems or taking medicines that make you bleed easily such as anticoagulants ("blood thinners")
- cigarette smoker

N

- diabetes
- drink more than three alcohol-containing beverages a day
- heart failure
- high blood pressure
- kidney disease
- liver disease
- stomach or duodenal ulcers
- systemic lupus erythematosus
- ulcerative colitis
- an unusual or allergic reaction to aspirin, other salicylates, other NSAIDs, other medicines, foods, dyes or preservatives
- pregnant or trying to get pregnant
- breast-feeding

How should I take this medicine?

Take naproxen tablets by mouth. Follow the directions on the prescription label. Swallow tablets whole with a full glass of water; take tablets in an upright or sitting position. Taking a sip of water first, before taking the tablets, may help you swallow them. If possible take bedtime doses at least 10 minutes before lying down. You can take naproxen with food to prevent stomach upset. If you are taking the delayed-release tablets swallow them whole; do not crush or chew. Take your doses at regular intervals. Do not take your medicine more often than directed. Contact your pediatrician or health care professional regarding the use of this medicine in children. Special care may be needed. Do not give to children less than 12 years unless directed by your health care provider.

What if I miss a dose?

If you miss a dose, take it as soon as you can. If it is almost time for your next dose, take only that dose. Do not take double or extra doses.

What other drug(s) may interact with naproxen?

- alcohol
- alendronate
- aspirin and aspirin-like medicines
- cidofovir
- cyclosporine
- entecavir
- herbal products that contain feverfew, garlic, ginger, or ginkgo biloba
- lithium
- medicines for high blood pressure
- medicines that affect platelets
- medicines that treat or prevent blood clots such as warfarin and other "blood thinners"
- methotrexate
- other anti-inflammatory drugs (such as ibuprofen or prednisone)
- pemetrexed
- water pills (diuretics)

Tell your prescriber or health care professional about all other medicines you are taking, including non-prescription medicines, nutritional supplements, or herbal products. Also tell your prescriber or health care professional if you are a frequent user of drinks with caffeine or alcohol, if you smoke, or if you use illegal drugs. These may affect the way your medicine works. Check with your health care professional before stopping or starting any of your medicines.

What should I watch for while I taking naproxen?

Let your prescriber or health care professional know if your pain continues. Do not take naproxen with other pain killers without advice. If you get flu-like symptoms (fever, chills, muscle aches and pains), call your prescriber or health care professional; do not treat yourself. Do not treat yourself for pain more than 10 days or for fever more than 3 days without consulting your health care provider. To reduce unpleasant effects on your throat and stomach, take naproxen with a full glass of water and never just before lying down. If you notice black, tarry stools or experience severe stomach pain and vomit blood or what looks like coffee grounds, notify your health care prescriber immediately. If you are taking medicines that affect the clotting of your blood, such as aspirin or blood thinners such as Coumadin®, talk to your health care provider or prescriber before taking this medicine. You may get dizzy. Do not drive, use machinery, or do anything that needs mental alertness until you know how naproxen affects you. Stand or sit up slowly, this reduces the risk of dizzy or fainting spells. These effects may be worse if you are an older patient. Do not smoke cigarettes or drink alcohol; these increase irritation to your stomach and can make it more susceptible to damage from naproxen. It is especially important not to use naproxen during the last 3 months of pregnancy unless specifically directed to do so by your health care provider. Naproxen may cause problems in the unborn child or complications during delivery. If you are going to have surgery, tell your prescriber or health care professional that you are taking naproxen. Problems can arise if you need dental work, and in the day-to-day care of your teeth. Try to avoid damage to your teeth and gums when you brush or floss your teeth.

What side effects may I notice from taking naproxen?

Side effects that you should report to your prescriber or health care professional as soon as possible:

- signs of bleeding—bruising, pinpoint red spots on the skin, black tarry stools, blood in the urine, unusual tiredness or weakness, vomiting blood or vomit that looks like coffee grounds
- signs of an allergic reaction—difficulty breathing or wheezing, skin rash, redness, blistering or peeling skin, hives, or itching, swelling of eyelids, throat, lips
- blurred vision
- change in the amount of urine passed
- difficulty swallowing, severe heartburn or burning, pain in throat

tion (report to your prescriber or health care professional if they continue or are bothersome):

Rare or less common:
- headache
- sexual difficulties

More common:
- constipation
- dry mouth
- feeling of dizziness

- drowsiness
- mild nausea or stomach upset

Where can I keep my medicine?

Keep out of the reach of children in a container that small children cannot open. Store at room temperature between 15 and 30 degrees C (59 and 86 degrees F). Throw away any unused medicine after the expiration date.

Nelfinavir tablets

VIRACEPT®;
250 mg; Tablet
Agouron Pharmaceuticals Inc

What are nelfinavir tablets?

NELFINAVIR (Viracept®) is an antiviral drug called a protease inhibitor. Nelfinavir is used to treat human immunodeficiency virus (HIV) infection. Nelfinavir may reduce the amount of HIV in the blood and increase the number of CD4 cells (T-cells) in the blood. Nelfinavir is used in combination with other drugs used to treat the HIV virus. Nelfinavir will not cure or prevent HIV infection or AIDS. You may still develop other infections or conditions associated with HIV. Generic nelfinavir tablets are not yet available.

What should my health care professional know before I take nelfinavir?

They need to know if you have any of these conditions:
- diabetes or high blood sugar
- hemophilia
- high cholesterol or lipids in your blood
- liver disease
- received other treatments for HIV or AIDS
- an unusual or allergic reaction to nelfinavir, other medicines, foods, dyes, or preservatives
- breast-feeding
- pregnancy or recent attempts to get pregnant

How should I take this medicine?

Take nelfinavir tablets by mouth with a meal or light snack, within 1 hour before or after a meal. Follow the directions on the prescription label. Fruit or fruit juice is not enough food to take with nelfinavir. Appropriate foods include cheese and crackers, cookies and milk, a granola bar, a bagel or a small sandwich. Take your doses at regular intervals. If you cannot swallow the tablets, put the whole or crushed tablets in a small amount of water to dissolve or mix crushed tablets in a small amount of food. The pills will dissolve in 1 to 2 minutes; there may still be some small pieces, but they should be easy to swallow. Once mixed with food or water, you must eat or drink the whole amount to get the full dose. Rinse the drinking glass and drink the rinse to ensure the entire dose is consumed. Avoid mixing nelfinavir with acidic foods or juices (like orange juice, apple juice, or apple sauce) because a bitter taste may occur. To help to make sure that your anti-HIV therapy works as well as possible, be very careful to take all of your medicine exactly as prescribed. Do not take your medicine more often than directed. Do not stop taking except on your prescriber's advice. Contact your pediatrician or health care professional regarding the use of this medicine in children. Special care may be needed.

What if I miss a dose?

If you miss a dose, take it as soon as you can. If it is almost time for your next dose, take only that dose. Do not take double or extra doses.

What may interact with nelfinavir?

Many medicines may interact with nelfinavir, if you have a question concerning other medicines you may be taking, talk with your pharmacist, prescriber or other health care professional.

Do not take nelfinavir with any of these medicines:

- amiodarone (Cordarone®)
- astemizole (Hismanal®)
- bepridil (Vascor®) or mibefradil (Posicor®)
- cerivastatin (Baycol®)
- cisapride (Propulsid®)
- ergotamine medicines (such as Cafergot®, Migranal®, D.H.E. 45®, and others)
- lovastatin (Mevacor®)
- midazolam (Versed®)
- pimozide (Orap®)
- quinidine (Quinaglute®, Cardioquin®, Quinidex®, and others)
- rifampin (Rimactane®, Rifadin®, Rifater®, or Rifamate®)
- simvastatin (Zocor®)
- St. John's wort or any herbal products containing St. John's wort
- terfenadine (Seldane®)
- triazolam (Halcion®)
- went yeast (Cholestin™)

Other medicines that may interact with nelfinavir:

- birth control pills or hormone-type birth control
- bosentan
- calcium-channel blockers, often used for high blood pressure or chest pain (examples: amlodipine, diltiazem, felodipine, nifedipine, nimodipine, nisoldipine, verapamil)

N

- certain medicines for anxiety or for difficulty sleeping
- certain medicines for fungal infections
- certain medicines for high cholesterol
- certain pain medicines
- cilostazol
- cyclosporine
- disopyramide
- dofetilide
- imatinib, STI-571
- levomethadyl
- medicines for seizures
- medicines for depression
- medicines for diabetes
- other antiviral medicines such as delavirdine, didanosine, ddI, efavirenz, indinavir, ritonavir, saquinavir
- rifabutin
- sildenafil
- sirolimus
- tacrolimus
- went yeast (Cholestin™)

Tell your prescriber or health care professional about all other medicines you are taking, including nonprescription medicines, nutritional supplements, or herbal products. Also tell your prescriber or health care professional if you are a frequent user of drinks with caffeine or alcohol, if you smoke, or if you use illegal drugs. These may affect the way your medicine works. Check with your health care professional before stopping or starting any of your medicines.

What should I watch for while taking nelfinavir?

Visit your prescriber or health care professional for regular checks on your progress. Discuss any new symptoms with your prescriber or health care professional. Nelfinavir will not cure HIV and you can still get other illnesses or complications associated with your disease.

Taking nelfinavir does not reduce the risk of passing HIV infection to others through sexual or blood contact. It is best to avoid sexual contact so that you do not spread the disease to others. For any sexual contact, use a condom. Be careful about cuts, abrasions and other possible sources of blood contact. Never share a needle or syringe with anyone. If you are a women of childbearing age and are using hormone contraceptives, then you should use another form of birth control while taking nelfinavir. Nelfinavir may decrease the effectiveness of hormone birth control agents, including birth control pills and injections.

What side effects might I notice from taking nelfinavir?

Side effects that you should report to your prescriber or health care professional as soon as possible:
- difficulty breathing
- severe dizziness
- severe rash with fever
- unusual tiredness or weakness

Side effects that usually do not require medical attention (report to your prescriber or health care professional if they continue or are bothersome):
- diarrhea
- gas
- headache
- nausea, vomiting
- stomach pain
- tiredness or weakness

Where can I keep my medicine?

Keep out of the reach of children in a container that small children cannot open. Store at room temperature between 15 and 30 degrees C (59 and 86 degrees F). Keep container tightly closed. Throw away any unused medicine after the expiration date.

Neomycin tablets

NEOMYCIN;
500 mg; Tablet
Teva Pharmaceuticals USA Inc

What are neomycin tablets?

NEOMYCIN is an aminoglycoside antibiotic. It will help to prevent bacterial infection during surgery on the bowel. Neomycin will also help reduce the symptoms of hepatic coma associated with liver disease. Generic neomycin tablets are available.

What should my health care professional know before I take neomycin?

They need to know if you have any of these conditions:
- botulism
- bowel disease, or intestinal blockage (obstruction)
- difficulty hearing
- kidney disease
- myasthenia gravis
- Parkinson's disease
- other chronic illness
- an unusual or allergic reaction to neomycin or other antibiotics, foods, dyes or preservatives
- pregnant or trying to get pregnant
- breast-feeding

How should I take this medicine?

Take neomycin tablets by mouth. Follow the directions on the prescription label. Take with a full glass of water. Take your doses at regular intervals. Do not take your medicine more often than directed. Finish the full course of tablets prescribed by your prescriber or health care professional even if you feel better.

What if I miss a dose?

If you miss a dose, take it as soon as you can. If it is almost time for your next dose, take only that dose. Do not take double or extra doses.

What may interact with neomycin?

- cisplatin
- digoxin
- dimenhydrinate
- lactulose
- oral contraceptives (birth control pills)
- other antibiotics
- warfarin
- water pills

Tell your prescriber or health care professional about all other medicines you are taking, including non-prescription medicines, nutritional supplements, or herbal products. Also tell your prescriber or health care professional if you are a frequent user of drinks with caffeine or alcohol, if you smoke, or if you use illegal drugs. These may affect the way your medicine works. Check with your health care professional before stopping or starting any of your medicines.

What should I watch for while taking neomycin?

Tell your prescriber or health care professional if your symptoms do not improve in a few days. You may get dizzy or have trouble keeping your balance. Until you know how neomycin affects you, do not drive, use machinery, or do anything that requires mental alertness.

What side effects may I notice from taking neomycin?

Elderly patients are more likely to get serious side effects. Serious side effects with neomycin include:
- difficulty hearing
- dizziness
- loss of balance
- increased thirst
- pain or difficulty passing urine
- muscle weakness
- ringing in the ears
- skin rash, itching
- unusual tiredness or weakness

Side effects that usually do not require medical attention (report to your prescriber or health care professional if they continue or are bothersome):
- diarrhea
- headache
- nausea, vomiting

Where can I keep my medicine?

Keep out of the reach of children in a container that small children cannot open. Store at room temperature between 15 and 30 degrees C (59 and 86 degrees F). Throw away any unused medicine after the expiration date.

Nevirapine tablets

VIRAMUNE®;
200 mg; Tablet
Boehringer Ingelheim
Pharmaceuticals Inc

This drug requires an FDA medication guide. See page xxxvii.

What are nevirapine tablets?

NEVIRAPINE (Viramune®) is an antiviral drug called a nonnucleoside reverse transcriptase inhibitor or NNRTI. Nevirapine is used to treat human immunodeficiency virus (HIV) infection. Nevirapine may reduce the amount of HIV in the blood and increase the number of CD4 cells (T-cells) in the blood. Nevirapine is used in combination with other drugs to treat the HIV virus. Nevirapine will not cure or prevent HIV infection or AIDS. You may still develop other infections or conditions associated with HIV. Generic nevirapine tablets are not yet available.

What should my health care professional know before I take nevirapine?

They need to know if you have any of these conditions:
- kidney disease requiring dialysis
- liver disease, including hepatitis
- an unusual or allergic reaction to nevirapine, other medicines, foods, dyes, or preservatives
- breast-feeding
- pregnant or trying to get pregnant

How should I take this medicine?

Take nevirapine tablets by mouth. Follow the directions on the prescription label. Swallow tablets with a drink of water. You may take nevirapine with or without food. Take your doses at regular intervals. Do not take your medicine more often than directed. To make sure that your medication works as well as possible to treat your condition, take all of your medicine exactly as prescribed. Do not stop taking except on your prescriber's advice. Before starting this medication, read the paper on your prescription provided by your pharmacist or health care professional. This paper will tell you about the specific product you are taking. Make certain you understand the instructions. Contact your pediatrician or health care professional regarding the use of this medicine in children. Special care may be needed.

What if I miss a dose?

If you miss a dose, take it as soon as you can. If it is almost time for your next dose, take only that dose. Do not take double or extra doses.

What may interact with nevirapine?

- birth control pills or other hormonal birth control medicines (like the patch, ring, or injections)
- cimetidine
- dronabinol, THC
- erythromycin
- ketoconazole

N

- medicines for anxiety or depression including alprazolam, triazolam, or zolpidem
- medicines for seizures including carbamazepine, phenobarbital, or phenytoin
- methadone
- rifabutin
- rifampin
- St. John's wort

Tell your prescriber or health care professional about all other medicines you are taking, including non-prescription medicines, nutritional supplements, or herbal products. Also tell your prescriber or health care professional if you are a frequent user of drinks with caffeine or alcohol, if you smoke, or if you use illegal drugs. These may affect the way your medicine works. Check with your health care professional before stopping or starting any of your medicines.

What should I watch for while taking nevirapine?

Severe liver reactions or skin rashes may be seen with nevirapine therapy. The risk of these reactions is greatest during the first 18 weeks of treatment, but can also occur later. If you develop a rash at any time while you are taking nevirapine, call your health care provider immediately. You must visit your prescriber or health care professional for regular checks on your progress and to watch for possible reactions. You will need to have your blood drawn regularly to monitor your therapy and your liver function. Discuss any new symptoms with your prescriber or health care professional. Nevirapine will not cure HIV infection and you can still get other illnesses or complications associated with your health condition. Taking nevirapine does not reduce the risk of passing HIV infection to others through sexual or blood contact. It is best to avoid sexual contact so that you do not spread the disease to others. For any sexual contact, use a condom. Be careful about cuts, abrasions, and other possible sources of blood contact. Never share a needle or syringe with anyone. If

you are a women of childbearing age and are using hormone contraceptives, then you should use another form of birth control while taking nevirapine. Nevirapine may decrease the effectiveness of hormone birth control agents, including oral contraceptives.

What side effects might I notice from taking nevirapine?

Side effects that you should report to your prescriber or health care professional as soon as possible:
- abdominal pain
- dark yellow or brown urine
- general ill feeling or "flu-like" symptoms
- hives
- loss of appetite
- mouth blisters or lesions
- muscle or joint aches
- pain, ache, or sensitivity to touch just below your ribs
- pale colored stools (bowel movements)
- redness, blistering, peeling or loosening of the skin, including inside the mouth
- severe dizziness
- skin rash or peeling skin
- swelling of the eyelids or face
- unusual tiredness or weakness
- yellow color of eyes or skin

Side effects that usually do not require medical attention (report to your prescriber or health care professional if they continue or are bothersome):
- diarrhea
- headache
- itching
- nausea, vomiting
- tingling or numbness in the hands or feet or around the mouth

Where can I keep my medicine?

Keep out of the reach of children in a container that small children cannot open. Store at room temperature between 15 and 30 degrees C (59 and 86 degrees F). Keep container tightly closed. Throw away any unused medicine after the expiration date.

Niacin, Niacinamide extended-release tablets or capsules

NIACIN;
250 mg; Capsule, Extended Release
Goldline Laboratories Inc/
IVAX Pharmaceuticals

What are niacin extended-release tablets or capsules?

NIACIN, also known as nicotinic acid or vitamin B_3 (Slo-Niacin®, Niaspan®), is a B-vitamin that occurs naturally in foods, such as meat, fish, milk, eggs, green vegetables, and enriched cereal grains. Proper amounts of niacin are obtained in our diets daily. Niacin supplements are occasionally prescribed to treat pellagra, a serious but rare niacin-deficiency disorder. Niacin is available in many multivitamins in small amounts. Generic niacin extended-release tablets and capsules are

available. However, check with your prescriber before changing the type of niacin you are taking. Large doses of nicotinic acid, a form of niacin, are prescribed to help decrease the amount of fatty substances in the blood, known as cholesterol and triglycerides. Nicotinic acid is used in patients who cannot control their blood fats by diet alone. Nicotinic acid is occasionally used to help people with poor blood circulation. Niacin should not be used to treat high cholesterol without a prescription. Niacinamide, a different form of niacin, is available without a prescription as a vitamin supplement, but it does not help lower cholesterol or treat blood circulation problems. Do not use niacinamide to treat these conditions.

What should my health care professional know before I take niacin?

They need to know if you have any of these conditions:
- low blood counts, platelets, or bleeding problems
- diabetes
- gallbladder disease
- gout
- heart disease or a history of heart attack
- liver disease
- low blood pressure or taking medications to lower blood pressure
- ulcers of intestine or stomach
- an unusual or allergic reaction to niacin, other medicines, foods, dyes, or preservatives
- pregnant or trying or get pregnant
- breast-feeding

How should I take this medicine?

Take niacin extended-release tablets or capsules by mouth. Follow the directions on the prescription label. Swallow the tablets or capsules whole with a drink of water; do not crush or chew. Take with meals or milk. Take your doses at regular intervals. Do not take your medicine more often than directed. If you are taking niacin for a medical condition (such as to lower cholesterol levels), your prescriber or health care professional may have you start with low doses, with slow increases in the dose to help your body become used to the medicine. If you also take cholestyramine or colestipol, you should take your niacin at least 1 hour before or 4 hours after a dose of these medications.

What if I miss a dose?

If you miss a dose, take it as soon as you can. If it is almost time for your next dose, take only that dose. Do not take double or extra doses.

What may interact with niacin?

- alcohol
- aspirin
- atorvastatin
- cerivastatin
- cholestyramine
- colestipol
- fluvastatin
- certain medicines that lower blood pressure (e.g., diltiazem, nifedipine, verapamil)
- clonidine
- lovastatin
- nitroglycerin
- pravastatin
- simvastatin
- warfarin

Tell your prescriber or health care professional about all other medicines you are taking, including non-prescription medicines. Also tell your prescriber or health

care professional if you are a frequent user of drinks with caffeine or alcohol, if you smoke, or if you use illegal drugs. These may affect the way your medicine works. Check with your health care professional before stopping or starting any of your medicines.

What should I watch for while taking niacin?

Do not take more niacin than prescribed. Visit your prescriber or health care professional for regular checks on your progress if you are taking niacin for medical reasons and not as a vitamin supplement. You may get dizzy, faint, or have blurred vision; until you know how niacin affects you, do not drive, use machinery, or do anything that needs mental alertness. To avoid dizzy or fainting spells, do not stand or sit up quickly, especially if you are an older person. Do not drink hot drinks or alcohol at the same time you take your niacin dose. Hot drinks and alcohol can increase the flushing caused by niacin, which can be uncomfortable. Alcohol also can increase possible dizziness. If you are taking niacin to reduce your cholesterol, remember that it is only part of a total cholesterol-lowering program. Your health care professional or dietician can suggest a low-cholesterol and low-fat diet that will reduce your risk of getting heart and blood vessel disease. Avoid alcohol and smoking, and keep a proper exercise schedule. You may notice the empty shell of the tablet in your stool; this is no cause for concern.

What side effects may I notice from taking niacin?

Side effects that you should report to your prescriber or health care professional as soon as possible:
- dark yellow or brown urine
- fainting spells
- grayish stool color
- nausea, vomiting
- palpitations
- severe stomach pain and loss of appetite
- shortness of breath, wheezing
- skin rash and itching
- weakness or tiredness
- yellowing of skin or eyes

Side effects that usually do not require medical attention (report to your prescriber or health care professional if they continue or are bothersome):
- diarrhea
- dizziness, lightheadedness
- dry skin
- flushing, warmth, and burning or tingling of the skin
- headache
- stomach discomfort or bloating

Where can I keep my medicine?

Keep out of the reach of children in a container that small children cannot open. Store at room temperature between 15 and 30 degrees C (59 and 86 degrees F). Throw away any unused medicine after the expiration date.

N

Niacin, Niacinamide tablets

What are niacin tablets?

NIACIN, also known as nicotinic acid or vitamin B₃ (Niacor®, Nicolar®), is a B-vitamin that occurs naturally in foods, such as meat, fish, milk, eggs, green vegetables, and enriched cereal grains. Proper amounts of niacin are obtained in our diets daily. Niacin supplements are occasionally prescribed to treat pellagra, a serious but rare niacin-deficiency disorder. Niacin is available in many multivitamins in small amounts. Generic niacin tablets are available. However, check with your prescriber before changing the type of niacin you are taking. Large doses of nicotinic acid, a form of niacin, are prescribed to help decrease the amount of fatty substances in the blood, known as cholesterol and triglycerides. Nicotinic acid is used in patients who cannot control their blood fats by diet alone. Nicotinic acid is occasionally used to help people with poor blood circulation. Niacin should not be used to treat high cholesterol without a prescription. Niacinamide, a different form of niacin, is available without a prescription as a vitamin supplement, but it does not help lower cholesterol or treat blood circulation problems. Do not use niacinamide to treat these conditions.

What should my health care professional know before I take niacin?

They need to know if you have any of these conditions:
- low blood counts, platelets, or bleeding problems
- diabetes
- gallbladder disease
- gout
- heart disease or a history of heart attack
- liver disease
- low blood pressure or taking medications to lower blood pressure
- ulcers of intestine or stomach
- an unusual or allergic reaction to niacin, other medicines, foods, dyes, or preservatives
- pregnant or trying or get pregnant
- breast-feeding

How should I take this medicine?

Take niacin tablets by mouth. Follow the directions on the prescription label. Swallow the tablets with a drink of water. Take niacin with food or milk. Take your doses at regular intervals. Do not take your medicine more often than directed. If you are taking niacin for a medical condition (such as to lower cholesterol levels), your prescriber or health care professional may have you start with low doses, with slow increases in the dose to help your body become used to the medicine. If you also take cholestyramine or colestipol to lower your cholesterol, you should take your niacin at least 1 hour before or 4 hours after a dose of these medications.

What if I miss a dose?

If you miss a dose, take it as soon as you can. If it is almost time for your next dose, take only that dose. Do not take double or extra doses.

What may interact with niacin?

- alcohol
- aspirin
- atorvastatin
- cerivastatin
- cholestyramine
- colestipol
- fluvastatin
- certain medicines that lower blood pressure (e.g., diltiazem, nifedipine, verapamil)
- clonidine
- lovastatin
- nitroglycerin
- pravastatin
- simvastatin
- warfarin

Tell your prescriber or health care professional about all other medicines you are taking, including non-prescription medicines. Also tell your prescriber or health care professional if you are a frequent user of drinks with caffeine or alcohol, if you smoke, or if you use illegal drugs. These may affect the way your medicine works. Check with your health care professional before stopping or starting any of your medicines.

What should I watch for while taking niacin?

Do not take more niacin than prescribed. Visit your prescriber or health care professional for regular checks on your progress if you are taking niacin for medical reasons and not as a vitamin supplement. You may get dizzy, faint, or have blurred vision; until you know how niacin affects you, do not drive, use machinery, or do anything that needs mental alertness. To avoid dizzy or fainting spells, do not stand or sit up quickly, especially if you are an older person. Do not drink hot drinks or alcohol at the same time you take your niacin dose. Hot drinks and alcohol can increase the flushing caused by niacin, which can be uncomfortable. Alcohol also can increase possible dizziness. If you are taking niacin to reduce your cholesterol, remember that it is only part of a total cholesterol-lowering program. Your health care professional or dietician can suggest a low-cholesterol and low-fat diet that will reduce your risk of getting heart and blood vessel disease. Avoid alcohol and smoking, and keep a proper exercise schedule.

What side effects may I notice from taking niacin?

Side effects that you should report to your prescriber or health care professional as soon as possible:

- dark yellow or brown urine
- fainting spells
- grayish stool color
- palpitations
- shortness of breath, wheezing
- skin rash and itching
- stomach pain or heartburn
- nausea, vomiting
- weakness or tiredness

Side effects that usually do not require medical attention (report to your prescriber or health care professional if they continue or are bothersome):

- diarrhea
- dizziness, lightheadedness
- dry skin
- flushing, warmth, and burning or tingling of the skin
- headache

Where can I keep my medicine?

Keep out of the reach of children in a container that small children cannot open. Store at room temperature between 15 and 30 degrees C (59 and 86 degrees F). Throw away any unused medicine after the expiration date.

Nicardipine capsules or sustained-release capsules

CARDENE SR®;
60 mg; Capsule,
Extended Release
Hoffmann La Roche
Inc

CARDENE®;
20 mg; Capsule
Hoffmann La Roche
Inc

What are nicardipine capsules or sustained-release capsules?

NICARDIPINE (Cardene®, Cardene SR®) is a calcium-channel blocker. It affects the amount of calcium found in your heart and muscle cells. This results in relaxation of blood vessels, which can reduce the amount of work the heart has to do. Nicardipine (regular capsules only) reduces attacks of chest pain (angina), and helps reduce high blood pressure (hypertension). It is not a cure. Generic nicardipine regular capsules are available. Generic nicardipine sustained-release capsules are not yet available.

What should my health care professional know before I take nicardipine?

They need to know if you have any of these conditions:
- heart problems, low blood pressure, slow or irregular heartbeat
- liver disease
- previous heart attack
- over 65 years old
- an unusual or allergic reaction to nicardipine, other medicines, foods, dyes, or preservatives
- pregnant or trying to get pregnant
- breast-feeding

How should I take this medicine?

Take nicardipine capsules by mouth. Follow the directions on the prescription label. Swallow the capsules whole with a drink of water, do not crush or chew the sustained-release capsules. Take on an empty stomach. Fatty foods can interfere with the action of nicardipine. Avoid taking nicardipine with grapefruit juice or grapefruit. Take your doses at regular intervals. Do not take your medicine more often then directed. Do not stop taking except on your prescriber's advice. Contact your pediatrician or health care professional regarding the use of this medicine in children. Special care may be needed. Elderly patients over 65 years old may have a stronger reaction to this medicine and need smaller doses.

What if I miss a dose?

If you miss a dose, take it as soon as you can. If it is almost time for your next dose (less than 6 to 8 hours if you are taking sustained-release capsules), take only that dose. Do not take double or extra doses.

What may interact with nicardipine?

Do not take nicardipine with any of the following:

- astemizole
- cisapride
- grapefruit juice
- pimozide
- terfenadine

Nicardipine may also interact with the following medications:

- alcohol
- alosetron
- antiinflammatory drugs (NSAIDs, such as ibuprofen)
- barbiturates such as phenobarbital
- bosentan
- certain antibiotics (clarithromycin, erythromycin, telithromycin, troleandomycin)
- certain medicines used to treat cancer
- certain medicines to treat migraine (ergotamine, dihydroergotamine, methysergide)
- cilostazol
- cimetidine
- cyclosporine
- female hormones, including contraceptive or birth control pills
- fentanyl
- galantamine
- herbal or dietary supplements such as gingko biloba, ginseng, hawthorn, ma huang (ephedra), melatonin, St. John's wort, went yeast
- local anesthetics or general anesthetics

N

- medicines for anxiety or difficulty sleeping (examples: alprazolam, buspirone, midazolam, triazolam)
- medicines for depression or mental problems (fluoxetine, fluvoxamine, nefazodone, ziprasidone)
- medicines for fungal infections (fluconazole, itraconazole, ketoconazole, voriconazole)
- medicines for heart-rhythm problems (amiodarone, digoxin, disopyramide, dofetilide, flecainide, quinidine)
- medicine for high blood pressure or heart problems
- medicines for high cholesterol (atorvastatin, cerivastatin, lovastatin, simvastatin)
- medicines for HIV infection or AIDS
- medicines for prostate problems
- medicines for seizures (carbamazepine, clonazepam, ethosuximide, phenobarbital, phenytoin, primidone, zonisamide)
- methadone
- rifampin, rifapentine, or rifabutin
- sildenafil
- sirolimus
- tacrolimus
- warfarin
- water pills (diuretics)
- yohimbine
- zafirlukast
- zileuton

Tell your prescriber or health care professional about all other medicines you are taking, including non-prescription medicines, nutritional supplements, or herbal products. Also tell your prescriber or health care professional if you are a frequent user of drinks with caffeine or alcohol, if you smoke, or if you use illegal drugs. These may affect the way your medicine works. Check with your health care professional before stopping or starting any of your medicines.

What should I watch for while taking nicardipine?

Check your blood pressure and pulse rate regularly; this is important while you are taking nicardipine. Ask your prescriber or health care professional what your blood pressure and pulse rate should be and when you should contact him or her. You may feel dizzy or lightheaded. Do not drive, use machinery, or do anything that needs mental alertness until you know how nicardipine affects you. To reduce the risk of dizzy or fainting spells, do not sit or stand up quickly, especially if you are an older patient. Alcohol can make you more dizzy, and increase flushing and rapid heartbeats. Avoid alcoholic drinks. Do not suddenly stop taking nicardipine. Ask your prescriber or health care professional how to gradually reduce the dose. If you are going to have surgery, tell your prescriber or health care professional that you are taking nicardipine.

What side effects may I notice from taking nicardipine?

Side effects that you should report to your prescriber or health care professional as soon as possible:

- fast heartbeat, palpitations, irregular heartbeat, chest pain
- difficulty breathing
- dizziness
- fainting spells, lightheadedness
- swelling of the legs and ankles

Side effects that usually do not require medical attention (report to your prescriber or health care professional if they continue or are bothersome):

- facial flushing
- headache
- weakness or tiredness

Where can I keep my medicine?

Keep out of the reach of children in a container that small children cannot open. Store at room temperature, approximately 25 degrees C (77 degrees F). Protect from light and moisture. Throw away any unused medicine after the expiration date.

Nicotine chewing gum

NICORETTE®;
2 mg; Gum, Chewing
SmithKline Beecham
Pharmaceuticals

What is nicotine chewing gum?

NICOTINE (Nicorette®) helps people stop smoking. By replacing nicotine found in cigarettes, physical withdrawal effects are less severe. Nicotine chewing gum is most effective when used in combination with a supervised stop-smoking program. Nicotine gum is for use over short periods of time (not more than 6 months). Generic nicotine chewing gum is available. NOTE: In some cases, Zyban® (also known as bupropion), a prescription medication, is used together with nicotine to help people stop smoking. You should only use Zyban® with nicotine skin patches or nicotine gum if these have been prescribed by your health care prescriber. Ask your prescriber for information and advice before purchasing any non-prescription nicotine products if you are currently on Zyban®. The use of the two medicines together requires special observation by your prescriber.

What should my health care professional know before I use nicotine?

They need to know if you have any of these conditions:

- angina
- dental disease
- diabetes
- high blood pressure
- irregular heartbeat
- overactive thyroid

N

- pheochromocytoma
- previous heart attack
- stomach problems or ulcers
- an unusual or allergic reaction to nicotine, other medicines, foods, dyes, or preservatives
- pregnant or trying to get pregnant
- breast-feeding

How should I use this medicine?

Chew nicotine gum in the mouth. Do not swallow the gum. Follow carefully the directions that come with the chewing gum. Use exactly as directed. When you feel an urgent desire for a cigarette, chew one piece of gum slowly. Continue chewing until you taste the gum or feel a slight tingling in your mouth. Then, stop chewing and place the gum between your cheek and gum. Wait until the taste or tingling is almost gone then start chewing again. Continue chewing in this manner for about 30 minutes. Do not use more than 30 pieces of gum a day. Too much gum can increase the risk of an overdose. As the urge to smoke gets less, gradually reduce the number of pieces each day over a period of 2 to 3 months. When you are only using 1 or 2 pieces a day, stop using the nicotine gum. Contact your pediatrician or health care professional regarding the use of this medicine in children. Special care may be needed.

What if I miss a dose?

This does not apply. Only use the chewing gum when you have a strong desire to smoke. Do not use more than one piece of gum at a time.

What may interact with nicotine?

- bupropion
- insulin
- propoxyphene
- propranolol
- theophylline
- warfarin

Tell your prescriber or health care professional about all other medicines you are taking, including nonprescription medicines, nutritional supplements, or herbal products. Also tell your prescriber or health care professional if you are a frequent user of drinks with caffeine or alcohol, or if you use illegal drugs. These may affect the way your medicine works. Check with your health care professional before stopping or starting any of your medicines.

What should I watch for while taking nicotine?

Always carry the nicotine gum with you. Do not smoke while you are using nicotine chewing gum. If your mouth gets sore from chewing the gum, suck hard sugarless candy between pieces of gum to help relieve the soreness. Brush your teeth regularly to reduce mouth irritation. If you wear dentures, contact your prescriber or health care professional if the gum sticks to your dental work. If you are a diabetic and you quit smoking, the effects of insulin may be increased and you may need to reduce your insulin dose. Check with your prescriber or health care professional about how you should adjust your insulin dose.

What side effects may I notice from using nicotine?

Side effects that you should report to your prescriber or health care professional as soon as possible:
- confusion
- damage to teeth or dental work
- dizziness
- fainting or lightheadedness
- fast or irregular heartbeat (palpitations), chest pain
- headache
- hearing changes
- increased saliva
- nausea, vomiting
- seizures (convulsions)
- stomach pain
- vision changes
- weakness

Side effects that usually do not require medical attention (report to your prescriber or health care professional if they continue or are bothersome):
- belching
- constipation or diarrhea
- flushing
- increased appetite
- irritability
- jaw ache
- joint or muscle ache
- sleep disturbance
- sore throat or mouth

Where can I keep my medicine?

Keep out of the reach of children. Store nicotine in a safe place where children and pets cannot reach it, and be careful about throwing gum away. If a child chews or swallows nicotine gum, call your prescriber or health care professional or a poison control center at once. Store below 30 degrees C (86 degrees F). All nicotine products are sensitive to heat. Store in manufacturers packaging until ready to use. Protect from light. Throw away unused medicine after the expiration date.

N

Nicotine lozenge

COMMIT®;
2 mg; Lozenge
GlaxoSmithKline Consumer
Health

What is nicotine lozenge?

NICOTINE (Commit®) helps people stop smoking. By replacing nicotine found in cigarettes, physical withdrawal effects are less severe. Nicotine lozenges are most effective when used in combination with a supervised stop-smoking program. Nicotine lozenge is for use over short periods of time (not more than 6 months). Generic nicotine lozenges are available. NOTE: In some cases, Zyban® (also known as bupropion), a prescription medication, is used together with nicotine to help people stop smoking. You should only use Zyban® with nicotine skin patches or nicotine gum if these have been prescribed by your healthcare prescriber. Ask your prescriber for information and advice before purchasing any non-prescription nicotine products if you are currently on Zyban®. The use of the two medicines together requires special observation by your prescriber.

What should my health care professional know before I use nicotine?

They need to know if you have any of these conditions:
- angina
- dental disease
- diabetes
- high blood pressure
- irregular heartbeat
- overactive thyroid
- pheochromocytoma
- previous heart attack
- stomach problems or ulcers
- an unusual or allergic reaction to nicotine, other medicines, foods, dyes, or preservatives
- pregnant or trying to get pregnant
- breast-feeding

How should I use this medicine?

Place nicotine lozenge in the mouth. Suck on the lozenge until it is completely dissolved. Do not swallow the lozenge. Follow carefully the directions that come with the lozenge. Use exactly as directed. Contact your pediatrician or health care professional regarding the use of this medicine in children. Special care may be needed.

What if I miss a dose?

This does not apply.

What may interact with nicotine?

- bupropion
- insulin
- propoxyphene
- propranolol
- theophylline
- warfarin

Tell your prescriber or health care professional about all other medicines you are taking, including non-prescription medicines, nutritional supplements, or herbal products. Also tell your prescriber or health care professional if you are a frequent user of drinks with caffeine or alcohol, or if you use illegal drugs. These may affect the way your medicine works. Check with your health care professional before stopping or starting any of your medicines.

What should I watch for while taking nicotine?

Always carry the nicotine lozenges with you. Do not smoke while you are using nicotine lozenges. Brush your teeth regularly to reduce mouth irritation. If you are a diabetic and you quit smoking, the effects of insulin may be increased and you may need to reduce your insulin dose. Check with your prescriber or health care professional about how you should adjust your insulin dose.

What side effects may I notice from using nicotine?

Side effects that you should report to your prescriber or health care professional as soon as possible:
- confusion
- damage to teeth or dental work
- dizziness
- fainting or lightheadedness
- fast or irregular heartbeat (palpitations), chest pain
- headache
- hearing changes
- increased saliva
- nausea, vomiting
- seizures (convulsions)
- stomach pain
- vision changes
- weakness

Side effects that usually do not require medical attention (report to your prescriber or health care professional if they continue or are bothersome):
- constipation or diarrhea
- flushing
- increased appetite
- irritability
- joint or muscle ache
- sleep disturbance
- sore throat or mouth

Where can I keep my medicine?

Keep out of the reach of children. Store nicotine in a safe place where children and pets cannot reach it. If a child eats a nicotine lozenge, call your prescriber or

N

health care professional or a poison control center at once. Store below 30 degrees C (86 degrees F). All nicotine products are sensitive to heat. Store in manu-facturers packaging until ready to use. Protect from light. Throw away unused medicine after the expiration date.

Nicotine skin patches

NICODERM® CQ; 21 mg/24 hr; Film, Extended Release GlaxoSmithKline Pharmaceuticals	NICOTINE PATCH; 21 mg/24 hr; Film, Extended Release Schein Pharmaceutical Inc

What are nicotine skin patches?

NICOTINE (Nicotrol®, ProStep®, Habitrol®, NicoDerm® CQ) helps people stop smoking. By replacing nicotine found in cigarettes, physical withdrawal effects are less severe. Nicotine patches are most effective when used in combination with a supervised stop-smoking program. Patches are most effective during the first six months of use. Do not use nicotine skin patches for more than 12 to 20 months, depending on your prescriber's advice. Generic nicotine skin patches are available. NOTE: In some cases, Zyban® (also known as bupropion), a prescription medication, is used together with nicotine to help people stop smoking. You should only use Zyban® with nicotine skin patches or nicotine gum if these have been prescribed by your healthcare prescriber. Ask your prescriber for information and advice before purchasing any non-prescription nicotine products if you are currently on Zyban®. The use of the two medicines together requires special observation by your prescriber.

What should my health care professional know before I use nicotine?

They need to know if you have any of these conditions:
- angina
- asthma
- depression
- diabetes
- heart disease
- high blood pressure
- irregular heartbeat
- overactive thyroid
- pheochromocytoma
- previous heart attack
- stomach ulcers
- an allergy to adhesive plasters or other skin problems
- an unusual or allergic reaction to nicotine, other medicines, foods, dyes, or preservatives
- pregnant or trying to get pregnant
- breast-feeding

How should I use this medicine?

Nicotine patches are for use on the skin. Follow carefully the directions that come with the patches. Use exactly as directed. Find an area of skin on your upper arm, chest, or back that is clean, dry, greaseless, undamaged and hairless. Wash hands in water; do not use soap. Remove the patch from the sealed pouch. Do not try to cut or trim the patch. Using your palm, press the patch firmly in place for 10 seconds to make sure that there is good contact with your skin. Wash your hands with water only. Change the patch every day, keeping to a regular schedule. When you apply a new patch, use a new area of skin. Wait at least 1 week before using the same area again.

What if I miss a dose?

If you forget to replace a patch, use it as soon as you can. Only use one patch at a time and do not leave on the skin for longer than directed. If a patch falls off, you can replace it, but keep to your schedule and remove the patch at the right time.

What may interact with nicotine?

- bupropion
- insulin
- propoxyphene
- propranolol
- theophylline
- warfarin

Tell your prescriber or health care professional about all other medicines you are taking, including non-prescription medicines, nutritional supplements, or herbal products. Also tell your prescriber or health care professional if you are a frequent user of drinks with caffeine or alcohol, or if you use illegal drugs. These may affect the way your medicine works. Check with your health care professional before stopping or starting any of your medicines.

What should I watch for while taking nicotine?

Do not smoke, chew nicotine gum, or use snuff while you are using nicotine skin patches. This reduces the chance of a nicotine overdose. You can keep the patch in place during swimming, bathing, and showering. If your patch falls off during these activities, replace it. When you first apply the patch, your skin may itch or burn; this should soon go away. When you remove a patch, the skin may look red, but this should only last for a day. Call your prescriber or health care professional if you get a permanent skin rash. If you are a diabetic and you quit smoking, the effects of insulin may be increased and you may need to reduce your insulin dose. Check with your prescriber or health care professional about how you should adjust your insulin dose. If you are going to have a MRI procedure, let your MRI technician know about the use of these patches. Some drug patches contain an aluminized backing that can become heated when exposed to MRI and may cause burns. You may need to temporarily remove the patch during the MRI procedure.

N

What side effects may I notice from using nicotine?

Side effects that you should report to your prescriber or health care professional as soon as possible:

- confusion
- dizziness
- fainting or lightheadedness
- fast or irregular heartbeat (palpitations), chest pain
- headache
- hearing changes
- increased saliva
- nausea, vomiting
- seizures (convulsions)
- skin redness that lasts more than 4 days
- skin rash or swelling
- stomach pain
- vision changes
- weakness

Side effects that usually do not require medical attention (report to your prescriber or health care professional if they continue or are bothersome):

- constipation or diarrhea
- flushing
- increased appetite
- irregular menstrual periods
- irritability
- joint or muscle ache
- mild itching, burning, or tingling for the first hour after applying
- sleep disturbance

Where can I keep my medicine?

Keep out of the reach of children. Store nicotine in a safe place where children and pets cannot reach it. When you remove a patch, fold with sticky sides together; put in an empty opened pouch and throw away. Store below 30 degrees C (86 degrees F). All nicotine products are sensitive to heat. Store in manufacturers packaging until ready to use. Protect from light. Throw away unused medicine after the expiration date.

Nifedipine capsules and extended-release tablets

PROCARDIA XL®; 60 mg; Tablet, Extended Release Pfizer Laboratories Div Pfizer Inc

ADALAT®; 10 mg; Capsule Bayer Corp Pharmaceutical Div

What are nifedipine capsules or extended-release tablets?

NIFEDIPINE (Adalat®, Adalat® CC, Procardia®, Procardia XL®) is a calcium-channel blocker. It affects the amount of calcium found in your heart and muscle cells. This results in relaxation of blood vessels, which can reduce the amount of work the heart has to do. Depending on the dosage form, nifedipine reduces attacks of chest pain (angina), and/or helps reduce high blood pressure (hypertension). It is not a cure. Generic nifedipine capsules and extended-release tablets are available.

What should my health care professional know before I take nifedipine?

They need to know if you have any of these conditions:

- difficulty swallowing
- heart problems, low blood pressure, slow or irregular heartbeat
- liver disease
- previous heart attack
- over 65 years old
- an unusual or allergic reaction to nifedipine, other medicines, foods, dyes, or preservatives
- pregnant or trying to get pregnant
- breast-feeding

How should I take this medicine?

Take nifedipine capsules or tablets by mouth. Follow the directions on the prescription label. Swallow the tablets whole with a drink of water; do not cut, crush or chew. Avoid taking nifedipine with grapefruit juice or grapefruit. Take your doses at regular intervals. Do not take your medicine more often then directed. Do not stop taking except on your prescriber's advice. Contact your pediatrician or health care professional regarding the use of this medicine in children. Special care may be needed. Elderly patients over 65 years old may have a stronger reaction to this medicine and need smaller doses.

What if I miss a dose?

If you miss a dose, take it as soon as you can. If it is almost time for your next dose, (less than 6 to 8 hours) take only that dose. Do not take double or extra doses.

What may interact with nifedipine?

Do not take nifedipine with any of the following:

- grapefruit juice

Nifedipine may also interact with the following medications:

- alcohol
- anti-inflammatory drugs (NSAIDs, such as ibuprofen)
- barbiturates such as phenobarbital
- bosentan
- calcium salts (intravenous)
- cimetidine
- cyclosporine
- female hormones, including contraceptive or birth control pills
- herbal or dietary supplements such as gingko biloba, ginseng, hawthorn, ma huang (ephedra), melatonin, St. John's wort, went yeast
- imatinib, STI-571

N

- local anesthetics or general anesthetics
- magnesium salts (intravenous)
- medicines for fungal infections (fluconazole, itraconazole, ketoconazole, voriconazole)
- medicines for high blood pressure
- medicines for HIV infection or AIDS
- medicines for prostate problems
- medicines for seizures (carbamazepine, phenobarbital, phenytoin, primidone)
- metformin
- rifampin, rifapentine, or rifabutin
- some antibiotics (clarithromycin, erythromycin, telithromycin, troleandomycin)
- some medicines for heart-rhythm problems (amiodarone, digoxin, diltiazem, disopyramide, flecainide, quinidine, verapamil)
- some medicines for depression or mental problems (fluoxetine, fluvoxamine, nefazodone)
- tacrolimus
- vincristine
- warfarin
- water pills (diuretics)
- yohimbine
- zafirlukast
- zileuton

Tell your prescriber or health care professional about all other medicines you are taking, including non-prescription medicines, nutritional supplements, or herbal products. Also tell your prescriber or health care professional if you are a frequent user of drinks with caffeine or alcohol, if you smoke, or if you use illegal drugs. These may affect the way your medicine works. Check with your health care professional before stopping or starting any of your medicines.

What should I watch for while taking nifedipine?

Check your blood pressure and pulse rate regularly; this is important while you are taking nifedipine. Ask your prescriber or health care professional what your blood pressure and pulse rate should be and when you should contact him or her. Do not suddenly stop taking nifedipine. Ask your prescriber or health care professional how to gradually reduce the dose. You may feel dizzy or lightheaded. Do not drive, use machinery, or do anything that needs mental alertness until you know how nifedipine affects you. To reduce the risk of dizzy or fainting spells, do not sit or stand up quickly, especially if you are an older patient. Alcohol can make you more dizzy, increase flushing and rapid heartbeats. Avoid alcoholic drinks. If you are going to have surgery, tell your prescriber or health care professional that you are taking nifedipine. If you are taking Procardia XL, you may notice the empty shell of the tablet in your stool.

What side effects may I notice from taking nifedipine?

Side effects that you should report to your prescriber or health care professional as soon as possible:
- blood in the urine
- fast heartbeat, palpitations, irregular heartbeat, chest pain
- difficulty breathing
- dizziness
- fainting spells, lightheadedness
- reduced amount of urine passed
- redness, blistering, peeling or loosening of the skin, including inside the mouth
- skin rash
- swelling of the legs and ankles

Side effects that usually do not require medical attention (report to your prescriber or health care professional if they continue or are bothersome):
- facial flushing
- headache
- weakness or tiredness

Where can I keep my medicine?

Keep out of the reach of children in a container that small children cannot open. Store at room temperature between 15 and 25 degrees C (59 and 77 degrees F). Protect from light and moisture. Keep container tightly closed. Throw away any unused medicine after the expiration date.

Nilutamide tablets

NILANDRON®;
150 mg; Tablet
Aventis Pharmaceuticals Inc

What are nilutamide tablets?

NILUTAMIDE (Nilandron®) blocks the effect of the male hormone called testosterone. Prostate cancer responds to the removal of androgens. Nilutamide is used in combination with surgical treatment. Generic nilutamide tablets are not yet available.

What should my health care professional know before I take nilutamide?

They need to know if you have any of these conditions:
- alcoholism
- anemia
- liver disease
- lung disease
- visual problems
- an unusual or allergic reaction to nilutamide, other medicines, foods, dyes, or preservatives

How should I take this medicine?

Take nilutamide tablets by mouth at the same time each day. Follow the directions on the prescription label. Swallow the tablets with a drink of water. Do not take your medicine more often than directed. Finish the full course prescribed by your doctor or health care professional, even if the tablets make you feel unwell. Do not stop taking except on your prescriber's advice. Contact your pediatrician or health care professional regarding the use of this medicine in children. Special care may be needed.

What if I miss a dose?

If you miss a dose, take it as soon as you can. If it is almost time for your next dose, take only that dose. Do not take double or extra doses. If you vomit after taking a dose, call your prescriber or health care professional for advice.

What may interact with nilutamide?

- ethanol
- phenytoin
- theophylline
- warfarin

Tell your prescriber or health care professional about all other medicines you are taking, including non-prescription medicines, nutritional supplements, or herbal products. Also tell your prescriber or health care professional if you are a frequent user of drinks with caffeine or alcohol, if you smoke, or if you use illegal drugs. These may affect the way your medicine works. Check with your health care professional before stopping or starting any of your medicines.

What should I watch for while taking nilutamide?

Visit your prescriber or health care professional for regular checks on your progress. At first your condition can get worse, but it will then improve as you continue your treatment. Improvement in your condition can take several days. Nilutamide may affect your vision. If you notice a change in how your eyes adjust to the dark after starting nilutamide, do not drive at night or through tunnels. This side effect usually goes away. Wearing tinted glasses may help. You should avoid alcohol while taking nilutamide. Mixing alcohol and nilutamide can cause more side effects.

What side effects may I notice from taking nilutamide?

Side effects that you should report to your prescriber or health care professional as soon as possible:
- difficulty breathing when exerting yourself
- chest pain
- fever
- persistent cough
- skin rash, hives, or itching
- swelling of the lips, tongue or face
- vomiting
- yellowing of the skin

Side effects that usually do not require medical attention (report to your prescriber or health care professional if they continue or are bothersome):
- constipation
- diarrhea
- dizziness
- hot flashes
- nausea
- vision disturbance (trouble adjusting to the dark)

Where can I keep my medicine?

Keep out of the reach of children in a container that small children cannot open. Store between 15 and 30 degrees C (59 and 86 degrees F). Protect from light. Throw away any unused medicine after the expiration date.

Nimodipine capsules

NIMOTOP®;
30 mg; Capsule
Bayer Corp Pharmaceutical
Div

What are nimodipine capsules?

NIMODIPINE (Nimotop®) is a calcium-channel blocker. It affects the flow of calcium in and out of certain cells in your body and relaxes blood vessels. Nimodipine is used to treat subarachnoid hemorrhage, a condition in which severe headaches and stiff neck are caused by bleeding into the space around the brain. Generic nimodipine capsules are not yet available.

What should my health care professional know before I take nimodipine?

They need to know if you have any of these conditions:
- heart problems, slow heart rate
- liver disease
- low blood pressure
- previous heart attack
- an unusual or allergic reaction to nimodipine, other medicines, foods, dyes, or preservatives
- pregnant or trying to get pregnant
- breast-feeding

How should I take this medicine?

Take nimodipine capsules by mouth. Follow the directions on the prescription label. Swallow the capsules with a drink of water. Avoid taking nimodipine with grapefruit juice or grapefruit. Take your doses at regular intervals. Do not take your medicine more often than directed. Continue to take your medicine even if you feel better. Do not stop taking except on your prescriber's advice. Contact your pediatrician or health care professional regarding the use of this medicine in children. Special care may be needed.

N

What if I miss a dose?

If you miss a dose, take it as soon as you can. If it is almost time for your next dose, take only that dose. Do not take double or extra doses.

What may interact with nimodipine?

Do not take nimodipine with any of the following:

- grapefruit juice

Nimodipine may also interact with the following medications:

- anti-inflammatory drugs (NSAIDs, such as ibuprofen)
- barbiturates such as phenobarbital
- bosentan
- calcium salts (intravenous)
- cimetidine
- herbal or dietary supplements such as gingko biloba, ginseng, hawthorn, ma huang (ephedra), melatonin, St. John's wort, went yeast
- imatinib, STI-571
- local anesthetics or general anesthetics
- medicines for fungal infections (fluconazole, itraconazole, ketoconazole, voriconazole)
- medicines for high blood pressure
- medicines for HIV infection or AIDS
- medicines for prostate problems
- medicines for seizures (carbamazepine, phenobarbital, phenytoin, primidone)
- rifampin, rifapentine, or rifabutin
- some antibiotics (clarithromycin, erythromycin, telithromycin, troleandomycin)
- some medicines for heart-rhythm problems (amiodarone, diltiazem, verapamil)
- some medicines for depression or mental problems (fluoxetine, fluvoxamine, nefazodone)
- valproic acid
- water pills (diuretics)
- yohimbine
- zafirlukast
- zileuton

Tell your prescriber or health care professional about all other medicines you are taking, including non-prescription medicines, nutritional supplements, or herbal products. Also tell your prescriber or health care professional if you are a frequent user of drinks with caffeine or alcohol, if you smoke, or if you use illegal drugs. These may affect the way your medicine works. Check with your health care professional before stopping or starting any of your medicines.

What should I watch for while taking nimodipine?

Visit your prescriber or health care professional for regular checks on your progress. Alcohol can increase the chance of getting low blood pressure. Avoid alcoholic drinks while you are taking nimodipine.

What side effects may I notice from taking nimodipine?

Side effects that you should report to your prescriber or health care professional as soon as possible:

- difficulty breathing
- dizziness or drowsiness
- irregular or fast heartbeats (palpitations)
- lightheadedness or fainting
- slow heartbeat
- swelling of the legs or ankles
- unusual bleeding or bruising, red spots on skin
- unusual weakness or tiredness

Side effects that usually do not require medical attention (report to your prescriber or health care professional if they continue or are bothersome):

- flushing
- headache
- nausea
- sweating

Where can I keep my medicine?

Keep out of reach of children in a container that small children cannot open. Store at room temperature between 15 and 30 degrees C (59 and 86 degrees F); do not freeze. Protect from light. Keep foil packaged capsules in their original foil until needed. Throw away any unused medicine after the expiration date.

Nisoldipine tablets

SULAR®;
20 mg; Tablet,
Extended Release
First Horizon
Pharmaceutical Corp

SULAR®;
10 mg; Tablet,
Extended Release
First Horizon
Pharmaceutical Corp

What are nisoldipine tablets?

NISOLDIPINE (Sular®) is a calcium-channel blocker. It relaxes blood vessels, which can lower blood pressure and reduce the amount of work the heart has to do. Nisoldipine reduces blood pressure and may reduce attacks of chest pain if you have angina. It is not a cure. Generic nisoldipine is not available.

What should my health care professional know before I take nisoldipine?

They need to know if you have any of these conditions:

- heart problems, including heart failure or aortic stenosis
- liver disease
- low blood pressure

N

- persistent chest pain
- previous heart attack
- slow or irregular heartbeat
- an unusual or allergic reaction to nisoldipine, nifedipine, dihydropyridines, other medicines, foods, dyes, or preservatives
- pregnant or trying to get pregnant
- breast-feeding

How should I take this medicine?

Take nisoldipine tablets by mouth. Follow the directions on the prescription label. Swallow the tablets whole with a drink of water. The tablets should not be chewed, divided, or crushed. Do not take nisoldipine with grapefruit juice, grapefruit, or with a high-fat meal. Take your doses at regular intervals. Do not take your medicine more often then directed. Do not stop taking except when advised by your prescriber. Older patients (over 65 years old) may have a stronger reaction to this medicine and need smaller doses.

What if I miss a dose?

If you miss a dose, take it as soon as you can. If it is almost time for your next dose, take only that dose. Do not take double or extra doses.

What may interact with nisoldipine?

Do not take nisoldipine with any of the following:

- grapefruit juice

Nisoldipine may also interact with the following medications:

- anti-inflammatory drugs (NSAIDs, such as ibuprofen)
- barbiturates such as phenobarbital
- bosentan
- cimetidine
- female hormones, including contraceptive or birth control pills
- herbal or dietary supplements such as gingko biloba, ginseng, hawthorn, ma huang (ephedra), melatonin, St. John's wort, went yeast
- imatinib, STI-571
- local anesthetics or general anesthetics
- medicines for fungal infections (fluconazole, itraconazole, ketoconazole, voriconazole)
- medicines for high blood pressure
- medicines for HIV infection or AIDS
- medicines for prostate problems
- medicines for seizures (carbamazepine, phenobarbital, phenytoin, primidone)
- rifampin, rifapentine, or rifabutin
- some antibiotics (clarithromycin, erythromycin, telithromycin, troleandomycin)
- some medicines for heart-rhythm problems (amiodarone, digoxin, diltiazem, disopyramide, flecainide, quinidine, verapamil)
- some medicines for depression or mental problems (fluoxetine, fluvoxamine, nefazodone)
- water pills (diuretics)
- yohimbine
- zafirlukast
- zileuton

Tell your prescriber or health care professional about all other medicines you are taking, including non-prescription medicines, nutritional supplements, or herbal products. Also tell your prescriber or health care professional if you are a frequent user of drinks with caffeine or alcohol, if you smoke, or if you use illegal drugs. These may affect the way your medicine works. Check with your health care professional before stopping or starting any of your medicines.

What should I watch for while taking nisoldipine?

Check your blood pressure and pulse rate regularly; this is important while you are taking nisoldipine. Ask your prescriber or health care professional what your blood pressure and pulse rate should be and when you should contact him or her. Do not stop taking nisoldipine except as advised by your prescriber. You may feel dizzy or lightheaded. Do not drive, use machinery, or do anything that needs mental alertness until you know how nisoldipine affects you. To reduce the risk of dizzy or fainting spells, do not sit or stand up quickly, especially if you are an older patient. Alcohol can make you more dizzy, increase flushing and rapid heartbeats. Avoid alcoholic drinks. If you are going to have surgery, tell your prescriber or health care professional that you are taking nisoldipine.

What side effects may I notice from taking nisoldipine?

Side effects that you should report to your prescriber or health care professional as soon as possible:

- fast heartbeat, palpitations, or irregular heartbeat
- chest pain
- difficulty breathing
- dizziness, fainting spells, confusion, or lightheadedness
- impaired sexual function
- muscle cramps
- reduced amount of urine passed
- swelling of the legs or ankles
- swelling of the gums
- unusual tiredness or fatigue
- unusual rash or skin reaction

Side effects that usually do not require medical attention (report to your prescriber or health care professional if they continue or are bothersome):

- facial or skin flushing
- headache
- nasal congestion
- nausea or vomiting
- weakness or tiredness

Where can I keep my medicine?

Keep out of the reach of children in a container that small children cannot open. Store at room temperature between 20 and 25 degrees C (68 and 77 degrees F). Protect from light and moisture. Keep container tightly closed. Throw away any unused medicine after the expiration date.

Nitrofurantoin tablets or capsules

MACROBID®;
75 mg/25 mg; Capsule
Procter and Gamble
Pharmaceuticals Inc Sub
Procter and Gamble Co

What are nitrofurantoin tablets or capsules?

NITROFURANTOIN (Furadantin®, Macrodantin®, Macrobid®) is an antibiotic. It is used to treat cystitis and other urinary tract infections. Generic nitrofurantoin tablets or capsules are available.

What should my health care professional know before I take nitrofurantoin?

They need to know if you have any of these conditions:
- anemia or other blood disorders
- dehydration or fluid or electrolyte problems (problems with the amount of water and salts in your body)
- diabetes
- glucose-6-phosphate dehydrogenase (G6PD) deficiency
- kidney disease
- liver disease
- lung disease
- vitamin B deficiency
- other chronic illness
- an unusual or allergic reaction to nitrofurantoin, furazolidone, nitrofurazone, or to any food, dye, or medicine
- pregnant or trying to get pregnant
- breast-feeding

How should I take this medicine?

Take nitrofurantoin tablets or capsules by mouth. Follow the directions on the prescription label. Take with food or milk if nitrofurantoin upsets your stomach. Do not take your medicine more often than directed. Finish the full course of medicine prescribed by your doctor or health care professional, even if you feel better. Take your doses at regular intervals and at the same time each day. Contact your pediatrician or health care professional regarding the use of this medicine in children. Special care may be needed.

What if I miss a dose?

If you miss a dose, take it as soon as you can. If it is almost time for your next dose, take only that dose. Do not take double doses. You must leave a suitable interval between doses. If you have to take a missed dose make sure there is at least 2 to 4 hours between doses.

What may interact with nitrofurantoin?

- antacids containing magnesium trisilicate
- certain antibiotics (such as ciprofloxacin, lomefloxacin, norfloxacin and ofloxacin)
- probenecid
- sulfinpyrazone

Tell your prescriber or health care professional about all other medicines you are taking, including non-prescription medicines, nutritional supplements, or herbal products. Also tell your prescriber or health care professional if you are a frequent user of drinks with caffeine or alcohol, if you smoke, or if you use illegal drugs. These may affect the way your medicine works. Check with your health care professional before stopping or starting any of your medicines.

What should I watch for while taking nitrofurantoin?

Tell your prescriber or health care professional if your symptoms do not improve in 3 or 4 days. If you are taking this medicine for a long time, you must visit your prescriber or health care professional for regular checks on your progress. Drink several glasses of water a day. This will help to reduce possible kidney damage. If you are diabetic you may get a false-positive result for sugar in your urine. Check with your prescriber or health care professional before you change your diet or the dose of your diabetic medicine.

What side effects may I notice from taking nitrofurantoin?

Side effects that you should report to your prescriber or health care professional as soon as possible:
- fever or chills, sore throat
- chest pain
- cough
- difficulty breathing or shortness of breath
- dizziness, drowsiness
- headache
- joint aches or pains
- pale skin
- redness, blistering, peeling or loosening of the skin, including inside the mouth
- skin rash, itching and swelling
- tingling, burning, pain, or numbness in hands or feet
- unusual bleeding or bruising
- unusual weakness or tiredness
- vomiting
- yellowing of eyes or skin

Side effects that usually do not require medical attention (report to your prescriber or health care professional if they continue or are bothersome):
- diarrhea
- loss of appetite
- nausea
- stomach pain
- dark yellow or brown urine

Where can I keep my medicine?

Keep out of the reach of children in a container that small children cannot open. Store at room temperature between 15 and 30 degrees C (59 and 86 degrees F). Protect from light. Throw away any unused medicine after the expiration date.

N

Nitroglycerin skin patches

NITROGLYCERIN
0.1 MG/HR;
Patch
Mylan
Pharmaceuticals Inc

NITROGLYCERIN
0.6 MG/HR;
Patch
Mylan
Pharmaceuticals Inc

What are nitroglycerin skin patches?

NITROGLYCERIN (Transderm-Nitro®, Nitro-Dur®, Nitrodisc®, Minitran®, Deponit®) is a type of vasodilator. It relaxes blood vessels, increasing the blood and oxygen supply to your heart. Nitroglycerin skin patches are used regularly to help reduce the number of angina attacks (chest pains). They are not suitable for immediate relief during an angina attack. Generic nitroglycerin skin patches are available.

What should my health care professional know before I use nitroglycerin?

They need to know if you have any of these conditions:
- anemia
- dizziness or fainting spells when rising from a sitting position
- fever
- glaucoma
- head injury, recent stroke, or bleeding in the brain
- liver disease
- low blood pressure, or low blood volume
- previous heart attack
- overactive thyroid
- stomach or intestinal disease
- an unusual or allergic reaction to nitroglycerin, other medicines, foods, dyes, or preservatives
- pregnant or trying to get pregnant
- breast-feeding

How should I use this medicine?

Nitroglycerin skin patches are for external use only. Follow the directions on the prescription label. Use exactly as directed. One patch contains a full day's supply of nitroglycerin. It is usually worn for up to 18 hours a day. Apply the patch to an area on the upper body that is clean, dry and hairless; avoid injured, irritated, calloused, or scarred areas. Use a different site each day to prevent skin irritation. Do not cut or trim the patch. Do not stop using except on your prescriber's advice. Do not use your medicine more often than directed. Contact your pediatrician or health care professional regarding the use of this medicine in children. Special care may be needed.

What if I miss a dose?

If you miss a dose, apply the patch as soon as you can. Do not wear two patches at the same time unless told to by your prescriber or health care professional.

What may interact with nitroglycerin?

Do not take nitroglycerin if you are taking the following medications:

- sildenafil (Viagra®)
- tadalafil (Cialis®)
- vardenafil (Levitra®)

Nitroglycerin may also interact with the following medications:

- alcohol
- bromocriptine
- hawthorn
- heparin
- medicines for anxiety or sleeping problems, such as diazepam or temazepam
- medicines for colds and breathing difficulties
- medicines for high blood pressure
- medicines for mental depression
- medicines for migraine
- medicines for pain
- procainamide
- quinidine
- water pills

Viagra® (sildenafil), Cialis® (tadalafil), or Levitra® (vardenafil) should not be taken with this medication to avoid severe side effects including very low blood pressure and other complications. Tell your prescriber or health care professional about all other medicines you are taking, including non-prescription medicines, nutritional supplements, or herbal products. Also tell your prescriber or health care professional if you are a frequent user of drinks with caffeine or alcohol, if you smoke, or if you use illegal drugs. These may affect the way your medicine works. Check with your health care professional before stopping or starting any of your medicines.

What should I watch for while taking nitroglycerin?

Check your heart rate and blood pressure regularly while you are using nitroglycerin. Ask your prescriber or health care professional what your heart rate and blood pressure should be and when you should contact him or her. Tell your prescriber or health care professional if you feel your medicine is no longer having any effect. You may get dizzy. Do not drive, use machinery, or do anything that needs mental alertness until you know how nitroglycerin affects you. To reduce the risk of dizzy or fainting spells, do not sit or stand up quickly, especially if you are an older patient. If you feel dizzy, take several deep breaths and lie down with your feet propped up, or bend forward with your head resting between your knees. Alcohol can make you more dizzy, increase flushing and rapid heartbeats. Avoid alcoholic drinks. Do not stop using nitroglycerin suddenly or your symptoms may get worse. Ask your prescriber or health care professional how to gradually reduce the dose. If the patch pulls loose or falls off, fold it in half (sticky side in) and throw away out of the reach of children or pets. Replace with a fresh patch. Avoid use of microwave ovens that are in bad

N

repair; leaking radiation can heat the patch, causing rare reports of burns or changes in the absorption and action of this medicine. If you are going to have a MRI procedure, let your MRI technician know about the use of these patches. Some drug patches contain an aluminized backing that can become heated when exposed to MRI and may cause burns. You may need to temporarily remove the patch during the MRI procedure.

What side effects may I notice from using nitroglycerin?

Side effects that you should report to your prescriber or health care professional as soon as possible:

- bluish discoloration of lips, fingernails, or palms of hands
- blurred vision
- dry mouth
- skin rash, or irritation from the skin patch

- sweating
- the feeling of extreme pressure in the head
- unusual tiredness or weakness

Side effects that usually do not require medical attention (report to your prescriber or health care professional if they continue or are bothersome):

- dizziness or fainting
- flushing of the face or neck
- headache, this is common after a dose, but usually only lasts for a short time
- irregular heartbeat, palpitations
- nausea, vomiting

Where can I keep my medicine?

Keep out of the reach of children. Store at room temperature between 15 and 25 degrees C (59 and 77 degrees F); do not refrigerate. Heat can reduce the effectiveness of this medicine. Throw away any unused medicine after the expiration date.

Nitroglycerin **sublingual tablets**	NITROSTAT®; 0.3 mg; Tablet Pfizer Pharmaceuticals Ltd		NITROQUICK®; 0.4 mg; Tablet Ethex Corporation	

What are nitroglycerin sublingual (under the tongue) tablets?

NITROGLYCERIN (Nitrostat®, Nitroquick®) is a type of vasodilator. It relaxes blood vessels, increasing the blood and oxygen supply to your heart. Nitroglycerin sublingual tablets are used to relieve chest pain (angina). They can be used to prevent chest pain before activities that can cause an angina attack (such as climbing stairs, going outdoors in cold weather, or having sex). Generic nitroglycerin sublingual tablets are available.

What should my health care professional know before I take nitroglycerin?

They need to know if you have any of these conditions:
- anemia
- dizziness or fainting spells when rising from a sitting position
- fever
- glaucoma
- head injury, recent stroke, or bleeding in the brain
- liver disease
- low blood pressure, or low blood volume
- previous heart attack
- overactive thyroid
- stomach or intestinal disease
- an unusual or allergic reaction to nitroglycerin, other medicines, foods, dyes, or preservatives
- pregnant or trying to get pregnant
- breast-feeding

How should I take this medicine?

You can take nitroglycerin sublingual tablets as needed. At the first sign of an angina attack (chest pain or tightness) place one tablet under your tongue. You can also use a nitroglycerin sublingual tablet 5 to 10 min-

utes before an event likely to produce chest pain. Follow the directions on the prescription label. Let the tablet dissolve under the tongue; do not swallow whole. Replace the dose if you accidentally swallow it. It will help if your mouth is not dry; saliva (fluid) around the tablet will help it to dissolve more quickly. Do not eat or drink, or smoke or chew tobacco while a tablet is dissolving. Your symptoms should improve in 1 to 5 minutes. You can repeat the dose every 5 minutes for up to three doses. If you are no better after 3 doses, contact your prescriber or health care professional immediately or have someone take you straight to an emergency room. Although it is acceptable to take more than 3 doses to treat an acute attack, do not take your medicine more often than directed. Contact your pediatrician or health care professional regarding the use of this medicine in children. Special care may be needed.

What if I miss a dose?

This does not apply because the nitroglycerin sublingual tablets are used as needed. Do not use double or extra doses. Extra doses will not take away chest pain.

What may interact with nitroglycerin?

Do not take nitroglycerin if you are taking the following medications:

- sildenafil (Viagra®)
- tadalafil (Cialis®)
- vardenafil (Levitra®)

Nitroglycerin may also interact with the following medications:

- alcohol
- bromocriptine

N

- hawthorn
- heparin
- medicines for anxiety or sleeping problems, such as diazepam or temazepam
- medicines for colds and breathing difficulties
- medicines for high blood pressure
- medicines for mental depression
- medicines for migraine
- medicines for pain
- procainamide
- quinidine
- water pills

Viagra® (sildenafil), Cialis® (tadalafil), or Levitra® (vardenafil) should not be taken with this medication to avoid severe side effects including very low blood pressure and other complications. Tell your prescriber or health care professional about all other medicines you are taking, including non-prescription medicines, nutritional supplements, or herbal products. Also tell your prescriber or health care professional if you are a frequent user of drinks with caffeine or alcohol, if you smoke, or if you use illegal drugs. These may affect the way your medicine works. Check with your health care professional before stopping or starting any of your medicines.

What should I watch for while taking nitroglycerin?

Tell your prescriber or health care professional if you feel your medicine is no longer having any effect. Keep this medicine with you at all times. At the first sign of an angina attack (chest pain or tightness) place a tablet under the tongue. Sit or lie down to prevent falling if you feel dizzy or faint after using nitroglycerin. Try to remain calm; this will help you to feel better faster. If you feel dizzy, take several deep breaths and lie down with your feet propped up, or bend forward with your head resting between your knees. If nitroglycerin does make you dizzy, do not drive, use machinery, or do anything that needs mental alertness. To reduce the risk of dizzy or fainting spells, do not sit or stand up quickly, especially if you are an older patient. Alcohol can make you more dizzy, increase flushing and rapid heartbeats. Avoid alcoholic drinks. Replace sublingual nitroglycerin tablets regularly. When exposed to heat, light, or moisture they can quickly lose their effectiveness. Keep the tablets in the original container. If the bottle is unopened the tablets will keep for 6 months. Once opened, replace after 2 months. Do not leave the tablets in the car, or in a warm place. Do not tip tablets out into your hand, but into the bottle lid and then try to handle only the tablet you are about to take.

What side effects may I notice from taking nitroglycerin?

Side effects that you should report to your prescriber or health care professional as soon as possible:
- blurred vision
- dry mouth
- skin rash
- sweating
- the feeling of extreme pressure in the head
- unusual tiredness or weakness

Side effects that usually do not require medical attention (report to your prescriber or health care professional if they continue or are bothersome):
- dizziness or fainting
- flushing of the face or neck
- headache, this is common after a dose, but usually only lasts for a short time
- irregular heartbeat, palpitations
- nausea, vomiting

Where can I keep my medicine?

Keep out of the reach of children. These tablets should be dispensed and stored in the original container; keep tightly closed. Remove the cotton from the bottle before the medicine is required for chest pain. Store at room temperature between 15 and 25 degrees C (59 and 77 degrees F). Heat and moisture can reduce the effectiveness of this medicine. Throw away any unused medicine after the expiration date.

Nitroglycerin sustained-release tablets or capsules

NITROGLYCERIN;
6.5 mg; Capsule,
Extended Release
Eon Labs Inc

NITROGLYCERIN;
6.5 mg; Capsule,
Extended Release
Ethex Corporation

What are nitroglycerin sustained release tablets or capsules?

NITROGLYCERIN (Nitro-Bid®, Nitroglyn®) is a type of vasodilator. It relaxes blood vessels, increasing the blood and oxygen supply to your heart. Nitroglycerin sustained-release products are taken regularly to help prevent or relieve chest pain (angina). They are not suitable for immediate relief during an angina attack. Generic nitroglycerin sustained-release tablets and capsules are available.

What should my health care professional know before I take nitroglycerin?

They need to know if you have any of these conditions:
- anemia
- dizziness or fainting spells when rising from a sitting position
- fever
- glaucoma
- head injury, recent stroke, or bleeding in the brain
- liver disease

N

- low blood pressure, or low blood volume
- previous heart attack
- overactive thyroid
- stomach or intestinal disease
- an unusual or allergic reaction to nitroglycerin, other medicines, foods, dyes, or preservatives
- pregnant or trying to get pregnant
- breast-feeding

How should I take this medicine?

Take nitroglycerin sustained-release tablets or capsules by mouth. Follow the directions on the prescription label. Swallow the tablets or capsules whole with a drink of water; do not crush or chew. Take on an empty stomach, at least 30 minutes before or 1 to 2 hours after meals. Take at regular intervals and try to take your doses at the same time each day, following the schedule prescribed by your prescriber or health care professional. Continue to take them even if you feel better. It can take several weeks or longer to see the full effects of this medicine. Do not stop taking except on your prescriber's advice. Do not take your medicine more often than directed. Contact your pediatrician or health care professional regarding the use of this medicine in children. Special care may be needed.

What if I miss a dose?

If you miss a dose, take it as soon as you can. If it is almost time for your next dose (less than 6 hours), take only that dose. Do not take double or extra doses. Extra doses will not take away chest pain.

What may interact with nitroglycerin?

Do not take nitroglycerin if you are taking the following medications:

- sildenafil (Viagra®)
- tadalafil (Cialis®)
- vardenafil (Levitra®)

Nitroglycerin may also interact with the following medications:

- alcohol
- bromocriptine
- hawthorn
- heparin
- medicines for anxiety or sleeping problems, such as diazepam or temazepam
- medicines for colds and breathing difficulties
- medicines for high blood pressure
- medicines for mental depression
- medicines for migraine
- medicines for pain
- procainamide
- quinidine
- water pills

Viagra® (sildenafil), Cialis® (tadalafil), or Levitra® (vardenafil) should not be taken with this medication to avoid severe side effects including very low blood pressure and other complications. Tell your prescriber or health care professional about all other medicines you are taking, including non-prescription medicines, nutritional supplements, or herbal products. Also tell your prescriber or health care professional if you are a frequent user of drinks with caffeine or alcohol, if you smoke, or if you use illegal drugs. These may affect the way your medicine works. Check with your health care professional before stopping or starting any of your medicines.

What should I watch for while taking nitroglycerin?

Check your heart rate and blood pressure regularly while you are taking nitroglycerin. Ask your prescriber or health care professional what your heart rate and blood pressure should be and when you should contact him or her. Tell your prescriber or health care professional if you feel your medicine is no longer having any effect. You may get dizzy. Do not drive, use machinery, or do anything that needs mental alertness until you know how nitroglycerin affects you. To reduce the risk of dizzy or fainting spells, do not sit or stand up quickly, especially if you are an older patient. If you feel dizzy, take several deep breaths and lie down with your feet propped up, or bend forward with your head resting between your knees. Alcohol can make you more dizzy, increase flushing and rapid heartbeats. Avoid alcoholic drinks. Do not stop taking nitroglycerin suddenly or your symptoms may get worse. Ask your prescriber or health care professional how to gradually reduce the dose.

What side effects may I notice from taking nitroglycerin?

Side effects that you should report to your prescriber or health care professional as soon as possible:

- bluish discoloration of lips, fingernails, or palms of hands
- blurred vision
- dry mouth
- skin rash
- sweating
- the feeling of extreme pressure in the head
- unusual tiredness or weakness

Side effects that usually do not require medical attention (report to your prescriber or health care professional if they continue or are bothersome):

- dizziness or fainting
- flushing of the face or neck
- headache, this is common after a dose, but usually only lasts for a short time
- irregular heartbeat, palpitations
- nausea, vomiting

Where can I keep my medicine?

Keep out of the reach of children, especially if you are not using a child-resistant container. Store at room temperature between 15 and 25 degrees C (59 and 77 degrees F). Keep dry in a tightly sealed container. Heat and moisture can reduce the effectiveness of this medicine. Throw away any unused medicine after the expiration date.

N

Nizatidine capsules

AXID®;
300 mg; Capsule
Reliant
Pharmaceuticals Llc

AXID®;
150 mg; Capsule
Reliant
Pharmaceuticals Llc

What are nizatidine capsules?

NIZATIDINE (Axid®) is a type of antihistamine that blocks the release of stomach acid. Nizatidine is used to treat gastric and duodenal ulcers. It can relieve ulcer pain and discomfort, and the heartburn from gastroesophageal reflux disease. Generic nizatidine capsules are available.

What should my health care professional know before I take nizatidine?

They need to know if you have any of these conditions:
- bloody or black stools
- frequently drink alcoholic beverages
- kidney disease
- liver disease
- other chronic illness
- difficulty or pain while swallowing
- an unusual or allergic reaction to nizatidine, other medicines, foods, dyes, or preservatives
- pregnant or trying to get pregnant
- breast-feeding

How should I take this medicine?

Take nizatidine capsules by mouth. Follow the directions on the prescription label. Swallow the capsules with a drink of water. If you only take nizatidine once a day take it at bedtime. Take your doses at regular intervals. Do not take your medicine more often than directed. Contact your pediatrician or health care professional regarding the use of this medicine in children. Special care may be needed.

What if I miss a dose?

If you miss a dose, take it as soon as you can. If it is almost time for your next dose, take only that dose. Do not take double or extra doses.

What may interact with nizatidine?

- aspirin and aspirin-like medicines
- cefditoren
- cefpodoxime
- cefuroxime
- delavirdine
- itraconazole
- ketoconazole
- metformin

Tell your prescriber or health care professional about all other medicines you are taking, including non-pre-scription medicines, nutritional supplements, or herbal products. Also tell your prescriber or health care professional if you are a frequent user of drinks with caffeine or alcohol, if you smoke, or if you use illegal drugs. These may affect the way your medicine works. Check with your health care professional before stopping or starting any of your medicines.

What should I watch for while taking nizatidine?

Tell your prescriber or health care professional if your ulcer pain does not improve or gets worse. You may need to take this medicine for several days as prescribed before your symptoms improve. Finish the full course of tablets prescribed by your prescriber or health care professional even if you feel better. Do not self-medicate with aspirin, ibuprofen or other antiinflammatory medicines; these can aggravate your ulcer and may make it bleed. Do not smoke cigarettes or drink alcohol; these increase irritation in your stomach and can lengthen the time it will take for your ulcers to heal. If you get black, tarry stools or vomit up what looks like coffee grounds, call your prescriber or health care professional at once. You may have a bleeding ulcer.

What side effects may I notice from taking nizatidine?

Side effects with nizatidine are infrequent but include:
- agitation, nervousness, depression, hallucinations
- breast swelling and tenderness, or sexual difficulties (impotence) in men
- dark yellow or brown urine
- diarrhea
- dizziness
- headache
- increased sweating
- nausea, vomiting
- skin rash, itching
- stomach pain
- yellowing of the skin or eyes

Let your prescriber or health care professional know if you get any of these side effects.

Where can I keep my medicine?

Keep out of the reach of children in a container that small children cannot open. Store at room temperature between 15 and 30 degrees C (59 and 86 degrees F). Throw away any unused medicine after the expiration date.

N

Norethindrone tablets

AYGESTIN®;
5 mg; Tablet
Duramed Pharmaceuticals Inc
Sub Barr Laboratories Inc

What are norethindrone tablets?

NORETHINDRONE (Ortho-Micronor® or Errin™ or Jolivette™, Nor-QD® or Camila™, Norlutin®, Aygestin®) is used as a birth control pill (to prevent an unwanted pregnancy) or a hormone treatment, depending on the brand you have been prescribed. Norethindrone acts like the natural hormone progesterone. Natural progesterone is essential to normal functioning of the female reproductive system. Norethindrone also helps to treat an irregular menstrual cycle, lack of menstrual periods, or abnormal uterine bleeding caused by a hormonal imbalance. Norethindrone tablets are available from several pharmaceutical manufacturers; however, not all brands are substitutable for one another.

What should my health care professional know before I take norethindrone?

They need to know if you have any of these conditions:
- blood vessel disease, blood clotting disorder, or suffered a stroke
- breast, cervical, or vaginal cancer
- diabetes
- heart, kidney or liver disease
- high blood lipids or cholesterol
- mental depression
- migraine
- seizures (convulsions)
- vaginal bleeding
- an unusual or allergic reaction to norethindrone, other hormones, medicines, foods, dyes, or preservatives
- pregnant or trying to get pregnant
- breast-feeding

How should I take this medicine?

Take norethindrone tablets by mouth. Follow the directions on the prescription label. Swallow the tablets with a drink of water. Take your doses at regular intervals. Do not take your medicine more often than directed. For treating absent or irregular menses or for controlling unusual bleeding: Take norethindrone from day 5 to day 25 of the cycle. For treating endometriosis: Before you start taking these pills decide what is a suitable time of day and always take them at the same time of day. Your doctor may instruct you to take norethindrone every day for 2 weeks, and from there may increase your dosage to get the proper effect. You will probably take the medication every day for 6 to 9 months. As a contraceptive (birth control method): Before you start taking these pills decide what is a suitable time of day and always take them at the same time of day. Norethindrone birth control tablets should be taken every day, without breaks between packs. For all uses of this medicine:

Read the paper on your prescription provided by your health care provider or pharmacist. This paper will tell you about the specific product you are taking. Make certain you understand the instructions. Contact your pediatrician or health care professional regarding the use of this medicine in children. Special care may be needed.

What if I miss a dose?

For general use: If you miss a dose, take it as soon as you can. If it is almost time for your next dose, take only that dose. Do not take double or extra doses. For contraceptive use: Every time you miss a dose, or take a dose late by > 3 hours, your chance of getting pregnant increases. Try not to miss a dose. When one pill is missed (even if only 3 hours late), take the missed pill as soon as possible and continue taking a pill each day at the regular time (a backup method of birth control, like a condom or spermicide, should be used for the next 48 hours). Whenever > 1 dose is missed, additional contraception should be used for the rest of your pill pack until menses occurs. You should also contact your health care professional for instruction whenever more than 1 dose has been missed.

What may interact with norethindrone?

- antibiotics or medicines for infections, especially rifampin, rifabutin, rifapentine, and griseofulvin
- aprepitant, a medicine used for chemotherapy-induced nausea and vomiting
- barbiturate medicines for inducing sleep or treating seizures (convulsions)
- bosentan
- carbamazepine
- modafinil
- phenytoin
- St. John's Wort
- topiramate
- troglitazone or pioglitazone

Tell your doctor or pharmacist about all other medicines you are taking, including non-prescription medicines; if you are a frequent user of drinks with caffeine or alcohol; if you smoke; or if you use illegal drugs. These may affect the way your medicine works. Check before stopping or starting any of your medicines.

What should I watch for while taking norethindrone?

You should have a complete check-up every 6 to 12 months. If you have any unusual bleeding contact your prescriber or health care professional for advice. If you are taking norethindrone as a contraceptive (birth control), use an additional form of contraception during the first 2 weeks of the first cycle (first pack). If you

N

have any reason to think you are pregnant, stop taking norethindrone at once and contact your doctor. Tobacco smoking increases the risk of getting a blood clot or having a stroke while you are taking norgestrel, especially if you are more than 35 years old. You are strongly advised not to smoke. If you wear contact lenses and notice visual changes, or if the lenses begin to feel uncomfortable, consult your eye prescriber or health care professional. Progestins may cause swelling, tenderness, or bleeding of the gums; be careful when brushing and flossing teeth, and visit your dentist regularly. Norethindrone tablets do not protect you against HIV infection (AIDS) or other sexually transmitted diseases.

What side effects may I notice from taking norethindrone?

Side effects that you should report to your prescriber or health care professional as soon as possible:
- breast tenderness or discharge
- numbness or pain in the arm or leg
- pain in the chest, groin or leg
- severe headache
- stomach pain
- sudden shortness of breath
- unusual weakness or tiredness
- vision or speech problems
- yellowing of skin or eyes

Call your doctor as soon as you can if you get any of these side effects.
Side effects that usually do not require medical attention (report to your prescriber or health care professional if they continue or are bothersome):
- changes in sexual desire or ability
- changes in vaginal bleeding
- facial hair growth
- fluid retention and swelling
- headache
- increased sweating or hot flashes
- loss of appetite or increase in appetite
- mood changes, anxiety, depression, frustration, anger, or emotional outbursts
- nausea, vomiting
- skin rash
- stomach discomfort
- weight gain or weight loss
- vaginal yeast infection (irritation and white discharge)

Let your doctor know about these side effects if they do not go away or if they annoy you.

Where can I keep my medicine?

Keep out of the reach of children in a container that small children cannot open. Store at room temperature between 15 and 30 degrees C (59 and 86 degrees F). Keep container tightly closed. Throw away any unused medicine after the expiration date.

Norfloxacin tablets

NOROXIN®;
400 mg; Tablet
Shire US Inc

What are norfloxacin tablets?

NORFLOXACIN (Noroxin®) is a fluoroquinolone antibiotic. Norfloxacin kills certain bacteria or stops their growth. It treats infections of the urinary tract and certain sexually transmitted disease. Generic norfloxacin tablets are not yet available.

What should my health care professional know before I take norfloxacin?

They need to know if you have any of these conditions:
- dehydration
- kidney disease
- long exposure to sunlight (working outdoors)
- seizures (convulsions)
- stomach problems (especially colitis)
- stroke
- pain or soreness in a tendon
- an unusual or allergic reaction to fluoroquinolone antibiotics, foods, dyes, or preservatives
- pregnant or trying to get pregnant
- breast-feeding

How should I take this medicine?

Take norfloxacin tablets by mouth. Follow the directions on the prescription label. Swallow tablets whole with a full glass of water. It is best to take norfloxacin

on an empty stomach, either 1 hour before or 2 hours after a meal and/or other dairy products. Take your doses at regular intervals. Do not take your medicine more often than directed. Finish the full course prescribed by your prescriber or health care professional even if you think your condition is better. Do not stop taking except on your prescriber's advice. Contact your pediatrician or health care professional regarding the use of this medicine in children. Special care may be needed.

What if I miss a dose?

If you miss a dose, take it as soon as you can. If it is almost time for your next dose, take only that dose. Do not take double or extra doses. There should be an interval of at least 10 to 12 hours between doses.

What may interact with norfloxacin?

- aluminum salts
- antacids
- caffeine
- calcium salts
- chloramphenicol
- cyclosporine
- dofetilide
- iron (ferrous sulfate) preparations

N

- magnesium salts
- manganese
- medicines for diabetes
- multivitamins containing iron, zinc, calcium, or manganese
- NSAIDs such as Advil® or Motrin® (ibuprofen), Aleve® (naproxen)
- rifampin
- sucralfate
- tetracycline
- theophylline, aminophylline
- warfarin
- zinc salts

Tell your prescriber or health care professional about all other medicines you are taking, including non-prescription medicines, nutritional supplements, or herbal products. Also tell your prescriber or health care professional if you are a frequent user of drinks with caffeine or alcohol, if you smoke, or if you use illegal drugs. These may affect the way your medicine works. Check with your health care professional before stopping or starting any of your medicines.

What should I watch for while taking norfloxacin?

Tell your prescriber or health care professional if your symptoms do not improve in 2 to 3 days. Stop taking norfloxacin immediately if you develop a skin rash or other allergic reaction. Contact your healthcare provider immediately. Keep out of the sun, or wear protective clothing outdoors and use a sunscreen. Do not use sun lamps or sun tanning beds or booths. You may get drowsy or dizzy. Do not drive, use machinery, or do anything that needs mental alertness until you know how norfloxacin affects you. To reduce the risk of dizzy or fainting spells, do not sit or stand up quickly, especially if you are an older patient. Drink several glasses of water a day. Cut down on drinks that contain caffeine. Norfloxacin can increase the stimulant effects of caffeine and cause heart, breathing and other problems. Antacids can stop norfloxacin from working. If you get an upset stomach and want to take an antacid, make sure there is an interval of at least 2 hours since you last took norfloxacin, or 6 hours before your next dose.

Calcium, iron and zinc preparations can also stop norfloxacin from working properly. Take calcium tablets, iron tablets, zinc tablets, or vitamins that contain calcium, iron, or zinc at least 6 hours before your dose of norfloxacin or at least 2 hours after your dose of norfloxacin. If you experience pain in a joint, stop taking norfloxacin. Call your healthcare provider. Rest the affected area. Do not exercise or take norfloxacin again until your healthcare provider tells you to do so. If you are going to have surgery, tell your prescriber or health care professional that you are taking norfloxacin.

What side effects may I notice from taking norfloxacin?

Side effects that you should report to your prescriber or health care professional as soon as possible:
- difficulty breathing
- confusion
- depression
- increased sensitivity to the sun or ultraviolet light
- joint, muscle or tendon pain
- nervousness, excitability, restlessness
- severe or watery diarrhea
- skin rash, itching
- seizures (convulsions)
- swelling of the face or neck
- tremors
- vomiting

Side effects that usually do not require medical attention (report to your prescriber or health care professional if they continue or are bothersome):
- constipation or diarrhea
- difficulty sleeping
- dizziness, drowsiness
- gas or heartburn
- headache
- nausea
- stomach pain

Where can I keep my medicine?

Keep out of the reach of children in a container that small children cannot open. Store at room temperature between 15 and 30 degrees C (59 and 86 degrees F). Throw away any unused medicine after the expiration date.

Norgestrel tablets

OVRETTE®;
0.075 mg; Tablet
Wyeth Div Wyeth
Pharmaceuticals Inc

What are norgestrel tablets?

NORGESTREL (Ovrette®) is a birth control pill (to prevent an unwanted pregnancy). This drug is discontinued in the United States. Norgestrel acts like the natural hormone progesterone. Natural progesterone is essential to normal functioning of the womb and reproductive system. Generic norgestrel tablets are not yet available.

What should my health care professional know before I take norgestrel?

They need to know if you have any of these conditions:
- blood vessel disease, blood clotting disorder, or suffered a stroke
- breast, uterine, vaginal or cervical cancer
- diabetes
- heart, kidney or liver disease

N

- high blood lipids or cholesterol
- incomplete abortion, or ectopic pregnancy
- mental depression
- migraine
- seizures (convulsions)
- vaginal bleeding
- an unusual or allergic reaction to norgestrel, other hormones, medicines, foods, dyes, or preservatives
- pregnant or trying to get pregnant
- breast-feeding

How should I take this medicine?

Take norgestrel tablets by mouth. Follow the directions on the prescription label. Before you start taking these pills decide what is a suitable time of day and always take them at the same time of day. Norgestrel tablets should be taken every day, without breaks between packs. Swallow the tablet with a drink of water. Take your doses at regular intervals. Do not take your medicine more often than directed. For all uses of this medicine:

Read the paper on your prescription provided by your health care provider or pharmacist. This paper will tell you about the specific product you are taking. Make certain you understand the instructions. Contact your pediatrician or health care professional regarding the use of this medicine in children. Special care may be needed.

What if I miss a dose?

For contraceptive use: Every time you miss a dose, or take a dose late by > 3 hours, your chance of getting pregnant increases. Try not to miss a dose. When one pill is missed (even if only 3 hours late), take the missed pill as soon as possible and continue taking a pill each day at the regular time (a backup method of birth control, like a condom or spermicide, should be used for the next 48 hours). Whenever > 1 dose is missed, additional contraception should be used for the rest of your pill pack until menses occurs. You should also contact your health care professional for instruction whenever more than 1 dose has been missed.

What may interact with norgestrel?

- aprepitant, a medicine used for chemotherapy-induced nausea and vomiting
- barbiturate medicines for inducing sleep or treating seizures (convulsions)
- bosentan
- carbamazepine
- griseofulvin
- modafinil
- oxcarbazepine
- phenytoin
- rifabutin
- rifampin
- rifapentine
- St. John's wort

- topiramate
- troglitazone or pioglitazone

Tell your prescriber or health care professional about all other medicines you are taking, including non-prescription medicines, nutritional supplements, or herbal products. Also tell your prescriber or health care professional if you are a frequent user of drinks with caffeine or alcohol, if you smoke, or if you use illegal drugs. These may affect the way your medicine works. Check with your health care professional before stopping or starting any of your medicines.

What should I watch for while taking norgestrel?

Visit your prescriber or health care professional for regular checks on your progress. You should have a complete check-up every 6 to 12 months. If you have any unusual bleeding contact your prescriber or health care professional for advice. If you are taking norgestrel as a contraceptive, use an additional form of contraception during the first 2 weeks of the first cycle (first pack). If you have any reason to think you are pregnant; stop taking norgestrel at once and contact your prescriber or health care professional. Tobacco smoking increases the risk of getting a blood clot or having a stroke while you are taking norgestrel, especially if you are more than 35 years old. You are strongly advised not to smoke. If you wear contact lenses and notice visual changes, or if the lenses begin to feel uncomfortable, consult your eye prescriber or health care professional. Progestins may cause swelling, tenderness, or bleeding of the gums; be careful when brushing and flossing teeth, and visit your dentist regularly. Norgestrel tablets do not protect you against HIV infection (AIDS) or other sexually transmitted diseases.

What side effects may I notice from taking norgestrel?

Side effects that you should report to your prescriber or health care professional as soon as possible:
- heavy vaginal bleeding
- breast pain or discharge
- numbness or pain in the arm or leg
- pain in the chest, groin or leg
- severe headache
- stomach pain
- sudden shortness of breath
- swelling of the hands, feet or ankles, or rapid weight gain
- unusual weakness or tiredness
- vision or speech problems
- yellowing of skin or eyes

Side effects that usually do not require medical attention (report to your prescriber or health care professional if they continue or are bothersome):
- breakthrough bleeding, spotting, irregular menstrual cycle, or no menstruation
- facial hair growth
- loss of appetite or increase in appetite

- mood changes, anxiety, depression, frustration, anger, or emotional outbursts
- nausea, vomiting, or stomach discomfort
- skin rash
- vaginal yeast infection (irritation and white discharge)
- weight change

Where can I keep my medicine?

Keep out of the reach of children in a container that small children cannot open. Store at room temperature between 15 and 30 degrees C (59 and 86 degrees F). Keep container tightly closed. Throw away any unused medicine after the expiration date.

Nortriptyline capsules

PAMELOR®;
50 mg; Capsule
Mallinckrodt Inc
Pharmaceuticals
Group

PAMELOR®;
25 mg; Capsule
Mallinckrodt Inc
Pharmaceuticals
Group

This drug requires an FDA medication guide. See page xxxvii.

What are nortriptyline capsules?

NORTRIPTYLINE (Pamelor®) is an antidepressant. Nortriptyline can help to lift your spirits by treating your depression. Generic nortriptyline capsules are not yet available.

What should my health care professional know before I take nortriptyline?

They need to know if you have any of these conditions:
- an alcohol problem
- asthma, difficulty breathing
- blood disorders or disease
- diabetes
- difficulty passing urine, prostate trouble
- glaucoma
- having intramuscular injections
- heart disease, or recent heart attack
- liver disease
- overactive thyroid
- Parkinson's disease
- schizophrenia
- seizures (convulsions)
- stomach disease
- an unusual or allergic reaction to nortriptyline, other medicines, foods, dyes, or preservatives
- pregnant or trying to get pregnant
- breast-feeding

How should I take this medicine?

Take nortriptyline capsules by mouth. Follow the directions on the prescription label. Swallow the capsules with a drink of water. Take your doses at regular intervals. Do not take your medicine more often than directed. Do not stop taking except on your prescriber's advice. Contact your pediatrician or health care professional regarding the use of this medicine in children. Special care may be needed. Elderly patients over 65 years old and adolescents may have a stronger reaction to this medicine and need smaller doses.

What if I miss a dose?

If you miss a dose, take it as soon as you can. If it is almost time for your next dose, take only that dose. Do not take double or extra doses.

What may interact with nortriptyline?

Nortriptyline can interact with many other medicines. Some interactions can be very important. Make sure your prescriber or health care professional knows about all other medicines you are taking. Many important interactions are listed below.

Do not take nortriptyline with any of the following medications:

- astemizole (Hismanal®)
- cisapride (Propulsid®)
- probucol
- terfenadine (Seldane®)
- thioridazine (Mellaril®)
- medicines called MAO inhibitors-phenelzine (Nardil®), tranylcypromine (Parnate®), isocarboxazid (Marplan®), selegiline (Eldepryl®)
- other medicines for mental depression (may be duplicate therapies or cause additive side effects)

Nortriptyline may also interact with any of the following:

- alcohol
- antacids
- atropine and related drugs like hyoscyamine, scopolamine, tolterodine and others
- barbiturate medicines for inducing sleep or treating seizures (convulsions), such as phenobarbital
- blood thinners, such as warfarin
- bromocriptine
- bupropion
- cimetidine
- clonidine
- cocaine
- delavirdine
- diphenoxylate
- disulfiram
- donepezil
- drugs for treating HIV infection
- female hormones, including contraceptive or birth control pills and estrogen
- galantamine
- herbs and dietary supplements like ephedra (Ma huang), kava kava, SAM-e, St. John's wort, valerian, or others
- imatinib, STI-571
- kaolin; pectin
- labetalol
- levodopa and other medicines for movement problems like Parkinson's disease
- lithium

N

- medicines for anxiety or sleeping problems
- medicines for colds, flu and breathing difficulties, like pseudoephedrine
- medicines for hay fever or allergies (antihistamines)
- medicines for weight loss or appetite control
- medicines used to regulate abnormal heartbeat or to treat other heart conditions (examples: amiodarone, bepridil, disopyramide, dofetilide, encainide, flecainide, ibutilide, mibefradil, procainamide, propafenone, quinidine, and others)
- metoclopramide
- muscle relaxants, like cyclobenzaprine
- other medicines for mental or mood problems and psychotic disturbances
- prescription pain medications like morphine, codeine, tramadol and others
- procarbazine
- seizure (convulsion) or epilepsy medicine such as carbamazepine or phenytoin
- stimulants like dexmethylphenidate or methylphenidate
- some antibiotics (examples: erythromycin, gatifloxacin, levofloxacin, linezolid, moxifloxacin, sotalol, sparfloxacin)
- tacrine
- thyroid hormones such as levothyroxine

Tell your prescriber or health care professional about all other medicines you are taking, including non-prescription medicines, nutritional supplements, or herbal products. Also tell your prescriber or health care professional if you are a frequent user of drinks with caffeine or alcohol, if you smoke, or if you use illegal drugs. These may affect the way your medicine works. Check with your health care professional before stopping or starting any of your medicines.

What should I watch for while taking nortriptyline?

Visit your prescriber or health care professional for regular checks on your progress. It can take several days or weeks before you feel the full effect of nortriptyline. If you have been taking nortriptyline regularly for some time, do not suddenly stop taking it. You must gradually reduce the dose or you may get severe side effects. Ask your prescriber or health care professional for advice. Even after you stop taking nortriptyline it can still affect your body for several days. You may get drowsy or dizzy. Do not drive, use machinery, or do anything that needs mental alertness until you know how nortriptyline affects you. Do not stand or sit up quickly, especially if you are an older patient. This reduces the risk of dizzy or fainting spells. Alcohol can increase dizziness and drowsiness. Avoid alcoholic drinks. Do not treat yourself for coughs, colds or allergies without asking your prescriber or health care professional for advice. Some ingredients can increase possible side effects. Your mouth may get dry. Chewing sugarless gum or sucking hard candy, and drinking plenty of water will help. Nortriptyline may cause dry eyes and blurred vision. If you wear contact lenses you may feel some discomfort. Lubricating drops may help. See your ophthalmologist if the problem does not go away or is severe. Nortriptyline may make your skin more sensitive to the sun. Keep out of the sun, or wear protective clothing outdoors and use a sunscreen. Do not use sun lamps or sun tanning beds or booths. Nortriptyline can affect blood glucose (sugar) levels. If you are a diabetic, check your blood sugar more often than usual, especially during the first few weeks of nortriptyline treatment. Call your prescriber or health care professional for advice if you notice a change in the results of blood or urine glucose tests. If you are going to have surgery or will need an x-ray procedure that uses contrast agents, tell your prescriber or health care professional that you are taking this medicine.

What side effects may I notice from taking nortriptyline?

Side effects that you should report to your prescriber or health care professional as soon as possible:
- abnormal production of milk in females
- blurred vision or eye pain
- breast enlargement in both males and females
- confusion, hallucinations (seeing or hearing things that are not really there)
- difficulty breathing
- fainting spells
- fever
- irregular or fast, pounding heartbeat, palpitations
- muscle stiffness, or spasms
- pain or difficulty passing urine, loss of bladder control
- seizures (convulsions)
- sexual difficulties (decreased sexual ability or desire)
- stomach pain
- swelling of the testicles
- tingling, pain, or numbness in the feet or hands
- tremor (shaking)
- unusual weakness or tiredness
- yellowing of the eyes or skin

Side effects that usually do not require medical attention (report to your prescriber or health care professional if they continue or are bothersome):
- anxiety
- constipation, or diarrhea
- drowsiness or dizziness
- dry mouth
- headache
- increased sensitivity of the skin to sun or ultraviolet light
- loss of appetite
- nausea, vomiting
- skin rash or itching
- weight gain or loss

Where can I keep my medicine?

Keep out of the reach of children in a container that small children cannot open. Store at room temperature below 30 degrees C (86 degrees F). Keep container tightly closed. Throw away any unused medicine after the expiration date.

N

Nystatin lozenges

MYCOSTATIN®;
200,000 unit; Lozenge
ER Squibb and Sons Inc

What are nystatin lozenges?

NYSTATIN (Mycostatin®) is an antifungal type of antibiotic. Nystatin lozenges treat oral thrush infections. Generic nystatin lozenges are not yet available.

What should my health care professional know before I take nystatin?

They need to know if you have any of these conditions:
- an unusual or allergic reaction to nystatin, other foods, dyes or preservatives
- pregnant or trying to get pregnant
- breast-feeding

How should I use this medicine?

Allow a nystatin lozenge to dissolve slowly in the mouth; this can take between 15 and 30 minutes. Do not chew or swallow the lozenge whole. Follow the directions on the prescription label. Do not take your medicine more often than directed. Take your doses at regular intervals. Finish the full course prescribed by your prescriber or health care professional even if you think your condition is better. Do not stop taking except on your prescriber's advice. Contact your pediatrician or health care professional regarding the use of this medicine in children. Special care may be needed.

What if I miss a dose?

If you miss a dose, take it as soon as you can. If it is almost time for your next dose, take only that dose. Do not take double or extra doses.

What may interact with nystatin?

Nystatin is poorly absorbed and is not known to interact with other medicines.

Tell your prescriber or health care professional about all other medicines you are taking, including non-prescription medicines, nutritional supplements, or herbal products. Also tell your prescriber or health care professional if you are a frequent user of drinks with caffeine or alcohol, if you smoke, or if you use illegal drugs. These may affect the way your medicine works. Check with your health care professional before stopping or starting any of your medicines.

What should I watch for while taking nystatin?

Tell your prescriber or health care professional if your symptoms do not improve after 3 days. Some fungal infections can take a long time to clear completely so finish your prescribed course. Dentures can be a source of candida (thrush) infection. To avoid reinfection you may need to soak your dentures in nystatin suspension. Ask your prescriber or health care professional for advice.

What side effects may I notice from taking nystatin?

Side effects with nystatin are rare, but include:
- diarrhea
- nausea, vomiting
- stomach pain

Where can I keep my medicine?

Keep out of the reach of children in a container that small children cannot open. Store in a refrigerator between 2 and 8 degrees C (36 and 46 degrees F); do not freeze. Protect from light. Protect powder from moisture. Throw away any unused medicine after the expiration date.

N

Ofloxacin tablets

FLOXIN®;
200 mg; Tablet
Ortho McNeil
Pharmaceutical Inc

FLOXIN®;
400 mg; Tablet
Ortho McNeil
Pharmaceutical Inc

What are ofloxacin tablets?

OFLOXACIN (Floxin®) is an antibiotic. Ofloxacin kills certain bacteria or stops their growth. It treats urinary tract, prostate, skin, urinary and respiratory tract infections, as well as certain sexually transmitted diseases. Generic ofloxacin tablets are available.

What should my health care professional know before I take ofloxacin?

They need to know if you have any of these conditions:
- arteriosclerosis
- dehydration
- heart disease
- kidney disease
- liver disease
- long exposure to sunlight (working outdoors)
- seizures (convulsions)
- stomach problems (especially colitis)
- stroke
- tendon or joint pain
- other chronic conditions
- an unusual or allergic reaction to fluoroquinolone antibiotics, foods, dyes, or preservatives
- pregnant or trying to get pregnant
- breast-feeding

How should I take this medicine?

Take ofloxacin tablets by mouth. Follow the directions on the prescription label. Swallow tablets whole with a full glass of water. Take ofloxacin on an empty stomach, 1 hour before, or at least 2 hours after eating. Take your doses at regular intervals. Do not take your medicine more often than directed. Finish the full course prescribed by your prescriber or health care professional even if you think your condition is better. Do not stop taking except on your prescriber's advice. Contact your pediatrician or health care professional regarding the use of this medicine in children. Special care may be needed.

What if I miss a dose?

If you miss a dose, take it as soon as you can. If it is almost time for your next dose, take only that dose. Do not take double or extra doses. There should be an interval of at least 10 to 12 hours between doses.

What may interact with ofloxacin?

- aluminum salts
- antacids
- arsenic trioxide
- astemizole
- bepridil
- calcium salts
- certain heart medications for irregular rhythm (e.g., amiodarone, disopyramide, dofetilide, flecainide, ibutilide, quinidine, procainamide, sotalol)
- certain medications for depression or other mental problems (e.g., tricyclic antidepressants, amoxapine, maprotiline, phenothiazines, haloperidol, pimozide, risperidone, sertindole, and ziprasidone)
- cisapride
- clarithromycin
- cyclobenzaprine
- cyclosporine
- didanosine (Videx® tablets or oral solution)
- iron (ferrous sulfate) preparations
- dolasetron
- droperidol
- erythromycin
- levomethadyl
- magnesium salts
- manganese
- medicines for diabetes
- multivitamins containing iron, calcium, zinc, or manganese
- NSAIDs such as Advil®, Aleve®, ibuprofen, Motrin®, naproxen
- pentamidine
- probucol
- terfenadine
- sucralfate
- theophylline
- troleandomycin
- warfarin
- zinc salts

Tell your prescriber or health care professional about all other medicines you are taking, including non-prescription medicines, nutritional supplements, or herbal products. Also tell your prescriber or health care professional if you are a frequent user of drinks with caffeine or alcohol, if you smoke, or if you use illegal drugs. These may affect the way your medicine works. Check with your health care professional before stopping or starting any of your medicines.

What should I watch for while taking ofloxacin?

Tell your prescriber or health care professional if your symptoms do not improve in 2 to 3 days. If you are a diabetic, monitor your blood glucose carefully. If you get an unusual reaction stop taking ofloxacin at once and call your prescriber or health care professional for advice. You may get drowsy or dizzy. Do not drive, use machinery, or do anything that needs mental alertness until you know how ofloxacin affects you. To reduce the risk of dizzy or fainting spells, do not sit or stand up quickly, especially if you are an older patient. Drink several glasses of water a day. Cut down on drinks that contain caffeine. Antacid can stop ofloxacin working. If you get an upset stomach and want to take an antacid, make sure there is an interval of at least 2 hours since you last took ofloxacin, or 6 hours before your next dose. Iron and zinc preparations can also stop ofloxacin from working properly. Keep out of the sun, or wear protective clothing outdoors and use a sunscreen. Do not use sun lamps or sun tanning beds or booths. If you notice pain or soreness of a tendon or around a joint, stop taking ofloxacin. Call your healthcare provider immediately. You must rest and stop exercise until your healthcare provider says it is okay to start again. If you are going to have surgery, tell your prescriber or health care professional that you are taking ofloxacin.

What side effects may I notice from taking ofloxacin?

Side effects that you should report to your prescriber or health care professional as soon as possible:
- difficulty breathing
- irregular heartbeat, palpitations or chest pain
- joint, muscle or tendon pain
- severe or watery diarrhea
- redness, blistering, peeling or loosening of the skin, including inside the mouth
- skin rash, itching
- swelling of the face or neck
- vomiting

Side effects that usually do not require medical attention (report to your prescriber or health care professional if they continue or are bothersome):
- diarrhea
- difficulty sleeping
- dizziness, drowsiness
- headache
- nausea

Where can I keep my medicine?

Keep out of the reach of children in a container that small children cannot open. Store at a temperature below 30 degrees C (85 degrees F). Throw away any unused medicine after the expiration date.

Olanzapine tablets and disintegrating tablets

ZYPREXA®;
10 mg; Tablet
Eli Lilly and Co

ZYPREXA® ZYDIS®;
15 mg; Tablet,
Orally disintegrating
Eli Lilly and Co

What are olanzapine tablets?

OLANZAPINE (Zyprexa®, Zyprexa® Zydis®) helps to treat emotional and mental problems like schizophrenia or psychosis. Olanzapine is also sometimes used for the treatment of other emotional or mental problems like manic-depressive illness, bipolar disorder, or behavioral problems that occur with dementia. Olanzapine can help you to keep in touch with reality and reduce your mental problems. It is not a cure. Generic olanzapine tablets are not yet available.

What should my health care professional know before I take olanzapine?

They need to know if you have any of these conditions:
- frequently drink alcoholic beverages
- breast cancer
- cigarette smoker
- diabetes mellitus, high blood sugar or a family history of diabetes
- difficulty passing urine
- glaucoma
- heart disease, irregular heartbeat, or previous heart attack
- high blood pressure treated with medication
- kidney or liver disease
- low blood pressure
- Parkinson's disease
- prostate trouble
- seizures (convulsions)
- an unusual or allergic reaction to olanzapine, other medicines, foods, dyes, or preservatives
- pregnant or trying to get pregnant
- breast-feeding

How should I take this medicine?

Take olanzapine tablets by mouth. Follow the directions on the prescription label.
Tablets:
Swallow the tablets with a drink of water. You can take olanzapine with food or meals if you want to.
Disintegrating tablets:
Leave the olanzapine disintegrating tablet in the foil package until you are ready to take it. Do not push the tablet through the blister pack. Peel open the package with dry hands and place the tablet on your tongue. The tablet will dissolve rapidly and be swallowed in your saliva. It is not necessary to drink any water to take this medicine, but you may drink some water if you would like to. You can also take olanzapine with food or meals if you want to.

Take your doses at regular intervals. Do not take your medicine more often than directed. Do not stop taking except on your prescriber's advice. Contact your pediatrician or health care professional regarding the use of this medicine in children. Special care may be needed.

What if I miss a dose?

If you miss a dose of olanzapine by a few hours, take the dose when you remember. If most of the day has passed, wait until your next scheduled dose. If it is almost time for your next dose, take only that dose. Do not take double or extra doses.

What may interact with olanzapine?

- alcohol
- carbamazepine

- cimetidine
- cisapride
- clozapine
- donepezil
- erythromycin or clarithromycin
- fluvoxamine
- ketoconazole
- levodopa and other medicines for Parkinson's disease
- lithium
- medicines for colds, hay fever, or allergies
- medicines for diabetes
- medicines for high blood pressure
- medicines for mental depression, anxiety, other mood disorders, or sleeping problems
- phenobarbital
- rifampin
- ritonavir
- some medicines for pain (examples: codeine, morphine)
- some medicines for gastrointestinal spasm
- tacrine
- tobacco in cigarettes

Tell your prescriber or health care professional about all other medicines you are taking, including non-prescription medicines, nutritional supplements, or herbal products. Also tell your prescriber or health care professional if you are a frequent user of drinks with caffeine or alcohol, if you smoke, or if you use illegal drugs. These may affect the way your medicine works. Check with your health care professional before stopping or starting any of your medicines.

What should I watch for while taking olanzapine?

Visit your prescriber or health care professional for regular checks on your progress. It may be several weeks before you see the full effects of olanzapine. Do notify your prescriber if your symptoms get worse or you have new symptoms, if you are having an unusual effect from olanzapine, or if you feel out of control, very discouraged or think you might harm yourself or others. Your prescriber can help you manage these problems. Do not suddenly stop taking olanzapine. You may need to gradually reduce the dose. Only stop taking olanzapine on your prescriber's advice. You may get dizzy or drowsy. Do not drive, use machinery, or do anything that needs mental alertness until you know how olanzapine affects you. Do not stand or sit up quickly, especially if you are an older patient. This reduces the risk of dizzy or fainting spells. Alcohol can increase dizziness and drowsiness with olanzapine. Avoid alcoholic drinks. Do not treat yourself for colds, diarrhea or allergies. Ask your prescriber or health care professional for advice, some nonprescription medicines may increase possible side effects. Your mouth may get dry. Chewing sugarless gum or sucking hard candy, and drinking plenty of water will help. Be careful when brushing and flossing your teeth to avoid mouth infections or damage

to your gums. See your dentist regularly. Sometimes olanzapine can make your mouth water a lot. Olanzapine can reduce the response of your body to heat or cold. Try not to get overheated or dehydrated from exercise. Avoid temperature extremes, such as saunas, hot tubs, or very hot or cold baths or showers. Dress warmly in cold weather. Olanzapine may make your skin more sensitive to sun or ultraviolet light. Limit your sun exposure; wear protective clothing outdoors and use a sunscreen (at least SPF 15). Avoid using sun lamps or sun tanning beds or booths. If you are going to have surgery, tell your prescriber or health care professional that you are taking olanzapine.

What side effects may I notice from taking olanzapine?

Side effects that you should report to your prescriber or health care professional as soon as possible:

More common:
- agitation or hostile, angry behavior
- changes in emotions or behavior, like a very depressed mood
- restlessness or need to keep moving
- stiffness, spasms
- tremors or trembling

Rare or less common:
- changes in vision, inability to control eye movements
- confusion
- difficulty breathing
- difficulty concentrating
- difficulty in speaking or swallowing
- excessive thirst and/or hunger
- fainting spells, loss of balance
- fast heartbeat (palpitations)
- frequently needing to urinate
- inability to control muscle movements in the face, hands, arms, or legs
- menstrual changes
- painful erections
- seizures (convulsions)
- skin rash
- swelling of face or legs
- uncontrollable tongue or chewing movements, smacking lips or puffing cheeks
- unusual tiredness or weakness

Side effects that usually do not require medical attention (report to your prescriber or health care professional if they continue or are bothersome):

Less common or rare:
- blurred or unclear vision
- changes in sexual desire
- excessive drainage from eyes
- excessive watering or drooling of mouth
- joint pain
- nausea or vomiting
- sensitivity of skin to sunlight

- tingling sensation in your hands, feet or other area of your body
- trouble in controlling urine

More common:
- constipation
- dizziness; especially on standing from a sitting or lying position
- drowsiness
- dry mouth
- lowered blood pressure

- runny nose
- weight gain

Where can I keep my medicine?

Keep out of the reach of children in a container that small children cannot open. Store at controlled room temperature between 20 and 25 degrees C (68 and 77 degrees F). Protect from light and moisture. Throw away any unused medicine after the expiration date.

Olmesartan tablets

BENICAR™;
20 mg; Tablet
Sankyo Pharma Inc

BENICAR™;
40 mg; Tablet
Sankyo Pharma Inc

What are olmesartan tablets?

OLMESARTAN (Benicar™) helps lower blood pressure to normal levels. It controls high blood pressure, but it is not a cure. High blood pressure can damage your kidneys, and may lead to a stroke or heart failure. Olmesartan helps prevent these things from happening. Generic olmesartan tablets are not yet available.

What should my health care professional know before I take olmesartan?

They need to know if you have any of these conditions:
- heart failure
- kidney disease
- liver disease
- if you are on a special diet, such as a low-salt diet
- an unusual or allergic reaction to olmesartan, other medicines, foods, dyes, or preservatives
- pregnant or trying to get pregnant
- breast-feeding

How should I take this medicine?

Take olmesartan tablets by mouth. Follow the directions on the prescription label. Swallow the tablets with a glass of water. Olmesartan can be taken with or without food. Take your doses at regular intervals. Do not take your medicine more often than directed.

What if I miss a dose?

If you miss a dose, take it as soon as you can. If it is almost time for your next dose, take only that dose. Do not take double or extra doses.

What may interact with olmesartan?

- blood pressure medications
- hawthorn
- lithium
- potassium supplements
- water pills (diuretics)

Tell your prescriber or health care professional about all other medicines you are taking, including non-prescription medicines, nutritional supplements, or herbal products. Also tell your prescriber or health care professional if you are a frequent user of drinks with caffeine or alcohol, if you smoke, or if you use illegal drugs. These may affect the way your medicine works. Check

with your health care professional before stopping or starting any of your medicines.

What should I watch for while taking olmesartan?

Check your blood pressure regularly while you are taking olmesartan. Ask your prescriber or health care professional what your blood pressure should be. When you check your blood pressure, write down the measurements to show your prescriber or health care professional. If you are taking this medicine for a long time, you must visit your prescriber or health care professional for regular checks on your progress. Make sure you schedule appointments on a regular basis. If you are going to have surgery, tell your prescriber or health care professional that you are taking olmesartan.

What side effects may I notice from taking olmesartan?

Side effects that you should report to your prescriber or health care professional as soon as possible:
Rare or uncommon:
- difficulty breathing or swallowing, hoarseness, or tightening of the throat
- swelling of your face, lips, tongue, hands, or feet
- unusual rash

Other:
- confusion, dizziness, lightheadedness or fainting spells
- decreased amount of urine passed
- fast or uneven heart beat, palpitations, or chest pain

Side effects that usually do not require medical attention (report to your prescriber or health care professional if they continue or are bothersome):
- back pain
- diarrhea
- dizziness
- sore throat
- stuffy nose or stuffy sinuses

Where can I keep my medicine?

Keep out of the reach of children and in a container that small children cannot open. Store your medicine at room temperature between 15 and 30 degrees C (59 and 86 degrees F). Throw away any unused medicine after the expiration date.

Olsalazine capsules

DIPENTUM®;
250 mg; Capsule
Celltech Pharmaceuticals, Inc

What are olsalazine capsules?

OLSALAZINE (Dipentum®) is an anti-inflammatory agent. It reduces inflammation inside the bowel and pain associated with ulcerative colitis and helps to prevent recurring inflammation. Generic olsalazine capsules are not yet available.

What should my health care professional know before I take olsalazine?

They need to know if you have any of these conditions:
- kidney disease
- an unusual or allergic reaction to olsalazine, aspirin, other medicines, foods, dyes, or preservatives
- pregnant or trying to get pregnant
- breast-feeding

How should I take this medicine?

Take olsalazine capsules by mouth. Follow the directions on the prescription label. Swallow the capsules whole with a drink of water. If olsalazine upsets your stomach, take it with food or milk. Take your doses at regular intervals. Do not take your medicine more often than directed. Contact your pediatrician or health care professional regarding the use of this medicine in children. Special care may be needed.

What if I miss a dose?

If you miss a dose, take it as soon as you can. If it is almost time for your next dose, take only that dose. Do not take double or extra doses.

What may interact with olsalazine?

- digoxin

Tell your prescriber or health care professional about all other medicines you are taking, including non-prescription medicines, nutritional supplements, or herbal products. Also tell your prescriber or health care professional if you are a frequent user of drinks with caffeine or alcohol, if you smoke, or if you use illegal drugs.

These may affect the way your medicine works. Check with your health care professional before stopping or starting any of your medicines.

What should I watch for while taking olsalazine?

Tell your prescriber or health care professional if your symptoms do not start to improve after several days. There is usually an improvement in 3 to 21 days. You may need about 6 weeks of treatment to get good results. It is important that you go on taking your medicine and only stop taking it on your prescriber's advice.

What side effects may I notice from taking olsalazine?

Side effects that you should report to your prescriber or health care professional as soon as possible:
- chest pain
- difficulty breathing, wheezing
- fever, chills, sore throat
- skin rash or itching
- unusual bleeding or bruising
- unusual weakness or tiredness
- yellowing of the eyes or skin

Side effects that usually do not require medical attention (report to your prescriber or health care professional if they continue or are bothersome):
- depression
- diarrhea
- dizziness
- headache
- muscle aches
- nausea, vomiting
- stomach pain or cramps

Where can I keep my medicine?

Keep out of the reach of children in a container that small children cannot open. Store at room temperature between 15 and 30 degrees C (59 and 86 degrees F). Throw away any unused medicine after the expiration date.

Omeprazole capsules

PRILOSEC®;
20 mg; Capsule, Delayed
Release Pellets
AstraZeneca LP

What are omeprazole capsules?

OMEPRAZOLE (Prilosec®) prevents the production of acid in the stomach. It reduces symptoms and prevents injury to the esophagus, stomach, or intestines in patients with gastroesophageal reflux disease (GERD) or ulcers. Omeprazole is also useful in conditions that cause excessive stomach acid production such as Zollinger-Ellison syndrome and certain cancers. Generic omeprazole capsules are available.

What should my health care professional know before I take omeprazole?

They need to know if you have any of these conditions:

- liver disease
- an unusual or allergic reaction to omeprazole, other medicines, foods, dyes, or preservatives
- pregnant or trying to get pregnant
- breast-feeding

How should I take this medicine?

Take omeprazole capsules by mouth. Follow the directions on the prescription label. Swallow the capsules whole with a drink of water; do not crush, break or chew. The capsules can be opened and the contents sprinkled on a small amount of applesauce or yogurt, given with fruit juices, or swallowed immediately with water. Omeprazole works best if taken on an empty stomach. It is best to take the capsules 30 to 60 minutes before breakfast. Take your doses at regular intervals. Do not take your medicine more often than directed. Contact your pediatrician or health care professional regarding the use of this medicine in children. Special care may be needed.

What if I miss a dose?

If you miss a dose, take it as soon as you can. If it is almost time for your next dose, take only that dose. Do not take double or extra doses.

What may interact with omeprazole?

- ampicillin
- diazepam
- digoxin
- iron salts
- itraconazole, ketoconazole, voriconazole or other prescription medicines for fungus or yeast infections
- phenytoin
- warfarin

Tell your prescriber or health care professional about all other medicines you are taking, including non-prescription medicines, nutritional supplements, or herbal products. Also tell your prescriber or health care professional if you are a frequent user of drinks with caffeine or alcohol, if you smoke, or if you use illegal drugs.

These may affect the way your medicine works. Check with your health care professional before stopping or starting any of your medicines.

What should I watch for while taking omeprazole?

It can take several days of therapy with omeprazole before your stomach condition improves. Check with your prescriber or health care professional if your condition does not improve, or if it gets worse. You can take antacids for the occasional relief of pain unless your prescriber or health care professional tells you otherwise.

What side effects may I notice from taking omeprazole?

Serious side effects are rare. Side effects that you should report to your prescriber or health care professional as soon as possible:

- blood in urine
- chest pain or tightness
- dark yellow or brown urine
- fever or sore throat
- pain or difficulty passing urine
- redness, blistering, peeling or loosening of the skin, including inside the mouth
- shortness of breath
- skin rash
- unusual bleeding or bruising
- yellowing of the eyes or skin

Side effects that usually do not require medical attention (report to your prescriber or health care professional if they continue or are bothersome):

- headache
- diarrhea or constipation

Where can I keep my medicine?

Keep out of the reach of children in a container that small children cannot open. Store at room temperature between 15 and 30 degrees C (59 and 86 degrees F). Protect from light and moisture. Throw away any unused medicine after the expiration date.

Omeprazole tablets

PRILOSEC OTC℠; 20 mg; Tablet, Delayed Release Procter and Gamble Pharmaceuticals Inc Sub Procter and Gamble Co

What are omeprazole tablets?

OMEPRAZOLE (Prilosec OTC℠) prevents the production of acid in the stomach. It helps to treat the symptoms of heartburn, the feeling of acid burning in your stomach or throat. You can buy omeprazole tablets without a prescription; however, this product is not for long-term use, unless otherwise directed by your health care provider. Generic omeprazole tablets are not yet available.

What should my health care professional know before I take omeprazole tablets?

They need to know if you have any of these conditions:

- black or bloody stools
- chest pain
- difficulty swallowing
- have had heartburn for over 3 months
- have heartburn with dizziness, lightheadedness or sweating

- liver disease
- stomach pain
- unexplained weight loss
- vomiting with blood
- wheezing
- an unusual or allergic reaction to omeprazole, other medicines, foods, dyes, or preservatives
- pregnant or trying to get pregnant
- breast-feeding

How should I take this medicine?

Take omeprazole tablets by mouth. Follow the directions on the product label. Take one tablet every day for 14 days in a row; do not skip any doses. Swallow the tablet whole with a drink of water; do not crush, break or chew. Omeprazole works best if taken on an empty stomach. It is best to take the tablet 30 minutes before breakfast. Take your dose at regular intervals every 24 hours. Do not take your medicine more often than directed. Do not take this product for heartburn for more than 2 weeks out of every 4 months. If your symptoms continue, visit your health care provider; you may need additional care or different treatments. Contact your pediatrician or health care professional regarding the use of this medicine in children. Special care may be needed.

What if I miss a dose?

If you miss a dose, take it as soon as you can. If it is almost time for your next dose, take only that dose. Do not take double or extra doses.

What may interact with omeprazole tablets?

- ampicillin
- diazepam
- digoxin
- iron salts
- itraconazole, ketoconazole, voriconazole, or other prescription medicines for fungus or yeast infections
- phenytoin
- warfarin

Tell your prescriber or health care professional about all other medicines you are taking, including non-prescription medicines, nutritional supplements, or herbal products. Also tell your prescriber or health care professional if you are a frequent user of drinks with caffeine or alcohol, if you smoke, or if you use illegal drugs. These may affect the way your medicine works. Check with your health care professional before stopping or starting any of your medicines.

What should I watch for while taking omeprazole?

It can take several days of therapy with omeprazole before your heartburn improves. Check with your prescriber or health care professional if your condition does not improve, or if it gets worse. Do not treat yourself for heartburn with non-prescription omeprazole for more than 14 days in a row. You should only self-medicate with omeprazole for a 2-week treatment period once every 4 months. If your symptoms return shortly after your therapy is complete, or within the 4-month time frame, seek the advice of your health care professional.

What side effects may I notice from taking omeprazole tablets?

Serious side effects are rare. Side effects that you should report to your prescriber or health care professional as soon as possible:

- blood in urine
- chest pain or tightness
- dark yellow or brown urine
- fever or sore throat
- pain or difficulty passing urine
- redness, blistering, peeling or loosening of the skin, including inside the mouth
- shortness of breath
- skin rash
- unusual bleeding or bruising
- yellowing of the eyes or skin

Side effects that usually do not require medical attention (report to your prescriber or health care professional if they continue or are bothersome):

- headache
- diarrhea or constipation

Where can I keep my medicine?

Keep out of the reach of children in a container that small children cannot open. Store at room temperature between 15 and 30 degrees C (59 and 86 degrees F). Protect from light and moisture. Throw away any unused medicine after the expiration date.

Ondansetron tablets

ZOFRAN®;
4 mg; Tablet
Glaxo Wellcome

ZOFRAN® ODT®;
4 mg; Tablet, Orally
Disintegrating
Glaxo Wellcome

What are ondansetron tablets?

ONDANSETRON (Zofran®, Zofran® ODT®) helps to relieve nausea and vomiting, especially when associated with the treatment of cancer (chemotherapy). Ondansetron may also be used to prevent or treat nausea and vomiting that occurs after surgery, and occasionally is used to treat severe vomiting during pregnancy. Generic ondansetron tablets are not yet available.

What should my health care professional know before I take ondansetron?

They need to know if you have any of these conditions:
- liver disease
- an unusual or allergic reaction to ondansetron, granisetron, other medicines, foods, dyes, or preservatives
- pregnant or trying to get pregnant
- breast-feeding

How should I take this medicine?

Ondansetron tablets are taken by mouth, refer to the directions below that match the type of tablets you were prescribed. Follow the directions on your prescription label. Take your doses at regular intervals. Do not take your medicine more often than directed.

If you are taking ondansetron to prevent nausea due to chemotherapy, the first dose of ondansetron is usually given 30 minutes before chemotherapy, followed by a dose at regular intervals for one or two days after chemotherapy. Contact your pediatrician or health care professional regarding the use of this medicine in children. Special care may be needed.

Zofran® tablets: Take regular ondansetron tablets by mouth. Swallow the tablets with a drink of water.

Zofran® ODT® tablets: These tablets are made to dissolve in the mouth without having to take them with water. Place the tablet in the mouth and allow it to dissolve, then swallow. While you may take these tablets with water, it is not necessary to do so.

What if I miss a dose?

If you miss a dose, take it as soon as you can. If it is almost time for your next dose, take only that dose. Do not take double or extra doses.

What may interact with ondansetron?

- alcohol and alcoholic beverages
- bosentan
- cisplatin
- cyclophosphamide
- delavirdine
- imatinib, STI-571
- rifabutin
- rifampin
- rifapentine
- ritonavir

Tell your prescriber or health care professional about all other medicines you are taking, including non-prescription medicines, nutritional supplements, or herbal products. Also tell your prescriber or health care professional if you are a frequent user of drinks with caffeine or alcohol, if you smoke, or if you use illegal drugs. These may affect the way your medicine works. Check with your health care professional before stopping or starting any of your medicines.

What should I watch for while taking ondansetron?

Check with your prescriber or health care professional as soon as you can if you have any sign of an allergic reaction. Do not take alcohol while taking ondansetron.

What side effects may I notice from taking ondansetron?

Side effects that you should report to your prescriber or health care professional as soon as possible:
- difficulty breathing, wheezing, shortness of breath
- fast or irregular heartbeat
- fever and chills
- tightness in the chest
- skin rash, itching
- swelling of the face, tongue, throat, hands and feet

Side effects that usually do not require medical attention (report to your prescriber or health care professional if they continue or are bothersome):
- constipation or diarrhea
- dry mouth
- fainting or lightheadedness
- headache
- stomach pain
- tiredness

Where can I keep my medicine?

Keep out of the reach of children. Store between 2 and 30 degrees C (36 and 86 degrees F). Protect from light. Throw away any unused medicine after the expiration date.

Orlistat capsules

XENICAL®;
120 mg; Capsule
Hoffmann La Roche Inc

What are orlistat capsules?

ORLISTAT (Xenical®) is a prescription drug used to help obese people lose weight and keep the weight off while eating a reduced-calorie diet. Orlistat decreases the amount of fat that is absorbed from your diet.

What should my health professional know before I take orlistat?

They need to know if you have any of these conditions:
- an eating disorder, such as anorexia or bulimia
- problems absorbing food (chronic malabsorption)
- gallbladder problems or gallstones
- diabetes
- an unusual or allergic reaction to orlistat, other medicines, foods, dyes, supplements or preservatives
- pregnant or trying to get pregnant
- breast-feeding
- if you are taking any other weight-loss medications

How should I take this medicine?

Orlistat is taken by mouth and swallowed with a drink of liquid. Follow the directions on the prescription label. You can take orlistat with each main meal that contains about 30% of the calories from fat, or you can take the capsule one hour after the meal. Do not take your medicine more often than directed. If you occasionally miss a meal or have a meal without fat, you can omit that dose of orlistat. Doses greater than 120 mg three times per day have not been shown to increase weight loss. You should use orlistat with a reduced-calorie diet that contains no more than about 30% of the calories from fat. Divide your daily intake of fat, carbohydrates, and protein evenly over your 3 main meals. You should try to follow a healthy eating plan as prescribed by your doctor such as the one developed by the American Heart Association. Following this eating plan can help reduce the possible GI side effects from orlistat.

Contact your pediatrician or health care professional regarding the use of this medicine in children. Special care may be needed.

What if I miss a dose?

If you miss a dose, take it within 1 hour following the meal that contains fat. If it is almost time for your next dose, take only that dose. Do not take double or extra doses.

What may interact with orlistat?

- Dietary supplements, such as beta-carotene and vitamins A, D, E, and K
- warfarin
- cyclosporine
- pravastatin
- drugs used to treat diabetes

Because orlistat can cause decreased absorption of some fat-soluble vitamins, you may need to take a daily multivitamin that contains normal amounts of vitamins D, E, K and beta-carotene. Take the multivitamin once per day at least 2 hours after your dose of orlistat unless otherwise directed by your physician or other healthcare professional. Tell your prescriber or other health care professional about all other medicines you are taking including non-prescription medicines, nutritional supplements, or herbal products. Also, tell your prescriber or health care professional if you are a frequent user of drinks with caffeine or alcohol, if you smoke or if you use illegal drugs. These may affect the way your medicine works. Check before stopping or starting any of your medications.

What should I watch for while taking orlistat?

Watch for any unusual changes in your body's normal function. You need to watch the amount of fat in your diet. Too much dietary fat can increase the side effects from orlistat. Also, watch for any changes in your eyesight, skin or hair that may be caused by a vitamin deficiency.

What side effects may I notice from taking orlistat?

The side effects seen with orlistat are related to the reduced absorption of fat from your diet. Gastrointestinal (GI) side effects may last for less than one week, but have occurred for up to 6 months or longer. Maintaining an appropriate diet can help decrease side effects. The use of orlistat for greater than 2 years has not been studied.

Side effects that you should report to your prescriber or health care professional as soon as possible:
- arthritis or joint pain/tenderness
- back pain

Side effects that usually do not require medical attention (report to your prescriber or health care professional if they continue or are bothersome):
- abdominal discomfort
- increased number of bowel movements
- loss of control of bowel movements
- urgent need to go to the bathroom
- gas with release of stool
- oily/fatty stools
- oily discharge
- clear, orange or brown-colored bowel movements

Where can I keep my medicine?

Keep out of the reach of children in a container that small children cannot open.

Storage at 25 degrees C (77 degrees F) is preferred. You may store at 15 to 30 degrees C (59 to 86 degrees F). Protect from moisture. Keep container tightly closed. Throw away any unused medicine after the expiration date.

Orphenadrine tablets

ORPHENADRINE;
100 mg; Tablet,
Extended Release
Eon Labs Inc

ORPHENADRINE;
100 mg; Tablet,
Extended Release
Sandoz
Pharmaceuticals

O

What is orphenadrine tablets?

ORPHENADRINE (Norflex®) is a muscle relaxant. It helps to relieve pain and stiffness in muscles and can treat muscle spasms. Generic orphenadrine tablets are available.

What should my health care professional know before I take orphenadrine?

They need to know if you have any of these conditions:

- bowel obstruction
- glaucoma
- heart disease
- kidney or liver disease
- myasthenia gravis
- peptic ulcer disease
- prostate disease
- an unusual or allergic reaction to orphenadrine, sulfites, other medicines, foods, dyes, or preservatives
- pregnant or trying to get pregnant
- breast-feeding

How should I take this medicine?

Take orphenadrine tablets by mouth. Follow the directions on the prescription label. Swallow the tablets with a drink of water. Take your doses at regular intervals. Do not take your medicine more often than directed. Contact your pediatrician or health care professional regarding the use of this medicine in children. Special care may be needed.

What if I miss a dose?

If you miss a dose, take it as soon as you can. If it is almost time for your next dose, take only the next dose. Do not take double or extra doses.

What may interact with orphenadrine?

- alcohol and alcoholic beverages
- barbiturate medicines for inducing sleep or treating seizures (convulsions), such as phenobarbital
- dronabinol, THC
- entacapone
- kava kava
- medicines for hay fever and other allergies
- medicines for mental depression, anxiety or psychotic disturbances
- medicines to treat sleeping problems (insomnia)
- other muscle relaxants
- prescription medicines for pain
- tolcapone
- valerian

Tell your prescriber or health care professional about all other medicines you are taking, including non-prescription medicines, nutritional supplements, or herbal products. Also tell your prescriber or health care professional if you are a frequent user of drinks with caffeine or alcohol, if you smoke, or if you use illegal drugs. These may affect the way your medicine works. Check with your health care professional before stopping or starting any of your medicines.

What should I watch for while taking orphenadrine?

You may get drowsy or dizzy. Do not drive, use machinery, or do anything that needs mental alertness until you know how orphenadrine affects you. To reduce the risk of dizzy or fainting spells, do not sit or stand up quickly, especially if you are an older patient. Alcohol can make you more drowsy; avoid alcoholic drinks.

What side effects may I notice from taking orphenadrine?

Side effects that you should report to your prescriber or health care professional as soon as possible:

- difficulty breathing
- fast heartbeat
- hallucinations
- lightheadedness, fainting spells
- skin itching or rash
- redness or swelling of the face or lips
- vomiting

Side effects that usually do not require medical attention (report to your prescriber or health care professional if they continue or are bothersome):

- agitation
- blurred vision
- dilated pupils
- dizziness
- drowsiness
- dry mouth
- headache
- nausea
- nervousness or confusion

Where can I keep my medicine?

Keep out of the reach of children in a container that small children cannot open. Store between 15 and 30 degrees C (59 and 86 degrees F). Keep container tightly closed. Throw away any unused medicine after the expiration date.

o

Oseltamivir capsules

TAMIFLU®;
75 mg; Capsule
Hoffmann La Roche Inc

What are oseltamivir capsules?

OSELTAMIVIR (Tamiflu®) is a drug used to treat infections caused by two of the most common flu viruses. Oseltamivir may decrease the length of time you experience symptoms of the flu by 1 to 2 days. Oseltamivir may also help to reduce the risk of spreading the flu to others. Generic oseltamivir capsules are not yet available.

What should my health care professional know before I take oseltamivir?

They need to know if you have any of the following conditions:

- decreased kidney function
- heart disease
- liver disease
- lung disease
- an unusual or allergic reaction to oseltamivir, other medicines, foods, dyes, or preservatives
- pregnant or trying to get pregnant
- breast-feeding

How should I take this medicine?

Oseltamivir capsules are taken by mouth. You may take oseltamivir with or without food. If oseltamivir upsets your stomach, take it with food. To treat the flu, oseltamivir is usually given two times per day for 5 days. Follow the instructions given to you by your prescriber or health care professional. Contact your pediatrician or health care professional regarding the use of this medicine in children. Special care may be needed.

What if I miss a dose?

If you miss a dose, take it as soon as you remember. If it is almost time for your next dose (within 2 hours), take only that dose and continue with your regular schedule, spacing doses evenly. Do not take double or extra doses. If you have missed several doses, call your prescriber or health care provider.

What may interact with oseltamivir?

There are no known drug interactions with oseltamivir. Tell your prescriber or health care professional about all other medicines that you are taking, including non-

prescription medicines, nutritional supplements, or herbal products. Also tell your prescriber or health care professional if you are a frequent user of drinks with caffeine or alcohol, if you smoke, or if you use illegal drugs. These may affect the way your medicine works. Check before starting or stopping any of your medicines.

What should I watch for while taking oseltamivir?

Treatment with oseltamivir should be started within 2 days of the beginning of flu symptoms to be effective. Finish the whole course of treatment even if you start to feel better sooner. The entire treatment is needed to make sure the infection is totally treated. Do not share oseltamivir with anyone, even if they have the same symptoms. Oseltamivir is not a substitute for the flu shot. You should continue receiving an annual flu shot based upon the advice of your primary health care provider.

What side effects may I notice from using oseltamivir?

Side effects due to oseltamivir are uncommon and are not usually severe.
Side effects that you should report to your prescriber or health care professional as soon as possible:

- difficulty breathing or shortness of breath
- infection and inflammation of the sinuses (nose) and chest
- skin rash

Side effects that usually do not require medical attention (report to your prescriber or health care professional if they continue or are bothersome):

- coughing
- difficulty sleeping
- dizziness
- headache
- nausea and vomiting

Where can I keep my medicine?

Keep out of the reach of children. Store at controlled room temperature between 15 and 30 degrees C (59 and 86 degrees F). Throw away any unused medicine after the expiration date.

Oxacillin capsules

What are oxacillin capsules?

OXACILLIN (Bactocill®, Prostaphlin®) is a penicillin antibiotic. Oxacillin kills certain bacteria that cause infection, or stops their growth. It treats many kinds of infections of the skin, central nervous system, heart, brain, bones, respiratory tract, sinuses, and urinary tract. Generic oxacillin capsules are available.

What should my health care professional know before I take oxacillin?

They need to know if you have any of these conditions:
- asthma
- eczema
- kidney disease
- liver disease
- stomach problems (especially colitis)
- other chronic illness
- an unusual or allergic reaction to oxacillin, other penicillins, cephalosporin antibiotics, foods, dyes, or preservatives
- breast-feeding

How should I take this medicine?

Take oxacillin capsules by mouth. Follow the directions on the prescription label. Take oxacillin 1 to 2 hours before or at least 2 hours after eating; taking it with food can make it less effective. Take with a full glass of water. Take your doses at regular intervals. Do not take your medicine more often than directed. Finish the full course prescribed by your prescriber or health care professional even if you think your condition is better. Do not stop taking except on your prescriber's advice. Contact your pediatrician or health care professional regarding the use of this medicine in children. Special care may be needed.

What if I miss a dose?

If you miss a dose, take it as soon as you can. If it is almost time for your next dose, take only that dose. Do not take double or extra doses. There should be an interval of at least 4 to 6 hours between doses.

What may interact with oxacillin?

- certain antibiotics given by injection
- probenecid
- rifampin

Tell your prescriber or health care professional about all other medicines you are taking, including non-prescription medicines, nutritional supplements, or herbal products. Also tell your prescriber or health care professional if you are a frequent user of drinks with caffeine or alcohol, if you smoke, or if you use illegal drugs. These may affect the way your medicine works. Check with your health care professional before stopping or starting any of your medicines.

What should I watch for while taking oxacillin?

Tell your prescriber or health care professional if your symptoms do not improve in 2 or 3 days. If you get severe or watery diarrhea, do not treat yourself. Call your prescriber or health care professional for advice. If you get a skin rash, do not treat yourself. Call your prescriber or health care professional for advice. If you are diabetic and taking large doses of oxacillin, you may get a false-positive result for sugar in your urine. Check with your prescriber or health care professional before you change your diet or the dose of your diabetic medicine.

What side effects may I notice from taking oxacillin?

Side effects that you should report to your prescriber or health care professional as soon as possible:
- dark yellow or brown urine
- difficulty breathing, wheezing
- fever or chills, sore throat
- headache
- less frequent passing of urine
- red spots on the skin
- redness, blistering, peeling or loosening of the skin, including inside the mouth
- seizures (convulsions)
- severe or watery diarrhea
- skin rash, itching
- swollen joints
- unusual bleeding or bruising
- unusual weakness or tiredness
- yellowing of the eyes or skin

Side effects that usually do not require medical attention (report to your prescriber or health care professional if they continue or are bothersome):
- diarrhea
- nausea, vomiting
- sore mouth

Where can I keep my medicine?

Keep out of the reach of children in a container that small children cannot open. Store at room temperature between 15 and 30 degrees C (59 and 86 degrees F). Keep container tightly closed. Throw away any unused medicine after the expiration date.

Oxandrolone tablets

OXANDRIN®;
2.5 mg; Tablet
BTG Pharmaceuticals
Corp Sub
Biotechnology
General Corp

OXANDRIN®;
10 mg; Tablet
BTG Pharmaceuticals
Corp Sub
Biotechnology
General Corp

What are oxandrolone tablets?

OXANDROLONE (Oxandrin®) helps promote weight gain, helps improve muscle strength in certain conditions, and helps promote growth in certain patients. Oxandrolone does not enhance athletic ability. Generic oxandrolone tablets are not available.

What should my health care professional know before I take oxandrolone?

They need to know if you have any of these conditions:
- breast cancer
- breast-feeding
- diabetes
- heart or blood vessel disease
- high blood calcium levels
- kidney disease
- liver disease
- pregnant or trying to get pregnant
- previous heart attack
- prostate disease
- an unusual or allergic reaction to oxandrolone, other medicines, foods, dyes, or preservatives

How should I take this medicine?

Take oxandrolone tablets by mouth. They can be taken with or without food. Follow the directions on the prescription label. Do not take your medicine more often than directed. Contact your pediatrician or health care professional regarding the use of this medicine in children. Special care may be needed.

What if I miss a dose?

Try not to miss a dose. If it is almost time for your next dose, take only that dose. Do not take double or extra doses.

What may interact with oxandrolone?

- blood thinners such as warfarin
- corticosteroids
- epoetin alfa
- finasteride
- goserelin
- leuprolide
- medicines for diabetes
- saw palmetto

Tell your prescriber or health care professional about all other medicines that you are taking, including nonprescription medicines, nutritional supplements, or herbal products. Also, tell your prescriber or health care professional if you are a frequent user of drinks with caffeine or alcohol, if you smoke, or if you use illegal drugs. These may affect the way your medicine works. Check with your health care professional before stopping or starting any of your medicines.

What should I watch for while taking oxandrolone?

Visit your prescriber or health care professional for regular checks on your progress. Do not stop taking oxandrolone except on your prescriber's advice. You should make sure you are eating enough calories if you are taking oxandrolone to help gain weight. Discuss your dietary needs with your health care professional or nutritionist. Oxandrolone can affect your liver. Promptly report any nausea, vomiting, ankle swelling, or skin color changes to your prescriber or health care professional. It is important to have any blood tests done that your health care professional may order. If you have diabetes, oxandrolone may affect your blood sugar levels. Check with your prescriber or health care professional before you change your diet or the dose of your medicine for diabetes. The Olympic Committee and other athletic organizations ban oxandrolone use by athletes.

What side effects may I notice from taking oxandrolone?

Side effects that you should report to your prescriber or health care professional as soon as possible:
- black, tarry stools or light-colored stools
- dark yellow or brown urine
- depression
- nausea, vomiting
- skin rash and itching (hives)
- stomach pain
- unusual bleeding
- unusual swelling
- weight gain
- yellowing of the eyes or skin

Additional side effects that can occur in men include:
- breast tenderness or enlargement
- frequent erections
- frequent or difficult passing of urine
- groin or scrotum pain

Additional side effects that can occur in women include:
- decrease in breast size
- enlarged clitoris
- facial hair growth
- hair loss
- irregular vaginal bleeding/spotting
- voice changes (deepening or hoarseness)

Side effects that usually do not require medical attention (report to your prescriber or health care professional if they continue or are bothersome):

- acne
- difficulty sleeping
- hair loss
- headache
- sexual difficulties; changes in sexual desire can occur in either male or female patients, and excessive doses can cause impotence in men

Oxaprozin caplets

DAYPRO®;
600 mg; Tablet
GD Searle LLC a
Subsidiary of
Pharmacia Company
Pfizer

OXAPROZIN;
600 mg; Tablet
Warrick
Pharmaceuticals
Corp

What are oxaprozin caplets?

OXAPROZIN (Daypro®) is a nonsteroidal anti-inflammatory drug (NSAID). Oxaprozin helps reduce inflammation and ease mild to moderate pain. It reduces fever and helps relieve the symptoms of rheumatoid arthritis, osteoarthritis, and other conditions associated with inflammation. Generic oxaprozin tablets are available.

What should my health care professional know before I take oxaprozin?

They need to know if you have any of these conditions:
- anemia
- asthma, especially aspirin sensitive asthma
- bleeding problems or taking medicines that make you bleed more easily such as anticoagulants ("blood thinners")
- cigarette smoker
- diabetes
- drink more than 3 alcohol-containing beverages a day
- heart failure
- high blood pressure
- kidney disease
- liver disease
- stomach or duodenal ulcers
- systemic lupus erythematosus
- ulcerative colitis
- an unusual or allergic reaction to aspirin, other salicylates, other NSAIDs, other medicines, foods, dyes or preservatives
- pregnant or trying to get pregnant
- breast-feeding

How should I take this medicine?

Take oxaprozin caplets by mouth. Follow the directions on the prescription label. Swallow caplets whole with a full glass of water; take caplets in an upright or sitting position. Taking a sip of water first, before taking the caplets, may help you swallow them. If possible take bedtime doses at least 10 minutes before lying down. It is better to take oxaprozin with food. Take your doses at regular intervals. Do not take your medicine more often than directed. Contact your pediatrician or health care professional regarding the use of oxaprozin

Where can I keep my medicine?

Keep out of the reach of children in a container that small children cannot open. Store between 15 and 26 degrees C (59 and 77 degrees F). Keep container tightly closed. Throw away any unused medicine after the expiration date.

in children. Special care may be needed. This medicine is usually not for children under 6 years of age.

What if I miss a dose?

If you miss a dose, take it as soon as you can. If it is almost time for your next dose, take only that dose. Do not take double or extra doses.

What may interact with oxaprozin?

- alcohol
- anti-inflammatory drugs (other NSAIDs, prednisone)
- aspirin and aspirin-like medicines
- cidofovir
- cyclosporine
- entecavir
- herbal products that contain feverfew, garlic, ginger, or ginkgo biloba
- lithium
- medicines for high blood pressure
- medicines that affect platelets
- medicines that treat or prevent blood clots such as warfarin and other "blood thinners"
- methotrexate
- pemetrexed
- water pills (diuretics)

Tell your prescriber or health care professional about all other medicines you are taking, including non-prescription medicines, nutritional supplements, or herbal products. Also tell your prescriber or health care professional if you are a frequent user of drinks with caffeine or alcohol, if you smoke, or if you use illegal drugs. These may affect the way your medicine works. Check with your health care professional before stopping or starting any of your medicines.

What should I watch for while taking oxaprozin?

Let your prescriber or health care professional know if your pain continues. Do not take oxaprozin with other pain killers or anti-inflammatory drugs without advice. If you get flu-like symptoms (fever, chills, muscle aches and pains), do not treat yourself; consult your health care provider. To reduce unpleasant effects on your throat and stomach, take oxaprozin with a full glass of

This drug requires an FDA medication guide. See page xxxvii.

water and never just before lying down. If you notice black, tarry stools or experience severe stomach pain and/or vomit blood or what looks like coffee grounds, notify your health care prescriber immediately. You may get drowsy. Do not drive, use machinery, or do anything that needs mental alertness until you know how oxaprozin affects you. Do not sit or stand up quickly, especially if you are an older patient. This reduces the risk of dizzy or fainting spells. Do not smoke cigarettes or drink alcohol; these increase irritation to your stomach and can make it more susceptible to damage from oxaprozin. If you are taking medicines that affect the clotting of your blood, such as aspirin or blood thinners such as Coumadin®, talk to your health care provider or prescriber before taking this medicine. If you are going to have surgery, tell your prescriber or health care professional that you are taking oxaprozin. Problems can arise if you need dental work, and in the day to day care of your teeth. Try to avoid damage to your teeth and gums when you brush or floss your teeth. It is especially important not to use oxaprozin during the last 3 months of pregnancy unless specifically directed to do so by your health care provider. Oxaprozin may cause problems in the unborn child or complications during delivery.

What side effects may I notice from taking oxaprozin?

Side effects that you should report to your prescriber or health care professional as soon as possible:
- signs of bleeding—bruising, pinpoint red spots on the skin, black tarry stools, blood in the urine, unusual tiredness or weakness, vomiting blood or vomit that looks like coffee grounds
- signs of an allergic reaction—difficulty breathing or wheezing, skin rash, redness, blistering or peeling skin, hives, or itching, swelling of eyelids, throat, lips
- blurred vision
- change in the amount of urine passed
- difficulty swallowing, severe heartburn or burning, pain in throat
- pain or difficulty passing urine
- stomach pain or cramps
- swelling of feet or ankles
- yellowing of eyes or skin

Side effects that usually do not require medical attention (report to your prescriber or health care professional if they continue or are bothersome):
- diarrhea or constipation
- dizziness
- drowsiness
- gas or heartburn
- headache
- nausea, vomiting

Where can I keep my medicine?

Keep out of the reach of children in a container that small children cannot open. Store at 25 degrees C (77 degrees F). Avoid temperature above 30 degrees C (86 degrees F) or below 15 degrees C (59 degrees F). Protect from light. Keep container tightly closed. Throw away any unused medicine after the expiration date.

Oxazepam tablets or capsules

OXAZEPAM; 30 mg; Capsule Ivax Pharmaceuticals Inc	OXAZEPAM; 30 mg; Capsule Purepac Pharmaceutical Co

What are oxazepam tablets or capsules?

OXAZEPAM (Serax®) is a benzodiazepine. Benzodiazepines belong to a group of medicines that slow down the central nervous system. Oxazepam relieves anxiety and nervousness, and can help patients cope with alcohol withdrawal. Federal law prohibits the transfer of oxazepam to any person other than the patient for whom it was prescribed. Do not share this medicine with anyone else. Generic oxazepam tablets and capsules are available.

What should my health care professional know before I take oxazepam?

They need to know if you have any of these conditions:
- an alcohol or drug abuse problem
- bipolar disorder, depression, psychosis or other mental health condition
- glaucoma
- kidney disease
- liver disease
- lung disease, such as chronic obstructive pulmonary disease (COPD), sleep apnea or other breathing difficulties
- myasthenia gravis
- porphyria
- Parkinson's disease
- seizures or a history of seizures
- shortness of breath
- snoring
- suicidal thoughts
- an unusual or allergic reaction to oxazepam, other benzodiazepines, foods, dyes, or preservatives
- pregnant or trying to get pregnant
- breast-feeding

How should I take this medicine?

Take oxazepam tablets or capsules by mouth. Follow the directions on the prescription label. Swallow the tablets or capsules with a drink of water. If oxazepam upsets your stomach, take it with food or milk. Take your doses at regular intervals. Do not take your medicine more often than directed. Do not stop taking except on your prescriber's advice. Contact your pediatrician or health care professional regarding the use of this medicine in children. Special care may be needed.

What if I miss a dose?

If you miss a dose, take it as soon as you can. If it is almost time for your next dose, take only that dose. Do not take double or extra doses.

What may interact with oxazepam?

- alcohol
- barbiturate medicines for inducing sleep or treating seizures (convulsions), like phenobarbital or primidone
- caffeine
- female hormones, including contraceptive or birth control pills
- herbal or dietary supplements such as kava kava, melatonin, or valerian
- medicines for anxiety or sleeping problems, such as alprazolam, diazepam, lorazepam or triazolam
- medicines for depression, mental problems or psychiatric disturbances
- phenytoin
- prescription pain medicines
- probenecid
- some medicines for colds, hay fever or other allergies
- theophylline

Tell your prescriber or health care professional about all other medicines you are taking, including non-prescription medicines, nutritional supplements, or herbal products. Also tell your prescriber or health care professional if you are a frequent user of drinks with caffeine or alcohol, if you smoke, or if you use illegal drugs. These may affect the way your medicine works. Check with your health care professional before stopping or starting any of your medicines.

What should I watch for while taking oxazepam?

Visit your prescriber or health care professional for regular checks on your progress. Your body can become dependent on oxazepam, ask your prescriber or health care professional if you still need to take it. However, if you have been taking oxazepam regularly for some time, do not suddenly stop taking it. You must gradually reduce the dose or you may get severe side effects. Ask your prescriber or health care professional for advice. Even after you stop taking oxazepam it can still affect your body for several days. You may get drowsy or dizzy. Do not drive, use machinery, or do anything that needs mental alertness until you know how oxazepam affects you. To reduce the risk of dizzy and fainting spells, do not stand or sit up quickly, especially if you are an older patient. Alcohol may increase dizziness and drowsiness. Avoid alcoholic drinks. Do not treat yourself for coughs, colds or allergies without asking your prescriber or health care professional for advice. Some ingredients can increase possible side effects. If you are going to have surgery, tell your prescriber or health care professional that you are taking oxazepam.

What side effects may I notice from taking oxazepam?

Side effects that you should report to your prescriber or health care professional as soon as possible:

- confusion
- depression
- lightheadedness or fainting spells
- mood changes, excitability or aggressive behavior
- movement difficulty, staggering or jerky movements
- muscle cramps
- restlessness
- tremors
- weakness or tiredness

Side effects that usually do not require medical attention (report to your prescriber or health care professional if they continue or are bothersome):

- difficulty sleeping, nightmares
- dizziness, drowsiness, clumsiness, or unsteadiness; a "hangover" effect
- headache
- nausea, vomiting

Where can I keep my medicine?

Keep out of the reach of children in a container that small children cannot open. Store at room temperature between 15 and 30 degrees C (59 and 86 degrees F). Keep container tightly closed. Throw away any unused medicine after the expiration date.

Oxcarbazepine tablets

TRILEPTAL®; 300 mg; Tablet Novartis Pharmaceuticals

TRILEPTAL®; 150 mg; Tablet Novartis Pharmaceuticals

What are oxcarbazepine tablets?

OXCARBAZEPINE (Trileptal®) can help to control partial seizures (convulsions) in people with epilepsy. Oxcarbazepine can also treat facial nerve pain from trigeminal neuralgia. Generic oxcarbazepine tablets are not yet available.

What should my health care professional know before I take oxcarbazepine?

They need to know if you have any of these conditions:
- an alcohol abuse problem
- kidney disease
- allergic reaction to carbamazepine

- any unusual or allergic reaction to oxcarbazepine, other medicines, foods, dyes, or preservatives
- pregnant or trying to get pregnant
- breast-feeding

How should I take this medicine?

Take oxcarbazepine tablets by mouth. Oxcarbazepine tablets may be taken with or without food. Follow the directions on the prescription label. Take your doses at regular intervals. Do not take your medicine more often than directed. Contact your pediatrician or health care professional regarding the use of this medicine in children. Special care may be needed.

What if I miss a dose?

If you miss a dose, take it as soon as you can. If it is almost time for your next dose, take only that dose. Do not take double or extra doses.

What may interact with oxcarbazepine?

- alcohol
- carbamazepine
- felodipine
- female hormones, including birth control pills, injections, patches or implants
- fosphenytoin
- lamotrigine
- phenobarbital
- phenytoin
- primidone
- valproic acid
- verapamil

Tell your prescriber or health care professional about all other medicines you are taking, including non-prescription medicines and herbal products. Also tell your prescriber or health care professional if you are a frequent user of drinks with caffeine or alcohol, if you smoke, or if you use illegal drugs. These may affect the way your medicine works. Check with your health care professional before stopping or starting any of your medicines.

What should I watch for while taking oxcarbazepine?

Visit your prescriber or health care professional for a regular check on your progress. Do not stop taking oxcarbazepine suddenly. This increases the risk of seizures. Wear a Medic Alert bracelet or necklace. Carry an identification card with information about your condition, medications, and prescriber or health care professional. You may get drowsy or dizzy when you first start taking this medicine. Do not drive, use ma-

chinery, or do anything that needs mental alertness until you know how oxcarbazepine affects you. Alcohol can increase drowsiness and dizziness. Avoid alcoholic drinks. If you are female and are taking birth control pills (contraceptive pills) or using other hormonal birth control methods (like injections), you should know that the birth control may not work as well while you are taking this drug. You may need to talk to your prescriber about effective ways to prevent pregnancy. Let your prescriber know if you experience any unusual menstrual-type bleeding or spotting or if you think you might be pregnant while on this medicine. If you are going to have surgery, tell your prescriber or health care professional that you are taking oxcarbazepine.

What side effects may I notice from taking oxcarbazepine?

Side effects that you should report to your prescriber or health care professional as soon as possible:
- allergic reaction (fever, rash, muscle aches or pain, hives, or difficulty breathing)
- confusion
- difficulty speaking or walking
- dizziness
- infection
- muscle incoordination
- nausea or vomiting
- redness, blistering, peeling or loosening of the skin, including inside the mouth
- swelling of the legs and ankles
- unexplained tiredness
- unusual bruising or bleeding
- vision changes
- weakness

Side effects that usually do not require medical attention (report to your prescriber or health care professional if they continue or are bothersome):
- constipation
- diarrhea
- difficulty sleeping
- drowsiness
- headache
- loss of appetite
- nervousness
- stomach upset, indigestion
- tremor

Where can I keep my medicine?

Keep out of reach of children in a container that small children cannot open. Store at room temperature between 20 and 25 degrees C (68 and 77 degrees F). Keep container tightly closed. Protect from light or moisture. Throw away any unused medicine after the expiration date

Oxybutynin tablets

DITROPAN®;
5 mg; Tablet
Ortho McNeil
Pharmaceutical Inc

DITROPAN® XL;
10 mg; Tablet,
Extended Release
Ortho McNeil
Pharmaceutical Inc

What are oxybutynin tablets?

OXYBUTYNIN (Ditropan®, Ditropan® XL) is an antispasmodic medicine that helps control overactive bladder, a chronic condition that can be improved with medication. Oxybutynin may reduce the frequency of bathroom visits and may help to control wetting accidents. Generic oxybutynin tablets are available.

What should my health care professional know before I take oxybutynin?

They need to know if you have any of these conditions:
- diarrhea
- glaucoma
- heart or blood vessel disease
- high blood pressure
- kidney disease
- liver disease
- myasthenia gravis
- nervous system disease
- overactive thyroid
- prostate trouble
- stomach problems, intestinal obstruction or ulcerative colitis
- an unusual or allergic reaction to oxybutynin, other medicines, foods, dyes, or preservatives
- pregnant or trying to get pregnant
- breast-feeding

How should I take this medicine?

Take oxybutynin tablets by mouth. Follow the directions on the prescription label. Swallow the tablets with a drink of water. Oxybutynin works best on an empty stomach. Take your medicine at regular intervals. Do not take your medicine more often than directed. Contact your pediatrician or health care professional regarding the use of this medicine in children. Special care may be needed. Elderly patients over 65 years old may have a stronger reaction to this medicine and need smaller doses.

What if I miss a dose?

If you miss a dose, take it as soon as you can. If it is almost time for your next dose, take only that dose. Do not take double or extra doses.

What may interact with oxybutynin?

- alcohol
- some medicines for gastrointestinal problems
- medicines for mental problems and psychotic disturbances
- medicines for movement abnormalities as in Parkinson's disease
- medicines for pain or sleep

Tell your prescriber or health care professional about all other medicines you are taking, including non-prescription medicines, nutritional supplements, or herbal products. Also tell your prescriber or health care professional if you are a frequent user of drinks with caffeine or alcohol, if you smoke, or if you use illegal drugs. These may affect the way your medicine works. Check with your health care professional before stopping or starting any of your medicines.

What should I watch for while taking oxybutynin?

You may get drowsy, dizzy, or have blurred vision. Do not drive, use machinery, or do anything that needs mental alertness until you know how oxybutynin affects you. To reduce the risk of dizzy or fainting spells, do not sit or stand up quickly, especially if you are an older patient. Alcohol can make you more drowsy, avoid alcoholic drinks. Your mouth may get dry. Chewing sugarless gum or sucking hard candy, and drinking plenty of water will help. If you are taking Ditropan® XL tablets, you may notice the shells of the tablets in your stool from time to time. This is normal. The medication is absorbed from this shell, but the shell does not dissolve. Avoid extreme heat (e.g., hot tubs, saunas). Oxybutynin can cause you to sweat less than normal. Your body temperature could increase to dangerous levels, which may lead to heat stroke.

What side effects may I notice from taking oxybutynin?

Side effects that you should report to your prescriber or health care professional as soon as possible:
- confusion, nervousness
- difficulty breathing
- eye pain
- fever
- flushing (reddening of the skin)
- memory loss
- palpitations
- skin rash (hives), itching

Side effects that usually do not require medical attention (report to your prescriber or health care professional if they continue or are bothersome):
- blurred vision
- constipation
- decreased sweating
- dizziness, drowsiness
- dry mouth
- pain or difficulty passing urine
- sexual difficulties (impotence)

Where can I keep my medicine?

Keep out of the reach of children in a container that small children cannot open. Store at room temperature between 15 and 30 degrees C (59 and 86 degrees F). Protect from light. Throw away any unused medicine after the expiration date.

Oxycodone sustained-release tablets

OXYCONTIN®;
10 mg; Tablet,
Extended Release
Purdue Pharma LP

OXYCONTIN®;
40 mg; Tablet,
Extended Release
Purdue Pharma LP

What are oxycodone sustained-release tablets?

OXYCODONE (OxyContin®) relieves moderate to severe pain. This type of oxycodone is for people who need pain medicine for more than a few days. These tablets are specially designed to release oxycodone over a period of time. Do not share this medicine with anyone else. Federal law prohibits the transfer of oxycodone to any person other than the patient for whom it was prescribed. Generic oxycodone sustained-release tablets are available.

What should my health care professional know before I take oxycodone?

They need to know if you have any of these conditions:
- if you frequently drink alcohol-containing beverages
- abnormal bladder function, difficulty urinating
- constipation
- diarrhea
- heart disease
- intestinal disease
- kidney disease
- liver disease
- lung disease, severe asthma, or breathing difficulties
- seizures
- an unusual or allergic reaction to oxycodone, codeine, hydrocodone, morphine, other medicines, foods, dyes, or preservatives
- pregnant or trying to get pregnant
- breast-feeding

How should I take this medicine?

Take oxycodone sustained-release tablets (OxyContin®) by mouth. Follow the directions on the prescription label. Do not take OxyContin® on an "as needed" basis; OxyContin® should be taken on a regular basis only for the condition for which it was prescribed. Swallow the tablets with a drink of water. Do not break, crush, or chew OxyContin® tablets; this will cause the release of a large amount of oxycodone to be absorbed into your body at once, which can be dangerous causing an overdose and serious adverse reactions. If oxycodone upsets your stomach, you can take it with food or milk. If you are taking OxyContin® 160 mg tablets, it is important to avoid high-fat foods around the time you are taking you medicine. Contact your pediatrician or health care professional regarding the use of this medicine in children. Special care may be needed. Do NOT share this medicine with anyone.

What if I miss a dose?

If you miss a dose, take it as soon as you can. If it is almost time for your next dose, take only that dose. Do not take double or extra doses.

What may interact with oxycodone?

- delavirdine
- imatinib, STI-571
- medicines for high blood pressure
- medicines for seizures
- rifampin
- ritonavir

Because oxycodone can cause drowsiness, other medicines that also cause drowsiness may increase this effect of oxycodone. Some medicines that cause drowsiness are:

- alcohol-containing medicines
- barbiturates such as phenobarbital
- certain antidepressants or tranquilizers
- muscle relaxants
- certain antihistamines used in cold medicines

Ask your prescriber or health care professional about other medicines that may increase the effect of oxycodone. Tell your prescriber or health care professional about all other medicines you are taking, including non-prescription medicines, nutritional supplements, or herbal products. Also tell your prescriber or health care professional if you are a frequent user of drinks with caffeine or alcohol, if you smoke, or if you use illegal drugs. These may affect the way your medicine works. Check with your health care professional before stopping or starting any of your medicines.

What should I watch for while taking oxycodone?

Tell your prescriber or health care professional if your pain does not go away, if it gets worse, or if you have new or different type of pain. Report episodes of breakthrough pain and adverse reactions to your health care provider. This will help your prescriber adjust your medication appropriately. Do not adjust the dose of your therapy without consulting your prescriber. Use exactly as directed by your prescriber or health care professional. If you are taking oxycodone on a regular basis, do not suddenly stop taking it. Your body becomes used to the oxycodone and when you suddenly stop taking it, you may develop a severe reaction. This does NOT mean you are "addicted" to oxycodone. Addiction is a behavior related to getting and using a drug for a non-medical reason. If you have pain, you have a medical reason to take pain medicine such as oxycodone to control your pain. If you do stop oxycodone treatment after several days, your prescriber will gradually decrease your dose over a period of time to avoid any adverse reactions. You may get drowsy or dizzy when you first start taking oxycodone or change doses.

Do not drive, use machinery, or do anything that needs mental alertness until you know how oxycodone affects you. Stand or sit up slowly as this reduces the risk of dizzy or fainting spells. These effects may be worse if you are an older patient. The drowsiness should decrease after taking oxycodone for a couple of days. If you have not slept because of your pain, you may sleep more the first few days your pain is controlled to catch-up on missed sleep. Be careful taking other medicines which may also make you tired. This effect may be worse when taking these medicines with oxycodone. Alcohol can increase possible drowsiness, dizziness, confusion and affect your breathing. Avoid alcohol while taking oxycodone. Oxycodone will cause constipation. Make sure to take a laxative and/or a stool softener while taking oxycodone. Try to have a bowel movement at least every 2 to 3 days. If you do not have a bowel movement for 3 days or more call your prescriber or health care professional. They may recommend using an enema or suppository to help you move your bowels. You may pass empty tablets (matrix "ghosts") in your colostomy or in your stool, this is of no concern since the active medication has already been absorbed. Your mouth may get dry. Drinking plenty of water, chewing sugarless gum or sucking on hard candy may help to relieve dry mouth symptoms. Have regular dental checks. Rarely, oxycodone may cause you to have hallucinations (to see things that are not really there) or cause your legs or arms to "jerk" or have spasms. If you experience these effects, call your prescriber or health care professional.

What side effects may I notice from taking oxycodone?

Side effects that you should report to your prescriber or health care professional as soon as possible:
Rare or uncommon:
- breathing difficulties, wheezing
- cold, clammy skin

- seizures
- slow or fast heartbeat
- severe rash
- unusual weakness

More common:
- confusion
- lightheadedness or fainting spells
- nervousness or restlessness

Side effects that usually do not require medical attention (report to your prescriber or health care professional if they continue or are bothersome):
- itching
- clumsiness, unsteadiness
- constipation
- decrease or difficulty passing urine
- dizziness, drowsiness
- dry mouth
- flushing
- headache
- nausea, vomiting
- pinpoint pupils
- sweating

Where can I keep my medicine?

Keep out of the reach of children in a container that small children cannot open. Do not share or give this medicine to anyone else. Avoid accidental swallowing of oxycodone by someone (especially children) other than the person for whom it was prescribed as this may result in severe effects and possibly death. OxyContin® contains oxycodone, which can be a target for people who abuse prescription medicines. Therefore, keep your tablets in a secure place, to protect them from theft. Never give them to anyone else. Selling or giving away this medicine is dangerous and against the law. Store at room temperature between 15 and 30 degrees C (59 and 86 degrees F). Protect from light. Keep container tightly closed. Throw away any unused medicine after the expiration date

Oxycodone tablets or capsules

OXYCODONE; 5 mg; Tablet Ethex Corporation

OXYCODONE; 5 mg; Capsule Mallinckrodt Inc Pharmaceuticals Group

What are oxycodone tablets or capsules?

OXYCODONE (Roxicodone®, OxyIR®, M-Oxy™, Percolone™) relieves moderate to severe pain. Federal law prohibits the transfer of oxycodone to any person other than the patient for whom it was prescribed. Do not share this medicine with anyone else. Generic oxycodone tablets are available.

What should my health care professional know before I take oxycodone?

They need to know if you have any of these conditions:
- abnormal bladder function

- diarrhea
- heart disease
- intestinal disease
- kidney disease
- liver disease
- lung disease or breathing difficulties
- seizures
- an unusual or allergic reaction to oxycodone, codeine, morphine, other medicines, foods, dyes, or preservatives
- pregnant or trying to get pregnant
- breast-feeding

O

How should I take this medicine?

Take oxycodone tablets by mouth. Follow the directions on the prescription label. Swallow the tablets with a drink of water. If oxycodone upsets your stomach, you can take it with food or milk. Contact your pediatrician or health care professional regarding the use of this medicine in children. Special care may be needed. Do not share this medicine with anyone.

What if I miss a dose?

If you miss a dose, take it as soon as you can. If it is almost time for your next dose, take only that dose. Do not take double or extra doses.

What may interact with oxycodone?

- medicines for high blood pressure
- medicines for seizures
- ritonavir

Because oxycodone can cause drowsiness, other medicines that also cause drowsiness may increase this effect of oxycodone. Some medicines that cause drowsiness are:

- alcohol and alcohol-containing medicines
- barbiturates such as phenobarbital
- certain antidepressants or tranquilizers
- muscle relaxants
- certain antihistamines used in cold medicines

Ask your prescriber or health care professional about other medicines that may increase the effect of oxycodone. Tell your prescriber or health care professional about all other medicines you are taking, including non-prescription medicines, nutritional supplements, or herbal products. Also tell your prescriber or health care professional if you are a frequent user of drinks with caffeine or alcohol, if you smoke, or if you use illegal drugs. These may affect the way your medicine works. Check with your health care professional before stopping or starting any of your medicines.

What should I watch for while taking oxycodone?

Tell your prescriber or health care professional if your pain does not go away, if it gets worse, or if you have new or different type of pain. Use exactly as directed by your prescriber or health care professional. If you are taking oxycodone on a regular basis, do not suddenly stop taking it. Your body becomes used to the oxycodone and when you suddenly stop taking it, you may develop a severe reaction. This does NOT mean you are "addicted" to oxycodone. Addiction is a behavior related to getting and using a drug for a non-medical reason. If you have pain, you have a medical reason to take pain medicine such as oxycodone to control your pain. If you do stop oxycodone treatment after several days, your prescriber will gradually decrease your dose over a period of time to avoid any adverse reactions. You may get drowsy or dizzy when you first start taking oxycodone or change doses. Do not drive, use machinery, or do anything that needs mental alertness until you know how oxycodone affects you. Stand or sit up slowly, this reduces the risk of dizzy or fainting spells. These effects may be worse if you are an older patient. The drowsiness should decrease after taking oxycodone for a couple of days. If you have not slept because of your pain, you may sleep more the first few days your pain is controlled to catch-up on missed sleep. Be careful taking other medicines which may also make you tired. This effect may be worse when taking these medicines with oxycodone. Alcohol can increase possible drowsiness, dizziness, confusion and affect your breathing. Avoid alcohol while taking oxycodone. Oxycodone will cause constipation. Make sure to take a laxative and/or a stool softener while taking oxycodone. Try to have a bowel movement at least every 2 to 3 days. If you do not have a bowel movement for 3 days or more call your prescriber or health care professional. They may recommend using an enema or suppository to help you move your bowels. Your mouth may get dry. Drinking plenty of water, chewing sugarless gum or sucking on hard candy may help to relieve dry mouth symptoms. Have regular dental checks. If you are going to have surgery tell your prescriber or health care professional that you are taking oxycodone. Rarely, oxycodone may cause you to have hallucinations (to see things that are not really there) or cause your legs or arms to "jerk" or have spasms. If you experience these effects, call your prescriber or health care professional.

What side effects may I notice from taking oxycodone?

Side effects that you should report to your prescriber or health care professional as soon as possible:
Rare or uncommon:
- breathing difficulties, wheezing
- cold, clammy skin
- seizures
- slow or fast heartbeat
- severe rash
- unusual weakness

More common:
- confusion
- lightheadedness or fainting spells
- nervousness or restlessness

Side effects that usually do not require medical attention (report to your prescriber or health care professional if they continue or are bothersome):
- itching
- clumsiness, unsteadiness
- constipation
- decrease or difficulty passing urine
- dizziness, drowsiness
- dry mouth
- flushing
- headache
- nausea, vomiting

- pinpoint pupils
- sweating

Where can I keep my medicine?

Keep out of the reach of children in a container that small children cannot open. Do not share or give this medicine to anyone else. Avoid accidental swallowing of oxycodone by someone (especially children) other than the person for whom it was prescribed as this may result in severe effects and possibly death. Store at room temperature between 15 and 30 degrees C (59 and 86 degrees F). Protect from light. Keep container tightly closed. Throw away any unused medicine after the expiration date.

O

Pancrelipase
tablets or capsules

PANCREASE®
MT 20;
56000 unit/20000
unit/44000 unit;
Capsule, Delayed
Release Pellets
Janssen Ortho, LLC

PANOKASE®;
30000 unit/8000
unit/30000 unit;
Tablet
Breckenridge Inc

What are pancrelipase tablets or capsules?

PANCRELIPASE (Cotazym®, Cotazym-S®, Creon®, Ilozyme®, Ku-Zyme® HP, Lipram®, Pancrecarb®, Pancrease®, Panokase®, Ultrase®, Viokase®, Zymase®) tablets or capsules improve your digestion of foods by replacing digestive enzymes. Digestive enzymes are substances produced by an organ called the pancreas; some health problems that cause the body to produce less of these enzymes. You may need to take pancrelipase if you have cystic fibrosis or chronic inflammation of your pancreas, have had your pancreas removed, or have had certain types of stomach or intestinal surgery. Generic pancrelipase tablets and capsules are not available.

What should my health care professional know before I take pancrelipase?

They need to know if you have any of these conditions:
- acute pancreatitis
- difficulty swallowing
- esophagitis (inflammation of the tube leading from the mouth to the stomach)
- history of bowel obstruction
- frequent surgeries of the stomach or bowel
- an unusual or allergic reaction to pancrelipase, pancreatin, pork, pork protein, other medicines, foods, dyes, or preservatives
- pregnant or trying to get pregnant
- breast-feeding

How should I take this medicine?

Take pancrelipase tablets or capsules by mouth. Follow the directions on the prescription label. Swallow the tablets or capsules with a drink of water, do not crush or chew the tablets or capsules. Take pancrelipase just before or with food. Drink plenty of water or juice after the dose. Take your doses at regular intervals. Do not take your medicine more often than directed. Some pancrelipase capsules may be opened and sprinkled on soft foods that do not require chewing such as applesauce, instant pudding or gelatin. Do not mix in milk, ice cream, or other dairy products. Pancrelipase is often prescribed for children with specific health problems that impair their digestion. Contact your pediatrician or health care professional regarding the use of this medicine in children. Special care may be needed.

What if I miss a dose?

If you miss a dose, take it as soon as you can. If it is almost time for your next dose, take only that dose. Do not take double or extra doses.

What may interact with pancrelipase?

- acarbose
- antacids containing calcium or magnesium
- iron salts
- miglitol

Tell your prescriber or health care professional about all other medicines you are taking, including non-prescription medicines, nutritional supplements, or herbal products. Also tell your prescriber or health care professional if you are a frequent user of drinks with caffeine or alcohol, if you smoke, or if you use illegal drugs. These may affect the way your medicine works. Check with your health care professional before stopping or starting any of your medicines.

What should I watch for while taking pancrelipase?

Ask your prescriber or health care professional before you change your brand of pancrelipase. Each brand of pancrelipase contains different amounts of enzymes and may not give the same results. Drink plenty of fluids while taking this medication. Follow the instructions of your health care professional regarding your diet. Do not hold the tablet or capsule in your mouth or chew it; the enzymes in the medicine may cause mouth sores. Do not take antacids containing calcium or magnesium.

What side effects may I notice from taking pancrelipase?

Side effects are rare at recommended doses.
Side effects that you should report to your prescriber or health care professional as soon as possible:
- diarrhea (severe or continuing)
- mouth irritation
- muscle aches or pains
- nausea, vomiting
- skin rash
- stomach pain
- swelling
- shortness of breath

Where can I keep my medicine?

Keep out of the reach of children in a container that small children cannot open. Store at room temperature below 25 degrees C (77 degrees F); do not freeze. Protect from moisture and do not refrigerate. Keep container tightly closed. Throw away any unused medicine after the expiration date.

Pantoprazole tablets

PROTONIX®;
40 mg; Tablet,
Delayed Release
Wyeth
Pharmaceuticals Inc

PROTONIX®;
20 mg; Tablet,
Delayed Release
Wyeth
Pharmaceuticals Inc

P

What are pantoprazole tablets?

PANTOPRAZOLE (Protonix®) prevents the production of acid in the stomach. It reduces symptoms and prevents injury to the esophagus or stomach in patients with gastroesophageal reflux disease (GERD) or ulcers. Pantoprazole is also useful in conditions that produce too much stomach acid such as Zollinger-Ellison syndrome. Generic pantoprazole tablets are not yet available.

What should my health care professional know before I take pantoprazole?

They need to know if you have any of these conditions:

- liver disease
- an unusual or allergic reaction to omeprazole, lansoprazole, pantoprazole, rabeprazole, other medicines, foods, dyes, or preservatives
- pregnant or trying to get pregnant
- breast-feeding

How should I take this medicine?

Take pantoprazole tablets by mouth. Follow the directions on the prescription label. Swallow the tablets whole with a drink of water; do not crush, break, or chew. Take your doses at regular intervals. Do not take your medicine more often than directed. Contact your pediatrician or health care professional regarding the use of this medicine in children. Special care may be needed.

What if I miss a dose?

If you miss a dose, take it as soon as you can. If it is almost time for your next dose, take only that dose. Do not take double or extra doses.

What may interact with pantoprazole?

- ampicillin
- delavirdine
- iron salts
- itraconazole
- ketoconazole

Tell your prescriber or health care professional about all other medicines you are taking, including non-prescription medicines, nutritional supplements, or herbal products. Also tell your prescriber or health care professional if you are a frequent user of drinks with caffeine or alcohol, if you smoke, or if you use illegal drugs. These may affect the way your medicine works. Check with your health care professional before stopping or starting any of your medicines.

What should I watch for while taking pantoprazole?

It can take several days of therapy with pantoprazole before your stomach pains improve. Check with your prescriber or health care professional if your condition does not improve, or if it gets worse. You can take antacids for the occasional relief of stomach pain unless your prescriber or health care professional tells you otherwise.

What side effects may I notice from taking pantoprazole?

Side effects that you should report to your prescriber or health care professional as soon as possible:

- fever or sore throat
- redness, blistering, peeling or loosening of the skin, including inside the mouth
- skin rash, itching
- unusual bleeding or bruising
- unusual weakness or tiredness
- yellowing of the eyes or skin

Side effects that usually do not require medical attention (report to your prescriber or health care professional if they continue or are bothersome):

- diarrhea
- dizziness
- dry skin
- headache
- nausea/vomiting
- stomach pain or gas
- tiredness

Where can I keep my medicine?

Keep out of the reach of children in a container that small children cannot open. Store at room temperature between 15 and 30 degrees C (59 and 86 degrees F). Protect from light and moisture. Throw away any unused medicine after the expiration date.

Papaverine extended-release capsules

PAPAVERINE;
150 mg; Capsule,
Extended Release
Mutual/United
Research
Laboratories

PARA-TIME™;
150 mg; Capsule,
Extended Release
Time Cap
Laboratories Inc

What are papaverine extended-release capsules?
PAPAVERINE (Pavabid®, Pavacot®) is a vasodilator that relaxes blood vessels and makes them wider and allows the blood to pass through them more easily. Generic papaverine extended-release capsules are available.

What should my health care professional know before I use papaverine?
They need to know if you have, or have had, any of these conditions:
- an alcohol problem
- heart disease or irregular heartbeats
- liver disease
- glaucoma
- Parkinson's disease
- any usual or allergic reaction to papaverine or other medicines, foods, dyes, or preservatives
- pregnant or trying to get pregnant
- breast-feeding

How should I use this medicine?
Take papaverine by mouth. Follow the directions on the prescription label. Swallow the capsules with a drink of water. Do not chew, open, break or crush the capsules. The capsules are formulated to release the drug slowly in your body. Take your doses at regular intervals. Do not take your medicine more often than directed.

What if I miss a dose?
If you miss a dose, take it as soon as you can. If it is almost time for your next dose, take only that dose. Do not take double or extra doses.

What may interact with papaverine?
- alcohol
- barbiturate medicines for inducing sleep or treating seizures (convulsions)
- medicines for anxiety or sleeping problems, such as diazepam or temazepam
- medicines for Parkinson's disease
- some medicines for pain (narcotic analgesics such as morphine, tramadol)

Tell your prescriber or health care professional about all other medicines you are taking, including non-prescription medicines, nutritional supplements, or herbal products. Also tell your prescriber or health care professional if you are a frequent user of drinks with caffeine or alcohol, if you smoke, or if you use illegal drugs. These may affect the way your medicine works. Check with your health care professional before stopping or starting any of your medicines.

What should I watch for while taking papaverine?
If you experience dizziness or feel faint, this may be due to the lowering of your blood pressure. Lie down immediately and raise your legs. If symptoms persist, call your prescriber or health care professional. Do not drive, use machinery, or do anything that requires mental alertness until you know how papaverine affects you.

What side effects may I notice from using papaverine?
Side effects that you should report to your prescriber or health care professional as soon as possible:
- fainting or falling spells
- fast or irregular heartbeat
- stomach pain
- yellowing or the eyes or skin

Side effects that usually do not require medical attention report to your prescriber or health care professional if they continue or are bothersome):
- nausea or vomiting, decreased appetite, diarrhea, constipation
- dizziness
- drowsiness
- headache
- sweating or flushing

Where can I keep my medicine?
Keep out of the reach of children in a container that small children cannot open. Store the bottle at room temperature at 15 and 30 degrees C (59 and 86 degrees F).

Paromomycin capsules

PAROMOMYCIN;
250 mg; Capsule
Caraco
Pharmaceutical
Laboratories Ltd

HUMATIN®;
250 mg; Capsule
Monarch
Pharmaceuticals Inc

What are paromomycin capsules?

PAROMOMYCIN (Aminosidiner®, Humatin®) is an antibiotic, which will help reduce the symptoms of confusion associated with liver disease. Paromomycin is also used for the treatment of various intestinal infections. Generic paromomycin capsules are available.

What should my health care professional know before I take paromomycin?

They need to know if you have any of these conditions:
- bowel disease, or intestinal blockage (obstruction)
- difficulty hearing
- inflammatory bowel disease
- kidney disease
- myasthenia gravis
- Parkinson's disease
- ulcerative colitis
- an unusual or allergic reaction to paromycin, other antibiotics, foods, dyes or preservatives
- pregnant or trying to get pregnant
- breast-feeding

How should I take this medicine?

Take paromomycin capsules by mouth. Follow the directions on the prescription label. Take with a full glass of water with a meal. Take your doses at regular intervals. Do not take your medicine more often than directed. Finish the full course of capsules prescribed by your prescriber or health care professional even if you feel better. Contact your pediatrician or health care professional regarding the use of this medicine in children. Special care may be needed.

What if I miss a dose?

If you miss a dose, use it as soon as you can. If it is almost time for your next dose, use only that dose. Do not use double or extra doses without advice.

What may interact with paromomycin?

- amphotericin B
- carboplatin
- cidofovir
- cisplatin
- cyclosporine
- digoxin
- foscarnet
- ganciclovir
- methotrexate
- oral contraceptives (birth control pills)
- tacrolimus
- warfarin

Tell your prescriber or health care professional about all other medicines you are taking, including non-prescription medicines, nutritional supplements, or herbal products. Also tell your prescriber or health care professional if you are a frequent user of drinks with caffeine or alcohol, if you smoke, or if you use illegal drugs. These may affect the way your medicine works. Check with your health care professional before stopping or starting any of your medicines.

What should I watch for while taking paromomycin?

Tell your prescriber or health care professional if your symptoms do not improve in a few days. You may get dizzy or have trouble keeping your balance. Until you know how paromomycin affects you, do not drive, use machinery, or do anything that requires mental alertness. Any loss or change in hearing should be reported to your physician immediately.

What side effects may I notice from taking paromomycin?

Side effects that you should report to your prescriber or health care professional as soon as possible:
- difficulty hearing
- increased thirst
- pain or difficulty passing urine
- muscle weakness
- ringing in the ears or hearing loss
- skin rash, itching
- unusual tiredness or weakness

Side effects that usually do not require medical attention (report to your prescriber or health care professional if they continue or are bothersome):
- diarrhea
- dizziness
- headache
- nausea, vomiting

Where can I keep my medicine?

Keep out of the reach of children. Store at room temperature between 5 and 30 degrees C (41 and 86 degrees F). Avoid excessive heat above 40 degrees C (104 degrees F); do not freeze. Throw away any unused medicine after the expiration date.

Paroxetine tablets or extended-release tablets

PAXIL®;
20 mg; Tablet
SmithKline Beecham
Corp

PAXIL® CR;
37.5 mg; Tablet,
Extended Release
SmithKline Beecham
Corp

This drug requires an FDA medication guide. See page xxxvii.

What are paroxetine tablets or extended-release tablets?

PAROXETINE (Paxil®, Paxil® CR™, Pexeva™) is classified as an antidepressant. It helps to improve a person's mood by treating depression. Paroxetine can also help people with anxiety problems like social anxiety, obsessive compulsive disorder, panic attacks, or post-traumatic stress. Paroxetine may also be prescribed for other purposes, like premenstrual dysphoric disorder (PMDD). Generic paroxetine tablets are available; the extended-release tablets are not yet available.

What should my health care professional know before I take paroxetine?

They need to know if you have any of these conditions:

- heart disease
- kidney disease
- liver disease
- receiving electroconvulsive therapy
- seizures (convulsions)
- suicidal thoughts or a previous suicide attempt
- an unusual or allergic reaction to paroxetine, other medicines, foods, dyes, or preservatives
- pregnant or trying to get pregnant
- breast-feeding

How should I take this medicine?

Take paroxetine tablets by mouth. Follow the directions on the prescription label. If you are taking Paxil® CR™, you should not chew, crush, or cut these tablets. You may take paroxetine with or without food. Swallow the tablets with a drink of water. Take your doses at regular intervals. Do not take your medicine more often than directed. Do not stop taking except on your prescriber's advice. Contact your pediatrician or health care professional regarding the use of this medicine in children. Special care may be needed.

What if I miss a dose?

If you miss a dose, take it as soon as you can. If it is almost time for your next dose, skip the missed dose and go back to your regular dosing schedule. Do not take double or extra doses.

What may interact with paroxetine?

Paroxetine has the potential to interact with a variety of medications, check with your healthcare professional. The following list contains some of these interactions.
Do not take paroxetine with any of the following medications:

- astemizole (Hismanal®)
- cisapride (Propulsid®)
- pimozide (Orap®)
- terfenadine (Seldane®)
- thioridazine (Mellaril®)
- medicines called MAO inhibitors-phenelzine (Nardil®), tranylcypromine (Parnate®), isocarboxazid (Marplan®), selegiline (Eldepryl®)

Paroxetine may also interact with the following medications:

- antacids (interacts with Paxil® CR™ only)
- alcohol
- amphetamine
- certain diet drugs (dexfenfluramine, fenfluramine, phentermine, sibutramine)
- certain migraine headache medicines (almotriptan, eletriptan, frovatriptan, naratriptan, rizatriptan, sumatriptan, zolmitriptan)
- cimetidine
- dextroamphetamine
- dextromethorphan
- digoxin
- fosphenytoin
- furazolidone
- linezolid
- lithium
- medicines for psychotic disturbances
- other medicines for mental depression, mania, anxiety, or difficulty sleeping
- medicines for regulating heart rhythm or blood pressure
- phenobarbital
- phenytoin
- prescription pain medications
- primidone
- procarbazine
- selegiline
- St. John's Wort, Hypericum perforatum
- theophylline
- tramadol
- warfarin

Tell your prescriber or health care professional about all other medicines you are taking, including non-prescription medicines, nutritional supplements, and herbal products. Also tell your prescriber or health care professional if you are a frequent user of drinks with caffeine or alcohol, if you smoke, or if you use illegal drugs. These may affect the way your medicine works. Check with your health care professional before stopping or starting any of your medicines.

What should I watch for while taking paroxetine?

Visit your prescriber or health care professional for regular checks on your progress. Continue to take your tablets even if you do not immediately feel better. It can take several weeks before you feel the full effect of paroxetine. Patients and their families should watch out for worsening depression or thoughts of suicide. Also watch out for sudden or severe changes in feelings such as feeling anxious, agitated, panicky, irritable, hostile, aggressive, impulsive, severely restless, overly excited and hyperactive, or not being able to sleep. If this happens, especially at the beginning of antidepressant treatment or after a change in dose, call your health care professional. If you have been taking paroxetine regularly for some time, do not suddenly stop taking it. You must gradually reduce the dose or your symptoms may get worse. Ask your prescriber or health care professional for advice. You may get drowsy or dizzy. Do not drive, use machinery, or do anything that needs mental alertness until you know how paroxetine affects you. Do not stand or sit up quickly, especially if you are an older patient. This reduces the risk of dizzy or fainting spells. Alcohol can increase or decrease the effects of paroxetine. Avoid alcoholic drinks. Do not treat yourself for coughs, colds or allergies without asking your prescriber or health care professional for advice. Some ingredients can increase possible side effects. Your mouth may get dry. Chewing sugarless gum or sucking hard candy, and drinking plenty of water will help. If you are going to have surgery, tell your prescriber or health care professional that you are taking paroxetine.

What side effects may I notice from taking paroxetine?

Side effects that you should report to your prescriber or health care professional as soon as possible:
- agitation, anxiety, or restlessness, especially in the first week of treatment or when doses are changed
- difficulty breathing
- dizziness or lightheadedness
- heart palpitations
- pain or difficulty passing urine
- painful or prolonged erection (men)
- passing urine more often than usual
- fast talking and excited feelings or actions that are out of control
- rash, itching (hives)
- tingling, pain or numbness in the hands or feet
- unusual tiredness or weakness
- vomiting

Side effects that usually do not require medical attention (report to your prescriber or health care professional if they continue or are bothersome):
- constipation or diarrhea
- difficulty sleeping
- drowsiness
- dry mouth
- headache
- increased or decreased appetite
- increased sweating
- muscle pain or weakness
- sexual difficulties (decreased sexual ability or desire)
- stomach gas, indigestion
- tremor (shaking)
- unusual taste
- weight gain or loss

Where can I keep my medicine?

Keep out of the reach of children in a container that small children cannot open. Store at room temperature between 15 and 30 degrees C (59 and 86 degrees F). Keep container tightly closed. Throw away any unused medicine after the expiration date.

Pemoline tablets or chewable tablets

CYLERT®;
37.5 mg; Tablet
Abbott Pharmaceutical
Product Division

What are pemoline tablets or chewable tablets?

PEMOLINE (Cylert®) is a stimulant. This drug is discontinued in the United States. Pemoline treated attention-deficit hyperactivity disorder (ADHD). It has been prescribed for other purposes. Federal law prohibits giving this medication to any person other than the person for whom it was prescribed. Do not share this medicine with anyone else.
NOTE: This drug is discontinued in the United States. Pemoline was removed from the U.S. drug market due to the possibility of liver toxicity. You cannot get this medication in the U.S. as of November 2005. Ask your health care provider regarding alternative medical treatments.

What should my health care professional know before I take pemoline?

They need to know if you have any of these conditions:
- regularly drink alcohol-containing beverages
- kidney disease
- liver disease
- psychotic or mental illness, depressed mood, or suicidal thoughts
- recent weight loss
- seizure disorder
- Tourette's syndrome
- an unusual or allergic reaction to pemoline, other medicines, foods, dyes, or preservatives
- pregnant or trying to get pregnant
- breast-feeding

How should I take this medicine?

Take pemoline tablets by mouth. Follow the directions on the prescription label. If you are taking the chewable tablets, they work best if you chew them before swallowing. Swallow the tablets or chewed tablets with a drink of water. Take your doses at regular intervals. Do not take your medicine more often than directed.

Remember: The prescription for pemoline is only for the person for whom it was prescribed. Never share or give your prescription to anyone else. Contact your pediatrician or health care professional regarding the use of this medicine in children. Pemoline has been prescribed for children 6 years of age and older for the treatment of attention-deficit disorder.

What if I miss a dose?

If you miss a dose, take it as soon as you can. If it is almost time for your next dose, take only that dose. Do not take double or extra doses.

What may interact with pemoline?

- amphetamine or dextroamphetamine
- bupropion
- caffeine
- lithium
- medicines for the treatment of mental conditions or depression
- medicines for the treatment of colds or weight loss
- modafinil
- seizure (convulsion) or epilepsy medicine

Tell your prescriber or health care professional about all other medicines you are taking, including non-prescription medicines, nutritional supplements, or herbal products. Also tell your prescriber or health care professional if you are a frequent user of drinks with caffeine or alcohol, if you smoke, or if you use illegal drugs. These may affect the way your medicine works. Check with your health care professional before stopping or starting any of your medicines.

What should I watch for while taking pemoline?

The use of pemoline needs careful supervision. Visit your prescriber or health care professional for regular checks on your progress. You will need to receive blood tests twice monthly to monitor the medication's effects on your liver. It may be the third or fourth week after you start therapy before you see the full effect of pemoline. Your prescriber or health care professional may want you to stop taking pemoline after a while to see if there is still a need for you to take it. Do not stop taking except on your prescriber's advice. Tell your prescriber or health care professional if you feel a need to take more tablets than prescribed, or to take them more often. Decreased appetite is a common side effect when starting this medicine. Eating small, frequent meals or snacks can help. Talk to your prescriber if you continue to have poor eating habits. Height, weight and growth of a child taking this medication will be monitored closely. Take your daily dose in the morning to prevent trouble sleeping at night. Avoid drinks that contain caffeine and try to stick to a regular bedtime every night. Do not take this medicine with other non-prescription medicines, especially cold and allergy medicines or weight-loss aides, without asking your prescriber or health care professional for advice. Pemoline can hide signs that you are tired, reduce your coordination, or make you dizzy. Do not drive, use machinery, or do anything that needs mental alertness until you know how this medicine affects you. Older adults may be more sensitive to these effects. If you are going to have surgery or other medical procedures, tell your prescriber, surgeon, or health care professional that you are taking pemoline.

What side effects may I notice from taking pemoline?

Side effects that you should report to your prescriber or health care professional as soon as possible:
Symptoms of liver trouble such as:
- dark yellow or brown urine
- severe nausea or vomiting
- unusual tiredness or weakness
- yellowing of the eyes or skin

Other rare side effects to report to your prescriber or health care professional as soon as possible:
- changes in vision or eye movements
- confusion
- depressed mood or sadness
- fever
- hallucinations (seeing and hearing things that are not really there)
- rapid heart beat or palpitations
- seizures (convulsions)
- skin rash, itching, or hives
- trembling, twitching
- uncontrollable movements, especially of face, tongue, lips, arms or legs
- unusual behavior or mood swings

Side effects that usually do not require medical attention (report to your prescriber or health care professional if they continue or are bothersome):
Less Common or Rare:
- a sense of well being
- dizziness or lightheadedness
- stomach-ache

More Common, especially in the first few weeks of treatment:
- decreased appetite or loss of appetite
- headache
- mild stomach upset
- nervousness, restlessness, or difficulty sleeping
- weight loss

Where can I keep my medicine?

Keep out of the reach of children in a container that small children cannot open. Store at room temperature below 30 degrees C (86 degrees F). Keep container tightly closed. Throw away any unused medicine after the expiration date.

Penicillamine
tablets or capsules

CUPRIMINE®;
250 mg; Capsule
Merck and Co Inc

CUPRIMINE®;
125 mg; Capsule
Merck and Co Inc

P

What are penicillamine tablets or capsules?

PENICILLAMINE (Cuprimine®, Depen®) helps to treat Wilson's disease (too much copper in the body); rheumatoid arthritis; and iron, mercury, arsenic, or lead poisoning. It can also help to prevent kidney stones. Generic penicillamine tablets and capsules are not yet available.

What should my health care professional know before I take penicillamine?

They need to know if you have any of these conditions:
- anemia or other blood disorders
- fever
- kidney disease
- liver disease
- passing blood in urine
- skin or mouth problems
- an unusual or allergic reaction to penicillamine, penicillin, other medicines, foods, dyes, or preservatives
- pregnant or trying to get pregnant
- breast-feeding

How should I take this medicine?

Take penicillamine tablets or capsules by mouth. Follow the directions on the prescription label. Swallow the tablets or capsules with a drink of water. Take penicillamine on an empty stomach, at least 1 hour before or 2 hours after food. Do not take your medicine more often than directed. Finish the full course prescribed by your prescriber or health care professional even if the tablets make you feel unwell. Do not stop taking except on your prescriber's advice. Contact your pediatrician or health care professional regarding the use of this medicine in children. Special care may be needed.

What if I miss a dose?

If you miss a dose, take it as soon as you can. If it is almost time for your next dose, take only that dose. Do not take double or extra doses.

What may interact with penicillamine?

- aluminum salts, like aluminum hydroxide
- antacids
- gold compounds, often used for arthritis
- iron supplements
- magnesium hydroxide (Milk of Magnesia)
- magnesium supplements
- medicines for cancer chemotherapy
- medicines for prevention or treatment of malaria
- medicines that suppress your immune response
- pyridoxine (vitamin B_6)

Tell your prescriber or health care professional about all other medicines you are taking, including non-prescription medicines, nutritional supplements, or herbal products. Also tell your prescriber or health care professional if you are a frequent user of drinks with caffeine or alcohol, if you smoke, or if you use illegal drugs. These may affect the way your medicine works. Check with your health care professional before stopping or starting any of your medicines.

What should I watch for while taking penicillamine?

Visit your prescriber or health care professional at regular intervals to check on your progress. Penicillamine takes some time to work. If you are treating rheumatoid arthritis or Wilson's disease, you may not notice an improvement in your condition for 2 or 3 months. Take your doses regularly and do not stop taking except on your prescriber's advice. If you are taking penicillamine for Wilson's disease or metal poisoning, you must follow any dietary restrictions given by your prescriber or health care professional. Foods you may need to avoid are those that contain copper (such as chocolate, nuts, liver, and broccoli). If you are taking penicillamine to prevent kidney stones you need to drink plenty of water. Drink 2 full glasses of water at bedtime and a further 2 full glasses of water during the night. Penicillamine makes your body need more pyridoxine (vitamin B_6). Check with your prescriber or health care professional to see if you need to take extra vitamin B_6. Antacids and iron preparations can stop penicillamine working properly. Check before taking vitamin and mineral supplements; they often contain iron. Avoid taking antacids. If you are going to have surgery, tell your prescriber or health care professional that you are taking penicillamine.

What side effects may I notice from taking penicillamine?

Side effects that you should report to your prescriber or health care professional as soon as possible:
- black, tarry stools
- blood in urine, or cloudy urine
- cough or hoarseness
- difficulty breathing, wheezing
- eye pain or vision problems, red or irritated eyes
- fever, chills, sore throat
- joint pain
- lower back or side pain
- mouth ulcers, sores, or white spots on the lips or in the mouth
- pain or difficulty passing urine
- ringing or buzzing in ears
- skin rash, hives or blisters, itching

- swelling of face, feet, or lower legs
- swollen or painful glands
- unusual bleeding or bruising, pinpoint red spots on skin
- unusual tiredness or weakness
- yellowing of your skin or eyes

Side effects that usually do not require medical attention (report to your prescriber or health care professional if they continue or are bothersome):
- anxiety or nervousness
- changes in taste

- diarrhea
- loss of appetite
- nausea, vomiting
- stomach pain

Where can I keep my medicine?

Keep out of the reach of children in a container that small children cannot open. Store at room temperature between 15 and 30 degrees C (59 and 86 degrees F). Protect from moisture. Throw away any unused medicine after the expiration date.

Penicillin V tablets

VEETIDS®; 500 mg; Tablet Sandoz Pharmaceuticals

PENICILLIN-VK; 250 mg (400,000 units); Tablet Geneva

What are penicillin V tablets?

PENICILLIN V (Pen-Vee® K, V-Cillin K®, Veetids®) is a penicillin antibiotic. Penicillin V kills certain bacteria that cause infection, or stops their growth. It treats many kinds of infections including those of the skin, brain, heart, respiratory tract, sinuses, and ears. Generic penicillin V tablets are available.

What should my health care professional know before I take penicillin V?

They need to know if you have any of these conditions:
- asthma
- eczema
- kidney disease
- stomach problems (especially colitis)
- an unusual or allergic reaction to penicillins, cephalosporin antibiotics, imipenem, foods, dyes, or preservatives
- breast-feeding

How should I take this medicine?

Take penicillin V tablets by mouth. Follow the directions on the prescription label. Take with a full glass of water; try to take while in a sitting or upright position. It is best to take penicillin V 1 to 2 hours before or at least 2 hours after eating; taking it with food can make it less effective. If penicillin V upsets your stomach you can take it with food. If possible, "bedtime" doses should be taken at least 10 minutes before actually reclining. Do not take your medicine more often than directed. Finish the full course prescribed by your prescriber or health care professional even if you think your condition is better. Do not stop taking except on your prescriber's advice.

What if I miss a dose?

If you miss a dose, take it as soon as you can. If it is almost time for your next dose, take only that dose. Do not take double or extra doses. There should be an interval of at least 4 to 6 hours between doses.

What may interact with penicillin V?

- certain antibiotics given by injection
- female hormones, including contraceptive or birth control pills
- probenecid

Tell your prescriber or health care professional about all other medicines you are taking, including non-prescription medicines, nutritional supplements, or herbal products. Also tell your prescriber or health care professional if you are a frequent user of drinks with caffeine or alcohol, if you smoke, or if you use illegal drugs. These may affect the way your medicine works. Check with your health care professional before stopping or starting any of your medicines.

What should I watch for while taking penicillin V?

Tell your prescriber or health care professional if your symptoms do not improve in 2 or 3 days. If you get severe or watery diarrhea, do not treat yourself. Call your prescriber or health care professional for advice. If you get a skin rash, do not treat yourself. Call your prescriber or health care professional for advice. If you are diabetic and taking large doses of penicillin, you may get a false-positive result for sugar in your urine. Check with your prescriber or health care professional before you change your diet or the dose of your diabetic medicine. Birth control pills (contraceptive pills) may not work properly while you are taking this medicine. Use an extra method of birth control for at least one month.

What side effects may I notice from taking penicillin V?

Side effects that you should report to your prescriber or health care professional as soon as possible:
- dark yellow or brown urine
- difficulty breathing, wheezing
- fever or chills, sore throat
- headache

- less frequent passing of urine
- pain on swallowing
- red spots on the skin
- redness, blistering, peeling or loosening of the skin, including inside the mouth
- seizures (convulsions)
- severe or watery diarrhea
- skin rash, itching
- swelling of face and neck
- unusual bleeding or bruising
- unusual weakness or tiredness

Side effects that usually do not require medical atten-

tion (report to your prescriber or health care professional if they continue or are bothersome):

- diarrhea
- nausea, vomiting
- sore mouth

Where can I keep my medicine?

Keep out of the reach of children in a container that small children cannot open. Store at room temperature between 15 and 30 degrees C (59 and 86 degrees F). Keep container tightly closed. Throw away any unused medicine after the expiration date.

Pentazocine tablets

TALWIN® NX;
50 mg; Tablet
Sanofi-Synthelabo
Inc

PENTAZOCINE;
0.5 mg/50 mg;
Tablet
Watson
Pharmaceuticals Inc

What are pentazocine tablets?

PENTAZOCINE (Talwin® Nx) relieves moderate to severe pain. Pentazocine tablets also contain naloxone, which is included to deter the misuse of this medicine. Naloxone does not affect how pentazocine tablets work. Do not share this medicine with anyone else. Federal law prohibits the transfer of pentazocine to any person other than the patient for whom it was prescribed. Generic pentazocine tablets are available.

What should my health care professional know before I take pentazocine?

They need to know if you have any of these conditions:

- if you frequently drink alcohol-containing beverages
- constipation
- head injury
- heart disease
- intestinal disease, such as inflammatory bowel disease or ulcerative colitis
- liver disease
- lung disease, such as asthma or COPD
- kidney disease
- seizures
- an unusual or allergic reaction to pentazocine, naloxone, codeine, morphine, other medicines, foods, dyes, or preservatives
- pregnant or trying to get pregnant
- breast-feeding

How should I take this medicine?

Take pentazocine tablets by mouth. Follow the directions on the prescription label. Swallow the tablets with a drink of water. If pentazocine upsets your stomach, you can take it with food or milk. Contact your pediatrician or health care professional regarding the use of this medicine in children. Special care may be needed. Do not share this medicine with any one.

What if I miss a dose?

If you miss a dose, take it as soon as you can. If it is almost time for your next dose, take only that dose. Do not take double or extra doses.

What may interact with pentazocine?

- medicines called MAO inhibitors—examples: phenelzine (Nardil®), tranylcypromine (Parnate®), isocarboxazid (Marplan®)
- medicines called SSRIs—examples: fluoxetine (Prozac®), paroxetine (Paxil®), sertraline (Zoloft®), and others

Because pentazocine can cause drowsiness, other medicines that also cause drowsiness may increase this effect of pentazocine. Some medicines that cause drowsiness are:

- alcohol and alcohol-containing medicines
- barbiturates such as phenobarbital
- certain antidepressants or tranquilizers
- muscle relaxants
- certain antihistamines used in cold medicines

Ask your prescriber or health care professional about other medicines that may increase the effect of pentazocine.

Tell your prescriber or health care professional about all other medicines that you are taking, including nonprescription medicines, nutritional supplements, or herbal products. Also, tell your prescriber or health care professional if you are a frequent user of drinks with caffeine or alcohol, if you smoke, or if you use illegal drugs. These may affect the way your medicine works. Check with your health care professional before stopping or starting any of your medicines.

What should I watch for while taking pentazocine?

Tell your prescriber or health care professional if your pain does not go away, if it gets worse, or if you have new or different type of pain. Use exactly as directed by your prescriber or health care professional. If you are taking pentazocine on a regular basis, do not suddenly stop taking it. Your body becomes used to the pentazocine, and when you suddenly stop taking it, you may develop a severe reaction. This DOES NOT mean you are "addicted" to pentazocine. Addiction is a behavior related to getting and using a drug for a non-medical reason. If you have pain, you have a medical reason to take pain medicine such as pentazocine to control your pain. You may get drowsy or dizzy when you first start taking pentazocine. Do not drive, use machinery, or do anything that needs mental alertness until you know how pentazocine affects you. Be careful taking other medicines that may also make you tired. This effect may be worse when taking these medicines with pentazocine. Alcohol can increase possible drowsiness, dizziness, confusion, and affect your breathing. Avoid alcohol while taking pentazocine. If you are going to have surgery, tell your prescriber or health care professional that you are taking pentazocine.

What side effects may I notice from taking pentazocine?

Side effects that you should report to your prescriber or health care professional as soon as possible:
Rare or uncommon:
- difficulty passing urine
- slow or fast heartbeat
- seizures
- severe rash
- unusual weakness

More common:
- confusion
- feeling disoriented

- hallucinations (seeing or hearing things that are not really there)
- lightheadedness or fainting spells
- nervousness or restlessness

Side effects that usually do not require medical attention (report to your prescriber or health care professional if they continue or are bothersome):
- clumsiness, unsteadiness
- constipation
- decrease or difficulty passing urine
- dizziness, drowsiness
- dry mouth
- flushing
- headache
- itching
- lightheadedness
- nausea/vomiting
- sweating

Where can I keep my medicine?

Keep out of the reach of children in a container that small children cannot open. Do not share or give this medicine to anyone else. Avoid accidental swallowing of pentazocine by someone (especially children) other than the person for whom it was prescribed as this may result in severe effects and possibly death. Store at room temperature between 15 and 30 degrees C (59 and 86 degrees F). Protect from light. Throw away any unused medicine after the expiration date.

Pentosan capsules

ELMIRON®;
100 mg; Capsule
Johnson and Johnson/Merck

What are pentosan capsules?

PENTOSAN (Elmiron®) is used to treat the pain or discomfort of a bladder disorder called interstitial cystitis. Pentosan is also a very weak blood thinner. Generic pentosan capsules are not yet available.

What should my health care professional know before I take pentosan?

They need to know if you have any of these conditions:
- bleeding disorders or blood problems
- high blood pressure
- liver disease
- previous stroke
- stomach, intestinal or bowel disease
- stomach or intestinal ulcers
- an unusual or allergic reaction to pentosan, other medicines, foods, dyes, or preservatives
- pregnant or trying to get pregnant
- breast-feeding

How should I take this medicine?

Take pentosan capsules by mouth on an empty stomach, 1 hour before or 2 hours after meals. Follow the directions on the prescription label. Swallow the capsules with a drink of water. Do not take your medicine more often than directed.

What if I miss a dose?

If you miss a dose, take it as soon as you can. If it is almost time for your next dose, take only that dose. Do not take double or extra doses.

What may interact with pentosan?

- agents that dissolve blood clots
- aspirin, especially in higher doses
- blood thinners, such as warafin
- clopidogrel
- dipyridamole
- fish oil (omega-3 fatty acids) supplements
- herbal supplements, like garlic, ginger, ginkgo biloba, or horse chestnut
- non-steroidal anti-inflammatory drugs (NSAIDs) such as ibuprofen
- ticlopidine

Tell your prescriber or health care professional about all other medicines you are taking, including non-prescription medicines. Tell your prescriber or health care professional if you are a frequent user of caffeine or alcohol, if you smoke, or if you use illegal drugs. These may affect the way your medicine works. Check with your health care professional before stopping or starting any of your medicines.

What should I watch for while taking pentosan?

Pentosan is a very weak blood thinner. Watch for any signs of blood in your urine or stools or for any unusual bruising or bleeding. If you take any other medications that may thin the blood (see drug interactions), be especially watchful. You may wish to check with your health care professional prior to taking any non-prescription (OTC) products containing aspirin. Read package labels carefully. Tell your prescriber or health care professional that you are taking pentosan if you are going to have a medical procedure or surgery.

What side effects may I notice from taking pentosan?

Side effects that you should report to your prescriber or health care professional as soon as possible:

Rare or uncommon:
- unusual bleeding
- nosebleeds
- coughing up blood
- blood in your urine or stools
- rash

More frequent:
- bruising
- diarrhea
- abdominal pain

Side effects that usually do not require medical attention (report to your prescriber or health care professional if they continue or are bothersome):
- hair loss
- nausea
- headache

Where can I keep my medicine?

Keep out of the reach of children and in a container that small children cannot open. Store your medicine at room temperature between 15 and 30 degrees C (59 and 86 degrees F). Keep your medicine container tightly closed and protect it from light.

Pentoxifylline extended-release tablets	TRENTAL®; 400 mg; Tablet, Extended Release Hoechst Roussel Pharmaceuticals Div		PENTOXIL™; 400 mg; Tablet, Extended Release Upsher-Smith Laboratories Inc	

What are pentoxifylline extended-release tablets?

PENTOXIFYLLINE (Pentoxil™, Trental®) improves blood flow by making the red blood cells more flexible and by thinning the blood. Pentoxifylline helps to decrease the pain, discomfort, or cramps you can get from having poor circulation in your leg veins. Generic pentoxifylline extended-release tablets are available.

What should my health care professional know before I take pentoxifylline?

They need to know if you have any of these conditions:
- kidney disease
- liver disease
- an unusual or allergic reaction to pentoxifylline, caffeine, theophylline, other medicines, foods, dyes, or preservatives
- pregnant or trying to get pregnant
- breast-feeding

How should I take this medicine?

Take pentoxifylline tablets by mouth. Follow the directions on the prescription label. Swallow the tablets whole with a drink of water; do not crush or chew. You can take pentoxifylline with food or antacids if it upsets your stomach. Take your doses at regular intervals. Do not take your medicine more often than directed. Contact your pediatrician or health care professional regarding the use of this medicine in children.

Special care may be needed. Elderly patients over 65 years old need smaller doses to reduce possible side effects.

What if I miss a dose?

If you miss a dose, take it as soon as you can. If it is almost time for your next dose, take only that dose. Do not take double or extra doses.

What may interact with pentoxifylline?

- cimetidine
- ciprofloxacin
- some herbal supplements, like garlic, ginger or ginkgo biloba
- theophylline
- warfarin

Tell your prescriber or health care professional about all other medicines you are taking, including non-prescription medicines, nutritional supplements, or herbal products. Also tell your prescriber or health care professional if you are a frequent user of drinks with caffeine or alcohol, if you smoke, or if you use illegal drugs. These may affect the way your medicine works. Check with your health care professional before stopping or starting any of your medicines.

What should I watch for while taking pentoxifylline?

Visit your prescriber or health care professional for regular checks on your progress. You may feel some benefit after 2 to 4 weeks of treatment, but it can take up to 8 weeks before you get the full benefit. Do not stop taking pentoxifylline except on your prescriber's advice. Smoking tobacco or marijuana can make your condition worse by further narrowing the blood vessels; do not smoke.

What side effects may I notice from taking pentoxifylline?

Side effects that you should report to your prescriber or health care professional as soon as possible:
- agitation
- chest pain, fast or irregular heartbeat (palpitations)
- drowsiness
- flushing
- seizures (convulsions)

Side effects that usually do not require medical attention (report to your prescriber or health care professional if they continue or are bothersome):
- dizziness
- headache
- indigestion
- nausea, vomiting

Where can I keep my medicine?

Keep out of the reach of children in a container that small children cannot open. Store at room temperature between 15 and 30 degrees C (59 and 86 degrees F). Protect from light. Keep container tightly closed. Throw away any unused medicine after the expiration date.

Pergolide tablets

PERMAX®;
0.25 mg; Tablet
Elan
Pharmaceuticals Inc

PERMAX®;
1 mg; Tablet
Elan
Pharmaceuticals Inc

What are pergolide tablets?

PERGOLIDE (Permax®) can help treat Parkinson's disease. Pergolide helps to improve muscle control and movement difficulties. Pergolide will not cure Parkinson's disease, but will help to control the symptoms. Pergolide tablets are taken together with other tablets that control parkinsonian symptoms. Generic pergolide tablets are available.

What should my health care professional know before I take pergolide?

They need to know if you have any of these conditions:
- dizzy or fainting spells
- history of heart disease or heart valve disease
- low blood pressure
- an unusual or allergic reaction to pergolide, ergot alkaloids (like ergonovine or ergotamine), other medicines, foods, dyes, or preservatives
- pregnant or trying to get pregnant
- breast-feeding

How should I take this medicine?

Take pergolide tablets by mouth. Follow the directions on the prescription label. Swallow the tablets with a drink of water. Take your doses at regular intervals. Do not take your medicine more often than directed. Contact your pediatrician or health care professional regarding the use of this medicine in children. Special care may be needed.

What if I miss a dose?

If you miss a dose, take it as soon as you can. If it is almost time for your next dose, take only that dose. Do not take double or extra doses.

What may interact with pergolide?

- metoclopramide
- medicines for mental problems and psychotic disturbances

Tell your prescriber or health care professional about all other medicines you are taking, including non-prescription medicines, nutritional supplements, or herbal products. Also tell your prescriber or health care professional if you are a frequent user of drinks with caffeine or alcohol, if you smoke, or if you use illegal drugs. These may affect the way your medicine works. Check with your health care professional before stopping or starting any of your medicines.

What should I watch for while taking pergolide?

Visit your prescriber or health care professional for regular checks on your progress. It may be several weeks or months before you feel the full effect of pergolide. Continue to take your medicine on a regular schedule and do not stop taking except on your prescriber's advice. You may get dizzy or have difficulty controlling your movements. Do not drive, use machinery, or do anything that needs mental alertness until you know how pergolide affects you. Pergolide may cause abrupt drowsiness or sleep. If you experience abrupt sleepiness without warning, do not drive or use machinery while taking pergolide, and do not perform other activities where falling asleep could result in an injury. If you experience sudden sleep without warning, contact your health care professional immediately. Do not stand or sit up quickly, especially if you are an older patient. This reduces the risk of dizzy or fainting spells. Alcohol can increase possible dizziness; avoid alcoholic drinks. Pergolide may make your mouth dry. Chewing sugarless gum, sucking hard candy and drinking plenty of water may help. Visit your dentist regularly. If you are going to have surgery, tell your prescriber or health care professional that you are taking pergolide.

What side effects may I notice from taking pergolide?

Side effects that you should report to your prescriber or health care professional as soon as possible:

Rare or uncommon:
- abrupt drowsiness or falling asleep without warning
- double vision, or other vision problems
- chest pain or abnormal heart beats (fast, slow or irregular)
- difficulty breathing or catching your breath
- fainting spells
- palpitations
- severe weakness
- lower back pain, or chest or neck pain

More common:
- anxiety, restlessness
- confusion
- hallucinations
- mental changes

- uncontrollable movements of the arms, face, hands, head, mouth, shoulders, or upper body
- dizziness

Side effects that usually do not require medical attention (report to your prescriber or health care professional if they continue or are bothersome):
- headache
- constipation or diarrhea
- difficulty sleeping
- drowsiness
- flu-like symptoms (fever/chills/muscle aches)
- loss of appetite
- nausea/vomiting
- runny or stuffy nose
- stomach pain
- mild weakness
- weight change

Where can I keep my medicine?

Keep out of the reach of children in a container that small children cannot open. Store at room temperature between 15 and 30 degrees C (59 and 86 degrees F). Keep container tightly closed. Throw away any unused medicine after the expiration date.

Perindopril tablets

ACEON®;
4 mg; Tablet
Solvay
Pharmaceuticals Inc

ACEON®;
8 mg; Tablet
Solvay
Pharmaceuticals Inc

What are perindopril tablets?

PERINDOPRIL (Aceon®) is a medication which lowers blood pressure by relaxing blood vessels; it is not a cure. High blood pressure levels can damage your kidneys, and may lead to a stroke or heart failure. Generic perindopril tablets are not yet available.

What should my health care professional know before I take perindopril?

They need to know if you have any of these conditions:
- autoimmune disease (such as lupus), or suppressed immune function
- previous swelling of the tongue, face, or lips with difficulty breathing, difficulty swallowing, hoarseness, or tightening of the throat (angioedema)
- bone marrow disease
- diabetes
- heart or blood vessel disease
- low blood pressure
- kidney disease
- if you are on a special diet, such as a low-salt diet
- an unusual or allergic reaction to perindopril, other ACE inhibitors, foods, dyes, or preservatives
- pregnant or trying to get pregnant
- breast-feeding

How should I take this medicine?

Take perindopril tablets by mouth one hour before meals. Follow the directions on the prescription label. Swallow the tablets with a drink of water. Take your doses at regular intervals. Do not take your medicine more often than directed. Do not stop taking perindopril except on your prescriber's advice. Contact your pediatrician or health care professional regarding the use of this medicine in children. Special care may be needed.

What if I miss a dose?

If you miss a dose, take it as soon as you can. If it is almost time for your next dose, take only that dose. Do not take double or extra doses. If you take only one dose a day and forget to take it that day, do not take a double dose the next day.

What may interact with perindopril?

- anti-inflammatory drugs (NSAIDs, such as ibuprofen)
- hawthorn
- heparin
- lithium
- medicines for high blood pressure
- potassium salts
- water pills

Tell your prescriber or health care professional about all other medicines you are taking, including non-prescription medicines, nutritional supplements, or herbal products. Also tell your prescriber or health care professional if you are a frequent user of drinks with caffeine or alcohol, if you smoke, or if you use illegal drugs. These may affect the way your medicine works. Check

with your health care professional before stopping or starting any of your medicines.

What should I watch for while taking perindopril?

Visit your prescriber or health care professional for regular checks on your progress. Check your blood pressure regularly while you are taking perindopril. Ask your prescriber or health care professional what your blood pressure should be and when you should contact him or her. Stop taking perindopril and call your prescriber or health care professional if you have difficulty breathing, or notice any swelling of the lips, tongue or face. Check with your prescriber or health care professional if you get an attack of severe diarrhea, nausea and vomiting, or if you sweat a lot. The loss of body fluid can make it dangerous to take perindopril. You may get dizzy. Do not drive, use machinery, or do anything that needs mental alertness until you know how perindopril affects you. To avoid dizzy or fainting spells, do not stand or sit up quickly, especially if you are an older person. Alcohol can make you more dizzy. Avoid alcoholic drinks. If you are going to have surgery, tell your prescriber or health care professional that you are taking perindopril. Avoid salt substitutes or other foods or substances high in potassium salts. Do not treat yourself for cough, sore throat, colds, or pain while you are using perindopril without asking your prescriber or health care professional for advice.

What side effects may I notice from taking perindopril?

Side effects that you should report to your prescriber or health care professional as soon as possible:
- decreased amount of urine passed
- difficulty breathing, or difficulty swallowing
- dizziness, lightheadedness or fainting spells
- fast or uneven heart beat, palpitations, or chest pain
- fever or chills
- numbness or tingling in your fingers or toes
- skin rash, itching
- swelling of your face, lips, or tongue
- sore throat

Side effects that usually do not require medical attention (report to your prescriber or health care professional if they continue or are bothersome):
- cough
- headache
- tiredness

Where can I keep my medicine?

Keep out of the reach of children in a container that small children cannot open. Store at room temperature between 20 and 25 degrees C (68 and 77 degrees F). Protect from moisture. Keep container tightly closed. Throw away any unused medicine after the expiration date.

Perphenazine tablets

PERPHENAZINE; 4 mg; Tablet Ivax Pharmaceuticals Inc

PERPHENAZINE; 4 mg; Tablet Sandoz Pharmaceuticals

What are perphenazine tablets?

PERPHENAZINE (Trilafon®) helps to treat disordered thoughts and some other emotional, nervous, and mental problems. It also is used to treat severe nausea and vomiting in adults. Generic perphenazine tablets are available.

What should my health care professional know before I take perphenazine?

They need to know if you have any of these conditions:
- blood disorders or disease
- difficulty passing urine
- glaucoma
- head injury
- heart or liver disease
- low blood level of calcium
- Parkinson's disease
- prostate trouble
- Reye's syndrome
- seizures (convulsions)
- stomach problems or peptic ulcer
- an unusual or allergic reaction to perphenazine, other medicines, foods, dyes, or preservatives
- pregnant or trying to get pregnant
- breast-feeding

How should I take this medicine?

Take perphenazine tablets by mouth. Follow the directions on the prescription label. Swallow the tablets with a drink of water. Take perphenazine with food or milk if it upsets your stomach. Take your doses at regular intervals. Do not take your medicine more often than directed. Contact your pediatrician or health care professional regarding the use of this medicine in children. Special care may be needed. Elderly patients over age 65 years may have a stronger reaction to this medicine and need smaller doses.

What if I miss a dose?

If you miss a dose, take it as soon as you can. If it is almost time for your next dose, take only that dose. Try to take your doses at the same time each day. Do not take double or extra doses.

What may interact with perphenazine?

- alcohol
- antacids
- some antibiotics
- antidiarrheal medications
- atropine

- bromocriptine
- cimetidine
- cisapride
- dextroamphetamine or amphetamine
- dronabinol or marijuana
- haloperidol or droperidol
- levodopa
- lithium
- medicines for an over-active thyroid gland
- medicines for colds and flu
- medicines for hay fever and other allergies
- medicines for mental depression
- medicines for movement abnormalities as in Parkinson's disease
- medicines to prevent or treat malaria
- medications for treating seizures (convulsions)
- medicines for pain or for use as muscle relaxants, including tramadol
- medicines to treat urine or bladder incontinence
- metoclopramide
- pimozide
- probucol
- some medications for high blood pressure or heart problems
- some weight loss medications

Tell your prescriber or health care professional about all other medicines you are taking, including non-prescription medicines, nutritional supplements, or herbal products. Also tell your prescriber or health care professional if you are a frequent user of drinks with caffeine or alcohol, if you smoke, or if you use illegal drugs. These may affect the way your medicine works. Check with your health care professional before stopping or starting any of your medicines.

What should I watch for while taking perphenazine?

Visit your prescriber or health care professional for regular checks on your progress. Do not stop taking perphenazine suddenly; this can cause nausea, vomiting, and dizziness. Ask your prescriber or health care professional for advice if you are to stop taking this medicine. You may get drowsy, dizzy, or have blurred vision. Do not drive, use machinery, or do anything that needs mental alertness until you know how perphenazine affects you. Do not stand or sit up quickly, especially if you are an older patient. This reduces the risk of dizzy or fainting spells. Alcohol can increase possible dizziness or drowsiness. Avoid alcoholic drinks. Perphenazine can reduce the response of your body to heat or cold. Try not to get overheated. Avoid temperature extremes, such as saunas, hot tubs, or very hot or cold baths or showers. Dress warmly in cold weather. Perphenazine can make your skin more sensitive to sun or ultraviolet light. Keep out of the sun, or wear protective clothing outdoors and use a sunscreen (at least SPF 15). Do not use sun lamps or sun tanning beds or booths. Wear sunglasses to protect your eyes. Perphenazine may make your mouth dry, chewing sugarless gum or sucking hard candy and drinking plenty of water will help. Do not treat yourself for coughs, colds, sore throat, indigestion, diarrhea, or allergies. Ask your prescriber or health care professional for advice. If you are going to have surgery or will need a procedure that uses contrast agents, tell your prescriber or health care professional that you are taking this medicine.

What side effects may I notice from taking perphenazine?

Side effects that you should report to your prescriber or health care professional as soon as possible:
- blurred vision
- breast enlargement in men or women
- breast milk in women who are not breast-feeding
- chest pain, fast or irregular heartbeat
- confusion, restlessness
- dark yellow or brown urine
- difficulty breathing or swallowing
- dizziness or fainting spells
- drooling, shaking, movement difficulty (shuffling walk) or rigidity
- fever, chills, sore throat
- hot, dry skin, unable to sweat
- involuntary or uncontrollable movements of the eyes, mouth, head, arms, and legs
- menstrual changes
- puffing cheeks, smacking lips, or worm-like movements of the tongue
- seizures (convulsions)
- slurred speech
- stomach area pain
- sweating
- unusual weakness or tiredness
- unusual bleeding or bruising
- yellowing of skin or eyes

Side effects that usually do not require medical attention (report to your prescriber or health care professional if they continue or are bothersome):
- constipation
- difficulty passing urine
- difficulty sleeping, agitation or restlessness
- drowsiness
- dry mouth
- headache
- increased sensitivity to the sun or ultraviolet light
- sexual difficulties (impotence in men; increased sexual desire in women)
- skin rash, or itching
- stuffy nose
- weight gain

Where can I keep my medicine?

Keep out of the reach of children in a container that small children cannot open. Store at room temperature between 2 and 25 degrees C (36 and 77 degrees F). Throw away any unused medicine after the expiration date.

Perphenazine; Amitriptyline tablets

PERPHENAZINE; AMITRIPTYLINE; 25 mg/2 mg; Tablet Watson Pharmaceuticals Inc

PERPHENAZINE; AMITRIPTYLINE; 2 mg/ 10 mg; Tablet Geneva

What are perphenazine; amitriptyline tablets?

PERPHENAZINE; AMITRIPTYLINE (Triavil®, Etrafon®, Etrafon Forte®) is used to treat depression that may be accompanied by anxiety or agitation. Your prescriber or health care professional may prescribe amitriptyline for other conditions, such as relief from pain. Generic perphenazine; amitriptyline tablets are available.

What should my health care professional know before I take perphenazine; amitriptyline?

They need to know if you have any of these conditions:
- an alcohol problem
- asthma, difficulty breathing
- blood disorders or disease
- diabetes
- difficulty passing urine, prostate trouble
- glaucoma
- having intramuscular injections
- head injury
- heart disease or previous heart attack
- liver disease
- low blood level of calcium
- overactive thyroid
- Parkinson's disease
- Reye's syndrome
- schizophrenia
- seizures (convulsions)
- stomach disease or peptic ulcers
- an unusual or allergic reaction to perphenazine, amitriptyline, other medicines, foods, dyes, or preservatives
- pregnant or trying to get pregnant
- breast-feeding

How should I take this medicine?

Take perphenazine; amitriptyline tablets by mouth. Follow the directions on the prescription label. Swallow the tablets with a drink of water. Take this drug with food or milk if it upsets your stomach. Take your doses at regular intervals. Do not take your medicine more often than directed. Do not stop taking except on your prescriber's advice. Contact your pediatrician or health care professional regarding the use of this medicine in children. Special care may be needed. Adolescents and elderly patients over 65 years old may have a stronger reaction to this medicine and may need smaller doses.

What if I miss a dose?

If it is almost time for your next dose, take only that dose. Do not take double or extra doses.

What may interact with perphenazine; amitriptyline?

Perphenazine; amitriptyline can interact with many other medicines. Some interactions can be very important. Make sure your prescriber or health care professional knows about all other medicines you are taking. Many important interactions are listed below:

Do not take perphenazine; amitriptyline with any of the following medications:

- astemizole (Hismanal®)
- cisapride (Propulsid®)
- probucol
- terfenadine (Seldane®)
- medicines called MAO inhibitors-phenelzine (Nardil®), tranylcypromine (Parnate®), isocarboxazid (Marplan®), selegiline (Eldepryl®)
- other medicines for mental depression (may be duplicate therapies or cause additive side effects)
- other medicines for mental or mood problems and psychotic disturbances (may be duplicate therapies or cause additive side effects)

Perphenazine; amitriptyline also interact with any of the following:

- alcohol
- antacids
- atropine and related drugs like hyoscyamine, scopolamine, tolterodine and others
- barbiturate medicines for inducing sleep or treating seizures (convulsions), such as phenobarbital
- blood thinners, such as warfarin
- bromocriptine
- bupropion
- cimetidine
- clonidine
- cocaine
- delavirdine
- diphenoxylate
- disulfiram
- donepezil
- drugs for treating HIV infection
- female hormones, including contraceptive or birth control pills and estrogen
- galantamine
- herbs and dietary supplements like ephedra (Ma huang), kava kava, SAM-e, St. John's wort, valerian, or others
- imatinib, STI-571
- kaolin; pectin
- labetalol
- levodopa and other medicines for movement problems like Parkinson's disease
- lithium
- medicines for anxiety or sleeping problems

- medicines for colds, flu and breathing difficulties, like pseudoephedrine
- medicines for hay fever or allergies (antihistamines)
- medicines for weight loss or appetite control
- medicines used to regulate abnormal heartbeat or to treat other heart conditions (examples: amiodarone, bepridil, disopyramide, dofetilide, flecainide, ibutilide, mibefradil, procainamide, quinidine, and others)
- metoclopramide
- muscle relaxants, like cyclobenzaprine
- prescription pain medications like morphine, codeine, tramadol and others
- procarbazine
- seizure (convulsion) or epilepsy medicine such as carbamazepine or phenytoin
- stimulants like dexmethylphenidate or methylphenidate
- some antibiotics (examples: erythromycin, gatifloxacin, levofloxacin, linezolid, moxifloxacin, sotalol, sparfloxacin)
- tacrine
- thyroid hormones such as levothyroxine

Tell your prescriber or health care professional about all other medicines you are taking, including non-prescription medicines, nutritional supplements, or herbal products. Also tell your prescriber or health care professional if you are a frequent user of drinks with caffeine or alcohol, if you smoke, or if you use illegal drugs. These may affect the way your medicine works. Check with your health care professional before stopping or starting any of your medicines.

What should I watch for while taking perphenazine; amitriptyline?

Visit your prescriber or health care professional for regular checks on your progress. It may take several weeks before you feel the full effect of this medicine. If you have been taking this medicine regularly for some time, do not suddenly stop taking it. You must gradually reduce the dose or you may get severe side effects. Ask your prescriber or health care professional for advice. Even after you stop taking perphenazine; amitriptyline it can still affect your body for several days. You may get drowsy or dizzy. Do not drive, use machinery, or do anything that needs mental alertness until you know how this drug affects you. Do not stand or sit up quickly, especially if you are an older patient. This reduces the risk of dizzy or fainting spells. Alcohol may increase dizziness and drowsiness. Avoid alcoholic drinks. Do not treat yourself for coughs, colds or allergies without asking your prescriber or health care professional for advice. Some ingredients can increase possible side effects. Your mouth may get dry. Chewing sugarless gum or sucking hard candy, and drinking plenty of water will help. This medicine may cause dry eyes and blurred vision. If you wear contact lenses you may feel some discomfort. Lubricating drops may help. See your ophthalmologist if the problem does not go away or is severe. This medicine may make your skin more sensitive to the sun. Keep out of the sun, or wear protective clothing outdoors and use a sunscreen. Do not use sun lamps or sun tanning beds or booths. If you are diabetic, check your blood sugar more often than usual, especially during the first few weeks of treatment with perphenazine; amitriptyline. Perphenazine; amitriptyline can affect blood glucose (sugar) levels. Call your prescriber or health care professional for advice if you notice a change in the results of blood or urine glucose tests. If you are going to have surgery or will need a procedure that uses contrast agents, tell your prescriber or health care professional that you are taking this medicine.

What side effects may I notice from taking perphenazine; amitriptyline?

Side effects that you should report to your prescriber or health care professional as soon as possible:

- abnormal production of milk in females
- blurred vision or eye pain
- breast enlargement in both males and females
- confusion, hallucinations (seeing or hearing things that are not really there)
- difficulty breathing
- fainting spells
- fever with increased sweating
- high or low blood pressure
- irregular or fast, pounding heartbeat, palpitations
- menstrual cycle changes
- muscle stiffness, or spasms
- pain or difficulty passing urine, loss of bladder control
- seizures (convulsions)
- sexual difficulties (decreased sexual ability or desire, difficulty ejaculating)
- stomach pain
- swelling of the testicles
- tingling, pain, or numbness in the feet or hands
- tremors or shakiness
- uncontrolled movements of the mouth, head, hands, feet, shoulders, eyelids or other unusual muscle movements
- unusual weakness or tiredness
- yellowing of the eyes or skin

Side effects that usually do not require medical attention (report to your prescriber or health care professional if they continue or are bothersome):

- anxiety
- constipation or diarrhea
- difficulties falling asleep
- drowsiness or dizziness
- dry mouth
- headache
- increased sensitivity of the skin to sun or ultraviolet light
- increased sweating
- loss of appetite
- nausea, vomiting
- skin rash or itching
- weight gain or loss

Where can I keep my medicine?

Keep out of the reach of children in a container that small children cannot open. Store at room temperature between 15 and 30 degrees C (59 and 86 degrees F). Throw away any unused medicine after the expiration date.

Phenazopyridine tablets

PHENAZOPYRIDINE;
200 mg; Tablet
Amide
Pharmaceutical Inc

PHENAZOPYRIDINE;
100 mg; Tablet
Qualitest
Pharmaceuticals Inc

What is phenazopyridine?

PHENAZOPYRIDINE (Pyridiate®, Pyridium®, Urodol®, Urogesic®, Viridium®) is used to relieve the pain, burning, or discomfort caused by infection or irritation of the urinary tract. Phenazopyridine is not an antibiotic and will not cure a urinary tract infection. Generic phenazopyridine tablets are available.

What should my health care professional know before I take phenazopyridine?

They need to know if you have any of these conditions:

- glucose-6-phosphate dehydrogenase (G6PD) deficiency
- kidney disease
- liver disease
- an unusual or allergic reaction to phenazopyridine, other medicines, foods, dyes, or preservatives
- pregnant or trying to get pregnant
- breast-feeding

How should I take this medicine?

Take phenazopyridine tablets by mouth. Follow the directions on the prescription label. Swallow the tablets with a drink of water. You should take phenazopyridine with or following food (or a snack) to reduce the chance of stomach upset. Take your doses at regular intervals. Do not take your medicine more often than directed. If you are being treated for a urinary tract infection, phenazopyridine should not be taken for more than 2 days. However, make sure you complete the full course of antibiotic therapy as directed by your prescriber or health care professional.

What if I miss a dose?

If you miss a dose, take it as soon as you can. If it is almost time for your next dose, skip the missed dose and go back to your regular dosing schedule. Do not take double or extra doses.

What may interact with phenazopyridine?

Tell your prescriber or health care professional about all other medicines you are taking, including non-prescription medicines. Also tell your prescriber or health care professional if you are a frequent user of drinks with caffeine or alcohol, if you smoke, or if you use illegal drugs. These may affect the way your medicine works. Check with your health care professional before stopping or starting any of your medicines.

What should I watch for while taking phenazopyridine?

Phenazopyridine produces an orange to red color in the urine. This is to be expected while you are taking this medicine. This effect is harmless and will go away after you stop taking phenazopyridine. Also, the medicine may stain clothing. Do not use any leftover medicine for future urinary tract problems without first checking with your prescriber or health care professional. If you have an infection, your prescriber or health care professional will need to prescribe additional medicine. Tell your prescriber or health care professional if symptoms such as bloody urine or painful urination appear or become worse while you are taking this medicine. Also tell your prescriber or health care professional if you have a sudden decrease in the amount of urine while you are taking this medicine. For patients who wear soft contact lenses: it is best not to wear soft contact lenses while taking this medicine. Phenazopyridine may cause discoloration or staining of the contact lenses. It may not be possible to remove the stain. For diabetic patients: this medicine may cause false test results with urine sugar tests and urine ketone tests. If you have questions about this, check with your health care professional.

What side effects may I notice from taking phenazopyridine?

Side effects that you should report to your prescriber or health care professional as soon as possible:
Rare or uncommon:

- blue or blue-purple color of the skin
- fever or confusion
- shortness of breath
- skin rash
- chest tightness, wheezing, or troubled breathing
- unusual tiredness or weakness
- vomiting
- yellow eyes or skin

Side effects that usually do not require medical attention (report to your prescriber or health care professional if they continue or are bothersome):

- headache
- indigestion
- stomach upset

Where can I keep my medicine?

Keep out of the reach of young children. Store away from heat and direct light. Do not store this medicine in the bathroom, near the kitchen sink, or in other damp places. Heat or moisture may cause the medicine to break down. Throw away any unused medicine after the expiration date.

Phendimetrazine capsules, tablets, and sustained-release capsules

BONTRIL® SR;
105 mg; Capsule,
Extended Release
Valeant
Pharmaceuticals

BONTRIL® PDM;
35 mg; Tablet
Valeant
Pharmaceuticals

What are phendimetrazine tablets and capsules?

PHENDIMETRAZINE (Adipost®, Bontril Sustained Release®, Bontril® PDM, Dital®, Dyrexan-OD®, Melfiat 105®, Phendiet-105®, Bontril® PDM, Phenzene®, Prelu-2®, Rexigen Forte®) helps you lose weight. Combined with a reduced calorie diet, it can help you reduce weight by decreasing your appetite. Generic phendimetrazine tablets and capsules are available.

What should my health care professional know before I take phendimetrazine?

They need to know if you have any of these conditions:
- diabetes
- glaucoma
- heart disease
- high blood pressure
- thyroid disease
- taken other medicines to lose weight in the past year
- an unusual or allergic reaction to phendimetrazine, other medicines, foods, dyes, or preservatives
- pregnant or trying to get pregnant
- breast-feeding

How should I take this medicine?

Take phendimetrazine tablets and capsules by mouth.
Tablets and capsules:
Take tablets and capsules at least 1 hour before eating.
Sustained-release capsules:
Swallow whole; do not open or chew the capsules. Sustained-release capsules should be taken in the morning.

What if I miss a dose?

If you miss a dose, take it as soon as you can. If it is late in the day, or near bedtime, do not take that dose. Do not take double or extra doses.

What may interact with phendimetrazine?

- linezolid
- medicines for blood pressure
- medicines for diabetes
- medicines for mental depression
- other medicines or herbal products for weight loss or to decrease appetite

Tell your prescriber or health care professional about all other medicines you are taking, including non-prescription medicines, nutritional supplements, or herbal products. Also tell your prescriber or health care professional if you are a frequent user of drinks with caffeine or alcohol, if you smoke, or if you use illegal drugs. These may affect the way your medicine works. Check with your health care professional before stopping or starting any of your medicines.

What should I watch for while taking phendimetrazine?

Notify your physician immediately if you become short of breath while doing your normal activities. Keep in mind that phendimetrazine was intended to be used in addition to a healthy diet and exercise. The best results are achieved this way. Although your prescriber or health care professional will most likely prescribe phendimetrazine for only a few months, some people have used it for longer periods. Eventually your weight loss may "level out." At that point, the drug will only help you maintain your new weight. Do not increase or in any way change your dose without consulting your prescriber. Do not drive, use machinery, or do anything that requires mental alertness or physical coordination until you know how phendimetrazine affects you. Alcohol can increase the possibility of experiencing side effects with phendimetrazine. Therefore, it is best to avoid alcoholic drinks.

What side effects may I notice from taking phendimetrazine?

Side effects that you should report to your prescriber or health care professional as soon as possible:
- breathlessness on exertion
- chest pain
- depression or severe changes in mood
- dry cough
- heart palpitations
- increased blood pressure
- severe dizziness
- problems urinating
- vomiting

Side effects that usually do not require medical attention (report to your prescriber or health care professional if they continue or are bothersome):
- a false sense of well being
- blurred vision or other eye problems
- changes in sexual ability or desire
- constipation
- diarrhea
- difficulty sleeping
- dizziness
- dry mouth
- fatigue
- flushing
- headache
- irritability
- nervousness or restlessness
- nausea
- sweating
- unpleasant taste

Where can I keep my medicine?

Keep out of the reach of children in a container that small children cannot open. Store at room temperature between 15 and 30 degrees C (59 and 86 degrees F). Throw away any unused medicine after the expiration date.

Phenelzine tablets

NARDIL®;
15 mg; Tablet
Parke Davis Division of Pfizer
Co.

P

!

This drug requires an FDA medication guide. See page xxxvii.

What are phenelzine tablets?

PHENELZINE (Nardil®) belongs to a class of drugs called monoamine oxidase inhibitors (MAOIs). Phenelzine increases the level of certain chemicals in the brain that help fight depression and other mood problems, including certain anxiety disorders. Phenelzine can interact with certain foods and other medicines to cause unpleasant side effects. You must know what foods and medicines to avoid (see below). Generic phenelzine tablets are not yet available.

What should my health care professional know before I take phenelzine?

They need to know if you have any of these conditions:
- frequently drink alcohol-containing beverages
- asthma or bronchitis
- attempted suicide
- bipolar disorder or mania
- diabetes
- headaches or migraine
- heart or blood vessel disease, or irregular heart beats
- high blood pressure
- kidney disease
- liver disease
- over-active thyroid
- Parkinson's disease
- pheochromocytoma
- recent head trauma
- seizures or convulsions
- schizophrenia or psychosis
- stroke or other cerebrovascular disease
- an unusual or allergic reaction to phenelzine, other medicines, foods, dyes, or preservatives
- pregnant or trying to get pregnant
- breast-feeding

How should I take this medicine?

Take phenelzine tablets by mouth. Follow the directions on the prescription label. Swallow the tablets with a drink of water. Take your doses at regular intervals. Do not take your medicine more often than directed. Do not stop taking the tablets except on your prescriber's advice. Contact your pediatrician or health care professional regarding the use of this medicine in children. Special care may be needed. Elderly patients over age 65 years may have a stronger reaction to this medicine and should use this medicine with caution.

What if I miss a dose?

If you miss a dose, take it as soon as you can. If it is less than two hours to your next dose, take only that dose and skip the missed dose. Do not take double or extra doses.

What may interact with phenelzine?

- alcohol
- barbiturates such as phenobarbital
- bupropion
- buspirone
- caffeine
- carbamazepine
- certain medicines for blood pressure (especially beta-blockers, methyldopa, reserpine, guanadrel, and guanethidine)
- cocaine
- dextromethorphan
- diet pills or stimulants, like amphetamines or ephedra
- furazolidone
- ginseng
- guarana
- kava kava
- levodopa
- linezolid
- local anesthetics
- medicines for allergies, colds, flu symptoms, sinus congestion and breathing difficulties
- medicines for diabetes
- medicines for migraine headaches
- medicines for movement abnormalities as in Parkinson's disease (examples: entacapone, levodopa, selegiline, tolcapone)
- muscle relaxants
- other medicines for mental depression, anxiety, or mood or mental problems
- meperidine
- procarbazine
- SAM-e
- seizure (convulsion) or epilepsy medicine
- St. John's wort
- tramadol
- tryptophan
- tyramine—see below for foods that contain tyramine
- valerian
- water pills (diuretics)
- yohimbine

Tell your prescriber or health care professional about all other medicines you are taking, including non-prescription medicines, nutritional supplements, or herbal products. Also tell your prescriber or health care professional if you are a frequent user of drinks with caffeine or alcohol, if you smoke, or if you use illegal drugs.

These may affect the way your medicine works. Check with your health care professional before stopping or starting any of your medicines.

What should I watch for while taking phenelzine?

Visit your prescriber or health care professional for regular checks on your progress. It can take up to 4 weeks to see the full effects of phenelzine. Do not suddenly stop taking your medicine; this may make your condition worse or give you withdrawal symptoms. Ask your prescriber or health care professional for advice about gradually reducing your dosage. Even after you stop taking phenelzine the effects can last for at least 2 weeks. Continue to take all precautions and avoid all food and medicine that interact with phenelzine. Phenelzine can interact with certain foods that contain tyramine to produce severe headaches, a rise in blood pressure, or irregular heart beat. Foods that contain significant amounts of tyramine include aged cheeses; meats and fish (especially aged, smoked, pickled, or processed such as bologna, pepperoni, salami, summer sausage); beer and ale; alcohol-free beer; wine (especially red); sherry; hard liquor; liqueurs; avocados; bananas; figs; raisins; soy sauce; miso soup; yeast/protein extracts; bean curd; fava or broad bean pods; or any over-ripe fruit. Also, avoid drinks containing caffeine, such as tea, coffee, chocolate, or cola. Ask your prescriber or health care professional, pharmacist, or nutritionist for a complete listing of foods to be limited or avoided. Call your prescriber or health care professional as soon as you can if you get headaches or other unusual symptoms, such as palpitations or a change in behavior. You may get drowsy, dizzy or have blurred vision. Do not drive, use machinery, or do anything that needs mental alertness until you know how phenelzine affects you. Do not stand or sit up quickly, especially if you are an older patient. This reduces the risk of dizzy or fainting spells. Alcohol may increase dizziness or drowsiness; avoid alcoholic drinks. Phenelzine can make your mouth dry. Chewing sugarless gum, sucking hard candy and drinking plenty of water will help. Do not treat yourself for coughs, colds, flu or allergies without asking your prescriber or health care professional for advice. Do not take any medications for weight loss without advice either. Some ingredients in these products may increase possible side effects. If you are diabetic there is a possibility that phenelzine may affect your blood sugar. Ask your prescriber or health care professional for advice if there is any change in your blood or urine sugar tests. Notify your health care professional if you are scheduled to have any surgery, procedure or medical testing (including myelography). You should usually stop taking this drug at least 10 days before elective surgery; tell your prescriber or health care professional that you have been taking phenelzine.

What side effects may I notice from taking phenelzine?

Side effects that you should report to your prescriber or health care professional as soon as possible:

- agitation
- chest pain
- confusion
- difficulty breathing
- difficulty passing urine
- enlarged pupils, sensitivity of the eyes to light
- fever, clammy skin, increased sweating
- headache
- lightheadedness or fainting spells
- muscle or neck stiffness or spasm
- sexual dysfunction
- slow, fast, or irregular heartbeat (palpitations)
- yellowing of the skin or eyes

Side effects that usually do not require medical attention (report to your prescriber or health care professional if they continue or are bothersome):

- blurred vision
- constipation
- difficulty sleeping
- drowsiness or dizziness
- dry mouth
- increased appetite; weight increase
- muscle aches or pains, trembling
- nausea, vomiting
- swelling of the feet or legs
- unusual tiredness or weakness

Where can I keep my medicine?

Keep out of the reach of children in a container that small children cannot open. Store at room temperature between 15 and 30 degrees C (59 and 86 degrees F). Keep container tightly closed. Throw away any unused medicine after the expiration date.

Phenobarbital tablets or capsules

PHENOBARBITAL;
16.2 mg; Tablet
Qualitest
Pharmaceuticals Inc

PHENOBARBITAL;
15 mg; Tablet
Excellium
Pharmaceutical Inc

What are phenobarbital tablets or capsules?

PHENOBARBITAL (Solfoton®) is a barbiturate that acts by slowing down the activity of the brain and nervous system. Phenobarbital has sedative and hypnotic properties, which will help make you relaxed and sleepy before surgery or help you to sleep. It also reduces or controls seizures or convulsions, except for absence (petit mal) seizures. Federal law prohibits the transfer of phenobarbital to any person other than the patient for whom it was prescribed. Do not share this medicine with any one else. Generic phenobarbital tablets are available, but not capsules.

P

What should my health care professional know before I take phenobarbital?

They need to know if you have any of these conditions:
- an alcohol or drug abuse problem
- heart disease
- kidney disease or undergoing dialysis
- liver disease
- low blood pressure
- lung disease, chest infection or breathing difficulties
- mental depression or mental problems
- osteoporosis or other bone diseases
- porphyria
- seizures or convulsions
- shock
- an unusual or allergic reaction to phenobarbital, other barbiturates or seizure medications, other medicines, foods, dyes, or preservatives
- pregnant or trying to get pregnant
- breast-feeding

How should I take this medicine?

Take phenobarbital tablets or capsules by mouth. Follow the directions on the prescription label. Swallow the tablets or capsules with a drink of water. If phenobarbital upsets your stomach, take it with food or milk. Take your doses at regular intervals. Do not take your medicine more often than directed. Elderly patients over age 65 years may have a stronger reaction to this medicine and need smaller doses. Contact your pediatrician or health care professional regarding the use of this medication in children. Special care may be needed.

What if I miss a dose?

If you are on a regular schedule and miss a dose, take it as soon as you can. If it is almost time for your next dose, take only that dose. Try not to miss doses if you are taking phenobarbital for epilepsy. Do not take double or extra doses.

What may interact with phenobarbital?

Phenobarbital can interact with many different types of medications. You should check with your prescriber or pharmacist before taking other medications with phenobarbital. The following list includes some of the types of medications that may interact:

- acetaminophen
- alcohol
- alosetron
- antifungal drugs like fluconazole, griseofulvin, itraconazole or ketoconazole
- caffeine
- cancer-treating medications
- chloramphenicol
- cyclophosphamide
- cyclosporine
- digoxin
- disopyramide
- doxycycline

- female hormones, including contraceptive or birth control pills
- hormones such a prednisone or cortisone
- levothyroxine
- medicines for sleeping problems
- medicines for mental depression, anxiety or other mood problems
- medicines for treating HIV infection or AIDS
- metronidazole
- mexiletine
- prescription pain medications
- quinidine
- quinine
- riluzole
- sirolimus
- tacrolimus
- tamoxifen
- other seizure (convulsion) or epilepsy medicine
- theophylline
- warfarin

Tell your prescriber or health care professional about all other medicines you are taking, including non-prescription medicines, nutritional supplements, or herbal products. Also tell your prescriber or health care professional if you are a frequent user of drinks with caffeine or alcohol, if you smoke, or if you use illegal drugs. These may affect the way your medicine works. Check with your health care professional before stopping or starting any of your medicines.

What should I watch for while taking phenobarbital?

Visit your prescriber or health care professional for regular checks on your progress. If you are taking phenobarbital for epilepsy, take it at the same time each day. It may be 2 to 3 weeks before the full effects in controlling seizures are apparent. If you have been taking phenobarbital regularly and suddenly stop taking it, you may increase the risk of seizures. Your prescriber or health care professional may want to gradually reduce the dose. Do not stop taking except on your prescriber's advice. If sleep medicine is taken every night for a long time it may no longer help you to sleep. In general phenobarbital should not be taken for longer than 1 or 2 weeks as a sleep aid. Consult your prescriber or health care professional if you still have difficulty in sleeping. If you are taking phenobarbital for epilepsy, wear a Medic Alert bracelet or necklace. Carry an identification card with information about your condition, medications, and prescriber or health care professional. After taking phenobarbital you may get a residual hangover effect that leaves you drowsy or dizzy. Do not drive, use machinery, or do anything that needs mental alertness until you know how phenobarbital affects you. To reduce dizzy or fainting spells, do not sit or stand up quickly, especially if you are an older patient. Alcohol can increase possible unpleasant effects. Avoid alcoholic drinks. Phenobarbital can reduce the effectiveness of birth control pills (oral contraceptives) or other hormonal birth control drugs. Talk to your prescriber about alternatives or use of additional birth control methods while taking this drug. If you are going to have surgery, tell your prescriber or health care professional that you are taking phenobarbital.

What side effects may I notice from taking phenobarbital?

Side effects that you should report to your prescriber or health care professional as soon as possible:
- bone tenderness
- changes in behavior, mood, or mental ability
- changes in the frequency or severity of seizures
- confusion, agitation
- difficulty breathing or shortness of breath
- eye problems, very small or enlarged centers to the eyes
- fever, sore throat
- hallucinations
- lightheadedness or fainting spells
- redness, blistering, peeling or loosening of the skin, including inside the mouth
- skin rash, itching, hives
- slow heartbeat
- swelling of the face or lips
- unusual bleeding or bruising, pinpoint red spots on the skin
- unusual tiredness or weakness
- weight loss
- yellowing of skin or eyes

Side effects that usually do not require medical attention (report to your prescriber or health care professional if they continue or are bothersome):
- constipation
- clumsiness, unsteadiness, or a "hang-over" effect
- difficulty sleeping or nightmares
- drowsiness, dizziness
- headache
- irritability, nervousness
- nausea or vomiting

Where can I keep my medicine?

Keep out of the reach of children in a container that small children cannot open. Store at room temperature between 15 and 30 degrees C (59 and 86 degrees F). Keep container tightly closed. Throw away any unused medicine after the expiration date.

Phenoxybenzamine capsules

DIBENZYLINE®;
10 mg; Capsule
Wellspring Pharmaceutical
Corp

What are phenoxybenzamine capsules?

PHENOXYBENZAMINE (Dibenzyline®) is an antihypertensive. Phenoxybenzamine blocks the effects of certain chemicals that cause high blood pressure. It helps to control the sweating and high blood pressure that occur with a disease called pheochromocytoma. Generic phenoxybenzamine capsules are not yet available.

What should my health care professional know before I take phenoxybenzamine?

They need to know if you have any of the following conditions:
- dental disease
- heart or circulation disease
- if you are over 65 years old
- kidney disease
- respiratory infection
- shock
- stroke
- an unusual or allergic reaction to phenoxybenzamine, other medicines, foods, dyes, or preservatives
- pregnant or trying to get pregnant
- breast-feeding

How should I take this medicine?

Take phenoxybenzamine capsules by mouth. Follow the directions on the prescription label. Swallow the capsules with a drink of water. If phenoxybenzamine upsets your stomach, take the capsules with food or milk. Take your doses at regular intervals even if you feel better. Do not take your medicine more often than directed. Do not stop taking except on your prescriber's advice. Contact your pediatrician or health care professional regarding the use of this medicine in children. Special care may be needed.

What if I miss a dose?

If you miss a dose, take it as soon as you can. If it is almost time for your next dose, take only that dose. Do not take double or extra doses.

What may interact with phenoxybenzamine?

- alcohol
- medicines for colds and breathing difficulties
- medicines for high blood pressure
- metaraminol
- methoxamine

Tell your prescriber or health care professional about all other medicines you are taking, including nonprescription medicines, nutritional supplements, or herbal products. Also tell your prescriber or health care professional if you are a frequent user of drinks with caffeine or alcohol, if you smoke, or if you use illegal drugs. These may affect the way your medicine works. Check

P

with your prescriber or health care professional before stopping or starting any of your medicines.

What should I watch for while taking phenoxybenzamine?

Visit your prescriber or health care professional for regular checks on your progress. You may feel drowsy or dizzy. Do not drive, use machinery, or do anything that requires mental alertness until you know how phenoxybenzamine affects you. To reduce the risk of dizzy or fainting spells, do not sit or stand up quickly. Avoid alcoholic drinks; they can make you more drowsy, and increase flushing and rapid heartbeats. Taking initial doses of phenoxybenzamine at bedtime can lessen the effects of drowsiness and dizziness, but be careful if you have to get up during the night. Drowsiness and dizziness are more likely to occur after the first dose of phenoxybenzamine, after an increase in dose, or during hot weather or exercise. Dizziness can decrease once your body adjusts to this medicine. Your mouth may get dry. Chewing sugarless gum or sucking hard candy, and drinking plenty of water, will help. Do not take nonprescription medicine for weight-loss without asking your prescriber or health care professional. Also, do not take cough and cold, hay fever or sinus medications without asking your prescriber or health care professional. If you are going to have surgery, tell your prescriber or health care professional that you are taking phenoxybenzamine.

What side effects may I notice from taking phenoxybenzamine?

Side effects that you should report to your prescriber or health care professional as soon as possible:
- dizziness or drowsiness
- fainting spells
- fast heartbeat
- vomiting

Side effects that usually do not require medical attention (report to your prescriber or health care professional if they continue or are bothersome):
- confusion
- dry mouth
- headache
- nasal stuffiness
- small pupils (constricted)
- nausea
- sexual difficulties for men
- unusual tiredness

Where can I keep my medicine?

Keep out of the reach of children in a container that small children cannot open. Store at room temperature between 15 and 30 degrees C (59 and 86 degrees F). Keep container tightly closed. Throw away any unused medicine after the expiration date.

Phentermine sustained-release capsules

IONAMIN®;
15 mg; Capsule, Extended Release
Celltech Pharmaceuticals, Inc

What are phentermine sustained-release capsules?

PHENTERMINE (Ionamin®) helps you lose weight. Combined with a reduced calorie diet, it can help you reduce weight by decreasing your appetite. Generic phentermine sustained-release capsules are available.

What should my health care professional know before I take phentermine?

They need to know if you have any of these conditions:
- diabetes
- glaucoma
- heart disease
- high blood pressure
- kidney disease
- thyroid disease
- taken other medicines to lose weight in the past year
- an unusual or allergic reaction to phentermine, other medicines, foods, dyes, or preservatives
- pregnant or trying to get pregnant
- breast-feeding

How should I take this medicine?

Take phentermine sustained-release capsules by mouth in the morning with a drink of water. Swallow whole; do not open or chew the capsules. Follow the specific directions on the prescription label. Do not take your medicine more often than directed.

What if I miss a dose?

If you miss a dose, take it as soon as you can. If it is late in the day, or near bedtime, do not take that dose. Do not take double or extra doses.

What may interact with phentermine?

- linezolid
- medicines for blood pressure
- medicines for diabetes
- medicines for mental depression
- other medicines or herbal products for weight loss or to decrease appetite

Tell your prescriber or health care professional about all other medicines you are taking, including nonprescription medicines, nutritional supplements, or herbal products. Also tell your prescriber or health care professional if you are a frequent user of drinks with caffeine or alcohol, if you smoke, or if you use illegal drugs. These may affect the way your medicine works. Check with your health care professional before stopping or starting any of your medicines.

What should I watch for while taking phentermine?

Notify your physician immediately if you become short of breath while doing your normal activities. Keep in mind that phentermine was intended to be used in addition to a healthy diet and exercise. The best results are achieved this way. While your prescriber or health care professional will most likely prescribe phentermine for only a few months, some people have used it for longer periods. Eventually your weight loss may "level out." At that point, the drug will only help you maintain your new weight. Do not increase or in any way change your dose without consulting your prescriber. Do not drive, use machinery, or do anything that requires mental alertness or physical coordination until you know how phentermine affects you. Alcohol can increase the possibility of experiencing side effects with phentermine. Therefore, it is best to avoid alcoholic drinks.

What side effects may I notice from taking phentermine?

Side effects that you should report to your prescriber or health care professional as soon as possible:
- breathlessness on exertion
- chest pain
- depression or severe changes in mood
- dry cough
- heart palpitations

- increased blood pressure
- severe dizziness
- problems urinating
- vomiting

Side effects that usually do not require medical attention (report to your prescriber or health care professional if they continue or are bothersome):
- a false sense of well being
- blurred vision or other eye problems
- changes in sexual ability or desire
- constipation
- diarrhea
- difficulty sleeping
- dizziness
- dry mouth
- fatigue
- flushing
- headache
- irritability
- nervousness or restlessness
- nausea
- sweating
- unpleasant taste

Where can I keep my medicine?

Keep out of the reach of children in a container that small children cannot open. Store at room temperature between 15 and 30 degrees C (59 and 86 degrees F). Throw away any unused medicine after the expiration date.

Phentermine tablets or capsules

ADIPEX-P®;
37.5 mg; Tablet
Gate
Pharmaceuticals

ADIPEX-P®;
37.5 mg; Capsule
Gate
Pharmaceuticals

What are phentermine capsules or tablets?

PHENTERMINE (Adipex-P®, Fastin®, Phentamine®, Zantryl®) helps you lose weight. Combined with a reduced calorie diet, it can help you reduce weight by decreasing your appetite. Generic phentermine is available.

What should my health care professional know before I take phentermine?

They need to know if you have any of these conditions:
- diabetes
- glaucoma
- heart disease
- high blood pressure
- kidney disease
- thyroid disease
- taken other medicines to lose weight in the past year
- an unusual or allergic reaction to phentermine, other medicines, foods, dyes, or preservatives
- pregnant or trying to get pregnant
- breast-feeding

How should I take this medicine?

Take phentermine capsules or tablets by mouth. Follow the specific directions on the prescription label. Swallow the capsules or tablets with a drink of water at least 30 minutes before eating. Do not take your medicine more often than directed.

What if I miss a dose?

If you miss a dose, take it as soon as you can. If it is almost time for your next dose, take only that dose. Do not take double or extra doses.

What may interact with phentermine?

- linezolid
- medicines for blood pressure
- medicines for diabetes
- medicines for mental depression
- other medicines or herbal products for weight loss or to decrease appetite

Tell your prescriber or health care professional about all other medicines you are taking, including non-prescription medicines, nutritional supplements, or herbal products. Also tell your prescriber or health care professional if you are a frequent user of drinks with caffeine or alcohol, if you smoke, or if you use illegal drugs. These may affect the way your medicine works. Check

with your health care professional before stopping or starting any of your medicines.

What should I watch for while taking phentermine?

Notify your physician immediately if you become short of breath while doing your normal activities. Keep in mind that phentermine was intended to be used in addition to a healthy diet and exercise. The best results are achieved this way. While your prescriber or health care professional will most likely prescribe phentermine for only a few months; however, some people have used it for longer periods. Eventually your weight loss may "level out." At that point, the drug will only help you maintain your new weight. Do not increase or in any way change your dose without consulting your prescriber. Do not drive, use machinery, or do anything that requires mental alertness or physical co-ordination until you know how phentermine affects you. Alcohol can increase the possibility of experiencing side effects with phentermine. Therefore, it is best to avoid alcoholic drinks.

What side effects may I notice from taking phentermine?

Side effects that you should report to your prescriber or health care professional as soon as possible:
- breathlessness on exertion
- chest pain
- depression or severe changes in mood
- dry cough
- heart palpitations
- increased blood pressure
- severe dizziness
- problems urinating
- vomiting

Side effects that usually do not require medical attention (report to your prescriber or health care professional if they continue or are bothersome):
- a false sense of well being
- blurred vision or other eye problems
- changes in sexual ability or desire
- constipation
- diarrhea
- difficulty sleeping
- dizziness
- dry mouth
- fatigue
- flushing
- headache
- irritability
- nervousness or restlessness
- nausea
- sweating
- unpleasant taste

Where can I keep my medicine?

Keep out of the reach of children in a container that small children cannot open. Store at room temperature between 15 and 30 degrees C (59 and 86 degrees F). Throw away any unused medicine after the expiration date.

Phenytoin capsules, extended-release capsules, and chewable tablets

DILANTIN®;
100 mg; Capsule,
Extended Release
Parke Davis Division
of Pfizer Co.

DILANTIN®
INFATABS®;
50 mg; Chewable
tablets
Parke Davis Division
of Pfizer Co.

What are phenytoin capsules, extended-release capsules, and chewable tablets?

PHENYTOIN (Dilantin® Kapseals®, Dilantin® Infatabs®, Phenytek™) helps to control seizures (convulsions) in certain types of epilepsy. Phenytoin can help to prevent seizures occurring during or after surgery. Phenytoin also treats nerve-related pain such as trigeminal neuralgia. It is not for common aches and pains. Generic phenytoin capsules are available; generic chewable tablets are not available.

What should my health care professional know before I take phenytoin?

They need to know if you have any of these conditions:
- an alcohol abuse problem
- blood disorders or disease
- diabetes
- fever
- heart problems
- kidney disease
- liver disease
- porphyria
- receiving intramuscular injections
- receiving radiation therapy
- skin problems
- thyroid disease
- an unusual or allergic reaction to phenytoin, other medicines, foods, dyes, or preservatives
- pregnant or trying to get pregnant
- breast-feeding

How should I take this medicine?

Take phenytoin capsules and tablets by mouth. Follow the directions on the prescription label. Swallow the capsules with a drink of water. If you are taking extended-release capsules, swallow them whole; do not crush or chew. Chewable tablets may be chewed and tablets may be swallowed whole with a drink of water.

Take phenytoin with food if it upsets your stomach. It may be best to take your phenytoin dose consistently with or without food. Take your doses at regular intervals. Do not take your medicine more often than directed.

What if I miss a dose?

Try not to miss a scheduled dosage, especially if you are taking phenytoin extended-release capsules just once per day. If you miss a dose, take it as soon as you can. If it is less than 4 hours to your next dose, take only that dose. If you only take a dose once a day and do not remember until the next day, skip the missed dose and resume your normal schedule. Do not take double or extra doses.

What may interact with phenytoin?

Many medicines can interact with phenytoin; check with your prescriber or health care professional if you regularly take other medications or over-the-counter products. Some of the medicines that can interact with phenytoin are listed:

- alcohol
- amphetamines
- antacids
- aspirin and aspirin-like medicines
- barbiturate medicines for inducing sleep or treating seizures (convulsions)
- bosentan
- calcium supplements
- carbamazepine
- cimetidine
- ciprofloxacin
- clopidogrel
- cyclosporine
- disulfiram
- enteral feedings (liquid nutritional drinks or tube feeding liquids)
- ethosuximide
- felbamate
- female hormones, including contraceptive or birth control pills
- fluconazole
- folic acid, vitamin B₉
- heart medicines such as digoxin or digitoxin
- chloramphenicol
- corticosteroid hormones such as prednisone or cortisone
- isoniazid
- itraconazole
- kava kava
- ketoconazole
- leucovorin
- levodopa
- lidocaine
- medicines for hay fever and other allergies
- medicines for mental depression, anxiety or other mood problems
- medicines to control heart rhythm
- medicines used to treat HIV infection or AIDS
- methadone or other medicines for pain
- methsuximide
- modafinil
- omeprazole
- oxcarbazepine
- rifampin, rifabutin or rifapentine
- sirolimus
- St. John's wort
- sucralfate
- tacrolimus
- theophylline
- tiagabine
- ticlopidine
- tramadol
- valproic acid
- voriconazole
- warfarin
- zonisamide

Tell your prescriber or health care professional about all other medicines you are taking, including non-prescription medicines. Also tell your prescriber or health care professional if you are a frequent user of drinks with caffeine or alcohol, if you smoke, or if you use illegal drugs. These may affect the way your medicine works. Check with your health care professional before stopping or starting any of your medicines.

What should I watch for while taking phenytoin?

Visit your prescriber or health care professional for regular checks on your progress. Your prescriber or health care professional may schedule regular blood tests, because phenytoin therapy needs careful monitoring. Do not stop taking phenytoin suddenly. If you take phenytoin for seizures, it is a good idea to carry an identification card, necklace or bracelet with details of your condition, medications and prescriber or health care professional. Do not change brands or dosage forms of phenytoin without discussing the change with your prescriber or health care professional. You may feel dizzy or drowsy. Do not drive, use machinery, or do anything that needs mental alertness until you know how phenytoin affects you. To reduce the risk of dizzy or fainting spells, do not sit or stand up quickly, especially if you are an older patient. Alcohol can make you more dizzy, increase flushing and rapid heartbeats. Avoid alcoholic drinks. If you are going to have surgery, tell your prescriber or health care professional that you are taking phenytoin. Birth control pills (contraceptive pills) may not work properly while you are taking phenytoin; talk with your prescriber about the use of other methods of birth control. Phenytoin can cause unusual growth of gum tissues; visit your dentist regularly. Problems can arise if you need dental work, and in the day to day care of your teeth. Try to avoid damage to your teeth and gums when you brush or floss your teeth. Do not take antacids at the same time as phenytoin. If you get an upset stomach and want to take an antacid or medicine for diarrhea, make sure there is an interval of 2 to 3 hours before or after you took phenytoin.

P

What side effects may I notice from taking phenytoin?

Side effects that you should report to your prescriber or health care professional as soon as possible:

- chest pain or tightness; fast or irregular heartbeat (palpitations)
- confusion, nervousness, hostility, or other behavioral changes (especially in children or elderly patients)
- dark yellow or brown urine
- difficulty breathing, wheezing or shortness of breath
- double vision or uncontrollable and rapid eye movement
- fainting spells or lightheadedness
- fever, sore throat
- headache
- loss of seizure control
- mouth ulcers
- poor control of body movements or difficulty walking
- redness, blistering, peeling or loosening of the skin, including inside the mouth
- sexual problems (painful erections, loss of sexual desire)
- skin rash, itching
- stomach pain
- swollen or painful glands

- unusual bleeding or bruising, pinpoint red spots on skin
- unusual tiredness or weakness
- unusual swelling
- vomiting
- yellowing of the eyes or skin

Side effects that usually do not require medical attention (report to your prescriber or health care professional if they continue or are bothersome):

- clumsiness or unsteadiness
- constipation
- difficulty sleeping
- dizziness or drowsiness
- excessive hair growth on the face or body
- loss of appetite
- nausea
- stomach upset
- unusual growth of gum tissue

Where can I keep my medicine?

Keep out of the reach of children in a container that small children cannot open. Store at room temperature between 15 and 30 degrees C (59 and 86 degrees F). Keep container tightly closed. Throw away any unused medicine after the expiration date.

Pilocarpine tablets

SALAGEN;
5 mg; Tablet
MGI Pharma

What are pilocarpine tablets?

PILOCARPINE (Salagen®) can increase the flow of saliva. Pilocarpine tablets relieve a dry mouth following radiotherapy treatment for cancer of the head and neck. Generic pilocarpine tablets are available.

What should my health care professional know before I take pilocarpine?

They need to know if you have any of these conditions:
- asthma, bronchitis
- gallstones or biliary tract disease
- glaucoma
- heart disease
- inflammation of the eye
- kidney stones
- liver disease
- mental problems
- an unusual or allergic reaction to pilocarpine, other medicines, foods, dyes, or preservatives
- breast-feeding
- pregnant or trying to get pregnant

How should I take this medicine?

Take pilocarpine tablets by mouth. Follow the directions on the prescription label. Swallow the tablets with a drink of water. Take your doses at regular intervals. Do not take your medicine more often than directed. Contact your pediatrician or health care profes-

sional regarding the use of this medicine in children. Special care may be needed.

What if I miss a dose?

If you miss a dose, take it as soon as you can. If it is almost time for your next dose, take only that dose. Do not take double or extra doses.

What may interact with pilocarpine?

- atropine
- acetazolamide
- epinephrine
- timolol

Tell your prescriber or health care professional about all other medicines you are taking, including non-prescription medicines, nutritional supplements, or herbal products. Also tell your prescriber or health care professional if you are a frequent user of drinks with caffeine or alcohol, if you smoke, or if you use illegal drugs. These may affect the way your medicine works. Check with your health care professional before stopping or starting any of your medicines.

What should I watch for while taking pilocarpine?

Pilocarpine can make your vision blur. You may find it is difficult to see, especially at night. Do not drive, use machinery, or do anything that needs clear vision until you know how pilocarpine affects you. While you are taking pilocarpine, have plenty to drink. You can get dehydrated if the tablets make you sweat a lot.

What side effects may I notice from taking pilocarpine?

Side effects that you should report to your prescriber or health care professional as soon as possible:
- difficulty breathing
- irregular heartbeat
- vomiting
- weakness or tiredness

Side effects that usually do not require medical attention (report to your prescriber or health care professional if they continue or are bothersome):
- blurred vision

- catarrh or runny nose
- chills
- dizziness
- flushing
- headache
- increased sweating
- nausea
- stomach upset
- trembling
- urgent need to pass urine

Where can I keep my medicine?

Keep out of the reach of children in a container that small children cannot open. Store at room temperature between 15 and 30 degrees C (59 and 86 degrees F). Throw away any unused medicine after the expiration date.

Pimozide tablets

ORAP®;
1 mg; Tablet
Gate
Pharmaceuticals

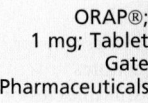

ORAP®;
2 mg; Tablet
Gate
Pharmaceuticals

What are pimozide tablets?

PIMOZIDE (Orap®) helps to lessen the muscle and speech tics that are caused by Tourette's syndrome. Pimozide can also treat conditions that may cause you to hear or see things that others do not. Generic pimozide tablets are not yet available.

What should my health care professional know before I take pimozide?

They need to know if you have any of these conditions:
- an alcohol abuse problem
- blood disease
- cancer
- difficulty urinating
- glaucoma
- heart, kidney, or liver disease
- low potassium or magnesium levels in your blood
- Parkinson's disease
- prostate trouble
- seizures (convulsions)
- an unusual or allergic reaction to pimozide, other medicines, foods, dyes, or preservatives
- pregnant or trying to get pregnant
- breast-feeding

How should I take this medicine?

Take pimozide tablets by mouth with or without food. Follow the directions on the prescription label. Swallow the tablets with a drink of water. If pimozide upsets your stomach you can take it with food. Take your doses at regular intervals. Do not take your medicine more often than directed. Do not stop taking except on your prescriber's advice. Do not drink alcoholic beverages or grapefruit juice products while taking pimozide. Contact your pediatrician or health care professional regarding the use of this medicine in children. Special care may be needed. Patients over age 65 years

may have a stronger reaction to this medicine and need smaller doses.

What if I miss a dose?

If you miss a dose, take it as soon as you can. If it is almost time for your next dose, take only that dose. Do not take double or extra doses.

What may interact with pimozide?

Pimozide has the potential to interact with many medications. The list below contains some of the drugs that can interact:
Do not take pimozide with any of the following medications:

- aprepitant
- astemizole
- bepridil
- certain antibiotics: clarithromycin, dirithromycin, erythromycin, gatifloxacin, grepafloxacin, moxifloxacin, sparfloxacin, or troleandomycin
- cimetidine
- cisapride
- diltiazem
- dolasetron
- grapefruit juice
- halofantrine
- medicines for fungal infections (examples—fluconazole, itraconazole, ketoconazole, voriconazole)
- medicines for treating HIV virus infection or AIDS (examples—amprenavir, indinavir, nelfinavir, saquinavir, ritonavir)
- mefloquine
- mibefradil
- nicardipine
- probucol
- quinine
- some medicines for treating depression or other mental problems (examples—amoxapine, fluoxetine, flu-

voxamine, maprotiline, nefazodone, sertraline, ziprasidone)
- some medicines for treating heart-rhythm problems (examples- amiodarone, flecainide, disopyramide, dofetilide, ibutilide, procainamide, quinidine, sotalol)
- tacrolimus
- terfenadine
- verapamil
- zileuton

Pimozide may also interact with the following medications:

- barbiturates, like phenobarbital
- bosentan
- carbamazepine
- ciprofloxacin
- citalopram
- enoxacin
- isoniazid (INH)
- levodopa
- medicines for sleep or anxiety
- medicines for treating seizures
- norfloxacin
- pain relievers
- paroxetine
- rifampin
- sertraline
- some medicines for treating asthma
- some medicines for treating pain
- tacrine

Tell your prescriber or health care professional about all other medicines you are taking, including non-prescription medicines. Also tell your prescriber or health care professional if you are a frequent user of drinks with caffeine or alcohol, if you smoke, or if you use illegal drugs. These may affect the way your medicine works. Check with your health care professional before stopping or starting any of your medicines.

What should I watch for while taking pimozide?

Visit your prescriber or health care professional for regular checks on your progress. It may be several weeks before you see the full effects of pimozide. Do not suddenly stop taking pimozide. You may need to gradually reduce the dose. Only stop taking pimozide on your prescriber's advice. You may get dizzy or drowsy. Do not drive, use machinery, or do anything that needs mental alertness until you know how pimozide affects you. Alcohol can increase dizziness and drowsiness. Avoid alcoholic drinks. Do not drink grapefruit juice products while taking pimozide. An ingredient in grapefruit juice can increase the chance of developing serious heart problems from pimozide. If you are going to have surgery tell your prescriber or health care professional that you are taking pimozide.

What side effects may I notice from taking pimozide?

Side effects that you should report to your prescriber or health care professional as soon as possible:
- change in emotion or behavior such as feeling depressed, angry, or anxious
- change in vision
- difficulty breathing
- difficulty swallowing
- fast, slow or irregular heartbeat (palpitations)
- fever
- inability to control muscle movements in the face, hands, arms, or legs
- increased thirst
- loss of balance or difficulty walking
- menstrual changes
- rash
- restlessness or need to keep moving
- seizures
- stiff muscles or jaw
- seizures
- sexual difficulties
- skin rash
- spasms of the face, tongue, or mouth
- tremors or trembling
- uncontrollable tongue or mouth movements

Side effects that usually do not require medical attention (report to your prescriber or health care professional if they continue or are bothersome):
Less common:
- changes in sexual desire
- constipation
- difficulty sleeping
- difficulty urinating
- excessive watering or drooling of mouth
- headache
- nausea or vomiting
- trouble in controlling urine
- weight gain

More common:
- dizziness; especially on standing from a sitting or lying position
- drowsiness
- dry mouth
- weight loss

Where can I keep my medicine?

Keep out of the reach of children in a container that small children cannot open. Store at room temperature between 20 degrees and 25 degrees C (68 degrees and 77 degrees F). Throw away any unused medicine after the expiration date.

Pindolol tablets

VISKEN®;
10 mg; Tablet
Novartis
Pharmaceuticals

PINDOLOL;
10 mg; Tablet
Ivax Pharmaceuticals
Inc

What are pindolol tablets?

PINDOLOL (Visken®) belongs to a group of medicines called beta-blockers. Beta-blockers reduce the workload on the heart and help it to beat more regularly. Pindolol controls, but does not cure, high blood pressure (hypertension). High blood pressure may not make you feel sick, but it can lead to serious heart problems. Pindolol also relieves chest pain (angina). Generic pindolol tablets are available.

What should my health care professional know before I take pindolol?

They need to know if you have any of these conditions:
- asthma, bronchitis or bronchospasm
- circulation problems, or blood vessel disease (such as Raynaud's disease)
- depression
- diabetes
- emphysema, or other lung disease
- history of heart attack or heart disease, vasospastic angina
- kidney disease
- liver disease
- muscle weakness or disease
- pheochromocytoma
- psoriasis
- thyroid disease
- an unusual or allergic reaction to pindolol, other beta-blockers, medicines, foods, dyes, or preservatives
- pregnant or trying to get pregnant
- breast-feeding

How should I take this medicine?

Take pindolol tablets by mouth. Follow the directions on the prescription label. Swallow the tablets with a drink of water. Take your doses at regular intervals. Do not take your medicine more often than directed. Do not stop taking except on your prescriber's advice. Contact your pediatrician or health care professional regarding the use of this medicine in children. Special care may be needed.

What if I miss a dose?

If you miss a dose, take it as soon as you can. If it is almost time for your next dose (less than 4 hours), take only that dose. Do not take double or extra doses.

What may interact with pindolol?

- anti-inflammatory drugs (NSAIDs, such as ibuprofen)
- cimetidine
- cocaine
- digoxin
- ergotamine
- hawthorn
- levodopa
- medicines for diabetes
- medicines for high blood pressure
- medicine for mental problems and psychotic disturbances
- reserpine
- water pills

Tell your prescriber or health care professional about all other medicines you are taking, including non-prescription medicines, nutritional supplements, or herbal products. Also tell your prescriber or health care professional if you are a frequent user of drinks with caffeine or alcohol, if you smoke, or if you use illegal drugs. These may affect the way your medicine works. Check with your health care professional before stopping or starting any of your medicines.

What should I watch for while taking pindolol?

Check your heart rate and blood pressure regularly while you are taking pindolol. Ask your prescriber or health care professional what your heart rate and blood pressure should be, and when you should contact him or her. It can be 2 weeks or longer before the full effect of pindolol in lowering blood pressure is seen. Do not stop taking this medicine suddenly. This could lead to serious heart-related effects. You may get drowsy or dizzy. Do not drive, use machinery, or do anything that requires mental alertness until you know how pindolol affects you. To reduce the risk of dizzy or fainting spells, do not sit or stand up quickly. Alcohol can make you more drowsy, and increase flushing and rapid heartbeats. Therefore, it is best to avoid alcoholic drinks. Pindolol can affect blood sugar levels. If you have diabetes, check with your prescriber or health care professional before you change your diet or the dose of your diabetic medicine. If you are going to have surgery, tell your prescriber or health care professional that you are taking pindolol.

What side effects may I notice from taking pindolol?

Side effects that you should report to your prescriber or health care professional as soon as possible:
- confusion, hallucinations (seeing and hearing things that are not really there)
- changes in blood sugar
- chest pain
- cold hands or feet
- difficulty breathing, wheezing
- difficulty sleeping, nightmares
- dizziness or fainting spells

- joint pain
- muscle cramps or weakness
- skin rash, itching, dry peeling skin
- slow heart rate (less than 50 beats per minute)
- swelling of the legs and ankles
- vomiting

Side effects that usually do not require medical attention (report to your prescriber or health care professional if they continue or are bothersome):

- diarrhea
- dry sore eyes

- hair loss
- nausea
- sexual difficulties (impotence or decreased sexual urges)
- weakness or tiredness

Where can I keep my medicine?

Keep out of the reach of children in a container that small children cannot open. Store at room temperature below 30 degrees C (86 degrees F). Protect from light, Keep container tightly closed. Throw away any unused medicine after the expiration date.

Pioglitazone tablets

ACTOS™;
30 mg; Tablet
Takeda
Pharmaceuticals
North America Inc

ACTOS™;
45 mg; Tablet
Takeda
Pharmaceuticals
North America Inc

What are pioglitazone tablets?

PIOGLITAZONE (Actos™) helps to treat type 2 diabetes mellitus. Pioglitazone helps your body to use insulin more efficiently and helps to lower high blood sugar. Generic pioglitazone tablets are not yet available.

What should my health care professional know before I take pioglitazone?

They need to know if you have any of these conditions:
- heart problems
- kidney or liver problems
- swelling of the arms, legs, or feet
- an unusual or allergic reaction to pioglitazone, other medicines, foods, dyes, or preservatives
- pregnant or trying to get pregnant
- breast-feeding

How should I take this medicine?

Take pioglitazone tablets by mouth. Follow the directions on the prescription label. Swallow the tablets with a drink of water with meals. Take your doses at the same time each day; do not take more often than directed. Contact your pediatrician or health care professional regarding the use of this medicine in children. Special care may be needed.

What if I miss a dose?

If you miss a dose, take it with the next meal. If it is almost time for your next dose, take only that dose. Do not take double or extra doses.

What may interact with pioglitazone?

- atorvastatin
- birth control pills or other hormonal methods of birth control
- bosentan
- itraconazole
- ketoconazole
- midazolam
- nifedipine

Many medications may cause changes (increase or decrease) in blood sugar; these include:

- alcohol-containing beverages
- aspirin and aspirin-like drugs
- beta-blockers, often used for high blood pressure or heart problems (examples include atenolol, metoprolol, propranolol)
- chromium
- female hormones, such as estrogens or progestins, birth control pills
- isoniazid
- male hormones or anabolic steroids
- medications to suppress appetite or for weight loss
- medicines for allergies, asthma, cold, or cough
- niacin
- other medicines for diabetes
- pentamidine
- phenytoin
- quinolone antibiotics (examples: ciprofloxacin, levofloxacin, ofloxacin)
- some herbal dietary supplements
- steroid medicines such as prednisone or cortisone
- thyroid hormones
- water pills (diuretics)

Tell your prescriber or health care professional about all other medicines you are taking, including non-prescription medicines, nutritional supplements, or herbal products. Also tell your prescriber or health care professional if you are a frequent user of drinks with caffeine or alcohol, if you smoke, or if you use illegal drugs. These may affect the way your medicine works. Check with your health care professional before stopping or starting any of your medicines.

What should I watch for while taking pioglitazone?

Visit your prescriber or health care professional for regular checks on your progress. Learn how to monitor blood or urine sugar and urine ketones regularly. Check with your prescriber or health care professional if your blood sugar is high, you may need a change of dose of pioglitazone. Do not skip meals. If you are exercising much more than usual you may need extra snacks to avoid side effects caused by low blood sugar. If you have mild symptoms of low blood sugar, eat or drink something containing sugar at once and contact your prescriber or health care professional. It is wise to check your blood sugar to confirm that it is low. It is important to recognize your own symptoms of low blood sugar so that you can treat them quickly. Make sure family members know that you can choke if you eat or drink when you have serious symptoms of low blood sugar, such as seizures or unconsciousness. They must get medical help at once. Your health care professional will have to check blood tests regularly to assess the effect of this medication on your liver. Pioglitazone may rarely cause changes in some of these measurements. If you are going to have surgery, tell your prescriber or health care professional that you are taking pioglitazone. Wear a medical identification bracelet or chain to say you have diabetes, and carry a card that lists all your medications.

What side effects may I notice from taking pioglitazone?

Side effects that you should report to your prescriber or health care professional as soon as possible:

- anxiety or nervousness, confusion, difficulty concentrating
- blurred vision
- breathing problems such as rapid, deep breathing or difficulty breathing with activity
- cold sweats, increased sweating
- cool, pale skin
- dark yellow or brown urine, or yellowing of the eyes or skin
- diarrhea
- drowsiness
- muscle pain
- nausea, vomiting
- skin rash or hives
- slow heartbeat
- tremors or shakiness
- unusual tiredness or weakness
- swelling of the hands, legs, and/or feet

Side effects that usually do not require medical attention (report to your prescriber or health care professional if they continue or are bothersome):

- headache
- weight gain

Where can I keep my medicine?

Keep out of the reach of children in a container that small children cannot open. Store at room temperature between 15 and 30 degrees C (59 and 86 degrees F). Keep container tightly closed and protect from moisture and humidity. Throw away any unused medicine after the expiration date.

Piroxicam capsules

FELDENE®;
20 mg; Capsule
Pfizer Laboratories
Div Pfizer Inc

FELDENE®;
10 mg; Capsule
Pfizer Laboratories
Div Pfizer Inc

This drug requires an FDA medication guide. See page xxxvii.

What are piroxicam capsules?

PIROXICAM (Feldene®) is a nonsteroidal anti-inflammatory drug (NSAID). It helps relieves pain and inflammation associated with rheumatoid arthritis and osteoarthritis. Generic piroxicam capsules are available.

What should my health care professional know before I take piroxicam?

They need to know if you have any of these conditions:

- anemia
- asthma, especially aspirin sensitive asthma
- bleeding problems or taking medicines that make you bleed more easily such as anticoagulants ("blood thinners")
- cigarette smoker
- diabetes
- drink more than three alcohol-containing beverages a day
- heart failure
- high blood pressure
- kidney disease
- liver disease
- stomach or duodenal ulcers
- systemic lupus erythematosus
- ulcerative colitis
- an unusual or allergic reaction to aspirin, other salicylates, other NSAIDs, other medicines, foods, dyes or preservatives
- pregnant or trying to get pregnant
- breast-feeding

How should I take this medicine?

Take piroxicam capsules by mouth. Follow the directions on the prescription label. Swallow capsules whole with a full glass of water; take capsules in an upright or sitting position. Taking a sip of water first, before taking the capsules, may help you swallow them. If possible take bedtime doses at least 10 minutes before lying down. You can take piroxicam with food to prevent stomach upset. Piroxicam is usually taken once a day. Do not take your medicine more often than directed. Contact your pediatrician or health care professional regarding the use of this medicine in children. Special care may be needed.

What if I miss a dose?

If you miss a dose, take it as soon as you can. If it is almost time for your next dose, take only that dose. Do not take double or extra doses.

What may interact with piroxicam?

- alcohol
- anti-inflammatory drugs (such as other NSAIDs or prednisone)
- aspirin and aspirin-like medicines
- cidofovir
- cyclosporine
- entecavir
- herbal products that contain feverfew, garlic, ginger, or ginkgo biloba
- lithium
- medicines for high blood pressure
- medicines that affect platelets
- medicines that treat or prevent blood clots such as warfarin and other "blood thinners"
- methotrexate
- pemetrexed
- water pills (diuretics)

Tell your prescriber or health care professional about all other medicines you are taking, including non-prescription medicines, nutritional supplements, or herbal products. Also tell your prescriber or health care professional if you are a frequent user of drinks with caffeine or alcohol, if you smoke, or if you use illegal drugs. These may affect the way your medicine works. Check with your health care professional before stopping or starting any of your medicines.

What should I watch for while taking piroxicam?

It can take 7 to 12 days of treatment with piroxicam before the full effects are felt. Let your prescriber or health care professional know if your pain continues after 2 weeks. Do not take other pain-killers with piroxicam without advice. If you get flu-like symptoms (fever, chills, muscle aches and pains), call your prescriber or health care professional; do not treat yourself. To reduce unpleasant effects on your throat and stomach, take piroxicam with a full glass of water and never just before lying down.. If you notice black, tarry stools or experience severe stomach pain and/or vomit blood or what looks like coffee grounds, notify your health care prescriber immediately. If you are taking medicines that affect the clotting of your blood, such as aspirin or blood thinners such as Coumadin®, talk to your health care provider or prescriber before taking piroxicam. You may get dizzy. Do not drive, use machinery, or do anything that needs mental alertness until you know how piroxicam affects you. Do not sit or stand up quickly, especially if you are an older patient. This reduces the risk of dizzy or fainting spells. Do not smoke cigarettes or drink alcohol; these increase irritation to your stomach and can make it more susceptible to damage from piroxicam. If you are going to have surgery, tell your prescriber or health care professional that you are taking this medicine. Problems can arise if you need dental work, and in the day to day care of your teeth. Try to avoid damage to your teeth and gums when you brush or floss your teeth. It is especially important not to use piroxicam during the last 3 months of pregnancy unless specifically directed to do so by your health care provider. Piroxicam may cause problems in the unborn child or complications during delivery.

What side effects may I notice from taking piroxicam?

Side effects that you should report to your prescriber or health care professional as soon as possible:

- signs of bleeding—bruising, red spots on the skin, black tarry stools, blood in the urine, unusual tiredness or weakness, vomiting blood or vomit that looks like coffee grounds
- signs of an allergic reaction—difficulty breathing or wheezing, skin rash, redness, blistering or peeling skin, hives, or itching, swelling of eyelids, throat, lips
- blurred vision
- change in the amount of urine passed
- difficulty swallowing, severe heartburn or burning, pain in throat
- pain or difficulty passing urine
- stomach pain or cramps
- swelling of feet or ankles
- yellowing of the eyes or skin

Side effects that usually do not require medical attention (report to your prescriber or health care professional if they continue or are bothersome):

- diarrhea or constipation
- dizziness, drowsiness
- gas or heartburn
- headache
- nausea, vomiting

Where can I keep my medicine?

Keep out of the reach of children in a container that small children cannot open. Store at room temperature between 15 and 30 degrees C (59 and 86 degrees F). Protect from light. Keep container tightly closed. Throw away any unused medicine after the expiration date.

Polysaccharide—Iron Complex tablets or capsules

NU-IRON® 150;
150 mg; Capsule
Merz
Pharmaceuticals LLC

NIFEREX FORTE;
150 mg; Capsule
Schwarz Pharma

What are polysaccharide-iron complex tablets or capsules?

POLYSACCHARIDE-IRON COMPLEX (Ferrex® 150, Fe-Tinic™, Hytinic™, Niferex Forte®, Nu-Iron 150® and others) is an iron supplement. Iron is a mineral needed by your body to make new red blood cells. Iron also helps red blood cells function. Red blood cells carry oxygen to all of your body tissues. There are many different kinds of iron supplements. However, extra iron should only be taken under the advice of a health care professional. Adults or kids with anemia due to low iron levels or a low red blood cell count may be prescribed iron. Pregnant women in their last 3 to 6 months of pregnancy may need to take extra iron, but should only take iron if their doctor tells them to. Do not treat yourself with iron if you are feeling tired or fatigued. Most healthy people get adequate iron in their diets, particularly if they regularly eat fortified cereals, meat, poultry, and fish. Generic polysaccharide-iron complex is available.

What should my health care professional know before I take polysaccharide-iron complex?

They need to know if you have any of these conditions:
- an alcohol problem
- blood transfusions
- bowel disease
- hemolytic anemia
- iron overload (hemochromatosis, hemosiderosis)
- liver disease
- stomach ulcers
- an unusual or allergic reaction to iron, other medicines, foods, dyes, or preservatives
- pregnant or trying to get pregnant
- breast-feeding

How should I take this medicine?

Take the tablets or capsules by mouth. Follow the directions on the prescription label. Swallow tablets or capsules whole with a full glass of water or fruit juice; take tablets or capsules in an upright or sitting position. Taking a sip of water first, before taking the tablets or capsules, may help you swallow them. If possible take bedtime doses at least 10 minutes before lying down. It is best to take iron on an empty stomach. Take at least 1 hour before or 2 hours after food. If the iron causes your stomach to be upset, you may take it with food. Take your doses at regular intervals. Do not take iron more often than directed. Contact your pediatrician or health care professional regarding the use of this medicine in children. Special care may be needed. Never give iron to a child or infant unless directed by a doctor to do so.

What if I miss a dose?

If you miss a dose, take it as soon as you can. However, if it is almost time for your next dose, take only that dose. Do not take double or extra doses.

What may interact with polysaccharide-iron complex?

If you are taking this iron product, you should not take iron in any other medicine or dietary supplement. *Other medications that may interact with iron:*

- alendronate
- antacids
- ascorbic acid (vitamin C)
- calcium carbonate
- cefdinir
- chloramphenicol
- cholestyramine
- deferoxamine
- dimercaprol
- etidronate
- levodopa or Sinemet®
- medicines for stomach ulcers or other stomach problems
- methyldopa
- pancreatic enzyme supplements
- penicillamine
- quinolone antibiotics (examples: Cipro®, Floxin®, Tequin® and others)
- risedronate
- tetracycline antibiotics (examples: doxycycline, tetracycline, minocycline, and others)
- tiludronate
- thyroid hormones
- zinc supplements

Tell your prescriber or health care professional about all other medicines you are taking, including non-prescription medicines. Also tell your prescriber or health care professional if you are a frequent user of drinks with caffeine or alcohol, if you smoke, or if you use illegal drugs. These may affect the way your medicine works. Check with your health care professional before stopping or starting any of your medicines.

What should I watch for while taking polysaccharide-iron complex?

You should only use iron supplements under the supervision of your health care professional. If you are told by your health care provider that you need iron supplements, you should visit your health care professional for regular blood checks. Do not use iron longer than prescribed, and do not take a higher dose than recommended. Long-term use may cause excess iron to build-up in the body. Once the cause of a low red blood cell

P

count is treated by your prescriber, it usually takes 3 to 6 months of iron therapy to reverse the problem. Pregnant women should follow the dose and length of iron treatment as directed by their doctors. Do not take iron with dairy products or antacids. If you need to take an antacid, take it 2 hours after a dose of iron. Alcohol can reduce the amount of iron taken in from your diet; avoid large amounts of alcohol.

What side effects may I notice from taking polysaccharide-iron complex?

Side effects that you should report to your prescriber or health care professional as soon as possible:
- blue lips, nails, or palms
- drowsiness
- pain on swallowing
- pale or clammy skin
- seizures (convulsions)

- stomach pain
- unusual tiredness
- vomiting
- weak, fast, or irregular heartbeat

Side effects that usually do not require medical attention (report to your prescriber or health care professional if they continue or are bothersome):
- constipation
- indigestion
- nausea or stomach upset

Where can I keep my medicine?

Keep out of the reach of children in a container that small children cannot open. Even small amounts of iron-containing products can be poisonous to a child or pet. Store at room temperature between 15 and 30 degrees C (59 and 86 degrees F). Keep container tightly closed. Throw away any unused medicine after the expiration date.

Potassium Citrate extended-release tablets

UROCIT®-K; 10 meq; Tablet, Extended Release Mission Pharmacal Co		UROCIT®-K; 5 meq; Tablet, Extended Release Mission Pharmacal Co	

What are potassium citrate extended-release tablets?

POTASSIUM CITRATE (Urocit®-K) is a medicine used to make the urine more alkaline (less acidic). This helps prevent the formation of certain kinds of kidney stones. In some cases, your health care professional may prescribe this medicine to balance the level of potassium in your body (when the potassium level is low). This medicine contains potassium, which is a naturally occurring salt that is important for the normal functioning of the heart, muscles, and nerves. Generic potassium citrate extended-release tablets are not yet available.

What should my health care professional know before I take potassium citrate?

They need to know if you have any of these conditions:
- dehydration
- diarrhea
- irregular heartbeat
- kidney disease
- liver disease
- stomach ulcers or other stomach or esophagus problems
- swallowing problems
- urinary tract infection
- an unusual reaction to potassium citrate, other medicines, foods, dyes, or preservatives
- pregnant or trying to get pregnant
- breast-feeding

How should I take this medicine?

Take potassium citrate tablets by mouth. Follow the directions on the prescription label. Swallow tablets whole with a full glass of water or juice. Do not crush or chew the tablets. Take tablets in an upright or sitting position. If possible take bedtime doses at least 10 minutes before lying down. Taking a sip of water first, before taking the tablets, may help you swallow them. Take this medicine with meals or a snack. In general, do not take this medicine with tomato juice. Tomato juice contains a high amount of sodium/salt that may not be beneficial to your medication regimen or health conditions. Take your doses at regular intervals. Do not take your medicine more often than directed. Contact your pediatrician or health care professional regarding the use of this medicine in children. Special care may be needed.

What if I miss a dose?

If you miss a dose, take it as soon as you can with food or liquids. If it is more than 2 hours since your missed dose, skip that dose and resume your normal schedule. Do not take double or extra doses.

What may interact with potassium citrate?

- ammonium chloride
- amphetamine, dextroamphetamine, or similar drugs
- antacids (especially those containing aluminum hydroxide or calcium carbonate)
- aspirin or aspirin-like drugs used for pain relief (salicylates)
- anti-inflammatory drugs (NSAIDs, such as ibuprofen)
- beta blockers, often used for high blood pressure or heart problems
- certain antibiotics such as ciprofloxacin or norfloxacin
- cisplatin

- digoxin
- ephedrine
- flecainide
- heparin
- lithium
- medicines for high blood pressure
- medicines for movement abnormalities as in Parkinson's disease, or for gastrointestinal problems
- methenamine
- penicillin G
- pseudoephedrine or phenylpropanolamine
- quinidine
- sodium polystyrene sulfonate
- water pills (diuretics)

Tell your prescriber or health care professional about all other medicines you are taking, including non-prescription medicines, nutritional supplements, or herbal products. Also tell your prescriber or health care professional if you are a frequent user of drinks with caffeine or alcohol, if you smoke, or if you use illegal drugs. These may affect the way your medicine works. Check with your health care professional before stopping or starting any of your medicines.

What should I watch for while taking potassium citrate?

Make sure to see your prescriber or health care professional for regular checks on your health condition. Potassium Citrate contains potassium. Your health care provider may monitor the level of potassium in your blood to make sure the level is not too high or too low. Too much potassium can be as dangerous as too little potassium. Potassium is a normal part of a regular diet and is found in beef, veal, ham, chicken, turkey, fish, shellfish, milk, bananas, dates, prunes, raisins, avocado, watermelon, molasses, beans, yams, broccoli, brussel sprouts, lentils, potatoes, and spinach. Salt substitutes and "low-salt" milks also contain large amounts of potassium. Ask your prescriber or health care professional

if you need to change your diet or avoid salt substitutes. Ask your health care provider about your fluid intake. If you are taking this medicine for kidney stones, it is suggested to drink plenty of water each day. Contact your health care professional if you have trouble swallowing potassium citrate tablets, or if the tablets seem to stick in your throat. If you notice tarry stools or signs of stomach bleeding, contact your health care provider right away. The shell of extended-release tablets (such as Urocit®-K) may appear intact in the stool; this is not cause for concern. The tablet will have released the medication.

What side effects may I notice from taking potassium citrate?

Side effects that you should report to your prescriber or health care professional as soon as possible:
- black, tarry stools
- blood in the stools
- confusion
- dizziness, lightheadedness, or fainting spells
- irregular heartbeat
- muscle weakness
- numbness or tingling in hands or feet
- pain on swallowing
- severe vomiting
- stomach pain or bloating
- unusual tiredness

Side effects that usually do not require medical attention (report to your prescriber or health care professional if they continue or are bothersome):
- diarrhea
- indigestion
- nausea, vomiting

Where can I keep my medicine?

Keep out of the reach of children in a container that small children cannot open. Store at room temperature between 15 and 30 degrees C (59 and 86 degrees F). Protect from light and moisture. Throw away any unused medicine after the expiration date.

| Potassium Salts effervescent tablets or powder | KLOR-CON® POWDER; 20 meq/pkt; Powder for Reconstitution Upsher-Smith Laboratories Inc | | K-LOR®; 1.5 g; Powder for Reconstitution Abbott Pharmaceutical Product Division | |

What are potassium effervescent tablets or powder?

POTASSIUM (Klorvess®, K-Lyte/Cl®, Effer-K®, Micro-K®, Klor-Con® Powder, K-Lor®) is a naturally occurring salt that is important for the normal functioning of the heart, muscles, and nerves. Too much or too little potassium in the body can cause serious problems. Potassium occurs naturally in many foods and is normally supplied by a balanced diet. Potassium supplements are used to treat potassium deficiency (hypokalemia) that occurs in certain illnesses or from use

of certain medicines. Generic effervescent tablets and powders are available.

What should my health care professional know before I take potassium salts?

They need to know if you have any of these conditions:
- dehydration
- diarrhea
- stomach ulcers or other stomach problems
- kidney disease
- irregular heartbeat

■ an unusual or allergic reaction to potassium salts, tartrazine, other medicines, foods, dyes, or preservatives

How should I take this medicine?

Dissolve potassium effervescent tablets or powders in a full glass of water and take by mouth. Always make sure the powder or tablet is fully dissolved in at least 4 fluid ounces of water or juice. Undissolved or undiluted potassium can damage your throat and stomach. Make sure the tablet or powder has stopped fizzing or is fully dissolved before you drink the liquid. Take it with or straight after food. Follow the directions on the prescription label. Take your doses at regular intervals. Do not take your medicine more often than directed.

What if I miss a dose?

If you miss a dose, take it as soon as you can with food or liquids. If it is more than 2 hours since your missed dose, skip that dose and resume your normal schedule. Do not take double or extra doses.

What may interact with potassium salts?

■ anti-inflammatory drugs (NSAIDs, such as ibuprofen)
■ beta blockers, often used for high blood pressure or heart problems
■ cisplatin
■ digoxin
■ heparin
■ medicines for high blood pressure
■ medicines for movement abnormalities as in Parkinson's disease, or for gastrointestinal problems
■ penicillin G
■ sodium polystyrene sulfonate
■ trimethoprim
■ water pills (diuretics)

Tell your prescriber or health care professional about all other medicines you are taking, including non-prescription medicines, nutritional supplements, or herbal products. Also tell your prescriber or health care professional if you are a frequent user of drinks with caffeine or alcohol, if you smoke, or if you use illegal drugs. These may affect the way your medicine works. Check with your health care professional before stopping or starting any of your medicines.

What should I watch for while taking potassium salts?

Changes in the potassium blood level can occur without symptoms, see your prescriber or health care professional for regular checks on your progress. Too much potassium can be as dangerous as too little potassium. Potassium is a normal part of a regular diet and is found in beef, veal, ham, chicken, turkey, fish, shellfish, milk, bananas, dates, prunes, raisins, avocado, watermelon, molasses, beans, yams, broccoli, brussel sprouts, lentils, potatoes, and spinach. Salt substitutes and "low-salt" milks also contain large amounts of potassium. Ask your prescriber or health care professional if you need to change your diet and avoid salt-substitutes unless otherwise directed.

What side effects may I notice from taking potassium salts?

Side effects that you should report to your prescriber or health care professional as soon as possible:
■ black, tarry stools
■ blood in the stools
■ confusion
■ dizziness, lightheadedness, or fainting spells
■ irregular heartbeat
■ muscle weakness
■ numbness or tingling in hands or feet
■ severe vomiting
■ stomach pain or bloating
■ unusual tiredness

Side effects that usually do not require medical attention (report to your prescriber or health care professional if they continue or are bothersome):
■ indigestion
■ nausea, vomiting

Where can I keep my medicine?

Keep out of the reach of children. Store at room temperature between 15 and 30 degrees C (59 and 86 degrees F). Protect from light and moisture. Throw away any unused medicine after the expiration date.

Potassium Salts tablets, extended-release tablets, or capsules

K-DUR®;
20 meq; Tablet,
Extended Release
Schering Corp

MICRO-K®;
8 meq; Capsule,
Extended Release
Ther-Rx Corp

What are potassium tablets, extended-release tablets or capsules?

POTASSIUM (K-Norm®, K-Dur®, Slow-K®, Micro-K®, and many others) is a naturally occurring salt that is important for the normal functioning of the heart, muscles, and nerves. Too much or too little potassium in the body can cause serious problems. Potassium occurs naturally in many foods and is normally supplied by a balanced diet. Potassium supplements are used to treat potassium deficiency (hypokalemia) that occurs in certain illnesses or from use of certain medicines. Potassium comes as different salts and generic potassium salts are available in tablet form.

What should my health care professional know before I take potassium salts?

They need to know if you have any of these conditions:
- dehydration
- diarrhea
- stomach ulcers or other stomach problems
- kidney disease
- irregular heartbeat
- an unusual or allergic reaction to potassium salts, other medicines, foods, dyes, or preservatives

How should I take this medicine?

Take potassium tablets or capsules by mouth. Follow the directions on the prescription label. Swallow tablets or capsules whole with a full glass of water or juice (In general, do not take this medicine with tomato juice; tomato juice contains a high amount of sodium/salt that may not be beneficial to your medication regimen or health conditions). Take tablets or capsules in an upright or sitting position. If possible take bedtime doses at least 10 minutes before lying down. Do not crush or chew the sustained-release tablets or capsules. Taking a sip of water first, before taking the tablets or capsules, may help you swallow them. If you have difficulty swallowing, you may be able to open the capsule and sprinkle the contents on applesauce or pudding, and swallow the dose without chewing. Check with your pharmacist if you are not sure whether you are taking an extended-release preparation. If potassium upsets your stomach take it with food or milk. Take your doses at regular intervals. Do not take your medicine more often than directed.

What if I miss a dose?

If you miss a dose, take it as soon as you can. If it is more than 2 hours since your missed dose, skip that dose and resume your normal schedule. Do not take double or extra doses.

What may interact with potassium salts?

- anti-inflammatory drugs (NSAIDs, such as ibuprofen)
- beta blockers, often used for high blood pressure or heart problems
- cisplatin
- digoxin
- heparin
- medicines for high blood pressure
- medicines for movement abnormalities as in Parkinson's disease, or for gastrointestinal problems
- penicillin G
- sodium polystyrene sulfonate
- water pills (diuretics)

Tell your prescriber or health care professional about all other medicines you are taking, including non-prescription medicines, nutritional supplements, or herbal products. Also tell your prescriber or health care professional if you are a frequent user of drinks with caffeine or alcohol, if you smoke, or if you use illegal drugs. These may affect the way your medicine works. Check with your health care professional before stopping or starting any of your medicines.

What should I watch for while taking potassium salts?

Changes in the potassium blood level can occur without symptoms, see your prescriber or health care professional for regular checks on your progress. Too much potassium can be as dangerous as too little potassium. Potassium is a normal part of a regular diet and is found in beef, veal, ham, chicken, turkey, fish, shellfish, milk, bananas, dates, prunes, raisins, avocado, watermelon, molasses, beans, yams, broccoli, brussel sprouts, lentils, potatoes, and spinach. Salt substitutes and "low-salt" milks also contain large amounts of potassium. Ask your prescriber or health care professional if you need to change your diet and avoid salt-substitutes unless otherwise directed. Contact your health care professional if you have trouble swallowing potassium tablets, or if the tablets seem to stick in your throat. If you notice tarry stools or signs of stomach bleeding, contact your health care provider right away. The shell of extended-release tablets (such as Slow-K®) may appear intact in the stool; this is not cause for concern. The tablet will have released the medication.

What side effects may I notice from taking potassium salts?

Side effects that you should report to your prescriber or health care professional as soon as possible:
- black, tarry stools
- blood in the stools
- confusion
- dizziness, lightheadedness, or fainting spells
- irregular heartbeat
- muscle weakness
- numbness or tingling in hands or feet
- pain on swallowing
- severe vomiting
- stomach pain or bloating
- unusual tiredness

Side effects that usually do not require medical attention (report to your prescriber or health care professional if they continue or are bothersome):
- indigestion
- nausea, vomiting

Where can I keep my medicine?

Keep out of the reach of children in a container that small children cannot open. Store at room temperature between 15 and 30 degrees C (59 and 86 degrees F). Protect from light and moisture. Throw away any unused medicine after the expiration date.

Pramipexole tablets

MIRAPEX®;
0.5 mg; Tablet
Boehringer
Ingelheim
Pharmaceuticals Inc

MIRAPEX®;
1.5 mg; Tablet
Boehringer
Ingelheim
Pharmaceuticals Inc

What are pramipexole tablets?

PRAMIPEXOLE (Mirapex®) can help treat the symptoms of Parkinson's disease. Pramipexole helps to improve muscle control and movement difficulties. Pramipexole will not cure Parkinson's disease. Pramipexole may be taken together with other medicines that control symptoms of Parkinson's. Generic pramipexole tablets are not yet available.

What should my health care professional know before I take pramipexole?

They need to know if you have any of these conditions:
- dizzy or fainting spells
- kidney disease
- heart disease
- low blood pressure
- sleeping problems
- an unusual or allergic reaction to other medicines, foods, dyes, or preservatives
- pregnant or trying to get pregnant
- breast-feeding

How should I take this medicine?

Take pramipexole tablets by mouth. Taking this medicine with food can decrease stomach upset. Follow the directions on the prescription label. Swallow the tablets with a drink of water. Take your doses at regular intervals. Do not take your medicine more often than directed. Do not stop taking pramipexole except on your prescriber's advice.

What if I miss a dose?

If you miss a dose, take it as soon as you can. If it is almost time for your next dose, take only that dose. Do not take double or extra doses.

What may interact with pramipexole?

- cimetidine (Tagamet®)
- diltiazem
- medicines for mental problems or psychotic disturbances
- medicines for sleep
- metoclopramide
- quinidine or quinine
- ranitidine (Zantac®)
- triamterene
- verapamil

Tell your prescriber or health care professional about all other medicines you are taking, including non-prescription medicines. Also tell your prescriber or health care professional if you are a frequent user of drinks with caffeine or alcohol, if you smoke, or if you use illegal drugs. These may affect the way your medicine

works. Check with your health care professional before stopping or starting any of your medicines.

What should I watch for while taking pramipexole?

Visit your prescriber or health care professional for regular checks on your progress. It may be several weeks or months before you feel the full effect of pramipexole. Continue to take your medicine on a regular schedule and do not stop taking except on your prescriber's advice. You may get dizzy or sleepy on this medication. Do not drive, use machinery, or do anything that needs mental alertness until you know how pramipexole affects you. If you find that you have sudden feelings of wanting to sleep during normal activities, like cooking, watching television, or while driving or riding in a car, you should contact your prescriber. Do not stand or sit up quickly, especially if you are an older patient. This reduces the risk of dizzy or fainting spells. Alcohol can increase possible dizziness; avoid alcoholic drinks. If you are going to have surgery, tell your prescriber or health care professional that you are taking pramipexole. Pramipexole may make your mouth dry. Chewing sugarless gum, sucking hard candy and drinking plenty of water may help. Visit your dentist regularly.

What side effects may I notice from taking pramipexole?

Side effects that you should report to your prescriber or health care professional as soon as possible:
Rare or uncommon:
- muscle pain or severe muscle weakness
- double vision or other vision problems
- fainting spells
- sudden loss of alertness or sudden feelings of sleepiness

More common:
- dizziness
- hallucinations
- mental changes
- confusion
- uncontrollable movements of the arms, face, hands, head, mouth, shoulders, or upper body
- dream disturbances or trouble with sleeping

Side effects that usually do not require medical attention (report to your prescriber or health care professional if they continue or are bothersome):
- constipation
- nausea
- drowsiness
- mild weakness
- dry mouth
- frequent urination

Where can I keep my medicine?

Keep out of the reach of children in a container that small children cannot open. Store at room temperature between 15 and 30 degrees C (59 and 86 degrees F). Keep container tightly closed. Throw away any unused medicine after the expiration date.

Pravastatin tablets

PRAVACHOL®;
20 mg; Tablet
ER Squibb and Sons
Inc

PRAVACHOL®;
40 mg; Tablet
ER Squibb and Sons
Inc

What are pravastatin tablets?

PRAVASTATIN (Pravachol®) blocks the body's ability to make cholesterol. Pravastatin can help lower blood cholesterol for patients who are at risk of getting heart disease or a stroke. It is only for patients whose cholesterol level is not controlled by diet. It is not a cure. Generic pravastatin tablets are available.

What should my health care professional know before I take pravastatin?

They need to know if you have any of these conditions:
- an alcohol problem
- any hormone disorder (such as diabetes, under-active thyroid)
- blood salt imbalance
- infection
- kidney disease
- liver disease
- low blood pressure
- muscle disorder or condition
- recent surgery
- seizures (convulsions)
- severe injury
- an unusual or allergic reaction to pravastatin, other medicines, foods, dyes, or preservatives
- pregnant or trying to get pregnant
- breast-feeding

How should I take this medicine?

Take pravastatin tablets by mouth. Follow the directions on the prescription label. Swallow the tablets with a drink of water. The usual pravastatin dose is taken once a day. You can take pravastatin with or without food. Take your doses at regular intervals. Do not take your medicine more often than directed. Contact your pediatrician or health care professional regarding the use of this medicine in children. Special care may be needed.

What if I miss a dose?

If you miss a dose, take it as soon as you can. If it is almost time for your next dose, take only that dose. Do not take double or extra doses.

What may interact with pravastatin?

- alcohol-containing beverages
- herbal medicines such as went yeast (Cholestin™)
- itraconazole
- medicines to lower cholesterol or triglycerides (examples: cholestyramine, clofibrate, colestipol, fenofibrate, gemfibrozil, niacin)
- cyclosporine
- orlistat

Tell your prescriber or health care professional about all other medicines you are taking, including non-prescription medicines, nutritional supplements, or herbal products. Also tell your prescriber or health care professional if you are a frequent user of drinks with caffeine or alcohol, if you smoke, or if you use illegal drugs. These may affect the way your medicine works. Check with your health care professional before stopping or starting any of your medicines.

What should I watch for while taking pravastatin?

Visit your prescriber or health care professional for regular checks on your progress. You will need to have regular tests to make sure your liver is working properly. Tell your prescriber or health care professional as soon as you can if you get any unexplained muscle pain, tenderness, or weakness, especially if you also have a fever and tiredness. Pravastatin is only part of a total cholesterol-lowering program. Your physician or dietician can suggest a low-cholesterol and low-fat diet that will reduce your risk of getting heart and blood vessel disease. Avoid alcohol and smoking, and keep a proper exercise schedule. If you are going to have surgery tell your prescriber or health care professional that you are taking pravastatin.

What side effects may I notice from taking pravastatin?

Side effects that you should report to your prescriber or health care professional as soon as possible:
Rare or uncommon:
- dark yellow or brown urine
- decreased urination, difficulty passing urine
- fever
- muscle pain, tenderness, cramps, or weakness
- redness, blistering, peeling or loosening of the skin, including inside the mouth
- skin rash, itching
- unusual tiredness or weakness
- yellowing of the skin or eyes

Side effects that usually do not require medical attention (report to your prescriber or health care professional if they continue or are bothersome):

- dizziness
- flu-like symptoms
- headache

Praziquantel tablets

BILTRICIDE®;
600 mg; Tablet
Schering Corp

What are praziquantel tablets?

PRAZIQUANTEL (Biltricide®) is an anthelmintic. Anthelmintics are used for treating worm infections. Praziquantel is used mainly to treat fluke and tapeworm infections. The fluke infections are also known as schistosomiasis, clonorchiasis, or opisthorchiasis. Praziquantel does not work for pinworm or other roundworm infections. Generic praziquantel tablets are not available.

What should my health care professional know before I take praziquantel?

They need to know if you have any of these conditions:

- liver disease
- worm cysts in the eye
- an unusual reaction to praziquantel, other medicines, foods, dyes, or preservatives
- pregnant or trying to get pregnant
- breast-feeding

How should I take this medicine?

Take praziquantel tablets by mouth. Follow the directions on the prescription label. Praziquantel tablets have a bitter taste that may cause gagging or vomiting. Do not chew, crush, or hold the tablets in the mouth before swallowing. Swallow the tablets whole with a small amount of liquid during meals. Take with food. Do not take your medicine more often than directed. Finish the full course of medicine prescribed by your prescriber or health care professional even if you feel better. Take at the prescribed intervals and do not miss any doses. Contact your pediatrician or health care professional regarding the use of this medicine in children. Special care may be needed. Praziquantel is not for use in children less than 4 years of age.

What if I miss a dose?

If you miss a dose, take it as soon as you can. If it is almost time for your next dose, take only that dose. Do not take double or extra doses.

What may interact with praziquantel?

- albendazole
- barbiturates, such as phenobarbital
- certain antiepileptic medications, such carbamazepine, phenytoin, fosphenytoin, oxcarbazepine
- chloroquine

Where can I keep my medicine?

Keep out of the reach of children in a container that small children cannot open. Store at room temperature below 30 degrees C (86 degrees F). Protect from light and moisture. Keep container tightly closed. Throw away any unused medicine after the expiration date.

- cimetidine
- dexamethasone
- grapefruit juice
- rifampin
- St. John's Wort, *Hypericum perforatum*

Tell your prescriber or health care professional about all other medicines you are taking, including non-prescription medicines, nutritional supplements, or herbal products. Also tell your prescriber or health care professional if you are a frequent user of drinks with caffeine or alcohol, if you smoke, or if you use illegal drugs. These may affect the way your medicine works. Check with your health care professional before stopping or starting any of your medicines.

What should I watch for while taking praziquantel?

Visit your prescriber or health care professional to check that your infection has gone. If your symptoms do not improve after you have taken finished the full course of praziquantel, or if your symptoms become worse, check with your healthcare provider. You may get dizzy, drowsy, or less alert while taking praziquantel. Do not drive, use machinery, or do anything that needs mental alertness while you are taking praziquantel and for 24 hours after you stop taking it. Practice good hygiene to prevent infection of others. Wash your hands, scrub your fingernails and shower often. Every day change and launder linens and undergarments. Scrub toilets often and keep floors clean. Other people in your house may need treatment. Check with your prescriber or health care professional. To prevent worm infections, treat pets regularly for worms. Keep children out of contact with animal feces (wastes).

What side effects may I notice from taking praziquantel?

Side effects that you should report to your prescriber or health care professional as soon as possible:

- difficulty breathing
- skin rash, hives, or itching

Side effects that usually do not require medical attention (report to your prescriber or health care professional if they continue or are bothersome):

- diarrhea
- dizziness

- drowsiness
- fever
- headache
- increased sweating
- loss of appetite
- nausea or vomiting
- stomach cramps

Where can I keep my medicine?
Keep out of the reach of children in a container that small children cannot open. Store below 86 degrees F (30 degrees C). Store away from heat and direct light. Do not store in the bathroom, near the kitchen sink, or in other damp places. Discard any unused or expired medication.

Prazosin capsules

| MINIPRESS®; 2 mg; Capsule Pfizer Laboratories Div Pfizer Inc | | MINIPRESS®; 5 mg; Capsule Pfizer Laboratories Div Pfizer Inc | |

What are prazosin capsules?
PRAZOSIN (Minipress®) is an antihypertensive. Prazosin lowers, but does not cure, high blood pressure. It works by relaxing the blood vessels. Prazosin is sometimes used for prostate problems. Generic prazosin capsules are available.

What should my health care professional know before I take prazosin?
They need to know if you have any of the following conditions:
- angina
- kidney disease
- an unusual or allergic reaction to prazosin, other medicines, foods, dyes, or preservatives
- pregnant or trying to get pregnant
- breast-feeding

How should I take this medicine?
Take prazosin capsules by mouth. Follow the directions on the prescription label. Swallow the capsules with a drink of water. Taking the capsules with food can help to reduce side effects. Take your doses at regular intervals. Do not take your medicine more often than directed. Do not stop taking except on your prescriber's advice. Contact your pediatrician or health care professional regarding the use of this medicine in children. Special care may be needed.

What if I miss a dose?
If you miss a dose, take it as soon as you can. If it is almost time for your next dose, take only that dose. Do not take double or extra doses.

What may interact with prazosin?
Do not take prazosin if you are taking the following medications: other alpha-blockers such as alfuzosin, doxazosin, phentolamine, phenoxybenzamine, tamsulosin, and terazosin.
Prazosin may interact with the following drugs:
- medicines for colds or breathing difficulty
- medicines for high blood pressure
- sildenafil (doses of sildenafil higher than 25 mg should be taken at least 4 hours apart from prazosin)
- tadalafil (Cialis®)
- vardenafil (Levitra®)
- water pills

Tell your prescriber or health care professional about all other medicines you are taking, including nonprescription medicines, nutritional supplements, or herbal products. Also tell your prescriber or health care professional if you are a frequent user of drinks with caffeine or alcohol, if you smoke, or if you use illegal drugs. These may affect the way your medicine works. Check with your prescriber or health care professional before stopping or starting any of your medicines.

What should I watch for while taking prazosin?
Check your blood pressure regularly. Ask your prescriber or health care professional what your blood pressure should be and when you should contact him or her. You may feel drowsy or dizzy. Do not drive, use machinery, or do anything that requires mental alertness until you know how prazosin affects you. To reduce the risk of dizzy or fainting spells, do not sit or stand up quickly. Avoid alcoholic drinks; they can make you more drowsy, and can increase flushing and rapid heartbeats. Taking initial doses of prazosin at bedtime can lessen the effects of drowsiness and dizziness, but be careful if you have to get up during the night. Drowsiness and dizziness are more likely to occur after the first dose, after an increase in dose, or during hot weather or exercise. These effects can decrease once your body adjusts to this medicine. Although extremely rare in men taking prazosin, contact you health care provider immediately if you experience prolonged and painful erection of the penis which is unrelated to sexual activity (priapism). If not brought to immediate medical attention, priapism can lead to permanent erectile dysfunction (impotence). Your mouth may get dry. Chewing sugarless gum or sucking hard candy, and drinking plenty of water, will help. Do not take nonprescription medicine for weight loss without asking your prescriber or health care professional. Also, do not take cough and cold, hay fever or sinus medications without asking your prescriber or health care professional. If you are going to have surgery, tell your prescriber or health care professional that you are taking prazosin.

What side effects may I notice from taking prazosin?
Side effects that you should report to your prescriber or health care professional as soon as possible:

Rare or uncommon:
- difficulty breathing, shortness of breath
- prolonged painful erection of the penis (priapism)

More common:
- blurred vision
- fainting spells, lightheadedness
- irregular heartbeat, palpitations or chest pain
- mental depression
- swelling of the legs and ankles
- vomiting

Side effects that usually do not require medical attention (report to your prescriber or health care professional if they continue or are bothersome):
- constipation or diarrhea
- drowsiness or dizziness

- dry mouth
- headache
- nausea
- sexual difficulties (impotence)
- stomach pain
- unusual weakness or tiredness

Where can I keep my medicine?

Keep out of the reach of children in a container that small children cannot open. Store at room temperature between 15 and 30 degrees C (59 and 86 degrees F). Protect from light. Keep container tightly closed. Throw away any unused medicine after the expiration date.

Prednisolone tablets

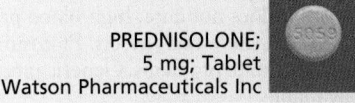

PREDNISOLONE;
5 mg; Tablet
Watson Pharmaceuticals Inc

What are prednisolone tablets?

PREDNISOLONE (Delta-Cortef®) is a corticosteroid. It helps to reduce swelling, redness, itching, and allergic reactions and can be used to treat severe allergies, skin problems, asthma, arthritis and other conditions. Generic prednisolone tablets are available.

What should my health care professional know before I take prednisolone?

They need to know if you have any of these conditions:
- cataracts or glaucoma
- Cushing's syndrome
- diabetes
- heart problems, or previous heart attack
- high blood pressure or blood clotting disorder
- infection, such as herpes, measles, tuberculosis or chickenpox
- myasthenia gravis
- psychosis
- osteoporosis
- recent surgery
- seizures (convulsions)
- stomach or intestinal disease, including colitis
- under-active thyroid
- an unusual or allergic reaction to prednisolone, other corticosteroids, medicines, foods, dyes, or preservatives
- pregnant or trying to get pregnant
- breast-feeding

How should I take this medicine?

Take prednisolone tablets by mouth. Follow the directions on the prescription label. Swallow the tablets with a drink of water. Take with food or milk to avoid stomach upset. If you are only taking prednisolone once a day, take it in the morning, which is the time your body normally secretes cortisol. Take your doses at regular intervals. Do not take your medicine more often than directed. Contact your pediatrician or health care professional regarding the use of this medicine in children. Special care may be needed.

What if I miss a dose?

If you miss a dose, take it a soon as you can. If it is almost time for your next dose, consult your prescriber or health care professional. You may need to miss a dose or take a double dose, depending on your condition and treatment. Do not take double or extra doses without advice.

What may interact with prednisolone?

- acetazolamide
- amphotericin B
- anti-inflammatory drugs (NSAIDs, such as ibuprofen)
- barbiturate medicines for inducing sleep or treating seizures
- blood thinners
- bosentan
- certain heart medicines
- female hormones, including contraceptives or birth control pills
- live virus vaccines, and other toxoids and vaccines
- medicines for diabetes
- phenytoin
- rifabutin
- rifampin
- water pills

Tell your prescriber or health care professional about all other medicines you are taking, including non-prescription medicines, nutritional supplements, or herbal products. Also tell your prescriber or health care professional if you are a frequent user of drinks with caffeine or alcohol, if you smoke, or if you use illegal drugs. These may affect the way your medicine works. Check with your health care professional before stopping or starting any of your medicines.

What should I watch for while taking prednisolone?

Visit your prescriber or health care professional for regular checks on your progress. If you are taking prednisolone over a prolonged period, carry an identification card with your name and address, the type and dose of your medicine, and your prescriber's name and address. Do not suddenly stop taking prednisolone. You may need to gradually reduce the dose, so that your body can adjust. Follow the advice of your prescriber or health care professional. If you are taking prednisolone regularly, avoid contact with people who have an infection. You will have an increased risk from infection while taking prednisolone. Do not receive any vaccinations as you may get a strong reaction, and avoid people who have recently taken oral polio vaccine. Tell your prescriber or health care professional if you are exposed to anyone with measles or chickenpox, or if you develop sores or blisters that do not heal properly. If you are going to have surgery, tell your prescriber or health care professional that you have received prednisolone within the last twelve months. If you receive prednisolone every day, you may need to watch your diet. Your body can lose potassium while you are taking this medicine. Ask your prescriber or health care professional about your diet. Prednisolone can affect your blood sugar. If you are diabetic check with your prescriber or health care professional if you need help adjusting the dose of your diabetic medicine. Alcohol can increase the risk of getting serious side effects while you are taking prednisolone. Avoid alcoholic drinks. Prednisolone can interfere with certain lab tests and can cause false skin test results. People who are taking certain dosages of prednisolone may need to avoid immunization with certain vaccines or may need to have changes in their vaccination schedules to ensure adequate protection from certain diseases. Make sure to tell your prescriber or health care professional that you are taking prednisolone before receiving any vaccine.

What side effects may I notice from taking prednisolone?

Side effects that you should report to your prescriber or health care professional as soon as possible:

- bloody or black, tarry stools
- confusion, excitement, restlessness, a false sense of well-being
- eye pain, decreased or blurred vision, or bulging eyes
- fever, sore throat, sneezing, cough, or other signs of infection, wounds that will not heal
- frequent passing of urine
- increased thirst
- irregular heartbeat
- menstrual problems
- mental depression, mood swings, mistaken feelings of self-importance or of being mistreated
- muscle cramps or weakness
- nausea, vomiting
- pain in hips, back, ribs, arms, shoulders, or legs
- rounding out of face
- skin problems, acne, thin and shiny skin
- stomach pain
- swelling of feet or lower legs
- unusual bruising, pinpoint red spots on the skin
- unusual tiredness or weakness
- weight gain or weight loss

Side effects that usually do not require medical attention (report to your prescriber or health care professional if they continue or are bothersome):

- diarrhea or constipation
- headache
- increased or decreased appetite
- increased sweating
- nervousness, restlessness, or difficulty sleeping
- upset stomach
- unusual increased growth of hair on the face or body

Where can I keep my medicine?

Keep out of the reach of children in a container that small children cannot open. Store at room temperature between 15 and 30 degrees C (59 and 86 degrees F). Throw away any unused medicine after the expiration date.

Prednisone tablets

PREDNISONE;
5 mg; Tablet
Mutual/United
Research
Laboratories

PREDNISONE;
10 mg; Tablet
West Ward
Pharmaceutical Corp

What are prednisone tablets?

PREDNISONE (Deltasone®) is a corticosteroid. It helps to reduce swelling, redness, itching, and allergic reactions and can be used to treat severe allergies, skin problems, asthma, arthritis and other conditions. Generic prednisone tablets are available.

What should my health care professional know before I take prednisone?

They need to know if you have any of these conditions:
- cataracts or glaucoma
- Cushing's syndrome
- diabetes
- heart problems, or previous heart attack
- high blood pressure or blood clotting disorder
- infection, such as herpes, measles, tuberculosis or chickenpox
- myasthenia gravis
- pschosis
- osteoporosis
- recent surgery
- seizures (convulsions)
- stomach or intestinal disease, including colitis
- under-active thyroid

P

- an unusual or allergic reaction to prednisone, other corticosteroids, medicines, foods, dyes, or preservatives
- pregnant or trying to get pregnant
- breast-feeding

How should I take this medicine?

Take prednisone tablets by mouth. Follow the directions on the prescription label. Swallow the tablets with a drink of water. Take with food or milk to avoid stomach upset. If you are only taking prednisone once a day, take it in the morning, which is the time your body normally secretes cortisol. Take your doses at regular intervals. Do not take your medicine more often than directed. Contact your pediatrician or health care professional regarding the use of this medicine in children. Special care may be needed.

What if I miss a dose?

If you miss a dose, take it a soon as you can. If it is almost time for your next dose, consult your prescriber or health care professional. You may need to miss a dose or take a double dose, depending on your condition and treatment. Do not take double or extra doses without advice.

What may interact with prednisone?

- acetazolamide
- anti-inflammatory drugs (NSAIDs, such as ibuprofen)
- barbiturate medicines for inducing sleep or treating seizures
- bosentan
- certain heart medicines
- female hormones, including contraceptives or birth control pills
- live virus vaccines, and other toxoids and vaccines
- medicines for diabetes
- phenytoin
- rifabutin
- rifampin
- water pills
- warfarin

Tell your prescriber or health care professional about all other medicines you are taking, including non-prescription medicines, nutritional supplements, or herbal products. Also tell your prescriber or health care professional if you are a frequent user of drinks with caffeine or alcohol, if you smoke, or if you use illegal drugs. These may affect the way your medicine works. Check with your health care professional before stopping or starting any of your medicines.

What should I watch for while taking prednisone?

Visit your prescriber or health care professional for regular checks on your progress. If you are taking prednisone over a prolonged period, carry an identification card with your name and address, the type and dose of your medicine, and your prescriber's name and address. Do not suddenly stop taking prednisone. You may need

to gradually reduce the dose, so that your body can adjust. Follow the advice of your prescriber or health care professional. If you are taking prednisone regularly, avoid contact with people who have an infection. You will have an increased risk from infection while taking prednisone. Tell your prescriber or health care professional if you are exposed to anyone with measles or chickenpox, or if you develop sores or blisters that do not heal properly. People who are taking certain dosages of prednisone may need to avoid immunization with certain vaccines or may need to have changes in their vaccination schedules to ensure adequate protection from certain diseases. Make sure to tell your prescriber or health care professional that you are taking prednisone before receiving any vaccine. If you are going to have surgery, tell your prescriber or health care professional that you have received prednisone within the last twelve months. If you receive prednisone every day, you may need to watch your diet. Your body can lose potassium while you are taking this medicine. Ask your prescriber or health care professional about your diet. Prednisone can affect your blood sugar. If you are diabetic check with your prescriber or health care professional if you need help adjusting the dose of your diabetic medicine. Alcohol can increase the risk of getting serious side effects while you are taking prednisone. Avoid alcoholic drinks. Prednisone can interfere with certain laboratory tests and can cause false skin test results.

What side effects may I notice from taking prednisone?

Side effects that you should report to your prescriber or health care professional as soon as possible:
- bloody or black, tarry stools
- confusion, excitement, restlessness, a false sense of well-being
- eye pain, decreased or blurred vision, or bulging eyes
- fever, sore throat, sneezing, cough, or other signs of infection, wounds that will not heal
- frequent passing of urine
- increased thirst
- irregular heartbeat
- menstrual problems
- mental depression, mood swings, mistaken feelings of self-importance or of being mistreated
- muscle cramps or weakness
- nausea, vomiting
- pain in hips, back, ribs, arms, shoulders, or legs
- rounding out of face
- skin problems, acne, thin and shiny skin
- stomach pain
- swelling of feet or lower legs
- unusual bruising, pinpoint red spots on the skin
- unusual tiredness or weakness
- weight gain or weight loss

Side effects that usually do not require medical attention (report to your prescriber or health care professional if they continue or are bothersome):

- diarrhea or constipation
- headache
- increased or decreased appetite
- increased sweating
- nervousness, restlessness, or difficulty sleeping
- upset stomach
- unusual increased growth of hair on the face or body

Primaquine tablets

What are primaquine tablets?

PRIMAQUINE is an antimalarial agent. Primaquine treats attacks of malaria; it may be used alone or together with another medicine. Primaquine is used together with an antibiotic to treat *Pneumocystis carinii* pneumonia. Generic primaquine tablets are available.

What should my health care professional know before I take primaquine?

They need to know if you have any of these conditions:
- anemia or other blood disorders
- glucose 6-phosphate dehydrogenase (G6PD) deficiency
- methemoglobin reductase deficiency
- rheumatoid arthritis
- systemic lupus erythematosus
- an unusual or allergic reaction to primaquine, iodoquinol, other medicines, foods, dyes, or preservatives
- pregnant or trying to get pregnant
- breast-feeding

How should I take this medicine?

Take primaquine tablets by mouth. Follow the directions on the prescription label. Swallow tablets whole with a drink of water. Do not crush or chew these tablets.

If primaquine upsets your stomach take it with food or milk. Take your doses at regular intervals. Do not take your medicine more often than directed.

What if I miss a dose?

If you miss a dose, take it as soon as you can. If it is almost time for your next dose, take only that dose. Do not take double or extra doses.

What may interact with primaquine?

- quinacrine

Tell your prescriber or health care professional about all other medicines you are taking, including non-prescription medicines, nutritional supplements, or herbal products. Also tell your prescriber or health care professional if you are a frequent user of drinks with caffeine or alcohol, if you smoke, or if you use illegal drugs.

Where can I keep my medicine?

Keep out of the reach of children in a container that small children cannot open. Store at room temperature between 15 and 30 degrees C (59 and 86 degrees F). Throw away any unused medicine after the expiration date.

These may affect the way your medicine works. Check with your health care professional before stopping or starting any of your medicines.

What should I watch for while taking primaquine?

Tell your prescriber or health care professional if your symptoms do not improve in 2 to 3 days. If you are taking primaquine for a long time, visit your prescriber or health care professional for regular checks on your progress. If your urine becomes a dark color, tell your prescriber or health care professional as soon as you can. Check with your pharmacist before you visit a new area where there are malaria-carrying mosquitoes. You may need to take a different antimalarial medicine. You may get drowsy. Do not drive, use machinery, or do anything that needs mental alertness until you know how primaquine affects you.

What side effects may I notice from taking primaquine?

Side effects that you should report to your prescriber or health care professional as soon as possible:
- back, leg, or stomach pains
- bluish fingernails, lips, or skin
- dark urine
- difficulty breathing
- dizziness or lightheadedness
- fever and sore throat
- loss of appetite
- pale skin
- unusual tiredness or weakness

Side effects that usually do not require medical attention (report to your prescriber or health care professional if they continue or are bothersome):
- stomach pain or cramps
- nausea, vomiting

Where can I keep my medicine?

Keep out of the reach of children in a container that small children cannot open. Store at room temperature between 15 and 30 degrees C (59 and 86 degrees F). Protect from light. Keep container tightly closed. Throw away any unused medicine after the expiration date.

Primidone tablets or chewable tablets

MYSOLINE®;
250 mg; Tablet
Xcel
Pharmaceuticals

MYSOLINE®;
250 mg; Tablet
Xcel
Pharmaceuticals

What are primidone tablets or chewable tablets?

PRIMIDONE (Mysoline®) slows down the brain and nervous system. Primidone (Thysoline®)is a barbiturate. Primidone reduces or controls seizures or convulsions in certain types of epilepsy, except for absence (petit mal) seizures. Generic primidone tablets are available, but not chewable tablets.

What should my health care professional know before I take primidone?

They need to know if you have any of these conditions:
- an alcohol or drug abuse problem
- kidney disease or undergoing dialysis
- liver disease
- low blood pressure
- lung disease, chest infection or breathing difficulties
- mental depression or other mental illnesses
- osteoporosis or other bone diseases
- porphyria
- seizures or convulsions
- an unusual or allergic reaction to primidone, phenobarbital, other barbiturates or seizure medications, other medicines, foods, dyes, or preservatives
- pregnant or trying to get pregnant
- breast-feeding

How should I take this medicine?

Take primidone tablets by mouth. Follow the directions on the prescription label. Swallow the tablets with a drink of water. Chewable tablets can be chewed, crushed, or swallowed whole. If primidone upsets your stomach, take it with food or milk. Take your doses at regular intervals. Do not take your medicine more often than directed. Elderly patients over age 65 years may have a stronger reaction to this medicine and need smaller doses. Contact your pediatrician or health care professional regarding the use of this medication in children. Special care may be needed.

What if I miss a dose?

If you miss a dose, take it as soon as you can if it is more than an hour to your next dose. If it is almost time for your next dose, take only that dose. Do not take double or extra doses.

What may interact with primidone?

- acetaminophen
- alcohol
- alosetron
- antifungal drugs like fluconazole, griseofulvin, itraconazole or ketoconazole
- caffeine
- cancer-treating medications
- chloramphenicol
- cyclophosphamide
- cyclosporine
- digoxin
- disopyramide
- doxycycline
- female hormones, including contraceptive or birth control pills
- hormones such a prednisone or cortisone
- levothyroxine
- medicines for sleeping problems
- medicines for mental depression, anxiety or other mood problems
- medicines for treating HIV infection or AIDS
- metronidazole
- mexiletine
- prescription pain medications
- quinidine
- quinine
- riluzole
- sirolimus
- tacrolimus
- tamoxifen
- other seizure (convulsion) or epilepsy medicine
- theophylline
- warfarin

Tell your prescriber or health care professional about all other medicines you are taking, including non-prescription medicines, nutritional supplements, or herbal products. Also tell your prescriber or health care professional if you are a frequent user of drinks with caffeine or alcohol, if you smoke, or if you use illegal drugs. These may affect the way your medicine works. Check with your health care professional before stopping or starting any of your medicines.

What should I watch for while taking primidone?

Visit your prescriber or health care professional for regular checks on your progress. Take primidone at the same time each day. It may be 2 to 3 weeks before the full effects in controlling seizures are apparent. Do not suddenly stop taking primidone, you may increase the risk of seizures. Your prescriber or health care professional may want to gradually reduce the dose. Do not stop taking except on your prescriber's advice. Wear a Medic Alert bracelet or necklace. Carry an identification card with information about your condition, medications, and prescriber or health care professional. After taking primidone you may get a residual hangover effect that leaves you drowsy or dizzy. Do not drive, use machinery, or do anything that needs mental alertness until you know how primidone affects you. To reduce dizzy or fainting spells, do not sit or stand up quickly, especially if you are an older patient. Alcohol can increase possible unpleasant effects. Avoid alcoholic drinks. Primidone can reduce the effectiveness of birth control pills (oral contraceptives) or other hormonal birth control drugs. Talk to your prescriber about alternatives or use of additional birth control methods while taking this drug. If you are going to have surgery, tell your prescriber or health care professional that you are taking primidone.

What side effects may I notice from taking primidone?

Side effects that you should report to your prescriber or health care professional as soon as possible:
- blurred, double vision, or uncontrollable rolling or movements of the eyes
- irritability or mood changes
- lightheadedness or fainting spells
- shortness of breath or difficulty breathing
- redness, blistering, peeling or loosening of the skin, including inside the mouth
- skin rash, or itching
- unusual excitement or restlessness, more likely in children and the elderly
- unusual weakness or tiredness

Side effects that usually do not require medical attention (report to your prescriber or health care professional if they continue or are bothersome):
- clumsiness, unsteadiness, or a "hang-over" effect
- decreased sexual ability
- dizziness, drowsiness
- loss of appetite
- nausea or vomiting

Where can I keep my medicine?

Keep out of the reach of children in a container that small children cannot open. Store at room temperature, approximately 25 degrees C (77 degrees F). Protect from light. Keep container tightly closed. Throw away any unused medicine after the expiration date.

Probenecid tablets

PROBENECID;
500 mg; Tablet
Ivax Pharmaceuticals
Inc

PROBENECID;
500 mg; Tablet
Mylan
Pharmaceuticals Inc

What are probenecid tablets?

PROBENECID (Benemid®, Probalan®) helps to remove excess uric acid from the body. Uric acid can cause gout or gouty arthritis. Probenecid is not a cure for gout, but can help to prevent recurring gouty attacks. It is not for use in treating an attack of gout, and can make an attack worse. Certain illnesses or medications can cause an increase in uric acid. Probenecid can help to reduce the risk of complications (such as kidney stones) that may arise as a result of an increase in uric acid levels (hyperuricemia). Probenecid can also help to prolong the action of certain antibiotics and make them more effective. Generic probenecid tablets are available.

What should my health care professional know before I take probenecid?

They need to know if you have any of these conditions:
- blood disorders or disease
- kidney disease, or kidney stones
- recent radiation therapy
- stomach ulcers
- an unusual or allergic reaction to probenecid, other medicines, foods, dyes, or preservatives
- pregnant or trying to get pregnant
- breast-feeding

How should I take this medicine?

Take probenecid tablets by mouth. Follow the directions on the prescription label. Swallow the tablets with a drink of water. Take your doses at regular intervals. Do not take your medicine more often than directed. Contact your pediatrician or health care profes-

sional regarding the use of this medicine in children. Special care may be needed.

What if I miss a dose?

If you miss a dose, take it as soon as you can. If it is almost time for your next dose, take only that dose. Do not take double or extra doses.

What may interact with probenecid?

- alcohol
- allopurinol
- anti-inflammatory drugs (NSAIDs, such as ibuprofen)
- antibiotics including penicillins
- antiviral medicines such as acyclovir, famciclovir, ganciclovir
- aspirin and aspirin-like medicines
- clofibrate
- diazoxide
- entacapone
- ethambutol
- heparin
- lorazepam
- mecamylamine
- methotrexate
- nitrofurantoin
- pyrazinamide, PZA
- water pills

Tell your prescriber or health care professional about all other medicines you are taking, including non-prescription medicines, nutritional supplements, or herbal products. Also tell your prescriber or health care professional if you are a frequent user of drinks with caffeine or alcohol, if you smoke, or if you use illegal drugs. These may affect the way your medicine works. Check

with your health care professional before stopping or starting any of your medicines.

What should I watch for while taking probenecid?

It may take several months before you see the full effect of probenecid. Do not stop taking except on your prescriber or health care professional's advice. Probenecid is only effective if you keep taking it regularly even if you have an attack of gout. Your prescriber or health care professional will prescribe other tablets to treat an acute attack. Aspirin and non-steroidal anti-inflammatory drugs like ibuprofen can make probenecid less effective. Do not treat yourself for headaches or pain; ask your prescriber or health care professional for advice. Alcohol can increase the amount of uric acid in your body and aggravate gout. Alcohol can also make probenecid less effective. Avoid alcoholic drinks. Drink 10 or more full glasses of water a day while taking probenecid. This will help to prevent formation of kidney stones and other possible kidney problems by removing excess uric acid. Probenecid works best when the urine is alkaline (non-acidic). Ask your prescriber or health care professional about which foods or juices to avoid, and about other foods, beverages or antacids that may help to make the urine alkaline. Probenecid can interfere with the results of copper sulfate urine tests (Clinitest®), but not with glucose enzymatic urine sugar tests (Clinistix®). Diabetic patients may get false results.

What side effects may I notice from taking probenecid?

Side effects that you should report to your prescriber or health care professional as soon as possible:
- blood in urine
- difficulty breathing, wheezing or shortness of breath
- fever, chills or sore throat
- lower back or side pain
- mouth sores
- pain or difficulty passing urine
- skin rash and itching (hives)
- swelling of the feet, ankles, face or lips
- unusual weakness or tiredness
- unusual bleeding or bruising

Side effects that usually do not require medical attention (report to your prescriber or health care professional if they continue or are bothersome):
- dizziness
- flushing
- frequent passing of urine
- hair loss
- headache
- loss of appetite
- nausea, vomiting
- painful or swollen joints

Where can I keep my medicine?

Keep out of the reach of children in a container that small children cannot open. Store at room temperature between 15 and 30 degrees C (59 and 86 degrees F). Keep container tightly closed. Throw away any unused medicine after the expiration date.

Procainamide capsules

PRONESTYL®;
500 mg; Capsule
ER Squibb and Sons
Inc

PROCAINAMIDE;
375 mg; Capsule
Ivax Pharmaceuticals
Inc

What are procainamide capsules?

PROCAINAMIDE (Pronestyl®) is an antiarrhythmic agent. Procainamide treats irregular heart rhythm and can slow rapid heartbeats (tachycardia). Procainamide can help your heart to return to and maintain a normal rhythm. Generic procainamide capsules are available.

What should my health care professional know before I take procainamide?

They need to know if you have any of these conditions:
- anemia or blood disease
- dental disease
- having intramuscular injections
- heart disease or heart rhythm disorders
- kidney disease
- liver disease
- low blood pressure
- myasthenia gravis
- neuropathy
- skin disease
- systemic lupus erythematosus

- an unusual or allergic reaction to procainamide, procaine, other medicines, foods, dyes, or preservatives
- pregnant or trying to get pregnant
- breast-feeding

How should I take this medicine?

Take procainamide capsules by mouth. Follow the directions on the prescription label. Swallow the capsules with a drink of water. Take procainamide on an empty stomach, 1 hour before or 2 hours after eating, and take with plenty of water. If stomach upset occurs, however, you can take procainamide with food. Take your doses at regular intervals. Do not take your medicine more often than directed. Contact your pediatrician or health care professional regarding the use of this medicine in children. Special care may be needed. Elderly patients over 65 years old may have a stronger reaction to this medicine and may need smaller doses.

What if I miss a dose?

If you miss a dose, take it as soon as you can if it is not more than two hours since your dose was due. If it is almost time for your next dose, take only that dose. Do not take double or extra doses.

What may interact with procainamide?

- alosetron
- arsenic trioxide
- bepridil
- beta-blockers, often used for high blood pressure or heart problems
- certain antibiotics (such as clarithromycin, erythromycin, gatifloxacin, grepafloxacin, levofloxacin, moxifloxacin, ofloxacin, sparfloxacin)
- cimetidine
- cisapride
- cyclobenzaprine
- ginger
- hawthorn
- maprotiline
- medicines for asthma or breathing difficulties
- medicines for mental depression such as tricyclic antidepressants
- medicines for mental problems or psychotic disturbances
- medicines for movement abnormalities as in Parkinson's disease, or for gastrointestinal problems
- medicines to control blood pressure
- medicines to control heart rhythm (examples: amiodarone, disopyramide, dofetilide, flecainide, sotalol, quinidine)
- metformin
- pilocarpine
- pimozide
- probucol
- ranitidine
- terfenadine
- tricyclic antidepressants
- trimethoprim
- water pills (diuretics)

Tell your prescriber or health care professional about all other medicines you are taking, including non-prescription medicines, nutritional supplements, or herbal products. Also tell your prescriber or health care professional if you are a frequent user of drinks with caffeine or alcohol, if you smoke, or if you use illegal drugs. These may affect the way your medicine works. Check with your health care professional before stopping or starting any of your medicines.

What should I watch for while taking procainamide?

Visit your prescriber or health care professional for regular checks on your progress. Do not stop taking procainamide suddenly; this may cause serious, heart-related side effects. Because your condition and the use of procainamide carry some risk, it is a good idea to carry an identification card, necklace or bracelet with details of your condition, medications and prescriber or health care professional. Check your heart rate (pulse) and blood pressure regularly while you are taking procainamide. Ask your prescriber or health care professional what your heart rate and blood pressure should be, and when you should contact him or her. Your prescriber or health care professional also may schedule regular blood tests and electrocardiograms to check your progress. You may feel dizzy or faint. Do not drive, use machinery, or do anything that needs mental alertness until you know how procainamide affects you. To reduce the risk of dizzy or fainting spells, do not sit or stand up quickly, especially if you are an older patient. Alcohol can make you more dizzy, increase flushing and rapid heartbeats. Avoid alcoholic drinks. If you are going to have surgery, tell your prescriber or health care professional that you are taking procainamide.

What side effects may I notice from taking procainamide?

Side effects that you should report to your prescriber or health care professional as soon as possible:
- changes in behavior, mood, or mental ability including mental depression
- chest pain or palpitations
- confusion
- dark yellow or brown urine
- decrease in the amount of urine passed
- difficulty breathing, shortness of breath, hoarseness, or tightening of the throat
- fainting spells, dizziness or lightheadedness
- fever, chills, or sore throat
- hallucinations (seeing, feeling, or hearing things that are not there)
- hives or flushing
- irregular or fast heartbeat
- joint or muscle pain or swelling
- skin rash, redness, blistering, or itching
- swelling of your face, lips, tongue, hands, or feet
- unusual bruising, bleeding, or pinpoint red spots on the skin
- unusual weakness or tiredness
- tingling or numbness in the hands or feet
- vomiting
- yellowing of the eyes or skin

Side effects that usually do not require medical attention (report to your prescriber or health care professional if they continue or are bothersome):
- diarrhea
- loss of appetite
- nausea
- stomach pain

Where can I keep my medicine?

Keep out of the reach of children in a container that small children cannot open. Store at room temperature between 15 and 30 degrees C (59 and 86 degrees F). Keep container tightly closed. Protect from moisture. Throw away any unused medicine after the expiration date.

Procainamide tablets, extended-release tablets, or sustained-release tablets

PROCANBID®; 500 mg; Tablet, Extended Release Monarch Pharmaceuticals Inc	
PRONESTYL-SR®; 500 mg; Tablet, Extended Release ER Squibb and Sons Inc	

What are procainamide extended-release or sustained-release tablets?

PROCAINAMIDE (Procanbid™ Pronestyl-SR®) is an antiarrhythmic agent. Procainamide treats irregular heart rhythm and can slow rapid heartbeats (tachycardia). Procainamide can help your heart to return to and maintain a normal rhythm. Some formulations of procainamide are not interchangeable. Make sure you keep to the same brand unless your prescriber or health care professional tells you otherwise. Generic procainamide extended-release tablets are available.

What should my health care professional know before I take procainamide?

They need to know if you have any of these conditions:
- anemia or blood disease
- dental disease
- having intramuscular injections
- heart disease or heart rhythm disorders
- kidney disease
- liver disease
- low blood pressure
- myasthenia gravis
- neuropathy
- skin disease
- systemic lupus erythematosus
- an unusual or allergic reaction to procainamide, procaine, other medicines, foods, dyes, or preservatives
- pregnant or trying to get pregnant
- breast-feeding

How should I take this medicine?

Take procainamide tablets by mouth. Follow the directions on the prescription label. Swallow the tablets whole with a drink of water; do not crush or chew. Take procainamide on an empty stomach, 1 hour before or 2 hours after eating, and take with plenty of water. If stomach upset occurs, however, you can take procainamide with food. Take your doses at regular intervals. Do not take your medicine more often than directed. Contact your pediatrician or health care professional regarding the use of this medicine in children. Special care may be needed. Elderly patients over 65 years old may have a stronger reaction to this medicine and may need smaller doses.

What if I miss a dose?

If you miss a dose, take it as soon as you can if it is not more than four hours since your dose was due (except for Procanbid™ tablets, which should not be taken unless 8 hours before the next dose.) If it is almost time for your next dose, take only that dose. Do not take double or extra doses. Consult your prescriber or health care professional if you are in doubt.

What may interact with procainamide?

- alosetron
- arsenic trioxide
- bepridil
- beta-blockers, often used for high blood pressure or heart problems
- certain antibiotics (such as clarithromycin, erythromycin, gatifloxacin, grepafloxacin, levofloxacin, moxifloxacin, ofloxacin, sparfloxacin)
- cimetidine
- cisapride
- cyclobenzaprine
- ginger
- hawth orn
- maprotiline
- medicines for asthma or breathing difficulties
- medicines for mental depression such as tricyclic antidepressants
- medicines for mental problems or psychotic disturbances
- medicines for movement abnormalities as in Parkinson's disease, or for gastrointestinal problems
- medicines to control blood pressure
- medicines to control heart rhythm (examples: amiodarone, disopyramide, dofetilide, flecainide, sotalol, quinidine)
- metformin
- pilocarpine
- pimozide
- probucol
- ranitidine
- terfenadine
- tricyclic antidepressants
- trimethoprim
- water pills (diuretics)

Tell your prescriber or health care professional about all other medicines you are taking, including non-prescription medicines, nutritional supplements, or herbal products. Also tell your prescriber or health care professional if you are a frequent user of drinks with caffeine or alcohol, if you smoke, or if you use illegal drugs. These may affect the way your medicine works. Check with your health care professional before stopping or starting any of your medicines.

What should I watch for while taking procainamide?

Visit your prescriber or health care professional for regular checks on your progress. Do not stop taking procainamide suddenly; this may cause serious, heart-related side effects. Because your condition and the use of procainamide carry some risk, it is a good idea to carry an identification card, necklace or bracelet with details of your condition, medications and prescriber or health care professional. Check your heart rate (pulse) and blood pressure regularly while you are taking procainamide. Ask your prescriber or health care professional what your heart rate and blood pressure should be, and when you should contact him or her. Your prescriber or health care professional also may schedule regular blood tests and electrocardiograms to check your progress. You may feel dizzy or faint. Do not drive, use machinery, or do anything that needs mental alertness until you know how procainamide affects you. To reduce the risk of dizzy or fainting spells, do not sit or stand up quickly, especially if you are an older patient. Alcohol can make you more dizzy, increase flushing and rapid heartbeats. Avoid alcoholic drinks. If you are going to have surgery, tell your prescriber or health care professional that you are taking procainamide. NOTE: The tablet shell for some brands of extended or sustained-release tablets may not dissolve; this is normal. The tablet shell may appear whole in the stool; this is not a cause for concern.

What side effects may I notice from taking procainamide?

Side effects that you should report to your prescriber or health care professional as soon as possible:
- changes in behavior, mood, or mental ability including mental depression
- chest pain or palpitations
- confusion

- dark yellow or brown urine
- decrease in the amount of urine passed
- difficulty breathing, shortness of breath, hoarseness, or tightening of the throat
- fainting spells, dizziness or lightheadedness
- fever, chills, or sore throat
- hallucinations (seeing, feeling, or hearing things that are not there)
- hives or flushing
- irregular or fast heartbeat
- joint or muscle pain or swelling
- skin rash, redness, blistering, or itching
- swelling of your face, lips, tongue, hands, or feet
- unusual bruising, bleeding, or pinpoint red spots on the skin
- unusual weakness or tiredness
- tingling or numbness in the hands or feet
- vomiting
- yellowing of the eyes or skin

Side effects that usually do not require medical attention (report to your prescriber or health care professional if they continue or are bothersome):
- diarrhea
- loss of appetite
- nausea
- stomach pain

Where can I keep my medicine?

Keep out of the reach of children in a container that small children cannot open. Store at room temperature between 15 and 30 degrees C (59 and 86 degrees F). Keep container tightly closed. Protect from moisture. Throw away any unused medicine after the expiration date.

Procarbazine capsules

MATULANE®;
50 mg; Capsule
Sigma Tau Pharmaceuticals Inc

What are procarbazine capsules?

PROCARBAZINE (Matulane®) is a type of chemotherapy for treating cancer. Procarbazine interferes with the growth of cells. It is used to treat a cancer of the blood called Hodgkin's disease. It is also sometimes used to treat other types of cancer. Generic procarbazine capsules are not yet available.

What should my health care professional know before I take procarbazine?

They need to know if you have any of these conditions:
- if you frequently drink alcohol-containing beverages
- bleeding problems or blood disorders
- dental disease
- heart disease, including irregular heart rate, heart failure, or coronary artery disease
- infection (especially virus infection such as chickenpox or herpes)
- kidney disease
- liver disease

- Parkinson's disease
- pheochromocytoma
- psychiatric disease such as bipolar disorder, mania, or paranoid schizophrenia
- recent radiation therapy
- seizures (convulsions)
- smoke tobacco
- stroke or other vascular disease
- thyroid disease
- an unusual or allergic reaction to procarbazine, other chemotherapy, other medicines, foods, dyes, or preservatives
- pregnant or trying to get pregnant
- breast-feeding

How should I take this medicine?

Take procarbazine capsules by mouth. Follow the directions on the prescription label. Swallow the capsules with a drink of water. Take your doses at regular intervals. Do not take your medicine more often than directed. Finish the full course prescribed by your doctor or health care professional, even if the capsules make you feel unwell. Do not stop taking except on your prescriber's advice.

What if I miss a dose?

If you miss a dose, take it as soon as you can. If it is almost time for your next dose, take only that dose. Do not take double or extra doses. If you vomit after taking a dose, call your prescriber or health care professional for advice.

What may interact with procarbazine?

- alcohol
- buproprion
- caffeine
- cocaine
- diet pills, stimulants, or amphetamine-like drugs
- furazolidone
- guarana
- linezolid
- medicines for allergies, colds, hayfever, sinus, and breathing difficulties
- medicines for headaches or migraine (such as naratriptan, rizatriptan, sumatriptan, zolmitriptan, or Midrin®)
- medicines for high blood pressure and heart medicines
- medicines called MAO inhibitors [such as phenelzine (Nardil®), tranylcypromine (Parnate®), isocarboxazid (Marplan®)]
- medicines for mental depression, anxiety, psychotic disturbances, or other mental problems
- meperidine
- phenytoin
- some medications for Parkinson's disease, such as entacapone, levodopa, or tolcapone
- tramadol
- tryptophan
- tyramine (present in some foods such as wine, yogurt, cheese, ripe bananas, yeast, meat extracts, smoked or pickled meats; ask your nutritionist for a complete list of foods to avoid)
- vaccines

Tell your prescriber or health care professional about all other medicines you are taking, including non-prescription medicines, nutritional supplements, or herbal products. Also tell your prescriber or health care professional if you are a frequent user of drinks with caffeine or alcohol, if you smoke, or if you use illegal drugs. These may affect the way your medicine works. Check with your health care professional before stopping or starting any of your medicines.

What should I watch for while taking procarbazine?

Visit your prescriber or health care professional for checks on your progress. You will need to have regular blood checks. The side effects of procarbazine can continue after you finish your treatment; report side effects promptly. Procarbazine may make you feel generally unwell. This is not uncommon because procarbazine affects good cells as well as cancer cells. Report any side effects as above, but continue your course of medicine even though you feel ill, unless your prescriber or health care professional tells you to stop. While you are using procarbazine, you will be more susceptible to infection. Try to avoid people with colds, flu, and bronchitis. Do not have any vaccinations without your prescriber's approval and avoid anyone who has recently had oral polio vaccine. Avoid taking aspirin, acetaminophen (Tylenol®), ibuprofen (Advil®), naproxen (Aleve®), or ketoprofen (Orudis® KT) products as these may hide a fever, unless instructed to by your prescriber or health care professional. Call your prescriber or health care professional for advice if you get a fever, chills or sore throat. Do not treat yourself. Do not take any nonprescription products for coughs, colds, nasal congestion, hay fever, bites or stings without asking your prescriber or health care professional. You may get dizzy. Do not drive, use machinery, or do anything that needs mental alertness until you know how procarbazine affects you. To reduce the risk of dizzy or fainting spells, do not sit or stand up quickly, especially if you are an older patient. Procarbazine can cause blood problems. This can mean slow healing and a risk of infection. Try to avoid cutting or injuring yourself. Problems can arise if you need dental work, and in the day to day care of your teeth. Try to avoid damage to your teeth and gums when you brush or floss your teeth. Alcohol and caffeine can cause serious reactions with procarbazine. Avoid alcoholic drinks and those containing caffeine, such as tea, coffee, cola or chocolate while you are taking procarbazine and for 14 days afterward. Avoid foods containing high amounts of tyramine (see interactions above), while you are taking procarbazine and for 14 days afterward. These foods might cause a serious reaction with procarbazine. Procarbazine can change male sperm or female eggs. Talk to your prescriber or health care professional about how this medicine can affect your ability to have normal babies. It is recommended that you stop smoking tobacco products (like cigarettes or cigars) while taking procarbazine. Smoking tobacco products while receiving treatment with procarbazine may increase your risk of developing lung cancer after completing therapy. If you are going to have surgery, tell your prescriber or health care professional if you have taken procarbazine within the last 2 weeks.

What side effects may I notice from taking procarbazine?

Side effects that you should report to your prescriber or health care professional as soon as possible:
- low blood counts—procarbazine may decrease the number of white blood cells, red blood cells and platelets. You may be at increased risk for infections and bleeding.
- signs of infection—fever or chills, cough, sore throat, pain or difficulty passing urine
- signs of decreased platelets or bleeding—bruising, pinpoint red spots on the skin, black, tarry stools, blood in the urine
- signs of decreased red blood cells—unusual weakness or tiredness, fainting spells, lightheadedness

- burning, tingling or pricking feeling in the skin
- difficulty breathing, wheezing or cough
- irregular heartbeat, palpitations or chest pain
- lower back pain
- missed menstrual periods
- mouth or throat sores
- nervousness, confusion, nightmares, hallucinations
- seizures (convulsions)
- stiff neck, sweating and severe headache
- swollen face
- trembling
- vomiting
- yellowing of the eyes or skin

Side effects that usually do not require medical attention (report to your prescriber or health care professional if they continue or are bothersome):

- change in skin color (darkening)

- diarrhea
- difficulty sleeping
- dizziness
- headache
- increased sensitivity to the sun or ultraviolet light
- loss of appetite
- mental depression
- muscle or joint aches and pains
- nausea

Where can I keep my medicine?

Keep out of the reach of children in a container that small children cannot open. Store at room temperature between 15 and 30 degrees C (59 and 86 degrees F). Protect from light. Keep container tightly closed. Throw away any unused medicine after the expiration date.

Prochlorperazine tablets and extended-release capsules

PROCHLORPERAZINE;
10 mg; Tablet
Breckenridge Inc

COMPAZINE®;
15 mg; Capsule,
Extended Release
SmithKline Beecham
Co

What are prochlorperazine tablets?

PROCHLORPERAZINE (Compazine®) helps to control nausea and vomiting that can occur after surgery, or with the treatment of cancer (chemotherapy). Prochlorperazine also treats psychological or mental disorders. Another use of prochlorperazine is the treatment of non-psychotic anxiety (nervousness). Generic prochlorperazine capsules and tablets are available.

What should my health care professional know before I take prochlorperazine?

They need to know if you have any of these conditions:

- blood disorders or disease
- difficulty passing urine
- glaucoma
- liver disease or jaundice
- Parkinson's disease
- pheochromocytoma
- prostate trouble
- seizures (convulsions)
- uncontrollable movement disorder
- an unusual or allergic reaction to prochlorperazine, other medicines, foods, dyes, or preservatives
- pregnant or trying to get pregnant
- breast-feeding

How should I take this medicine?

Take prochlorperazine capsules and tablets by mouth. Follow the directions on the prescription label. Swallow capsules and tablets with a drink of water. Do not crush or chew capsules. Take your doses at regular intervals. Do not take your medicine more often than directed. Contact your pediatrician or health care professional regarding the use of this medicine in children. Special care may be needed. Elderly patients over

age 65 years may have a stronger reaction to this medicine and need smaller doses.

What if I miss a dose?

If you miss a dose, take it as soon as you can. If it is almost time for your next dose, take only that dose. Do not take double or extra doses.

What may interact with prochlorperazine?

- alcohol
- bromocriptine
- dofetilide
- lithium
- medicines for movement abnormalities as in Parkinson's disease, or for gastrointestinal problems
- medicines for pain
- seizure (convulsion) or epilepsy medicine

Tell your prescriber or health care professional about all other medicines you are taking, including non-prescription medicines, nutritional supplements, or herbal products. Also tell your prescriber or health care professional if you are a frequent user of drinks with caffeine or alcohol, if you smoke, or if you use illegal drugs. These may affect the way your medicine works. Check with your health care professional before stopping or starting any of your medicines.

What should I watch for while taking prochlorperazine?

Visit your prescriber or health care professional for regular checks on your progress. Do not stop taking prochlorperazine suddenly; this can cause nausea, vomiting, and dizziness. Ask your prescriber or health care professional for advice if you are to stop taking this medicine. You may get drowsy, dizzy, or have blurred vision. Do not drive, use machinery, or do anything that needs mental alertness until you know how prochlorperazine affects you. Do not stand or sit up quickly, especially if you are an older patient. This reduces the risk of dizzy or fainting spells. Alcohol can increase possible dizziness or drowsiness. Avoid alcoholic drinks. Prochlorperazine can reduce the response of your body to heat or cold. Try not to get overheated. Avoid temperature extremes, such as saunas, hot tubs, or very hot or cold baths or showers. Dress warmly in cold weather. Prochlorperazine can make your skin more sensitive to sun or ultraviolet light. Keep out of the sun, or wear protective clothing outdoors and use a sunscreen (at least SPF 15). Do not use sun lamps or sun tanning beds or booths. Wear sunglasses to protect your eyes. Your mouth may get dry, chewing sugarless gum or sucking hard candy and drinking plenty of water will help. Do not treat yourself for coughs, colds, sore throat, or allergies. Ask your prescriber or health care professional for advice. If you are going to have surgery, tell your prescriber or health care professional that you are taking prochlorperazine.

What side effects may I notice from taking prochlorperazine?

Side effects that you should report to your prescriber or health care professional as soon as possible:
- blurred vision
- breast enlargement in men or women
- breast milk in women who are not breast-feeding
- chest pain, fast or irregular heartbeat
- confusion, restlessness
- dark yellow or brown urine
- difficulty breathing or swallowing

- dizziness or fainting spells
- drooling, shaking, movement difficulty (shuffling walk) or rigidity
- fever, chills, sore throat
- involuntary or uncontrollable movements of the eyes, mouth, head, arms, and legs
- menstrual changes
- seizures (convulsions)
- sexual difficulties (decreased sexual desire or impotence)
- slurred speech
- stomach area pain
- sweating
- unusual weakness or tiredness
- unusual bleeding or bruising
- yellowing of skin or eyes

Side effects that usually do not require medical attention (report to your prescriber or health care professional if they continue or are bothersome):
- constipation
- difficulty passing urine
- difficulty sleeping
- drowsiness
- dry mouth
- headache
- increased sensitivity to the sun or ultraviolet light
- nasal congestion
- skin rash, or itching
- weight gain

Where can I keep my medicine?

Keep out of the reach of children in a container that small children cannot open. Store at room temperature between 15 and 30 degrees C (59 and 86 degrees F). Protect from light. Keep container tightly closed. Throw away any unused medicine after the expiration date.

Progesterone capsules

PROMETRIUM®; 200 mg; Capsule Solvay Pharmaceuticals Inc

PROMETRIUM®; 100 mg; Capsule Solvay Pharmaceuticals Inc

What are progesterone capsules?

PROGESTERONE (Prometrium®) is a female hormone that is produced naturally in the body. These progesterone capsules are used to prevent the overgrowth of the uterine lining in post-menopausal women who are taking estrogens for menopausal symptoms. Progesterone is also used for the treatment of secondary amenorrhea (absence of menstrual periods in women who have previously had a menstrual period) due to progesterone deficiency. Generic progesterone capsules are not yet available.

What should my health care professional know before I take progesterone?

They need to know if you have any of these conditions:
- blood vessel disease, blood clotting disorder, or suffered a stroke
- breast, cervical or vaginal cancer

- diabetes
- heart, kidney or liver disease
- high blood lipids or cholesterol
- hysterectomy
- mental depression
- migraine
- seizures (convulsions)
- vaginal bleeding
- an unusual or allergic reaction to progesterone, other hormones, peanut oil, medicines, foods, dyes or preservatives
- recent miscarriage
- pregnant or trying to get pregnant
- breast-feeding

How should I take this medicine?

Progesterone capsules are taken by mouth. Use exactly as directed. Do not use more often than prescribed. Your prescriber or health care professional will tell you how long you must use these capsules, and which days you should take them. Contact your pediatrician or health care professional regarding the use of this medicine in children. Special care may be needed.

What if I miss a dose?

If you miss a dose, use it as soon as you can. If it is almost time for your next dose, use only that dose. Do not use double or extra doses.

What may interact with progesterone?

- barbiturate medicines for inducing sleep or treating seizures (convulsions)
- bromocriptine
- carbamazepine
- ketoconazole
- phenytoin
- rifampin
- voriconazole

Tell your prescriber or health care professional about all other medicines you are taking, including non-prescription medicines, nutritional supplements, or herbal products. Also tell your prescriber or health care professional if you are a frequent user of drinks with caffeine or alcohol, if you smoke, or if you use illegal drugs. These may affect the way your medicine works. Check with your health care professional before stopping or starting any of your medicines.

What should I watch for while taking progesterone?

Visit your prescriber or health care professional for a regular check on your progress. Progestins can cause swelling, tenderness, or bleeding of the gums; be careful when brushing and flossing teeth. See your dentist regularly for routine dental care You may get dizzy while taking progesterone. Do not drive, use machinery, or do anything that needs mental alertness until you know how progesterone affects you.

What side effects may I notice from taking progesterone?

Side effects that you should report to your prescriber or health care professional as soon as possible:
- abdominal pain
- breast tenderness or discharge
- dizziness
- muscle or bone pain
- numbness or pain in the arm or leg
- pain in the chest, groin or leg
- severe headache
- stomach pain
- sudden shortness of breath
- unusual weakness or tiredness
- vision or speech problems
- yellowing of skin or eyes

Side effects that usually do not require medical attention (report to your prescriber or health care professional if they continue or are bothersome):
- changes in sexual desire or ability
- changes in vaginal bleeding
- facial hair growth
- fluid retention and swelling
- headache
- increased sweating or hot flashes
- loss of appetite or increase in appetite
- mood changes, anxiety, depression, frustration, anger, or emotional outbursts
- nausea, vomiting
- skin rash
- stomach discomfort
- weight gain or weight loss
- vaginal yeast infection (irritation and white discharge)

Where can I keep my medicine?

Keep out of the reach of children. Store at room temperature 25 degrees C (77 degrees F). Throw away any unused medicine after the expiration date.

Promethazine tablets

PROMETHAZINE; 25 mg; Tablet Watson Pharmaceuticals Inc

PHENERGAN®; 25 mg; Tablet Wyeth Pharmaceuticals Inc

What are promethazine tablets?

PROMETHAZINE (Phenergan®) is an antihistamine. It relieves moderate to severe allergic reactions, reduces or prevents nausea and vomiting from illness or motion sickness, helps to make you sleep before surgery, and may help with pain relief or nausea after surgery. Generic promethazine tablets are available.

What should my health care professional know before I take promethazine?

They need to know if you have any of these conditions:
- asthma or congestive lung disease
- diabetes
- glaucoma
- high blood pressure or heart disease
- kidney disease
- liver disease
- prostate trouble
- pain or difficulty passing urine
- seizures (convulsions)
- an unusual or allergic reaction to promethazine or phenothiazines, other medicines, foods, dyes, or preservatives
- pregnant or trying to get pregnant
- breast-feeding

How should I take this medicine?

Take promethazine tablets by mouth. Follow the directions on the prescription label. Take your doses at regular intervals. Do not take your medicine more often than directed. If you are taking promethazine to stop you getting car (travel) sick, take the first dose 30 to 60 minutes before you leave. Contact your pediatrician or health care professional regarding the use of this medicine in children. Special care may be needed. This medicine should not be given to infants and children younger than 2 years old.

What if I miss a dose?

If you miss a dose, take it as soon as you can. If it is almost time for your next dose, take only that dose. Do not take double doses.

What may interact with promethazine?

- bromocriptine
- doxercalciferol
- epinephrine
- levodopa
- metoclopramide
- metrizamide
- medicines for diabetes that are taken by mouth
- medicines for mental problems and psychotic disturbances
- medicines for movement abnormalities as in Parkinson's disease, or for gastrointestinal problems

Because promethazine causes drowsiness, other medicines that also cause drowsiness may increase this effect of promethazine. Some medicines that cause drowsiness are:

- alcohol and alcohol containing medicines
- barbiturates such as phenobarbital
- certain antidepressants
- certain antihistamines used in allergy or cold medicines
- medicines for sleep
- muscle relaxants
- prescription pain medicines

Tell your prescriber or health care professional about all other medicines you are taking, including non-prescription medicines, nutritional supplements, or herbal products. Also tell your prescriber or health care professional if you are a frequent user of drinks with caffeine or alcohol, if you smoke, or if you use illegal drugs. These may affect the way your medicine works. Check with your health care professional before stopping or starting any of your medicines.

What should I watch for while taking promethazine?

Tell your prescriber or health care professional if your symptoms do not improve in 1 to 2 days. You may get drowsy or dizzy. Do not drive, use machinery, or do anything that needs mental alertness until you know how promethazine affects you. To reduce the risk of dizzy or fainting spells, do not stand or sit up quickly, especially if you are an older patient. Alcohol may increase dizziness and drowsiness. Avoid alcoholic drinks. Your mouth may get dry. Chewing sugarless gum or sucking hard candy, and drinking plenty of water will help. Promethazine may cause dry eyes and blurred vision. If you wear contact lenses you may feel some discomfort. Lubricating drops may help. See your ophthalmologist if the problem does not go away or is severe. Keep out of the sun, or wear protective clothing outdoors and use a sunscreen. Do not use sun lamps or sun tanning beds or booths. If you are diabetic, check your blood-sugar levels regularly.

What side effects may I notice from taking promethazine?

Side effects that you should report to your prescriber or health care professional as soon as possible:

- blurred vision
- fainting spells
- irregular heartbeat, palpitations or chest pain
- muscle or facial twitches
- nightmares, agitation, nervousness, excitability, not able to sleep (these are more likely in children)
- pain or difficulty passing urine
- seizures (convulsions)
- skin rash
- slowed or shallow breathing
- sore mouth, gums, or throat
- unusual bleeding or bruising
- unusual tiredness
- yellowing of the eyes or skin

Side effects that usually do not require medical attention (report to your prescriber or health care professional if they continue or are bothersome):

- drowsiness, dizziness
- dry mouth
- headache
- increased sensitivity to the sun or ultraviolet light
- stuffy nose

Where can I keep my medicine?

Keep out of the reach of children in a container that small children cannot open. Store at room temperature, between 15 and 25 degrees C (59 and 77 degrees F). Protect from light. Throw away any unused medicine after the expiration date.

Propafenone tablets and extended-release capsules

RYTHMOL® SR;
225 mg; Capsule,
Extended Release
Reliant
Pharmaceuticals LLc

RYTHMOL®;
150 mg; Tablet
Abbott
Pharmaceutical
Product Division

What are propafenone tablets and extended-release capsules?

PROPAFENONE (Rythmol® SR, Rythmol®) is an antiarrhythmic agent. Propafenone treats irregular heart rhythm and can slow rapid heartbeats (tachycardia). Propafenone can help your heart to return to and maintain a normal rhythm. Generic propafenone tablets are available; however, generic extended-release capsules are not yet available.

What should my health care professional know before I take propafenone?

They need to know if you have any of these conditions:
- asthma, chronic bronchitis, or emphysema
- heart disease
- high blood levels of potassium
- kidney disease
- liver disease
- an unusual or allergic reaction to propafenone, other medicines, foods, dyes, or preservatives
- pregnant or trying to get pregnant
- breast-feeding

How should I take this medicine?

Take propafenone tablets or extended-release capsules by mouth. Follow the directions on the prescription label. Swallow the tablets or capsules with a drink of water. Do not break or crush the capsules. Take your doses at regular intervals. Do not take your medicine more often than directed. Contact your pediatrician or health care professional regarding the use of this medicine in children. Special care may be needed.

What if I miss a dose?

If you miss a dose, take it as soon as you can. There should be an interval of at least 8 hours between doses of capsules and at least 4 hours between tablet doses. If it is almost time for your next dose, take only that dose. Do not take double or extra doses.

What may interact with propafenone?

- arsenic trioxide
- astemizole
- bepridil
- certain antibiotics (such as clarithromycin, erythromycin, gatifloxacin, gemifloxacin, grepafloxacin, levofloxacin, moxifloxacin, sparfloxacin)
- cisapride
- digoxin
- ginger
- hawthorn
- medicines for angina or high blood pressure
- medicines for asthma or breathing difficulties (such as formoterol or salmeterol)
- some medicines for treating depression or mental illness (amoxapine, maprotiline, pimozide, phenothiazines, tricyclic antidepressants)
- medicines to control heart rhythm
- pimozide
- probucol
- terfenadine
- warfarin

Tell your prescriber or health care professional about all other medicines you are taking, including non-prescription medicines, nutritional supplements, or herbal products. Also tell your prescriber or health care professional if you are a frequent user of drinks with caffeine or alcohol, if you smoke, or if you use illegal drugs. These may affect the way your medicine works. Check with your health care professional before stopping or starting any of your medicines.

What should I watch for while taking propafenone?

Visit your prescriber or health care professional for regular checks on your progress. Do not stop taking propafenone suddenly; this may cause serious, heart-related side effects. Because your condition and the use of propafenone carry some risk, it is a good idea to carry an identification card, necklace or bracelet with details of your condition, medications and prescriber or health care professional. Check your heart rate (pulse) and blood pressure regularly while you are taking propafenone. Ask your prescriber or health care professional what your heart rate and blood pressure should be, and when you should contact him or her. Your prescriber or health care professional also may schedule regular blood tests and electrocardiograms to check your progress. You may feel dizzy or faint. Do not drive, use machinery, or do anything that needs mental alertness until you know how propafenone affects you. To reduce the risk of dizzy or fainting spells, do not sit or stand up quickly, especially if you are an older patient. Alcohol can make you more dizzy, increase flushing and rapid heartbeats. Avoid alcoholic drinks. If you are going to have surgery, tell your prescriber or health care professional that you are taking propafenone.

What side effects may I notice from taking propafenone?

Side effects that you should report to your prescriber or health care professional as soon as possible:
- chest pain, palpitations
- fever or chills

- shortness of breath
- swelling of feet or legs
- trembling or shaking

Side effects that usually do not require medical attention (report to your prescriber or health care professional if they continue or are bothersome):
- blurred vision
- changes in taste (a metallic or bitter taste)
- constipation or diarrhea
- dizziness

- dry mouth
- headache
- nausea or vomiting
- tiredness or weakness

Where can I keep my medicine?

Keep out of the reach of children in a container that small children cannot open. Store at room temperature between 15 and 30 degrees C (59 and 86 degrees F). Keep container tightly closed. Throw away any unused medicine after the expiration date.

Propantheline tablets

PROPANTHELINE;
15 mg; Tablet
Roxane Laboratories Inc

What are propantheline tablets?

PROPANTHELINE (Norpanth®, Pro-Banthine®) helps relieve spasms in the stomach. It helps treat peptic ulcer disease and other stomach problems. Generic propantheline tablets are available.

What should my health care professional know before I take propantheline?

They need to know if you have any of these conditions:
- difficulty passing urine
- heart or blood vessel disease
- hiatal hernia
- glaucoma
- liver disease
- overactive thyroid
- stomach obstruction
- ulcerative colitis
- an unusual or allergic reaction to propantheline, other medicines, foods, dyes, or preservatives
- pregnant or trying to get pregnant
- breast-feeding

How should I take this medicine?

Take propantheline tablets by mouth. Follow the directions on the prescription label. Swallow the tablets with a drink of water. It is best to take the tablets 30 minutes before meals. Take your medicine at regular intervals. Do not take your medicine more often than directed. Contact your pediatrician or health care professional regarding the use of this medicine in children. Special care may be needed.

What if I miss a dose?

If you miss a dose, take it as soon as you can. If it is almost time for your next dose, take only that dose. Do not take double or extra doses.

What may interact with propantheline?

- amantadine
- benztropine
- bethanechol
- cisapride
- disopyramide

- donepezil
- erythromycin
- galantamine
- glutethimide
- ketoconazole
- levodopa
- medicines for hay fever and other allergies
- meperidine
- metformin
- metoclopramide
- medicines for mental depression
- medicines for mental problems and psychotic disturbances
- potassium salts
- rivastigmine
- tacrine
- tegaserod

Tell your prescriber or health care professional about all other medicines you are taking, including nonprescription medicines, nutritional supplements, or herbal products. Also tell your prescriber or health care professional if you are a frequent user of drinks with caffeine or alcohol, if you smoke, or if you use illegal drugs. These may affect the way your medicine works. Check with your health care professional before stopping or starting any of your medicines.

What should I watch for while taking propantheline?

You may get drowsy, dizzy, or have blurred vision. Do not drive, use machinery, or do anything that needs mental alertness until you know how propantheline affects you. To reduce the risk of dizzy or fainting spells, do not sit or stand up quickly, especially if you are an older patient. Alcohol can make you more drowsy; avoid alcoholic drinks. Avoid extreme heat (e.g., hot tubs, saunas). Propantheline can cause you to sweat less than normal. Your body temperature could increase to dangerous levels, which may lead to heat stroke. Your mouth may get dry. Chewing sugarless gum or sucking hard candy, and drinking plenty of water will help.

What side effects may I notice from taking propantheline?

Side effects that you should report to your prescriber or health care professional as soon as possible:

- agitation, nervousness, confusion
- blurred vision and other eye problems
- decreased sweating
- dizziness, drowsiness
- fever
- irregular heartbeat (palpitations)
- pain or difficulty passing urine
- skin rash, itching
- unusual weakness or tiredness
- vomiting

Side effects that usually do not require medical attention (report to your prescriber or health care professional if they continue or are bothersome):

- constipation
- difficulty sleeping
- difficulty swallowing
- dry mouth
- headache
- nausea
- sexual difficulty (impotence)

Where can I keep my medicine?

Keep out of the reach of children in a container that small children cannot open. Store at room temperature below 30 degrees C (86 degrees F). Throw away any unused medicine after the expiration date.

Propoxyphene capsules or tablets

DARVON®; 65 mg; Capsule AAI Pharma Inc

PROPOXYPHENE; 65 mg; Capsule Mylan Pharmaceuticals Inc

What are propoxyphene capsules or tablets?

PROPOXYPHENE (Darvon®, Darvon-N®) relieves moderate to severe pain. Propoxyphene can be combined in tablets with acetaminophen. Federal law prohibits the transfer of propoxyphene to any person other than the patient for whom it was prescribed. Do not share this medicine with anyone else. Generic propoxyphene tablets and capsules are available.

What should my health care professional know before I take propoxyphene?

They need to know if you have any of these conditions:

- diarrhea
- liver disease
- depression or emotional difficulties
- heart disease
- kidney disease
- lung disease or breathing difficulties
- seizures
- an unusual or allergic reaction to propoxyphene, methadone, other medicines, foods, dyes, or preservatives
- pregnant or trying to get pregnant
- breast-feeding

How should I take this medicine?

Take propoxyphene tablets or capsules by mouth. Follow the directions on the prescription label. Swallow the tablets or capsules with a drink of water. If propoxyphene upsets your stomach, you can take it with food or milk. Do not take more than 6 tablets or capsules a day. Do not share this medicine with anyone. Contact your pediatrician or health care professional regarding the use of this medicine in children. Special care may be needed.

What if I miss a dose?

If you miss a dose, take it as soon as you can. If it is almost time for your next dose, take only that dose. Do not take double or extra doses.

What may interact with propoxyphene?

- medicines for high blood pressure
- medicines for seizures, especially carbamazepine

Because propoxyphene can cause drowsiness, other medicines that also cause drowsiness may increase this effect of propoxyphene. Some medicines that cause drowsiness are:

- alcohol and alcohol-containing medicines
- barbiturates such as phenobarbital
- certain antidepressants or tranquilizers
- muscle relaxants
- certain antihistamines used in cold medicines

Tell your prescriber or health care professional about all other medicines you are taking, including non-prescription medicines, nutritional supplements, or herbal products. Also tell your prescriber or health care professional if you are a frequent user of drinks with caffeine or alcohol, if you smoke, or if you use illegal drugs. These may affect the way your medicine works. Check with your health care professional before stopping or starting any of your medicines.

What should I watch for while taking propoxyphene?

Tell your prescriber or health care professional if your pain does not go away. Use exactly as directed by your prescriber or health care professional. If you are being prescribed propoxyphene continuously around-the-clock for pain, do not stop taking except on your prescriber's advice. You may get drowsy or dizzy when you first start taking propoxyphene. Do not drive, use machinery, or do anything that needs mental alertness until you know how propoxyphene affects you. Stand or sit up slowly, this reduces the risk of dizzy or fainting spells. These effects may be worse if you are an older patient. The drowsiness should decrease after taking propoxyphene for a couple of days. Be careful taking other medicines which may also make you tired. This effect may be worse when taking these medicines with propoxyphene. Alcohol can increase possible drowsiness, dizziness, confusion and affect your breathing. Avoid alcohol while taking propoxyphene. Propoxyphene may cause constipation with long-term use. Try to have a bowel movement at least every 2 to 3 days. If you do not have a bowel movement for 3 days or more call your prescriber or health care professional. Your mouth may get dry. Chewing sugarless gum or sucking hard candy, and drinking plenty of water may help. Visit the dentist regularly. If you are going to have surgery tell your prescriber or health care professional that you are taking propoxyphene.

What side effects may I notice from taking propoxyphene?

Side effects that you should report to your prescriber or health care professional as soon as possible:
Rare or uncommon:
- breathing difficulties, wheezing
- seizures
- slow or fast heartbeat
- severe rash

More common:
- confusion
- lightheadedness or fainting spells
- nervousness or restlessness

Side effects that usually do not require medical attention (report to your prescriber or health care professional if they continue or are bothersome):
- clumsiness, unsteadiness
- constipation
- dizziness, drowsiness
- headache
- nausea, vomiting

Where can I keep my medicine?

Keep out of the reach of children in a container that small children cannot open. Do not share or give this medicine to anyone else. Avoid accidental swallowing of propoxyphene by someone (especially children) other than the person for whom it was prescribed as this may result in severe effects and possibly death. Store at room temperature between 15 and 30 degrees C (59 and 86 degrees F). Protect from light. Keep container tightly closed. Throw away any unused medicine after the expiration date.

Propranolol tablets or extended-release capsules

INDERAL®;
80 mg; Tablet
Wyeth
Pharmaceuticals Inc

INDERAL® LA;
160 mg; Capsule,
Extended Release
Wyeth
Pharmaceuticals Inc

What are propranolol tablets or extended-release capsules?

PROPRANOLOL (Inderal®, Inderal® LA) belongs to a group of medicines called beta-blockers. Beta-blockers reduce the workload on the heart and help it to beat more regularly. Propranolol controls, but does not cure, high blood pressure (hypertension). High blood pressure may not make you feel sick, but it can lead to serious heart problems. Propranolol has a number of other uses; for some of these the sustained-release capsules are not suitable. Propranolol steadies irregular heart rhythms (arrhythmias) and relieves chest pain (angina), and it may be helpful after a heart attack. Propranolol can help prevent migraine headaches, relieve serious tremors (uncontrollable shaking), and help certain problems related to the thyroid gland and adrenal gland. Generic propranolol tablets and extended-release capsules are available.

What should my health care professional know before I take propranolol?

They need to know if you have any of these conditions:
- asthma, bronchitis or bronchospasm
- circulation problems, or blood vessel disease (such as Raynaud's disease)
- depression
- diabetes
- emphysema, or other lung disease
- history of heart attack or heart disease, vasospastic angina
- liver disease
- low blood pressure
- muscle weakness or disease
- pheochromocytoma
- psoriasis
- thyroid disease
- an unusual or allergic reaction to propranolol, other beta-blockers, medicines, foods, dyes, or preservatives
- pregnant or trying to get pregnant
- breast-feeding

How should I take this medicine?

Take propranolol tablets or extended-release capsules by mouth. Follow the directions on the prescription label. Swallow the tablets or capsules with a drink of water; do not crush or chew the capsules. Take your doses at regular intervals. Do not take your medicine more often than directed. Do not stop taking except on your prescriber's advice.

What if I miss a dose?

If you miss a dose, take it as soon as you can. If it is almost time for your next dose (less than 4 hours for regular tablets, or less than 8 hours for extended-release capsules), take only that dose. Do not take double or extra doses.

What may interact with propranolol?

- anti-inflammatory drugs (NSAIDs, such as ibuprofen)
- atropine
- barbiturate medicines for inducing sleep or treating seizures (convulsions)
- cimetidine
- cocaine
- ergotamine
- hawthorn
- levodopa
- medicines for colds and breathing difficulties
- medicines for diabetes
- medicines for high blood pressure
- medicines for mental depression
- medicines for mental problems and psychotic disturbances
- medicines to control heart rhythm
- rifampin
- theophylline
- tubocurarine
- water pills

Tell your prescriber or health care professional about all other medicines you are taking, including nonprescription medicines, nutritional supplements, or herbal products. Also tell your prescriber or health care professional if you are a frequent user of drinks with caffeine or alcohol, if you smoke, or if you use illegal drugs. These may affect the way your medicine works. Check with your health care professional before stopping or starting any of your medicines.

What should I watch for while taking propranolol?

Check your heart rate and blood pressure regularly while you are taking propranolol. Ask your prescriber or health care professional what your heart rate and blood pressure should be, and when you should contact him or her. Do not stop taking this medicine suddenly. This could lead to serious heart-related effects. You may get drowsy or dizzy. Do not drive, use machinery, or do anything that requires mental alertness until you

know how propranolol affects you. To reduce the risk of dizzy or fainting spells, do not sit or stand up quickly. Alcohol can make you more drowsy, and increase flushing and rapid heartbeats. Therefore, it is best to avoid alcoholic drinks. Propranolol can affect blood sugar levels. If you have diabetes, check with your prescriber or health care professional before you change your diet or the dose of your diabetic medicine. If you are going to have surgery, tell your prescriber or health care professional that you are taking propranolol.

What side effects may I notice from taking propranolol?

Side effects that you should report to your prescriber or health care professional as soon as possible:
- changes in blood sugar
- cold hands or feet
- difficulty breathing, wheezing
- difficulty sleeping, nightmares
- dizziness or fainting spells
- hallucinations (seeing and hearing things that are not really there)
- muscle cramps or weakness
- skin rash, itching, dry peeling skin
- slow heart rate (less than 50 beats per minute)
- swelling of the legs and ankles
- vomiting

Side effects that usually do not require medical attention (report to your prescriber or health care professional if they continue or are bothersome):
- dark coloration of skin
- diarrhea
- dry sore eyes
- hair loss
- nausea
- sexual difficulties (impotence or decreased sexual urges)
- weakness or tiredness

Where can I keep my medicine?

Keep out of the reach of children in a container that small children cannot open. Store at room temperature approximately 25 degrees C (77 degrees F). Protect from light and moisture. Throw away any unused medicine after the expiration date.

Propylthiouracil, PTU tablets

PROPYLTHIOURACIL, PTU; 50 mg; Tablet Purepac Pharmaceutical Co

PROPYLTHIOURACIL, PTU; 50 mg; Tablet West Ward Pharmaceutical Corp

What are propylthiouracil tablets?

PROPYLTHIOURACIL, PTU prevents the thyroid gland from producing too much thyroid hormone. Propylthiouracil is used to treat a condition known as hyperthyroidism (over-active thyroid). Generic propylthiouracil tablets are available.

What should my health care professional know before I take propylthiouracil?

They need to know if you have any of these conditions:
- blood disorder
- liver disease
- an unusual or allergic reaction to propylthiouracil, other medicines, foods, dyes, or preservatives

- pregnant or trying to get pregnant
- breast-feeding

How should I take this medicine?

Take propylthiouracil tablets by mouth. Follow the directions on the prescription label. Swallow the tablets with a drink of water. Take your doses at regular intervals. Do not take your medicine more often than directed.

What if I miss a dose?

If you miss a dose, take it as soon as you can. If it is almost time for your next dose, take only that dose. Do not take double or extra doses.

What may interact with propylthiouracil?

- amiodarone
- digoxin
- potassium iodide
- sodium iodide
- theophylline
- thyroid hormones
- warfarin

Tell your prescriber or health care professional about all other medicines you are taking, including non-prescription medicines, nutritional supplements, or herbal products. Also tell your prescriber or health care professional if you are a frequent user of drinks with caffeine or alcohol, if you smoke, or if you use illegal drugs. These may affect the way your medicine works. Check with your health care professional before stopping or starting any of your medicines.

What should I watch for while taking propylthiouracil?

Visit your prescriber or health care professional for regular checks on your progress, and to make sure your body is producing the right amount of thyroid hormone. If you are going to have surgery, tell your prescriber or health care professional that you are taking propylthiouracil. Propylthiouracil can reduce your resistance to infection. Contact your prescriber or health care professional if you have any infection or injury. Do not have any vaccinations without your prescriber's approval.

What side effects may I notice from taking propylthiouracil?

Side effects that you should report to your prescriber or health care professional as soon as possible:

- backache
- black, tarry stools
- decrease in the amount of urine passed
- fever, sore throat, hoarseness
- goiter (enlarged thyroid gland causing swelling in the throat)
- menstrual changes
- mouth sores
- numbness or tingling in the hands or feet
- severe redness or itching of the skin
- stomach pain
- swelling of the feet or legs
- unusual bleeding or bruising, red spots on the skin
- unusual or sudden weight gain
- unusual tiredness or weakness
- yellowing of skin or eyes

Side effects that usually do not require medical attention (report to your prescriber or health care professional if they continue or are bothersome):

- fever
- muscle aches and pains
- nausea, vomiting
- skin rashes, itching

Where can I keep my medicine?

Keep out of the reach of children in a container that small children cannot open. Store at room temperature between 15 and 30 degrees C (59 and 86 degrees F). Keep container tightly closed. Throw away any unused medicine after the expiration date.

This drug requires an FDA medication guide. See page xxxvii.

Protriptyline tablets

VIVACTIL;
10 mg; Tablet
Odyssey
Pharmaceuticals Inc

VIVACTIL;
5 mg; Tablet
Odyssey
Pharmaceuticals Inc

What are protriptyline tablets?

PROTRIPTYLINE (Vivactil®) is an antidepressant. Protriptyline can help to lift your spirits by treating your depression. Generic protriptyline tablets are available.

What should my health care professional know before I take protriptyline?

They need to know if you have any of these conditions:

- an alcohol problem
- asthma, difficulty breathing
- blood disorders or disease
- diabetes
- difficulty passing urine, prostate trouble
- glaucoma
- having intramuscular injections
- heart disease, or recent heart attack
- liver disease
- overactive thyroid
- Parkinson's disease
- schizophrenia
- seizures (convulsions)
- stomach disease

- an unusual or allergic reaction to protriptyline, other medicines, foods, dyes, or preservatives
- pregnant or trying to get pregnant
- breast-feeding

How should I take this medicine?

Take protriptyline tablets by mouth. Follow the directions on the prescription label. Swallow the tablets with a drink of water. Take your doses at regular intervals. Do not take your medicine more often than directed. Do not stop taking except on your prescriber's advice. Contact your pediatrician or health care professional regarding the use of this medicine in children. Special care may be needed. Elderly patients over 65 years old and adolescents may have a stronger reaction to this medicine and need smaller doses.

What if I miss a dose?

If you miss a dose, take it as soon as you can. If it is almost time for your next dose, take only that dose. Do not take double or extra doses.

What may interact with protriptyline?

Protriptyline can interact with many other medicines. Some interactions can be very important. Make sure your prescriber or health care professional knows about all other medicines you are taking. Many important interactions are listed below:

Do not take protriptyline with any of the following medications:

- astemizole (Hismanal®)
- cisapride (Propulsid®)
- probucol
- terfenadine (Seldane®)
- thioridazine (Mellaril®)
- medicines called MAO inhibitors-phenelzine (Nardil®), tranylcypromine (Parnate®), isocarboxazid (Marplan®), selegiline (Eldepryl®)
- other medicines for mental depression (may be duplicate therapies or cause additive side effects)

Protriptyline may also interact with any of the following medications:

- alcohol
- antacids
- atropine and related drugs like hyoscyamine, scopolamine, tolterodine and others
- barbiturate medicines for inducing sleep or treating seizures (convulsions), such as phenobarbital
- blood thinners, such as warfarin
- bromocriptine
- bupropion
- cimetidine
- clonidine
- cocaine
- delavirdine
- diphenoxylate
- disulfiram
- donepezil
- drugs for treating HIV infection

- female hormones, including contraceptive or birth control pills and estrogen
- galantamine
- herbs and dietary supplements like ephedra (Ma huang), kava kava, SAM-e, St. John's wort, valerian, or others
- imatinib, STI-571
- kaolin; pectin
- labetalol
- levodopa and other medicines for movement problems like Parkinson's disease
- lithium
- medicines for anxiety or sleeping problems
- medicines for colds, flu and breathing difficulties, like pseudoephedrine
- medicines for hay fever or allergies (antihistamines)
- medicines for weight loss or appetite control
- medicines used to regulate abnormal heartbeat or to treat other heart conditions (examples: amiodarone, bepridil, disopyramide, dofetilide, encainide, flecainide, ibutilide, mibefradil, procainamide, propafenone, quinidine, and others)
- metoclopramide
- muscle relaxants, like cyclobenzaprine
- other medicines for mental or mood problems and psychotic disturbances
- prescription pain medications like morphine, codeine, tramadol and others
- procarbazine
- seizure (convulsion) or epilepsy medicine such as carbamazepine or phenytoin
- stimulants like dexmethylphenidate or methylphenidate
- some antibiotics (examples: erythromycin, gatifloxacin, levofloxacin, linezolid, moxifloxacin, sotalol, sparfloxacin)
- tacrine
- thyroid hormones such as levothyroxine

Tell your prescriber or health care professional about all other medicines you are taking, including non-prescription medicines, nutritional supplements, or herbal products. Also tell your prescriber or health care professional if you are a frequent user of drinks with caffeine or alcohol, if you smoke, or if you use illegal drugs. These may affect the way your medicine works. Check with your health care professional before stopping or starting any of your medicines.

What should I watch for while taking protriptyline?

Visit your prescriber or health care professional for regular checks on your progress. It can take several days or weeks before you feel the full effect of protriptyline. If you have been taking protriptyline regularly for some time, do not suddenly stop taking it. You must gradually reduce the dose or you may get severe side effects. Ask your prescriber or health care professional for advice. Even after you stop taking protriptyline it can still affect your body for several days. You may get drowsy or dizzy. Do not drive, use machinery, or do anything that needs mental alertness until you know how propriptyline affects you. Do not stand or sit up quickly, especially if you are an older patient. This reduces the risk of dizzy or fainting spells. Alcohol can increase dizziness and drowsiness. Avoid alcoholic drinks. Do not treat yourself for coughs, colds or allergies without asking your prescriber or health care professional for advice. Some ingredients can increase possible side effects. Your mouth may get dry. Chewing sugarless gum or sucking hard candy, and drinking plenty of water will help. Protriptyline may cause dry eyes and blurred vision. If you wear contact lenses you may feel some discomfort. Lubricating drops may help. See your ophthalmologist if the problem does not go away or is severe. Protriptyline may make your skin more sensitive to the sun. Keep out of the sun, or wear protective clothing outdoors and use a sunscreen. Do not use sun lamps or sun tanning beds or booths. Protriptyline can affect blood glucose (sugar) levels. If you are a diabetic, check your blood sugar more often than usual, especially during the first few weeks of protriptyline treatment. Call your prescriber or health care professional for advice if you notice a change in the results of blood or urine glucose tests. If you are going to have surgery or will need an x-ray procedure that uses contrast agents, tell your prescriber or health care professional that you are taking this medicine.

What side effects may I notice from taking protriptyline?

Side effects that you should report to your prescriber or health care professional as soon as possible:
- abnormal production of milk in females
- blurred vision or eye pain
- breast enlargement in both males and females
- confusion, hallucinations (seeing or hearing things that are not really there)
- difficulty breathing
- fainting spells
- fever
- irregular or fast, pounding heartbeat, palpitations
- muscle stiffness, or spasms
- pain or difficulty passing urine, loss of bladder control
- seizures (convulsions)
- sexual difficulties (decreased sexual ability or desire)
- stomach pain
- swelling of the testicles
- tingling, pain, or numbness in the feet or hands
- tremor (shaking)
- unusual weakness or tiredness
- yellowing of the eyes or skin

Side effects that usually do not require medical attention (report to your prescriber or health care professional if they continue or are bothersome):
- anxiety
- constipation, or diarrhea
- drowsiness or dizziness
- dry mouth
- headache
- increased sensitivity of the skin to sun or ultraviolet light
- loss of appetite
- nausea, vomiting
- skin rash or itching
- weight gain or loss

Where can I keep my medicine?

Keep out of the reach of children in a container that small children cannot open. Store at room temperature between 15 and 30 degrees C (59 and 86 degrees F). Keep container tightly closed. Throw away any unused medicine after the expiration date.

Pseudoephedrine tablets and extended-release tablets

SUDAFED®;
30 mg; Tablet
Pfizer Consumer Healthcare

What are pseudoephedrine tablets and extended-release tablets?

PSEUDOEPHEDRINE tablets and extended-release tablets (Sudafed® and others) is a decongestant. It can help relieve nasal or sinus congestion (stuffiness). Extended-release tablets can give day-long relief. Generic pseudoephedrine tablets and extended-release tablets are available.

What should my health care professional know before I take pseudoephedrine?

They need to know if you have any of the following conditions:
- blood vessel disease
- diabetes
- difficulty urinating (urinary retention)
- glaucoma
- heart disease or heart rhythm problems
- high blood pressure
- kidney disease
- overactive thyroid
- phenylketonuria (products containing aspartame such as the chewable tablets)
- prostate trouble
- an unusual or allergic reaction to pseudoephedrine, other medicines, foods, dyes, or preservatives
- pregnant or trying to get pregnant
- breast-feeding

How should I take this medicine?

Take pseudoephedrine tablets by mouth. Swallow with a drink of water. Do not crush or chew extended-release tablets. Follow the directions on the prescription label. Take your doses at regular intervals. Do not take your medicine more often than directed. Contact your pediatrician or health care professional regarding the use of this medicine in children. Special care may be needed. Elderly patients over 60 years old may have a stronger reaction to this medicine and need smaller doses.

What if I miss a dose?

If you miss a dose, and you are taking it on a regular schedule, take it as soon as you can. If it is almost time for your next dose (less than 2 hours for regular release or 12 hours for extended-release tablets), take only that dose. Do not take double or extra doses.

What may interact with pseudoephedrine?

- ammonium chloride
- amphetamine or other stimulant drugs
- bicarbonate, citrate, or acetate products (such as sodium bicarbonate, sodium acetate, sodium citrate, sodium lactate, and potassium citrate)
- bromocriptine
- caffeine
- cocaine
- furazolidone
- linezolid
- medicines for colds and breathing difficulties
- medicines for diabetes
- medicines known as MAO inhibitors, such as phenelzine (Nardil®), tranylcypromine (Parnate®), isocarboxazid (Marplan®), and selegiline (Carbex®, Eldepryl®)
- medicines for mental depression
- medicines for migraine
- procarbazine
- some medicines for chest pain, heart disease, high blood pressure or heart rhythm problems
- some medicines for weight loss (including some herbal products, ephedrine, dextroamphetamine)
- St. John's wort
- theophylline
- thyroid hormones

Tell your prescriber or health care professional about all other medicines you are taking, including non-prescription medicines, nutritional supplements, or herbal products. Also tell your prescriber or health care professional if you are a frequent user of drinks with caffeine or alcohol, if you smoke, or if you use illegal drugs. These may affect the way your medicine works. Check before starting or stopping any of your medicines.

What should I watch for while taking pseudoephedrine?

Check with your prescriber or health care professional if your congestion has not improved within 7 days, or if you have a high fever. If pseudoephedrine (regular-release product) makes it difficult for you to sleep at night; take your last dose a few hours before bedtime. If nervousness, dizziness, or sleeplessness occur, stop using pseudoephedrine and consult a health care professional. If you are going to have surgery, tell your prescriber you are taking pseudoephedrine.

What side effects may I notice from taking pseudoephedrine?

Side effects that you should report to your prescriber or health care professional as soon as possible:
Rare or uncommon:
- bloody diarrhea and abdominal pain
- chest pain
- confusion
- dizziness, or fainting spells
- hallucinations
- numbness or tingling in the hands or feet
- rapid or troubled breathing
- seizures (convulsions)
- severe, persistent, or worsening headache

More common:
- anxiety
- fast or irregular heartbeat, palpitations
- increased blood pressure
- increased sweating
- pain or difficulty passing urine
- sleeplessness (insomnia)
- tremor
- vomiting

Side effects that usually do not require medical attention (report to your prescriber or health care professional if they continue or are bothersome):
- difficulty sleeping
- headache (mild)
- loss of appetite
- nausea, stomach upset
- restlessness or nervousness

Where can I keep my medicine?

Keep out of the reach of children in a container that small children cannot open. Store at room temperature, between 15 and 30 degrees C (59 and 86 degrees F), unless otherwise specified on the product label. Protect from heat and moisture. Throw away any unused medicine after the expiration date.

P

Pyrazinamide, PZA tablets

PYRAZINAMIDE, PZA; 500 mg; Tablet Versapharm Incorporated

PYRAZINAMIDE, PZA; 500 mg; Tablet Lederle Laboratories

What are pyrazinamide tablets?

PYRAZINAMIDE, PZA is an antibiotic that is used to treat or prevent tuberculosis infections. Other medicines for tuberculosis are used in combination with pyrazinamide; it should never be used alone. Generic pyrazinamide tablets are available.

What should my health care professional know before I take pyrazinamide?

They need to know if you have any of these conditions:
- if you frequently drink alcohol-containing beverages
- gout
- liver disease, including hepatitis
- previously experienced side effects to isoniazid (INH) treatment
- an unusual or allergic reaction to pyrazinamide, other medicines, foods, dyes or preservatives
- pregnant or trying to get pregnant
- breast-feeding

How should I take this medicine?

Take pyrazinamide tablets by mouth. Follow the directions on the prescription label. Swallow tablets whole with a full glass of water. Pyrazinamide can be taken with or without food. Take your doses at regular intervals and try not to miss any doses. Do not take your medicine more often than directed. Finish the full course prescribed by your prescriber or health care professional even if you think your condition is better. Do not stop taking except on your prescriber's advice.

What if I miss a dose?

If you miss a dose, take it as soon as you can. If it is almost time for your next dose, take only that dose. Do not take double or extra doses.

What may interact with pyrazinamide?

- alcohol
- allopurinol
- colchicine
- probenecid
- sulfinpyrazone

Tell your prescriber or health care professional about all other medicines you are taking, including non-prescription medicines, nutritional supplements, or herbal products. Also tell your prescriber or health care professional if you are a frequent user of drinks with caffeine or alcohol, if you smoke, or if you use illegal drugs. These may affect the way your medicine works. Check with your health care professional before stopping or starting any of your medicines.

What should I watch for while taking pyrazinamide?

Pyrazinamide can cause serious liver problems, especially if you are also taking rifampin (Rifadin® or Rimactane®). Make sure you understand the risks for liver problems and how to identify the symptoms. If you have any questions, talk with your prescriber or other health care provider. Visit your prescriber or health care professional for regular checks and report any serious side effects promptly. Keep taking your pyrazinamide even if you feel better. You may need to take this medicine for an extended period of time for a complete cure. Avoid alcoholic drinks while you are taking pyrazinamide. Drinking alcohol during treatment with pyrazinamide increases the risk of serious liver problems. Your skin may become more sensitive to sunlight. Keep out of the sun, or wear protective clothing outdoors and use a sunscreen. Do not use sun lamps or sun tanning beds or booths. If you are diabetic note that pyrazinamide can interfere with urine ketone determination tests, such as Acetest® and Ketostix®, causing a pink-brown result. Check with your prescriber or health care professional before you change your diet or the dose of your diabetic medicine.

What side effects may I notice from taking pyrazinamide?

Side effects that you should report to your prescriber or health care professional as soon as possible:
- dark yellow or brown urine
- fever
- loss of appetite
- unusual bleeding or bruising
- unusual tiredness or weakness
- yellowing of the eyes or skin

Side effects that usually do not require medical attention (report to your prescriber or health care professional if they continue or are bothersome):
- sensitivity to sun or ultraviolet light
- skin rash, itching

Where can I keep my medicine?

Keep out of the reach of children in a container that small children cannot open. Store at room temperature between 15 and 30 degrees C (59 and 86 degrees F). keep container tightly closed. Throw away any unused medicine after the expiration date.

Pyridostigmine tablets or extended-release tablets

MESTINON®;
60 mg; Tablet
Valeant
Pharmaceuticals

MESTINON®
TIMESPAN;
180 mg; Extended-Release Tablets
Valeant
Pharmaceuticals

What are pyridostigmine tablets or extended-release tablets?

PYRIDOSTIGMINE (Mestinon®, Mestinon Timespan®) can improve muscle strength. It can help to treat myasthenia gravis, a disease that affects your muscles. Pyridostigmine tablets may also be used by the military before an anticipated threat of exposure to certain nerve gas agents. Generic pyridostigmine regular-release tablets are available. Extended-release tablets are not yet available.

What should my health care professional know before I take pyridostigmine?

They need to know if you have any of these conditions:
- asthma
- difficulty passing urine
- heart disease or irregular heartbeat
- kidney disease
- over active thyroid
- seizures (convulsions)
- stomach obstruction or ulcers
- an unusual or allergic reaction to pyridostigmine, bromides, other medicines, foods, dyes, or preservatives
- pregnant or trying to get pregnant
- breast-feeding

How should I take this medicine?

Take pyridostigmine tablets by mouth. Follow the directions on the prescription label. Swallow the tablets with a drink of water. If pyridostigmine upsets your stomach, take it with food or milk. If you are taking the extended-release tablets, swallow them whole; do not crush or chew. Take your doses regularly. The interval between doses is very important. You must take your tablets day and night. Do not take your medicine more often than directed. If you are in the military and instructed to use pyridostigmine in case of threatened exposure to Soman nerve gas, be sure to get instructions on the use of the antidote atropine and pralidoxime. In this case, you will need to get an adequate supply of these drugs. Pyridostigmine tablets are only to be used prior to exposure to Soman. Pyridostigmine should not be used during or after exposure to Soman.

What if I miss a dose?

Try to keep to your prescribed medication schedule to get the best effects. If you miss a dose, take it as soon as you can. If it is almost time for your next dose, take only that dose. Do not take double or extra doses.

What may interact with pyridostigmine?

- atropine
- certain antibiotics given by injection
- disopyramide
- mecamylamine
- medicines that cause muscle relaxation
- other medicines that improve muscle strength or tone for conditions like myasthenia gravis
- quinine
- trimethaphan

Tell your prescriber or health care professional about all other medicines you are taking, including nonprescription medicines, nutritional supplements, or herbal products. Also tell your prescriber or health care professional if you are a frequent user of drinks with caffeine or alcohol, if you smoke, or if you use illegal drugs. These may affect the way your medicine works. Check with your health care professional before stopping or starting any of your medicines.

What should I watch for while taking pyridostigmine?

Each patient can take pyridostigmine tablets on a schedule that best suits their individual needs. These needs can increase at certain times of the day. Your prescriber or health care professional may want you to keep a record of when you take your tablets, how you feel after taking them, and if you get any side effects. This information will help your prescriber or health care professional to plan a schedule and dose best suited to your condition. Always carry an identification card describing your disease and the details of your medication regimen. If you are in the military and are asked to use or carry pyridostigmine in the event of threatened exposure to Soman nerve gas, be sure to get adequate instructions on the use and administration of this drug.

What side effects may I notice from taking pyridostigmine?

Side effects that you should report to your prescriber or health care professional as soon as possible:
- changes in vision
- diarrhea
- difficulty breathing
- dizziness
- difficulty moving
- headache
- increase in the need to pass urine
- increased saliva
- increased sweating
- muscle cramps or spasms
- nausea, vomiting
- skin rash
- slow or irregular heartbeat
- stomach pain
- unusual weakness or tiredness

Where can I keep my medicine?

Keep out of the reach of children in a container that small children cannot open. Store at room temperature between 15 and 30 degrees C (59 and 86 degrees F). Keep container tightly closed. Throw away any unused medicine after the expiration date.

Pyridoxine, Vitamin B₆ tablets or capsules

VITAMIN B-6;
100 mg; Tablet
Goldline Laboratories Inc/
IVAX Pharmaceuticals

What are pyridoxine, vitamin B6 tablets or capsules?

PYRIDOXINE (Vitamin B6) is a naturally occurring vitamin found in beans, grains, vegetables, liver, meat, and eggs. Pyridoxine treats or prevents vitamin B6 deficiency resulting from certain medications and medical conditions. The vitamin is also used to supplement a poor diet. Generic pyridoxine tablets or capsules are available.

What should my health care professional know before I take pyridoxine?

They need to know if you have any of the following conditions:

- heart disease
- an unusual or allergic reaction to B vitamins, other medicines, foods, dyes, or preservatives
- pregnant or trying to get pregnant
- breast-feeding

How should I take this medicine?

Take pyridoxine tablets or capsules by mouth. Follow the directions on the prescription label. Swallow the tablets or capsules with a glass of water. If you are taking a sustained-release form of tablet or capsule, swallow whole; do not crush or chew.

What if I miss a dose?

If you miss a dose, skip that dose. Continue with your next scheduled dose.

What may interact with pyridoxine?

- levodopa

Tell your prescriber or health care professional about all other medicines you are taking, including non-prescription medicines, nutritional supplements, or herbal products. Also tell your prescriber or health care professional if you are a frequent user of drinks with caffeine or alcohol, if you smoke, or if you use illegal drugs. These may affect the way your medicine works. Check with your health care professional before stopping or starting any of your medicines.

What should I watch for while taking pyridoxine?

Make sure you have a proper diet. Taking pyridoxine tablets or capsules does not replace the need for a balanced diet. Some foods that contain pyridoxine include: beans, grains, vegetables, liver, meat, and eggs.

What side effects may I notice from taking pyridoxine?

The recommended daily allowance of pyridoxine does not cause any side effects.
Side effects related to overdose include:

- headache
- nausea, vomiting
- seizures (convulsions)
- tingling, pain, or numbness in the hands or feet

Call your prescriber or health care professional as soon as you can if you think you have taken an overdose and have any of these side effects.

Where can I keep my medicine?

Keep out of the reach of children in a container that small children cannot open. Store at room temperature between 15 and 30 degrees C (59 and 86 degrees F). Protect from light. Throw away any unused medicine after the expiration date.

Pyrimethamine tablets

DARAPRIM®;
25 mg; Tablet
Glaxo Wellcome Division

What are pyrimethamine tablets?

PYRIMETHAMINE (Daraprim®) is an antiparasitic agent. It is used to help prevent or treat malaria and can be used to treat toxoplasmosis. Pyrimethamine can also be used to treat Pneumocystis carinii pneumonia, if you cannot take more standard treatment. Generic pyrimethamine tablets are not yet available.

What should my health care professional know before I take pyrimethamine?

They need to know if you have any of these conditions:
- an alcohol problem
- anemia or other blood disorders
- asthma
- dental disease
- folic acid deficiency
- kidney disease
- liver disease
- seizures (convulsions)
- an unusual or allergic reaction to pyrimethamine, other medicines, foods, dyes, or preservatives
- pregnant or trying to get pregnant
- breast-feeding

How should I take this medicine?

Take pyrimethamine tablets by mouth. Follow the directions on the prescription label. Swallow tablets whole with a drink of water. If pyrimethamine upsets your stomach take it with food or milk. Take your doses at regular intervals. Do not take your medicine more often than directed.

What if I miss a dose?

If you miss a weekly dose, take it as soon as you can. If you miss a daily dose, take it as soon as you remember, but miss that dose if it is nearly time for your next dose. Do not take double or extra doses.

What may interact with pyrimethamine?

- medicines for HIV infection
- carbamazepine
- folic acid, folinic acid
- p-aminobenzoic acid, PABA
- lorazepam
- medicines for cancer chemotherapy
- medicines for mental problems and psychotic disturbances
- medicines for an over-active thyroid gland
- procainamide
- some antibiotics

Tell your prescriber or health care professional about all other medicines you are taking, including non-prescription medicines, nutritional supplements, or herbal products. Also tell your prescriber or health care professional if you are a frequent user of drinks with caffeine or alcohol, if you smoke, or if you use illegal drugs. These may affect the way your medicine works. Check with your health care professional before stopping or starting any of your medicines.

What should I watch for while taking pyrimethamine?

Tell your prescriber or health care professional if your symptoms do not improve in 2 to 3 days. High doses of pyrimethamine for toxoplasmosis can cause blood problems; visit your prescriber or health care professional for regular checks on your blood. If you get a skin rash, stop taking your medicine and consult your prescriber or health care professional as soon as you can. Pyrimethamine can cause blood problems. This can mean slow healing and a risk of infection. Try to avoid cutting or injuring yourself. Problems can arise if you need dental work, and in the day to day care of your teeth. Try to avoid damage to your teeth and gums when you brush or floss your teeth. Check with your pharmacist before you visit a new area where there are malaria-carrying mosquitoes. You may need to take a different antimalarial medicine.

What side effects may I notice from taking pyrimethamine?

Side effects that you should report to your prescriber or health care professional as soon as possible:
- difficulty breathing
- fever or chills, sore throat
- increased sensitivity to the sun or ultraviolet light
- sore mouth or odd taste, swollen tongue
- seizures (convulsions)
- redness, blistering, peeling, or loosening of skin, including skin inside the mouth
- skin rash, itching
- stomach pain
- unusual bleeding or bruising
- unusual tiredness or weakness

Side effects that usually do not require medical attention (report to your prescriber or health care professional if they continue or are bothersome):
- diarrhea
- loss of appetite
- nausea, vomiting

Where can I keep my medicine?

Keep out of the reach of children in a container that small children cannot open. It is important to keep pyrimethamine out of reach of children; overdose is dangerous. Store at room temperature between 15 and 25 degrees C (59 and 77 degrees F). Protect from light and moisture. Keep container tightly closed. Throw away any unused medicine after the expiration date.

Quazepam tablets

DORAL®;
15 mg; Tablet
Medpointe
Pharmaceuticals

DORAL®;
7.5 mg; Tablet
Medpointe
Pharmaceuticals

What are quazepam tablets?

QUAZEPAM (Doral®) is a benzodiazepine used to treat insomnia (trouble sleeping). Benzodiazepines are a family of medicines that have a relaxing effect on the central nervous system. This effect allows an individual to fall asleep and stay asleep more easily. Generic quazepam is not available.

What should my health care professional know before I take quazepam?

Your health care professional should know if you have any of the following conditions:

- an alcohol or drug abuse problem
- bipolar disorder, depression, psychosis or other mental health condition
- glaucoma
- kidney disease
- liver disease
- lung disease, such as chronic obstructive pulmonary disease (COPD), sleep apnea or other breathing difficulties
- myasthenia gravis
- Parkinson's disease
- porphyria
- seizures or a history of seizures
- shortness of breath
- snoring
- suicidal thoughts
- uncontrolled pain
- an unusual or allergic reaction to quazepam, other benzodiazepines, other medicines, foods, dyes, or preservatives
- pregnant or trying to get pregnant
- breast-feeding

How should I take this medication?

Quazepam tablets are taken by mouth just before you go to bed at night.

What if I miss a dose?

Take the missed dose when you remember, however, if it is the next day when you remember, wait until bedtime to take your medicine and skip the missed dose. Do not take two doses at the same time.

What may interact with quazepam?

- alcohol
- bosentan
- caffeine
- cimetidine
- disulfiram
- female hormones, including contraceptive or birth control pills
- herbal or dietary supplements such as kava kava, melatonin, St. John's Wort or valerian
- imatinib, STI-571
- isoniazid
- medicines for anxiety or sleeping problems, such as alprazolam, diazepam, lorazepam or triazolam
- medicines for depression, mental problems or psychiatric disturbances
- medicines for fungal infections (fluconazole, itraconazole, ketoconazole, voriconazole)
- medicines for HIV infection or AIDS
- prescription pain medicines
- probenecid
- rifampin, rifapentine, or rifabutin
- some antibiotics (clarithromycin, erythromycin, troleandomycin)
- some medicines for colds, hay fever or other allergies
- some medicines for blood pressure or heart problems (amiodarone, diltiazem, nicardipine, verapamil)
- some medicines for seizures (carbamazepine, phenobarbital, phenytoin, primidone)
- theophylline
- zafirlukast
- zileuton

Tell your doctor or other health professional about all other medicines you are taking, including vitamins, herbal supplements and over-the-counter medicines. Notify your prescriber if you use alcohol or illegal drugs frequently as they may affect how your medicine works. Check with your doctor before starting or stopping any of your medicines.

What should I watch for while taking quazepam?

See your doctor or other healthcare professional regularly to assess your response to quazepam and to determine if you still need it. Quazepam may make you drowsy or dizzy and you should not operate machinery, drive or do anything that requires mental alertness until you see how quazepam affects you. Quazepam can have these effects even the day after you take it. Avoid alcoholic drinks because they can increase the dizziness and drowsiness that you experience. Check with your doctor or healthcare professional before taking other medicines that could make you drowsy such as sedatives, tranquilizers, narcotic pain medicine, other sleeping pills, or cold or allergy medicines.

What side effects may I notice from taking quazepam?

Side effects you should report to your doctor or other health care professional immediately:

- confusion
- depression
- seizures

- change in behavior (mood swings, aggressiveness)
- difficulty walking
- muscle cramps or spasms
- trouble with speech
- skin rash
- tremors

Side effects that do not usually require medical attention:
- dizziness, drowsiness, feeling of a hangover
- headache

- stomach upset, vomiting
- dry mouth
- trouble sleeping, nightmares

Where can I keep my medicine?

Keep out of reach of children in a container that small children cannot open. Store between 2 and 30 degrees C (36 and 86 degrees F). Keep container tightly closed. Throw away any unused medicine after the expiration date.

Quetiapine tablets

  SEROQUEL®; 200 mg; Tablet AstraZeneca Pharmaceuticals LP SEROQUEL®; 300 mg; Tablet AstraZeneca Pharmaceuticals LP

What are quetiapine tablets?

QUETIAPINE (Seroquel®) helps to treat schizophrenia or bipolar disorder, also known as manic depression. Quetiapine can help you to keep in touch with reality, stabilize the mood, and reduce your mental problems. Generic quetiapine tablets are not yet available.

What should my health care professional know before I take quetiapine?

They need to know if you have any of these conditions:
- an alcohol abuse problem
- brain tumor or head injury
- breast cancer
- cataracts
- diabetes (increased blood sugar) or a family history of diabetes
- difficulty swallowing
- heart disease
- kidney disease
- liver disease
- low blood pressure (hypotension) or dizziness when standing up
- Parkinson's disease
- previous heart attack
- seizures (convulsions)
- thyroid problems
- an unusual or allergic reaction to quetiapine, other medicines, foods, dyes, or preservatives
- pregnant or trying to get pregnant
- breast-feeding

How should I take this medicine?

Take quetiapine tablets by mouth with or without food. Follow the directions on the prescription label. Swallow the tablets with a drink of water. If quetiapine upsets your stomach you can take it with food. Take your doses at regular intervals. Do not take your medicine more often than directed. Do not stop taking except on your prescriber's advice. Contact your pediatrician or health care professional regarding the use of this medicine in children. Special care may be needed. Patients over age 65 years may have a stronger reaction to this medicine and need smaller doses.

What if I miss a dose?

If you miss a dose, take it as soon as you can. If it is almost time for your next dose, take only that dose. Do not take double or extra doses.

What may interact with quetiapine?

- alcohol
- antifungal medicines, such as fluconazole, itraconazole, ketoconazole, or voriconazole
- barbiturates
- carbamazepine
- cimetidine
- erythromycin
- levodopa
- lorazepam
- medicines for diabetes
- medicines for mental problems and psychotic disturbances
- oxcarbazepine
- phenobarbital
- phenytoin
- rifampin
- thioridazine

Tell your prescriber or health care professional about all other medicines you are taking, including non-prescription medicines. Also tell your prescriber or health care professional if you are a frequent user of drinks with caffeine or alcohol, if you smoke, or if you use illegal drugs. These may affect the way your medicine works. Check with your health care professional before stopping or starting any of your medicines.

What should I watch for while taking quetiapine?

Visit your prescriber or health care professional for regular checks on your progress. It may be several weeks before you see the full effects of quetiapine. Do not suddenly stop taking quetiapine. You may need to gradually reduce the dose. Only stop taking quetiapine on your prescriber's advice. Your health care provider may suggest that you have your eyes examined prior to starting quetiapine, and every 6 months thereafter. You may get dizzy or drowsy. Do not drive, use machinery, or do anything that needs mental alertness until you know how quetiapine affects you. Do not stand or sit up quickly, especially if you are an older patient. This reduces the risk of dizzy or fainting spells. Alcohol can increase dizziness and drowsiness. Avoid alcoholic drinks. If you notice an increased hunger or thirst, different from your normal hunger or thirst, or if you find that you must frequently use the restroom (excessive urination), you should contact your health care provider as soon as possible. You may need to have your blood sugar monitored. Do not treat yourself for colds, diarrhea or allergies. Ask your prescriber or health care professional for advice, some nonprescription medicines may increase possible side effects. If you are going to have surgery tell your prescriber or health care professional that you are taking quetiapine.

What side effects may I notice from taking quetiapine?

Side effects that you should report to your prescriber or health care professional as soon as possible:
Rare or uncommon:
- difficulty swallowing
- severe weakness
- fainting spells
- inability to control muscle movements in the face, hands, arms, or legs
- increased thirst or hunger
- increased need to pass urine
- loss of balance or difficulty walking
- rash
- restlessness or need to keep moving
- seizures
- stiff muscles
- sexual difficulties

More common:
- dizziness or lightheadedness
- fast or irregular heartbeat (palpitations)

Side effects that usually do not require medical attention (report to your prescriber or health care professional if they continue or are bothersome):
- constipation
- drowsiness or dizziness
- dry mouth
- nausea
- runny nose
- stomach pain
- unusual tiredness
- weight gain

Where can I keep my medicine?

Keep out of the reach of children in a container that small children cannot open. Store at room temperature between 20 degrees and 25 degrees C (68 degrees and 77 degrees F). Throw away any unused medicine after the expiration date.

Quinapril tablets

ACCUPRIL®;
10 mg; Tablet
Parke Davis Division
of Pfizer Co.

ACCUPRIL®;
20 mg; Tablet
Parke Davis Division
of Pfizer Co.

What are quinapril tablets?

QUINAPRIL (Accupril®) is an antihypertensive (blood pressure lowering agent) known as an ACE inhibitor. Quinapril controls high blood pressure (hypertension) by relaxing blood vessels; it is not a cure. High blood pressure levels can damage your kidneys, and may lead to a stroke or heart failure. Quinapril also helps to treat patients with heart failure (heart does not pump strongly enough). Generic quinapril tablets are available.

What should my health care professional know before I take quinapril?

They need to know if you have any of these conditions:
- autoimmune disease (such as lupus), or suppressed immune function
- previous swelling of the tongue, face, or lips with difficulty breathing, difficulty swallowing, hoarseness, or tightening of the throat (angioedema)
- bone marrow disease
- heart or blood vessel disease
- liver disease
- low blood pressure
- kidney disease
- if you are on a special diet, such as a low-salt diet
- an unusual or allergic reaction to quinapril, other ACE inhibitors, foods, dyes, or preservatives
- pregnant or trying to get pregnant
- breast-feeding

How should I take this medicine?

Take quinapril tablets by mouth. Follow the directions on the prescription label. Swallow the tablets with a drink of water. It is best to take quinapril on an empty stomach, at least 1 hour before or 2 hours after meals. Take your doses at regular intervals. Do not take your medicine more often than directed. Do not stop taking quinapril except on your prescriber's advice. Contact your pediatrician or health care professional regarding the use of this medicine in children. Special care may be needed.

What if I miss a dose?

If you miss a dose, take it as soon as you can. If it is almost time for your next dose, take only that dose. Do not take double or extra doses. If you take only one dose a day and forget to take it that day, do not take a double dose the next day.

What may interact with quinapril?

- anti-inflammatory drugs (NSAIDs, such as ibuprofen)
- hawthorn

- heparin
- lithium
- medicines for high blood pressure
- potassium salts
- tetracycline
- water pills

Tell your prescriber or health care professional about all other medicines you are taking, including non-prescription medicines, nutritional supplements, or herbal products. Also tell your prescriber or health care professional if you are a frequent user of drinks with caffeine or alcohol, if you smoke, or if you use illegal drugs. These may affect the way your medicine works. Check with your health care professional before stopping or starting any of your medicines.

What should I watch for while taking quinapril?

Visit your prescriber or health care professional for regular checks on your progress. Check your blood pressure regularly while you are taking quinapril. Ask your prescriber or health care professional what your blood pressure should be and when you should contact him or her. Call your prescriber or health care professional if you notice an uneven or fast heart beat. Do not treat yourself for a fever or sore throat; check with your prescriber or health care professional as these may be the result of a quinapril side effect. Check with your prescriber or health care professional if you get an attack of severe diarrhea, nausea and vomiting, or if you sweat a lot. The loss of body fluid can make it dangerous to take quinapril. You may get dizzy. Do not drive, use machinery, or do anything that needs mental alertness until you know how quinapril affects you. To avoid

dizzy or fainting spells, do not stand or sit up quickly, especially if you are an older person. Alcohol can make you more dizzy. Avoid alcoholic drinks. If you are going to have surgery, tell your prescriber or health care professional that you are using quinapril. Avoid salt substitutes or other foods or substances high in potassium salts. Do not treat yourself for coughs, colds, or pain while you are using quinapril without asking your prescriber or health care professional for advice.

What side effects may I notice from taking quinapril?

Side effects that you should report to your prescriber or health care professional as soon as possible:
- decreased amount of urine passed
- difficulty breathing, or difficulty swallowing
- dizziness, lightheadedness or fainting spells
- fast or uneven heart beat, palpitations, or chest pain
- fever or chills
- numbness or tingling in your fingers or toes
- skin rash, itching
- swelling of your face, lips, or tongue

Side effects that usually do not require medical attention (report to your prescriber or health care professional if they continue or are bothersome):
- change in taste
- cough
- tiredness

Where can I keep my medicine?

Keep out of the reach of children in a container that small children cannot open. Store at room temperature between 15 and 30 degrees C (59 and 86 degrees F). Throw away any unused medicine after the expiration date.

Quinidine tablets, capsules, and extended-release tablets

QUINIDEX®;
300 mg; Tablet,
Extended Release
A H Robins Co Div
American Home
Products Corp

QUINIDEX®;
324 mg; Tablet
URL/Mutual Pharm.

What are quinidine tablets, capsules, and extended-release tablets?

QUINIDINE (Quinidex®) is an antiarrhythmic agent. Quinidine treats irregular heart rhythm and can slow rapid heartbeats (tachycardia). Quinidine can help your heart to return to and maintain a normal rhythm. Generic quinidine tablets, capsules, and extended-release tablets are available.

What should my health care professional know before I take quinidine?

They need to know if you have any of these conditions:
- asthma, chronic bronchitis, or emphysema
- fever
- kidney disease
- liver disease

- low blood pressure
- myasthenia gravis
- other heart problems
- an unusual or allergic reaction to quinidine, quinine, other medicines, foods, dyes, or preservatives
- pregnant or trying to get pregnant
- breast-feeding

How should I take this medicine?

Take quinidine tablets, capsules, and extended-release tablets by mouth. Follow the directions on the prescription label. Swallow tablets and capsules whole with a full glass of water; take tablets or capsules in an upright or sitting position. Taking a sip of water first, before taking the tablets, may help you swallow them. Do not crush or chew extended-release tablets. If possible take bedtime doses at least 10 minutes before lying down.

Take your doses at regular intervals. Do not take your medicine more often than directed. Contact your pediatrician or health care professional regarding the use of this medicine in children. Special care may be needed.

What if I miss a dose?

If you miss a dose, take it as soon as you can. If the dose is more than two hours late or almost time for your next dose, take only that dose. Do not take double or extra doses.

What may interact with quinidine?

- acetazolamide
- antacids
- arsenic trioxide
- astemizole
- barbiturate medicines for inducing sleep or treating seizures
- bepridil
- beta-blockers, often used for high blood pressure or heart problems
- bosentan
- certain antibiotics (such as clarithromycin, erythromycin, gatifloxacin, grepafloxacin, levofloxacin, moxifloxacin, sparfloxacin)
- cevimeline
- cimetidine
- cisapride
- citrate salts (examples: Bicitra®, Oracit®, Cytra-2, Polycitra®, Urocit®-K)
- cyclobenzaprine
- dalfopristin; quinupristin
- galantamine
- ginger
- grapefruit juice
- hawthorn
- itraconazole
- ketoconazole
- loperamide
- medicines for asthma or breathing difficulties
- medicines for diabetes such as metformin
- medicines for high blood pressure or angina
- medicines for mental depression, behavioral problems, or psychotic disturbances
- medicines for pain such as codeine, methadone, tramadol
- medicines for surgery that relax muscles or block pain
- medicines to control heart rhythm (examples: amiodarone, digoxin, diltiazem, disopyramide, dofetilide, flecainide, propafenone, procainamide, sotalol, verapamil)
- mefloquine
- methazolamide
- neostigmine
- phenytoin
- probucol
- rifampin
- ritonavir
- sodium bicarbonate
- tacrolimus
- terfenadine
- warfarin
- water pills (diuretics)

Tell your prescriber or health care professional about all other medicines you are taking, including non-prescription medicines, nutritional supplements, or herbal products. Also tell your prescriber or health care professional if you are a frequent user of drinks with caffeine or alcohol, if you smoke, or if you use illegal drugs. These may affect the way your medicine works. Check with your health care professional before stopping or starting any of your medicines.

What should I watch for while taking quinidine?

Visit your prescriber or health care professional for regular checks on your progress. Do not stop taking quinidine suddenly; this may cause serious, heart-related side effects. Because your condition and the use of quinidine carry some risk, it is a good idea to carry an identification card, necklace or bracelet with details of your condition, medications and prescriber or health care professional. Check your heart rate (pulse) and blood pressure regularly while you are taking quinidine. Ask your prescriber or health care professional what your heart rate and blood pressure should be, and when you should contact him or her. Your prescriber or health care professional also may schedule regular blood tests and electrocardiograms to check your progress. You may feel dizzy, faint, or have trouble seeing clearly. Do not drive, use machinery, or do anything that needs mental alertness until you know how quinidine affects you. To reduce the risk of dizzy or fainting spells, do not sit or stand up quickly, especially if you are an older patient. Alcohol can make you more dizzy, increase flushing and rapid heartbeats. Avoid alcoholic drinks. Quinidine may make your skin and eyes more sensitive to sun or ultraviolet light. Keep out of the sun, or wear protective clothing and sunglasses outdoors; use a sunscreen (at least SPF 15). Do not use sun lamps or sun tanning beds or booths. If you are going to have surgery, tell your prescriber or health care professional that you are taking quinidine.

What side effects may I notice from taking quinidine?

Side effects that you should report to your prescriber or health care professional as soon as possible:

- blurred vision or other change in vision
- difficulty breathing, wheezing
- dizziness or fainting spells
- fever
- headache
- irregular heartbeat (palpitations)
- pain on swallowing
- skin rash, peeling or loose skin
- ringing in the ears
- unusual bruising or bleeding
- unusual tiredness or weakness

Side effects that usually do not require medical attention (report to your prescriber or health care professional if they continue or are bothersome):

- changes in taste (bitter or metallic taste)
- confusion

- diarrhea
- flushing of the skin with intense itching
- heartburn, stomach pain or cramps
- increased sensitivity of the skin to sun or ultraviolet light
- loss of appetite
- nausea, vomiting

Where can I keep my medicine?

Keep out of the reach of children in a container that small children cannot open. Store at room temperature between 15 and 30 degrees C (59 and 86 degrees F). Protect from light. Keep container tightly closed. Throw away any unused medicine after the expiration date.

Q

Rabeprazole tablets

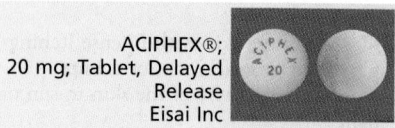

ACIPHEX®;
20 mg; Tablet, Delayed
Release
Eisai Inc

What are rabeprazole tablets?

RABEPRAZOLE (AcipHex™) prevents the production of acid in the stomach. It reduces symptoms and prevents injury to the esophagus or stomach in patients with gastroesophageal reflux disease (GERD) or ulcers. Rabeprazole is also useful in conditions that produce too much stomach acid such as Zollinger-Ellison syndrome. Rabeprazole may also be used with antibiotics to get rid of bacteria that are associated with some ulcers. Generic rabeprazole tablets are not yet available.

What should my health care professional know before I take rabeprazole?

They need to know if you have any of these conditions:
- liver disease
- an unusual or allergic reaction to omeprazole, lansoprazole, rabeprazole, other medicines, foods, dyes, or preservatives
- pregnant or trying to get pregnant
- breast-feeding

How should I take this medicine?

Take rabeprazole tablets by mouth. Follow the directions on the prescription label. Swallow the tablets whole with a drink of water; do not crush, break, or chew. You may take this medicine with or without food. Take your doses at regular intervals. Do not take your medicine more often than directed. Contact your pediatrician or health care professional regarding the use of this medicine in children. Special care may be needed.

What if I miss a dose?

If you miss a dose, take it as soon as you can. If it is almost time for your next dose, take only that dose. Do not take double or extra doses.

What may interact with rabeprazole?

- ampicillin
- cyclosporine
- diazepam
- digoxin
- iron salts
- itraconazole
- ketoconazole

Tell your prescriber or health care professional about all other medicines you are taking, including non-prescription medicines, nutritional supplements, or herbal products. Also tell your prescriber or health care professional if you are a frequent user of drinks with caffeine or alcohol, if you smoke, or if you use illegal drugs. These may affect the way your medicine works. Check with your health care professional before stopping or starting any of your medicines.

What should I watch for while taking rabeprazole?

It can take several days of therapy with rabeprazole before your stomach pains improve. Check with your prescriber or health care professional if your condition does not improve, or if it gets worse. You can take antacids for the occasional relief of stomach pain unless your prescriber or health care professional tells you otherwise.

What side effects may I notice from taking rabeprazole?

Side effects that you should report to your prescriber or health care professional as soon as possible:
- fever or sore throat
- persistent skin rash
- unusual bleeding or bruising
- yellowing of the eyes or skin

Side effects that usually do not require medical attention (report to your prescriber or health care professional if they continue or are bothersome):
- diarrhea
- dizziness
- headache
- nausea/vomiting
- rash
- tiredness

Where can I keep my medicine?

Keep out of the reach of children in a container that small children cannot open. Store at room temperature between 15 and 30 degrees C (59 and 86 degrees F). Protect from light and moisture. Throw away any unused medicine after the expiration date.

Raloxifene tablets

EVISTA®;
60 mg; Tablet
Eli Lilly and Co

What are raloxifene tablets?

RALOXIFENE (Evista®) reduces the amount of calcium lost from bones. It helps to prevent bone loss and to increase normal healthy bone formation in patients with osteoporosis. Raloxifene does not reduce hot flashes associated with estrogen deficiency. Generic raloxifene tablets are not yet available.

What should my health care professional know before I take raloxifene?

They need to know if you have any of these conditions:
- cancer
- a history of blood clots
- low level of blood calcium
- heart failure
- high level of blood triglycerides
- liver disease
- vitamin D deficiency
- an unusual or allergic reaction to raloxifene, other medicines, foods, dyes, or preservatives
- pregnant or trying to get pregnant
- breast-feeding

How should I take this medicine?

Raloxifene tablets are taken by mouth. They can be taken with or without food. Follow the directions on the prescription label. Swallow the tablets with a full glass of water. Do not take your medicine more often than directed. Contact your pediatrician or health care professional regarding the use of this medicine in children. Special care may be needed.

What if I miss a dose?

If you miss a dose, take it as soon as you can. If it is almost time for your next dose, take only that dose. Do not take double or extra doses.

What may interact with raloxifene?

- ampicillin
- thyroid hormones like levothyroxine
- herbal or dietary supplements like black cohosh or soy

Tell your prescriber or health care professional about all other medicines you are taking including non-prescription medicines. Also tell your prescriber or health care professional if you are a frequent user of drinks with caffeine or alcohol, if you smoke, or if you use illegal drugs. These can affect the way your medicine works. Check with your health care professional before stopping or starting any of your medicines.

What should I watch for while taking raloxifene?

Visit your prescriber or health care professional for regular checks on your progress. Do not stop taking raloxifene except on your prescriber's advice. You should make sure you get enough calcium and vitamin D in your diet while you are taking raloxifene. Discuss your dietary needs with your health care professional or nutritionist. Exercise may help to prevent bone loss. Discuss your exercise needs with your prescriber or health care professional. Raloxifene can rarely cause blood clots. You should avoid long periods of bed rest while taking raloxifene. If you are going to have surgery, tell your prescriber or health care professional that you are taking raloxifene. Raloxifene should be stopped at least 3 days before surgery. After surgery, it should be restarted only after you are walking again. It should not be restarted while you still need long periods of bed rest. You should not smoke while taking raloxifene. Smoking may also increase your risk of blood clots. Smoking can also decrease the effects of raloxifene on bone.

What side effects might I notice from taking raloxifene?

Side effects that you should report to your prescriber or health care professional as soon as possible:
Rare or uncommon:
- difficulty breathing
- leg pain or swelling
- skin rash, itching

Side effects that usually do not require medical attention (report to your prescriber or health care professional if they continue or are bothersome):
- difficulty sleeping
- fluid build-up
- hot flashes
- leg cramps
- muscle aches
- sinus pressure or drainage
- stomach or intestinal gas
- stomach pain
- sweating
- weight gain

Where can I keep my medicine?

Keep out of the reach of children in a container that small children cannot open. Store at room temperature between 15 and 30 degrees C (59 and 86 degrees F). Throw away any unused medicine after the expiration date.

R

Ramipril capsules

ALTACE®;
5 mg; Capsule
Monarch
Pharmaceuticals Inc

ALTACE®;
2.5 mg; Capsule
Monarch
Pharmaceuticals Inc

What are ramipril capsules?

RAMIPRIL (Altace®) is an antihypertensive (blood pressure lowering agent) known as an ACE inhibitor. Ramipril controls high blood pressure (hypertension) by relaxing blood vessels; it is not a cure. High blood pressure levels can damage your kidneys, and may lead to a stroke or heart failure. Generic ramipril capsules are not yet available.

What should my health care professional know before I take ramipril?

They need to know if you have any of these conditions:
- autoimmune disease (such as lupus) or suppressed immune function
- previous swelling of the tongue, face, or lips with difficulty breathing, difficulty swallowing, hoarseness, or tightening of the throat (angioedema)
- bone marrow disease
- heart or blood vessel disease
- liver disease
- low blood pressure
- kidney disease
- if you are on a special diet, such as a low-salt diet
- an unusual or allergic reaction to ramipril, other ACE inhibitors, foods, dyes, or preservatives
- pregnant or trying to get pregnant
- breast-feeding

How should I take this medicine?

Take ramipril capsules by mouth. Follow the directions on the prescription label. Swallow the capsules with a drink of water. Take your doses at regular intervals. Do not take your medicine more often than directed. Do not stop taking ramipril except on your prescriber's advice. Contact your pediatrician or health care professional regarding the use of this medicine in children. Special care may be needed.

What if I miss a dose?

If you miss a dose, take it as soon as you can. If it is almost time for your next dose, take only that dose. Do not take double or extra doses. If you take only one dose a day and forget to take it that day, do not take a double dose the next day.

What may interact with ramipril?

- anti-inflammatory drugs (NSAIDs, such as ibuprofen)
- hawthorn
- heparin
- lithium
- medicines for high blood pressure
- potassium salts
- water pills

Tell your prescriber or health care professional about all other medicines you are taking, including non-prescription medicines, nutritional supplements, or herbal products. Also tell your prescriber or health care professional if you are a frequent user of drinks with caffeine or alcohol, if you smoke, or if you use illegal drugs. These may affect the way your medicine works. Check with your health care professional before stopping or starting any of your medicines.

What should I watch for while taking ramipril?

Visit your prescriber or health care professional for regular checks on your progress. Check your blood pressure regularly while you are taking ramipril. Ask your prescriber or health care professional what your blood pressure should be and when you should contact him or her. Call your prescriber or health care professional if you notice an uneven or fast heart beat. Do not treat yourself for a fever or sore throat; check with your prescriber or health care professional as these may be the result of a ramipril side effect. Check with your prescriber or health care professional if you get an attack of severe diarrhea, nausea and vomiting, or if you sweat a lot. The loss of body fluid can make it dangerous to take ramipril. You may get dizzy. Do not drive, use machinery, or do anything that needs mental alertness until you know how ramipril affects you. To avoid dizzy or fainting spells, do not stand or sit up quickly, especially if you are an older person. Alcohol can make you more dizzy. Avoid alcoholic drinks. If you are going to have surgery, tell your prescriber or health care professional that you are using ramipril. Avoid salt substitutes or other foods or substances high in potassium salts. Do not treat yourself for coughs, colds, or pain while you are using ramipril without asking your prescriber or health care professional for advice.

What side effects may I notice from taking ramipril?

Side effects that you should report to your prescriber or health care professional as soon as possible:
- decreased amount of urine passed
- difficulty breathing, or difficulty swallowing
- dizziness, lightheadedness or fainting spells
- fast or uneven heart beat, palpitations, or chest pain
- fever or chills
- numbness or tingling in your fingers or toes
- skin rash, itching
- swelling of your face, lips, or tongue

Side effects that usually do not require medical attention (report to your prescriber or health care professional if they continue or are bothersome):
- change in taste
- cough
- headache
- tiredness

Where can I keep my medicine?

Keep out of the reach of children in a container that small children cannot open. Store at room tempera ture between 15 and 30 degrees C (59 and 86 degrees F). Keep container tightly closed. Throw away any unused medicine after the expiration date.

Ranitidine Bismuth Citrate tablets

TRITEC;
400 mg; Tablet
Glaxo Wellcome Division

What are ranitidine bismuth citrate tablets?

RANITIDINE BISMUTH CITRATE (Tritec®) is used in combination with the antibiotic clarithromycin (Biaxin®) to treat active duodenal ulcers associated with *Helicobacter pylori*. This drug is discontinued in the United States. Generic ranitidine bismuth citrate tablets are not available.

What should my health care professional know before I take ranitidine bismuth citrate?

They need to know if you have any of these conditions:
- kidney disease
- porphyria
- an unusual or allergic reaction to ranitidine bismuth citrate, other medicines, foods, dyes, or preservatives
- pregnant or trying to get pregnant
- breast-feeding

How should I take this medicine?

Take ranitidine bismuth citrate tablets by mouth. Follow the directions on the prescription label. Swallow the tablets with a drink of water. Take your medicine at regular intervals. Do not take your medicine more often than directed. Contact your pediatrician or health care professional regarding the use of this medicine in children. Special care may be needed.

What if I miss a dose?

If you miss a dose, take it as soon as you can. If it is almost time for your next dose, take only that dose. Do not take double or extra doses.

What may interact with ranitidine bismuth citrate?

- antacids
- cefditoren
- cefpodoxime
- cefuroxime
- delavirdine
- enoxacin
- itraconazole
- ketoconazole
- propantheline
- certain antibiotics such as tetracyclines or fluoroquinolones

Tell your prescriber or health care professional about all other medicines you are taking, including non-prescription medicines, nutritional supplements, or herbal products. Also tell your prescriber or health care professional if you are a frequent user of drinks with caffeine or alcohol, if you smoke, or if you use illegal drugs. These may affect the way your medicine works. Check with your health care professional before stopping or starting any of your medicines.

What should I watch for while taking ranitidine bismuth citrate?

Tell your prescriber or health care professional if your ulcer pain does not improve or gets worse. You may need to take this medicine for several days as prescribed before your symptoms improve. Finish the full course of tablets prescribed by your prescriber or health care professional even if you feel better. Do not self-medicate with aspirin, ibuprofen or other anti-inflammatory medicines; these can aggravate your ulcer and may make it bleed. Do not smoke cigarettes or drink alcohol; these increase ulcer irritation and can lengthen the time it will take for your ulcers to heal. If you need to take an antacid you should take it at least 1 hour before or 1 hour after ranitidine bismuth citrate. Ranitidine bismuth citrate will not be as effective if taken at the same time as an antacid. If you get black, tarry stools or vomit up what looks like coffee grounds, call your prescriber or health care professional at once. You may have a bleeding ulcer.

What side effects may I notice from taking ranitidine bismuth citrate?

Side effects that you should report to your prescriber or health care professional as soon as possible:
- agitation, nervousness, depression, hallucinations
- breast swelling and tenderness, or sexual difficulties (impotence) in men
- redness, blistering, peeling or loosening of the skin, including inside the mouth
- skin rash, itching
- unusual weakness or tiredness
- vomiting
- yellowing of the skin or eyes

Side effects that usually do not require medical attention (report to your prescriber or health care professional if they continue or are bothersome):
- constipation or diarrhea
- dizziness
- headache
- nausea

Where can I keep my medicine?

Keep out of the reach of children in a container that small children cannot open. Store at room temperature between 2 and 30 degrees C (36 and 86 degrees F) in a dry place. Protect from light and moisture. Keep container tightly closed. Throw away any unused medicine after the expiration date.

R

Ranitidine tablets
or capsules

ZANTAC®;
150 mg; Tablet
Glaxo Wellcome
Division

RANITIDINE;
150 mg; Capsule
Sandoz
Pharmaceuticals

What are ranitidine tablets or capsules?

RANITIDINE (Zantac®) is a type of antihistamine that blocks the release of stomach acid. Ranitidine is used to treat stomach or intestinal ulcers. It can relieve ulcer pain and discomfort, and the heartburn from acid reflux. Generic ranitidine tablets and capsules are available.

What should my health care professional know before I take ranitidine?

They need to know if you have any of these conditions:
- frequently drink alcohol-containing beverages
- kidney disease
- liver disease
- other chronic illness
- porphyria
- an unusual or allergic reaction to ranitidine, other medicines, foods, dyes, or preservatives
- pregnant or trying to get pregnant
- breast-feeding

How should I take this medicine?

Take ranitidine tablets or capsules by mouth. Follow the directions on the prescription label. Swallow the tablets or capsules with a drink of water. If you only take ranitidine once a day, take it at bedtime. Take your medicine at regular intervals. Do not take your medicine more often than directed. Contact your pediatrician or health care professional regarding the use of this medicine in children. Special care may be needed.

What if I miss a dose?

If you miss a dose, take it as soon as you can. If it is almost time for your next dose, take only that dose. Do not take double or extra doses.

What may interact with ranitidine?

- alcohol-containing beverages
- alendronate
- antacids
- cefditoren
- cefpodoxime
- cefuroxime
- delavirdine
- enoxacin
- glipizide
- glyburide
- iron supplements
- itraconazole
- ketoconazole
- metformin
- nifedipine
- propantheline
- theophylline
- triazolam
- warfarin

Tell your prescriber or health care professional about all other medicines you are taking, including non-prescription medicines, nutritional supplements, or herbal products. Also tell your prescriber or health care professional if you are a frequent user of drinks with caffeine or alcohol, if you smoke, or if you use illegal drugs. These may affect the way your medicine works. Check with your health care professional before stopping or starting any of your medicines.

What should I watch for while taking ranitidine?

Tell your prescriber or health care professional if your condition does not improve or gets worse. You may need to take this medicine for several days as prescribed before your symptoms improve. Finish the full course of tablets prescribed, even if you feel better. Do not self-medicate with aspirin, ibuprofen or other anti-inflammatory medicines; these can aggravate your condition. Do not smoke cigarettes or drink alcohol; these increase irritation in your stomach and can lengthen the time it will take for ulcers to heal. Cigarettes and alcohol can also worsen acid reflux or heartburn. If you need to take an antacid you should take it at least 1 hour before or 1 hour after ranitidine. Ranitidine will not be as effective if taken at the same time as an antacid. If you get black, tarry stools or vomit up what looks like coffee grounds, call your prescriber or health care professional at once. You may have a bleeding ulcer.

What side effects may I notice from taking ranitidine?

Side effects with ranitidine are infrequent but include:
- agitation, nervousness, hallucinations
- constipation or diarrhea
- dark yellow or brown urine
- diarrhea
- dizziness
- headache
- nausea, vomiting
- redness, blistering, peeling or loosening of the skin, including inside the mouth
- skin rash, itching
- sore throat, fever
- stomach pain
- unusual weakness or tiredness
- unusual bleeding or bruising
- yellowing of the skin or eyes

Let your prescriber or health care professional know if you get any of these side effects or any other unusual symptoms.

Where can I keep my medicine?

Keep out of the reach of children in a container that small children cannot open. Store at room temperature between 2 and 25 degrees C (36 and 77 degrees F). Protect from light and moisture. Keep container tightly closed. Throw away any unused medicine after the expiration date.

Ranolazine extended-release tablets

What are Ranolazine extended-release tablets?

RANOLAZINE (Ranexa®) is a medicine used to treat chronic angina. Ranolazine relieves chest pain (angina) when taking regularly. Ranolazine does not relieve an acute episode of angina or chest pain. Ranolazine should only be taken by patients who have tried other medicines for angina, and still do not have adequate relief of symptoms.

What should my health care professional know before I receive Ranolazine?

They need to know if you have any of these conditions:
- heart disease
- heart rhythm problems (fast heartbeat, family history of QT prolongation, congenital long QT syndrome)
- low blood levels of potassium or magnesium
- kidney disease
- liver disease
- an unusual reaction to Ranolazine, other medicines, foods, dyes, or preservatives
- pregnant or trying to get pregnant
- breast-feeding

How should this medicine be used?

Take ranolazine tablets by mouth. Follow the directions on the prescription label. Swallow the tablets whole. Do not cut, break, crush, or chew the tablets. The tablets can be taken with or without food. Do not take your medication with grapefruit juice. Take your doses at regular intervals. Do not take your medicine more often then directed. Contact your pediatrician or health care professional regarding the use of this medicine in children. Special care may be needed.

What if I miss a dose?

If you miss a dose, take it as soon as you can. If it is almost time for your next dose, take only that dose. Do not take double or extra doses.

What drug(s) may interact with Ranolazine?

Do not take ranolazine with any of the following:

- abarelix
- aprepitant
- certain antibiotics (chloramphenicol, clarithromycin, dalfopristin; quinupristin, erythromycin, telithromycin, troleandomycin)
- certain chemotherapy drugs used to treat cancer (arsenic trioxide, imatinib, STI-571)
- certain medicines for depression or mental problems (chlorpromazine, fluvoxamine, haloperidol, mesoridazine, thioridazine, pimozide, ziprasidone)
- certain medicines to control heart rhythm (amiodarone, disopyramide, dofetilide, flecainide, procainamide, propafenone, quinidine, sotalol)
- certain medicines to treat malaria (chloroquine, halofantrine, quinidine)
- cisapride
- conivaptan
- cyclosporine
- danazol
- diltiazem
- droperidol
- fluvoxamine
- grapefruit or grapefruit juice
- isoniazid (INH)
- medicines for fungal infections (fluconazole, itraconazole, ketoconazole, voriconazole)
- medicines for HIV infection (amprenavir, atazanavir, delavirdine, fosamprenavir, indinavir, nelfinavir, ritonavir, saquinavir, tipranavir)
- methadone
- mifepristone, RU-486
- pentamidine
- verapamil

Ranolazine may also interact with the following medications:

- alfuzosin
- certain antibiotics (ciprofloxacin, gatifloxacin, gemifloxacin, levofloxacin, moxifloxacin, norfloxacin, ofloxacin)
- digoxin
- efavirenz
- eplerenone
- ergot alkaloids used for migraine (such as ergotamine, dihydroergotamine)
- herbal or dietary supplements such as St. John's wort or red yeast rice
- local anesthetics or general anesthetics
- medicines for depression
- medicines for erectile dysfunction
- medicines for seizures (carbamazepine, phenobarbital, phenytoin, primidone)
- medicines for high cholesterol (atorvastatin, lovastatin, simvastatin)
- nicardipine
- some medicines for malaria (mefloquine, quinine)
- some medicines for mental problems (fluphenazine, perphenazine, risperidone, trifluoperazine)
- some medicines for pain (codeine, hydrocodone, oxycodone, propoxyphene)
- some medicines for stomach problems (octreotide, palonosetron, prochlorperazine)
- rifampin, rifapentine, or rifabutin
- sirolimus
- tacrolimus
- zafirlukast

Tell your prescriber or health care professional about all other medicines you are taking, including non-prescription medicines, nutritional supplements, or herbal products. Also tell your prescriber or health care professional if you are a frequent user of drinks with caffeine or alcohol, if you smoke, or if you use illegal drugs. These may affect the way your medicine works. Check

R

with your health care professional before stopping or starting any of your medicines.

What should I watch for while taking Ranolazine?

Ranolazine does not relieve an acute attack of angina or chest pain. Symptoms of an angina attack might include chest pain, reduced tolerance of exercise or walking, and/or shortness of breath. Contact your doctor if you feel palpitations or if you have fainting spells. Ranolazine may produce changes in the electrocardiogram (ECG). Your health care provider may check your heart rhythm by ordering an ECG while taking ranolazine. You may feel dizzy or lightheaded while taking ranolazine. Do not drive, use machinery, or do anything that needs mental alertness until you know how this medicine affects you. To reduce the risk of dizzy or fainting spells, do not sit or stand up quickly, especially if you are an older patient. Avoid alcoholic drinks; they can make you dizzy or increase flushing and rapid heartbeats. If you are going to have surgery, tell your prescriber or health care professional that you are taking ranolazine.

What side effects may I notice from receiving Ranolazine?

Side effects that you should report to your prescriber or health care professional as soon as possible:

- blurred vision
- difficulty breathing or shortness of breath
- fainting spells
- fast, irregular or pounding heartbeat (palpitations)
- low or high blood pressure
- numbness or tingling feelings
- persistent nausea or vomiting
- ringing in the ears
- tremor or shakiness
- slow heartbeat (fewer than 50 beats per minute)
- swelling of the legs or feet

Side effects that usually do not require medical attention (report to your prescriber or health care professional if they continue or are bothersome):

- constipation
- drowsiness
- dry mouth
- headache
- mild dizziness
- mild nausea or vomiting
- stomach upset

Where can I keep my medicine?

Keep out of the reach of children. Store at room temperature between 15 and 30 degrees C (59 and 86 degrees F). Throw away any unused medicine after the expiration date.

Repaglinide tablets

PRANDIN®;
1 mg; Tablet
Novo Nordisk
Pharmaceutical
Industries Inc

PRANDIN®;
2 mg; Tablet
Novo Nordisk
Pharmaceutical
Industries Inc

What are repaglinide tablets?

REPAGLINIDE (Prandin®) helps to treat type 2 diabetes mellitus. Treatment is combined with a balanced diet and suitable exercise. Repaglinide increases the amount of insulin released from the pancreas, which helps to control blood sugar. Generic repaglinide tablets are not available at this time.

What should my health care professional know before I take repaglinide?

They need to know if you have any of these conditions:
- kidney disease
- liver disease
- severe infection or injury
- an unusual or allergic reaction to repaglinide or other medicines, foods, dyes, or preservatives
- pregnant or trying to get pregnant
- breast-feeding

How should I take this medicine?

Take repaglinide tablets by mouth. Follow the directions on the prescription label. Swallow the tablets with a drink of water. The dose should be taken no earlier than 30 minutes before every meal. If a meal is added, take a tablet before that meal. Do not take more often than directed or without a meal. Contact your pediatrician or health care professional regarding the use of this medicine in children. Special care may be needed. Elderly patients over 65 years old may have a stronger reaction and need a smaller dose.

What if I miss a dose?

If you miss a dose before a meal, skip that dose. If it is almost time for your next dose, take only that dose with the next scheduled meal as directed. Do not take double or extra doses.

What may interact with repaglinide?

- barbiturates like phenobarbital or primidone
- carbamazepine
- erythromycin
- ketoconazole
- miconazole
- other medicines for diabetes
- rifampin

Many medications may cause changes (increase or decrease) in blood sugar; these include:

- alcohol containing beverages
- aspirin and aspirin-like drugs
- beta-blockers, often used for high blood pressure or heart problems (examples include atenolol, metoprolol, propranolol)
- chromium

- female hormones, such as estrogens, progestins, or contraceptive pills
- isoniazid
- male hormones or anabolic steroids
- medications to suppress appetite or for weight loss
- medicines for allergies, asthma, cold, or cough
- niacin
- pentamidine
- phenytoin
- some herbal dietary supplements
- steroid medicines such as prednisone or cortisone
- thyroid hormones
- water pills (diuretics)

Tell your prescriber or health care professional about all other medicines you are taking, including non-prescription medicines. Also tell your prescriber or health care professional if you are a frequent user of drinks with caffeine or alcohol, if you smoke, or if you use illegal drugs. These may affect the way your medicine works. Check with your health care professional before stopping or starting any of your medicines.

What should I watch for while taking repaglinide?

Visit your prescriber or health care professional for regular checks on your progress. Learn how to monitor your blood sugar. Check with your prescriber or health care professional if your blood sugar is high, you may need a change of dose of repaglinide. Do not skip meals. If you are exercising much more than usual you may need extra snacks to avoid side effects caused by low blood sugar. Alcohol can increase possible side effects of repaglinide. Ask your prescriber or health care professional if you should avoid alcohol. If you have mild symptoms of low blood sugar, eat or drink something containing sugar at once and contact your prescriber or health care professional. It is wise to check your blood sugar to confirm that it is low. It is important to recognize your own symptoms of low blood sugar so that you can treat them quickly. Make sure family members know that you can choke if you eat or drink

when you develop serious symptoms of low blood sugar, such as seizures or unconsciousness. They must get medical help at once. If you are going to have surgery, tell your prescriber or health care professional that you are taking repaglinide. Wear a medical identification bracelet or chain to say you have diabetes, and carry a card that lists all your medications.

What side effects may I notice from taking repaglinide?

Side effects that you should report to your prescriber or health care professional as soon as possible:

- hypoglycemia—contact your health care professional if you experience symptoms of low blood sugar, which may include: anxiety or nervousness, confusion, difficulty concentrating, hunger, pale skin, nausea, fatigue, sweating, headache, palpitations, numbness of the mouth, tingling in the fingers, tremors, muscle weakness, blurred vision, cold sensations, uncontrolled yawning, irritability, rapid heartbeat, shallow breathing, and loss of consciousness.
- breathing difficulties, severe skin reactions or excessive phlegm, which may indicate that you are having an allergic reaction to the drug
- dark yellow or brown urine, or yellowing of the eyes or skin, indicating that the drug is affecting your liver
- fever, chills, sore throat, which means the drug may be affecting your immune system
- unusual bleeding or bruising, which occurs when the drug is affecting your blood clotting system
- vomiting

Side effects that usually do not require medical attention (report to your prescriber or health care professional if they continue or are bothersome):

- headache
- nausea

Where can I keep my medicine?

Keep out of the reach of children in a container that small children cannot open. Store at room temperature between 15 and 30 degrees C (59 and 86 degrees F). Keep container tightly closed. Throw away any unused medicine after the expiration date.

Reserpine tablets

RESERPINE;
0.1 mg; Tablet
Eon Labs Inc

RESERPINE;
0.25 mg; Tablet
Eon Laboratories

What are reserpine tablets?

RESERPINE is an antihypertensive. It helps lower high blood pressure (hypertension) to normal levels. High blood pressure levels can cause you to have a stroke, get heart failure, or damage your kidneys. Reserpine is not a cure for high blood pressure. Generic reserpine tablets are available.

What should my health care professional know before I take reserpine?

They need to know if you have any of these conditions:
- depression

- gallstones
- heart disease
- kidney disease
- Parkinson's disease
- peptic ulcer
- pheochromocytoma
- receiving electroconvulsive therapy
- seizures (convulsions)
- ulcerative colitis
- an unusual or allergic reaction to reserpine, tartrazine dye, other medicines, foods, dyes, or preservatives
- pregnant or trying to get pregnant
- breast-feeding

How should I take this medicine?

Take reserpine tablets by mouth. Follow the directions on the prescription label. Swallow the tablets with a drink of water. If reserpine upsets your stomach you can take it with food or milk. Take your doses at regular intervals. Do not take your medicine more often than directed. Contact your pediatrician or health care professional regarding the use of this medicine in children. Special care may be needed.

What if I miss a dose?

If you miss a dose, take it as soon as you can. If it is almost time for your next dose, take only that dose. Do not take double or extra doses.

What may interact with reserpine?

- alcohol
- barbiturate medicines for inducing sleep or treating seizures (convulsions)
- hawthorn
- heart medicine such as digoxin or digitoxin
- levodopa
- linezolid
- medicines for colds and breathing difficulties
- medicines for high blood pressure
- medicine for mental depression
- procainamide
- quinidine
- water pills

Tell your prescriber or health care professional about all other medicines you are taking, including non-prescription medicines, nutritional supplements, or herbal products. Also tell your prescriber or health care professional if you are a frequent user of drinks with caffeine or alcohol, if you smoke, or if you use illegal drugs. These may affect the way your medicine works. Check with your health care professional before stopping or starting any of your medicines.

What should I watch for while taking reserpine?

Visit your prescriber or health care professional for regular checks on your progress. Check your heart rate and blood pressure regularly while you are taking reserpine. Ask your prescriber or health care professional what your heart rate should be and when you should contact him or her. You may get drowsy or dizzy. Do not drive, use machinery, or do anything that needs mental alertness until you know how reserpine affects you. To avoid dizzy or fainting spells, do not stand or sit up quickly, especially if you are an older person. Alcohol can make you more drowsy and dizzy. Avoid alcoholic drinks. Your mouth may get dry. Chewing sugarless gum or sucking hard candy, and drinking plenty of water will help.

What side effects may I notice from taking reserpine?

Side effects that you should report to your prescriber or health care professional as soon as possible:

- blurred vision
- confusion, nervousness, or excitability. nightmares
- depression
- difficulty breathing
- dizziness or fainting spells
- pain or difficulty passing urine
- irregular heartbeat or palpitations, chest pain
- stomach pain
- swelling of feet or legs
- unusual tiredness

Side effects that usually do not require medical attention (report to your prescriber or health care professional if they continue or are bothersome):

- dry mouth
- headache
- loss of appetite
- nausea, vomiting
- sexual difficulties (impotence)
- stuffy nose

Where can I keep my medicine?

Keep out of the reach of children in a container that small children cannot open. Store at room temperature between 15 and 30 degrees C (59 and 86 degrees F). Protect from light. Keep container tightly closed. Throw away any unused medicine after the expiration date.

This drug requires an FDA medication guide. See page xxxvii.

Ribavirin capsules and tablets

REBETOL;
200 mg; Capsule
Schering Corp

COPEGUS;
200 mg; Tablet
Hoffmann La Roche
Inc

What are ribavirin capsules and tablets?

RIBAVIRIN (Rebetol®, Copegus®) is an antiviral agent used to treat hepatitis C in combination with interferon alfa (capsules) or peginterferon alfa (tablets). It is not for the treatment of simple viral infections or other types of hepatitis infections. Generic ribavirin capsules and tablets are available.

What should my health care professional know before I take ribavirin capsules?

They need to know if you have any of these conditions:

- anemia
- breathing problems
- heart disease such as angina or history of a heart attack
- high blood pressure
- human immunodeficiency virus (HIV) infection
- kidney disease
- liver disease (other than hepatitis C)
- pancreatitis
- past interferon treatment for hepatitis C that did not work
- prior organ transplant
- sickle-cell disease

- thalassemia
- an unusual or allergic reaction to ribavirin, interferons, other medicines, foods, dyes, or preservatives
- pregnant or trying to get pregnant
- breast-feeding

How should I use this medicine?

Ribavirin capsules or tablets are taken by mouth. Swallow the capsules or tablets with a drink of water. You can take ribavirin capsules with or without food, but you should take it the same way every day as directed. Ribavirin tablets should be taken with food. Follow the directions on the prescription label. Take your doses at regular intervals.

Do not take your medicine more often than directed. Finish the full course prescribed by your prescriber or health care professional even if you think your condition is better. Do not stop taking except on your prescriber's advice. Do NOT share this medicine with anyone else. Contact your pediatrician or health care professional regarding the use of this medicine in children. Special care may be needed.

What if I miss a dose?

If you miss a dose, take it as soon as you can. If it is almost time for your next dose, take only that dose. Do not take double or extra doses.

What may interact with ribavirin?

- medicines to treat HIV, especially zidovudine, ZDV (AZT), lamivudine, or stavudine (d4T)

Tell your prescriber or other health care professional about all other medicines you are taking including non-prescription medicines, nutritional supplements, or herbal products. Also, tell your prescriber or health care professional if you are a frequent user of drinks with caffeine or alcohol, if you smoke or if you use illegal drugs. These may affect the way your medicine works. Check before stopping or starting any of your medications.

What should I watch for while taking ribavirin capsules?

Treatment with ribavirin may last for 24 to 48 weeks. It is important not to stop treatment even if you are feeling better. You may need to have blood tests done

during therapy to evaluate your progress. Ribavirin may cause severe birth defects or death to the unborn child if taken during pregnancy; therefore if you are pregnant, you must not take ribavirin. Women who can still have children must have a negative pregnancy test before starting treatment then monthly pregnancy tests until 6 months after stopping ribavirin. Female patients and female partners of men taking ribavirin must use 2 forms of effective birth control methods during treatment with ribavirin and for 6 months after stopping ribavirin therapy. If you think you may have become pregnant and are taking ribavirin, contact your prescriber or health care professional right away. There is no information regarding whether treatment with ribavirin and interferon will prevent the spread of hepatitis C to others. Also, it is not known if this combination can cure hepatitis C or prevent other complications of hepatitis C infection such as cirrhosis, liver failure, or liver cancer. Ribavirin therapy may cause anemia (low red blood counts). You will need to have frequent blood checks during the first month of treatment with ribavirin to follow your counts.

What side effects may I notice from taking ribavirin capsules?

Side effects that you should report to your prescriber or health care professional as soon as possible:

- changes in your heart rate
- coughing or wheezing
- difficulty breathing
- dizziness or light-headedness
- increased weakness, fatigue or tiredness
- missed menstrual cycle

Side effects that usually do not require medical attention (report to your prescriber or health care professional if they continue or are bothersome):

- headache
- heartburn
- itching
- nausea
- skin rash
- vomiting

Where can I keep my medicine?

Keep out of the reach of children. NEVER share this medicine with anyone. Ribavirin capsules should be kept at room temperature between 59 and 86 degrees F (15 and 30 degrees C).

Riboflavin, Vitamin B$_2$ tablets

VITAMIN B$_2$;
100 mg; Capsule
Twin Laboratories, Inc

What are riboflavin tablets?

RIBOFLAVIN (Vitamin B$_2$) is a naturally occurring vitamin found in milk, meat, eggs, nuts, enriched flour, and green vegetables. Riboflavin treats vitamin B$_2$ deficiency. Riboflavin deficiency can cause itching, burning eyes; increased sensitivity of the eyes to light;

mouth sores; and peeling of the skin on the nose and scrotum. Generic riboflavin tablets are available.

What should my health care professional know before I take riboflavin?

They need to know if you have any of the following conditions:

- an unusual or allergic reaction to B vitamins, other medicines, foods, dyes, or preservatives
- pregnant or trying to get pregnant
- breast-feeding

How should I take this medicine?

Take riboflavin tablets by mouth. Follow the directions on the prescription label. Swallow the tablets with a glass of water.

What if I miss a dose?

If you miss a dose, skip that dose. Continue with your next scheduled dose.

What may interact with riboflavin?

- propantheline

Tell your prescriber or health care professional about all other medicines you are taking, including non-prescription medicines, nutritional supplements, or herbal products. Also tell your prescriber or health care professional if you are a frequent user of drinks with caffeine or alcohol, if you smoke, or if you use illegal drugs. These may affect the way your medicine works. Check with your health care professional before stopping or starting any of your medicines.

What should I watch for while taking riboflavin?

Make sure you have a proper diet. Taking riboflavin tablets does not replace the need for a balanced diet. Some foods that contain riboflavin include: milk, meat, eggs, nuts, enriched flour, and green vegetables.

What side effects may I notice from taking riboflavin?

The recommended daily allowance of riboflavin does not cause any serious side effects.
A minor side effect of riboflavin:
- bright yellow urine

This is no cause for alarm.

Where can I keep my medicine?

Keep out of the reach of children in a container that small children cannot open. Store at room temperature between 15 and 30 degrees C (59 and 86 degrees F). Protect from light. Keep container tightly closed. Throw away any unused medicine after the expiration date.

Rifabutin capsules

MYCOBUTIN®;
150 mg; Capsule
Pharmacia and Upjohn Div
Pfizer

What are rifabutin capsules?

RIFABUTIN (Mycobutin®) is an antibacterial agent. It is effective in preventing the tuberculosis-like infection and illness known as mycobacterium avium complex (MAC) in patients with human immunodeficiency virus (HIV) infection. Rifabutin will not cure or prevent HIV infection or AIDS. Generic rifabutin capsules are not yet available.

What should my health care professional know before I take rifabutin?

They need to know if you have any of these conditions:
- dental disease
- tuberculosis
- wear contact lens
- an unusual or allergic reaction to rifabutin, rifamycin, other medicines, foods, dyes or preservatives
- pregnant or trying to get pregnant
- breast-feeding

How should I take this medicine?

Take rifabutin capsules by mouth. Follow the directions on the prescription label. Swallow capsules whole with a full glass of water. You can take rifabutin with or without food. Opening the capsule and mixing the contents with food, such as applesauce, is an easy way to give to children. Take your doses at regular intervals and try not to miss any doses. Do not take your medicine more often than directed. Finish the full course prescribed by your prescriber or health care professional even if you think your condition is better. Do not stop taking except on your prescriber's advice.

What if I miss a dose?

If you miss a dose, take it as soon as you can. If it is almost time for your next dose, take only that dose. Do not take double or extra doses.

What may interact with rifabutin?

Rifabutin has the potential to interact with many other drugs. Some of the possible interactions are listed:

- bosentan
- cyclosporine
- female hormones, including contraceptive or birth control pills
- fluconazole
- itraconazole
- levomethadyl
- medicines for lowering cholesterol (example: atorvastatin, lovastatin, simvastatin)
- medicines for the treatment of HIV infection or AIDS
- methadone
- sirolimus
- some medicines for seizures (convulsions)
- some medicines for depression, anxiety, psychosis or problems with sleep (insomnia)
- some prescription pain medications

- tacrolimus
- voriconazole

Tell your prescriber or health care professional about all other medicines you are taking, including non-prescription medicines, nutritional supplements, or herbal products. Also tell your prescriber or health care professional if you are a frequent user of drinks with caffeine or alcohol, if you smoke, or if you use illegal drugs. These may affect the way your medicine works. Check with your health care professional before stopping or starting any of your medicines.

What should I watch for while taking rifabutin?

Keep taking your rifabutin even if you feel better. Visit your prescriber or health care professional for regular checks and report any serious side effects promptly. Alcohol can increase possible damage to your liver. Avoid alcoholic drinks while you are taking rifabutin. If you get a persistent cough, chest pain, or have difficulty breathing do not treat yourself. Call your prescriber or health care professional for advice. These could be symptoms of tuberculosis. Birth control pills (contraceptive pills) may not work properly while you are taking this medicine. Use a different method of birth control while you are taking rifabutin. Ask your prescriber or health care professional for advice if necessary. This medicine can color your urine, feces (stool), perspiration (sweat), tears, sputum, skin or saliva reddish-orange to reddish-brown. This color can last for as long as you take rifabutin and is not a cause for alarm. Talk to your prescriber or health care professional about it if it concerns you. However, this color in tears may permanently stain soft contact lenses. It is better not to wear soft contact lenses while you are taking rifabutin. Rifabutin can cause blood problems. This can mean slow healing and a risk of infection. Problems can arise if you need dental work, and in the day to day care of your teeth. Try to avoid damage to your teeth and gums when you brush or floss your teeth.

What side effects may I notice from taking rifabutin?

Side effects that you should report to your prescriber or health care professional as soon as possible:
- dark yellow or brown urine
- difficulty breathing
- cough
- eye pain or loss of vision
- fever or chills, sore throat
- loss of appetite
- muscle aches or pains
- unusual tiredness or weakness
- yellowing of the eyes or skin

Side effects that usually do not require medical attention (report to your prescriber or health care professional if they continue or are bothersome):
- discoloration of soft contact lens
- nausea, vomiting
- reddish-orange to reddish-brown coloration of urine, stools, saliva, tears, and sweat
- skin rash, itching
- stomach pain

Where can I keep my medicine?

Keep out of the reach of children in a container that small children cannot open. Store at room temperature between 15 and 30 degrees C (59 and 86 degrees F). Keep container tightly closed. Throw away any unused medicine after the expiration date.

Rifampin capsules

RIFADIN®;
300 mg; Capsule
Aventis Pharmaceuticals Inc

What are rifampin capsules?

RIFAMPIN (Rifadin®, Rimactane®) is an antibiotic and is used for the prevention or treatment of tuberculosis infections. It is never used alone, but in combination with at least one other agent that treats tuberculosis. Rifampin also treats other infections, including carriers of meningitis and for this purpose it is given alone. Generic rifampin capsules are available.

What should my health care professional know before I take rifampin?

They need to know if you have any of these conditions:
- if you frequently drink alcohol-containing beverages
- liver disease, including hepatitis
- porphyria
- previously experienced side effects to isoniazid (INH) treatment
- wear contact lens
- an unusual or allergic reaction to rifampin, rifabutin, other medicines, foods, dyes or preservatives
- pregnant or trying to get pregnant
- breast-feeding

How should I take this medicine?

Take rifampin capsules by mouth. Follow the directions on the prescription label. Swallow capsules whole with a full glass of water. It is best to take rifampin on an empty stomach, 1 to 2 hours before food, or at least 2 hours after food. If rifampin upsets your stomach you can take it with food. Opening the capsule and mixing the contents with food, such as applesauce, is an easy way to give to children. Take your doses at regular intervals and try not to miss any doses. Do not take your medicine more often than directed. Finish the full course prescribed by your prescriber or health care professional even if you think your condition is better. Do not stop taking except on your prescriber's advice.

Contact your pediatrician or health care professional regarding the use of this medicine in children. Special care may be needed.

What if I miss a dose?

If you miss a dose, take it as soon as you can. If it is almost time for your next dose, take only that dose. Do not take double or extra doses.

What may interact with rifampin?

Many medicines can interact with rifampin. Make sure to tell your prescriber you are taking rifampin before starting any new medicines and to discuss all the medicines you are taking before starting rifampin therapy. The list below contains some, but not all, of the drugs that can interact with rifampin. If have any questions about the medicines you are taking talk to your prescriber or pharmacist.

- acetaminophen
- alcohol
- bosentan
- caspofungin
- certain medicines for diabetes
- clofibrate
- corticosteroids such as prednisone
- cyclosporine
- digoxin
- doxycycline
- entacapone
- female hormones, including contraceptive or birth control pills
- fluconazole
- imatinib, STI-571
- itraconazole
- levomethadyl
- levothyroxine
- medicines for lowering cholesterol (example: atorvastatin, lovastatin, simvastatin)
- medicines for the treatment of HIV infection or AIDS
- methadone
- sildenafil
- sirolimus
- some medicines for heart rhythm problems
- some medicines for high blood pressure, chest pain, or other heart problems
- some medicines for seizures (convulsions)
- some medicines for anxiety, psychosis or problems with sleep (insomnia)
- some prescription pain medications
- tacrolimus
- theophylline
- voriconazole
- warfarin

Tell your prescriber or health care professional about all other medicines you are taking, including non-prescription medicines, nutritional supplements, or herbal products. Also tell your prescriber or health care professional if you are a frequent user of drinks with caffeine or alcohol, if you smoke, or if you use illegal drugs. These may affect the way your medicine works. Check with your health care professional before stopping or starting any of your medicines.

What should I watch for while taking rifampin?

Rifampin can cause serious liver problems, especially if you are also taking pyrazinamide (PZA). Make sure you understand the risks for liver problems and how to identify the symptoms. If you have any questions, talk with your prescriber or other health care provider. Visit your prescriber or health care professional for regular checks and report any serious side effects promptly. Keep taking your rifampin even if you feel better. You may need to take this medicine for an extended period of time for a complete cure. Avoid alcoholic drinks while you are taking rifampin. Drinking alcohol during treatment with rifampin increases the risk of serious liver problems. Birth control pills (contraceptive pills) may not work properly while you are taking this medicine. Use a different method of birth control while you are taking rifampin. This medicine can color your urine, feces (stool), perspiration (sweat), tears, sputum, skin or saliva reddish-orange to reddish-brown. This color can last for as long as you take rifampin and is not a cause for alarm. Talk to your prescriber or health care professional about it if it concerns you. However, this color in tears may permanently stain soft contact lenses. It is better not to wear soft contact lenses while you are taking rifampin. If you are going to have surgery, tell your prescriber or health care professional that you are taking rifampin.

What side effects may I notice from taking rifampin?

Side effects that you should report to your prescriber or health care professional as soon as possible:
- difficulty breathing
- fever or chills, sore throat
- reduced amount of urine passed
- skin rash, itching, hives
- stomach pain
- unusual tiredness or weakness
- yellowing of the eyes or skin

Side effects that usually do not require medical attention (report to your prescriber or health care professional if they continue or are bothersome):
- diarrhea
- discoloration of soft contact lens
- dizziness
- headache
- loss of appetite
- nausea, vomiting
- reddish-orange to reddish-brown coloration of urine, stools, saliva, tears, and sweat

Where can I keep my medicine?

Keep out of the reach of children in a container that small children cannot open. Store at room temperature between 15 and 30 degrees C (59 and 86 degrees F). Protect from light and moisture. Throw away any unused medicine after the expiration date.

Rifapentine tablets

What are rifapentine tablets?

RIFAPENTINE (Priftin®) is an antibacterial agent. It is used to treat tuberculosis. For this purpose it is never used alone, but in combination with at least one other agent that treats tuberculosis. Generic rifapentine tablets are not yet available.

What should my health care professional know before I take rifapentine?

They need to know if you have any of these conditions:

- an unusual or allergic reaction to rifapentine, rifamycin, other medicines, foods, dyes or preservatives
- pregnant or trying to get pregnant
- breast-feeding

How should I take this medicine?

Take rifapentine tablets by mouth. Follow the directions on the prescription label. Swallow tablets whole with a full glass of water. If rifapentine upsets your stomach you can take it with food. Take your doses at regular intervals and do not miss any doses. Do not take your medicine more often than directed. Finish the full course prescribed by your prescriber or health care professional even if you think your condition is better. Do not stop taking except on your prescriber's advice. Contact your pediatrician or health care professional regarding the use of this medicine in children. Special care may be needed.

What if I miss a dose?

It is very important that you not miss any doses. If you miss a dose, take it as soon as you can. If it is almost time for your next dose, take only that dose. Do not take double or extra doses.

What may interact with rifapentine?

Rifapentine has the potential to interact with many other drugs. Some of the possible interactions are listed:

- caspofungin
- certain medicines for diabetes
- clofibrate
- corticosteroids such as prednisone
- cyclosporine
- digoxin
- doxycycline
- female hormones, including contraceptive or birth control pills
- fluconazole
- itraconazole
- levomethadyl
- levothyroxine
- medicines for lowering cholesterol (example: atorvastatin, lovastatin, simvastatin)
- medicines for the treatment of HIV infection or AIDS

- methadone
- sildenafil
- sirolimus
- some medicines for heart rhythm problems
- some medicines for high blood pressure, chest pain, or other heart problems
- some medicines for seizures (convulsions)
- some medicines for anxiety, psychosis or problems with sleep (insomnia)
- some prescription pain medications
- tacrolimus
- theophylline
- voriconazole
- warfarin

Tell your prescriber or health care professional about all other medicines you are taking, including non-prescription medicines, nutritional supplements, or herbal products. Also tell your prescriber or health care professional if you are a frequent user of drinks with caffeine or alcohol, if you smoke, or if you use illegal drugs. These may affect the way your medicine works. Check with your health care professional before stopping or starting any of your medicines.

What should I watch for while taking rifapentine?

Tell your prescriber or health care professional if your symptoms do not improve in 2 to 3 weeks. Keep taking your rifapentine even if you feel better. Visit your prescriber or health care professional for regular checks and report any serious side effects promptly. Alcohol can increase possible damage to your liver. Avoid alcoholic drinks while you are taking rifapentine. Birth control pills (contraceptive pills) may not work properly while you are taking this medicine. Use a different method of birth control while you are taking rifapentine. This medicine can color your urine, feces (stool), perspiration (sweat), tears (including contact lenses), breast milk, sputum, skin or saliva (including dentures) reddish-orange to reddish-brown. This color can last for as long as you take rifapentine and is not a cause for alarm. Talk to your prescriber or health care professional about it if it concerns you. However, this color may permanently stain soft contact lenses. It is better not to wear soft contact lenses while you are taking rifapentine. Dentures may also become permanently stained. Rifapentine can cause blood problems. This can mean slow healing and a risk of infection. Problems can arise if you need dental work, and in the day to day care of your teeth. Try to avoid damage to your teeth and gums when you brush or floss your teeth. If you are going to have surgery, tell your prescriber or health care professional that you are taking rifapentine.

What side effects may I notice from taking rifapentine?

Side effects that you should report to your prescriber or health care professional as soon as possible:

- darkened urine
- diarrhea
- difficulty breathing
- fever
- headache
- loss of appetite
- nausea and vomiting
- pain or swelling of the joints

- reduced amount of urine passed
- unusual tiredness or weakness
- yellowing of the eyes or skin

Side effects that usually do not require medical attention (report to your prescriber or health care professional if they continue or are bothersome):

- discoloration of soft contact lenses
- reddish-orange to reddish-brown coloration of urine, stools, saliva, tears, breast milk, and sweat
- skin rash, itching

Where can I keep my medicine?

Keep out of the reach of children in a container that small children cannot open. Store at room temperature between 15 and 30 degrees C (59 and 86 degrees F). Protect from excessive heat and moisture. Throw away any unused medicine after the expiration date.

Rifaximin tablets

XIFAXAN™;
200 mg; Tablet
Salix Pharmaceuticals Inc

What are rifaximin tablets?

RIFAXIMIN (Xifaxan™) is an antibiotic used for the treatment of traveler's diarrhea or other gastrointestinal infections. It is possible your health care provider may prescribe rifaximin to treat other conditions. Generic rifaximin tablets are not available.

What should my health care professional know before I take rifaximin?

They need to know if you have any of these conditions:

- bloody or tarry stools
- fever
- an unusual reaction to rifaximin, rifampin, rifabutin, other medicines, foods, dyes, or preservatives
- pregnant or trying to get pregnant
- breast-feeding

How should I take this medicine?

Take rifaximin tablets by mouth. Follow the directions on the prescription label. Swallow tablets whole with a full glass of water. Rifaximin may be taken with or without food. Take your doses at regular intervals and try not to miss any doses. Do not take your medicine more often than directed. Finish the full course prescribed by your prescriber or health care professional even if you think your condition is better. Do not stop taking except on your prescriber's advice. Contact your pediatrician or health care professional regarding the use of this medicine in children. Special care may be needed.

What if I miss a dose?

If you miss a dose, take it as soon as you can. If it is almost time for your next dose, take only that dose. Do not take double or extra doses.

What may interact with rifaximin?

- no drug interactions have been reported with rifaximin

Tell your prescriber or health care professional about all other medicines you are taking, including non-prescription medicines, nutritional supplements, or herbal products. Also tell your prescriber or health care professional if you are a frequent user of drinks with caffeine or alcohol, if you smoke, or if you use illegal drugs. These may affect the way your medicine works. Check with your health care professional before stopping or starting any of your medicines.

What should I watch for while taking rifaximin?

Keep taking your rifaximin even if you feel better. Contact your health care provider if you do not feel better or if your symptoms persist or get worse after 24 to 48 hours. Contact your health care provider immediately if you develop a fever or have bloody stools.

What side effects may I notice from taking rifaximin?

Side effects that you should report to your prescriber or health care professional as soon as possible:

- difficulty breathing
- fever
- skin rash, itching, or hives
- stomach pain
- worsening diarrhea during or after treatment or blood in the stool

Side effects that usually do not require medical attention (report to your prescriber or health care professional if they continue or are bothersome):

- constipation
- flatulence
- headache
- nausea/vomiting
- sensation of needing to empty the bowel
- urgent bowel movements

Where can I keep my medicine?

Keep out of the reach of children in a container that small children cannot open. Store at room temperature between 20 and 25 degrees C (68 and 77 degrees F). Protect from light and moisture. Throw away any unused medicine after the expiration date.

Riluzole tablets

RILUTEK®;
50 mg; Tablet
Aventis Pharmaceutical
Products Inc

R

What are riluzole tablets?

RILUZOLE (Rilutek®) slows down the progression of amyotrophic lateral sclerosis (also known as Lou Gehrig's disease). Riluzole helps to delay the loss of muscle strength and limb function for several months; it is not a cure. It can slow the loss of respiratory function. Generic riluzole tablets are approved, but are not yet marketed in the US.

What should my health care professional know before I take riluzole?

They need to know if you have any of these conditions:
- heart disease or high blood pressure
- kidney disease
- liver disease
- lung disease
- tobacco smoker
- an unusual or allergic reaction to riluzole, other medicines, foods, dyes, or preservatives
- pregnant or trying to get pregnant
- breast-feeding

How should I take this medicine?

Take riluzole tablets by mouth. Follow the directions on the prescription label. Swallow the tablets with a drink of water. It is best to take riluzole on an empty stomach, at least 1 hour before or 2 hours after meals. Take your doses at regular intervals. Do not take your medicine more often than directed. Do not stop taking except on your prescriber's advice. Contact your pediatrician or health care professional regarding the use of this medicine in children. Special care may be needed.

What if I miss a dose?

If you miss a dose, take it as soon as you can. If it is almost time for your next dose, take only that dose. Do not take double or extra doses.

What may interact with riluzole?

- allopurinol
- amitriptyline
- barbiturate medicines for inducing sleep or treating seizures (convulsions)
- caffeine
- carbamazepine
- certain antibiotics called quinolones
- methyldopa
- omeprazole
- rifampin
- sulfasalazine
- tacrine
- theophylline

Tell your prescriber or health care professional about all other medicines you are taking, including non-prescription medicines, nutritional supplements, or herbal products. Also tell your prescriber or health care professional if you are a frequent user of drinks with caffeine or alcohol, if you smoke, or if you use illegal drugs. These may affect the way your medicine works. Check with your health care professional before stopping or starting any of your medicines.

What should I watch for while taking riluzole?

Visit your prescriber or health care professional for regular checks on your progress. Check with your prescriber or health care professional if your symptoms get worse. Tell your prescriber or health care professional if you have a fever, chills, or other signs of infection; do not treat yourself. Avoid alcohol and tobacco while you are taking riluzole. They can increase the risk of getting liver damage. Ask your prescriber or health care professional for ways to help you stop smoking or drinking. You may get dizzy or lose your balance. Do not drive, use machinery, or do anything that needs mental alertness until you know how riluzole affects you.

What side effects may I notice from taking riluzole?

Side effects that you should report to your prescriber or health care professional as soon as possible:
- fever, chills or infection
- breathing difficulty, or shortness of breath
- yellowing of the skin or eyes

Side effects that usually do not require medical attention (report to your prescriber or health care professional if they continue or are bothersome):
- back pain
- cough
- diarrhea
- dizziness
- drowsiness
- increased blood pressure
- loss of appetite
- loss of balance from dizziness
- nausea, vomiting

- stomach pain
- tingling, pricking, or burning sensation around the mouth
- weakness and tiredness

Where can I keep my medicine?

Keep out of reach of children in a container that small children cannot open. Store at room temperature between 20 and 25 degrees C (68 and 77 degrees F). Protect from light. Throw away any unused medicine after the expiration date.

Rimantadine tablets

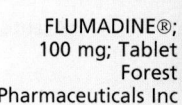
FLUMADINE®;
100 mg; Tablet
Forest
Pharmaceuticals Inc

RIMANTADINE;
100 mg; Tablet
Sandoz
Pharmaceuticals

What are rimantadine tablets?

RIMANTADINE (Flumadine®) is an antiviral agent. It treats or prevents certain influenza (flu) infections. Rimantadine is not an effective treatment for colds or for other viruses. Generic rimantadine tablets are not yet available.

What should my health care professional know before I take rimantadine?

They need to know if you have any of these conditions:
- kidney disease
- liver disease
- seizures (convulsions)
- an unusual or allergic reaction to rimantadine, amantadine, other medicines, foods, dyes, or preservatives
- pregnant or trying to get pregnant
- breast-feeding

How should I take this medicine?

Take rimantadine tablets by mouth. Follow the directions on the prescription label. Swallow tablets with a drink of water. Take rimantadine with food if it upsets your stomach. Take your doses at regular intervals. Do not take your medicine more often than directed. Finish the full course prescribed by your prescriber or health care professional even if you think your condition is better. Do not stop taking except on your prescriber's advice. Contact your pediatrician or health care professional regarding the use of this medicine in children. Special care may be needed.

What if I miss a dose?

If you miss a dose, take it as soon as you can. If it is almost time for your next dose, take only that dose. Do not take double or extra doses.

What may interact with rimantadine?

- acetaminophen
- aspirin
- cimetidine

Tell your prescriber or health care professional about all other medicines you are taking, including non-prescription medicines, nutritional supplements, or herbal products. Also tell your prescriber or health care professional if you are a frequent user of drinks with caffeine or alcohol, if you smoke, or if you use illegal drugs. These may affect the way your medicine works. Check with your health care professional before stopping or starting any of your medicines.

What should I watch for while taking rimantadine?

Tell your prescriber or health care professional if your symptoms do not improve within a few days, if you are being treated for influenza. You may get dizzy. Do not drive, use machinery, or do anything that needs mental alertness until you know how rimantadine affects you. Your mouth may get dry. Chewing sugarless gum or sucking hard candy, and drinking plenty of water will help.

What side effects may I notice from taking rimantadine?

Side effects that usually do not require medical attention (report to your prescriber or health care professional if they continue or are bothersome):
- difficulty sleeping
- dizziness, nervousness
- dry mouth
- headache
- loss of appetite
- nausea, vomiting
- stomach pain
- unusual tiredness or weakness

Where can I keep my medicine?

Keep out of the reach of children in a container that small children cannot open. Store at room temperature between 15 degrees and 30 degrees C (59 degrees and 86 degrees F). Throw away any unused medicine after the expiration date.

Risedronate tablets

ACTONEL®;
5 mg; Tablet
Procter and Gamble
Pharmaceuticals Inc Sub
Procter and Gamble Co

ACTONEL®;
35 mg; Tablet
Procter and Gamble
Pharmaceuticals Inc Sub
Procter and Gamble Co

What are risedronate tablets?

RISEDRONATE (Actonel®) reduces calcium loss from bones. It helps prevent bone loss and increases production of normal healthy bone in patients with Paget's disease, osteoporosis, and other conditions which place someone at risk for bone loss, including after menopause in females or from the long-term use of corticosteroids (like prednisone) in men or women. Generic risedronate tablets are not yet available.

What should my health care professional know before I take risedronate?

They need to know if you have any of these conditions:
- kidney disease
- low level of blood calcium
- stomach, intestinal, or esophageal problems, like acid-reflux or GERD
- problems swallowing
- vitamin D deficiency
- an unusual or allergic reaction to risedronate, other medicines, foods, dyes, or preservatives
- pregnant or trying to get pregnant
- breast-feeding

How should I take this medicine?

Follow the directions on the prescription label. Some patients take risedronate every day. Other patients may only take a dose of risedronate once a week. If you take risedronate only once a week, take the medicine on the same day every week. Take risedronate tablets by mouth in the morning, after you have risen for the day. Swallow the tablets with a full glass (6 to 8 fluid ounces) of plain water first thing in the morning. Do not take the tablets with any other type of liquid except plain water. Do not chew or suck the tablets. Do not eat or drink anything before you take your tablets and do not eat breakfast, drink, or take any other medicines for at least 30 minutes after taking risedronate. If you can wait for 2 hours before eating, your body will absorb even more of the medicine. After taking this medicine, remain sitting or standing upright (do not lie down) for at least 30 minutes to avoid irritation of your throat and esophagus (tube connecting mouth to stomach). Do not take this medicine at the same time as antacids, calcium, magnesium or iron supplements, or vitamins with minerals; if you take these medications, take them later in the day. Do not take your medicine more often than directed. Contact your pediatrician or health care professional regarding the use of this medicine in children. Special care may be needed.

What if I miss a dose?

If you take a daily dose of risedronate: If you have not already eaten, take your dose as soon as you can. Do not eat for at least 30 minutes after taking risedronate. If you have already eaten, wait at least 4 hours after eating to take your dose. Do not take double or extra doses.

If you take a once-weekly dose of risedronate: If you miss a dose of risedronate 35-mg once a week, take your dose on the morning after you remember. Then return to taking your dose just once a week, as originally scheduled on your regular chosen day of the week. Do not eat for at least 30 minutes after taking risedronate. If you have already eaten, wait at least 4 hours after eating to take your dose. Never take 2 tablets on the same day. Do not take double or extra doses.

What may interact with risedronate?

- aluminum hydroxide
- antacids
- anti-inflammatory drugs like ibuprofen, naproxen, and others
- aspirin
- calcium supplements
- iron supplements
- magnesium supplements
- parathyroid hormone
- teriparatide
- vitamins with minerals

Tell your prescriber or other health care professional about all other medicines you are taking including non-prescription medicines, nutritional supplements, or herbal products. Also tell your prescriber or health care professional if you are a frequent user of drinks with caffeine or alcohol, if you smoke or if you use illegal drugs. These may affect the way your medicine works. Check before stopping or starting any of your medications.

What should I watch for while taking risedronate?

Visit your prescriber or health care professional for regular checks on your progress. If you have Paget's disease it may be some time before you see the benefit from risedronate. Your prescriber or health care professional may order regular blood tests or other tests to check on your progress. It is very important to take risedronate with a full glass of plain water (6 to 8 ounces). Do not take with other fluids as these may decrease the absorption of risedronate. Do not take risedronate with food. Wait at least 30 minutes or longer after taking risedronate before you eat, drink or take other medicines. Because risedronate may irritate your throat, remain sitting or standing upright for at least 30 minutes after taking this medicine; do not lie down. If you begin to have pain when swallowing, difficulty swallowing, heartburn or stomach pain, call your pre-

R

scriber or health care professional right away. You should make sure you get enough calcium and vitamin D in your diet while you are taking risedronate, unless directed otherwise by your health care provider. Discuss your dietary needs with your health care professional or nutritionist. If you get bone pain, or a worsening of bone pain, check with your doctor. However, many patients have improvement in their bone pain during and after treatment with risedronate. If you are taking an antacid, a mineral supplement like calcium or iron, or a vitamin with minerals, make sure that you wait at least 2 hours before or after taking risedronate. Do not take them at same time.

What side effects might I notice from taking risedronate?

Side effects that you should report to your doctor as soon as possible:

- black or tarry stools
- eye inflammation, pain, or vision change

- low levels of calcium in the blood (may cause symptoms like confusion, severe fatigue or weakness)
- pain or difficulty when swallowing
- skin rash, itching
- stomach pain
- swelling of the lips, face, tongue, or throat

Side effects that usually do not require medical attention (report to your doctor if they continue or are bothersome):

- bone pain
- diarrhea
- headache
- indigestion or stomach gas
- mild heartburn
- nausea

Where can I keep my medicine?

Keep out of the reach of children in a container that small children cannot open. Store at room temperature between 68 and 77 degrees F (20 and 25 degrees C). Throw away any unused medicine after the expiration date.

Risperidone tablets or orally disintegrating tablets

RISPERDAL®;
2 mg; Tablet
Janssen Pharmaceuticals Inc

What are risperidone tablets or orally disintegrating tablets?

RISPERIDONE (Risperdal®, Risperdal® M-tab™) helps to treat schizophrenia. Risperidone can help you to keep in touch with reality and reduce your mental problems. Occasionally risperidone is used to treat other mood disturbances. Generic risperidone tablets or orally disintegrating tablets are not yet available.

What should my health care professional know before I take risperidone?

They need to know if you have any of these conditions:

- frequently drink alcohol or alcohol-containing beverages
- blood disorder or disease
- dementia
- diabetes (increased blood sugar) or a family history of diabetes
- difficulty swallowing
- heart disease
- history of brain tumor or head injury
- history of breast cancer
- irregular heartbeat
- kidney disease
- liver disease
- low blood pressure
- Parkinson's disease
- previous heart attack
- seizures (convulsions)
- an unusual or allergic reaction to risperidone, other medicines, foods, dyes, or preservatives
- pregnant or trying to get pregnant
- breast-feeding

How should I take this medicine?

Take risperidone tablets or orally disintegrating tablets by mouth. Follow the directions on the prescription label. If risperidone upsets your stomach you can take it with food. Take your doses at regular intervals. Do not take your medicine more often than directed. Do not stop taking except on your prescriber's advice. **Risperdal® tablets:** Take regular risperidone tablets by mouth. Swallow the tablets with a drink of water. **Risperdal® M-tab™ disintegrating tablets:** These tablets are made to dissolve in the mouth without having to take them with water. After removing the tablet from the package, place the tablet in the mouth on the tongue and allow it to dissolve, then swallow. Do not chew the tablet. While you may take these tablets with water, it is not necessary to do so. Contact your pediatrician or health care professional regarding the use of this medicine in children. Special care may be needed.

What if I miss a dose?

If you miss a dose, take it as soon as you can. If it is almost time for your next dose, take only that dose. Do not take double or extra doses.

What may interact with risperidone?

- alcohol
- arsenic trioxide
- astemizole
- bromocriptine
- cabergoline
- carbamazepine

- clarithromycin
- cimetidine
- cisapride
- droperidol
- erythromycin
- halofantrine
- imatinib, STI-571
- levodopa and other medications for Parkinson's disease
- levomethadyl
- medicines for high blood pressure
- medicines for irregular heartbeats
- medicines for sleep or sedation
- medicines for treating seizures (convulsions)
- other medicines for mental anxiety, depression or psychotic disturbances
- pentamidine
- prescription pain medications
- probucol
- rifampin
- ritonavir
- some medicines for infertility
- some medicines for the hormonal treatment of cancer
- some quinolone antibiotics for treating infections (gatifloxacin, levofloxacin, moxifloxacin, sparfloxacin
- terfenadine

Tell your prescriber or health care professional about all other medicines you are taking, including non-prescription medicines, nutritional supplements, or herbal products. Also tell your prescriber or health care professional if you are a frequent user of drinks with caffeine or alcohol, if you smoke, or if you use illegal drugs. These may affect the way your medicine works. Check with your health care professional before stopping or starting any of your medicines.

What should I watch for while taking risperidone?

Visit your prescriber or health care professional for regular checks on your progress. It may be several weeks before you see the full effects of risperidone. Do not suddenly stop taking risperidone. You may need to gradually reduce the dose. Only stop taking risperidone on your prescriber's advice. If you notice and increased thirst or hunger, different from your normal hunger or thirst, or if you find that you must frequently use the restroom (excessive urination), you should contact your health care provider as soon as possible. You may need to have your blood sugar monitored. You may get dizzy or drowsy. Do not drive, use machinery, or do anything that needs mental alertness until you know how risperidone affects you. Do not stand or sit up

quickly, especially if you are an older patient. This reduces the risk of dizzy or fainting spells. Alcohol can increase dizziness and drowsiness. Avoid alcoholic drinks. You can get a hangover effect the morning after a bedtime dose. Do not treat yourself for colds, diarrhea or allergies. Ask your prescriber or health care professional for advice, some nonprescription medicines may increase possible side effects. Risperidone may make you more sensitive to sun or ultraviolet light. Keep out of the sun, or wear protective clothing outdoors and use a sunscreen (at least SPF 15). Do not use sun lamps, or sun tanning beds or booths. To protect your eyes wear sunglasses even on cloudy days. If you are going to have surgery tell your prescriber or health care professional that you are taking risperidone.

What side effects may I notice from taking risperidone?

Side effects that you should report to your prescriber or health care professional as soon as possible:
- aching muscles and joints
- changes in vision
- confusion
- fast or irregular heartbeat (palpitations)
- fainting spells
- increased thirst or hunger
- increased need to pass urine
- inner restlessness, unable to keep still
- loss of balance, difficulty walking or falls
- stiffness, spasms, trembling

Side effects that usually do not require medical attention (report to your prescriber or health care professional if they continue or are bothersome):
- constipation
- decreased sexual ability
- difficulty sleeping
- drowsiness or dizziness
- headache
- increase or decrease in saliva
- increased sensitivity to the sun
- menstrual irregularity
- nausea, vomiting
- stomach pain
- stuffy or runny nose, cough
- unusual tiredness
- weight gain

Where can I keep my medicine?

Keep out of the reach of children in a container that small children cannot open. Store at room temperature between 15 to 25 degrees C (59 and 77 degrees F). Protect the tablets from exposure to bright light. Throw away any unused medicine after the expiration date.

Ritonavir capsules

NORVIR®;
100 mg; Capsule
Abbott Pharmaceutical
Product Division

What are ritonavir capsules?

RITONAVIR (Norvir®) is a type of antiviral drug called a protease inhibitor. Ritonavir is used to treat human immunodeficiency virus (HIV) infection. Ritonavir may reduce the amount of HIV in the blood and increase the number of CD4 cells (T-cells) in the blood. Ritonavir is used in combination with other drugs to treat the HIV virus. Ritonavir will not cure or prevent HIV infection or AIDS. You may still develop other infections or conditions associated with HIV. Generic ritonavir capsules are not available.

What should my health care professional know before I take ritonavir?

They need to know if you have any of these conditions:
- diabetes mellitus or high blood sugar
- hemophilia
- high cholesterol levels
- high triglyceride levels
- liver disease, including hepatitis
- an unusual or allergic reaction to ritonavir, other medicines, foods, dyes, or preservatives
- breast-feeding
- pregnancy or trying to get pregnant

How should I take this medicine?

Take ritonavir capsules by mouth. Follow the directions on the prescription label exactly. Take the capsules with meals, if possible. Take your doses at regular intervals. Do not take your medicine more often than directed. To help to make sure that your anti-HIV therapy works as well as possible, be very careful to take all of your medicine exactly as prescribed. Do not stop taking except on your prescriber's advice. Contact your pediatrician or health care professional regarding the use of this medicine in children. Special care may be needed.

What if I miss a dose?

If you miss a dose, take it as soon as you can. If it is almost time for your next dose, take only that dose. Do not take double or extra doses.

What may interact with ritonavir?

Many medicines may interact with ritonavir, if you have a question concerning other medicines you may be taking, talk with your pharmacist, prescriber or other health care professional.
Do not take ritonavir with any of these medicines:

- alfuzosin (Uroxatral®)
- amiodarone (Cordarone®)
- astemizole (Hismanal®)
- bepridil (Vascor®)
- cisapride (Propulsid®)

- dofetilide (Tykosin®)
- ergotamine medicines (Cafergot®, Migranal®, D.H.E. 45®, and others)
- flecainide (Tambocor®)
- lovastatin (Mevacor®)
- midazolam (Versed®)
- pimozide (Orap®)
- propafenone (Rythmol®)
- quinidine (Quinaglute®, Cardioquin®, Quinidex®, and others)
- simvastatin (Zocor®)
- St. John's wort or products containing St. John's wort
- terfenadine (Seldane®)
- triazolam (Halcion®)
- went yeast (Cholestin™)
- zolpidem (Ambien®)

Other medicines that may interact with ritonavir:

- atovaquone
- birth control pills or other hormonal birth control medicines (like the patch, ring, or injections)
- bosentan
- certain medicines for anxiety or difficulty sleeping
- certain medicines for fungal infections
- certain medicines for high cholesterol (e.g., atorvastatin or cerivastatin)
- certain medicines for high blood pressure
- certain pain medicines
- clarithromycin
- cyclosporine
- erythromycin
- medicines for depression
- medicines for diabetes
- medicines for seizures
- other antiviral medicines such as didanosine, ddI, saquinavir, or zidovudine
- rifabutin
- rifampin
- rifapentine
- theophylline
- sildenafil
- warfarin

Tell your prescriber or health care professional about all other medicines you are taking, including nonprescription medicines, nutritional supplements, or herbal products. Also tell your prescriber or health care professional if you are a frequent user of drinks with caffeine or alcohol, if you smoke, or if you use illegal drugs. These may affect the way your medicine works. Check with your health care professional before stopping or starting any of your medicines.

What should I watch for while taking ritonavir?

Visit your prescriber or health care professional for regular checks on your progress. Discuss any new symptoms with your prescriber or health care professional. Ritonavir will not cure HIV and you can still get other illnesses or complications associated with your disease. Taking ritonavir does not reduce the risk of passing HIV infection to others through sexual or blood contact. It is best to avoid sexual contact so that you do not spread the disease to others. For any sexual contact, use a condom. Be careful about cuts, abrasions and other possible sources of blood contact. Never share a needle or syringe with anyone. Ritonavir may cause abnormal liver function tests, changes in your cholesterol or triglyceride levels, and may increase the level of your blood sugar. Visit your health care professional or prescriber regularly to check for any of these side effects. Some of these effects may become serious. If you are a woman of childbearing age and are using hormone contraceptives, then you should use another form of birth control while taking ritonavir. Ritonavir may decrease the effectiveness of hormone birth control agents, including birth control pills and injections.

What side effects might I notice from taking ritonavir?

Side effects of ritonavir may be temporary and decrease after 2 weeks of treatment. Try to stay on ritonavir for at least 2 weeks. When you start taking ritonavir, your prescriber may slowly increase your dose to minimize the potential side effects.

Side effects that you should report to your prescriber or health care professional as soon as possible:
- signs of a severe allergic reaction including difficulty breathing, tightness in throat, or swelling of your tongue
- increases in your blood sugar

- redness, blistering, peeling or loosening of the skin, including inside the mouth
- severe dizziness
- skin rash, hives
- unusual tiredness or weakness
- vomiting
- yellow color of eyes or skin

Side effects that usually do not require medical attention (report to your prescriber or health care professional if they continue or are bothersome):
- changes in taste
- diarrhea
- difficulty sleeping
- dizziness
- headache
- heartburn
- loss of appetite
- nausea
- stomach pain
- tingling or numbness in the hands or feet or around the mouth
- tiredness or weakness

Where can I keep my medicine?

Keep out of the reach of children in a container that small children cannot open. Store the capsules in the refrigerator between 2 and 8 degrees C (36 and 46 degrees F). You do not need to keep them in the refrigerator if you use them all within 30 days and keep them below 77 degrees F. Do not expose the capsules to very hot or cold temperatures. Keep the container tightly closed. Throw away any unused medicine after the expiration date.

Rivastigmine capsules

EXELON®; 3 mg; Capsule Novartis Pharmaceuticals	EXELON®; 6 mg; Capsule Novartis Pharmaceuticals

What are rivastigmine capsules?

RIVASTIGMINE (Exelon®) helps treat the symptoms associated with Alzheimer's disease or dementia. It is not a cure for Alzheimer's disease but offers improvement in memory, attention, reason, language, and the ability to perform simple tasks. Benefits are greater in the early stages of the disease. Generic rivastigmine capsules are not yet available.

What should my health care professional know before I take rivastigmine?

They need to know if you have any of these conditions:
- asthma or other lung disease
- difficulty passing urine
- head injury
- heart disease, or irregular or slow heartbeat

- kidney disease
- liver disease
- low blood pressure
- Parkinson's disease
- seizures (convulsions)
- stomach or intestinal disease, ulcers, or stomach bleeding
- tobacco smoker
- an unusual or allergic reaction to rivastigmine, other medicines, foods, dyes, or preservatives
- pregnant or trying to get pregnant
- breast-feeding

How should I take this medicine?

Take rivastigmine capsules by mouth. Follow the directions on the prescription label. Swallow the capsules with a drink of water. Rivastigmine is usually administered twice daily with food, and is recommended to be taken with the morning and evening meals. Take your doses at regular intervals. Do not take your medicine more often than directed. Do not stop taking except on your prescriber's advice. If your prescriber asks you to stop taking rivastigmine; do not restart this medicine until your prescriber tells you to. Follow the special instructions given by your prescriber for restarting this medicine. Contact your pediatrician or health care professional regarding the use of this medicine in children. Special care may be needed.

What if I miss a dose?

If you miss a dose, take it as soon as you can. If it is almost time for your next dose, take only that dose. Do not take double or extra doses.

What may interact with rivastigmine?

- atropine
- benztropine
- dicyclomine
- digoxin
- donepezil
- galantamine
- glycopyrrolate
- hyoscyamine
- medications for motion sickness (examples: dimenhydrinate, scopolamine)
- medicines that relax your muscles for surgery
- non-steroidal anti-inflammatory drugs (NSAIDs, such as ibuprofen)
- oxybutynin
- propantheline
- tacrine

Tell your prescriber or health care professional about all other medicines you are taking, including non-prescription medicines, nutritional supplements, or herbal products. Also tell your prescriber or health care professional if you are a frequent user of drinks with caffeine or alcohol, if you smoke, or if you use illegal drugs. These may affect the way your medicine works. Check with your health care professional before stopping or starting any of your medicines.

What should I watch for while taking rivastigmine?

Visit your prescriber or health care professional for regular checks on your progress. Check with your prescriber or health care professional if there is no improvement in your symptoms or if they get worse. You may get dizzy or feel faint. Do not drive, use machinery, or do anything that needs mental alertness until you know how rivastigmine affects you. If you are going to have surgery tell your prescriber or health care professional that you are taking rivastigmine.

What side effects may I notice from taking rivastigmine?

Side effects that you should report to your prescriber or health care professional as soon as possible:
- changes in vision or balance
- diarrhea, if it is severe or does not stop
- dizziness, fainting spells, or falls
- increase in frequency of passing urine, or incontinence
- nervousness, agitation, or increased confusion
- redness, blistering, peeling or loosening of the skin, including inside the mouth
- skin rash or hives
- slow heartbeat, or palpitations
- stomach pain
- sweating
- uncontrollable movements
- vomiting
- weight loss

Side effects that usually do not require medical attention (report to your prescriber or health care professional if they continue or are bothersome):
- mild diarrhea, especially when starting treatment
- indigestion or heartburn
- loss of appetite
- nausea

Where can I keep my medicine?

Keep out of reach of children in a container that small children cannot open. Store at room temperature between 15 degrees and 30 degrees C (59 degrees and 86 degrees F). Throw away any unused medicine after the expiration date.

Rizatriptan tablets and disintegrating tablets

MAXALT®;
10 mg; Tablet
Merck and Co Inc

MAXALT-MLT™;
10 mg; Tablet,
Orally
Disintegrating
Merck and Co Inc

What are rizatriptan tablets?

RIZATRIPTAN (Maxalt®, Maxalt-MLT®) helps to relieve a migraine attack that starts with or without aura (a peculiar feeling or visual disturbance that warns you of an attack). Generic rizatriptan tablets and disintegrating tablets are not yet available.

What should my health care professional know before I take rizatriptan?

They need to know if you have any of these conditions:
- bowel disease or colitis
- diabetes
- family history of heart disease

- fast or irregular heartbeat
- headaches that are different from your usual migraine
- heart or blood vessel disease, angina (chest pain), or previous heart attack
- high blood pressure
- high cholesterol
- history of stroke, transient ischemic attacks (TIAs or "mini-strokes"), or intracranial bleeding
- kidney disease
- liver disease
- overweight
- poor circulation
- postmenopausal or surgical removal of uterus and ovaries
- Raynaud's syndrome
- seizure disorder
- tobacco smoker
- an unusual or allergic reaction to rizatriptan other medicines, foods, dyes, or preservatives
- unable to take aspartame-containing products
- pregnant or trying to get pregnant
- breast-feeding

How should I take this medicine?

Rizatriptan is taken by mouth. Follow the directions on the prescription label. Rizatriptan is taken at the first symptoms of a migraine attack; it is not for everyday use.

Tablets: Swallow the tablet whole with a drink of water.

Disintegrating tablets: Leave the rizatriptan disintegrating tablet in the foil package until you are ready to take it. Do not push the tablet through the blister pack. Peel open the blister pack with dry hands and place the tablet on your tongue. The tablet will dissolve rapidly and be swallowed in your saliva. It is not necessary to drink any water to take this medicine.

If your migraine headache returns after one dose, you can take another dose anytime after 2 hours of taking the first dose. Do not take more than 30 mg of rizatriptan in 24 hours. If there is no improvement at all after the first dose, do not take a second dose without talking to your prescriber or health care professional. Do not take your medicine more often than directed. Contact your pediatrician or health care professional regarding the use of this medicine in children. Special care may be needed.

What if I miss a dose?

This does not apply, rizatriptan is not for regular use.

What may interact with rizatriptan?

Do not take rizatriptan with any of the following medicines:

- amphetamine or cocaine
- dihydroergotamine, ergotamine, ergoloid mesylates, methysergide, or ergot-type medication—do not take within 24 hours of taking rizatriptan.
- almotriptan, eletriptan, naratriptan, sumatriptan, zolmitriptan—do not take within 24 hours of taking rizatriptan.

- medicines for weight loss such as dexfenfluramine, dextroamphetamine, fenfluramine, or sibutramine
- monoamine oxidase inhibitors (MAOIs) such as phenelzine (Nardil®), tranylcypromine (Parnate®), isocarboxazid (Marplan®), and selegiline (Carbex®, Eldepryl®)—do not take rizatriptan within 2 weeks of stopping MAOI therapy.

Check with your doctor or pharmacist if you take any of these medications:

- cough syrup or other products containing dextromethorphan
- feverfew
- lithium
- medicines for mental depression, anxiety or mood problems such as buspirone, citalopram, fluoxetine, fluvoxamine, mirtazapine, nefazodone, paroxetine, sertraline, trazodone, tricyclic antidepressants, or venlafaxine
- meperidine
- propranolol
- St. John's wort
- tryptophan

Tell your prescriber or other health care professional about all other medicines you are taking including nonprescription medicines, nutritional supplements, or herbal products. Also, tell your prescriber or health care professional if you are a frequent user of drinks with caffeine or alcohol, if you smoke or if you use illegal drugs. These may affect the way your medicine works. Check before stopping or starting any of your medications.

What should I watch for while taking rizatriptan?

Only take rizatriptan tablets for a migraine headache. Take it if you get warning symptoms or at the start of a migraine attack. Rizatriptan is not for regular use to prevent migraine attacks. Do not take migraine products that contain ergotamine or while you are taking rizatriptan; this combination can affect your heart. You may get drowsy, dizzy. Do not drive, use machinery, or do anything that needs mental alertness until you know how rizatriptan affects you. To reduce dizzy or fainting spells, do not sit or stand up quickly. Alcohol can increase drowsiness, dizziness and flushing. Avoid alcoholic drinks. Smoking cigarettes may increase the risk of heart-related side effects from using rizatriptan.

What side effects may I notice from taking rizatriptan?

Side effects that you should report to your prescriber as soon as possible:
Rare or uncommon:
- chest, neck, or throat pain or tightness
- dizziness or faintness
- fast or irregular heart beat, palpitations
- feeling of chest heaviness or pressure
- severe stomach pain and cramping, bloody diarrhea
- shortness of breath, wheezing, or difficulty breathing

R

- tingling, pain, or numbness in the face, hands or feet
- unusual reaction or swelling of the skin, eyelids, face, or lips

Side effects that usually do not require medical attention (report to your prescriber or health care professional if they continue or are bothersome):
- change in taste
- diarrhea
- drowsiness
- dry mouth

- hot flashes, feeling warm, flushing, or redness of the face
- nausea, vomiting, or stomach upset
- shakiness or tremor
- tiredness or weakness

Where can I keep my medicine?

Keep out of the reach of children. Store at room temperature between 59 and 86 degrees F (15 and 30 degrees C). Protect from light and moisture. Throw away any unused medicine after the expiration date.

Rofecoxib tablets

VIOXX®;
12.5 mg; Tablet
Merck and Co Inc

VIOXX®;
25 mg; Tablet
Merck and Co Inc

What are rofecoxib tablets?

ROFECOXIB (Vioxx®) is a drug used to reduce inflammation and ease mild to moderate pain for such conditions as arthritis, painful menstrual cycles, or pain after dental or surgical procedures. Generic rofecoxib tablets are not available. NOTE: This drug is discontinued in the United States. Patients currently taking Rofecoxib should contact their prescriber regarding discontinuation and alternative therapies. If you have unused tablets, you may return the product to NNC Group, Merck Returns, 2670 Executive Drive, Indianapolis, IN 46241 for a refund. Send any unused product in its original pharmacy packaging, the pharmacy receipt for the product you are returning, and your name, address, and phone number by regular, first-class U.S. mail. You will receive a full refund of the price paid, as reflected on your pharmacy receipt. You will also receive a refund of the cost of shipping via regular U.S. mail. If you have questions about the discontinuation of Rofecoxib or about the refund, you may call 1-800-805-9542 or 1-888-368-4699.

What should my health care professional know before I take rofecoxib?

They need to know if you have any of these conditions:
- anemia
- asthma
- cigarette smoker
- dehydrated
- drink more than 3 alcohol-containing beverages a day
- heart or circulation problems such as heart failure, angina, blocked artery in heart, or leg edema
- high blood pressure
- history of a heart attack
- kidney disease
- liver disease
- nasal polyps
- stomach bleeding or ulcers
- taking blood thinners
- taking hormones such as prednisone (steroids)
- pregnant or trying to get pregnant

- an unusual or allergic reaction to aspirin, other salicylates, rofecoxib, other NSAIDs, foods, dyes or preservatives
- breast-feeding

How should I take this medicine?

Take rofecoxib tablets by mouth. Follow the directions on the prescription label. Swallow tablets whole with a full glass of water; take tablets in an upright or sitting position. Taking a sip of water first, before taking the tablets, may help you swallow them. If possible take bedtime doses at least 10 minutes before laying down. If rofecoxib upsets your stomach, take it with food or milk. Take your doses at regular intervals. Do not take your medicine more often than directed. Contact your pediatrician or health care professional regarding the use of this medicine in children. Special care may be needed.

What if I miss a dose?

If you miss a dose, take it as soon as you can. If it is almost time for your next dose, take only that dose. Do not take double or extra doses.

What may interact with rofecoxib?

- alcohol
- alendronate
- aspirin and aspirin-like medicines
- cidofovir
- cyclosporine
- drospirenone; ethinyl estradiol (Yasmin®)
- herbal products that contain feverfew, garlic, ginger, or ginkgo biloba
- lithium
- medicines for high blood pressure
- methotrexate
- other anti-inflammatory drugs (such as ibuprofen or prednisone)
- pemetrexed
- probenecid
- theophylline
- warfarin
- water pills (diuretics)

Tell your prescriber or health care professional about all other medicines you are taking, including non-prescription medicines, nutritional supplements, or herbal products. Also tell your prescriber or health care professional if you are a frequent user of drinks with caffeine or alcohol, if you smoke, or if you use illegal drugs. These may affect the way your medicine works. Check with your health care professional before stopping or starting any of your medicines.

What should I watch for while taking rofecoxib?

Let your prescriber or health care professional know if your pain continues; do not take with other pain-killers without advice. If you get flu-like symptoms (fever, chills, muscle aches and pains), call your prescriber or health care professional; do not treat yourself. To reduce unpleasant effects on your stomach, take rofecoxib with a full glass of water. Do not smoke cigarettes or drink alcohol; these increase irritation to your stomach and can make it more susceptible to damage from rofecoxib. If you notice black, tarry stools or experience severe stomach pain and/or vomit blood or what looks like coffee grounds, notify your health care prescriber immediately. Avoid taking other prescription or over-the-counter non-steroidal anti-inflammatory drugs (NSAIDs), such as ibuprofen (Advil®), naproxen (Aleve®), or ketoprofen (Orudis® KT), while taking rofecoxib. Side effects including stomach upset, heartburn, nausea, vomiting or serious side effects such as ulcers are more likely if rofecoxib is given with other NSAIDs. Many non-prescription products contain NSAIDs; closely read labels before taking any medicines with rofecoxib. Rofecoxib cannot take the place of aspirin for the prevention of heart attack or stroke. If you are currently taking aspirin for this purpose, you should not discontinue taking aspirin without checking with your prescriber or health care professional. It is especially important not to use rofecoxib during the last 3 months of pregnancy unless specifically directed to do so by your health care provider. Rofecoxib may cause problems in the unborn child or complications during delivery.

What side effects may I notice from taking rofecoxib?

Patients should seek immediate emergency help in the case of a serious allergic reaction. Side effects that you should report to your prescriber or health care professional as soon as possible:
- black, tarry stools
- blurred vision
- decrease in the amount of urine passed
- difficulty breathing
- fainting or passing out
- fast heartbeat
- fatigue, weakness, or sleepiness
- skin rash, hives, redness, blistering, peeling or itching
- stomach tenderness, pain, bleeding, or cramps
- swelling of eyelids, throat, lips, legs, ankles, or feet
- unexplained weight gain or edema
- unusual headache with stiff neck
- severe nausea or vomiting
- yellowing of eyes or skin

Side effects that usually do not require medical attention (report to your prescriber or health care professional if they continue or are bothersome):
- constipation or diarrhea
- difficulty swallowing
- dizziness
- gas or heartburn
- minor upset stomach
- nausea or vomiting

Where can I keep my medicine?

Keep out of the reach of children in a container that small children cannot open. Store at room temperature between 15 and 30 degrees C (59 and 86 degrees F). Protect from moisture. Keep container tightly closed. Throw away any unused medicine after the expiration date.

Ropinirole tablets

REQUIP®;
0.5 mg; Tablet
SmithKline Beecham
Pharmaceuticals Div
SmithKline Beecham
Co

REQUIP®;
3 mg; Tablet
SmithKline Beecham
Pharmaceuticals Div
SmithKline Beecham
Co

What are ropinirole tablets?

ROPINIROLE (Requip™) can help treat Parkinson's disease. Ropinirole helps to improve muscle control and movement difficulties. Ropinirole will not cure Parkinson's disease, but will help to control the symptoms of the disease. Ropinirole tablets may be taken together with other medicines that control symptoms of Parkinson's. Ropinirole is also used for the treatment of Restless Legs Syndrome. Generic ropinirole tablets are not yet available.

What should my health care professional know before I take ropinirole?

They need to know if you have any of these conditions:
- dizzy or fainting spells
- kidney disease
- heart disease
- low blood pressure
- an unusual or allergic reaction to ropinirole, other medicines, foods, dyes, or preservatives
- pregnant or trying to get pregnant
- breast-feeding

How should I take this medicine?

Take ropinirole tablets by mouth. Taking this medicine with food can decrease your chance of developing nausea. Follow the directions on the prescription label. Swallow the tablets with a drink of water. Take your doses at regular intervals. Do not take your medicine more often than directed. Do not stop taking ropinirole except on your prescriber's advice.

What if I miss a dose?

If you miss a dose, take it as soon as you can. If it is almost time for your next dose, take only that dose. Do not take double or extra doses.

What may interact with ropinirole?

- cimetidine
- ciprofloxacin
- clarithromycin
- diltiazem
- droperidol
- entacapone
- erythromycin
- estrogens
- medicines for mental problems or psychotic disturbances
- metoclopramide
- mexiletine
- norfloxacin
- omeprazole
- phenobarbital
- phenytoin
- quinidine or quinine
- ranitidine
- rifampin
- triamterene
- verapamil

Tell your prescriber or health care professional about all other medicines that you are taking, including nonprescription medicines. Also, tell your prescriber or health care professional if you are a frequent user of drinks with caffeine or alcohol, if you smoke, or if you use illegal drugs. These may affect the way your medicine works. Check with your health care professional before stopping or starting any of your medicines.

What should I watch for while taking ropinirole?

Visit your prescriber or health care professional for regular checks on your progress. It may be several weeks or months before you feel the full effect of ropinirole. Continue to take your medicine on a regular schedule and do not stop taking except on your prescriber's advice. You may get dizzy or have difficulty controlling your movements. Do not drive, use machinery, or do anything that needs mental alertness until you know how ropinirole affects you. Ropinirole has been associated with a sudden urge to fall asleep; sometimes while driving. Contact your health care professional for advice if you have a sudden sleep episode. Do not stand or sit up quickly, especially if you are an older patient. Rise slowly if you have been sitting or lying down, especially if you

have been in this position for a long time. Also, if you have just recently started taking ropinirole, or if your prescriber has recently increased your dose, be careful when you stand or sit up. This reduces the risk of dizzy or fainting spells. The dizziness that sometimes occurs with ropinirole is called postural hypotension. You may also feel nauseous (sick to your stomach) or sweaty. Alcohol can increase possible dizziness; avoid alcoholic drinks. If you are going to have surgery, tell your prescriber or health care professional that you are taking ropinirole. Ropinirole may make your mouth dry. Chewing sugarless gum, sucking hard candy and drinking plenty of water may help. Visit your dentist regularly.

What side effects may I notice from taking ropinirole?

Side effects that you should report to your prescriber or health care professional as soon as possible:
Rare or Less common:
- chest pain
- fainting
- falling
- fast or irregular heartbeat
- increase or decrease in blood pressure
- joint or muscle pain
- loss of bladder control
- mental depression, anxiety, nervousness or other changes in behavior or mood
- numbness, tingling, or prickly sensations
- shortness of breath, troubled breathing, tightness in chest, or wheezing
- sudden sleep episodes, even while doing normal activities
- trouble swallowing
- uncontrollable movements of the arms, face, hands, head, mouth, shoulders, or upper body
- vision changes

More common:
- confusion
- drowsiness
- hallucinations (seeing or hearing things that are not there)
- vomiting

Side effects that usually do not require medical attention (report to your prescriber or health care professional if they continue or are bothersome):
- clumsiness, feeling unsteady, or dizziness, especially early in treatment
- dry mouth
- flushing
- headache
- increased sweating
- nausea
- tremor
- yawning

Where can I keep my medicine?

Keep out of the reach of children in a container that small children cannot open. Store at controlled room temperature between 20 degrees and 25 degrees C (68 degrees and 77 degrees F). Protect from light. Keep container tightly closed. Throw away any unused medicine after the expiration date.

Rosiglitazone tablets

AVANDIA®;
4 mg; Tablet
Beecham Div
SmithKline Beecham
Corp

AVANDIA®;
8 mg; Tablet
Beecham Div
SmithKline Beecham
Corp

What are rosiglitazone tablets?

ROSIGLITAZONE (Avandia®) helps to treat type 2 diabetes mellitus. Rosiglitazone helps your body to use insulin more efficiently and helps to lower high blood sugar. Generic rosiglitazone tablets are not yet available.

What should my health care professional know before I take rosiglitazone?

They need to know if you have any of these conditions:
- heart problems
- history of diabetic ketoacidosis
- kidney or liver problems
- swelling of the arms, legs, or feet
- an unusual or allergic reaction to rosiglitazone, other medicines, foods, dyes, or preservatives
- pregnant or trying to get pregnant
- breast-feeding

How should I take this medicine?

Take rosiglitazone tablets by mouth. Follow the directions on the prescription label. Swallow the tablets with a drink of water with meals. Take your doses at the same time each day; do not take more often than directed. Contact your pediatrician or health care professional regarding the use of this medicine in children. Special care may be needed.

What if I miss a dose?

If you miss a dose, take it with the next meal. If it is almost time for your next dose, take only that dose. Do not take double or extra doses.

What may interact with rosiglitazone?

- some diuretics (water pills)

Many medications may cause changes (increase or decrease) in blood sugar, these include:
- alcohol-containing beverages
- aspirin and aspirin-like drugs
- beta-blockers, often used for high blood pressure or heart problems (examples include atenolol, metoprolol, propranolol)
- chromium
- female hormones, such as estrogens or progestins, birth control pills
- fibric acid derivatives, often used for high cholesterol (examples gemfibrozil and fenofibrate)
- isoniazid
- male hormones or anabolic steroids
- medications to suppress appetite or for weight loss
- medicines for allergies, asthma, cold, or cough
- niacin
- other medicines for diabetes (like insulin, metformin, glipizide, or glyburide)
- pentamidine
- phenytoin
- quinolone antibiotics (examples: ciprofloxacin, levofloxacin, ofloxacin)
- some herbal dietary supplements
- steroid medicines such as prednisone or cortisone
- thyroid hormones
- water pills (diuretics)

Tell your prescriber or health care professional about all other medicines you are taking, including non-prescription medicines, nutritional supplements, or herbal products. Also tell your prescriber or health care professional if you are a frequent user of drinks with caffeine or alcohol, if you smoke, or if you use illegal drugs. These may affect the way your medicine works. Check with your health care professional before stopping or starting any of your medicines.

What should I watch for while taking rosiglitazone?

Visit your prescriber or health care professional for regular checks on your progress. Learn how to monitor blood or urine sugar and urine ketones regularly. Check with your prescriber or health care professional if your blood sugar is high, you may need a change of dose of rosiglitazone. Do not skip meals. If you are exercising much more than usual you may need extra snacks to avoid side effects caused by low blood sugar. If you have mild symptoms of low blood sugar, eat or drink something containing sugar at once and contact your prescriber or health care professional. It is wise to check your blood sugar to confirm that it is low. It is important to recognize your own symptoms of low blood sugar so that you can treat them quickly. Make sure family members know that you can choke if you eat or drink when you have serious symptoms of low blood sugar, such as seizures or unconsciousness. They must get medical help at once. If you are going to have surgery, tell your prescriber or health care professional that you are taking rosiglitazone. Wear a medical identification bracelet or chain to say you have diabetes, and carry a card that lists all your medications.

What side effects may I notice from taking rosiglitazone?

Side effects that you should report to your prescriber or health care professional as soon as possible:
- anxiety or nervousness, confusion, difficulty concentrating
- blurred vision
- breathing problems such as rapid, deep breathing or difficulty breathing with activity
- cold sweats, increased sweating

R

- cool, pale skin
- dark yellow or brown urine, or yellowing of the eyes or skin
- diarrhea
- drowsiness
- muscle pain
- nausea, vomiting
- rapid gain in weight
- skin rash or hives
- slow heartbeat
- tremors or shakiness
- unusual tiredness or weakness
- swelling of the hands, legs, and/or feet

Side effects that usually do not require medical atten-tion (report to your prescriber or health care profes-sional if they continue or are bothersome):

- back ache
- diarrhea
- headache
- slow weight gain

Where can I keep my medicine?

Keep out of the reach of children in a container that small children cannot open. Store at room temperature between 20 and 25 degrees C (68 and 77 degrees F). Keep container tightly closed and protect from light. Throw away any unused medicine after the expiration date.

R

Rosuvastatin tablets

CRESTOR®;
20 mg; Tablet
AstraZeneca
Pharmaceuticals LP

CRESTOR®;
5 mg; Tablet
AstraZeneca
Pharmaceuticals LP

What are rosuvastatin tablets?

ROSUVASTATIN (Crestor®) tablets block the body's ability to make cholesterol. Rosuvastatin can help lower blood cholesterol for patients who are at risk of getting heart disease or a stroke. It is only for patients whose cholesterol level is not controlled by diet. It is not a cure. Generic rosuvastatin tablets are not yet available.

What should my health care professional know before I take Rosuvastatin?

They need to know if you have any of these conditions:

- an alcohol problem
- diabetes mellitus
- infection
- kidney disease
- liver disease
- low blood pressure
- muscle disorder or condition
- recent surgery
- seizures (convulsions)
- severe injury
- an unusual reaction to rosuvastatin, medicines, foods, dyes, or preservatives
- pregnant or trying to get pregnant
- breast-feeding

How should I take this medicine?

Take rosuvastatin tablets by mouth. Follow the direc-tions on the prescription label. Swallow the tablets with a drink of water. You may take rosuvastatin with or without food. Take your doses at regular intervals. Do not take your medicine more often than directed. Contact your pediatrician or health care professional regarding the use of this medicine in children. Special care may be needed.

What if I miss a dose?

If you miss a dose, take it as soon as you can. If it is almost time for your next dose, take only that dose. Do not take double or extra doses.

What may interact with rosuvastatin?

- alcohol
- antacids
- birth control pills
- cyclosporine
- itraconazole
- medicines to lower cholesterol or triglycerides (exam-ples: fenofibrate, gemfibrozil, niacin)
- went yeast (Cholestin™, dietary supplement)
- warfarin

Tell your prescriber or health care professional about all other medicines you are taking, including non-pre-scription medicines, nutritional supplements, or herbal products. Also tell your prescriber or health care profes-sional if you are a frequent user of drinks with caffeine or alcohol, if you smoke, or if you use illegal drugs. These may affect the way your medicine works. Check with your health care professional before stopping or starting any of your medicines.

What should I watch for while taking rosuvastatin?

Visit your prescriber or health care professional for regu-lar checks on your progress. You will need to have regular tests to make sure your liver is working properly. Tell your prescriber or health care professional as soon as you can if you get any unexplained muscle pain, tenderness, or weakness, especially if you also have a fever and tired-ness. Rosuvastatin is only part of a total cholesterol-low-ering program. Your physician or dietician can suggest a low-cholesterol and low-fat diet that will reduce your risk of getting heart and blood vessel disease. Avoid alcohol and smoking, and keep a proper exercise schedule. If you are going to have surgery, tell your prescriber or health care professional that you are taking rosuvastatin.

What side effects may I notice from taking rosuvastatin?

Side effects that you should report to your prescriber or health care professional as soon as possible:

Rare or uncommon:
- blurred vision, or vision changes
- dark yellow or brown urine
- decreased urination, difficulty passing urine
- fever
- muscle pain, tenderness, cramps, or weakness
- skin rash, itching
- unusual tiredness or weakness
- yellowing of the skin or eyes

Side effects that usually do not require medical attention (report to your prescriber or health care professional if they continue or are bothersome):
- constipation or diarrhea
- difficulty sleeping
- dizziness
- headache
- nausea, vomiting
- stomach pain or indigestion

Where can I keep my medicine?

Keep out of the reach of children in a container that small children cannot open. Store at room temperature between 20 and 25 degrees C (68 and 77 degrees F). Protect from light. Throw away any unused medicine after the expiration date.

R

Salsalate tablets or capsules

AMIGESIC™;
750 mg; Tablet
Amide Pharmaceutical Inc

What are salsalate tablets or capsules?

SALSALATE (Amigesic®, Argesic-SA®, Disalcid®, Marthritic®, Mono-Gesic®, Salflex®, Salsitab®) relieves the mild to moderate pain caused by a variety of conditions including arthritis, bursitis, tendinitis, headaches, menstrual cramps or pain, minor injuries, and others. Salsalate reduces fever, pain, and inflammation (swelling and redness). Generic salsalate tablets are available.

What should my health care professional know before I take salsalate?

They need to know if you have any of these conditions:
- anemia
- bleeding or clotting problems
- drink more than 3 alcohol-containing beverages a day
- gout
- heart disease, including heart failure
- high blood pressure
- kidney disease
- liver disease
- smoke tobacco
- stomach ulcers, or other stomach problems
- systemic lupus erythematosus (SLE)
- thrombotic thrombocytopenic purpura (TTP)
- ulcerative colitis
- vitamin K deficiency
- an unusual or allergic reaction to salsalate, other salicylates, tartrazine dye, other medicines, dyes, or preservatives
- pregnant or trying to get pregnant
- breast-feeding

How should I take this medicine?

Take tablets or capsules of salsalate by mouth with a large glass of water. You may take the tablets with food to help decrease stomach upset. Follow the directions on the prescription label. Take your doses at regular intervals. Do not take your medicine more often than directed. Contact your pediatrician or health care professional regarding the use of this medicine in children. Special care may be needed.

What if I miss a dose?

If you are taking salsalate on a regular schedule and miss a dose, take it as soon as you can. If it is almost time for your next dose, take only that dose. Do not take double or extra doses.

What may interact with salsalate?

- alcohol
- antacids (in large doses)
- anti-inflammatory drugs (NSAIDs, such as ibuprofen)
- hormones such as prednisone or cortisone
- medicines used to treat or prevent blood clots
- medicines for diabetes that are taken by mouth
- medicines for gout
- methotrexate
- seizure (convulsion) or epilepsy medicine

Tell your prescriber or health care professional about all other medicines you are taking, including non-prescription medicines, nutritional supplements, or herbal products. Also tell your prescriber or health care professional if you are a frequent user of drinks with caffeine or alcohol, if you smoke, or if you use illegal drugs. These may affect the way your medicine works. Check with your health care professional before stopping or starting any of your medicines.

What should I watch for while taking salsalate?

Many non-prescription medicines contain aspirin as an ingredient. To prevent accidental overdose, read labels carefully and do not combine salsalate with aspirin or other medicines unless your prescriber or health care professional tells you to. If you are taking salsalate for arthritis or other types of pain, it can take up to 3 weeks to get the maximum effect. Do not stop taking without asking your prescriber or health care professional. If you are taking oral medicines to decrease your blood sugar, large doses of magnesium salicylate may increase the levels of these drugs. Check with your prescriber or health care professional before you change your diet or the dose of your diabetic medicine. Choline salicylate can irritate your stomach. Do not smoke cigarettes or drink alcohol; these increase irritation in your stomach and may cause ulcers or bleeding problems. Do not lie down for 30 minutes after taking choline salicylate to prevent irritation to your throat.

What side effects may I notice from taking salsalate?

Side effects that you should report to your prescriber or health care professional as soon as possible:
- signs or symptoms of bleeding from the stomach or intestine such as black, tarry stools, stomach pain, vomiting up blood or what looks like coffee grounds
- confusion
- difficulty breathing, wheezing
- ringing in the ears or changes in hearing
- skin rash, hives
- unusual bleeding or bruising, red or purple spots on the skin

Side effects that usually do not require medical attention (report to your prescriber or health care professional if they continue or are bothersome):

- diarrhea or constipation
- nausea, vomiting
- stomach gas, heartburn

Saquinavir capsules

This drug is no longer on the market

INVIRASE®;
200 mg; Capsule
Roche

FORTOVASE®;
200 mg; Capsule
Roche

What are saquinavir capsules?

SAQUINAVIR (Invirase®, Fortovase®) is an antiviral drug called a protease inhibitor. Saquinavir is used to treat human immunodeficiency virus (HIV) infection. Saquinavir may reduce the amount of HIV in the blood and increase the number of CD4 cells (T-cells) in the blood. Saquinavir is used in combination with other drugs to treat the HIV virus. You may still develop other infections or conditions associated with HIV. Saquinavir will not cure or prevent HIV infection or AIDS. Generic saquinavir capsules are not yet available. NOTE: In the U.S., the Fortovase® brand of saquinavir will not be available after February 2006. Talk to your health care professional about what other treatment options are available for you.

What should my health care professional know before I take saquinavir?

They need to know if you have any of these conditions:

- diabetes mellitus or high blood sugar
- hemophilia
- high cholesterol levels
- high triglyceride levels
- liver disease, including hepatitis
- an unusual or allergic reaction to saquinavir, other medicines, foods, dyes, or preservatives
- breast-feeding
- pregnant or trying to get pregnant

How should I take this medicine?

Take saquinavir capsules by mouth. Follow the directions on the prescription label. Swallow capsules with a drink of water. Take saquinavir within 2 hours after a full meal. Take your doses at regular intervals. Do not take your medicine more often than directed. To help to make sure that your anti-HIV therapy works as well as possible, be very careful to take all of your medicine exactly as prescribed. Do not stop taking except on your prescriber's advice. Contact your pediatrician or health care professional regarding the use of this medicine in children. Special care may be needed.

What if I miss a dose?

If you miss a dose, take it as soon as you can. If it is almost time for your next dose, take only that dose. Do not take double or extra doses.

Where can I keep my medicine?

Keep out of the reach of children in a container that small children cannot open. Store between 15 and 30 degrees C (59 and 86 degrees F). Throw away any unused medicine after the expiration date.

What may interact with saquinavir?

Do not take saquinavir with the following medicines:

- astemizole (Hismanal®)
- cisapride (Propulsid®)
- dofetilide (Tykosin®)
- ergot alkaloids (e.g., dihydroergotamine, ergotamine, methysergide)
- garlic supplements
- lovastatin (Mevacor®)
- midazolam (Versed®)
- simvastatin (Zocor®)
- St. John's wort or any herbal products containing St. John's wort
- terfenadine (Seldane®)
- triazolam (Halcion®)
- went yeast (Cholestin™)

Other medicines that may interact with saquinavir include:

- bosentan
- certain medicines for anxiety or difficulty sleeping
- carbamazepine
- clarithromycin
- dexamethasone
- grapefruit juice
- ketoconazole
- medicines for diabetes
- medicines for high cholesterol
- phenobarbital
- phenytoin
- pimozide
- ranitidine
- rifabutin
- rifampin
- sildenafil

Tell your prescriber or health care professional about all other medicines you are taking, including nonprescription medicines, nutritional supplements, or herbal products. Also tell your prescriber or health care professional if you are a frequent user of drinks with caffeine or alcohol, if you smoke, or if you use illegal drugs. These may affect the way your medicine works. Check with your health care professional before stopping or starting any of your medicines.

What should I watch for while taking saquinavir?

Visit your prescriber or health care professional for regular checks on your progress. Discuss any new symptoms with your prescriber or health care professional. Saquinavir will not cure HIV and you can still get other illnesses or complications associated with your disease. Taking saquinavir does not reduce the risk of passing HIV infection to others through sexual or blood contact. It is best to avoid sexual contact so that you do not spread the disease to others. For any sexual contact, use a condom. Be careful about cuts, abrasions and other possible sources of blood contact. Never share a needle or syringe with anyone.

What side effects may I notice from taking saquinavir?

Side effects that you should report to your prescriber or health care professional as soon as possible:
- severe dizziness
- unusual tiredness or weakness
- yellow color of skin or eyes

Side effects that usually do not require medical attention (report to your prescriber or health care professional if they continue or are bothersome):

- depression
- diarrhea
- stomach or intestinal gas
- headache
- nausea, vomiting
- stomach pain
- tiredness

Where can I keep my medicine?

Keep out of the reach of children in a container that small children cannot open. Store at Invirase® at room temperature between 15 and 30 degrees C (59 and 86 degrees F). Keep container tightly closed. Throw away any unused medicine after the expiration date. Store Fortovase® in the refrigerator at 2 to 8 degrees C (36 to 42 degrees F); discard after the expiration date on the label. If Fortovase® is kept at room temperature (15 to 30 degrees C or 59 to 86 degrees F), discard after 3 months.

Scopolamine tablets

SCOPACE®;
0.4 mg; Tablet
Hope Pharmaceuticals

What are scopolamine tablets?

SCOPOLAMINE (Scopace®) tablets help prevent nausea and vomiting associated with motion sickness. They are also used to help with symptoms of irritable bowel or other intestinal problems. Generic scopolamine tablets are not yet available.

What should my health care professional know before I take scopolamine?

They need to know if you have any of these conditions:
- abnormal heart rhythm
- asthma
- difficulty passing urine
- heart or blood vessel disease, high blood pressure
- hiatal hernia
- glaucoma
- liver disease
- nervous system disease
- over active thyroid
- stomach obstruction
- ulcerative colitis
- an unusual or allergic reaction to scopolamine, atropine, other medicines, foods, dyes, or preservatives
- pregnant or trying to get pregnant
- breast-feeding

How should I take this medicine?

Take scopolamine tablets by mouth. Follow the directions on the prescription label. If scopolamine is being used to prevent motion sickness, take on an empty stomach one hour before travel or before the event that causes motion sickness. Drink plenty of fluids after

taking a dose of scopolamine. Contact your pediatrician or health care professional regarding the use of this medicine in children. Special care may be needed.

What if I miss a dose?

If you are taking scopolamine for motion sickness, make sure you take the tablet(s) one hour before you need it. If you are taking scopolamine on a regular schedule for a reason other than motion sickness and you miss a dose, take it as soon as your remember. If it is almost time for your next dose, take only that dose. Do not take double or extra doses.

What may interact with scopolamine?

- alcohol
- amantadine
- benztropine
- bethanechol
- cisapride
- digoxin
- donepezil
- erythromycin
- galantamine
- glutethimide
- ketoconazole
- levodopa
- medicines for hay fever and other allergies
- medicines for mental depression
- medicines for mental problems and psychotic disturbances
- medicine for anxiety or sleeping problems (such as diazepam, or temazepam)

- meperidine
- metoclopramide
- quinidine
- rivastigmine
- tacrine
- tegaserod

Tell your prescriber or health care professional about all other medicines you are taking, including nonprescription medicines, nutritional supplements, or herbal products. Also tell your prescriber or health care professional if you are a frequent user of drinks with caffeine or alcohol, if you smoke, or if you use illegal drugs. These may affect the way your medicine works. Check with your health care professional before stopping or starting any of your medicines.

What should I watch for while taking scopolamine?

Check with your prescriber or health care professional as soon as you can if you get pain in your eye, or reddening of the whites of your eye. You may get drowsy, dizzy, or have blurred vision. Do not drive, use machinery, or do anything that requires mental alertness until you know how scopolamine affects you. To reduce the risk of dizzy or fainting spells, do not sit or stand up quickly, especially if you are an older patient. Alcohol can make you more drowsy, avoid alcoholic drinks. Your mouth may get dry. Chewing sugarless gum or sucking hard candy, and drinking plenty of water will help. Scopolamine may cause dry eyes and blurred vision. If you

wear contact lenses, you may feel some discomfort. Lubricating drops may help. See your ophthalmologist if the problem does not go away or is severe.

What side effects may I notice from taking scopolamine?

Side effects that you should report to your prescriber or health care professional as soon as possible:
- agitation, nervousness, confusion
- severe dizziness
- hallucinations (seeing and hearing things that are not really there)
- pain or difficulty passing urine
- palpitations
- skin rash, itching
- vomiting

Side effects that usually do not require medical attention (report to your prescriber or health care professional if they continue or are bothersome):
- blurred vision
- dry mouth
- flushing
- headache
- mild dizziness or lightheadedness
- nausea
- tiredness

Where can I keep my medicine?

Keep out of the reach of children. Store at room temperature between 15 and 30 degrees C (59 and 86 degrees F). Throw away any unused medicine after the expiration date.

Secobarbital capsules

SECONAL®;
100 mg; Capsule
Ranbaxy Pharmaceuticals Inc

What are secobarbital capsules?

SECOBARBITAL (Seconal®) is a barbiturate that slows down activity of the brain and nervous system. Secobarbital has sedative and hypnotic properties, which will help make you feel relaxed and sleepy when used before surgery. For short periods of 2 weeks or less, secobarbital can help treat insomnia (difficulty sleeping). Federal law prohibits the transfer of secobarbital to any person other than the patient for whom it was prescribed. Generic secobarbital capsules are not available.

What should my health care professional know before I take secobarbital?

They need to know if you have any of these conditions:
- an alcohol or substance abuse problem
- kidney disease
- low blood pressure
- lung disease or breathing difficulties
- mental depression or mental problems, suicidal thoughts

- porphyria
- an unusual or allergic reaction to secobarbital, other barbiturates, medicines, foods, dyes, or preservatives
- pregnant or trying to get pregnant
- breast-feeding

How should I take this medicine?

Take secobarbital capsules by mouth. Follow the directions on the prescription label. Swallow the capsules with a drink of water. If secobarbital upsets your stomach, take it with food or milk. Take your doses at regular intervals. Do not take your medicine more often than directed. Elderly patients over age 65 years may have a stronger reaction to this medicine and need smaller doses.

What if I miss a dose?

If you are on a regular schedule and miss a dose, take it as soon as you can. If it is almost time for your next dose, take only that dose. Do not take double or extra doses.

What may interact with secobarbital?

- alcohol
- caffeine
- chloramphenicol
- cyclophosphamide
- cyclosporine
- doxorubicin
- doxycycline
- metronidazole
- female hormones, including contraceptive or birth control pills
- hormones such a prednisone or cortisone
- medicines for anxiety or sleeping problems, such as diazepam or temazepam
- medicines for hay fever and other allergies
- medicines for high blood pressure
- medicines for mental depression
- medicines for mental problems and psychotic disturbances
- medicines for pain
- medicines to control heart rhythm or other heart problems
- quinine
- seizure (convulsion) or epilepsy medicine
- theophylline
- warfarin

Tell your prescriber or health care professional about all other medicines you are taking, including non-prescription medicines, nutritional supplements, or herbal products. Also tell your prescriber or health care professional if you are a frequent user of drinks with caffeine or alcohol, if you smoke, or if you use illegal drugs. These may affect the way your medicine works. Check with your health care professional before stopping or starting any of your medicines.

What should I watch for while taking secobarbital?

Visit your prescriber or health care professional for regular checks on your progress. If you have been taking secobarbital regularly and suddenly stop taking it, you may increase the risk of seizures. Your prescriber or health care professional may want to gradually reduce the dose. Do not stop taking except on your prescriber's advice. If sleep medicine is taken every night for a long time it may no longer help you to sleep. In general secobarbital should not be taken for longer than 1 or 2 weeks as a sleep aid. Consult your prescriber or health care professional if you still have difficulty in sleeping. After taking secobarbital you may get a residual hangover effect that leaves you drowsy or dizzy. Do not drive, use machinery, or do anything that needs mental alertness until you know how secobarbital affects you. To reduce dizzy or fainting spells, do not sit or stand up quickly, especially if you are an older patient. Alcohol can increase possible unpleasant effects. Avoid alcoholic drinks. Secobarbital can stop birth control pills (oral contraceptives) working properly. Use another method of birth control while you are taking phenobarbital. If you are going to have surgery, tell your prescriber or health care professional that you are taking secobarbital.

What side effects may I notice from taking secobarbital?

Side effects that you should report to your prescriber or health care professional as soon as possible:

- bone tenderness
- changes in behavior, mood, or mental ability
- changes in the frequency or severity of seizures
- confusion, agitation
- difficulty breathing or shortness of breath
- eye problems, very small or enlarged centers to the eyes
- fever, sore throat
- hallucinations
- lightheadedness or fainting spells
- redness, blistering, peeling or loosening of the skin, including inside the mouth
- skin rash, itching, hives
- slow heartbeat
- swelling of the face or lips
- unusual bleeding or bruising, pinpoint red spots on the skin
- unusual tiredness or weakness
- weight loss
- yellowing of skin or eyes

Side effects that usually do not require medical attention (report to your prescriber or health care professional if they continue or are bothersome):

- constipation
- clumsiness, unsteadiness, or a "hang-over" effect
- difficulty sleeping or nightmares
- drowsiness, dizziness
- headache
- irritability, nervousness
- nausea or vomiting

Where can I keep my medicine?

Keep out of the reach of children in a container that small children cannot open. Store at room temperature between 15 and 30 degrees C (59 and 86 degrees F). Throw away any unused medicine after the expiration date.

Selegiline tablets or capsules

ELDEPRYL®;
5 mg; Capsule
Somerset
Pharmaceuticals Inc

SELEGILINE;
5 mg; Tablet
Mylan
Pharmaceuticals Inc

What is selegiline?

SELEGILINE (Carbex®, Eldepryl®) helps to increase or extend the effects of levodopa or carbidopa, and slow the progression of Parkinson's disease. Selegiline belongs to a class of drugs, called monoamine oxidase inhibitors (MAOIs), that block certain enzymes in the brain and change the balance of certain chemicals in the brain. Generic selegiline is available.

What should my health care professional know before I take selegiline?

They need to know if you have any of these conditions:
- dementia
- peptic ulcer
- psychosis
- unusual movements of the face, lips or tongue
- an unusual or allergic reaction to selegiline, other medicines, foods, dyes, or preservatives
- pregnant or trying to get pregnant
- breast-feeding

How should I take this medicine?

Take selegiline by mouth. Follow the directions on the prescription label. Swallow the tablets or capsules with a drink of water. Do not open the capsules; swallow whole. Take your doses at regular intervals. Do not take doses in the late afternoon or evening. Do not take your medicine more often than directed. Do not stop taking the tablets except on your prescriber's advice. Contact your pediatrician or health care professional regarding the use of this medicine in children. Special care may be needed.

What if I miss a dose?

If you miss a dose, take it as soon as you can. If it is almost time for your next dose, take only that dose. Do not take double or extra doses.

What may interact with selegiline?

- birth control pills
- caffeine
- carbamazepine
- dextromethorphan
- ephedra, Ma huang
- ephedrine
- estrogens
- furazolidone
- guarana
- linezolid
- medicines for mental depression
- meperidine
- phenylpropanolamine
- procarbazine
- sumatriptan
- tyramine—see below

Tell your prescriber or health care professional about all other medicines you are taking, including non-prescription medicines, nutritional supplements, or herbal products. Also tell your prescriber or health care professional if you are a frequent user of drinks with caffeine or alcohol, if you smoke, or if you use illegal drugs. These may affect the way your medicine works. Check with your health care professional before stopping or starting any of your medicines.

What should I watch for while taking selegiline?

Visit your prescriber or health care professional for regular checks on your progress. It can take up to 4 weeks to see the full effects of selegiline. Do not suddenly stop taking your medicine; this may make your condition worse or give you withdrawal symptoms. Ask your prescriber or health care professional for advice about gradually reducing your dosage. Even after you stop taking selegiline the effects can last for at least two weeks. If your prescriber or health care professional increases the dose of selegiline to more than 10 mg a day, ask him/her about possible interactions with foods that contain tyramine. At higher doses, selegiline may interact with these foods to produce severe headaches, a rise in blood pressure, or irregular heart beat. Call your prescriber or health care professional as soon as you can if you get frequent headaches or have palpitations. You may get drowsy, dizzy or have blurred vision. Do not drive, use machinery, or do anything that needs mental alertness until you know how selegiline affects you. Do not stand or sit up quickly, especially if you are an older patient. This reduces the risk of dizzy or fainting spells. Alcohol may increase dizziness or drowsiness; avoid alcoholic drinks. Selegiline can make your mouth dry. Chewing sugarless gum, sucking hard candy and drinking plenty of water will help. Do not treat yourself for coughs, colds, or allergies without asking your prescriber or health care professional for advice. Some ingredients may increase possible side effects to selegiline. If you are going to have surgery, tell your prescriber or health care professional that you are taking selegiline.

What side effects may I notice from taking selegiline?

Side effects that you should report to your prescriber or health care professional as soon as possible:
- black, tarry stools
- changes in behavior: mood swings, irritability, confusion, agitation
- chest pain
- difficulty breathing
- difficulty speaking
- enlarged pupils

- fever, clammy skin, increased sweating
- hallucinations (seeing and hearing things that are not really there)
- headaches
- lightheadedness or fainting spells; loss of balance
- muscle or neck stiffness or spasms
- slow, fast, or irregular heartbeat (palpitations)
- uncontrollable muscle movements or spasms of the head, face, arms, or legs

Side effects that usually do not require medical attention (report to your prescriber or health care professional if they continue or are bothersome):
- anxiety or nervousness
- blurred vision, increased sensitivity of the eyes to light
- changes in taste

- constipation or diarrhea
- difficulty sleeping
- drowsiness or dizziness
- dry mouth
- loss of appetite, weight loss
- muscle aches or pains
- nausea/vomiting
- ringing in the ears
- stomach discomfort or pain
- unusual tiredness or weakness

Where can I keep my medicine?

Keep out of the reach of children in a container that small children cannot open. Store at room temperature between 15 and 30 degrees C (59 and 86 degrees F). Throw away any unused medicine after the expiration date.

Sertraline tablets

ZOLOFT®;
100 mg; Tablet
Roerig Division of
Pfizer

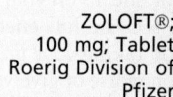

ZOLOFT®;
50 mg; Tablet
Roerig Division of
Pfizer

S

This drug requires an FDA medication guide. See page xxxvii.

What are sertraline tablets?

SERTRALINE (Zoloft®) is an antidepressant. It helps to improve a depressed person's mood. Sertraline can also help people with an obsessive compulsive disorder, panic attacks, post-trauma stress, or social anxiety. Sertraline may also be prescribed for other purposes, like premenstrual dysphoric disorder (PMDD), a severe type of premenstrual syndrome. Generic sertraline tablets are not yet available.

What should my health care professional know before I take sertraline?

They need to know if you have any of these conditions:
- bipolar disorder or a family history of bipolar disorder
- diabetes
- heart disease
- liver disease
- receiving electroconvulsive therapy
- seizures (convulsions)
- suicidal thoughts, plans, or attempt; a previous suicide attempt by you or a family member
- an unusual or allergic reaction to sertraline, other medicines, foods, dyes, or preservatives
- pregnant or trying to get pregnant
- breast-feeding

How should I take this medicine?

Take sertraline tablets by mouth. Follow the directions on the prescription label. Swallow the tablets with a drink of water. You may take sertraline with or without food. Take your doses at regular intervals. Do not take your medicine more often than directed. Do not stop taking except on your prescriber's advice. Do not use this medication in children unless you have been specifically instructed to do so by your health care provider. Contact your pediatrician or health care professional regarding the use of this medicine in children.

Special care may be needed. The *Medication Guide About Using Antidepressants in Children and Teenagers* is available from your health care professional and should be read and discussed with the health care provider if this drug is being used in a child or adolescent.

What if I miss a dose?

If you miss a dose, take it as soon as you can. If it is almost time for your next dose, skip the missed dose and go back to your regular dosing schedule. Do not take double or extra doses.

What may interact with sertraline?

Sertraline has the potential to interact with a variety of medications, check with your healthcare professional. The following list contains some of these interactions. *Do not take sertraline with any of the following medications:*

- astemizole (Hismanal®)
- cisapride (Propulsid®)
- pimozide (Orap®)
- terfenadine (Seldane®)
- thioridazine (Mellaril®)
- medicines called MAO inhibitors-phenelzine (Nardil®), tranylcypromine (Parnate®), isocarboxazid (Marplan®), selegiline (Eldepryl®)

Sertraline may also interact with the following medications:

- amphetamine
- bosentan
- carbamazepine
- certain diet drugs (dexfenfluramine, fenfluramine, phentermine, sibutramine)
- certain migraine headache medicines (almotriptan, eletriptan, frovatriptan, naratriptan, rizatriptan, sumatriptan, zolmitriptan)
- cimetidine

- cyclosporine
- dextroamphetamine
- dextromethorphan
- diazepam
- furazolidone
- linezolid
- other medicines for mental depression, mania, anxiety, psychosis or difficulty sleeping
- phenobarbital
- prescription pain medications
- procarbazine
- rifabutin
- rifampin
- rifapentine
- selegiline
- St. John's wort
- tolbutamide
- tramadol
- warfarin

Tell your prescriber or health care professional about all other medicines you are taking, including non-prescription medicines, nutritional supplements, and herbal products. Also tell your prescriber or health care professional if you are a frequent user of drinks with caffeine or alcohol, if you smoke, or if you use illegal drugs. These may affect the way your medicine works. Check with your health care professional before stopping or starting any of your medicines.

What should I watch for while taking sertraline?

Visit your prescriber or health care professional for regular checks on your progress. Continue to take your medicine even if you do not immediately feel better. It can take several weeks before you feel the full effect of sertraline. If you notice any unusual effects, such as restlessness, worsening of depression, agitation, difficulty sleeping, irritability, anger, acting on dangerous impulses, or thoughts of suicide or suicidal attempts, you should call your health care provider immediately. If you have been taking sertraline regularly for some time, do not suddenly stop taking it. You must gradually reduce the dose or your symptoms may get worse. Ask your prescriber for advice on slowly stopping sertraline. You may get drowsy or dizzy. Do not drive, use machinery, or do anything that needs mental alertness until you know how sertraline affects you. Do not stand or sit up quickly, especially if you are an older patient. This reduces the risk of dizzy or fainting spells. Alcohol may interfere with the effect of sertraline. Avoid alcoholic drinks. Do not treat yourself for coughs, colds or

allergies without asking your prescriber or health care professional for advice. Some ingredients can increase possible side effects. Your mouth may get dry. Chewing sugarless gum or sucking hard candy, and drinking plenty of water will help. If you are going to have surgery, tell your prescriber or health care professional that you are taking sertraline.

What side effects may I notice from taking sertraline?

Side effects that you should report to your prescriber or health care professional as soon as possible:
- anxiety, agitation, panic attacks, inability to sleep, irritability, hostility or extreme anger, aggressiveness, engaging in unusual or dangerous activities, restlessness or inability to sit still, fast talking, actions that are out of control, extreme elation or feeling of happiness that may switch back and forth with a depressed or sad mood
- fast heart rate, palpitations
- dizziness or lightheadedness
- skin rash, itching (hives)
- unusual tiredness or weakness
- vomiting

Side effects that usually do not require medical attention (report to your prescriber or health care professional if they continue or are bothersome):
- agitation or restlessness
- blurred vision
- constipation (less common) or diarrhea (more common)
- difficulty sleeping
- drowsiness
- dry mouth
- flushing (redness of skin)
- headache
- indigestion, nausea
- increased or decreased appetite
- increased sweating
- intestinal gas
- sexual difficulties (decreased sexual ability or desire)
- tremor (shaking)

Where can I keep my medicine?

Keep out of the reach of children in a container that small children cannot open. Store at room temperature between 15 and 30 degrees C (59 and 86 degrees F). Throw away any unused medicine after the expiration date.

Sevelamer capsules or tablets

RENAGEL®;
400 mg; Tablet
Genzyme Corp

What are sevelamer capsules?

SEVELAMER (Renagel®) is a polymer that binds phosphates in the stomach and prevents them from being absorbed into the body. For this reason, sevelamer also can help to prevent dangerous increases in phosphates that tend to occur in patients with end-stage kidney disease. Generic sevelamer capsules are not available.

What should my health care professional know before I take sevelamer?

They need to know if you have any of these conditions:
- an unusual or allergic reaction to sevelamer, other medicines, foods, dyes, or preservatives
- difficulty swallowing
- constipation or bowel obstruction
- prior gastrointestinal surgery
- scheduled for surgery
- low blood phosphate levels
- stomach bleeding or obstruction
- pregnant or trying to get pregnant
- breast-feeding

How should I take this medicine?

Take sevelamer capsules by mouth with meals. Follow the directions on the prescription label. Do not take the capsules apart or chew the capsules. Swallow the whole capsules with a drink of water. Take your doses regularly with meals and adhere to the diet prescribed by your health care professional. Do not take your medicine more often than directed. Contact your pediatrician or health care professional regarding the use of this medicine in children. Special care may be needed.

What if I miss a dose?

If you miss a dose, take it with your next meal. If it is almost time for your next dose, take only that dose. Do not take double or extra doses.

What may interact with sevelamer?

Due to its binding capacity in the stomach, sevelamer could possibly interact with any of the following medicines. If you are taking any of these medications, take them at least one hour before or 3 hours after you take sevelamer capsules.

- antibiotics
- medicines for an irregular heartbeat
- levothyroxine and other thyroid hormones
- seizure (convulsion) medications
- theophylline
- warfarin

Tell your prescriber or health care professional about all other medicines you are taking, including non-prescription medicines, nutritional supplements, or herbal products. Also tell your prescriber or health care professional if you are a frequent user of drinks with caffeine or alcohol, if you smoke, or if you use illegal drugs. These may affect the way your medicine works. Check with your health care professional before stopping or starting any of your medicines.

What should I watch for while taking sevelamer?

Check with your prescriber or health care professional if you have bothersome stomach problems; if you get black tarry stools; notice any rectal bleeding; experience confusion; if you are scheduled for surgery; or if you feel unusually tired or weak. If you are taking other medications, take them at least 1 hour before or 3 hours after taking sevelamer. Make sure to take this medicine with meals and adhere to the diet prescribed by your physician. This will help to provide you with the phosphate-lowering benefits of this medicine.

What side effects may I notice from taking sevelamer?

Side effects that you should report to your prescriber or health care professional as soon as possible:
- bone or joint aches and pains
- confusion or irritability
- headache
- loss of appetite
- muscle weakness or numbness
- severe or frequent constipation
- unusual weakness or tiredness
- vomiting

Side effects that usually do not require medical attention (report to your prescriber or health care professional if they continue or are bothersome):
- constipation
- diarrhea
- nausea
- stomach indigestion or gas

Where can I keep my medicine?

Keep out of the reach of children in a container that small children cannot open. Store at room temperature between 15 and 30 degrees C (59 and 86 degrees F). Throw away any unused medicine after the expiration date.

Sibutramine capsules

MERIDIA®; 15 mg; Capsule Abbott Pharmaceutical Product Division	MERIDIA®; 5 mg; Capsule Abbott Pharmaceutical Product Division

What are sibutramine capsules?

SIBUTRAMINE (Meridia®) is used to control hunger in patients who are overweight. Sibutramine is prescribed along with a reduced-calorie diet and, if appropriate, an exercise program. Do not share this medicine with anyone else. Generic sibutramine capsules are not yet available.

What should my health care professional know before I take sibutramine?

They need to know if you have or have had any of these conditions:
- anorexia nervosa, bulimia or other eating disorder
- bleeding disorder
- depression or other mood disorder
- gallstones
- glaucoma
- heart disease, such as congestive heart failure or a previous heart attack
- heart rhythm problems or palpitations, chest pain
- high blood pressure
- kidney disease
- liver disease
- lung disease
- migraine headaches
- osteoporosis
- Parkinson's disease
- previous use of other weight loss drugs
- sleeplessness
- seizures (epilepsy or convulsions)
- stroke or symptoms of a stroke (i.e., transient ischemic attacks or TIAs)
- thyroid disease
- an unusual or allergic reaction to sibutramine, other medicines, foods, dyes, or preservatives
- pregnant or trying to get pregnant
- breast-feeding

How should I take this medicine?

Take sibutramine capsules by mouth. Follow the directions on the prescription label. Swallow with a drink of water. You may take this medicine with meals or food. Do not take your medicine more often than directed. Do not stop taking except on your prescriber's advice. Contact your pediatrician or health care professional regarding the use of this medicine in children. Special care may be needed.

What if I miss a dose?

If you miss a dose, take it as soon as you can. If it is almost time for your next dose, take only that dose. Do not take double or extra doses.

What may interact with sibutramine?

Do not take sibutramine with the following medications:
- medicines called MAO Inhibitors-phenelzine (Nardil®), tranylcypromine (Parnate®), isocarboxazid (Marplan®), selegiline (Eldepryl®)
- other medicines for weight loss, including herbal and nonprescription weight-loss drugs, like Ma huang or ephedra
- some medicines for migraines (such as dihydroergotamine, ergotamine, eletriptan, naratriptan, rizatriptan, sumatriptan, zolmitriptan)
- tryptophan

Sibutramine may also interact with:
- bosentan
- bupropion
- dextromethorphan
- fentanyl
- grapefruit juice
- ketoconazole
- linezolid
- lithium
- medicines for high blood pressure
- medicines for allergy, cold or flu symptoms (decongestants, cough suppressants)
- medicines for anxiety, depression or other mental problems
- meperidine
- procarbazine
- St. John's wort
- voriconazole

Tell your prescriber or other health care provider about all other medicines you are taking, including non-prescription medicines and illegal drugs. These may affect the way your medicine works. Check with your health care professional before stopping or starting any of your medicines.

What should I watch for while taking sibutramine?

Visit your prescriber regularly to have your blood pressure and heart rate checked. Contact your prescriber if you think you are experiencing any unusual side effects. Keep in mind that sibutramine was intended to be used in addition to a healthy diet and appropriate exercise. The best results are achieved this way. Do not increase or in any way change your dose without consulting your prescriber. A weight loss of 4 pounds or more during your first month of treatment is a good indicator of success with sibutramine. Most of the weight you will lose will be lost gradually during 6 to 12 months. Many people who lose weight and remain on sibutramine therapy maintain their weight loss.

You should not use herbal or over-the-counter weight-loss products while taking sibutramine. Non-drug nutritional supplements, like vitamins, minerals, and proteins or amino acids (with the exception of tryptophan), can be used with sibutramine. You should make sure your prescriber knows what nutritional supplements you are taking and why you are taking them.

What side effects may I notice from taking sibutramine?

Side effects that you should report to your prescriber or health care professional as soon as possible:
Rare or uncommon:
- bleeding, easy bruising, nose bleeds, bleeding of gums
- chest pain
- difficulty breathing
- fever
- heart palpitations
- seizures
- severe dizziness

Stop using sibutramine and call your prescriber or health care professional as soon as possible if you experience any of these side effects.
More common:
- increased heart rate
- increased blood pressure
- menstrual problems
- muscle or joint pain
- pain, burning or tingling in the hands or feet
- unusual swelling of the arms or legs

- unusual tiredness or weakness
- visual problems

Side effects that usually do not require medical attention (report to your prescriber or health care professional if they continue or are bothersome):
- agitation or irritability
- anxiety
- back pain
- constipation
- diarrhea
- difficulty sleeping
- dizziness
- drowsiness
- dry mouth
- gas
- headache
- nausea or vomiting
- skin problems
- stomach problems
- sweating
- taste disturbance
- throat irritation or pain

Where can I keep my medicine?

Keep out of the reach of children in a container that small children cannot open. Store at controlled room temperature between 15 and 30 degrees C (59 and 86 degrees F). Keep container tightly closed. Protect capsules from heat, light and moisture. Throw away any unused medicine after the expiration date.

Sildenafil tablets

VIAGRA®; 25 mg; Tablet Pfizer Laboratories Div Pfizer Inc		
VIAGRA®; 50 mg; Tablet Pfizer Laboratories Div Pfizer Inc		

What are sildenafil tablets?

SILDENAFIL (Viagra®) is used to treat erection problems in men. Generic sildenafil tablets are not yet available.

What should my health care professional know before I take sildenafil?

They need to know if you have any of these conditions:
- anatomical deformity of the penis, Peyronie's disease, or ever had an erection that lasted more than 4 hours
- benign prostatic hypertrophy (BPH)
- bleeding disorder
- cancer
- diabetes
- frequent heartburn or gastroesophageal reflux disease (GERD)
- heart disease, angina, high or low blood pressure, a history of heart attack, or other heart problems
- high cholesterol
- kidney disease
- liver disease
- sickle cell disease
- stomach or intestinal ulcer

- stroke
- eye or vision problems, including a rare inherited eye disease called retinitis pigmentosa
- an unusual or allergic reaction to sildenafil, other medicines, foods, dyes, or preservatives
- pregnant or trying to get pregnant
- breast-feeding

How should I take this medicine?

Take sildenafil tablets by mouth. Follow the directions on the prescription label. The dose is usually taken 1 hour before sexual activity. You should not take this dose more than once per day. Swallow the tablets with a drink of water. Do not take double or extra doses. Contact your pediatrician or health care professional regarding the use of this medicine in children. Special care may be needed.

What if I miss a dose?

This does not apply.

What may interact with sildenafil?

Do not take sildenafil if you are taking the following medications:

- nitroglycerin-type drugs for the heart or chest pain such as amyl nitrite, isosorbide dinitrate, isosorbide mononitrate, nitroglycerin, even if these are only taken occasionally

Sildenafil may also interact with the following medications:

- alpha blockers, used for high blood pressure or an enlarged prostate. NOTE: Do not take doses of sildenafil higher than 25 mg within 4 hours of taking alpha blockers, such as alfuzosin (Uroxatral®), doxazosin (Cardura®), prazosin (Minipress®), or terazosin (Hytrin®).
- bosentan
- certain drugs used for seizures such as carbamazepine, phenytoin, and phenobarbital
- certain drugs used for fungal or yeast infections, such as fluconazole, ketoconazole, and voriconazole
- certain drugs for the treatment of HIV infection or AIDS
- cimetidine
- cisapride
- clarithromycin
- diltiazem
- erythromycin
- grapefruit juice
- mibefradil
- nitroprusside
- rifabutin
- rifampin
- quinidine
- some drugs for treating depression, anxiety or other mood problems (examples: fluoxetine, fluvoxamine, nefazodone)
- verapamil

Tell your prescriber or health care professional about all other medicines you are taking, including non-prescription medicines, nutritional supplements, or herbal products. Also tell your prescriber or health care professional if you are a frequent user of drinks with caffeine or alcohol, if you smoke, or if you use illegal drugs. These may affect the way your medicine works. Check with your health care professional before stopping or starting any of your medicines.

What should I watch for while taking sildenafil?

Contact you physician immediately if the erection lasts longer than 4 hours or if it becomes painful. This may

be a sign of priapism and must be treated immediately to prevent permanent damage. If you experience symptoms of nausea, dizziness, chest pain or arm pain upon initiation of sexual activity after sildenafil use, you should refrain from further activity and should discuss the episode with your prescriber or health care professional as soon as possible. If you notice any changes in your vision while taking this drug, notify your prescriber or health care professional as soon as possible. Do not change the dose of your medication. Please call your prescriber or health care professional to determine if your dose needs to be reevaluated. Using Viagra® (sildenafil) does not protect you or your partner against HIV infection (the virus that causes AIDS) or other sexually transmitted diseases.

What side effects may I notice from taking sildenafil?

Side effects that you should report to your prescriber or health care professional as soon as possible:

- changes in vision such as blurred vision, eyes being more sensitive to light, or trouble telling the difference between blue and green objects or objects having a blue color tinge to them
- difficulty breathing, shortness of breath
- chest pain or palpitations
- prolonged erection (lasting longer than 4 hours)
- skin rash, itching

Side effects that usually do not require medical attention (report to your prescriber or health care professional if they continue or are bothersome):

- diarrhea
- dizziness
- flushing
- headache
- indigestion
- nasal congestion

Where can I keep my medicine?

Keep out of reach of children in a container that small children cannot open. Store at room temperature between 15 and 30 degrees C (59 and 86 degrees F). Throw away any unused medicine after the expiration date.

Simethicone capsules, tablets, or chewable tablets

GAS-X®;
80 mg; Tablet,
Chewable
Novartis Consumer
Health

MAXIMUM
STRENGTH
GASAID®;
125 mg; Capsule
McNeil Consumer
Healthcare Div
McNeil Ppc Inc

What are simethicone capsules, tablets or chewable tablets?

SIMETHICONE (Gas-X®, Maximum Strength GasAid®, Phazyme®-125, Mylanta® Gas Relief and others) is an antiflatulent used to treat too much gas in the stomach and intestines. Swallowing too much air or eating foods that disagree often causes gas. Generic simethicone capsules, tablets, and chewable tablets are available.

What should my health care professional know before I take simethicone?

They need to know if you have any of these conditions:
- phenylketonuria
- an unusual or allergic reaction to simethicone, other medicines, foods, dyes, or preservatives
- pregnant or trying to get pregnant
- breast-feeding

How should I take this medicine?

Take simethicone capsules, tablets and chewable tablets by mouth. Swallow the tablets with a drink of water. If you are prescribed chewable tablets, crush or chew them; do not swallow them whole. The capsules (also known as softgels) should be swallowed whole with water; do not chew them. Follow the directions on the label. If your health care provider has given you special instructions, follow these directions instead of what is on the label. Do not take your medicine more often than directed. Contact your pediatrician or health care professional regarding the use of this medicine in children. Special care may be needed. Do not administer adult simethicone preparations to infants.

What if I miss a dose?

If it is almost time for your next dose, take only that dose. Do not take double or extra doses.

What may interact with simethicone?

- none reported

Tell your prescriber or health care professional about all other medicines you are taking, including non-prescription medicines, nutritional supplements, or herbal products. Also tell your prescriber or health care professional if you are a frequent user of drinks with caffeine or alcohol, if you smoke, or if you use illegal drugs. These may affect the way your medicine works. Check with your health care professional before stopping or starting any of your medicines.

What should I watch for while taking simethicone?

In general, simethicone is a very safe drug. Tell your health care prescriber if your symptoms get worse, or if you have severe pain, diarrhea, constipation, or blood in your stool.

What side effects may I notice from taking simethicone?

There are no reported side effects with simethicone.

Where can I keep my medicine?

Keep out of the reach of children in a container that small children cannot open. Store at room temperature between 15 and 30 degrees C (59 and 86 degrees F). Keep container tightly closed. Throw away any unused medicine after the expiration date.

Simvastatin tablets

ZOCOR®;
20 mg; Tablet
Merck and Co Inc

ZOCOR®;
40 mg; Tablet
Merck and Co Inc

What are simvastatin tablets?

SIMVASTATIN (Zocor®) blocks the body's ability to make cholesterol. Simvastatin can help lower blood cholesterol for patients who are at risk of getting heart disease or a stroke. It is only for patients whose cholesterol level is not controlled by diet. Generic simvastatin tablets are available.

What should my health care professional know before I take simvastatin?

They need to know if you have any of these conditions:
- an alcohol problem
- any hormone disorder (such as diabetes, under-active thyroid)
- blood salt imbalance
- infection
- kidney disease
- liver disease
- low blood pressure
- muscle disorder or condition
- recent surgery
- seizures (convulsions)
- severe injury

- an unusual or allergic reaction to simvastatin, other medicines, foods, dyes, or preservatives
- pregnant or trying to get pregnant
- breast-feeding

How should I take this medicine?

Take simvastatin tablets by mouth. Follow the directions on the prescription label. Swallow the tablets with a drink of water. If you take the tablets once a day, it is best to take your dose in the evening hours (like with the evening meal) or at bedtime. You may take this medicine with or without food. Do not take simvastatin with grapefruit juice; orange juice may be used instead. Take your doses at regular intervals. Do not take your medicine more often than directed. Contact your pediatrician or health care professional regarding the use of this medicine in children. Special care may be needed.

What if I miss a dose?

If you miss a dose, take it as soon as you can. If it is almost time for your next dose, take only that dose. Do not take double or extra doses.

What may interact with simvastatin?

Do not take Simvastatin with any of the following:

- amprenavir
- atazanavir
- clarithromycin
- delavirdine
- erythromycin
- grapefruit juice
- indinavir
- itraconazole
- ketoconazole
- lopinavir; ritonavir
- mibefradil
- nefazodone
- nelfinavir
- ritonavir
- saquinavir
- went yeast

Simvastatin may also interact with the following medications:

- alcohol
- amiodarone
- barbiturates (examples: phenobarbital, butalbital, primidone)
- bosentan
- carbamazepine
- cyclosporine
- digoxin
- diltiazem
- efavirenz
- fluconazole
- medicines to lower cholesterol or triglycerides (examples: fenofibrate, gemfibrozil, niacin)
- medicine used to stop early pregnancy (mifepristone, RU-486)

- nicardipine
- oxcarbazepine
- phenytoin
- rifampin, rifabutin, or rifapentine
- St. John's Wort
- telithromycin
- troleandomycin
- verapamil
- voriconazole
- warfarin

Tell your prescriber or health care professional about all other medicines you are taking, including non-prescription medicines, nutritional supplements, or herbal products. Also tell your prescriber or health care professional if you are a frequent user of drinks with caffeine or alcohol, if you smoke, or if you use illegal drugs. These may affect the way your medicine works. Check with your health care professional before stopping or starting any of your medicines.

What should I watch for while taking simvastatin?

Visit your prescriber or health care professional for regular checks on your progress. You may need to have blood tests drawn to make sure your liver is working properly. Tell your prescriber or health care professional as soon as you can if you get any unexplained muscle pain, tenderness, or weakness, especially if you also have a fever and tiredness. Some medicines increase the risk of muscle side effects while taking simvastatin. Discuss your drug regimen with your health care provider if you are prescribed certain antibiotics or antifungals which are not recommended to be taken with simvastatin (examples: clarithromycin, erythromycin, itraconazole, ketoconazole). Your prescriber may decide to temporarily stop taking simvastatin while you are taking a short course of the antibiotic or antifungal therapy. Alternatively, your health care provider may prescribe another antibiotic or antifungal medicine for your condition. Simvastatin is only part of a total cholesterol-lowering program. Your physician or dietician can suggest a low-cholesterol and low-fat diet that will reduce your risk of getting heart and blood vessel disease. Avoid alcohol and smoking, and keep a proper exercise schedule. If you are going to have surgery tell your prescriber or health care professional that you are taking simvastatin.

What side effects may I notice from taking simvastatin?

Side effects that you should report to your prescriber or health care professional as soon as possible:
Rare or uncommon:
- dark yellow or brown urine
- decreased urination, difficulty passing urine
- fever
- muscle pain, tenderness, cramps, or weakness
- redness, blistering, peeling or loosening of the skin, including inside the mouth

- skin rash, itching
- unusual tiredness or weakness
- yellowing of the skin or eyes

Side effects that usually do not require medical attention (report to your prescriber or health care professional if they continue or are bothersome):

- constipation
- headache

- upset stomach, indigestion, gas, heartburn

Where can I keep my medicine?

Keep out of the reach of children in a container that small children cannot open. Store at room temperature between 5 and 30 degrees C (41 and 86 degrees F). Throw away any unused medicine after the expiration date.

Sirolimus tablets

RAPAMUNE®;
1 mg; Tablet
Wyeth Div Wyeth
Pharmaceuticals Inc

What are sirolimus tablets?

SIROLIMUS (Rapamune®) is a medication used to decrease the immune system's response to a transplanted organ, which the body would otherwise see as foreign. Sirolimus helps to reduce immune responses and prevent organ rejection in patients who have received a kidney or other organ transplant. Generic sirolimus tablets are not yet available.

What should my health care professional know before I take sirolimus?

They need to know if you have any of these conditions:
- heart disease, heart failure, or heart rhythm problems (fast or slow heartbeat)
- high cholesterol or triglycerides
- an active infection
- liver disease
- an unusual or allergic reaction to sirolimus, other medicines, foods, dyes, or preservatives
- pregnant or trying to get pregnant
- breast-feeding

How should I take this medicine?

Take sirolimus tablets by mouth once daily. Follow the directions on the prescription label. You may take sirolimus with or without food, but make sure to take it the same way all the time. Do not take your medicine more often than directed. If you are also taking cyclosporine, make sure to take sirolimus at least 4 hours after taking your dose of cyclosporine. Contact your pediatrician or health care professional regarding the use of this medicine in children. Special care may be needed.

What if I miss a dose?

If you miss a dose, take it as soon as you can. Remember if you are taking cyclosporine, you should wait at least 4 hours after taking cyclosporine before taking your sirolimus dose. Do not take double-doses. Contact your prescriber or health care professional if you miss more than one dose, or if you vomit after a dose.

What may interact with sirolimus?

- amiodarone
- bosentan
- carbamazepine

- cimetidine
- cisapride
- clarithromycin
- cyclosporine
- diltiazem
- erythromycin
- fluoxetine
- fluvoxamine
- grapefruit juice
- imatinib
- medicines for fungal infections (antifungal medicines applied to the skin should not interact)
- medicines for HIV infection including protease inhibitors, delavirdine, efavirenz, and nevirapine
- metoclopramide
- mifepristone
- nefazodone
- nicardipine
- oxcarbazepine
- phenobarbital
- phenytoin
- rifabutin
- rifampin
- rifapentine
- St. John's wort
- telithromycin
- vaccines
- verapamil

Talk to your prescriber or health care professional before taking any of these medicines:

- aspirin
- acetaminophen
- ibuprofen
- ketoprofen
- naproxen

Tell your prescriber or health care professional about all other medicines that you are taking, including non-prescription medicines, nutritional supplements, or herbal products. Also tell your prescriber or health care professional if you are a frequent user of drinks with caffeine or alcohol, if you smoke, or if you use illegal drugs. These may affect the way your medicine works. Check with your health care professional before stopping or starting any of your medicines.

S

What should I watch for while taking sirolimus?

Sirolimus increases your cholesterol or lipid levels. This may require additional treatment in some cases. Your prescriber will check your blood levels on a regular basis while you are taking sirolimus to check for this effect. You will need to visit your prescriber or health care professional for regular checks on your progress. Sirolimus will decrease your body's ability to fight infections. Call your prescriber or health care professional if you have a fever, chills, sore throat or other symptoms of a cold or flu. Do not treat these symptoms yourself. Try to avoid being around people who are sick. Sirolimus may increase your risk to bruise or bleed. Call your prescriber or health care professional if you notice any unusual bruising or bleeding. After you stop taking this medication, side effects can continue. Some side effects may not occur until years after the medicine was taken. These effects can include the development of certain types of cancer. Discuss this possibility with your prescriber or health care professional. Avoid taking aspirin, acetaminophen (Tylenol®), ibuprofen (Advil®), ketoprofen (Orudis KT®), or naproxen (Aleve®) products as these may mask a fever, unless instructed to by your prescriber or health care professional. Patients who are able to have children should use effective birth control methods before, during, and for 12 weeks following sirolimus therapy.

What side effects may I notice from taking sirolimus?

Contact your prescriber or health care professional about any unusual effects. Side effects that you should report to your prescriber or health care professional as soon as possible:

- difficulty breathing
- rapid heart beat or chest pain
- signs of infection—fever or chills, cough, sore throat, pain or difficulty passing urine
- signs of decreased platelets or bleeding—bruising, pinpoint red spots on the skin, black, tarry stools, and blood in the urine
- signs of decreased red blood cells—unusual weakness or tiredness, fainting spells, lightheadedness
- skin rash or hives

Side effects that usually do not require medical attention (report to your prescriber or health care professional if they continue or are bothersome):

- acne
- aches
- diarrhea
- difficulty sleeping
- headache
- nausea, vomiting

Where can I keep my medicine?

Keep out of the reach of children. Store sirolimus tablets at room temperature.

Sodium Fluoride tablets or chewable tablets

SODIUM FLUORIDE;
1 mg; Tablet, Chewable
Mutual/United Research
Laboratories

What are sodium fluoride tablets or chewable tablets?

SODIUM FLUORIDE (Flura®, Karidium®, Fluoritab®, Fluorodex®, Luride®) is a mineral that strengthens tooth enamel and helps to prevent dental decay. Fluoride also helps to decrease sensitivity of the teeth. Fluoride, in small amounts, also helps maintain healthy bones. Most natural water supplies contain some fluoride and fluoride may be added to the water. Additional fluoride may be necessary in some cases. Generic fluoride tablets and chewable tablets are available.

What should my health care professional need to know before I take sodium fluoride?

They need to know if you have any of these conditions:

- arthritic joints
- stomach or intestinal disease
- kidney disease
- stained, mottled, or pitted teeth
- an unusual or allergic reaction to fluoride, tartrazine, other medicines, foods, dyes, or preservatives
- pregnant or trying to get pregnant
- breast-feeding

How should I take this medicine?

Take sodium fluoride tablets by mouth. Follow the directions on the prescription label. If taking the chewable tablets, chew well before swallowing, preferably after brushing the teeth at night. Do not drink or eat for 15 minutes after chewing the tablets. Do not take the tablets more often than directed. Contact your pediatrician or health care professional regarding the use of this medicine in children. Special care may be needed.

What if I miss a dose?

If you miss a dose, take it as soon as you can. If it is almost time for your next dose, take only that dose. Do not take double or extra doses.

What may interact with sodium fluoride?

- aluminum salts
- calcium salts
- magnesium salts

Tell your prescriber or health care professional about all other medicines you are taking, including non-prescription medicines, nutritional supplements, or herbal

products. Also tell your prescriber or health care professional if you are a frequent user of drinks with caffeine or alcohol, if you smoke, or if you use illegal drugs. These may affect the way your medicine works. Check with your health care professional before stopping or starting any of your medicines.

What should I watch for while taking sodium fluoride?

Do not take these tablets unless you are sure you need extra fluoride. Ask your dentist or health care professional for advice, especially if you move to a new area where the amount of fluoride in the water may be different. Do not take calcium supplements, or antacids containing calcium, aluminum, or magnesium, at the same time as sodium fluoride. There should be an interval of at least 2 hours to make sure the sodium fluoride works properly. If more than the recommended amount of the tablets is accidently swallowed, contact a Poison Control Center immediately. Also, prolonged daily ingestion can cause abnormal tooth enamel or brittle bones. Enamel is the hard part on the outside of the tooth. Immediately report any signs of abnormal tooth color or staining or spotting of the teeth.

What side effects may I notice from taking sodium fluoride?

Recommended doses of sodium fluoride produce few side effects. Serious side effects can occur with overuse of sodium fluoride and include:

- aches and pains in the bones or joints
- black, tarry stools
- blood in vomit
- mottled or discolored teeth
- nausea, vomiting
- skin rash, itching
- sores in the mouth or on the lips
- stomach pain
- unusual weakness

Call your prescriber or health care professional for advice if you get any of these side effects.

Where can I keep my medicine?

Keep out of the reach of children in a container that small children cannot open. Store at room temperature between 15 and 30 degrees C (59 and 86 degrees F). Keep container tightly closed. Throw away any unused medicine after the expiration date.

Solifenacin tablets

VESICARE®;
10 mg; Tablet
GlaxoSmithKline

VESICARE®;
5 mg; Tablet
GlaxoSmithKline

What are Solifenacin tablets?

SOLIFENACIN (Vesicare®) helps to control an overactive bladder, a chronic condition that can be improved with medication. Solifenacin may reduce the frequency of bathroom visits and may help to control wetting accidents. Generic solifenacin tablets are not yet available.

What should my health care professional know before I take solifenacin?

They need to know if you have any of these conditions:

- difficulty passing urine
- glaucoma
- intestinal obstruction
- kidney disease
- liver disease
- stomach problems like pyloric stenosis or reflux, or other problems with proper emptying of the contents of the stomach
- an unusual or allergic reaction to solifenacin, other medicines, foods, dyes, or preservatives
- pregnant or trying to get pregnant
- breast-feeding

How should I take this medicine?

Take solifenacin tablets by mouth. Follow the directions on the prescription label. Swallow the tablets whole with a drink of water. Solifenacin can be taken with or without food. Take your doses at regular intervals. Do not take your medicine more often than directed. Do not stop taking except on your doctor's advice. Contact your pediatrician or health care professional regarding the use of this medicine in children. Special care may be needed.

What if I miss a dose?

If it is almost time for your next dose, take only that dose on the regular schedule. Do not take double or extra doses.

What may interact with solifenacin?

- alcohol-containing beverages
- atropine
- bosentan
- caffeine
- cisapride
- clarithromycin
- clozapine
- diltiazem
- erythromycin
- fluvoxamine
- grapefruit juice
- medicines for fungal infections, like fluconazole, itraconazole, ketoconazole or voriconazole
- medicines for treating HIV infection or AIDS
- metoclopramide
- nefazodone
- omeprazole
- oxybutynin

- quinidine
- quinine
- scopolamine
- tegaserod
- troleandomycin
- verapamil
- water pills (diuretics)
- zafirlukast

Tell your prescriber or health care professional about all other medicines you are taking, including non-prescription medicines, nutritional supplements, or herbal products. Also tell your prescriber or health care professional if you are a frequent user of drinks with caffeine or alcohol, if you smoke, or if you use illegal drugs. These may affect the way your medicine works. Check with your health care professional before stopping or starting any of your medicines.

What should I watch for while taking solifenacin?

It may take 2 or 3 months to notice the maximum benefit from this medication. Your health care professional may also recommend techniques that may help improve control of your bladder and sphincter muscles. Such techniques will help train you to need the bathroom less frequently. You may need to limit your intake tea, coffee, caffeinated sodas, and alcohol; these drinks may aggravate your symptoms. Keeping healthy bowel habits may lessen bladder symptoms. If you currently smoke, quitting smoking may help reduce irritation to the bladder muscle. You may get dizzy or have blurred vision. Do not drive, use machinery, or do anything that requires mental alertness until you know how solifenacin affects you. Your mouth may get dry. Chewing sugarless gum or sucking hard candy, and drinking plenty of water, will help. Solifenacin may cause dry eyes and blurred vision. If you wear contact lenses, you may feel some discomfort. Lubricating drops may help. See your ophthalmologist if the problem does not go away or is severe.

What side effects may I notice from taking solifenacin?

Serious side effects are not common. Side effects that you should report to your doctor as soon as possible:
- blurred vision or difficulty focusing vision
- confusion
- difficulty passing urine
- palpitations
- severe dizziness

Side effects that usually do not require medical attention (report to your doctor if they continue or are bothersome):
- constipation
- dry eyes
- dry mouth
- headache
- mild dizziness or drowsiness
- upset stomach

Where can I keep my medicine?

Keep out of the reach of children. Store at room temperature between 15 and 30 degrees C (59 and 86 degrees F). Protect from light. Throw away any unused medicine after the expiration date.

Sotalol tablets

BETAPACE AF™;
160 mg; Tablet
Berlex Laboratories
Inc

BETAPACE AF™;
120 mg; Tablet
Berlex Laboratories
Inc

What are sotalol tablets (Betapace AF™)?

SOTALOL (Betapace AF™) belongs to a group of medicines called beta-blockers. Betapace AF™ is a brand of sotalol tablets given only to patients with an atrial heart arrhythmia (irregular heartbeat) such as atrial fibrillation. Atrial fibrillation happens when certain heart chambers beat too fast or irregularly. When this happens, you may feel weak and tired, or get out of breath easily. You may get an uncomfortable feeling in your chest and "fluttering" or "palpitations." Sotalol can help your heart return to and maintain a normal rhythm. Generic sotalol AF tablets are available.

What should my health care professional know before I take sotalol?

They need to know if you have any of these conditions:
- asthma, bronchitis or bronchospasm
- circulation problems, or blood vessel disease (such as Raynaud's disease)
- depression
- diabetes
- emphysema, or other lung disease
- heart disease or heart failure
- heart rhythm problems
- heart valve problems
- history of low levels of potassium or magnesium
- kidney disease
- low blood pressure
- muscle weakness or disease (such as myasthenia gravis)
- pheochromocytoma
- psoriasis
- thyroid disease
- an unusual or allergic reaction to sotalol, other beta-blockers, medicines, foods, dyes, or preservatives
- pregnant or trying to get pregnant
- breast-feeding

How should I take this medicine?

Take sotalol tablets by mouth. Follow the directions on the prescription label. Swallow the tablets with a drink of water. You may take sotalol tablets with or without food. Take your doses at regular intervals. Do not take your medicine more often than directed. Do not stop taking except on your prescriber's advice. Contact your pediatrician or health care professional regarding the use of this medicine in children. Special care may be needed. Elderly patients over 65 years old may have a stronger reaction to this medicine and need smaller doses.

What if I miss a dose?

If you miss a dose, do not try to make up the missed dose. Take your normal dose at the next scheduled time. Do not take double or extra doses.

What may interact with sotalol?

- amphetamine or other stimulant drugs
- antacids (such as Tums®, Rolaids®, Maalox®, and others)
- astemizole
- certain antibiotics such as clarithromycin, erythromycin, gatifloxacin, grepafloxacin, levofloxacin, moxifloxacin, sparfloxacin
- cevimeline
- cisapride
- clonidine
- digoxin
- dofetilide
- furazolidone
- hawthorn or ginger
- linezolid
- liothyronine
- medicines for angina or high blood pressure
- medicines for colds and breathing difficulties
- medicines for diabetes
- medicines for mental depression or other mental problems
- medicines known as MAO inhibitors, such as phenelzine (Nardil®), tranylcypromine (Parnate®), isocarboxazid (Marplan®), and selegiline (Carbex®, Eldepryl®)
- medicines to control heart rhythm
- procarbazine
- some medicines for weight loss (including some herbal products, ephedrine, dextroamphetamine)
- terfenadine
- water pills (diuretics)

Tell your prescriber or health care professional about all other medicines you are taking, including nonprescription medicines, nutritional supplements, or herbal products. Also tell your prescriber or health care professional if you are a frequent user of drinks with caffeine or alcohol, if you smoke, or if you use illegal drugs. These may affect the way your medicine works. Check with your health care professional before stopping or starting any of your medicines.

What should I watch for while taking sotalol?

You will be started on Betapace AF™ in a specialized facility for the first two or more days of treatment for your heart rhythm problem. After this, visit your prescriber or health care professional for regular checks on your progress. Check your heart rate and blood pressure regularly while you are taking sotalol. Ask your prescriber or health care professional what your heart rate and blood pressure should be, and when you should contact him or her. Your prescriber or health care professional also may schedule regular blood tests and electrocardiograms to check your progress. Do not stop taking this medicine suddenly. This could lead to serious, heart-related problems. Because your condition and the use of sotalol carry some risk, it is a good idea to carry an identification card, necklace or bracelet with details of your condition, medications, and prescriber or health care professional. If you have fast or irregular beating of the heart with lightheadedness or fainting, contact your health care professional immediately for evaluation. You may get drowsy or dizzy. Do not drive, use machinery, or do anything that requires mental alertness until you know how sotalol affects you. To reduce the risk of dizzy or fainting spells, do not sit or stand up quickly. Alcohol can make you more drowsy, and increase flushing and rapid heartbeats. Therefore, it is best to avoid alcoholic drinks. Sotalol can affect blood sugar levels. If you have diabetes, check with your prescriber or health care professional before you change your diet or the dose of your diabetic medicine. If you are going to have surgery (including dental surgery), tell your prescriber or health care professional that you are taking sotalol.

What side effects may I notice from taking sotalol?

Side effects that you should report to your prescriber or health care professional as soon as possible:
- chest pain
- confusion
- changes in blood sugar if you have diabetes
- cold hands or feet
- difficulty breathing, wheezing, or shortness of breath
- dizziness or fainting spells
- fast or irregular heartbeat, palpitations, chest pain
- less appetite or more thirst than normal
- slow heart rate (fewer than 50 beats per minute)
- swelling of legs or ankles
- unusual sweating
- unusual weakness or tiredness
- vomiting

Side effects that usually do not require medical attention (report to your prescriber or health care professional if they continue or are bothersome):
- diarrhea
- mental depression
- nausea
- sexual difficulties (impotence or decreased sexual urges)
- weakness or tiredness

Where can I keep my medicine?

Keep out of the reach of children in a container that small children cannot open. Store at room temperature between 15 and 30 degrees C (59 and 86 degrees F). Throw away any unused medicine after the expiration date.

Sotalol tablets (Betapace®)

 BETAPACE®;
160 mg; Tablet
Berlex Laboratories
Inc

 BETAPACE®;
240 mg; Tablet
Berlex Laboratories
Inc

What are sotalol tablets (Betapace®)?

SOTALOL (Betapace®) belongs to a group of medicines called beta-blockers. Betapace® is a brand of sotalol tablets given to patients with heart arrhythmias (rapid, irregular heartbeats) such as ventricular tachycardia. Betapace® treats irregular heart rhythm and can slow rapid heartbeats (tachycardia). Sotalol can help your heart to return to and maintain a normal rhythm. Generic sotalol tablets are available.

What should my health care professional know before I take sotalol?

They need to know if you have any of these conditions:
- asthma, bronchitis or bronchospasm
- circulation problems, or blood vessel disease (such as Raynaud's disease)
- depression
- diabetes
- emphysema, or other lung disease
- heart disease or heart failure
- heart rhythm problems
- heart valve problems
- history of low levels of potassium or magnesium
- kidney disease
- low blood pressure
- muscle weakness or disease (such as myasthenia gravis)
- pheochromocytoma
- psoriasis
- thyroid disease
- an unusual or allergic reaction to sotalol, other beta-blockers, medicines, foods, dyes, or preservatives
- pregnant or trying to get pregnant
- breast-feeding

How should I take this medicine?

Take sotalol tablets by mouth. Follow the directions on the prescription label. Swallow the tablets with a drink of water. You may take sotalol tablets with or without food. Take your doses at regular intervals. Do not take your medicine more often than directed. Do not stop taking except on your prescriber's advice. Contact your pediatrician or health care professional regarding the use of this medicine in children. Special care may be needed. Elderly patients over 65 years old may have a stronger reaction to this medicine and need smaller doses.

What if I miss a dose?

If you miss a dose, take it as soon as possible. However, if it is within 8 hours of your next dose, skip the missed dose and go back to your regular dosing schedule. Do not take double or extra doses.

What may interact with sotalol?

- amphetamine or other stimulant drugs
- antacids (such as Tums®, Rolaids®, Maalox®, and others)
- astemizole
- certain antibiotics such as clarithromycin, erythromycin, gatifloxacin, grepafloxacin, levofloxacin, moxifloxacin, sparfloxacin
- cevimeline
- cisapride
- clonidine
- digoxin
- dofetilide
- furazolidone
- hawthorn or ginger
- linezolid
- liothyronine
- medicines for angina or high blood pressure
- medicines for colds and breathing difficulties
- medicines for diabetes
- medicines for mental depression or other mental problems
- medicines known as MAO inhibitors, such as phenelzine (Nardil®), tranylcypromine (Parnate®), isocarboxazid (Marplan®), and selegiline (Carbex®, Eldepryl®)
- medicines to control heart rhythm
- procarbazine
- some medicines for weight loss (including some herbal products, ephedrine, dextroamphetamine)
- terfenadine
- water pills (diuretics)

Tell your prescriber or health care professional about all other medicines you are taking, including nonprescription medicines, nutritional supplements, or herbal products. Also tell your prescriber or health care professional if you are a frequent user of drinks with caffeine or alcohol, if you smoke, or if you use illegal drugs. These may affect the way your medicine works. Check with your health care professional before stopping or starting any of your medicines.

What should I watch for while taking sotalol?

Visit your prescriber or health care professional for a regular check on your progress. Check your heart rate and blood pressure regularly while you are taking sotalol. Ask your prescriber or health care professional what your heart rate and blood pressure should be, and when you should contact him or her. Your prescriber or health care professional also may schedule regular blood tests and electrocardiograms to check your progress. Do not stop taking this medicine suddenly. This could lead to serious, heart-related problems. Because your condition and the use of sotalol carry some

S

risk, it is a good idea to carry an identification card, necklace or bracelet with details of your condition, medications, and prescriber or health care professional. You may get drowsy or dizzy. Do not drive, use machinery, or do anything that requires mental alertness until you know how sotalol affects you. To reduce the risk of dizzy or fainting spells, do not sit or stand up quickly. Alcohol can make you more drowsy, and increase flushing and rapid heartbeats. Therefore, it is best to avoid alcoholic drinks. Sotalol can affect blood sugar levels. If you have diabetes, check with your prescriber or health care professional before you change your diet or the dose of your diabetic medicine. If you are going to have surgery (including dental surgery), tell your prescriber or health care professional that you are taking sotalol.

What side effects may I notice from taking sotalol?

Side effects that you should report to your prescriber or health care professional as soon as possible:

- chest pain
- confusion
- changes in blood sugar if you have diabetes
- cold hands or feet
- difficulty breathing, wheezing, or shortness of breath
- dizziness or fainting spells
- fast or irregular heartbeat, palpitations, chest pain
- less appetite or more thirst than normal
- slow heart rate (fewer than 50 beats per minute)
- swelling of legs or ankles
- unusual sweating
- unusual weakness or tiredness
- vomiting

Side effects that usually do not require medical attention (report to your prescriber or health care professional if they continue or are bothersome):

- diarrhea
- mental depression
- nausea
- sexual difficulties (impotence or decreased sexual urges)
- weakness or tiredness

Where can I keep my medicine?

Keep out of the reach of children in a container that small children cannot open. Store at room temperature between 15 and 30 degrees C (59 and 86 degrees F). Throw away any unused medicine after the expiration date.

Sparfloxacin tablets

What are sparfloxacin tablets?

SPARFLOXACIN (Zagam®) is a quinolone antibiotic. Sparfloxacin kills certain bacteria or stops their growth. It treats lung infections such as bronchitis or pneumonia. It also treats sinus infections and some other types of infection. Generic sparfloxacin tablets are not yet available.

What should my health care professional know before I take sparfloxacin?

They need to know if you have any of these conditions:

- abnormal heart rhythm
- heart disease
- kidney disease
- low potassium blood levels
- prolonged exposure to sunlight or severe sunburn
- seizures (convulsions)
- slow heart beat
- stroke
- an unusual or allergic reaction to other medicines, foods, dyes, or preservatives
- pregnant or trying to get pregnant
- breast-feeding

How should I take this medicine?

Take sparfloxacin tablets by mouth. Follow the directions on the prescription label. Swallow tablets whole with a full glass of water. Sparfloxacin may be taken with or without food. Do not take with magnesium/ aluminum antacids, sucralfate, Videx® (didanosine) chewable/buffered tablets or pediatric powder, or with other products containing iron or zinc. These products may be taken 4 hours after taking sparfloxacin. Take your doses at regular intervals; preferably at the same time each day. Do not take your medicine more often than directed. Finish the full course prescribed by your prescriber or health care professional even if you think your condition is better. Do not stop taking except on your prescriber's advice. Contact your pediatrician or health care professional regarding the use of this medicine in children. Special care may be needed.

What if I miss a dose?

If you miss a dose, take it as soon as you can. If it is almost time for your next dose, take only that dose. Do not take double or extra doses.

What may interact with sparfloxacin?

- aluminum or magnesium salts
- astemizole
- antacids
- bepridil
- calcium salts
- cisapride
- clarithromycin
- erythromycin
- iron preparations

- certain heart medications for irregular rhythm (e.g., amiodarone, disopyramide, dofetilide, flecainide, ibutilide, quinidine, procainamide, sotalol)
- certain medications for depression or other mental problems (e.g., tricyclic antidepressants, amoxapine, maprotiline, phenothiazines, haloperidol, pimozide, risperidone, and sertindole)
- magnesium salts
- manganese
- medicines for diabetes
- multivitamins containing iron or zinc
- NSAIDs such as Advil®, Aleve®, ibuprofen, Motrin®, naproxen
- pentamidine
- quinapril
- sevelamer
- sucralfate
- terfenadine
- warfarin
- zinc salts

Tell your physician or health care professional about all other medicines you are taking, including non-prescription medicines. Also tell your physician or health care professional if you are a frequent user of drinks with caffeine or alcohol, if you smoke, or if you use illegal drugs. These may affect the way your medicine works. Check with your health care professional before stopping or starting any of your medicines.

What should I watch for while taking sparfloxacin?

Tell your prescriber or health care professional if your symptoms do not improve in 2 to 3 days. You may get drowsy or dizzy. Do not drive, use machinery, or do anything that needs mental alertness until you know how sparfloxacin affects you. To reduce the risk of dizzy or fainting spells, do not sit or stand up quickly, especially if you are an older patient. It is important that you stay out of the sun (even during cloudy weather) while taking sparfloxacin and for five days after treatment. You should also avoid sunlight coming through windows. Do not go out in the sun even if you are using a sunscreen. Also, do not use artificial light such as sunlamps. If you must be in the sun for a brief time, make sure you cover as much of your skin as possible with clothing. Stop taking sparfloxacin and contact your physician if you develop a skin rash, burning, redness, swelling, blisters, or itching. Antacids can stop sparfloxacin from working. If you get an upset stomach and want to take an antacid, make sure there is an interval of at least 4 hours since you last took sparfloxacin. Iron and zinc preparations can also stop sparfloxacin from working properly. If you are taking mineral supplements or vitamins containing zinc or iron, make sure there is an interval of at least 4 hours since you last took sparfloxacin. Discontinue sparfloxacin and contact your physician if you notice pain or swelling of a tendon or around a joint. If you notice any of these symptoms while taking sparfloxacin, do not exercise until you have been checked by a prescriber or health care professional.

What side effects may I notice from taking sparfloxacin?

Side effects that you should report to your prescriber or health care professional as soon as possible:
Rare or uncommon:
- confusion
- convulsions (seizures)
- difficulty breathing
- hallucinations
- joint, muscle or tendon pain
- nightmares
- redness, blistering, peeling or loosening of the skin, including inside the mouth
- severe or watery diarrhea
- skin rash or hives
- swelling of the face or neck
- tremor
- weakness
- vomiting
- yellowing of the skin

More common:
- increased sensitivity to the sun
- skin redness, swelling, or burning

Side effects that usually do not require medical attention (report to your prescriber or health care professional if they continue or are bothersome):
- diarrhea
- difficulty sleeping
- dizziness or drowsiness
- dry mouth
- headache
- heartburn
- intestinal gas
- nausea or stomach upset
- nervousness

Where can I keep my medicine?

Keep out of the reach of children in a container that small children cannot open. Store at room temperature between 20 and 25 degrees C (68 and 77 degrees F). Throw away any unused medicine after the expiration date.

S

Spironolactone tablets

ALDACTONE®;
100 mg; Tablet
GD Searle LLC a
Subsidiary of
Pharmacia Company
Pfizer

ALDACTONE®;
50 mg; Tablet
GD Searle LLC a
Subsidiary of
Pharmacia Company
Pfizer

What are spironolactone tablets?

SPIRONOLACTONE (Aldactone®) is a diuretic. Diuretics increase the amount of urine passed, which causes the body to lose water and salt. Spironolactone helps to treat high blood pressure (hypertension). It is not a cure. It also reduces the swelling and water retention caused by various medical conditions, such as heart, liver, or kidney disease. Spironolactone is a potassium-sparing diuretic. It does not make your body lose potassium; it can help patients who have a low blood potassium. Generic spironolactone tablets are available.

What should my health care professional know before I take spironolactone?

They need to know if you have any of these conditions:
- diabetes
- heart disease
- high blood level of potassium
- liver disease
- low blood level of sodium
- kidney disease
- menstrual irregularity
- an unusual or allergic reaction to spironolactone, other medicines, foods, dyes, or preservatives
- pregnant or trying to get pregnant
- breast-feeding

How should I take this medicine?

Take spironolactone tablets by mouth. Follow the directions on the prescription label. Swallow the tablets with a drink of water. If spironolactone upsets your stomach, take it with food or milk. Take your doses at regular intervals. Do not take your medicine more often than directed. Remember that you will need to pass urine frequently after taking spironolactone. Do not take your doses at a time of day that will cause you problems. Do not take at bedtime.

What if I miss a dose?

If you miss a dose, take it as soon as you can. If it is almost time for your next dose, take only that dose. Do not take double or extra doses.

What may interact with spironolactone?

- anti-inflammatory drugs (NSAIDs, such as ibuprofen)
- cyclosporine
- digoxin
- heparin
- lithium
- medicines for high blood pressure
- potassium salts
- water pills

Tell your prescriber or health care professional about all other medicines you are taking, including non-prescription medicines, nutritional supplements, or herbal products. Also tell your prescriber or health care professional if you are a frequent user of drinks with caffeine or alcohol, if you smoke, or if you use illegal drugs. These may affect the way your medicine works. Check with your health care professional before stopping or starting any of your medicines.

What should I watch for while taking spironolactone?

Visit your prescriber or health care professional for regular checks on your progress. Check your blood pressure regularly. Ask your prescriber or health care professional what your blood pressure should be, and when you should contact him or her. You must not get dehydrated, ask your prescriber or health care professional how much fluid you need to drink a day. Do not stop taking spironolactone except on your prescriber's advice. Watch your diet while you are taking spironolactone. Ask your prescriber or health care professional about both potassium and sodium intake. Spironolactone can make your body retain potassium and you may have too much. Elderly patients, the severely ill, diabetics, or patients with kidney problems are more likely to suffer from the effects of too much potassium. Avoid salt-substitutes and nutritional supplements which contain potassium, unless your prescriber or health care professional tells you otherwise. Too much potassium can be very harmful. You may need to avoid foods that are high in potassium such as bananas, coconuts, dates, figs, prunes, apricots, peaches, grapefruit juice, tomato juice, and orange juice. If you are going to have surgery, tell your prescriber or health care professional that you are taking spironolactone.

What side effects may I notice from taking spironolactone?

Side effects that you should report to your prescriber or health care professional as soon as possible:
- confusion
- cough, hoarseness
- dry mouth, increased thirst
- enlarged breasts in males
- fast or irregular heartbeat, palpitations, chest pain
- fever, chills
- lower back or side pain
- nervousness
- numbness or tingling in hands, feet, or lips
- pain or difficulty passing urine
- shortness of breath; difficult breathing
- skin rash, itching
- unusual bleeding
- unusual tiredness or weakness
- weakness or heaviness of legs

Side effects that usually do not require medical attention (report to your prescriber or health care professional if they continue or are bothersome):

- breast tenderness in females
- deepening of voice in females
- diarrhea
- dizziness, drowsiness
- headache
- increased hair growth in females

- irregular menstrual periods
- nausea, vomiting
- sexual difficulty, inability to have an erection
- stomach pain or cramps, indigestion

Where can I keep my medicine?

Keep out of the reach of children in a container that small children cannot open. Store at room temperature below 30 degrees C (86 degrees F). Throw away any unused medicine after the expiration date.

Stavudine, d4T capsules

ZERIT®;
30 mg; Capsule
ER Squibb and Sons Inc

What are stavudine capsules?

STAVUDINE, d4T (Zerit®) is an antiviral drug called a nucleoside reverse transcriptase inhibitor or NRTI. Stavudine is used to treat human immunodeficiency virus (HIV) infection. Stavudine may reduce the amount of HIV in the blood and increase the number of CD4 cells (T-cells) in the blood. Stavudine is used in combination with other drugs to treat the HIV virus. Stavudine will not cure or prevent HIV infection or AIDS. You may still develop other infections or conditions associated with HIV. Generic stavudine capsules are not yet available.

What should my health care professional know before I take stavudine?

They need to know if you have any of these conditions:

- If you frequently drink alcohol-containing beverages
- kidney disease
- liver disease
- muscle weakness
- tingling or numbness in the hands or feet
- an unusual or allergic reaction to stavudine, other medicines, foods, dyes, or preservatives
- pregnant or trying to get pregnant
- breast-feeding

How should I take this medicine?

Take stavudine capsules by mouth. Follow the directions on the prescription label. Swallow capsules with a drink of water. Stavudine can be taken with or without food. Take your doses at regular intervals. Do not take your medicine more often than directed. To help to make sure that your anti-HIV therapy works as well as possible, be very careful to take all of your medicine exactly as prescribed. Do not stop taking except on your prescriber's advice. Contact your pediatrician or health care professional regarding the use of this medicine in children. Special care may be needed.

What if I miss a dose?

If you miss a dose, take it as soon as you can. If it is almost time for your next dose, take only that dose. Do not take double or extra doses.

What may interact with stavudine?

- didanosine, ddI
- hydroxyurea
- probenecid
- ribavirin
- zalcitabine, ddC
- zidovudine, ZDV (AZT)

Tell your prescriber or health care professional about all other medicines you are taking, including nonprescription medicines, nutritional supplements, or herbal products. Also tell your prescriber or health care professional if you are a frequent user of drinks with caffeine or alcohol, if you smoke, or if you use illegal drugs. These may affect the way your medicine works. Check with your health care professional before stopping or starting any of your medicines.

What should I watch for while taking stavudine?

Visit your prescriber or health care professional for regular checks on your progress. Discuss any new symptoms with your prescriber or health care professional. Alcohol can increase the risk of developing severe side effects when taken with stavudine. Avoid alcoholic drinks while you are taking stavudine. Do not treat yourself for nausea, vomiting, or stomach pain. Call your prescriber or health care professional for advice. Tell your prescriber or health care professional if you get tingling, pain or numbness in your hands or feet or develop muscle weakness. Stavudine will not cure HIV and you can still get other illnesses or complications associated with your disease. Taking stavudine does not reduce the risk of passing HIV infection to others through sexual or blood contact. It is best to avoid sexual contact so that you do not spread the disease to others. For any sexual contact, use a condom. Be careful about cuts, abrasions and other possible sources of blood contact. Never share a needle or syringe with anyone.

What side effects may I notice from taking stavudine?

Side effects that you should report to your prescriber or health care professional as soon as possible:

- difficulty breathing or shortness of breath
- muscle weakness in arms and legs
- nausea, vomiting; or unusual or unexpected stomach discomfort
- severe stomach or abdominal pain
- signs of low platelet counts such as unusual bleeding or bruising
- signs of low red blood cell counts such as increased tiredness or weakness
- signs of an infection such as fever, chills or sore throat
- tingling, pain, burning, or numbness in the hands or feet
- very tired or weak

Side effects that usually do not require medical atten-tion (report to your prescriber or health care professional if they continue or are bothersome):
- diarrhea
- difficulty sleeping
- headache
- loss of appetite
- muscle and joint pain
- stomach upset
- skin rash, itching

Where can I keep my medicine?

Keep out of the reach of children in a container that small children cannot open. Store at room temperature between 15 and 30 degrees C (59 and 86 degrees F). Keep container tightly closed. Throw away any unused medicine after the expiration date.

Sucralfate tablets

SUCRALFATE;
1 g; Tablet
Teva
Pharmaceuticals
USA Inc

SUCRALFATE;
1 g; Tablet
Watson
Pharmaceuticals Inc

What are sucralfate tablets?

SUCRALFATE (Carafate®) helps to treat or prevent the recurrence of stomach or duodenal (intestinal) ul-cers. Sucralfate coats and protects ulcers or irritated stomach lining from the effects of acid. Sucralfate is sometimes prescribed for other gastrointestinal prob-lems like acid-reflux, esophagitis, or mouth ulceration. Generic sucralfate tablets are available.

What should my health care professional know before I take sucralfate?

They need to know if you have any of these conditions:
- kidney disease
- an unusual or allergic reaction to sucralfate, other medicines, foods, dyes, or preservatives
- pregnant or trying to get pregnant
- breast-feeding

How should I take this medicine?

Take sucralfate tablets by mouth. Follow the directions on the prescription label. Swallow the tablets with a drink of water. Sucralfate works best if taken on an empty stomach, usually 1 hour before meals. Take your doses at regular intervals. Do not take your medicine more often than directed. Contact your pediatrician or health care professional regarding the use of this medicine in children. Special care may be needed.

What if I miss a dose?

If you miss a dose, take it as soon as you can. If it is almost time for your next dose, take only that dose. Do not take double or extra doses.

What may interact with sucralfate?

- antacids
- antibiotics
- digoxin
- ketoconazole
- levothyroxine and other thyroid hormones
- omeprazole or lansoprazole
- phenytoin
- ranitidine
- theophylline

Tell your prescriber or health care professional about all other medicines you are taking, including non-pre-scription medicines, nutritional supplements, or herbal products. Also tell your prescriber or health care profes-sional if you are a frequent user of drinks with caffeine or alcohol, if you smoke, or if you use illegal drugs. These may affect the way your medicine works. Check with your health care professional before stopping or starting any of your medicines.

What should I watch for while taking sucralfate?

Check with your prescriber or health care professional if your condition does not improve, or if it gets worse. Although healing with sucralfate may begin to occur within two weeks, you should continue treatment until your prescriber or health care professional has made sure healing is complete. If you need to take antacid, take it at least 2 hours after a dose of sucralfate or more than 30 minutes before.

What side effects may I notice from taking sucralfate?

Side effects that you should report to your prescriber or health care professional as soon as possible:
Rare:
- difficulty breathing
- drowsiness or dizziness
- skin rash
- swelling of the face and lips

Side effects that usually do not require medical attention (report to your prescriber or health care professional if they continue or are bothersome):

- constipation
- dry mouth
- headache
- indigestion, gas (flatulence)

Sulfadiazine tablets

SULFADIAZINE;
500 mg; Tablet
Eon Labs Inc

What are sulfadiazine tablets?

SULFADIAZINE is a sulfa antibiotic. Sulfadiazine stops the growth of certain bacteria and other organisms. It treats toxoplasmosis, urinary tract infections, and some other types of infections. Generic sulfadiazine tablets are available.

What should my health care professional know before I take sulfadiazine?

They need to know if you have any of these conditions:

- blood disorders
- glucose-6-phosphate dehydrogenase deficiency (G6PD deficiency)
- kidney disease
- liver disease
- porphyria
- an unusual or allergic reaction to "sulfa drugs," sulfite preservatives, furosemide or thiazide diuretics (water pills), or oral (by mouth) diabetes medicines, foods, dyes, or preservatives
- pregnant or trying to get pregnant
- breast-feeding

How should I take this medicine?

Take sulfadiazine tablets by mouth. Follow the directions on the prescription label. Swallow tablets whole with a full glass of water. You can take this medicine with or without food. Take your doses at regular intervals. Do not take your medicine more often than directed. Finish the full course prescribed by your prescriber or health care professional even if you think your condition is better. Do not stop taking except on your prescriber's advice. Special precautions for use in infants: This medicine is not for use in infants under 2 months old.

What if I miss a dose?

If you miss a dose, take it as soon as you can. If it is almost time for your next dose, take only that dose. Do not take double or extra doses.

What may interact with sulfadiazine?

- cyclosporine
- medicines for diabetes
- methotrexate
- phenytoin
- voriconazole
- warfarin
- water pills

Tell your prescriber or health care professional about all other medicines you are taking, including non-prescription medicines. Also tell your prescriber or health care professional if you are a frequent user of drinks with caffeine or alcohol, if you smoke, or if you use illegal drugs. These may affect the way your medicine works. Check with your health care professional before stopping or starting any of your medicines.

What should I watch for while taking sulfadiazine?

Tell your prescriber or health care professional if your symptoms do not improve in 2 or 3 days, or if you develop a skin rash. If you are taking this medicine for a long time you must visit your prescriber or health care professional for regular blood checks. Sulfadiazine can cause blood problems. This can mean slow healing and a risk of infection. Problems can arise if you need dental work, and in the day to day care of your teeth. Try to avoid damage to your teeth and gums when you brush or floss your teeth. If you are a diabetic using insulin or other medicines to lower blood sugar (like glyburide) monitor your blood sugar carefully. If you get an unusual reaction, stop using sulfadiazine at once and call your prescriber or health care professional for advice. Drink several glasses of water a day. This will help to reduce possible kidney problems. Keep out of the sun, or wear protective clothing outdoors and use a sunscreen. Do not use sun lamps or sun tanning beds or booths. You may get dizzy. Do not drive, use machinery, or do anything that needs mental alertness until you know how sulfadiazine affects you. To reduce the risk of dizzy or fainting spells, do not sit or stand up quickly, especially if you are an older patient. If you are going to have surgery, tell your prescriber or health care professional that you are using sulfadiazine.

What side effects may I notice from taking sulfadiazine?

Side effects that you should report to your prescriber or health care professional as soon as possible:

- difficulty breathing or tightening of the throat
- blood in urine
- bluish fingernails or lips

Where can I keep my medicine?

Keep out of the reach of children in a container that small children cannot open. Store at room temperature between 15 and 30 degrees C (59 and 86 degrees F). Keep container tightly closed. Throw away any unused medicine after the expiration date.

S

- dark yellow or brown urine
- fever or chills
- eye redness or irritation
- increased sensitivity to the sun or ultraviolet light
- joint aches or pains
- less urine passed
- muscle aches or pains
- pain or difficulty passing urine
- redness, blistering, peeling or loosening of the skin, including inside the mouth
- skin rash, hives, or itching
- sore mouth
- sore throat, fever
- swelling of the neck
- unusual bruising or bleeding
- unusual tiredness or weakness
- vomiting
- yellowing of the eyes or skin

Side effects that usually do not require medical atten-tion (report to your prescriber or health care professional if they continue or are bothersome):

- diarrhea
- difficulty sleeping
- mild dizziness
- headache
- loss of appetite
- nausea
- ringing in the ears
- stomach pain

Where can I keep my medicine?

Keep out of the reach of children in a container that small children cannot open. Store at room temperature between 15 and 30 degrees C (59 and 86 degrees F). Protect from light. Keep container tightly closed. Throw away any unused medicine after the expiration date.

Sulfamethoxazole tablets

What are sulfamethoxazole tablets?

SULFAMETHOXAZOLE (Gantanol®) is a sulfon-amide antibiotic. Sulfamethoxazole stops the growth of certain bacteria. It treats urinary tract infections and some other infections. Generic sulfamethoxazole tab-lets are available.

What should my health care professional know before I take sulfamethoxazole?

They need to know if you have any of these conditions:

- asthma
- blood disorders
- dental disease
- glucose-6-phosphate dehydrogenase deficiency (G6PD deficiency)
- kidney disease
- liver disease
- porphyria
- vitamin deficiency
- other chronic illness
- an unusual or allergic reaction to "sulfa drugs," sulfite preservatives, furosemide or thiazide diuretics (water pills), or oral (by mouth) diabetes or glaucoma medi-cines, foods, dyes, or preservatives
- pregnant or trying to get pregnant
- breast-feeding

How should I take this medicine?

Take sulfamethoxazole tablets by mouth. Follow the directions on the prescription label. Swallow tablets whole with a full glass of water. Take your doses at regular intervals. Do not take your medicine more often than directed. Finish the full course prescribed by your prescriber or health care professional even if you think your condition is better. Do not stop taking except on your prescriber's advice. Contact your pediatrician or health care professional regarding the use of this medi-cine in children. Special care may be needed.

What if I miss a dose?

If you miss a dose, take it as soon as you can. If it is almost time for your next dose, take only that dose. Do not take double or extra doses. There should be an interval of at least 6 to 8 hours between doses.

What may interact with sulfamethoxazole?

- cyclosporine
- medicines for diabetes that are taken by mouth
- methenamine
- methotrexate
- phenylbutazone
- phenytoin
- sulfinpyrazone
- voriconazole
- warfarin
- water pills

Tell your prescriber or health care professional about all other medicines you are taking, including non-pre-scription medicines, nutritional supplements, or herbal products. Also tell your prescriber or health care profes-sional if you are a frequent user of drinks with caffeine or alcohol, if you smoke, or if you use illegal drugs. These may affect the way your medicine works. Check with your health care professional before stopping or starting any of your medicines.

What should I watch for while taking sulfamethoxazole?

Tell your prescriber or health care professional if your symptoms do not improve in 2 or 3 days, or if you develop a skin rash. If you are taking this medicine for a long time you must visit your prescriber or health care professional for regular blood checks. Sulfamethoxazole can cause blood problems. This can mean slow healing and a risk of infection. Problems can arise if you need dental work, and in the day to day care of your teeth. Try to avoid damage to your teeth and gums when you brush or floss your teeth. If you are a diabetic using insulin or oral hypoglycemics (like glyburide) monitor your blood glucose carefully. If you get an unusual reaction stop using sulfamethoxazole at once and call your prescriber or health care professional for advice. Drink several glasses of water a day. This will help to reduce possible kidney problems. Keep out of the sun, or wear protective clothing outdoors and use a sunscreen. Do not use sun lamps or sun tanning beds or booths. You may get drowsy or dizzy. Do not drive, use machinery, or do anything that needs mental alertness until you know how sulfamethoxazole affects you. To reduce the risk of dizzy or fainting spells, do not sit or stand up quickly, especially if you are an older patient. If you are going to have surgery, tell your prescriber or health care professional that you are using sulfamethoxazole.

What side effects may I notice from taking sulfamethoxazole?

Side effects that you should report to your prescriber or health care professional as soon as possible:
- blood in urine
- bluish fingernails or lips
- dark yellow or brown urine
- cough
- difficulty breathing
- increased sensitivity to the sun or ultraviolet light
- joint aches or pains
- less urine passed
- muscle aches or pains
- pain or difficulty passing urine
- redness, blistering, peeling or loosening of the skin, including inside the mouth
- skin rash, hives, or itching
- sore mouth
- sore throat, fever
- swelling of the neck
- unusual bruising or bleeding
- unusual tiredness or weakness
- yellowing of the eyes or skin

Side effects that usually do not require medical attention (report to your prescriber or health care professional if they continue or are bothersome):
- diarrhea
- drowsiness, dizziness
- headache
- loss of appetite
- nausea, vomiting
- stomach pain

Where can I keep my medicine?

Keep out of the reach of children in a container that small children cannot open. Store at room temperature between 15 and 30 degrees C (59 and 86 degrees F). Protect from light. Keep container tightly closed. Throw away any unused medicine after the expiration date.

Sulfamethoxazole; Trimethoprim; SMX-TMP tablets

BACTRIM™ DS; 800 mg/160 mg; Tablet Hoffmann La Roche Inc

SEPTRA® DS; 800 mg/160 mg; Tablet Monarch Pharmaceuticals Inc

What are sulfamethoxazole; trimethoprim tablets?

SULFAMETHOXAZOLE; TRIMETHOPRIM or SMX-TMP (Septra®, Bactrim™ DS, Co-Trimoxazole and others) is a combination of two antibiotics. It is used to treat infections of the urinary tract, middle ear, and respiratory tract (bronchitis). This drug is also used for traveler's diarrhea, and *Pneumocystis carinii* pneumonia in AIDS or cancer patients. Generic tablets are available.

What should my health care professional know before I take sulfamethoxazole; trimethoprim?

They need to know if you have any of these conditions:
- anemia or other blood disorders
- high blood levels of potassium
- kidney disease
- liver disease
- porphyria
- glucose-6-phosphate dehydrogenase (G6PD) deficiency
- an unusual or allergic reaction to sulfamethoxazole or other sulfa antibiotics, trimethoprim, other sulfa drugs, other medicines, foods, dyes or preservatives
- pregnant or trying to get pregnant
- breast-feeding

How should I take this medicine?

Take SMX-TMP by mouth. Follow the directions on the prescription label. Take SMX-TMP with a full glass of water. Take your doses at regular intervals. Do not take your medicine more often than directed. Finish the full course of medicine prescribed by your prescriber or health care professional even if you feel better. Contact your pediatrician or health care professional re-

S

garding the use of this medicine in children. Special care may be needed.

What if I miss a dose?

If you miss a dose, take it as soon as you can. If it is almost time for your next dose, take only that dose. Do not take double or extra doses. You must leave a suitable interval between doses. If you are taking one dose a day and have to take a missed dose, make sure there is at least 10 to 12 hours between doses. If you are taking two doses a day and have to take a missed dose, make sure there is at least 5 to 6 hours between doses.

What may interact with sulfamethoxazole; trimethoprim?

- amiloride
- cyclosporine
- dapsone
- digoxin
- divalproex
- dofetilide
- medicines for diabetes
- methenamine
- methotrexate
- metronidazole
- phenytoin
- potassium salts (potassium chloride, potassium phosphate)
- procainamide
- pyrimethamine
- rifampin
- some medicines used to treat blood pressure and/or heart failure (ACE inhibitors such as benazepril, enalapril, lisinopril, moexipril, quinapril, ramipril, and others)
- spironolactone
- sulfinpyrazone
- tolbutamide
- triamterene
- trimetrexate
- valproic acid
- warfarin

Tell your prescriber or health care professional about all other medicines you are taking, including non-prescription medicines, nutritional supplements, or herbal products. Also tell your prescriber or health care professional if you are a frequent user of drinks with caffeine or alcohol, if you smoke, or if you use illegal drugs. These may affect the way your medicine works. Check with your health care professional before stopping or starting any of your medicines.

What should I watch for while taking sulfamethoxazole; trimethoprim?

Tell your prescriber or health care professional if your symptoms do not improve in 2 to 3 days. You may get dizzy. Do not drive, use machinery, or do anything that needs mental alertness until you know how SMX-TMP affects you. Keep out of the sun, or wear protective clothing outdoors and use a sunscreen. Do not use sun lamps or sun tanning beds or booths. Drink several glasses of water a day. This will help to reduce possible kidney problems.

What side effects may I notice from taking sulfamethoxazole; trimethoprim?

Side effects that you should report to your prescriber or health care professional as soon as possible:
- anemia or other blood disorders
- allergic reactions
- bluish fingernails or lips
- difficulty breathing
- fast or irregular heartbeat, palpitations, chest pain
- fever or chills, sore throat
- increased sensitivity to the sun or ultraviolet light
- joint aches or pains
- lower back pain
- muscle aches or pains
- pain or difficulty passing urine
- redness, blistering, peeling or loosening of the skin, including inside the mouth
- skin rash, hives, or itching
- unusual bleeding or bruising
- unusual weakness or tiredness
- yellowing of the eyes or skin

Side effects that usually do not require medical attention (report to your prescriber or health care professional if they continue or are bothersome):
- diarrhea
- dizziness
- headache
- loss of appetite
- nausea, vomiting

Where can I keep my medicine?

Keep out of the reach of children in a container that small children cannot open. Store at room temperature between 15 and 25 degrees C (59 and 77 degrees F). Protect from light and moisture. Throw away any unused medicine after the expiration date.

Sulfasalazine tablets or enteric-coated tablets

AZULFIDINE® EN-TABS®;
500 mg; Tablet,
Delayed Release
Pharmacia and
Upjohn Div Pfizer

AZULFIDINE®;
500 mg; Tablet
Pharmacia and
Upjohn Div Pfizer

What are sulfasalazine tablets or enteric-coated tablets?

SULFASALAZINE (Azulfidine®, Azulfidine® En-tabs®) is an anti-inflammatory agent. It is used to prevent and treat inflammatory bowel disease such as ulcerative colitis. It is also used to improve symptoms of rheumatoid arthritis or juvenile rheumatoid arthritis (JRA). Sulfasalazine works to reduce inflammation and other symptoms of these diseases. Generic sulfasalazine tablets are available.

What should my health care professional know before I take sulfasalazine?

They need to know if you have any of these conditions:

- asthma
- blood disorders or anemia
- glucose-6-phosphate dehydrogenase (G6PD) deficiency
- intestinal obstruction
- kidney disease
- liver disease
- porphyria
- severe allergies
- urinary tract obstruction
- an unusual or allergic reaction to sulfasalazine, sulfonamides, salicylates, sulfonylurea, thiazide diuretics (water pills), other medicines, foods, dyes, or preservatives
- pregnant or trying to get pregnant
- breast-feeding

How should I take this medicine?

Take sulfasalazine tablets or enteric-coated tablets by mouth. Follow the directions on the prescription label. Swallow the tablets whole with a drink of water; do not suck or chew enteric-coated tablets. If sulfasalazine upsets your stomach, take it with food or milk. Take your doses at regular intervals. Do not take your medicine more often than directed. Contact your pediatrician or health care professional regarding the use of this medicine in children. Special care may be needed. In general, children less than 2 years of age should not receive sulfasalazine.

What if I miss a dose?

If you miss a dose, take it as soon as you can. If it is almost time for your next dose, take only that dose. Do not take double or extra doses.

What may interact with sulfasalazine?

- digoxin
- female hormones, including contraceptives or birth control pills
- fosphenytoin
- medicines for diabetes
- methotrexate
- other medicines that make you sensitive to the sun including some antibiotics, retinoids (vitamin A analogs), or certain kinds of water pills (diuretics)
- phenytoin
- voriconazole
- warfarin

Tell your prescriber or health care professional about all other medicines you are taking, including non-prescription medicines, nutritional supplements, or herbal products. Also tell your prescriber or health care professional if you are a frequent user of drinks with caffeine or alcohol, if you smoke, or if you use illegal drugs. These may affect the way your medicine works. Check with your health care professional before stopping or starting any of your medicines.

What should I watch for while taking sulfasalazine?

Tell your prescriber or health care professional if your symptoms do not improve. There is usually an improvement within a month. You may need about 6—12 weeks of treatment to get good results. It is important that you go on taking your medicine and only stop taking it on your prescriber's advice. Sulfasalazine can make your skin more sensitive to sun or ultraviolet light. Keep out of the sun, or wear protective clothing outdoors and use a sunscreen (at least SPF 15). Do not use sun lamps or sun tanning beds or booths. Sulfasalazine can cause blood problems. You will need to have your blood checked while you are taking sulfasalazine. Notify your health care provider if you notice sores that do not heal, unusual bleeding or bruising, or get a cold that does not improve. Make sure to drink plenty of fluids while taking sulfasalazine.

What side effects may I notice from taking sulfasalazine?

Side effects that you should report to your prescriber or health care professional as soon as possible:

- bloody diarrhea
- chest pain
- difficulty breathing, wheezing
- difficulty swallowing
- fever, chills, or sore throat
- joint or muscle aches
- painful, difficult or reduced urination
- pale skin
- redness, blistering, peeling or loosening of the skin, including inside the mouth

S

- skin rash, itching
- stomach cramps or pain
- unusual bleeding or bruising
- unusual weakness or tiredness
- yellowing of the eyes or skin

Side effects that usually do not require medical attention (report to your prescriber or health care professional if they continue or are bothersome):

- diarrhea
- discolored urine or skin (orange-yellow color)
- dizziness
- headache

- increased sensitivity of the skin to sun or ultraviolet light
- indigestion
- loss of appetite
- nausea, vomiting
- reduced sperm count (loss of male fertility)

Where can I keep my medicine?

Keep out of the reach of children in a container that small children cannot open. Store at room temperature between 15 and 30 degrees C (59 and 86 degrees F). Keep container tightly closed. Throw away any unused medicine after the expiration date.

Sulfinpyrazone capsules and tablets

ANTURANE®;
200 mg; Capsule
Novartis
Pharmaceuticals

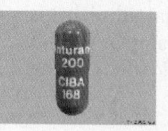

ANTURANE®;
100 mg; Tablet
Novartis
Pharmaceuticals

What are sulfinpyrazone capsules and tablets?

SULFINPYRAZONE (Anturane®) helps to remove excess uric acid from the body. Too much uric acid can cause gout or gouty arthritis. Sulfinpyrazone is not a cure for gout, and it is not used to treat an attack of gout once it has started. Sulfinpyrazone can prevent future gouty attacks as long as you continue to take it. Certain illnesses or medications can cause an increase in uric acid. Sulfinpyrazone can help to reduce the risk of complications (such as kidney stones) that can occur if uric acid levels in the blood are too high (hyperuricemia). Generic sulfinpyrazone capsules are available.

What should my health care professional know before I take sulfinpyrazone?

They need to know if you have any of these conditions:

- blood disorders or disease
- hepatic disease
- kidney disease, or kidney stones
- recent chemotherapy or radiation therapy
- stomach ulcers
- an unusual reaction to sulfinpyrazone, salicylates such as aspirin, phenylbutazone, nonsteroidal anti-inflammatory drugs (NSAIDs) such as ibuprofen, other medicines, foods, dyes, or preservatives
- pregnant or trying to get pregnant
- breast-feeding

How should I take this medicine?

Take sulfinpyrazone capsules or tablets by mouth. Follow the directions on the label. This medicine is usually taken twice daily. Take sulfinpyrazone with food, milk, or antacids if it upsets your stomach. Take your doses at regular intervals. Do not take your medicine more often than directed. Drink at least 8 to 10 glasses of water a day while taking sulfinpyrazone. This will help to prevent kidney stones from forming and other problems caused by an increased amount of uric acid in the kidneys. Sulfinpyrazone does not treat gouty attacks. However, if you have already been taking the drug when an attack occurs, you should continue taking it to help keep your uric acid levels under control, unless otherwise directed by your health care professional. Contact your pediatrician or health care professional regarding the use of this medicine in children. Special care may be needed.

What if I miss a dose?

If you miss a dose, take it as soon as you can. If it is almost time for your next dose, take only that dose. Do not take double or extra doses.

What may interact with sulfinpyrazone?

- acetaminophen
- alcohol
- alosetron
- aspirin or aspirin-like medicines such as bismuth subsalicylate, choline salicylate, magnesium salicylate, or salsalate
- drugs that prevent or treat blood clots such as warfarin, heparin, or enoxaparin
- cholestyramine
- cisplatin
- colchicine
- ethambutol
- mecamylamine
- medicines for diabetes
- nitrofurantoin
- probenecid
- pyrazinamide
- sulfamethoxazole
- sulfisoxazole
- theophylline
- verapamil
- water pills (diuretics)
- zonisamide

Tell your prescriber or health care professional about all other medicines you are taking, including non-prescription medicines, nutritional supplements, or herbal products. Also tell your prescriber or health care professional if you are a frequent user of drinks with caffeine or alcohol, if you smoke, or if you use illegal drugs. These may affect the way your medicine works. Check with your health care professional before stopping or starting any of your medicines.

What should I watch for while taking sulfinpyrazone?

Sulfinpyrazone helps to prevent gout attacks. It will not help an attack of gout once it has started. Take this medicine regularly as prescribed by your health care provider, even if you have an attack of gout. Other medicines can be prescribed for you to treat an attack of gout while you are taking sulfinpyrazone. Sulfinpyrazone is only effective in preventing gout if you keep taking it regularly. Do not stop taking this medicine except on the advice of your prescriber or health care professional. It may take several months before you see the full effect of sulfinpyrazone. Alcohol can increase the amount of uric acid in your body and aggravate gout. Avoid alcoholic drinks while taking this medicine. Do not take aspirin or aspirin-containing products while taking sulfinpyrazone, unless approved by your health care provider. Check with your pharmacist or doctor before taking any nonprescription medicines to be sure they do not contain aspirin or aspirin-like ingredients, since these medicines can make sulfinpyrazone less effective. Drink plenty of water (8 to 10 glasses per day) while taking this medicine. Sulfinpyrazone works best when the urine is alkaline (non-acidic). Ask your prescriber or health care professional about which foods or juices to avoid, and about other foods, beverages, or antacids that may help to keep the urine alkaline.

What side effects may I notice from taking sulfinpyrazone?

Side effects that you should report to your prescriber or health care professional as soon as possible:

- blood in urine or stool, or black tarry stools
- difficulty breathing, wheezing or shortness of breath
- fever, chills or sore throat
- lower back or side pain
- pain or difficulty passing urine
- skin rash and itching (hives)
- swelling of the feet, ankles, face or lips
- unusual bleeding or bruising
- unusual weakness or tiredness

Side effects that usually do not require medical attention (report to your prescriber or health care professional if they continue or are bothersome):

- heartburn
- nausea, vomiting
- painful, red, or swollen joints
- upset stomach

Where can I keep my medicine?

Keep out of the reach of children in a container that small children cannot open. Store at room temperature, between 15 and 30 degrees C (59 and 86 degrees F). Do not freeze. Protect from light. Throw away any unused medicine after the expiration date.

Sulfisoxazole tablets

SULFISOXAZOLE;
500 mg; Tablet
Ivax Pharmaceuticals Inc

What are sulfisoxazole tablets?

SULFISOXAZOLE (Gantrisin®) is a sulfonamide antibiotic. Sulfisoxazole stops the growth of certain bacteria. It treats urinary tract and some other infections. Generic sulfisoxazole tablets are available.

What should my health care professional know before I take sulfisoxazole?

They need to know if you have any of these conditions:

- asthma
- blood disorders
- dental disease
- glucose-6-phosphate dehydrogenase deficiency (G6PD deficiency)
- kidney disease
- liver disease
- porphyria
- vitamin deficiency
- other chronic illness
- an unusual or allergic reaction to "sulfa drugs," sulfite preservatives, furosemide or thiazide diuretics (water pills), or oral diabetes medicines, other medicines, foods, dyes, or preservatives
- pregnant or trying to get pregnant
- breast-feeding

How should I take this medicine?

Take sulfisoxazole tablets by mouth. Follow the directions on the prescription label. Swallow tablets whole with a full glass of water. Take your doses at regular intervals. Do not take your medicine more often than directed. Finish the full course prescribed by your prescriber or health care professional even if you think your condition is better. Do not stop taking except on your prescriber's advice. Contact your pediatrician or health care professional regarding the use of this medicine in children. Special care may be needed.

What if I miss a dose?

If you miss a dose, take it as soon as you can. If it is almost time for your next dose, take only that dose. Do not take double or extra doses. There should be an interval of at least 3 to 4 hours between doses.

What may interact with sulfisoxazole?

- cyclosporine
- medicines for diabetes

- methenamine
- methotrexate
- phenylbutazone
- phenytoin
- sulfinpyrazone
- voriconazole
- warfarin
- water pills

Tell your prescriber or health care professional about all other medicines you are taking, including nonprescription medicines, nutritional supplements, or herbal products. Also tell your prescriber or health care professional if you are a frequent user of drinks with caffeine or alcohol, if you smoke, or if you use illegal drugs. These may affect the way your medicine works. Check with your health care professional before stopping or starting any of your medicines.

What should I watch for while taking sulfisoxazole?

Tell your prescriber or health care professional if your symptoms do not improve in 2 or 3 days, or if you develop a skin rash. If you are taking this medicine for a long time you must visit your prescriber or health care professional for regular blood checks. Sulfisoxazole can cause blood problems. This can mean slow healing and a risk of infection. Problems can arise if you need dental work, and in the day to day care of your teeth. Try to avoid damage to your teeth and gums when you brush or floss your teeth. If you are a diabetic using insulin or oral hypoglycemics (like glyburide) monitor your blood glucose carefully. If you get an unusual reaction, stop using sulfisoxazole at once and call your prescriber or health care professional for advice. Drink several glasses of water a day. This will help to reduce possible kidney problems. Keep out of the sun, or wear protective clothing outdoors and use a sunscreen. Do not use sun lamps or sun tanning beds or booths. You may get drowsy or dizzy. Do not drive, use machinery, or do anything that needs mental alertness until you know how sulfisoxazole affects you. To reduce the risk of dizzy or fainting spells, do not sit or stand up quickly, especially if you are an older patient. If you are going to have surgery, tell your prescriber or health care professional that you are using sulfisoxazole.

What side effects may I notice from taking sulfisoxazole?

Side effects that you should report to your prescriber or health care professional as soon as possible:
- blood in urine
- bluish fingernails or lips
- dark yellow or brown urine
- cough
- difficulty breathing
- increased sensitivity to the sun or ultraviolet light
- joint aches or pains
- less urine passed
- muscle aches or pains
- pain or difficulty passing urine
- severe or watery diarrhea
- skin rash, redness, blistering, peeling or loosening of the skin, including inside the mouth
- sore mouth
- sore throat, fever
- swelling of the neck
- unusual bruising or bleeding
- unusual tiredness or weakness
- yellowing of the eyes or skin

Side effects that usually do not require medical attention (report to your prescriber or health care professional if they continue or are bothersome):
- diarrhea
- drowsiness, dizziness
- headache
- loss of appetite
- nausea, vomiting
- stomach pain

Where can I keep my medicine?

Keep out of the reach of children in a container that small children cannot open. Store at room temperature between 15 and 30 degrees C (59 and 86 degrees F). Protect from light.

This drug requires an FDA medication guide. See page xxxvii.

Sulindac tablets

CLINORIL®;
150 mg; Tablet
Merck and Co Inc

CLINORIL®;
200 mg; Tablet
Merck and Co Inc

What are sulindac tablets?

SULINDAC (Clinoril®) is a nonsteroidal anti-inflammatory drug (NSAID). It helps relieves pain and inflammation associated with rheumatoid arthritis, osteoarthritis, and gouty arthritis, as well as bursitis and tendinitis. Generic sulindac tablets are available.

What should my health care professional know before I take sulindac?

They need to know if you have any of these conditions:
- anemia
- asthma, especially aspirin sensitive asthma
- bleeding problems or taking medicines that make you bleed more easily such as anticoagulants ("blood thinners")
- cigarette smoker
- diabetes
- drink more than 3 alcohol-containing beverages a day
- heart failure
- high blood pressure
- kidney disease
- liver disease

- stomach or duodenal ulcers
- systemic lupus erythematosus
- ulcerative colitis
- an unusual or allergic reaction to aspirin, other salicylates, other NSAIDs, other medicines, foods, dyes or preservatives
- pregnant or trying to get pregnant
- breast-feeding

How should I take this medicine?

Take sulindac tablets by mouth. Follow the directions on the prescription label. Swallow tablets whole with a full glass of water; take tablets in an upright or sitting position. Taking a sip of water first, before taking the tablets, may help you swallow them. If possible take bedtime doses at least 10 minutes before lying down. You can take sulindac with food to prevent stomach upset. Take your doses at regular intervals. Do not take your medicine more often than directed. Contact your pediatrician or health care professional regarding the use of this medicine in children. Special care may be needed.

What if I miss a dose?

If you miss a dose, take it as soon as you can. If it is almost time for your next dose, take only that dose. Do not take double or extra doses.

What may interact with sulindac?

- alcohol
- anti-inflammatory drugs (such as other NSAIDs or prednisone)
- aspirin and aspirin-like medicines
- cidofovir
- cyclosporine
- entecavir
- herbal products that contain feverfew, garlic, ginger, or ginkgo biloba
- lithium
- medicines for high blood pressure
- medicines that affect platelets
- medicines that treat or prevent blood clots such as warfarin and other 'blood thinners'
- methotrexate
- pemetrexed
- water pills (diuretics)

Tell your prescriber or health care professional about all other medicines you are taking, including non-prescription medicines, nutritional supplements, or herbal products. Also tell your prescriber or health care professional if you are a frequent user of drinks with caffeine or alcohol, if you smoke, or if you use illegal drugs. These may affect the way your medicine works. Check with your health care professional before stopping or starting any of your medicines.

What should I watch for while taking sulindac?

Let your prescriber or health care professional know if your pain continues after 7 days. Do not take other pain-killers with sulindac without advice. If you get flu-like symptoms (fever, chills, muscle aches and pains), call your prescriber or health care professional; do not treat yourself. To reduce unpleasant effects on your throat and stomach, take sulindac with a full glass of water and never just before lying down. If you notice black, tarry stools or experience severe stomach pain and/or vomit blood or what looks like coffee grounds, notify your health care prescriber immediately. If you are taking medicines that affect the clotting of your blood, such as aspirin or blood thinners such as Coumadin®, talk to your health care provider or prescriber before taking this medicine. You may get dizzy. Do not drive, use machinery, or do anything that needs mental alertness until you know how sulindac affects you. Do not sit or stand up quickly, especially if you are an older patient. This reduces the risk of dizzy or fainting spells. Do not smoke cigarettes or drink alcohol; these increase irritation to your stomach and can make it more susceptible to damage from sulindac. It is especially important not to use sulindac during the last 3 months of pregnancy unless specifically directed to do so by your health care provider. Sulindac may cause problems in the unborn child or complications during delivery. If you are going to have surgery, tell your prescriber or health care professional that you are taking sulindac. Problems can arise if you need dental work, and in the day to day care of your teeth. Try to avoid damage to your teeth and gums when you brush or floss your teeth.

What side effects may I notice from taking sulindac?

Side effects that you should report to your prescriber or health care professional as soon as possible:

- signs of bleeding—bruising, pinpoint red spots on the skin, black tarry stools, blood in the urine, unusual tiredness or weakness, vomiting blood or vomit that looks like coffee grounds
- signs of an allergic reaction—difficulty breathing or wheezing, skin rash, redness, blistering or peeling skin, hives, or itching, swelling of eyelids, throat, lips
- blurred vision
- change in the amount of urine passed
- difficulty swallowing, severe heartburn or burning, pain in throat
- pain or difficulty passing urine
- stomach pain or cramps
- swelling of feet or ankles
- yellowing of the eyes or skin

Side effects that usually do not require medical attention (report to your prescriber or health care professional if they continue or are bothersome):

- diarrhea or constipation
- dizziness
- drowsiness
- gas or heartburn
- headache
- nausea, vomiting

Where can I keep my medicine?

Keep out of the reach of children in a container that small children cannot open. Store at room temperature between 15 and 30 degrees C (59 and 86 degrees F). Keep container tightly closed. Throw away any unused medicine after the expiration date.

S

Sumatriptan tablets

IMITREX®;
50 mg; Tablet
GlaxoSmithKline Inc

IMITREX®;
100 mg; Tablet
GlaxoSmithKline Inc

What are sumatriptan tablets?

SUMATRIPTAN (Imitrex®) helps to relieve a migraine attack that starts with or without aura (a peculiar feeling or visual disturbance that warns you of an attack). Sumatriptan is not used to prevent migraine attacks. Generic sumatriptan tablets are not yet available.

What should my health care professional know before I take sumatriptan?

They need to know if you have any of these conditions:
- bowel disease or colitis
- diabetes
- family history of heart disease
- fast or irregular heart beat
- headaches that are different from your usual migraine
- heart or blood vessel disease, angina (chest pain), or previous heart attack
- high blood pressure
- high cholesterol
- history of stroke, transient ischemic attacks (TIAs or "mini-strokes"), or intracranial bleeding
- postmenopausal or surgical removal of uterus and ovaries
- liver disease
- overweight
- poor circulation
- Raynaud's disease
- seizure disorder
- shortness of breath
- tobacco smoker
- an unusual or allergic reaction to sumatriptan, other medicines, foods, dyes, or preservatives
- pregnant or trying to get pregnant
- breast-feeding

How should I take this medicine?

Take sumatriptan tablets by mouth. Follow the directions on the prescription label. Sumatriptan is taken at the first symptoms of a migraine attack; it is not for everyday use. Swallow the tablets with a drink of water. If your migraine headache returns after one dose, you can take another dose as directed. You must leave at least 2 hours between doses, and do not take more than 100 mg as a single dose. Do not take more than 200 mg total in any 24 hour period. If there is no improvement at all after the first dose, do not take a second dose without talking to your prescriber or health care professional. Do not take your medicine more often than directed. Contact your pediatrician or health care professional regarding the use of this medicine in children. Special care may be needed.

What if I miss a dose?

This does not apply, sumatriptan is not for regular use.

What may interact with sumatriptan?

Do not take sumatriptan with any of the following medicines:
- amphetamine or cocaine
- dihydroergotamine, ergotamine, ergoloid mesylates, methysergide, or ergot-type medication—do not take within 24 hours of taking sumatriptan.
- almotriptan, eletriptan, naratriptan, rizatriptan, zolmitriptan—do not take within 24 hours of taking sumatriptan.
- medicines for weight loss such as dexfenfluramine, dextroamphetamine, fenfluramine, or sibutramine
- monoamine oxidase inhibitors (MAOIs) such as phenelzine (Nardil®), tranylcypromine (Parnate®), isocarboxazid (Marplan®), and selegiline (Carbex®, Eldepryl®)—do not take sumatriptan within 2 weeks of stopping MAOI therapy.

Check with your doctor or pharmacist if you take any of these medications:
- cough syrup or other products containing dextromethorphan
- feverfew
- lithium
- medicines for mental depression, anxiety or mood problems such as buspirone, citalopram, fluoxetine, fluvoxamine, mirtazapine, nefazodone, paroxetine, sertraline, trazodone, tricyclic antidepressants, or venlafaxine
- meperidine
- propranolol
- St. John's wort
- tryptophan

Tell your prescriber or health care professional about all other medicines you are taking, including non-prescription medicines, nutritional supplements, or herbal products. Also tell your prescriber or health care professional if you are a frequent user of drinks with caffeine or alcohol, if you smoke, or if you use illegal drugs. These may affect the way your medicine works. Check with your health care professional before stopping or starting any of your medicines.

What should I watch for while taking sumatriptan?

Only take sumatriptan tablets for a migraine headache. Take it if you get warning symptoms or at the start of a migraine attack. Sumatriptan is not for regular use to prevent migraine attacks. Do not take migraine products that contain ergotamine while you are taking sumatriptan; this combination can affect your heart.

You may get drowsy, dizzy. Do not drive, use machinery, or do anything that needs mental alertness until you know how sumatriptan affects you. To reduce dizzy or fainting spells, do not sit or stand up quickly, especially if you are an older patient. Alcohol can increase drowsiness, dizziness and flushing. Avoid alcoholic drinks. Smoking cigarettes may increase the risk of heart-related side effects from using sumatriptan.

What side effects may I notice from taking sumatriptan?

Side effects that you should report to your prescriber or health care professional as soon as possible:
Rare or uncommon:
- chest or throat pain, tightness
- dizziness or faintness
- fast, slow, or irregular heart beat
- feeling of chest heaviness or pressure
- increased or decreased blood pressure
- loss of vision or vision changes
- palpitations
- seizures (convulsions)
- severe stomach pain and cramping, bloody diarrhea
- shortness of breath, wheezing, or difficulty breathing
- tingling, pain, or numbness in the face, hands or feet
- unusual reaction or swelling of the skin, eyelids, face, or lips

Side effects that usually do not require medical attention (report to your prescriber or health care professional if they continue or are bothersome):
- change in taste
- diarrhea
- drowsiness
- feeling warm, flushing, or redness of the face
- muscle pain or cramps
- nausea, vomiting, or stomach upset
- tiredness or weakness

Where can I keep my medicine?

Keep out of the reach of children in a container that small children cannot open. Store at room temperature between 15 and 30 degrees C (59 and 86 degrees F). Throw away any unused medicine after the expiration date.

S

Tacrine capsules

COGNEX®;
20 mg; Capsule
First Horizon
Pharmaceutical Corp

COGNEX®;
30 mg; Capsule
First Horizon
Pharmaceutical Corp

What are tacrine capsules?

TACRINE (Cognex®) helps treat the symptoms associated with Alzheimer's disease or dementia. It is not a cure for Alzheimer's disease but offers improvement in memory, attention, reason, language, and the ability to perform simple tasks. Benefits are greater for mild to moderate symptoms seen in the early stages of the disease. Generic tacrine capsules are not yet available.

What should my health care professional know before I take tacrine?

They need to know if you have any of these conditions:
- asthma or other lung disease
- difficulty passing urine
- head injury
- heart disease, slow heartbeat
- jaundice
- liver disease
- low blood pressure
- Parkinson's disease
- seizures (convulsions)
- severe headaches
- stomach or intestinal disease, ulcers or stomach bleeding
- an unusual or allergic reaction to tacrine, other medicines, foods, dyes, or preservatives
- pregnant or trying to get pregnant
- breast-feeding

How should I take this medicine?

Take tacrine capsules by mouth. Follow the directions on the prescription label. Swallow the capsules with a drink of water. It is best to take tacrine on an empty stomach, at least 1 hour before or 2 hours after meals. Take your doses at regular intervals. Do not take your medicine more often than directed. Continue to take your medicine even if you feel better. Do not stop taking except on your prescriber's advice. Contact your pediatrician or health care professional regarding the use of this medicine in children. Special care may be needed.

What if I miss a dose?

If you miss a dose, take it as soon as you can. If it is almost time for your next dose, take only that dose. Do not take double or extra doses.

What may interact with tacrine?

- atropine
- benztropine
- caffeine
- cimetidine
- dicyclomine
- digoxin
- donepezil
- female hormones, like estrogens
- fluvoxamine
- galantamine
- glycopyrrolate
- guarana
- haloperidol
- ipratropium
- leflunomide
- medications for motion sickness (examples: dimenhydrinate, meclizine, scopolamine)
- medicines that relax your muscles for surgery
- methotrexate
- non-steroidal anti-inflammatory drugs (NSAIDs, such as ibuprofen)
- oxybutynin
- propantheline
- riluzole
- rivastigmine
- theophylline
- trihexyphenidyl
- warfarin
- zileuton

Tell your prescriber or health care professional about all other medicines you are taking, including non-prescription medicines, nutritional supplements, or herbal products. Also tell your prescriber or health care professional if you are a frequent user of drinks with caffeine or alcohol, if you smoke, or if you use illegal drugs. These may affect the way your medicine works. Check with your health care professional before stopping or starting any of your medicines.

What should I watch for while taking tacrine?

Visit your prescriber or health care professional for regular checks on your progress. Your prescriber will need to regularly check your blood to monitor the effect of the medication on your liver. Check with your prescriber or health care professional if there is no improvement in your symptoms or if they get worse. Avoid alcohol while you are taking tacrine. Alcohol may increase the risk of getting liver damage. Also try to avoid smoking. Smoking tobacco may lessen tacrine's effectiveness. Ask your prescriber or health care professional for ways to help you stop smoking or drinking. Drinking too much caffeine may make you feel nervous or may give you nausea while on this medication. Try to avoid caffeinated beverages like coffee and colas whenever you can. You may get dizzy or feel faint. Do not drive, use machinery, or do anything that needs mental alertness until you know how tacrine affects you. If you are going to have surgery tell your prescriber or health care professional that you are taking tacrine.

What side effects may I notice from taking tacrine?

Side effects that you should report to your prescriber or health care professional as soon as possible:

- changes in vision or balance
- dark yellow or brown urine
- diarrhea, if it is severe or does not stop
- dizziness, fainting spells, or falls
- increase in frequency of passing urine, or incontinence
- muscle pains
- nervousness, agitation, or increased confusion
- pain in the stomach or abdomen
- skin rash or hives
- slow heartbeat, or palpitations
- sweating
- uncontrollable movements

- vomiting
- yellowing of eyes or skin

Side effects that usually do not require medical attention (report to your prescriber or health care professional if they continue or are bothersome):

- diarrhea
- dry mouth
- indigestion
- loss of appetite
- nausea

Where can I keep my medicine?

Keep out of reach of children in a container that small children cannot open. Store at room temperature between 15 and 30 degrees C (59 and 86 degrees F). Throw away any unused medicine after the expiration date.

Tacrolimus capsules

PROGRAF®;
1 mg; Capsule
Fujisawa Healthcare
Inc

PROGRAF®;
5 mg; Capsule
Fujisawa Healthcare
Inc

What are tacrolimus capsules?

TACROLIMUS (Prograf®) is a medication used to decrease the immune system response. Tacrolimus is used to reduce immune responses and prevent rejection in patients who receive organ or bone marrow transplants. Tacrolimus may be used to treat other conditions such as dermatitis, eczema, or psoriasis. Generic tacrolimus capsules are not yet available.

What should my health care professional know before I take tacrolimus capsules?

They need to know if you have any of these conditions:

- diabetes
- heart disease or heart failure
- high blood pressure
- infection
- kidney disease
- an unusual or allergic reaction to tacrolimus, castor oil, other medicines, foods, dyes, or preservatives
- pregnant or trying to get pregnant
- breast-feeding

How should I take this medicine?

Take tacrolimus capsules by mouth. Follow the directions on the prescription label. Swallow the capsules with a drink of water. Take with food or milk or take at bedtime to reduce stomach upset. Do not take with grapefruit juice. Taking tacrolimus with food can decrease the amount absorbed, but if you take every dose in the same way this will be acceptable. Take your doses at regular intervals. Do not take your medicine more often than directed.

What if I miss a dose?

If you miss a dose, take it as soon as you can. If it is almost time for your next dose, take only that dose. Do not take double or extra doses. Contact your prescriber or health care professional if you miss more than one dose, or if you vomit after a dose.

What may interact with tacrolimus capsules?

- aluminum hydroxide
- amiodarone
- bosentan
- bromocriptine
- certain medicines for HIV-infection such as protease inhibitors
- cimetidine
- corticosteroids
- cyclosporine
- diltiazem
- entecavir
- erythromycin
- grapefruit juice
- medicines for diabetes
- medicines for fungal infections
- medicines for seizures
- medicines to control the heart rhythm
- metoclopramide
- pamidronate
- rifabutin
- rifampin
- St. John's wort
- theophylline or aminophylline
- vaccines
- verapamil
- water pills (diuretics)
- ziprasidone
- zoledronic acid

Talk to your prescriber or health care professional before taking any of these medicines:

- aspirin
- acetaminophen

- ibuprofen
- ketoprofen
- naproxen

Tell your prescriber or health care professional about all other medicines you are taking, including non-prescription medicines, nutritional supplements, or herbal products. Also tell your prescriber or health care professional if you are a frequent user of drinks with caffeine or alcohol, if you smoke, or if you use illegal drugs. These may affect the way your medicine works. Check with your health care professional before stopping or starting any of your medicines.

What should I watch for while taking tacrolimus capsules?

Tacrolimus is a strong medication and can produce serious side effects. Discuss the potential risks and benefits with your prescriber or health care professional before you begin taking tacrolimus. Visit your prescriber or health care professional for regular checks on your progress. You will need to have laboratory tests to monitor your therapy with tacrolimus. After you stop taking this medication, side effects can continue. Some side effects may not occur until years after the medicine was taken. These effects can include the development of certain types of cancer. Discuss this possibility with your prescriber or health care professional. Tacrolimus will decrease your body's ability to fight infections. Call your prescriber or health care professional if you have a fever, chills, sore throat or other symptoms of a cold or flu. Do not treat these symptoms yourself. Try to avoid being around people who are sick. Do not have any vaccinations without your prescriber's approval. Avoid people who have recently received the oral polio vaccine. Your blood sugar may increase while you are taking tacrolimus. Call your prescriber or health care professional for advice if you have any of the following symptoms: increased thirst, dry mouth, pass urine frequently, notice a fruity odor on your breath, or feel tired and lose your appetite. Avoid taking aspirin, acetaminophen (Tylenol®), ibuprofen (Advil®), ketoprofen (Orudis KT®), or naproxen (Aleve®) products as these may mask a fever, unless instructed to by your prescriber or health care professional.

What side effects may I notice from taking tacrolimus capsules?

Tacrolimus therapy can produce many side effects. These mainly affect the urinary system and the nervous system. Contact your prescriber or health care professional about any unusual effects. Side effects that you should report to your prescriber or health care professional as soon as possible:

- signs of infection—fever or chills, cough, sore throat, pain or difficulty passing urine
- signs of decreased red blood cells—unusual weakness or tiredness, fainting spells, lightheadedness
- blurred vision, increased sensitivity of the eyes to light
- burning or tingling in the hands or feet
- difficulty breathing, wheezing
- frequent urination
- increased thirst or hunger
- ringing in the ears
- skin rash or itching (hives)
- seizures (convulsions)
- stomach, back or general pain
- swelling of the feet or legs, unusual or sudden weight gain
- yellowing of skin or eyes

Side effects that usually do not require medical attention (report to your prescriber or health care professional if they continue or are bothersome):

- diarrhea or constipation
- difficulty sleeping, nightmares
- dizziness or drowsiness
- hair loss or unusual hair growth
- headache
- loss of appetite
- mood changes, depression, confusion
- muscle cramps
- nausea, vomiting
- tremor
- unusual sensitivity to touch

Where can I keep my medicine?

Keep out of the reach of children in a container that small children cannot open. Store at room temperature between 15 and 30 degrees C (59 and 86 degrees F). Throw away any unused medicine after the expiration date.

Tadalafil tablets

CIALIS®;
10 mg; Tablet
Eli Lilly and Co

CIALIS®;
20 mg; Tablet
Eli Lilly and Co

What are tadalafil tablets?

TADALAFIL (Cialis®) is used to treat erectile dysfunction (ED) in men. Tadalafil does not cure ED or increase a man's sexual desire. Tadalafil is only for men with ED and is not for women or children. Tadalafil should only be used under a healthcare provider's care. Generic tadalafil is not yet available.

What should my health care professional know before I take tadalafil?

They need to know if you have any of these conditions:
- anatomical deformity of the penis, Peyronie's disease, or ever had an erection that lasted more than 4 hours
- bleeding disorder

- diabetes
- frequent heartburn or gastroesophageal reflux disease (GERD)
- heart disease, angina, a history of heart attack, irregular heart beats, or other heart problems
- high or low blood pressure
- high cholesterol
- HIV infection
- kidney disease or require dialysis
- liver disease
- sickle cell disease
- stroke
- stomach or intestinal ulcers
- eye or vision problems or a rare genetic eye disease called retinitis pigmentosa
- an unusual or allergic reaction to tadalafil, other medicines, foods, dyes, or preservatives
- pregnant or trying to get pregnant
- breast-feeding

How should I take this medicine?

Take tadalafil tablets by mouth. Follow the directions on the prescription label. The dose is usually taken 30 minutes to 1 hour before sexual activity. You should not take this dose more than once per day. Swallow the tablets with a drink of water. You may take tadalafil with or without meals. Do not take double or extra doses. Do not change your dose without talking to your prescriber. Your prescriber may lower or raise your dose, depending on how your body reacts to tadalafil. If you have kidney or liver problems or are taking certain medications, your prescriber may limit your dose of tadalafil. Contact your pediatrician or health care professional regarding the use of this medicine in children. Special care may be needed. At this time, this medicine is not for use in children.

What if I miss a dose?

This does not apply.

What may interact with tadalafil?

Do not take tadalafil if you are taking the following medications:

- nitroglycerin-type drugs for the heart or chest pain such as amyl nitrite, isosorbide dinitrate, isosorbide mononitrate, nitroglycerin, even if these are only taken occasionally

Tadalafil may also interact with the following medications:

- alpha blockers, such as alfuzosin (Uroxatral®), doxazosin (Cardura®), prazosin (Minipress®), or terazosin (Hytrin®), used to treat high blood pressure or an enlarged prostate.
- bosentan
- certain antibiotics such as clarithromycin, erythromycin, troleandomycin
- certain drugs used for seizures such as carbamazepine, phenytoin, and phenobarbital
- cimetidine
- cisapride

- diltiazem
- grapefruit juice
- medicines for fungal infections (fluconazole, itraconazole, ketoconazole, voriconazole)
- mibefradil
- nicardipine
- certain medicines for the treatment of HIV infection or AIDS
- quinidine
- rifabutin, rifampin or rifapentine
- some drugs for treating depression, anxiety or other mood problems (examples: fluoxetine, fluvoxamine, nefazodone)
- verapamil

Tell your prescriber or health care professional about all other medicines you are taking, including non-prescription medicines, nutritional supplements, or herbal products. Also tell your prescriber or health care professional if you are a frequent user of drinks with caffeine or alcohol, if you smoke, or if you use illegal drugs. These may affect the way your medicine works. Check with your health care professional before stopping or starting any of your medicines.

What should I watch for while taking tadalafil?

Contact your physician immediately if the erection lasts longer than 4 hours or if it becomes painful. This may be a sign of priapism and must be treated immediately to prevent permanent damage. If you experience symptoms of nausea, dizziness, chest pain or arm pain upon initiation of sexual activity after tadalafil use, you should refrain from further activity and should discuss the episode with your prescriber or health care professional as soon as possible. Do not drink alcohol to excess (examples, 5 glasses of wine or 5 shots of whiskey) when taking tadalafil. When taken in excess, alcohol can increase your chances of getting a headache or getting dizzy, increasing your heart rate or lowering your blood pressure. If you notice any changes in your vision while taking this drug, notify your prescriber or health care professional as soon as possible. Do not change the dose of your medication. Please call your prescriber or health care professional to determine if your dose needs to be reevaluated. Using tadalafil does not protect you or your partner against HIV infection (the virus that causes AIDS) or other sexually transmitted diseases.

What side effects may I notice from taking tadalafil?

Side effects that you should report to your prescriber or health care professional as soon as possible:
- changes in vision
- chest pain or palpitations
- difficulty breathing, shortness of breath
- dizziness
- eyelid swelling

- prolonged erection (lasting longer than 4 hours)
- skin rash, itching

Side effects that usually do not require medical attention (report to your prescriber or health care professional if they continue or are bothersome):
- back pain
- flushing
- headache
- indigestion

- muscle aches
- stuffy or runny nose

Where can I keep my medicine?

Keep out of the reach of children in a container that small children cannot open. Store at room temperature between 15 and 30 degrees C (59 and 86 degrees F). Throw away any unused medicine after the expiration date.

This drug requires an FDA medication guide. See page xxxvii.

Tamoxifen tablets

NOLVADEX®; 20 mg; Tablet AstraZeneca Pharmaceuticals LP

NOLVADEX®; 10 mg; Tablet AstraZeneca Pharmaceuticals LP

What are tamoxifen tablets?

TAMOXIFEN (Nolvadex®) blocks the effects of estrogen hormone in the body. Tamoxifen is most commonly used to treat breast cancer in women or men. This drug may reduce the chance of breast cancer coming back in women previously treated with surgery, radiation, or chemotherapy. This drug may also help prevent breast cancer in certain women with a high risk of developing breast cancer. Occasionally this drug is used for other conditions. Generic tamoxifen tablets are available.

What should my health care professional know before I take tamoxifen?

They need to know if you have any of these conditions:
- blood clots
- blood disorders
- cataracts or impaired eyesight
- endometriosis, uterine fibroids
- high calcium levels
- high cholesterol
- irregular menstrual cycles
- an unusual or allergic reaction to tamoxifen, other medicines, foods, dyes, or preservatives
- pregnant or trying to get pregnant
- breast-feeding

How should I take this medicine?

Take tamoxifen tablets by mouth. Follow the directions on the prescription label. Swallow the tablets with a drink of water. You may take tamoxifen with or without food. Take your doses at regular intervals. Do not stop taking except on your prescriber's advice. Contact your pediatrician or health care professional regarding the use of this medicine in children. Special care may be needed.

What if I miss a dose?

If you miss a dose, take it as soon as you remember, and then take the next dose as usual. Do not take double or extra doses. If you vomit after taking a dose call your prescriber or health care professional for advice.

What may interact with tamoxifen?

- aminogluthemide
- bosentan
- bromocriptine
- chemotherapy drugs
- cyclosporine
- delavirdine
- dietary supplements like black cohosh, chasteberry, melatonin, or soy isoflavones
- efavirenz
- estrogen hormones, including some birth control products
- nevirapine
- protease inhibitors
- rifampin
- warfarin

Tell your prescriber or health care professional about all other medicines you are taking, including nonprescription medicines, nutritional supplements, or herbal products. Also, tell your prescriber or health care professional if you are a frequent user of drinks with caffeine or alcohol, if you smoke, or if you use illegal drugs. These may affect the way your medicine works. Check with your health care professional before stopping or starting any of your medicines.

What should I watch for while taking tamoxifen?

Visit your prescriber or health care professional for regular checks on your progress. You may need to have blood drawn to check your blood counts, calcium, and/or cholesterol. Serious side effects to tamoxifen occur rarely. However, you should contact your health care professional if you think you are having any problems with your tamoxifen therapy. Some side effects of tamoxifen may occur soon after starting the drug, but others may first appear at any time during your treatment. When you start taking tamoxifen to treat breast cancer, bone or tumor pain may increase. This means that tamoxifen is working and the pain should soon decrease. If the pain is severe, call your prescriber or health care professional. During this initial time, if you experience confusion or increased nausea, thirst, urination, or vomiting call your health care professional immediately. If you are taking tamoxifen to reduce your risk of getting breast cancer, you should know that tamoxifen does not prevent all types of breast cancer. You should have regular gynecological check-ups, including breast exams and mammograms, and follow your prescriber's recommendations. If breast cancer or other problem occurs, there is no guarantee that it will be detected at an early stage. This is why it is important to continue with regular check-ups. Women who are or have taken tamoxifen should inform their prescriber or health care professional of any irregular menstrual cycles, abnormal vaginal bleeding, changes in vaginal discharge, or pelvic pain or pressure. Women should not become pregnant while taking tamoxifen or for 2 months after tamoxifen therapy has stopped. You should see your prescriber immediately if you think you may have become pregnant while taking tamoxifen. Use of tamoxifen early in pregnancy may harm your unborn child. Women who can have children should use barrier birth control (condoms) or other methods of birth control that do not use hormones. Talk with your health care provider for birth control advice. Because tamoxifen may cause women ovulate, it may increase the risk of getting pregnant if appropriate birth control is not used. Women who take tamoxifen are at increased risk for developing blood clots. Some women may develop more than one clot, even if tamoxifen is stopped. If you experience pain or swelling in your calves, sudden chest pain, shortness of breath, or coughing up blood, call your prescriber or health care professional right away. Tamoxifen may increase the chance of having a stroke. If you experience symptoms of a stroke such as weakness, difficulty walking or talking, or numbness, contact your prescriber immediately. Tamoxifen may cause cataracts or changes to parts of the eye known as the cornea or retina. If you experience any changes in your vision, including difficulty in telling colors apart, tell your prescriber or health care professional immediately. Men who take tamoxifen may notice decreased sexual desire and impotence.

What side effects may I notice from taking tamoxifen?

Some side effects will only apply to women.

Side effects that you should report to your prescriber or health care professional as soon as possible:

- changes in your menstrual cycle
- changes in vaginal discharge
- changes in vision
- confusion
- difficulty walking or talking
- difficulty breathing
- excessive thirst
- new breast lumps
- numbness
- pelvic pain or pressure
- redness, blistering, peeling or loosening of the skin, including inside the mouth
- shortness of breath
- skin rash
- swelling, pain or tenderness in your calf or leg
- swelling of lips, face, or tongue
- sudden chest pain
- unusual bruising or bleeding
- weakness
- vaginal bleeding
- yellowing of the whites of the eyes or skin

Side effects that usually do not require medical attention (report to your prescriber or health care professional if they continue or are bothersome):

- bone pain
- fatigue
- headache
- hair loss, although uncommon and is usually mild
- hot flashes
- impotence (in men)
- nausea, vomiting
- pain at tumor site
- weight loss

Where can I keep my medicine?

Keep out of the reach of children in a container that small children cannot open. Store at room temperature between 15 and 30 degrees C (59 and 86 degrees F). Protect from light. Keep container tightly closed. Throw away any unused medicine after the expiration date.

Tamsulosin capsules

FLOMAX®;
0.4 mg; Capsule
Boehringer Ingelheim
Pharmaceuticals Inc

What are tamsulosin capsules?

TAMSULOSIN (Flomax®) is used to treat enlargement of the prostate gland in men (benign prostatic hyperplasia or BPH). It is not for use in women. Tamsulosin works by relaxing muscles in the prostate and bladder neck at the site of the obstruction. This imp-roves urine flow and reduces BPH symptoms. Generic tamsulosin capsules are not yet available.

What should my health care professional know before I take tamsulosin?

They need to know if you have any of the following conditions:

- kidney disease
- liver disease
- low blood pressure
- prostate cancer
- an unusual or allergic reaction to tamsulosin, other medicines, foods, dyes, or preservatives

How should I take this medicine?

Always take tamsulosin capsules by mouth after a meal, about 30 minutes after the same meal every day. Follow the directions on the prescription label. Swallow the capsules whole with a drink of water; do not crush, chew, or open capsules. Do not take your medicine more often than directed. Do not stop taking except on your prescriber's advice. Contact your pediatrician or health care professional regarding the use of this medicine in children. Special care may be needed.

What if I miss a dose?

If you miss a dose, take it as soon as you can. If it is almost time for your next dose, take only that dose. Do not take double or extra doses. If you stop taking tamsulosin for several days or more, restart treatment at one capsule a day, after consulting with your prescriber or health care professional.

What may interact with tamsulosin?

Do not take tamsulosin if you are taking the following medications:

- other alpha-blockers such as alfuzosin, doxazosin, phentolamine, phenoxybenzamine, prazosin, terazosin

Tamsulosin may also interact with the following medications:

- cimetidine
- medicines for high blood pressure
- sildenafil (doses of sildenafil higher than 25 mg should be taken at least 4 hours apart from taking tamsulosin)
- tadalafil
- vardenafil
- warfarin

Tell your prescriber or health care professional about all other medicines you are taking, including nonprescription medicines, nutritional supplements, or herbal products. Also tell your prescriber or health care professional if you are a frequent user of drinks with caffeine or alcohol, if you smoke, or if you use illegal drugs. These may affect the way your medicine works. Check with your prescriber or health care professional before stopping or starting any of your medicines.

What should I watch for while taking tamsulosin?

You must see your physician regularly. While taking tamsulosin, you must have regular checkups. Follow your physician's advice about when to have these checkups. You may feel drowsy or dizzy. Do not drive, use machinery, or do anything that requires mental alertness until you know how tamsulosin affects you. To reduce the risk of dizzy or fainting spells, do not sit or stand up quickly. If you begin to feel dizzy, sit down until you feel better. Avoid alcoholic drinks; they can make you more drowsy, increase flushing, and cause rapid heartbeats. Take tamsulosin at bedtime to lessen the effects of drowsiness and dizziness, but be careful if you have to get up during the night. Drowsiness and dizziness are more likely to occur after the first dose, after an increase in dose, or during hot weather or exercise. These effects can decrease once your body adjusts to this medicine. Although extremely rare in men taking tamsulosin, contact you health care provider immediately if you experience prolonged and painful erection of the penis which is unrelated to sexual activity (priapism). If not brought to immediate medical attention, priapism can lead to permanent erectile dysfunction (impotence). If you are going to have surgery, tell your prescriber or health care professional that you are taking tamsulosin.

What side effects may I notice from taking tamsulosin?

Side effects that you should report to your prescriber or health care professional as soon as possible:
Rare or uncommon:
- difficulty breathing, shortness of breath
- prolonged painful erection of the penis (priapism)

More common:
- fainting spells
- visual problems
- weakness

Side effects that usually do not require medical attention (report to your prescriber or health care professional if they continue or are bothersome):
- back pain
- diarrhea
- dizziness
- drowsiness
- sexual problems (ejaculation problems or decreased sex drive)
- headache
- insomnia
- nausea
- runny or stuffy nose

Where can I keep my medicine?

Keep out of the reach of children in a container that small children cannot open. Store at room temperature below 20 and 25 degrees C (68 and 77 degrees F). Throw away any unused medicine after the expiration date.

Tegaserod tablets

ZELNORM®;
2 mg; Tablet
Novartis
Pharmaceuticals

ZELNORM®;
6 mg; Tablet
Novartis
Pharmaceuticals

What are tegaserod tablets?

TEGASEROD (Zelnorm®) is used to treat women who have irritable bowel syndrome (IBS) and who have constipation as their main bowel problem. IBS is a disorder of the intestines that causes constipation, diarrhea, or both. Gas, bloating and stomach pain may also be present. Tegaserod helps to relieve the symptoms of stomach pain, bloating and constipation; it is not a cure. Tegaserod may also be used for relief of chronic constipation in patients (men and women) less than 65 years of age. Your health care provider may use tegaserod for other conditions. Generic tegaserod tablets are not available.

What should my health care professional know before I take tegaserod?

They need to know if you have any of these conditions:
- diarrhea or often have diarrhea
- gallbladder disease
- heart disease or a history of a heart attack
- kidney disease
- liver disease, like cirrhosis
- rectal bleeding
- stomach or intestinal disease, including bowel obstruction or abdominal adhesions
- an unusual or allergic reaction to tegaserod, other medicines, foods, dyes, or preservatives
- pregnant or trying to get pregnant
- breast-feeding

How should I take this medicine?

Take tegaserod tablets by mouth shortly before you eat a meal. Follow the directions on the prescription label. Take your doses at regular intervals. Tegaserod is not intended to be used only as needed. Do not take your medicine more often than directed.

What if I miss a dose?

If you miss a dose of tegaserod, just skip that dose. Wait until your next dose, and take only that dose. Do not take double or extra doses.

What may interact with tegaserod?

- medicines for bowel problems or bladder incontinence (these can cause constipation)

Tell your prescriber or health care professional about all other medicines you are taking, including non-prescription medicines, nutritional supplements, or herbal products. Also tell your prescriber or health care professional if you are a frequent user of drinks with caffeine or alcohol, if you smoke, or if you use illegal drugs. These may affect the way your medicine works. Check with your health care professional before stopping or starting any of your medicines.

What should I watch for while taking tegaserod?

Diarrhea is a common side effect of tegaserod that usually occurs in the first week of starting the medicine. Typically the diarrhea caused by tegaserod will last only a few days and will not recur. You should not start taking tegaserod if you already have diarrhea or have diarrhea most of the time. Severe or prolonged diarrhea can lead to dehydration, a lack of fluids within your body. If you experience severe cramping, stomach pain, lightheadedness, dizziness or fainting accompanied by diarrhea, notify your prescriber immediately. If you get new or worsening stomach pain with or without blood in your stools, call your prescriber immediately. Tegaserod may not work for all patients who take it. It may take several weeks for you notice any relief from your symptoms. If tegaserod is stopped, it is likely that that your symptoms will return within 1–2 weeks. Your diet and stress levels may affect your course of therapy. If you eat something that seems to worsen your constipation or if you have significant levels of stress in your life, be sure to discuss this with your health care professional. If you are going to have surgery, tell your prescriber or health care professional that you are taking tegaserod.

What side effects may I notice from taking tegaserod?

Side effects that you should report to your prescriber or health professional as soon as possible:
- sudden onset of chest pain
- diarrhea accompanied by severe stomach cramps with or without rectal bleeding, other stomach pain or dizziness
- new or worsening stomach pain
- worsening or prolonged diarrhea

Side effects that usually do not require medical attention (report to your prescriber or health care professional if they continue or are bothersome):
- mild dizziness
- gas
- headache
- heartburn
- nausea or vomiting

Where can I keep my medicine?

Keep out of the reach of small children in a container that small children cannot open. Store at room temperature between 15 and 30 degrees C (59 and 86 degree F). Protect from heat and moisture. Throw away any unused medicine after the expiration date.

T

Telithromycin tablets

KETEK™;
400 mg; Tablet
Aventis Pharmaceuticals Inc

What are telithromycin tablets?

TELITHROMYCIN (Ketek™) is an antibiotic. Telithromycin kills certain bacteria or stops their growth. It treats lung, sinus, and throat infections. Telithromycin will not work for colds, flu, or other viral infections. Generic telithromycin tablets are not yet available.

What should my health care professional know before I take telithromycin?

They need to know if you have any of these conditions:
- diarrhea
- heart disease
- irregular heart beat or abnormal heart beat
- kidney disease
- liver disease
- low blood potassium (hypokalemia) or magnesium (hypomagnesemia)
- myasthenia gravis
- stomach problems (especially colitis)
- other chronic illness
- taking cisapride (Propulsid®), pimozide (Orap®), or certain medicines known as antiarrhythmics (such as quinidine, procainamide, or dofetilide)
- an unusual or allergic reaction to telithromycin or macrolide antibiotics (such as erythromycin, azithromycin, clarithromycin, or dirithromycin), foods, dyes, or preservatives
- pregnant or trying to get pregnant
- breast-feeding

How should I take this medicine?

Take telithromycin tablets by mouth. Follow the directions on the prescription label. Take the tablets with a full glass of water. You may take telithromycin tablets with or without food. Take your doses at regular intervals. Do not take your medicine more often than directed. Finish the full course prescribed by your prescriber or health care professional even if you think your condition is better. Do not stop taking except on your prescriber's advice. Contact your pediatrician or health care professional regarding the use of this medicine in children. Special care may be needed.

What if I miss a dose?

If you miss a dose, take it as soon as you can. If it is almost time for your next dose, take only that dose. Do not take double or extra doses.

What may interact with telithromycin?

- alfentanil
- alosetron
- astemizole
- carbamazepine
- certain benzodiazepines (alprazolam, diazepam, midazolam, triazolam)
- certain heart medications (digoxin, diltiazem, disopyramide, dofetilide, felodipine, metoprolol, nifedipine, procainamide, quinidine, verapamil)
- certain medicines to treat fungal or yeast infections (itraconazole, ketoconazole, voriconazole)
- cisapride
- cyclosporine
- donepezil
- ergot alkaloid medicines, like ergotamine
- lidocaine
- medicines to treat viral infections (delavirdine, indinavir, nevirapine, ritonavir, saquinavir)
- methylprednisolone
- norethindrone
- phenytoin
- pimozide
- rifampin
- sirolimus
- some "statin" medicines for reducing cholesterol (examples: atorvastatin, lovastatin, simvastatin)
- tacrolimus
- terfenadine
- theophylline
- trimetrexate
- zonisamide

Tell your prescriber or health care professional about all other medicines that you are taking, including nonprescription medicines, nutritional supplements, or herbal products. Also tell your prescriber or health care professional if you are a frequent user of drinks with caffeine or alcohol, if you smoke, or if you use illegal drugs. These may affect the way your medicine works. Check with your health care professional before stopping or starting any of your medicines.

What should I watch for while taking telithromycin?

Tell your prescriber or health care professional if your symptoms do not improve in 2 to 3 days. Make sure to take all of this medicine as prescribed, even if you begin to feel better. If you get severe or watery diarrhea, do not treat yourself. Call your prescriber or health care professional for advice. If you have vision problems while taking telithromycin, avoid driving, operating heavy machinery, or engaging in otherwise hazardous activities. You should also avoid quickly looking between objects in the distance and nearby; this may help to decrease these visual difficulties. If these vision problems interfere with your daily activities, contact you healthcare provider. Telithromycin has been reported to cause liver problems. If you notice a yellowing of the skin or eyes, stop taking telithromycin immediately and contact your healthcare provider. If you have fainting spells while taking telithromycin, contact your healthcare provider. Telithromycin may be affecting the way your heart beats. If you have a disease called myasthenia gravis, telithromycin may worsen your symptoms. If you experience any worsening of your symptoms (such as muscle weakness, difficulty breathing) while taking telithromycin, stop taking telithromycin and contact your healthcare provider immediately. If you are going to have surgery, tell your prescriber or health care professional that you are taking telithromycin.

What side effects may I notice from taking telithromycin?

Side effects that you should report to your prescriber or health care professional as soon as possible:
- difficulty breathing
- fainting spells
- jaundice (yellowing of the skin and/or eyes)
- redness, blistering, peeling or loosening of the skin, including inside the mouth

- severe or watery diarrhea or persistent diarrhea
- skin rash, itching
- swelling of tongue or throat
- vomiting

Side effects that usually do not require medical attention (report to your prescriber or health care professional if they continue or are bothersome):
- diarrhea
- dizziness
- headache
- nausea
- vision problems such as blurred vision, difficulty focusing, and objects doubled

Where can I keep my medicine?

Keep out of the reach of children in a container that small children cannot open. Store at room temperature between 15 and 30 degrees C (59 and 86 degrees F). Keep container tightly closed. Protect from light. Throw away any unused medicine after the expiration date.

Telmisartan tablets

MICARDIS®;
40 mg; Tablet
Boehringer
Ingelheim
Pharmaceuticals Inc

MICARDIS®;
80 mg; Tablet
Boehringer
Ingelheim
Pharmaceuticals Inc

What are telmisartan tablets?

TELMISARTAN (Micardis®) helps lower blood pressure to normal levels. It controls high blood pressure, but it is not a cure. High blood pressure can damage your kidneys, and may lead to a stroke or heart failure. Telmisartan helps prevent these things from happening. Generic telmisartan tablets are not yet available.

What should my health care professional know before I take telmisartan?

They need to know if you have any of these conditions:
- heart failure
- kidney disease
- liver disease
- if you are on a special diet, such as a low-salt diet
- an unusual or allergic reaction to telmisartan, other medicines, foods, dyes, or preservatives
- pregnant or trying to get pregnant
- breast-feeding

How should I take this medicine?

Take telmisartan tablets by mouth. Follow the directions on the prescription label. Swallow the tablets with a drink of water. Telmisartan can be taken with or without food. Take your doses at regular intervals. Do not take your medicine more often than directed.

What if I miss a dose?

If you miss a dose, take it as soon as you can. If it is almost time for your next dose, take only that dose. Do not take double or extra doses.

What may interact with telmisartan?

- blood pressure medications
- digoxin
- hawthorn
- lithium
- potassium salts or potassium supplements
- warfarin
- water pills (especially potassium-sparing diuretics such as triamterene or amiloride)

Tell your prescriber or health care professional about all other medicines you are taking, including nonprescription medicines, nutritional supplements, or herbal products. Also tell your prescriber or health care professional if you are a frequent user of drinks with caffeine or alcohol, if you smoke, or if you use illegal drugs. These may affect the way your medicine works. Check with your health care professional before stopping or starting any of your medicines.

What should I watch for while taking telmisartan?

Check your blood pressure regularly while you are taking telmisartan. Ask your prescriber or health care professional what your blood pressure should be. When you check your blood pressure, write down the measurements to show your prescriber or health care professional. If you are taking this medicine for a long time, you must visit your prescriber or health care professional for regular checks on your progress. Make sure you schedule appointments on a regular basis. If you are going to have surgery, tell your prescriber or health care professional that you are taking telmisartan.

What side effects may I notice from taking telmisartan?

Side effects that you should report to your prescriber or health care professional as soon as possible:
Rare or uncommon:
- difficulty breathing or tightening of the throat
- swelling of lips or tongue

Side effects that usually do not require medical attention (report to your prescriber or health care professional if they continue or are bothersome):

- back pain
- diarrhea
- dizziness
- sore throat
- stuffy nose or stuffy sinuses

Where can I keep my medicine?

Keep out of the reach of children and in a container that small children cannot open. Store your medicine at room temperature between 15 and 30 degrees C (59 and 86 degrees F). Tablets should not be removed from the blisters until right before use. Throw away any unused medicine after the expiration date.

Temazepam tablets or capsules	RESTORIL®; 15 mg; Capsule Mallinckrodt Inc Pharmaceuticals Group		RESTORIL®; 30 mg; Capsule Mallinckrodt Inc Pharmaceuticals Group	

What are temazepam tablets or capsules?

TEMAZEPAM (Restoril®) is a benzodiazepine. Benzodiazepines belong to a group of medicines that slow down the central nervous system. Temazepam helps to treat insomnia (difficulty sleeping at night). Federal law prohibits the transfer of temazepam to any person other than the patient for whom it was prescribed. Do not share this medicine with anyone else. Generic temazepam tablets and capsules are available.

What should my health care professional know before I take temazepam?

They need to know if you have any of these conditions:
- an alcohol or drug abuse problem
- bipolar disorder, depression, psychosis or other mental health condition
- glaucoma
- kidney disease
- liver disease
- lung disease, such as chronic obstructive pulmonary disease (COPD), sleep apnea or other breathing difficulties
- myasthenia gravis
- Parkinson's disease
- porphyria
- seizures or a history of seizures
- shortness of breath
- snoring
- suicidal thoughts
- uncontrolled pain
- an unusual or allergic reaction to temazepam, other benzodiazepines, other medicines, foods, dyes, or preservatives
- pregnant or trying to get pregnant
- breast-feeding

How should I take this medicine?

Take temazepam tablets or capsules by mouth. Temazepam is only for use at bedtime. Follow the directions on the prescription label. Swallow the tablets or capsules with a drink of water. If temazepam upsets your stomach, take it with food or milk. Do not take your medicine more often than directed. Do not stop taking except on your prescriber's advice. Contact your pediatrician or health care professional regarding the use of this medicine in children. Special care may be needed.

What if I miss a dose?

If you miss a dose, take it as soon as you can. It can take up to 2 hours for drowsiness to occur; never repeat the dose before 2 hours have passed. Do not take double or extra doses.

What may interact with temazepam?

- alcohol
- barbiturate medicines for inducing sleep or treating seizures (convulsions), like phenobarbital
- caffeine
- female hormones, including contraceptive or birth control pills
- herbal or dietary supplements such as kava kava, melatonin, or valerian
- medicines for anxiety or sleeping problems, such as alprazolam, diazepam, lorazepam or triazolam
- medicines for depression, mental problems or psychiatric disturbances
- phenytoin
- prescription pain medicines
- probenecid
- some medicines for colds, hay fever or other allergies
- theophylline

Tell your prescriber or health care professional about all other medicines you are taking, including non-prescription medicines, nutritional supplements, or herbal products. Also tell your prescriber or health care professional if you are a frequent user of drinks with caffeine or alcohol, if you smoke, or if you use illegal drugs. These may affect the way your medicine works. Check with your health care professional before stopping or starting any of your medicines.

What should I watch for while taking temazepam?

Visit your prescriber or health care professional for regular checks on your progress. Temazepam is for short-term periods of use. If sleep medicine is taken every night for a long time it may no longer help you to sleep. Your body can become dependent on temazepam, ask your prescriber or health care professional if you still need to take it. However, if you have been taking temazepam regularly for some time, do not suddenly stop taking it. You must gradually reduce the dose or you may get severe side effects. Ask your prescriber or health care professional for advice. Even after you stop taking temazepam it can still affect your body for several days. You may get drowsy or dizzy. Do not drive, use machinery, or do anything that needs mental alertness until you know how temazepam affects you. To reduce the risk of dizzy and fainting spells, do not stand or sit up quickly, especially if you are an older patient. Alcohol may increase dizziness and drowsiness. Avoid alcoholic drinks. Do not treat yourself for coughs, colds or allergies without asking your prescriber or health care professional for advice. Some ingredients can increase possible side effects. If you are going to have surgery, tell your prescriber or health care professional that you are taking temazepam.

What side effects may I notice from taking temazepam?

Side effects that you should report to your prescriber or health care professional as soon as possible:

- confusion
- depression
- lightheadedness or fainting spells
- mood changes, excitability or aggressive behavior
- movement difficulty, staggering or jerky movements
- muscle cramps
- tremors
- weakness or tiredness

Side effects that usually do not require medical attention (report to your prescriber or health care professional if they continue or are bothersome):

- dizziness, drowsiness, clumsiness, or unsteadiness; a "hangover" effect
- headache
- increased dreaming
- nausea, vomiting

Where can I keep my medicine?

Keep out of the reach of children in a container that small children cannot open. Store at room temperature below 30 degrees C (86 degrees F). Protect from light. Keep container tightly closed. Throw away any unused medicine after the expiration date.

Temozolomide capsules

TEMODAR®;
100 mg; Capsule
Schering Corp

TEMODAR®;
20 mg; Capsule
Schering Corp

What are temozolomide capsules?

TEMOZOLOMIDE (Temodar®) is chemotherapy agent used to treat certain types of brain cancer and melanoma. Temozolomide interferes with the growth of rapidly dividing cells, like cancer cells, and eventually causes these cells to die. Generic temozolomide capsules are not yet available.

What should my health care professional know before I take temozolomide?

They need to know if you have any of these conditions:

- blood disorders
- an active infection
- an unusual or allergic reaction to temozolomide, dacarbazine (DTIC), other chemotherapy agents, other medicines, foods, dyes, or preservatives
- pregnant or trying to get pregnant
- breast-feeding

How should I take this medicine?

Temozolomide capsules are usually taken once a day by mouth with a glass of water for 5 days. Take each day's dose of capsules at one time. The capsules should be swallowed whole and never chewed. Try to take your medicine at the same time every day in relation to meals. To decrease any nausea, take the capsules on an empty stomach or at bedtime. Make sure to follow the instructions given to you by your health care provider. Your doses of temozolomide will be packaged in separate packages labeled "Day 1," "Day 2," etc. On the first day of treatment, you should take all the capsules in the package labeled Day 1, then on the second day, take all the capsules in the package labeled Day 2, and so on. Do not worry that the capsules you take on a given day are different size or colors; different capsules may be needed to make sure you get the right dose over the 5 days. If you think your medication has been packaged incorrectly, contact your prescriber or pharmacist immediately. Do not open or split the capsules. If the capsules are accidentally opened or damaged, you should be extremely careful to avoid breathing in the powder or getting the powder on your skin, nose, or mouth. Contact your pediatrician or health care professional regarding the use of this medicine in children. Special care may be needed.

What if I miss a dose?

It is important not to miss a dose. If it is the same day, take your missed dose as soon as possible, then continue your regular schedule. If you miss a whole day, call your prescriber or health care provider.

What may interact with temozolomide?

- other chemotherapy agents may increase the side effects seen with temozolomide.

Talk to your prescriber or health care professional before taking any of these medicines:

- aspirin
- acetaminophen
- ibuprofen
- ketoprofen
- naproxen

Tell your prescriber or health care professional about all other medicines that you are taking, including nonprescription medicines, nutritional supplements, or herbal products. Also tell your prescriber or health care professional if you are a frequent user of drinks with caffeine or alcohol, if you smoke, or if you use illegal drugs. These may affect the way your medicine works. Check with your health care professional before stopping or starting any of your medicines.

What should I watch for while taking temozolomide?

Visit your prescriber or health care professional for regular checks on your progress. You will need to have regular blood checks. It is extremely important not to open the temozolomide capsules. Breathing in the powder or other contact with the powder may be harmful. If the powder accidentally gets on your skin, wash the area thoroughly. If you have difficulty swallowing all of the capsules, contact your prescriber or health care professional. Temozolomide may make you feel generally unwell. This is because temozolomide affects good cells as well as cancer cells. Report any side effects as above, but continue your course of medicine even though you feel ill, unless your prescriber or health care professional tells you to stop. Temozolomide may decrease your body's ability to fight infections. Call your prescriber or health care professional if you have a fever, chills, sore throat or other symptoms of a cold or flu. Do not treat these symptoms yourself. Try to avoid being around people who are sick. Temozolomide may increase your risk to bruise or bleed. Call your prescriber or health care professional if you notice any unusual bleeding. Be careful not to cut, bruise or injure yourself because you may get an infection and bleed more than usual. Avoid taking aspirin, acetaminophen (Tylenol®), ibuprofen (Advil®), naproxen (Aleve®), or ketoprofen (Orudis® KT) products as these may hide a fever, unless instructed to by your prescriber or health care professional. Call your prescriber or health care professional if you get diarrhea. Do not treat yourself. Be careful brushing and flossing your teeth or using a toothpick while receiving temozolomide because you may get an infection or bleed more easily. If you have

any dental work done, tell your dentist you are received temozolomide. Temozolomide may cause birth defects; therefore, both men and women who are taking temozolomide should use effective birth control, if indicated. Women should avoid becoming pregnant if they or their partner is taking temozolomide. Talk to your health care professional about preventing pregnancy. Women should not nurse while taking temozolomide because there is a possibility of harm to the nursing infant.

What side effects may I notice from taking temozolomide?

The side effects you may experience with temozolomide therapy depend upon the dose, other types of chemotherapy or radiation therapy given, and the disease being treated. Not all of these effects occur in all patients. Discuss any concerns or questions with your prescriber or health care professional.
Side effects that you should report to your prescriber or health care professional as soon as possible:

- abnormal coordination
- abnormal walking or difficulty walking
- low blood counts—temozolomide may decrease the number of white blood cells, red blood cells and platelets. You may be at increased risk for infections and bleeding.
- signs of infection—fever or chills, cough, sore throat, pain or difficulty passing urine
- signs of decreased platelets or bleeding—bruising, pinpoint red spots on the skin, black, tarry stools, blood in the urine
- signs of decreased red blood cells—unusual weakness or tiredness, fainting spells, lightheadedness
- nausea and vomiting
- paralysis of legs or arms
- skin rash
- seizures
- vision changes

Side effects that usually do not require medical attention (report to your prescriber or health care professional if they continue or are bothersome):

- back pain
- constipation
- decreased appetite
- diarrhea
- difficulty sleeping
- dizziness
- easily tire
- headache
- itching

Where can I keep my medicine?

Keep this medicine out of reach of children and pets. Store capsules at room temperature, between 59 and 85 degrees F (15 and 30 degrees C).

Tenofovir, PMPA
tablets

VIREAD®;
300 mg; Tablet
Gilead Sciences Inc

What are tenofovir tablets?

TENOFOVIR, PMPA (Viread®) is a drug used to treat human immunodeficiency virus (HIV) infection. Tenofovir is an antiviral drug called a nucleotide reverse transcriptase inhibitor. Tenofovir may reduce the amount of HIV in the blood and increase the number of CD4 cells (T-cells) in the blood. Tenofovir is used in combination with other drugs to treat the HIV virus. Tenofovir will not cure or prevent HIV infection or AIDS. You may still develop other infections or conditions associated with HIV. Generic tenofovir capsules are not yet available.

What should my health care professional know before I take tenofovir?

They need to know if you have any of these conditions:
- bone disease or osteoporosis
- kidney disease or a history of kidney disease
- liver disease
- an unusual or allergic reaction to tenofovir, other medicines, foods, dyes, or preservatives
- pregnant or trying to get pregnant
- breast-feeding

How should I take this medicine?

Take tenofovir tablets by mouth. You may take this medicine with or without food. Follow the directions on the prescription label. Take your doses at regular intervals. Do not take your medicine more often than directed. To help to make sure that your anti-HIV therapy works as well as possible, be very careful to take all of your medicine exactly as prescribed. Do not stop taking except on your prescriber's advice. Contact your pediatrician or health care professional regarding the use of this medicine in children. Special care may be needed.

What if I miss a dose?

If you miss a dose, take it as soon as you can. If it is almost time for your next dose, take only that dose. Do not take double or extra doses.

What may interact with tenofovir?

- amphotericin B
- antiviral agents (such as acyclovir, cidofovir, foscarnet, ganciclovir, valacyclovir, valganciclovir)
- cyclosporine
- didanosine, ddI
- hydroxyurea
- lopinavir
- probenecid
- tacrolimus

Tell your prescriber or health care professional about all other medicines you are taking, including nonprescription medicines, nutritional supplements, or herbal products. Also tell your prescriber or health care professional if you are a frequent user of drinks with caffeine or alcohol, if you smoke, or if you use illegal drugs. These may affect the way your medicine works. Check with your health care professional before stopping or starting any of your medicines.

What should I watch for while taking tenofovir?

Visit your prescriber or health care professional for regular checks on your progress. Discuss any new symptoms with your prescriber or health care professional. Tenofovir will not cure HIV and you can still get other illnesses or complications associated with your disease. Taking tenofovir does not reduce the risk of passing HIV infection to others through sexual or blood contact. It is best to avoid sexual contact so that you do not spread the disease to others. For any sexual contact, use a condom. Be careful about cuts, abrasions and other possible sources of blood contact. Never share a needle or syringe with anyone.

What side effects may I notice from taking tenofovir?

Side effects that you should report to your prescriber or health care professional as soon as possible:
- breathing difficulties or shortness of breath
- changes in body appearance (weight gain around waist and/or face)
- dizziness
- muscle aches, pains, or weakness
- passing out or fainting
- severe vomiting or diarrhea
- slow or irregular heartbeat
- symptoms of high blood sugar: dizziness, dry mouth, flushed dry skin, fruit-like breath odor, loss of appetite, nausea, stomach ache, unusual thirst, frequent passing of urine
- unusual stomach pain or discomfort
- unusual weakness, fatigue or discomfort

Side effects that usually do not require medical attention (report to your prescriber or health care professional if they continue or are bothersome):
- diarrhea
- gas
- headache
- loss of appetite
- nausea, vomiting
- stomach pain
- tiredness

Where can I keep my medicine?

Keep out of the reach of children in a container that small children cannot open. Store at room temperature between 15 and 25 degrees C (59 and 77 degrees F). Protect from light and moisture. Throw away any unused medicine after the expiration date.

Terazosin capsules

HYTRIN®;
1 mg; Capsule
Abbott
Pharmaceutical
Product Division

HYTRIN®;
10 mg; Capsule
Abbott
Pharmaceutical
Product Division

What are terazosin capsules?

TERAZOSIN (Hytrin®) is an antihypertensive. Terazosin lowers, but does not cure, high blood pressure. It works by relaxing the blood vessels. Terazosin is sometimes used for prostate problems. Generic terazosin capsules are available.

What should my health care professional know before I take terazosin?

They need to know if you have any of the following conditions:
- angina
- kidney disease
- an unusual or allergic reaction to terazosin, other medicines, foods, dyes, or preservatives
- pregnant or trying to get pregnant
- breast-feeding

How should I take this medicine?

Take terazosin capsules by mouth. Follow the directions on the prescription label. Swallow the capsules with a drink of water. Taking the capsules with food can help to reduce side effects. Take your doses at regular intervals. Do not take your medicine more often than directed. Do not stop taking except on your prescriber's advice. Contact your pediatrician or health care professional regarding the use of this medicine in children. Special care may be needed.

What if I miss a dose?

If you miss a dose, take it as soon as you can. If it is almost time for your next dose, take only that dose. Do not take double or extra doses.

What may interact with terazosin?

Do not take terazosin if you are taking the following medications: other alpha-blockers such as alfuzosin, doxazosin, phentolamine, phenoxybenzamine, prazosin, tamsulosin
Terazosin may also interact with the following medications:

- medicines for colds and breathing difficulties, medicines for high blood pressure, hawthorn, sildenafil (doses of sildenafil higher than 25 mg should be taken at least 4 hours apart from taking terazosin)
- tadalafil
- vardenafil
- water pills

Tell your prescriber or health care professional about all other medicines you are taking, including nonprescription medicines, nutritional supplements, or herbal products. Also tell your prescriber or health care professional if you are a frequent user of drinks with caffeine or alcohol, if you smoke, or if you use illegal drugs.

These may affect the way your medicine works. Check with your prescriber or health care professional before stopping or starting any of your medicines.

What should I watch for while taking terazosin?

Check your blood pressure regularly. Ask your prescriber or health care professional what your blood pressure should be and when you should contact him or her. Do not take capsules that show evidence of melting or breakage. Terazosin capsules must be stored at a controlled room temperature (see below). You may feel drowsy or dizzy. Do not drive, use machinery, or do anything that requires mental alertness until you know how terazosin affects you. To reduce the risk of dizzy or fainting spells, do not sit or stand up quickly. Avoid alcoholic drinks; they can make you more drowsy, increase flushing, and cause rapid heartbeats. Taking initial doses of terazosin at bedtime can lessen the effects of drowsiness and dizziness, but be careful if you have to get up during the night. Drowsiness and dizziness are more likely to occur after the first dose, after an increase in dose, or during hot weather or exercise. These effects can decrease once your body adjusts to this medicine. Although extremely rare in men taking terazosin, contact you health care provider immediately if you experience prolonged and painful erection of the penis which is unrelated to sexual activity (priapism). If not brought to immediate medical attention, priapism can lead to permanent erectile dysfunction (impotence). If you are going to have surgery, tell your prescriber or health care professional that you are taking terazosin.

What side effects may I notice from taking terazosin?

Side effects that you should report to your prescriber or health care professional as soon as possible:
Rare or uncommon:
- difficulty breathing, shortness of breath
- prolonged painful erection of the penis (priapism)

More common:
- blurred vision
- fainting spells, lightheadedness
- fast or irregular heartbeat, palpitations or chest pain
- swelling of the legs and ankles

Side effects that usually do not require medical attention (report to your prescriber or health care professional if they continue or are bothersome):
- constipation or diarrhea
- drowsiness or dizziness
- headache
- nausea
- nasal stuffiness
- unusual weakness or tiredness

Where can I keep my medicine?

Keep out of the reach of children in a container that small children cannot open. Store at room temperature between 20 and 25 degrees C (68 and 77 degrees F). Higher temperatures may cause the capsules to soften or melt. Protect from light and moisture. Throw away any unused medicine after the expiration date.

Terbinafine tablets

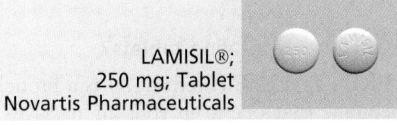

LAMISIL®;
250 mg; Tablet
Novartis Pharmaceuticals

What are terbinafine tablets?

TERBINAFINE (Lamisil®) is a medication used to treat infections caused by certain types of fungus. It is most commonly used for skin and nail infections. Generic terbinafine tablets are not yet available.

What should my health care professional know before I take terbinafine tablets?

They need to know if you have any of these conditions:
- frequently drink alcoholic beverages
- kidney disease
- liver disease (acute or chronic), including cirrhosis or hepatitis
- an unusual or allergic reaction to terbinafine, other medications, dyes, or preservatives
- pregnant or trying to get pregnant
- breast-feeding

How should I take this medicine?

Terbinafine tablets are taken by mouth. Follow the directions on the prescription label. You can take the tablets with food. If terbinafine upsets your stomach it may help to take it with food. Take your doses at regular intervals. Do not use your medicine more often than directed. Use your doses at regular intervals. Finish the full course prescribed by your prescriber or health care professional even if you think your condition is better. Do not stop using except on your prescriber's advice. Contact your pediatrician or health care professional regarding the use of this medicine in children. Special care may be needed.

What if I miss a dose?

If you miss a dose, use it as soon as you can. If it is almost time for your next dose, use only that dose. Do not use double or extra doses.

What may interact with terbinafine?

- caffeine
- cimetidine
- cyclosporine
- medicines for depression including amitriptyline, imipramine, or nortriptyline
- rifampin
- terfenadine
- theophylline
- warfarin

Tell your prescriber or health care professional about all other medicines you are taking, including non-prescription medicines, nutritional supplements, or herbal products. Also tell your prescriber or health care professional if you are a frequent user of drinks with caffeine or alcohol, if you smoke, or if you use illegal drugs. These may affect the way your medicine works. Check with your health care professional before stopping or starting any of your medicines.

What should I watch for while taking terbinafine?

Your prescriber may monitor your liver function. Tell your health care professional immediately if you develop symptoms of persistent nausea or vomiting, loss of appetite, fatigue, right upper abdominal pain or yellowing of the skin, dark urine, or pale stools. Some fungal infections need many weeks or months of treatment to cure. Take your medicine regularly for as long as your prescriber or health care professional tells you to. If you are taking this medication for nail fungus, it may still take time for the healthy nail to grow completely out after your course of therapy is complete. If you have a fungal infection of your skin or nails, dry your skin well after bathing. Most types of fungus live in moist environments. Wear clean socks and clothing every day.

What side effects may I notice from taking terbinafine?

Side effects that you should report to your prescriber or health care professional as soon as possible:
- dark yellow or brown urine
- fever or chills, cough, or sore throat
- loss of appetite
- nausea and vomiting
- redness, blistering, peeling or loosening of the skin, including inside the mouth
- skin rash, itching
- stomach or abdominal pain
- swelling, fluid retention
- unusual tiredness
- yellowing of skin or eyes

Side effects that usually do not require medical attention (report to your prescriber or health care professional if they continue or are bothersome):
- headache
- changes in taste
- stomach upset

Where can I keep my medicine?

Keep out of the reach of children. Store at room temperature between 5 and 30 degrees C (41 and 77 degrees F). Discard any unused medicine after the expiration date.

Terbutaline tablets

TERBUTALINE;
5 mg; Tablet
Global
Pharmaceuticals Div
of Impax Labs. Inc.

TERBUTALINE;
2.5 mg; Tablet
Global
Pharmaceuticals Div
of Impax Labs. Inc.

What are terbutaline tablets?

TERBUTALINE (Brethine®) is a bronchodilator, a medicine that opens up your air passages and makes breathing easier. It is a medicine for people with lung problems such as severe asthma and bronchospasm. Generic terbutaline tablets are available.

What should my health care professional know before I take terbutaline?

They need to know if you have any of the following conditions:
- diabetes
- heart disease
- high blood pressure
- over active thyroid
- seizures (convulsions)
- an unusual or allergic reaction to terbutaline, other medicines, foods, dyes, or preservatives
- pregnant or trying to get pregnant
- breast-feeding

How should I take this medicine?

Take terbutaline tablets by mouth. Follow the directions on the prescription label. Swallow the tablets with a drink of water. It is best to take terbutaline on an empty stomach, about 1 hour before or 2 hours after meals. Take your doses at regular intervals. Do not take your medicine more often than directed. Contact your pediatrician or health care professional regarding the use of this medicine in children. Special care may be needed.

What if I miss a dose?

If you miss a dose, take it as soon as you can. If it is almost time for your next dose, take only that dose. Do not take double or extra doses.

What may interact with terbutaline?

- beta-blockers, often used for high blood pressure or heart problems
- cocaine
- heart medicine (such as digoxin, digitoxin)
- levodopa
- maprotiline
- medicines for chest pain
- medicines for colds and breathing difficulties
- medicines for high blood pressure
- medicines for mental depression
- thyroid hormones
- water pills

Tell your prescriber or health care professional about all other medicines you are taking, including non-prescription medicines, nutritional supplements, or herbal products. Also tell your prescriber or health care professional if you are a frequent user of drinks with caffeine or alcohol, if you smoke, or if you use illegal drugs. These may affect the way your medicine works. Check before starting or stopping any of your medicines.

What should I watch for while taking terbutaline?

Tell your prescriber or health care professional if your symptoms so not improve in 1 or 2 days. Do not treat yourself for coughs, colds or allergies without checking with your pharmacist or prescriber or health care professional. Non-prescription medicines may contain ingredients that will increase the effects of your medicine.

What side effects may I notice from taking terbutaline?

Side effects that you should report to your prescriber or health care professional as soon as possible:
- chest pain, fast heartbeat, irregular heartbeat or palpitations
- difficulty breathing, wheezing
- dizziness, lightheadedness
- muscle cramps
- seizures (convulsions)
- skin rash, hives
- swelling of the face

Side effects that usually do not require medical attention (report to your prescriber or health care professional if they continue or are bothersome):
- change in taste
- dry mouth
- drowsiness
- flushing
- headache
- increased sweating
- nausea, vomiting
- nervousness, restlessness
- tremor
- weakness or tiredness

Where can I keep my medicine?

Keep out of the reach of children in a container that small children cannot open. Store at room temperature between 15 and 30 degrees C (59 and 86 degrees F). Protect from light. Throw away any unused medicine after the expiration date.

Tetracycline tablets or capsules

TETRACYCLINE;
250 mg; Capsule
Ivax Pharmaceuticals
Inc

TETRACYCLINE;
250 mg; Capsule
Barr Laboratories
Inc

What are tetracycline tablets or capsules?

TETRACYCLINE (Achromycin®, Sumycin®) is an antibiotic. It kills certain bacteria that cause infection, or stops their growth. Tetracycline treats many kinds of infections of the skin, bone, stomach, respiratory tract, sinuses, ear, and urinary tract. It also treats certain sexually transmitted diseases. Generic tablets and capsules are available.

What should my health care professional know before I take tetracycline?

They need to know if you have any of these conditions:
- kidney disease
- liver disease
- other chronic illness
- an unusual or allergic reaction to tetracycline antibiotics, foods, dyes, or preservatives
- pregnant or trying to get pregnant
- breast-feeding

How should I take this medicine?

Take tetracycline tablets or capsules by mouth. Follow the directions on the prescription label. Take tetracycline 1 hour before or at least 2 hours after eating. Swallow tablets or capsules whole with a full glass of water; take tablets or capsules in an upright or sitting position. Taking a sip of water first, before taking the tablets or capsules, may help you swallow them. If possible take bedtime doses at least 10 minutes before lying down. It is best to take tetracycline without food, but if it upsets your stomach take it with food. Avoid having dairy products, such as yogurt, milk, or cheese with your medicine; they can reduce the effect of tetracycline. Take your doses at regular intervals. Do not take your medicine more often than directed. Finish the full course prescribed by your prescriber or health care professional even if you think your condition is better. Do not stop taking except on your prescriber's advice. Contact your pediatrician or health care professional regarding the use of this medicine in children. Special care may be needed.

What if I miss a dose?

If you miss a dose, take it as soon as you can. If it is almost time for your next dose, take only that dose. Do not take double or extra doses. There should be an interval of at least 4 to 6 hours between doses.

What may interact with tetracycline?

- antacids
- calcium salts
- cholestyramine
- colestipol
- digoxin
- female hormones, including contraceptive or birth control pills
- ferrous sulfate
- magnesium salts
- methoxyflurane
- other antibiotic medicines
- sodium bicarbonate
- vitamin A
- warfarin
- zinc salts

Tell your prescriber or health care professional about all other medicines you are taking, including non-prescription medicines, nutritional supplements, or herbal products. Also tell your prescriber or health care professional if you are a frequent user of drinks with caffeine or alcohol, if you smoke, or if you use illegal drugs. These may affect the way your medicine works. Check with your health care professional before stopping or starting any of your medicines.

What should I watch for while taking tetracycline?

Tell your prescriber or health care professional if your symptoms do not improve in 2 to 3 days. Do not take tetracycline just before going to bed. It may not dissolve properly when you are lying down and can cause pain in your throat. Keep out of the sun, or wear protective clothing outdoors and use a sunscreen. Do not use sun lamps or sun tanning beds or booths. Make sure your diet provides vitamin B. Ask your prescriber or health care professional for advice if you think you are short of this vitamin. Birth control pills (contraceptive pills) may not work properly while you are taking this medicine. Use an extra method of birth control for at least one month. If you are being treated for a sexually transmitted disease, avoid sexual contact until you have finished your treatment. Your sexual partner may also need treatment. If you are going to have surgery, tell your prescriber or health care professional that you are taking tetracycline. Antacids can stop the effects of tetracycline. If you get an upset stomach and want to take an antacid, make sure there is an interval of at least 2 hours since you last took tetracycline, or 4 hours before your next dose. Iron and zinc preparations can also stop tetracycline from working properly. Never use tetracycline if it is past the expiration date; it can make you seriously ill.

What side effects may I notice from taking tetracycline?

Side effects that you should report to your prescriber or health care professional as soon as possible:
- dark yellow or brown urine
- decrease in the amount of urine

T

- difficulty breathing
- fever
- headache
- increased sensitivity to the sun or ultraviolet light
- itching in the rectal or genital area
- pain on swallowing
- redness, blistering, peeling or loosening of the skin, including inside the mouth
- skin rash, itching
- stomach pain or cramps
- unusual weakness or tiredness
- yellowing of the eyes or skin

Side effects that usually do not require medical atten-

tion (report to your prescriber or health care professional if they continue or are bothersome):

- diarrhea
- discolored tongue
- loss of appetite
- nausea, vomiting
- sore mouth

Where can I keep my medicine?

Keep out of the reach of children in a container that small children cannot open. Store at room temperature between 15 and 30 degrees C (59 and 86 degrees F). Protect from light. Throw away any unused medicine after the expiration date.

Thalidomide capsules

THALOMID®;
200 mg; Capsule
Celgene Corp

THALOMID®;
50 mg; Capsule
Celgene Corp

What are thalidomide capsules?

THALIDOMIDE (Thalomid®) alters the body's immune response. Thalidomide is used to treat diseases and symptoms of diseases caused by abnormalities in the immune system. Thalidomide is also used to treat multiple myeloma. Thalidomide causes severe, life-threatening birth defects or death to an unborn child and is only available under strict guidelines. Both women and men must commit to strict guidelines when receiving thalidomide. To receive thalidomide, you, your physician, and your pharmacy must be registered in the System for Thalidomide Education and Prescribing Safety (STEPS) Program. You may only receive up to a 28-day supply of thalidomide at a time, and you will need a new prescription for each refill. Your prescription must be filled within 7 days of your doctor's office visit.

What should my health care professional know before I take thalidomide?

They need to know if you have any of these conditions:

- pregnant or planning to get pregnant
- breast-feeding or planning to breast-feed
- tingling or numbness in hands or feet or other nerve pain
- low white blood cell count
- low blood pressure
- seizure disorder (epilepsy)
- an unusual or allergic reaction to thalidomide other medicines, foods, dyes, or preservatives

How should I use this medicine?

Thalidomide capsules are taken by mouth with water. Make sure to follow the directions on your prescription bottle. If you are only taking thalidomide once a day, take your dose at bedtime at least 1 hour after the evening meal to decrease the drowsiness effects. NEVER give this medicine to anyone else.

What if I miss a dose?

If you miss a dose, take it as soon as you can. If it is almost time for your next dose, consult your prescriber or health

care professional. You may need to miss a dose or take a double dose, depending on your condition and treatment. Do not take double or extra doses without advice.

What may interact with thalidomide?

- any medicines that may decrease the effectiveness of birth control pills
- any medicines which may cause tingling, numbness or nerve pain

Because thalidomide can cause drowsiness, other medicines that also cause drowsiness may increase this effect of thalidomide. Some medicines that cause drowsiness are:

- alcohol-containing medicines
- barbiturates such as phenobarbital
- certain antidepressants or tranquilizers
- muscle relaxants
- certain antihistamines used in cold medicines

Ask your prescriber or health care professional about other medicines that may increase the effect of thalidomide.

Tell your prescriber or other health care professional about all other medicines you are taking including nonprescription medicines, nutritional supplements, or herbal products. Also, tell your prescriber or health care professional if you are a frequent user of drinks with caffeine or alcohol, if you smoke or if you use illegal drugs. These may affect the way your medicine works. Check before stopping or starting any of your medications.

What should I watch for while taking thalidomide?

Thalidomide causes severe birth defects or death to an unborn child even after just ONE capsule. Both men and women must agree to take precautions against exposure of thalidomide to an unborn child. All patients will receive counseling about the potential birth defects and must agree to follow the conditions outlined in the System for Thalidomide Education and Prescribing Safety (STEPS) Program. The STEPS Program is a program to prevent exposure of thalidomide to an unborn child. The program involves required pregnancy testing, required birth control measures for men and women, doctor and patient education, registration of doctors, pharmacies and patients, and patient consent forms. You may not donate blood while taking thalidomide. Men are not permitted to donate sperm while taking thalidomide. Thalidomide has been associated with blood clots, especially when taken for multiple myeloma. Notify your healthcare provider immediately if develop shortness of breath, chest pain, or swelling in arms or legs. In some cases you may be given other medicine to help prevent blood clots while receiving thalidomide. Thalidomide causes drowsiness that will decrease as you continue taking the medicine. Be careful driving or operating machinery while taking thalidomide. Take thalidomide at bedtime to decrease this effect. Thalidomide may cause dizziness. Make sure to sit upright for a few minutes before standing up from a lying or seated position to avoid falling. You should take a stool softener (docusate) or fiber-product to avoid constipation while taking thalidomide.

What side effects may I notice from receiving thalidomide?

Side effects that you should report to your prescriber or health care professional as soon as possible:

- chest pain
- irregular menstrual bleeding
- missed menstrual cycle
- new or increased tingling or numbness in hands or feet
- muscle cramps
- rash associated with itching, blisters or open sores
- seizures
- shortness of breath
- numbness or tingling in arms or legs
- unusual swelling or pain in arms or legs

Side effects that usually do not require medical attention (report to your prescriber or health care professional if they continue or are bothersome):

- constipation
- drowsiness
- dizziness
- headache

Where can I keep my medicine?

Thalidomide may only be prescribed and dispensed by doctors and pharmacies registered in the STEPS program. Pharmacies may only fill a prescription if it is less than 7 days old and may only give you a 28-day supply. Keep thalidomide out of reach of children and never share this medication with anyone. Return any unused thalidomide to the pharmacy where your prescription was filled. Your pharmacy will accept all unused thalidomide as part of the controlled distribution program. Do not use beyond the expiration date on the package. Store this medicine at room temperature 59–86 degrees F (15–30 degrees C) and protect from light.

Theophylline, Aminophylline extended-release tablets or capsules

THEO-24®; 300 mg; Capsule, Extended Release UCB Pharma Inc

THEOCHRON®; 300 mg; Tablet, Extended Release Forest Pharmaceuticals Inc

What are theophylline extended-release tablets or capsules?

THEOPHYLLINE (Slo-bid ™, Slo-Phyllin®, Theo-bid®, Theo-24®, Theochron®, Theo-Dur®, Theo-lair™ SR, Uni-Dur®) is a bronchodilator, or medicine that helps to make breathing easier. It relaxes the bronchial airways, improving the flow of air through the lungs. Theophylline helps to reduce coughing, wheezing, shortness of breath, or difficulty breathing in patients with chronic (long-term) lung disorders such as asthma, bronchitis, or emphysema. Theophylline occurs naturally in teas and is chemically similar to caffeine or theobromine (found in cocoa). Generic theophylline extended-release tablets and capsules are available.

What should my health care professional know before I take theophylline?

They need to know if you have any of these conditions:
- fever, flu or respiratory infection
- heart or blood vessel disease, or previous heart attack
- liver disease
- prostate trouble
- stomach disease, such as ulcers
- an unusual or allergic reaction to theophylline, aminophylline, caffeine, theobromine, other medicines, foods, dyes, or preservatives
- pregnant or trying to get pregnant
- breast-feeding

How should I take this medicine?

Take theophylline extended-release tablets or capsules by mouth. Follow the directions on the prescription label. Swallow the tablets or capsules whole with a drink of water; do not crush or chew. (Theo-Dur® Sprinkle capsules can be opened and the contents sprinkled on soft food, such as applesauce, before swallowing without chewing). Take your doses at regular intervals; try to take doses at the same time each day. Do not take your medicine more often than directed.

What if I miss a dose?

If you miss a dose, take it as soon as you can. If it is almost time for your next dose, take only that dose.

There should be at least 6 hours between doses if you take theophylline twice a day, and at least 12 hours between doses if you only take theophylline once a day. Do not take double or extra doses.

What may interact with theophylline?

- beta-blockers, often used for high blood pressure or heart problems
- allopurinol
- barbiturate medicines for inducing sleep or treating seizures (convulsions)
- caffeine
- certain antibiotics given by injection
- diltiazem
- disulfiram
- ephedrine
- erythromycin
- fluvoxami ne
- guarana
- influenza virus vaccine
- ketoconazole
- lansoprazole
- lithium
- medicines for colds and breathing difficulties
- medicine for stomach ulcers and other stomach problems
- methotrexate
- mexiletine
- prednisone
- rifampin
- seizure (convulsion) or epilepsy medicine
- St. John's wort
- tacrolimus
- thyroid hormones, such as levothyroxine and liothyronine
- verapamil
- zafirlukast
- zileuton

Tell your prescriber or health care professional about all other medicines you are taking, including non-prescription medicines, nutritional supplements, or herbal products. Also tell your prescriber or health care professional if you are a frequent user of drinks with caffeine or alcohol, if you smoke, or if you use illegal drugs. These may affect the way your medicine works. Check with your health care professional before stopping or starting any of your medicines.

What should I watch for while taking theophylline?

Visit your prescriber or health care professional for regular checks on your progress. Your prescriber or health care professional may schedule regular blood tests, especially at first, to check how much theophylline is in your blood. There are many different brands of theophylline. Do not change your brand without checking with the prescriber or health care professional. Different brands may act differently in your body. Do not treat yourself for coughs, colds and allergies. Some non-prescription medicines contain ingredients that can interact with theophylline. Also check with your prescriber or health care professional if you get diarrhea. This can mean that you are having too much theophylline. Watch your diet while you are taking theophylline. Drinks with caffeine (like coffee, tea or cola) and food containing theobromine (like chocolate), can increase possible side effects to theophylline. Also charcoal-broiled food can stop theophylline from working properly. If you smoke tobacco or marijuana you may affect the level of theophylline in your body. Ask your prescriber or health care professional for help to give up smoking. If you are going to have surgery, tell your prescriber or health care professional that you are taking theophylline.

What side effects may I notice from taking theophylline?

Side effects that you should report to your prescriber or health care professional as soon as possible:

- anxiety, nervousness, restlessness
- diarrhea
- fainting spells, lightheadedness
- fast or irregular breathing or heartbeat (palpitations)
- flushing of the face
- nausea, vomiting (especially if the vomit looks like coffee grounds)
- seizures (convulsions)
- skin rash and itching (hives)
- unusual thirst
- unusual weakness or tiredness

Side effects that usually do not require medical attention (report to your prescriber or health care professional if they continue or are bothersome):

- difficulty sleeping
- dizziness
- headache
- increase in the need to pass urine
- irritability
- loss of appetite
- stomach cramps

Where can I keep my medicine?

Keep out of the reach of children in a container that small children cannot open. Store at room temperature between 15 and 30 degrees C (59 and 86 degrees F). Keep container tightly closed. Protect from light and moisture. Throw away any unused medicine after the expiration date.

Theophylline, Aminophylline tablets or capsules

QUIBRON® T;
300 mg; Tablet
Monarch
Pharmaceuticals Inc

AMINOPHYLLINE;
100 mg; Tablet
West Ward
Pharmaceutical Corp

What are theophylline tablets or capsules?

THEOPHYLLINE (Aminophylline, Quibron® T, Theo-24®, Theolair™, Bronkodyl®) is a bronchodilator, or medicine that helps to make breathing easier. It relaxes the bronchial airways, improving the flow of air through the lungs. Theophylline helps to reduce coughing, wheezing, shortness of breath, or difficulty breathing in patients with chronic (long-term) lung disorders such as asthma, bronchitis, or emphysema. Theophylline occurs naturally in teas and is chemically similar to caffeine or theobromine (found in cocoa). Generic theophylline tablets and capsules are available.

What should my health care professional know before I take theophylline?

They need to know if you have any of these conditions:
- fever, flu or respiratory infection
- heart or blood vessel disease, or previous heart attack
- liver disease
- prostate trouble
- stomach disease, such as ulcers
- an unusual or allergic reaction to theophylline, aminophylline, caffeine, theobromine, other medicines, foods, dyes, or preservatives
- pregnant or trying to get pregnant
- breast-feeding

How should I take this medicine?

Take theophylline tablets or capsules by mouth. Follow the directions on the prescription label. Swallow the tablets or capsules with a drink of water. It is best to take theophylline on an empty stomach about 30 minutes before a meal. If it upsets your stomach ask your prescriber or health care professional if you can take theophylline with food. Take your doses at regular intervals; try to take doses at the same time each day. Do not take your medicine more often than directed.

What if I miss a dose?

If you miss a dose, take it as soon as you can. If it is almost time for your next dose, take only that dose. There should be at least 2 to 3 hours between your doses. Do not take double or extra doses.

What may interact with theophylline?

- beta-blockers, often used for high blood pressure or heart problems
- allopurinol
- barbiturate medicines for inducing sleep or treating seizures (convulsions)
- caffeine
- certain antibiotics given by injection
- diltiazem
- disulfiram
- ephedrine
- erythromycin
- fluvoxamine
- guarana
- influenza virus vaccine
- ketoconazole
- lansoprazole
- lithium
- medicines for colds and breathing difficulties
- medicine for stomach ulcers and other stomach problems
- methotrexate
- mexiletine
- prednisone
- rifampin
- seizure (convulsion) or epilepsy medicine
- St. John's wort
- tacrolimus
- thyroid hormones, such as levothyroxine or liothyronine
- verapamil
- zafirlukast
- zileuton

Tell your prescriber or health care professional about all other medicines you are taking, including non-prescription medicines, nutritional supplements, or herbal products. Also tell your prescriber or health care professional if you are a frequent user of drinks with caffeine or alcohol, if you smoke, or if you use illegal drugs. These may affect the way your medicine works. Check with your health care professional before stopping or starting any of your medicines.

What should I watch for while taking theophylline?

Visit your prescriber or health care professional for regular checks on your progress. Your prescriber or health care professional may schedule regular blood tests, especially at first, to check how much theophylline is in your blood. There are many different brands of theophylline. Do not change your brand without checking with the prescriber or health care professional. Different brands may act differently in your body. Do not treat yourself for coughs, colds and allergies. Some non-prescription medicines contain ingredients that can interact with theophylline. Also check with your prescriber or health care professional if you get diarrhea. This can mean that you are having too much theophylline. Watch your diet while you are taking theophylline. Drinks with caffeine (like coffee, tea or cola) and food containing theobromine (like chocolate), can increase possible side effects to theophylline. Also charcoal-broiled food can stop theophylline from working properly. If you smoke tobacco or marijuana you may affect the level of theophylline in your body. Ask your prescriber or health care professional for help to give up smoking. If you are going to have surgery, tell your prescriber or health care professional that you are taking theophylline.

What side effects may I notice from taking theophylline?

Side effects that you should report to your prescriber or health care professional as soon as possible:

- anxiety, nervousness, restlessness
- diarrhea
- fainting spells, lightheadedness
- fast or irregular breathing or heartbeat (palpitations)
- flushing of the face
- nausea, vomiting (especially if the vomit looks like coffee grounds)
- seizures (convulsions)
- skin rash and itching (hives)

- unusual thirst
- unusual weakness or tiredness

Side effects that usually do not require medical attention (report to your prescriber or health care professional if they continue or are bothersome):

- difficulty sleeping
- dizziness
- headache
- increase in the need to pass urine
- irritability
- loss of appetite
- stomach cramps

Where can I keep my medicine?

Keep out of the reach of children in a container that small children cannot open. Store at room temperature between 15 and 30 degrees C (59 and 86 degrees F). Keep container tightly closed. Throw away any unused medicine after the expiration date.

Thiabendazole tablets

MINTEZOL®;
500 mg; Tablet, Chewable
Merck and Co Inc

What are thiabendazole tablets?

THIABENDAZOLE (Mintezol®) is an anthelmintic. This medicine treats parasitic (worm) infections from roundworms, hookworms, pinworms, whipworms, or threadworms. Generic thiabendazole tablets are not yet available.

What should my health care professional know before I take thiabendazole?

They need to know if you have any of these conditions:

- anemia
- dehydration
- kidney disease
- liver disease
- malnutrition
- other chronic illness
- an unusual or allergic reaction to thiabendazole or other substances, such as foods, preservatives or dyes
- pregnant or trying to get pregnant
- breast-feeding

How should I take this medicine?

Take thiabendazole tablets by mouth. Follow the directions on the prescription label. Chew or crush the tablets before swallowing. Take after meals. You can mix thiabendazole with juice or semi-solid food (such as applesauce or pudding), which is an easy way to give it to children. Do not take your medicine more often than directed. Finish the full course of medicine prescribed by your prescriber or health care professional even if you feel better. Take at regular intervals. Parasite (worm) death can be slow. To remove all parasites (worms) from the intestines can take several days. Contact your pediatrician or health care professional re-

garding the use of this medicine in children. Special care may be needed.

What if I miss a dose?

If you miss a dose, take it as soon as you can. If it is almost time for your next dose, take only that dose. Do not take double or extra doses. If you have to take a missed dose, make sure there is at least 10 to 12 hours between doses.

What may interact with thiabendazole?

- aminophylline
- caffeine
- theophylline

Tell your prescriber or health care professional about all other medicines you are taking, including non-prescription medicines, nutritional supplements, or herbal products. Also tell your prescriber or health care professional if you are a frequent user of drinks with caffeine or alcohol, if you smoke, or if you use illegal drugs. These may affect the way your medicine works. Check with your health care professional before stopping or starting any of your medicines.

What should I watch for while taking thiabendazole?

Visit your prescriber or health care professional to check that your infection has gone. If you have a severe infection you may need a second course of tablets. Wash your hands, scrub your fingernails and shower often. Every day change and launder bedclothes, linens, and undergarments. This will help keep other family members from getting infected. Disinfect the toilet every day, and damp mop the floors often to reduce the number of worm eggs. Other people in your house may need treatment. Check with your prescriber or health care professional as some worms are spread easily. Treat cats and dogs regularly for worms. Keep children out of contact with animal feces (wastes). Never eat undercooked (pink) pork meat. You can kill pork worm larvae (trichinosis) by cooking pork meat until it is well done. You may get dizzy; until you know how thiabendazole affects you, do not drive, use machinery, or do anything that needs mental alertness.

What side effects may I notice from taking thiabendazole?

Side effects that you should report to your prescriber or health care professional as soon as possible:
- blurred vision
- diarrhea (severe)
- difficulty breathing
- fever or chills, sore throat
- joint aches and pains
- lower back pain
- muscle aches and pains
- pain or difficulty passing urine
- redness, blistering, peeling or loosening of the skin, including inside the mouth
- seizures (convulsions)
- skin rash, hives, or itching
- unusual weakness or tiredness
- yellowing of eyes or skin

Side effects that usually do not require medical attention (report to your prescriber or health care professional if they continue or are bothersome):
- dizziness
- loss of appetite
- nausea, vomiting
- ringing in the ears
- stomach pain, which can occur when large numbers of parasites (worms) are present

Where can I keep my medicine?

Keep out of the reach of children in a container that small children cannot open. Store at room temperature between 15 and 30 degrees C (59 and 86 degrees F). Keep container tightly closed. Throw away any unused medicine after the expiration date.

Thioridazine tablets

THIORIDAZINE;
50 mg; Tablet
UDL Laboratories Inc

What are thioridazine tablets?

THIORIDAZINE (Mellaril®) helps to treat disordered thoughts and some other emotional, nervous, and mental problems. It also treats behavioral problems in children. Generic thioridazine tablets are available.

What should my health care professional know before I take thioridazine?

They need to know if you have any of these conditions:
- blood disorders or disease
- difficulty passing urine
- glaucoma
- head injury
- heart or liver disease
- low blood level of calcium
- Parkinson's disease
- prostate trouble
- Reye's syndrome
- seizures (convulsions)
- stomach problems or peptic ulcer
- an unusual or allergic reaction to thioridazine, other medicines foods, dyes, or preservatives
- pregnant or trying to get pregnant
- breast-feeding

How should I take this medicine?

Take thioridazine tablets by mouth. Follow the directions on the prescription label. Swallow the tablets with a drink of water. Take thioridazine with food or milk if it upsets your stomach. Take your doses at regular intervals. Do not take your medicine more often than directed. Contact your pediatrician or health care professional regarding the use of this medicine in children. Special care may be needed. Elderly patients over age 65 years may have a stronger reaction to this medicine and need smaller doses.

What if I miss a dose?

If you miss a dose, take it as soon as you can. If it is almost time for your next dose, take only that dose. Try to take your doses at the same time each day. Do not take double or extra doses.

What may interact with thioridazine?

- alcohol
- antacids
- some antibiotics
- antidiarrheal medications
- atropine
- bromocriptine
- cimetidine
- cisapride
- dextroamphetamine or amphetamine
- dronabinol or marijuana
- haloperidol or droperidol
- levodopa
- lithium
- medicines for an over-active thyroid gland
- medicines for colds and flu
- medicines for hay fever and other allergies
- medicines for mental depression
- medicines for movement abnormalities as in Parkinson's disease

- medicines to prevent or treat malaria
- medications for treating seizures (convulsions)
- medicines for pain or for use as muscle relaxants, including tramadol
- medicines to treat urine or bladder incontinence
- metoclopramide
- pimozide
- probucol
- some medications for high blood pressure or heart problems
- some weight loss medications

Tell your prescriber or health care professional about all other medicines you are taking, including non-prescription medicines, nutritional supplements, or herbal products. Also tell your prescriber or health care professional if you are a frequent user of drinks with caffeine or alcohol, if you smoke, or if you use illegal drugs. These may affect the way your medicine works. Check with your health care professional before stopping or starting any of your medicines.

What should I watch for while taking thioridazine?

Visit your prescriber or health care professional for regular checks on your progress. Do not stop taking thioridazine suddenly; this can cause nausea, vomiting, and dizziness. Ask your prescriber or health care professional for advice if you are to stop taking this medicine. You may get drowsy, dizzy, or have blurred vision. Do not drive, use machinery, or do anything that needs mental alertness until you know how thioridazine affects you. Do not stand or sit up quickly, especially if you are an older patient. This reduces the risk of dizzy or fainting spells. Alcohol can increase possible dizziness or drowsiness. Avoid alcoholic drinks. Thioridazine can reduce the response of your body to heat or cold. Try not to get overheated. Avoid temperature extremes, such as saunas, hot tubs, or very hot or cold baths or showers. Dress warmly in cold weather. Thioridazine can make your skin more sensitive to sun or ultraviolet light. Keep out of the sun, or wear protective clothing outdoors and use a sunscreen (at least SPF 15). Do not use sun lamps or sun tanning beds or booths. Wear sunglasses to protect your eyes. Thioridazine may make your mouth dry, chewing sugarless gum or sucking hard candy and drinking plenty of water will help. Do not treat yourself for coughs, colds, sore throat, indigestion, diarrhea, or allergies. Ask your prescriber or health care professional for advice. If you are going to have surgery or will need a procedure that uses contrast agents, tell your prescriber or health care professional that you are taking this medicine.

What side effects may I notice from taking thioridazine?

Side effects that you should report to your prescriber or health care professional as soon as possible:
- blurred vision
- breast enlargement in men or women
- breast milk in women who are not breast-feeding
- chest pain, fast or irregular heartbeat
- confusion, restlessness
- dark yellow or brown urine
- difficulty breathing or swallowing
- dizziness or fainting spells
- drooling, shaking, movement difficulty (shuffling walk) or rigidity
- fever, chills, sore throat
- hot, dry skin, unable to sweat
- involuntary or uncontrollable movements of the eyes, mouth, head, arms, and legs
- menstrual changes
- puffing cheeks, smacking lips, or worm-like movements of the tongue
- seizures (convulsions)
- slurred speech
- stomach area pain
- sweating
- unusual weakness or tiredness
- unusual bleeding or bruising
- yellowing of skin or eyes

Side effects that usually do not require medical attention (report to your prescriber or health care professional if they continue or are bothersome):
- constipation
- difficulty passing urine
- difficulty sleeping, agitation or restlessness
- drowsiness
- dry mouth
- headache
- increased sensitivity to the sun or ultraviolet light
- sexual difficulties (impotence in men; increased sexual desire in women)
- skin rash, or itching
- stuffy nose
- weight gain

Where can I keep my medicine?

Keep out of the reach of children in a container that small children cannot open. Store at room temperature below 30 degrees C (86 degrees F). Keep container tightly closed. Throw away any unused medicine after the expiration date.

Thiothixene capsules

| THIOTHIXENE;
2 mg; Capsule
UDL Laboratories
Inc | | THIOTHIXENE;
2 mg; Capsule
Sandoz
Pharmaceuticals | |

What are thiothixene capsules?

THIOTHIXENE (Navane®) helps to treat schizophrenia. Thiothixene can help you to keep in touch with reality and reduce your mental problems. Generic thiothixene capsules are available.

What should my health care professional know before I take thiothixene?

They need to know if you have any of these conditions:
- blood disorder or disease
- brain tumor or head injury
- breast cancer
- heart, kidney, or liver disease
- low blood pressure
- low level of calcium in the blood
- Parkinson's disease
- prostate trouble
- seizures (convulsions)
- thyroid disease
- an unusual or allergic reaction to thiothixene, other medicines, foods, dyes, or preservatives
- pregnant or trying to get pregnant
- breast-feeding

How should I take this medicine?

Take thiothixene capsules by mouth. Follow the directions on the prescription label. Swallow the capsules with a drink of water. If thiothixene upsets your stomach you can take it with food. Take your doses at regular intervals. Do not take your medicine more often than directed. Do not stop taking except on your prescriber's advice. Contact your pediatrician or health care professional regarding the use of this medicine in children. Special care may be needed.

What if I miss a dose?

If you miss a dose, take it as soon as you can. If it is almost time for your next dose, take only that dose. If you take only one dose a day at bedtime and forget, do not take it in the morning without calling your prescriber or health care professional for advice. Do not take double or extra doses.

What may interact with thiothixene?

- alcohol
- antacids
- bromocriptine
- dextroamphetamine
- guanadrel
- guanethidine
- levodopa
- medicine for colds and breathing difficulties
- medicines for movement abnormalities as in Parkinson's disease, or for gastrointestinal problems
- medicines for pain
- medicines for hay fever and other allergies
- medicines for mental depression
- quinidine

Tell your prescriber or health care professional about all other medicines you are taking, including non-prescription medicines, nutritional supplements, or herbal products. Also tell your prescriber or health care professional if you are a frequent user of drinks with caffeine or alcohol, if you smoke, or if you use illegal drugs. These may affect the way your medicine works. Check with your health care professional before stopping or starting any of your medicines.

What should I watch for while taking thiothixene?

Visit your prescriber or health care professional for regular checks on your progress. It may be several weeks before you see the full effects of thiothixene. Do not suddenly stop taking thiothixene. You may need to gradually reduce the dose. Only stop taking thiothixene on your prescriber's advice. You may get dizzy or drowsy. Do not drive, use machinery, or do anything that needs mental alertness until you know how thiothixene affects you. Do not stand or sit up quickly, especially if you are an older patient. This reduces the risk of dizzy or fainting spells. Alcohol can increase dizziness and drowsiness. Avoid alcoholic drinks. You can get a hangover effect the morning after a bedtime dose. Do not treat yourself for colds, diarrhea or allergies. Ask your prescriber or health care professional for advice, some nonprescription medicines may increase possible side effects. Thiothixene may make you more sensitive to sun or ultraviolet light. Keep out of the sun, or wear protective clothing outdoors and use a sunscreen (at least SPF 15). Do not use sun lamps, or sun tanning beds or booths. To protect your eyes wear sunglasses even on cloudy days. Avoid extreme heat or cold. Thiothixene can stop you sweating and increase your body temperature. It can also make your body unable to stand extreme cold. Avoid hot baths and saunas. Be careful about exercising especially in hot weather. Dress warmly in cold weather and do not stay out long in the cold. Thiothixene may make your mouth dry. Chewing sugarless gum or sucking hard candy, and drinking plenty of water will help. Be careful when brushing and flossing your teeth to avoid mouth infections or damage to your gums. See your dentist regularly. Do not take antacids or medicine for diarrhea within 2 hours of taking thiothixene. If you are going to have surgery tell your prescriber or health care professional that you are taking thiothixene.

What side effects may I notice from taking thiothixene?

Side effects that you should report to your prescriber or health care professional as soon as possible:

- changes in vision
- confusion
- difficulty breathing
- difficulty in speaking or swallowing
- difficulty passing urine, or sudden loss of bladder control
- dizziness or lightheadedness, fainting spells
- fast or irregular heartbeat (palpitations)
- fever, chills, or sore throat
- hot, dry skin or lack of sweating
- increased sweating
- loss of balance or difficulty walking
- seizures (convulsions)
- stiffness, spasms, trembling
- uncontrollable tongue or chewing movements, smacking lips or puffing cheeks
- uncontrollable muscle spasms, in the face hands, arms, or legs, twisting body movements
- unusual weakness or tiredness

Side effects that usually do not require medical attention (report to your prescriber or health care professional if they continue or are bothersome):

- anxiety or agitation
- breast pain or swelling
- constipation
- decreased sexual ability
- drowsiness
- dry mouth
- increased sensitivity to the sun (severe sunburn)
- menstrual changes
- nausea or vomiting
- pain or irritation at the injection site
- skin rash
- unusual production of breast milk
- weight gain

Where can I keep my medicine?

Keep out of the reach of children in a container that small children cannot open. Store at room temperature between 15 and 30 degrees C (59 and 86 degrees F). Protect from light. Throw away any unused medicine after the expiration date.

Tiagabine tablets

GABITRIL®;
12 mg; Tablet
Cephalon Inc

GABITRIL®;
4 mg; Tablet
Cephalon Inc

What are tiagabine tablets?

TIAGABINE (Gabitril®) can help to control partial seizures (convulsions) in people with epilepsy. Generic tiagabine tablets are not yet available.

What should my health care professional know before I take tiagabine?

They need to know if you have any of these conditions:
- an alcohol abuse problem
- liver disease
- any unusual or allergic reaction to tiagabine, other medicines, foods, dyes, or preservatives
- pregnant or trying to get pregnant
- breast-feeding

How should I take this medicine?

Take tiagabine tablets by mouth. Tiagabine tablets should be taken with food. Follow the directions on the prescription label. Swallow the tablets with a drink of water. Take your doses at regular intervals. Do not take your medicine more often than directed. Contact your pediatrician or health care professional regarding the use of this medicine in children. Special care may be needed.

What if I miss a dose?

If you miss a dose, take it as soon as you can. If it is almost time for your next dose, take only that dose. Do not take double or extra doses.

What may interact with tiagabine?

- alcohol
- carbamazepine
- medicines used for anxiety or to relax muscles (example: diazepam)
- phenobarbital
- phenytoin
- valproic acid

Tell your prescriber or health care professional about all other medicines you are taking, including non-prescription medicines. Also tell your prescriber or health care professional if you are a frequent user of drinks with caffeine or alcohol, if you smoke, or if you use illegal drugs. These may affect the way your medicine works. Check with your health care professional before stopping or starting any of your medicines.

What should I watch for while taking tiagabine?

Visit your prescriber or health care professional for a regular check on your progress. Do not stop taking tiagabine suddenly. This increases the risk of seizures. Wear a Medic Alert bracelet or necklace. Carry an identification card with information about your condition, medications, and prescriber or health care professional. You may get drowsy or dizzy when you first start taking this medicine. Do not drive, use machinery, or do anything that needs mental alertness until you know how tiagabine affects you. To reduce dizzy or fainting spells, do not sit or stand up quickly, especially if you are an older patient. Alcohol can increase drowsiness and dizziness. Avoid alcoholic drinks. If you are going to have surgery, tell your prescriber or health care professional that you are taking tiagabine.

What side effects may I notice from taking tiagabine?

Side effects that you should report to your prescriber or health care professional as soon as possible:

- confusion
- depression
- difficulty remembering things
- difficulty speaking
- difficulty with movements or with walking
- tingling of the hands or feet
- redness, blistering, peeling or loosening of the skin, including inside the mouth
- skin rash or itching
- sore throat or pain on swallowing
- vomiting
- weakness

Side effects that usually do not require medical attention (report to your prescriber or health care professional if they continue or are bothersome):

- diarrhea
- difficulty concentrating
- difficulty sleeping
- dizziness, drowsiness
- nausea
- nervousness
- skin rash, itching
- stomach upset, indigestion
- tremor

Where can I keep my medicine?

Keep out of reach of children in a container that small children cannot open. Store at room temperature between 20 and 25 degrees C (68 and 77 degrees F). Protect from light or moisture. Throw away any unused medicine after the expiration date.

Ticlopidine tablets

TICLID®;
250 mg; Tablet
Hoffmann La Roche
Inc

TICLOPIDINE;
250 mg; Tablet
Major
Pharmaceuticals Inc

What are ticlopidine tablets?

TICLOPIDINE (Ticlid®) helps to prevent blood clots. Ticlopidine helps to prevent strokes in patients who have already had a stroke, or those who are at high risk of having a stroke. However, ticlopidine should not used in patients who can take aspirin to prevent a stroke. Ticlopidine is also sometimes used to prevent a heart attack in patients who have already had unstable chest pain or a heart attack. It is also sometimes given with aspirin after certain procedures used to open blocked blood vessels leading to the heart. Generic ticlopidine tablets are available.

What should my health care professional know before I take ticlopidine?

They need to know if you have any of the following conditions:

- anemia
- bleeding disorder currently or history of one (including aplastic anemia, hemophilia, or thrombotic thrombocytopenic purpura [TTP])
- blood disease
- high level of cholesterol
- kidney disease
- liver disease
- recent surgery
- stomach ulcer
- an unusual or allergic reaction to ticlopidine, other medicines, foods, dyes, or preservatives
- pregnant or trying to get pregnant
- breast-feeding

How should I take this medicine?

Take ticlopidine tablets by mouth. Follow the directions on the prescription label. Swallow the tablets with a drink of water. Take with food or milk to help absorb ticlopidine into the body and reduce stomach upset. Avoid antacids for 2 hours before and after the dose of ticlopidine. Take your doses at regular intervals. Do not take your medicine more often than directed. Contact your pediatrician or health care professional regarding the use of this medicine in children. Special care may be needed.

What if I miss a dose?

If you miss a dose, take it as soon as you can. If it is almost time for your next dose, take only that dose. Do not take double or extra doses.

What may interact with ticlopidine?

- agents that dissolve blood clots
- antacids
- anti-inflammatory agents (NSAIDs such as ibuprofen)
- aspirin
- blood thinners such as warfarin
- cimetidine
- cilostazol
- clopidogrel
- cyclosporine
- digoxin
- dipyridamole
- fish oil (omega-3 fatty acids) supplements
- herbal or dietary supplements like feverfew, garlic, ginger, ginkgo biloba, and horse chestnut
- phenytoin
- prasterone, dehydroepiandrosterone, DHEA supplements
- theophylline

Tell your prescriber or health care professional about all other medicines you are taking, including non-prescription medicines. Also tell your prescriber or health care professional if you are a frequent user of drinks with caffeine or alcohol, if you smoke, or if you use illegal drugs. These may affect the way your medicine works. Check with your health care professional before stopping or starting any of your medicines.

What should I watch for while taking ticlopidine?

Visit your prescriber or health care professional for regular checks on your progress. Side effects to ticlopidine occur most frequently during the first 3 months of therapy. To make sure you do not develop any problems your health care provider will arrange for you to have blood tests before you start ticlopidine and then every 2 weeks for the first 3 months. It is essential that you keep your appointments for the blood tests. Do not stop taking ticlopidine without your prescriber's advice. If your prescriber decides to stop ticlopidine within the first 3 months, you will still need to have you blood tested for an additional 2 weeks after you have stopped taking ticlopidine. Ticlopidine can cause serious blood problems. This can mean risk of infection or bleeding. Avoid activities that increase your risk of bleeding. Tell your prescriber or health care professional at once if you have any unusual bleeding or bruise easily or an infection that will not get better. Problems can arise if you need dental work, and in the day to day care of your teeth. Try to avoid damage to your teeth and gums when you brush or floss your teeth. Inform your dentist you are taking ticlopidine prior to any appointment or procedure. Ask your prescriber or health care professional before you take non-prescription pain relievers. Do not take aspirin, aspirin-containing products, or anti-inflammatory drugs such as ibuprofen, ketoprofen, naproxen unless directed to do so by your prescriber or health care professional. If you are going to have sur-gery, tell your prescriber or health care professional that you are taking ticlopidine.

What side effects may I notice from taking ticlopidine?

Side effects that you should report to your prescriber or health care professional as soon as possible:
- low blood counts—ticlopidine may decrease the number of white blood cells and/or platelets. You may be at increased risk for infections and bleeding.
- signs of infection—fever or chills, cough, sore throat, pain or difficulty passing urine
- signs of decreased platelets or bleeding—bruising, pinpoint red spots on the skin, black, tarry stools, blood in the urine, nose bleeds, bleeding gums
- dark yellow or brown urine
- difficulty breathing or wheezing
- joint pain or swelling
- paleness
- ringing in the ears
- skin rash or itching (hives)
- stomach pain
- unusually heavy menstrual bleeding
- unusual tiredness or weakness
- weakness on a side of the body
- yellowing of skin or eyes

Side effects that usually do not require medical attention (report to your prescriber or health care professional if they continue or are bothersome):
- decreased appetite
- diarrhea
- headache
- indigestion
- nausea, vomiting
- stomach pain, bloating, or discomfort

Where can I keep my medicine?
Keep out of the reach of children in a container that small children cannot open. Store at room temperature between 15 and 30 degrees C (59 and 86 degrees F). Throw away any unused medicine after the expiration date.

Tiludronate tablets

What are tiludronate tablets?
TILUDRONATE (Skelid®) reduces the release and breakdown of calcium from bone. It helps to prevent bone loss and to increase normal healthy bone production in patients with Paget's disease. Generic tiludronate tablets are not available.

What should my health care professional know before I take tiludronate?
They need to know if you have any of these conditions:
- kidney disease
- stomach, intestinal, or esophageal problems
- an unusual or allergic reaction to tiludronate, other medicines, foods, dyes, or preservatives

- pregnant or trying to get pregnant
- breast-feeding

How should I take this medicine?
Take tiludronate tablets by mouth. Follow the directions on the prescription label. Swallow the tablets with 6 to 8 fluid ounces of water. Do not eat or drink anything before you take your tablets and do not eat food for at least 2 hours afterward. To avoid irritation of the esophagus (tube connecting mouth to stomach), do not lay down for at least 30 minutes after taking this drug. Do not take at the same time as vitamins with minerals such as iron or calcium, or antacids containing calcium, magnesium, or aluminum. Try to take your

tablets at the same time each day. Do not take your medicine more often than directed. Contact your pediatrician or health care professional regarding the use of this medicine in children. Special care may be needed.

What if I miss a dose?

If you miss a dose, take it as soon as you can if you have not already eaten. If you have already eaten, call your prescriber or health care professional for advice. Do not take double or extra doses.

What may interact with tiludronate?

- aluminum salts
- antacids
- aspirin
- calcium supplements
- indomethacin
- iron supplements
- magnesium supplements
- parathyroid hormone
- teriparatide

Tell your prescriber or health care professional about all other medicines you are taking including non-prescription medicines. Also tell your prescriber or health care professional if you are a frequent user of drinks with caffeine or alcohol, if you smoke, or if you use illegal drugs. These can affect the way your medicine works. Check with your health care professional before stopping or starting any of your medicines.

What should I watch for while taking tiludronate?

Visit your prescriber or health care professional for regular checks on your progress. If you have Paget's disease it may be some time before you see the benefit from tiludronate. Your prescriber or health care professional may order regular blood tests or other tests to check on your progress. You should make sure you get enough calcium and vitamin D in your diet while you are taking tiludronate, unless directed otherwise by your health care provider. Discuss your dietary needs with your prescriber or health care professional or nutritionist. If you get bone pain or a worsening of bone pain, check with your prescriber or health care professional. If you are taking an antacid, a mineral supplement, aspirin, or indomethacin, make sure that there is an interval of at least 2 hours before or after taking tiludronate. Do not take at the same time.

What side effects might I notice from taking tiludronate?

Side effects that you should report to your prescriber or health care professional as soon as possible:
Rare or uncommon:
- black or tarry stools
- difficulty swallowing
- eye inflammation, pain, or vision change
- numbness or tingling in the hands or feet
- redness, blistering, peeling or loosening of the skin, including inside the mouth
- skin rash, itching (hives)
- swelling of the lips, arms, legs, face, tongue, or throat
- vomiting
- worsening of bone pain

Side effects that usually do not require medical attention (report to your prescriber or health care professional if they continue or are bothersome):
- diarrhea or constipation
- headache
- indigestion or stomach gas
- nausea

Where can I keep my medicine?

Keep out of the reach of children in a container that small children cannot open. Store at room temperature between 15 and 30 degrees C (59 and 86 degrees F). Throw away any unused medicine after the expiration date.

Timolol tablets

BLOCADREN®;
5 mg; Tablet
Merck and Co Inc

BLOCADREN®;
10 mg; Tablet
Merck and Co Inc

What are timolol tablets?

TIMOLOL (Blocadren®) belongs to a group of medicines called beta-blockers. Beta-blockers reduce the workload on the heart and help it to beat more regularly. Timolol controls, but does not cure, high blood pressure (hypertension). High blood pressure may not make you feel sick, but it can lead to serious heart problems. Timolol can be used to improve symptoms in patients with heart disease. It is sometimes given after a heart attack to reduce heart-related adverse events. Timolol is also used to prevent migraine headaches. Generic timolol tablets are available.

What should my health care professional know before I take timolol?

They need to know if you have any of these conditions:
- angina (chest pain)
- asthma, bronchitis or bronchospasm
- circulation problems, or blood vessel disease (such as Raynaud's disease)
- depression
- diabetes
- emphysema, or other lung disease
- history of heart attack or heart failure
- kidney disease
- liver disease

- low blood pressure
- muscle weakness or disease
- pheochromocytoma
- psoriasis
- thyroid disease
- an unusual or allergic reaction to timolol, other beta-blockers, medicines, foods, dyes, or preservatives
- pregnant or trying to get pregnant
- breast-feeding

How should I take this medicine?

Take timolol tablets by mouth. Follow the directions on the prescription label. Swallow the tablets with a drink of water. Take your doses at regular intervals. Do not take your medicine more often than directed. Do not stop taking except on your prescriber's advice. This medicine is not for use in children.

What if I miss a dose?

If you miss a dose, take it as soon as you can. If it is almost time for your next dose (less than 4 hours), take only that dose. Do not take double or extra doses.

What may interact with timolol?

- anti-inflammatory drugs (NSAIDs, such as ibuprofen)
- atropine
- cimetidine
- clonidine
- cocaine
- ergotamine
- hawthorn
- levodopa
- medicines for high blood pressure
- medicines for colds and breathing difficulties
- medicines for diabetes
- medicines for mental depression
- medicines for mental problems and psychotic disturbances
- medicines to control heart rhythm
- theophylline
- water pills

Tell your prescriber or health care professional about all other medicines you are taking, including nonprescription medicines, nutritional supplements, or herbal products. Also tell your prescriber or health care professional if you are a frequent user of drinks with caffeine or alcohol, if you smoke, or if you use illegal drugs. These may affect the way your medicine works. Check with your health care professional before stopping or starting any of your medicines.

What should I watch for while taking timolol?

Check your heart rate and blood pressure regularly while you are taking timolol. Ask your prescriber or health care professional what your heart rate and blood pressure should be while taking this drug. Do not stop taking this medicine suddenly. This could lead to serious heart-related effects. You may get drowsy or dizzy. Do not drive, use machinery, or do anything that requires mental alertness until you know how timolol affects you. To reduce the risk of dizzy or fainting spells, do not sit or stand up quickly. Alcohol can make you more drowsy, and increase flushing and rapid heartbeats. Therefore, it is best to avoid alcoholic drinks. Timolol can affect blood sugar levels. If you have diabetes, check with your prescriber or health care professional before you change your diet or the dose of your diabetic medicine. If you are going to have surgery, tell your prescriber or health care professional that you are taking timolol.

What side effects may I notice from taking timolol?

Side effects that you should report to your prescriber or health care professional as soon as possible:

- changes in blood sugar
- cold hands or feet
- confusion, hallucinations (seeing and hearing things that are not really there)
- difficulty breathing, wheezing
- difficulty sleeping, nightmares
- dizziness or fainting spells
- irregular heartbeat, palpitations, chest pain
- skin rash, itching, peeling skin
- slow heart rate (less than 50 beats per minute)
- swelling of the legs or ankles
- vomiting

Side effects that usually do not require medical attention (report to your prescriber or health care professional if they continue or are bothersome):

- dark colored skin
- diarrhea
- dry sore eyes
- hair loss
- nausea
- sexual difficulties (impotence or decreased sexual urges)
- weakness or tiredness

Where can I keep my medicine?

Keep out of the reach of children in a container that small children cannot open. Store at room temperature between 15 and 30 degrees C (59 and 86 degrees F). Protect from light. Keep container tightly closed. Throw away any unused medicine after the expiration date.

Tinidazole tablets

TINDAMAX®;
250 mg; Tablet
Presutti
Laboratories, Inc

TINDAMAX®;
500 mg; Tablet
Presutti
Laboratories, Inc

What are tinidazole tablets?

TINIDAZOLE (Tindamax®) kills or prevents the growth of certain bacteria and protozoa (single cell organisms). Tinidazole is used to treat trichomoniasis (a sexually transmitted disease), giardiasis, and amebiasis. It is also prescribed for other types of infections. Generic tinidazole tablets are not available.

What should my health care professional know before I take tinidazole?

They need to know if you have any of these conditions:
- if you drink alcoholic beverages
- anemia or other blood disorders
- liver disease
- nervous system disease
- seizures (convulsions)
- other chronic illness
- an unusual reaction to tinidazole, other medicines, foods, dyes, or preservatives
- pregnant or trying to get pregnant
- breast-feeding

How should I take this medicine?

Take tinidazole tablets by mouth. Follow the directions on the prescription label. Swallow tablets whole with a full glass of water. Take this medicine with food to prevent stomach upset. Take your doses at regular intervals. Do not take your medicine more often than directed. Finish the full course prescribed by your prescriber or health care professional even if you think your condition is better. Do not stop taking except on your prescriber's advice. Contact your pediatrician or health care professional regarding the use of this medicine in children. Special care may be needed.

What if I miss a dose?

If you miss a dose, take it as soon as you can. If it is almost time for your next dose, take only that dose. Do not take double or extra doses.

What may interact with tinidazole?

- alcohol or alcohol-containing beverages or medicines
- amprenavir
- barbiturate medicines for inducing sleep or treating seizures (convulsions)
- carbamazepine
- cimetidine
- disulfiram
- fluorouracil
- lithium
- phenytoin
- sirolimus
- tacrolimus
- warfarin

Tell your prescriber or health care professional about all other medicines you are taking, including non-prescription medicines, nutritional supplements, or herbal products. Also tell your prescriber or health care professional if you are a frequent user of drinks with caffeine or alcohol, if you smoke, or if you use illegal drugs. These may affect the way your medicine works. Check with your health care professional before stopping or starting any of your medicines.

What should I watch for while taking tinidazole?

Tell your prescriber or health care professional if your symptoms do not improve in 2 or 3 days. If you are taking this medicine for a long time you must visit your prescriber or health care professional for regular blood checks. Avoid alcoholic drinks while you are taking tinidazole and for 3 days afterward. Alcohol may make you dizzy, feel sick, and flushed; give you headaches and stomach pains. You may get drowsy or dizzy. Do not drive, use machinery, or do anything that needs mental alertness until you know how tinidazole affects you. To reduce the risk of dizzy or fainting spells, do not sit or stand up quickly, especially if you are an older patient. Your mouth may get dry. Chewing sugarless gum or sucking hard candy, and drinking plenty of water will help. If you are being treated for a sexually transmitted disease, your sexual partner may also need treatment. You can use a condom to stop reinfection of you or your sexual partner. If you are going to have surgery, tell your prescriber or health care professional that you are using tinidazole.

What side effects may I notice from taking tinidazole?

Side effects that you should report to your prescriber or health care professional as soon as possible:
Rare or uncommon:
- clumsiness, dizziness, or unsteadiness
- fever
- numbness, tingling, pain or weakness in the hands or feet
- seizures (convulsions)
- skin rash, itching
- vomiting or severe stomach pain

More common:
- unusual tiredness or weakness
- increased vaginal discharge

Side effects that usually do not require medical attention (report to your prescriber or health care professional if they continue or are bothersome):

- dark brown or reddish urine
- change in taste (metal taste in mouth)
- diarrhea
- headache
- loss of appetite
- nausea
- mild stomach pain or cramps

Where can I keep my medicine?

Keep out of the reach of children in a container that small children cannot open. Store at room temperature between 15 and 30 degrees C (59 and 86 degrees F). Protect from light. Keep container tightly closed. Throw away any unused medicine after the expiration date.

Tizanidine tablets or capsules

ZANAFLEX®; 4 mg; Tablet Elan Pharmaceuticals Inc		TIZANIDINE; 4 mg; Tablet Par Pharmaceutical Inc	

What are tizanidine tablets or capsules?

TIZANIDINE (Zanaflex®) is a drug used to relax certain muscles. It can help to relieve, but not cure muscle spasms (or muscle tightening) caused by medical problems such as multiple sclerosis or injuries to the brain or spine. Generic tizanidine tablets or capsules are available.

What should my health care professional know before I take tizanidine?

They need to know if you have any of these conditions:
- heart or blood vessel disease
- kidney disease
- liver disease
- low blood pressure
- mental disorder
- an unusual or allergic reaction to tizanidine, other medicines, foods, dyes, or preservatives
- pregnant or trying to get pregnant
- breast-feeding

How should I take this medicine?

Take tizanidine tablets or capsules by mouth. Follow the directions on the prescription label. Swallow the tablets or capsules with a drink of water. Do not take with food until you have talked with your health care provider. Food can change the amount of tizanidine absorbed by the body. This can cause tizanidine not to work for you or to cause more side effects. Take your doses at regular intervals. Do not take your medicine more often than directed. Check with your prescriber or health care professional before stopping your medicine; gradual dosage reduction may be needed. Contact your pediatrician or health care professional regarding the use of this medicine in children. Special care may be needed. Older patients (>65 years) may have a stronger reaction to this medicine and may need smaller doses.

What if I miss a dose?

If you miss a dose, take it as soon as you can. If it is almost time for your next dose, take only that dose. Do not take double or extra doses.

What may interact with tizanidine?

- acetaminophen
- alcohol
- antihistamine medicines for colds, hay fever, or allergies
- baclofen
- benzodiazepine or sedative medicines for treating anxiety or to induce sleep
- barbiturate medicines for inducing sleep or treating seizures (convulsions)
- birth control pills
- medicines for high blood pressure
- medicines for mental depression or other mental disorders
- medicines for pain such codeine, morphine, hydrocodone and others
- phenytoin or fosphenytoin
- rofecoxib

Tell your prescriber or health care professional about all other medicines you are taking, including non-prescription medicines, nutritional supplements, or herbal products. Also tell your prescriber or health care professional if you are a frequent user of drinks with caffeine or alcohol, if you smoke, or if you use illegal drugs. These may affect the way your medicine works. Check with your health care professional before stopping or starting any of your medicines.

What should I watch for while taking tizanidine?

Visit your prescriber or health care professional for regular checks on your progress.

Do not suddenly stop taking tizanidine. Ask your prescriber or health care professional for advice on how to gradually reduce the dose of your medicine, before stopping completely. You may get drowsy or dizzy. Do not drive, use machinery, or do anything that needs mental alertness until you know how tizanidine affects you. To avoid dizzy or fainting spells, do not stand or sit up quickly, especially if you are an older person. Alcohol can make you more drowsy and dizzy. Avoid alcoholic drinks. Your mouth may get dry. Chewing sugarless gum or sucking hard candy, and drinking plenty of water will help. Do not treat yourself for coughs, colds or allergies without asking your prescriber or health care professional for advice. Some ingredients (antihistamines) can cause drowsiness which may be additive with tizanidine. If you are going to have surgery tell your prescriber or health care professional that you are taking tizanidine.

What side effects may I notice from taking tizanidine?

Taking too high of a dose of tizanidine can cause side effects. Ask your prescriber or health care professional before you reduce your dose, or stop taking tizanidine. Side effects that you should report to your prescriber or health care professional as soon as possible:
- confusion
- dizziness or fainting spells
- excitability, nervousness
- low blood pressure
- nausea or vomiting
- slow or irregular heartbeat, palpitations, or chest pain
- stomach pain

- unusual or persistent rash
- unusual tiredness or weakness
- yellowing of the skin or eyes

Side effects that usually do not require medical attention (report to your prescriber or health care professional if they continue or are bothersome):
- blurred vision
- constipation
- drowsiness
- dry mouth
- tiredness or weakness

Where can I keep my medicine?

Keep out of the reach of children in a container that small children cannot open. Store at room temperature between 15 and 30 degrees C (59 and 86 degrees F). Protect from light. Keep container tightly closed. Throw away any unused medicine after the expiration date.

Tolazamide tablets

TOLINASE®;
100 mg; Tablet
Pharmacia and
Upjohn Div Pfizer

TOLINASE®;
500 mg; Tablet
Pharmacia and
Upjohn Div Pfizer

What are tolazamide tablets?

TOLAZAMIDE (Tolinase®) helps to treat type 2 diabetes mellitus. Treatment is combined with a suitable diet and balanced exercise. Tolazamide increases the amount of insulin released from the pancreas and helps your body to use insulin more efficiently. Generic tolazamide tablets are available.

What should my health care professional know before I take tolazamide?

They need to know if you have any of these conditions:
- kidney disease
- liver disease
- major surgery
- severe infection or injury
- thyroid disease
- an unusual or allergic reaction to tolazamide, sulfonylureas, other medicines, foods, dyes, or preservatives
- pregnant or trying to get pregnant
- breast-feeding

How should I take this medicine?

Take tolazamide tablets by mouth. Follow the directions on the prescription label. Swallow the tablets with a drink of water. If you take tolazamide once a day, take it with breakfast or the first main meal. Take your doses at the same time each day; do not take more often than directed. Contact your pediatrician or health care professional regarding the use of this medicine in children. Special care may be needed. Elderly patients over 65 years old may have a stronger reaction and need a smaller dose.

What if I miss a dose?

If you miss a dose, take it as soon as you can. If it is almost time for your next dose, take only that dose. Do not take double or extra doses

What may interact with tolazamide?

- alcohol
- beta-blockers (used for high blood pressure or heart conditions)
- bosentan
- cisapride
- clofibrate
- diazoxide
- medicines for fungal or yeast infections (examples: itraconazole, miconazole, voriconazole)
- metoclopramide
- rifampin
- warfarin (a blood thinner)

Many medications may cause changes (increase or decrease) in blood sugar, these include:

- alcohol containing beverages
- aspirin and aspirin-like drugs
- beta-blockers, often used for high blood pressure or heart problems (examples include atenolol, metoprolol, propranolol)
- chromium
- female hormones, such as estrogens or progestins, birth control pills
- isoniazid
- male hormones or anabolic steroids
- medications for weight loss
- medicines for allergies, asthma, cold, or cough
- niacin
- pentamidine
- phenytoin
- quinolone antibiotics (examples: ciprofloxacin, levofloxacin, ofloxacin)
- some herbal dietary supplements
- steroid medicines such as prednisone or cortisone
- thyroid hormones
- water pills (diuretics)

Tell your prescriber or health care professional about all other medicines you are taking, including non-prescription medicines, nutritional supplements, or herbal products. Also tell your prescriber or health care professional if you are a frequent user of drinks with caffeine or alcohol, if you smoke, or if you use illegal drugs. These may affect the way your medicine works. Check with your health care professional before stopping or starting any of your medicines.

What should I watch for while taking tolazamide?

Visit your prescriber or health care professional for regular checks on your progress. Learn how to monitor blood or urine sugar and urine ketones regularly. Check with your prescriber or health care professional if your blood sugar is high; you may need a change of dose of tolazamide. Do not skip meals. If you are exercising much more than usual you may need extra snacks to avoid side effects caused by low blood sugar. If you have mild symptoms of low blood sugar, eat or drink something containing sugar at once and contact your prescriber or health care professional. It is wise to check your blood sugar to confirm that it is low. It is important to recognize your own symptoms of low blood sugar so that you can treat them quickly. Make sure family members know that you can choke if you eat or drink when you have serious symptoms, such as seizures or coma. They must get medical help at once. Alcohol can increase possible side effects of tolazamide. Ask your prescriber or health care professional if you should avoid alcohol. Tolazamide can increase the sensitivity of your skin to the sun. Keep out of the sun, or wear protective clothing outdoors and use a sunscreen. Do not use sun lamps or sun tanning beds or booths. If you are going to have surgery, tell your prescriber or health care professional that you are taking tolazamide. Wear a medical identification bracelet or chain to say you have diabetes, and carry a card that lists all your medications.

What side effects may I notice from taking tolazamide?

Side effects that you should report to your prescriber or health care professional as soon as possible:
- hypoglycemia (low blood glucose) which can cause symptoms such as anxiety or nervousness, confusion, difficulty concentrating, hunger, pale skin, nausea, fatigue, perspiration, headache, palpitations, numbness of the mouth, tingling in the fingers, tremors, muscle weakness, blurred vision, cold sensations, uncontrolled yawning, irritability, rapid heartbeat, shallow breathing, and loss of consciousness.
- breathing difficulties, severe skin reactions or excessive phlegm, which may indicate that you are having an allergic reaction to the drug.
- dark yellow or brown urine, or yellowing of the eyes or skin, indicating that the drug is affecting your liver.
- fever, chills, sore throat; which means the drug may be affecting your immune system.
- unusual bleeding or bruising; which occurs when the drug is affecting your blood clotting system.

Side effects that usually do not require medical attention (report to your prescriber or health care professional if they continue or are bothersome):
- dizziness
- fatigue
- headache
- heartburn, stomach discomfort
- increased sensitivity to the sun
- nausea, vomiting
- skin rash, redness, swelling or itching

Where can I keep my medicine?

Keep out of the reach of children in a container that small children cannot open. Store at room temperature between 15 and 30 degrees C (59 and 86 degrees F). Keep container tightly closed. Throw away any unused medicine after the expiration date.

Tolbutamide tablets

ORINASE®;
500 mg; Tablet
Pharmacia and
Upjohn Div Pfizer

TOLBUTAMIDE;
500 mg; Tablet
Mylan
Pharmaceuticals Inc

What are tolbutamide tablets?

TOLBUTAMIDE (Orinase®) helps to treat type 2 diabetes mellitus. Treatment is combined with a suitable diet and balanced exercise. Tolbutamide increases the amount of insulin released from the pancreas and helps your body to use insulin more efficiently. Generic tolbutamide tablets are available.

What should my health care professional know before I take tolbutamide?

They need to know if you have any of these conditions:
- kidney disease
- liver disease
- major surgery
- severe infection or injury
- thyroid disease
- an unusual or allergic reaction to tolbutamide or other medicines, foods, dyes, or preservatives
- pregnant or trying to get pregnant
- breast-feeding

How should I take this medicine?

Take tolbutamide tablets by mouth. Follow the directions on the prescription label. Swallow the tablets with a drink of water. It is best to take tolbutamide after meals. Take your doses at the same time each day; do not take more often than directed. Contact your pediatrician or health care professional regarding the use of this medicine in children. Special care may be needed. Elderly patients over 65 years old may have a stronger reaction and need a smaller dose.

What if I miss a dose?

If you miss a dose, take it as soon as you can. If it is almost time for your next dose, take only that dose. Do not take double or extra doses.

What may interact with tolbutamide?

- alcohol
- beta-blockers (used for high blood pressure or heart conditions)
- bosentan
- chloramphenicol
- cisapride
- clofibrate
- diazoxide
- medicines for fungal or yeast infections (examples: itraconazole, miconazole, voriconazole)
- metoclopramide
- rifampin
- warfarin (a blood thinner)

Many medications may cause changes (increase or decrease) in blood sugar, these include:

- alcohol containing beverages
- aspirin and aspirin-like drugs
- beta-blockers, often used for high blood pressure or heart problems (examples include atenolol, metoprolol, propranolol)
- chromium
- female hormones, such as estrogens or progestins, birth control pills
- isoniazid
- male hormones or anabolic steroids
- medications for weight loss
- medicines for allergies, asthma, cold, or cough
- niacin
- pentamidine
- phenytoin
- quinolone antibiotics (examples: ciprofloxacin, levofloxacin, ofloxacin)
- some herbal dietary supplements
- steroid medicines such as prednisone or cortisone
- thyroid hormones
- water pills (diuretics)

Tell your prescriber or health care professional about all other medicines you are taking, including non-prescription medicines, nutritional supplements, or herbal products. Also tell your prescriber or health care professional if you are a frequent user of drinks with caffeine or alcohol, if you smoke, or if you use illegal drugs. These may affect the way your medicine works. Check with your health care professional before stopping or starting any of your medicines.

What should I watch for while taking tolbutamide?

Visit your prescriber or health care professional for regular checks on your progress. Learn how to monitor blood or urine sugar and urine ketones regularly. Check with

your prescriber or health care professional if your blood sugar is high; you may need a change of dose of tolbutamide. Do not skip meals. If you are exercising much more than usual you may need extra snacks to avoid side effects caused by low blood sugar. If you have mild symptoms of low blood sugar, eat or drink something containing sugar at once and contact your prescriber or health care professional. It is wise to check your blood sugar to confirm that it is low. It is important to recognize your own symptoms of low blood sugar so that you can treat them quickly. Make sure family members know that you can choke if you eat or drink when you have serious symptoms, such as seizures or coma. They must get medical help at once. Alcohol can increase possible side effects of tolbutamide. Ask your prescriber or health care professional if you should avoid alcohol. Tolbutamide can increase the sensitivity of your skin to the sun. Keep out of the sun, or wear protective clothing outdoors and use a sunscreen. Do not use sun lamps or sun tanning beds or booths. If you are going to have surgery, tell your prescriber or health care professional that you are taking tolbutamide. Wear a medical identification bracelet or chain to say you have diabetes, and carry a card that lists all your medications.

What side effects may I notice from taking tolbutamide?

Side effects that you should report to your prescriber or health care professional as soon as possible:

- hypoglycemia (low blood glucose) which can cause symptoms such as anxiety or nervousness, confusion, difficulty concentrating, hunger, pallor, nausea, fatigue, perspiration, headache, palpitations, numbness of the mouth, tingling in the fingers, tremors, muscle weakness, blurred vision, cold sensations, uncontrolled yawning, irritability, rapid heartbeat, shallow breathing, and loss of consciousness.
- breathing difficulties or excessive phlegm, which may indicate that you are having an allergic reaction to the drug.
- dark yellow or brown urine, or yellowing of the eyes or skin, indicating that the drug is affecting your liver.
- fever, chills, sore throat; which means the drug may be affecting your immune system.
- unusual bleeding or bruising; which occurs when the drug is affecting your blood clotting system.

Side effects that usually do not require medical attention (report to your prescriber or health care professional if they continue or are bothersome):

- diarrhea
- headache
- heartburn, stomach discomfort
- increased sensitivity to the sun
- nausea, vomiting
- skin rash, redness, swelling or itching

Where can I keep my medicine?

Keep out of the reach of children in a container that small children cannot open. Store at room temperature between 15 and 30 degrees C (59 and 86 degrees F). Keep container tightly closed. Throw away any unused medicine after the expiration date.

Tolcapone tablets

TASMAR®;
100 mg; Tablet
Valeant
Pharmaceuticals

TASMAR®;
200 mg; Tablet
Valeant
Pharmaceuticals

What are tolcapone tablets?

TOLCAPONE (Tasmar®) is used in combination with levodopa-carbidopa (Sinemet® or others) to treat Parkinson's disease. Generic tolcapone tablets are not yet available.

What should my health care professional know before I take tolcapone?

They need to know if you have any of these conditions:
- anorexia
- dizzy or fainting spells
- kidney or liver disease
- low blood pressure
- an unusual or allergic reaction to other medicines, foods, dyes, or preservatives
- pregnant or trying to get pregnant
- breast-feeding

How should I take this medicine?

Take tolcapone tablets by mouth. Follow the directions on the prescription label. Swallow the tablets with a drink of water. Take your doses at regular intervals. Do not take your medicine more often than directed. Do not stop taking tolcapone except on your prescriber's advice.

What if I miss a dose?

If you miss a dose, take it as soon as you can. If it is almost time for your next dose, take only that dose. Do not take double or extra doses.

What may interact with tolcapone?

- apomorphine
- dobutamine
- furazolidone
- isocarboxazid
- isoproterenol
- linezolid
- methyldopa
- phenelzine
- procarbazine
- tranylcypromine
- warfarin

Tell your prescriber or health care professional about all other medicines you are taking, including non-prescription medicines. Also tell your prescriber or health care professional if you are a frequent user of drinks with caffeine or alcohol, if you smoke, or if you use illegal drugs. These may affect the way your medicine works. Check with your health care professional before stopping or starting any of your medicines.

What should I watch for while taking tolcapone?

Tolcapone may also increase the side effects caused by levodopa-carbidopa such as nausea or restless movements. If you notice an increase in or the appearance of certain side effects that occurred only while you were taking levodopa-carbidopa, contact your physician. The dose of levodopa-carbidopa may need to be lowered. Visit your prescriber or health care professional for regular checks on your progress. Your health care professional will need to frequently monitor blood tests to check the effects of tolcapone on the function of your liver. In rare cases tolcapone has caused liver injury. Your health care professional will monitor you closely and will want any unusual side effects reported to them as soon as possible. It may be several weeks before you feel the full effect of tolcapone. Continue to take your medicine on a regular schedule and do not stop taking except on your prescriber's advice. You may get dizzy or have difficulty controlling your movements. Do not drive, use machinery, or do anything that needs mental alertness until you know how tolcapone affects you. Do not stand or sit up quickly, especially if you are an older patient. This reduces the risk of dizzy or fainting spells. Alcohol can increase possible dizziness; avoid alcoholic drinks. If you are going to have surgery, tell your prescriber or health care professional that you are taking tolcapone. Tolcapone may make your mouth dry. Chewing sugarless gum, sucking hard candy and drinking plenty of water may help. Visit your dentist regularly.

What side effects may I notice from taking tolcapone?

Side effects that you should report to your prescriber or health care professional as soon as possible:
- abdominal pain
- anorexia or loss of appetite
- confusion
- fainting spells or lightheadedness
- fever
- hallucinations
- involuntary muscle movements
- severe diarrhea
- urine that is dark yellow or brown in color
- vomiting or nausea that does not go away
- yellowing of the skin or eyes

Side effects that usually do not require medical attention (report to your prescriber or health care professional if they continue or are bothersome):
- constipation
- difficulty sleeping or excessive dreaming
- dizziness
- drowsiness
- dry mouth

- fatigue
- headache
- increased sweating
- muscle cramping
- nausea
- upset stomach

Tolmetin tablets or capsules

TOLECTIN®;
600 mg; Tablet
OMP Div, Ortho-
McNeil
Pharmaceuticals

TOLECTIN®;
400 mg; Capsule
OMP Div, Ortho-
McNeil
Pharmaceuticals

This drug requires an FDA medication guide. See page xxxvii.

What are tolmetin tablets or capsules?

TOLMETIN (Tolectin®) is a nonsteroidal anti-inflammatory drug (NSAID). It helps relieve pain and inflammation associated with rheumatoid arthritis, osteoarthritis, and juvenile (childhood) arthritis. Generic tolmetin tablets and capsules are available.

What should my health care professional know before I take tolmetin?

They need to know if you have any of these conditions:
- anemia
- asthma, especially aspirin sensitive asthma
- bleeding problems or taking medicines that make you bleed more easily such as anticoagulants ("blood thinners")
- cigarette smoker
- diabetes
- drink more than 3 alcohol-containing beverages a day
- heart failure
- high blood pressure
- kidney disease
- liver disease
- stomach or duodenal ulcers
- systemic lupus erythematosus
- ulcerative colitis
- an unusual or allergic reaction to aspirin, other salicylates, other NSAIDs, other medicines, foods, dyes or preservatives
- pregnant or trying to get pregnant
- breast-feeding

How should I take this medicine?

Take tolmetin tablets or capsules by mouth. Follow the directions on the prescription label. Swallow tablets or capsules whole with a full glass of water; take tablets or capsules in an upright or sitting position. Taking a sip of water first, before taking the tablets or capsules, may help you swallow them. If possible take bedtime doses at least 10 minutes before lying down. You can take tolmetin with food to prevent stomach upset. Take your doses at regular intervals. Do not take your medicine more often than directed. Contact your pediatrician or health care professional regarding the use of this medicine in children. Special care may be

Where can I keep my medicine?

Keep out of the reach of children in a container that small children cannot open. Store at room temperature between 20 and 25 degrees C (68 and 77 degrees F) in tight containers. Throw away any unused medicine after the expiration date.

needed. Do not give to children less than 2 years of age unless directed by your health care provider.

What if I miss a dose?

If you miss a dose, take it as soon as you can. If it is almost time for your next dose, take only that dose. Do not take double or extra doses.

What may interact with tolmetin?

- alcohol
- anti-inflammatory drugs (such as other NSAIDs or prednisone)
- aspirin and aspirin-like medicines
- cidofovir
- cyclosporine
- entecavir
- herbal products that contain feverfew, garlic, ginger, or ginkgo biloba
- lithium
- medicines for high blood pressure
- medicines that affect platelets
- medicines that treat or prevent blood clots such as warfarin and other "blood thinners"
- methotrexate
- pemetrexed
- sodium bicarbonate-containing antacid
- water pills (diuretics)

Tell your prescriber or health care professional about all other medicines you are taking, including non-prescription medicines, nutritional supplements, or herbal products. Also tell your prescriber or health care professional if you are a frequent user of drinks with caffeine or alcohol, if you smoke, or if you use illegal drugs. These may affect the way your medicine works. Check with your health care professional before stopping or starting any of your medicines.

What should I watch for while taking tolmetin?

Let your prescriber or health care professional know if your pain continues. Do not take other pain-killers with tolmetin without advice. If you get flu-like symptoms (fever, chills, muscle aches and pains), call your prescriber or health care professional; do not treat yourself. To reduce unpleasant effects on your throat and stomach, take tolmetin with a full glass of water and never just before lying down. If you notice black, tarry stools or experience severe stomach pain and/or vomit blood or what looks like coffee grounds, notify your health care prescriber immediately. You may get dizzy. Do not drive, use machinery, or do anything that needs mental alertness until you know how tolmetin affects you. Do not sit or stand up quickly, especially if you are an older patient. Standing and sitting up slowly reduces the risk of dizzy or fainting spells. Do not smoke cigarettes or drink alcohol; these increase irritation to your stomach and can make it more susceptible to damage from tolmetin. If you are taking medicines that affect the clotting of your blood, such as aspirin or blood thinners such as Coumadin®, talk to your health care provider or prescriber before taking tolmetin. It is especially important not to use tolmetin during the last 3 months of pregnancy unless specifically directed to do so by your health care provider. Tolmetin may cause problems in the unborn child or complications during delivery. If you are going to have surgery, tell your prescriber or health care professional that you are taking tolmetin. Problems can arise if you need dental work, and in the day to day care of your teeth. Try to avoid damage to your teeth and gums when you brush or floss your teeth.

What side effects may I notice from taking tolmetin?

Side effects that you should report to your prescriber or health care professional as soon as possible:

- signs of bleeding—bruising, pinpoint red spots on the skin, black tarry stools, blood in the urine, unusual tiredness or weakness, vomiting blood or vomit that looks like coffee grounds
- signs of an allergic reaction—difficulty breathing or wheezing, skin rash, redness, blistering or peeling skin, hives, or itching, swelling of eyelids, throat, lips
- blurred vision
- change in the amount of urine passed
- difficulty swallowing, severe heartburn or burning, pain in throat
- pain or difficulty passing urine
- stomach pain or cramps
- swelling of feet or ankles
- yellowing of the eyes or skin

Side effects that usually do not require medical attention (report to your prescriber or health care professional if they continue or are bothersome):

- diarrhea or constipation
- dizziness
- drowsiness
- gas or heartburn
- headache
- nausea, vomiting

Where can I keep my medicine?

Keep out of the reach of children in a container that small children cannot open. Store at room temperature between 15 and 30 degrees C (59 and 86 degrees F). Protect from light. Keep container tightly closed. Throw away any unused medicine after the expiration date.

Tolterodine tablets or extended-release capsules

DETROL®; 2 mg; Tablet Pharmacia and Upjohn Div Pfizer

DETROL® LA; 4 mg; Capsule, Extended Release Pharmacia and Upjohn Div Pfizer

What are tolterodine tablets or extended-release capsules?

TOLTERODINE (Detrol® tablets and Detrol® LA extended-release capsules) help to control an overactive bladder, a chronic condition that can be improved with medication. Tolterodine may reduce the frequency of bathroom visits and may help to control wetting accidents. Generic tolterodine tablets and capsules are not yet available.

What should my health care professional know before I take tolterodine?

They need to know if you have any of these conditions:
- difficulty passing urine
- glaucoma
- intestinal obstruction
- kidney disease
- liver disease
- stomach problems like pyloric stenosis or reflux, or other problems with proper emptying of the contents of the stomach

- an unusual or allergic reaction to tolterodine, other medicines, foods, dyes, or preservatives
- pregnant or trying to get pregnant
- breast-feeding

How should I take this medicine?

Take tolterodine tablets by mouth. Follow the directions on the prescription label. Swallow the tablets with a drink of water. If you are taking the extended-release capsules, swallow them whole, do not crush, cut, or chew. Take your doses at regular intervals. Do not take your medicine more often than directed. Do not stop taking except on your doctor's advice. Contact your pediatrician or health care professional regarding the use of this medicine in children. Special care may be needed.

What if I miss a dose?

If it is almost time for your next dose, take only that dose on the regular schedule. Do not take double or extra doses.

What may interact with tolterodine?

- alcohol-containing beverages
- atropine
- bosentan
- caffeine
- cisapride
- clarithromycin
- cyclosporine
- diltiazem
- erythromycin
- fluvoxamine
- grapefruit juice
- hyoscyamine
- medicines for fungal infections, like fluconazole, itraconazole, ketoconazole or voriconazole
- medicines for treating HIV infection or AIDS
- metoclopramide
- nefazodone
- norfloxacin
- omeprazole
- oxybutynin
- quinidine
- quinine
- scopolamine
- tegaserod
- troleandomycin
- verapamil
- vinblastine
- warfarin
- water pills (diuretics)
- zafirlukast

Tell your prescriber or health care professional about all other medicines you are taking, including nonprescription medicines, nutritional supplements, or herbal products. Also tell your prescriber or health care professional if you are a frequent user of drinks with caffeine or alcohol, if you smoke, or if you use illegal drugs. These may affect the way your medicine works. Check before stopping or starting any of your medicines.

What should I watch for while taking tolterodine?

It may take 2 or 3 months to notice the maximum benefit from this medication. Your health care professional may also recommend techniques that may help improve control of your bladder and sphincter muscles. Such techniques will help train you to need the bathroom less frequently. You may need to limit your intake tea, coffee, caffeinated sodas, and alcohol; these drinks may aggravate your symptoms. Keeping healthy bowel habits may lessen bladder symptoms. If you currently smoke, quitting smoking may help reduce irritation to the bladder muscle. You may get dizzy or have blurred vision. Do not drive, use machinery, or do anything that requires mental alertness until you know how tolterodine affects you. Your mouth may get dry. Chewing sugarless gum or sucking hard candy, and drinking plenty of water, will help. Tolterodine may cause dry eyes and blurred vision. If you wear contact lenses, you may feel some discomfort. Lubricating drops may help. See your ophthalmologist if the problem does not go away or is severe.

What side effects may I notice from taking tolterodine?

Serious side effects are not common. Side effects that you should report to your doctor as soon as possible:
- any signs of an allergic reaction, like itching or hives
- blurred vision or difficulty focusing vision
- confusion
- difficulty passing urine
- severe dizziness

Side effects that usually do not require medical attention (report to your doctor if they continue or are bothersome):
- constipation
- dry eyes
- dry mouth
- headache
- mild dizziness or drowsiness
- indigestion or stomach discomfort

Where can I keep my medicine?

Keep out of the reach of children. Store at room temperature between 15 and 30 degrees C (59 and 86 degrees F). Protect from light. Throw away any unused medicine after the expiration date.

Topiramate tablets or sprinkle capsules

TOPAMAX®;
100 mg; Tablet
OMP Div, Ortho-
McNeil
Pharmaceuticals

TOPAMAX®;
25 mg; Capsule,
Coated Pellets
OMP Div, Ortho-
McNeil
Pharmaceuticals

What are topiramate tablets or sprinkle capsules?

TOPIRAMATE (Topamax®) is effective in helping to control seizures (convulsions) in adults or children with various forms of epilepsy. Topiramate may also be prescribed for other conditions, such as prevention of migraine headaches. Generic topiramate tablets or sprinkle capsules are not yet available.

What should my health care professional know before I take topiramate?

They need to know if you have any of these conditions:
- cirrhosis of the liver or other liver disease
- glaucoma
- kidney stones
- kidney disease
- an unusual or allergic reaction to topiramate, other medicines, foods, dyes, or preservatives
- pregnant or trying to get pregnant
- breast-feeding

How should I take this medicine?

Take topiramate tablets and capsules by mouth. Swallow the tablets whole with a drink of water; do not crush or chew. The capsules can be swallowed whole or opened carefully and the contents sprinkled on about on a small amount of soft food, such as applesauce, pudding, ice cream, oatmeal, or yogurt. This mixture must be swallowed immediately; do not chew or store the sprinkles on the food for later use. Be sure to take the entire dose. You may take topiramate with meals. Take your doses at regular intervals. Do not take your medicine more often than directed. Topiramate should be taken on a daily basis as prescribed by your health care professional for the prevention of migraine headaches. Topiramate should not be used to 'abort' or stop a migraine once it has started. Contact your pediatrician or health care professional regarding the use of this medicine in children. Special care may be needed. Topiramate has been used in children for the treatment of various seizure disorders.

What if I miss a dose?

If you miss a dose, take it as soon as you can. If it is almost time for your next dose, take only that dose. Do not take double or extra doses.

What may interact with topiramate?

- acetazolamide
- birth control pills or other hormones for birth control, including implants or injections
- bosentan
- carbamazepine
- dichlorphenamide
- digoxin
- ethanol
- medications for pain, sleep, or muscle relaxation
- methazolamide
- phenobarbital or primidone
- phenytoin
- probenecid
- valproic acid

Tell your prescriber or health care professional about all other medicines you are taking, including non-prescription medicines, nutritional supplements, or herbal products. Also tell your prescriber or health care professional if you are a frequent user of drinks with caffeine or alcohol, if you smoke, or if you use illegal drugs. These may affect the way your medicine works. Check with your health care professional before stopping or starting any of your medicines.

What should I watch for while taking topiramate?

Visit your prescriber or health care professional for a regular check on your progress. Do not stop taking topiramate suddenly. This increases the risk of seizures. Wear a Medic Alert bracelet or necklace. Carry an identification card with information about your condition, medications, and prescriber or health care professional. You should drink plenty of fluids while taking topiramate. If you have had kidney stones in the past, this will help to reduce your chances of forming kidney stones. If you have stomach pain, with nausea or vomiting and yellowing of your eyes or skin, call your health care provider immediately. You may get drowsy, dizzy, or have blurred vision. Do not drive, use machinery, or do anything that needs mental alertness until you know how topiramate affects you. To reduce dizziness, do not sit or stand up quickly, especially if you are an older patient. Alcohol can increase drowsiness and dizziness. Avoid alcoholic drinks. If you take birth control pills, topiramate may reduce their effectiveness at preventing pregnancy. Notify your prescriber or health care professional if you notice changes in your monthly cycles or bleeding patterns. You may want to discuss birth control options with your health care provider. If you notice blurred vision, eye pain, or other eye problems, seek medical attention at once for an eye exam. If you are going to have surgery, tell your prescriber or health care professional that you are taking topiramate.

What side effects may I notice from taking topiramate?

Side effects that you should report to your prescriber or health care professional as soon as possible:

- agitation, restlessness, irritability, or other changes in mood
- decreased sweating and/or rise in body temperature
- depression, or mood changes
- difficulty breathing; fast or irregular breathing patterns
- difficulty speaking
- difficulty walking or controlling muscle movements
- eye pain, redness or swelling
- hearing impairment
- kidney stones (severe pain in the side or back, or on urination)
- nose bleeds
- redness, blistering, peeling or loosening of the skin, including inside the mouth
- skin rash, itching
- stomach pain with nausea or vomiting
- swelling of the face, lips or tongue
- tingling, pain or numbness in the hands or feet
- unusual weakness or tiredness
- vision problems, like blurred vision
- vomiting
- yellowing of the skin or eyes

Side effects that usually do not require medical attention (report to your prescriber or health care professional if they continue or are bothersome):

- back pain, joint aches and pains
- breast pain
- diarrhea, or constipation
- difficulty sleeping
- dizziness, drowsiness
- dry mouth
- headache
- hot flashes
- loss of appetite
- menstrual disorder
- muscle aches or pains
- nausea
- swelling of the gums
- stomach upset, indigestion
- stuffy, runny nose
- sweating
- tiredness or weakness
- tremor

Where can I keep my medicine?

Keep out of reach of children in a container that small children cannot open. Store at room temperature between 15 and 30 degrees C (59 and 86 degrees F) in a tightly closed container. Protect from moisture. Throw away any unused medicine after the expiration date.

Toremifene tablets

FARESTON®;
60 mg; Tablet
Shire US Inc

What are toremifene tablets?

TOREMIFENE (Fareston®) is an "antiestrogen." Estrogens are female hormones. Toremifene blocks the effects of estrogen in the body and is used to treat and prevent breast cancer in both men and women. Generic toremifene tablets are not available.

What should my health care professional know before I take toremifene?

They need to know if you have any of these conditions:
- bleeding problems
- blood disorders
- receiving intramuscular injections
- vision problems
- an unusual or allergic reaction to toremifene, other medicines, foods, dyes, or preservatives
- pregnant or trying to get pregnant
- breast-feeding

How should I take this medicine?

Take toremifene tablets by mouth. Follow the directions on the prescription label. Swallow the tablets with a drink of water. Take your doses at regular intervals. Do not stop taking except on your prescriber's advice. Contact your pediatrician or health care professional regarding the use of this medicine in children. Special care may be needed.

What if I miss a dose?

If you miss a dose, skip that dose unless your prescriber or health care professional tells you otherwise. Do not take double or extra doses. If you vomit after taking a dose, call your prescriber or health care professional for advice.

What may interact with toremifene?

- antifungal agents
- carbamazepine
- certain types of diuretics
- clonazepam
- phenobarbital
- phenytoin
- rifampin
- warfarin

Tell your prescriber or health care professional about all other medicines you are taking, including nonprescription medicines, nutritional supplements, or herbal products. Also tell your prescriber or health care professional if you are a frequent user of drinks with caffeine or alcohol, if you smoke, or if you use illegal drugs. These may affect the way your medicine works. Check with your health care professional before stopping or starting any of your medicines.

What should I watch for while taking toremifene?

Visit your prescriber or health care professional for regular checks on your progress. Let your prescriber or health care professional know about any changes in your vision, or (for women) unusual vaginal bleeding. When you start taking toremifene, bone or tumor pain may increase. This means that toremifene is working and the pain should soon decrease.

What side effects may I notice from taking toremifene?

Side effects that you should report to your prescriber or health care professional as soon as possible:
- changes in vision
- chest pain
- dark yellow or brown urine
- difficulty breathing
- loss of appetite
- mood changes
- pain in the joints or legs
- swelling of the legs and feet
- unusual bruising or bleeding
- vaginal bleeding or discharge
- vomiting
- yellowing of the eyes or skin

Side effects that usually do not require medical attention (report to your prescriber or health care professional if they continue or are bothersome):
- dizziness
- fatigue
- hot flashes
- nausea
- sweating

Where can I keep my medicine?

Keep out of the reach of children in a container that small children cannot open. Store at 25 degrees C (77 degrees F). Protect from heat and light. Keep container tightly closed. Throw away any unused medicine after the expiration date.

Torsemide tablets

DEMADEX®; 10 mg; Tablet Hoffmann La Roche Inc		DEMADEX®; 20 mg; Capsule Hoffmann La Roche Inc	

What are torsemide tablets?

TORSEMIDE (Demadex®) is a diuretic (water or fluid pill). Diuretics increase the amount of urine passed, which causes the body to lose water and salt. Torsemide helps to treat high blood pressure (hypertension). It is not a cure. It also reduces the swelling and water retention caused by various medical conditions, such as heart, liver, or kidney disease. Generic torsemide tablets are available.

What should my health care professional know before I take torsemide?

They need to know if you have any of these conditions:
- diabetes
- gout
- hearing problems
- irregular heart beat
- kidney disease
- liver disease
- low blood levels of potassium, chloride, sodium or magnesium
- previous heart attack
- small amount of urine, or difficulty passing urine
- an unusual or allergic reaction to torsemide or furosemide, other medicines, foods, dyes, or preservatives
- pregnant or trying to get pregnant
- breast-feeding

How should I take this medicine?

Take torsemide tablets by mouth. Follow the directions on the prescription label. Swallow the tablets with a drink of water. Take your doses at regular intervals. Do not take your medicine more often than directed.

Contact your pediatrician or health care professional regarding the use of this medicine in children. Special care may be needed.

What if I miss a dose?

If you miss a dose, take it as soon as you can. If it is almost time for your next dose, take only that dose. Do not take double or extra doses.

What may interact with torsemide?

- alcohol
- amphotericin B
- anti-inflammatory drugs (NSAIDs, such as ibuprofen)
- cholestyramine
- cisplatin
- dofetilide
- heart medicines such as digoxin
- hormones such as cortisone, fludrocortisone, or hydrocortisone
- indomethacin
- lithium
- medicines for high blood pressure
- water pills

Tell your prescriber or health care professional about all other medicines you are taking, including non-prescription medicines, nutritional supplements, or herbal products. Also tell your prescriber or health care professional if you are a frequent user of drinks with caffeine or alcohol, if you smoke, or if you use illegal drugs. These may affect the way your medicine works. Check with your health care professional before stopping or starting any of your medicines.

What should I watch for while taking torsemide?

Visit your prescriber or health care professional for regular checks on your progress. Check your blood pressure regularly. Ask your prescriber or health care professional what your blood pressure should be, and when you should contact him or her. Check with your prescriber or health care professional if you get severe nausea, vomiting or diarrhea. You must not get dehydrated, ask your prescriber or health care professional how much fluid you need to drink a day. Torsemide will increase the amount of urine you pass. Take at a time of day that will not make this a problem. Avoid taking torsemide at bedtime. Do not stop taking torsemide except on your prescriber's advice. If you are diabetic, torsemide may increase your blood sugar levels. Check with your prescriber or health care professional before you change the dose of your diabetic medicine. You may get dizzy or lightheaded; until you know how torsemide affects you, do not drive, use machinery, or do anything that needs mental alertness. To reduce the risk of dizzy or fainting spells, do not sit or stand up quickly, especially if you are an older patient. Alcohol can make you lightheaded, dizzy and increase confusion. Avoid or limit intake of alcoholic drinks. Watch your diet while you are taking torsemide. Ask your prescriber or health care professional about both potassium and sodium intake. Torsemide can make your body lose potassium and you may need an extra supply. Some foods have a high potassium content such as bananas, coconuts, dates, figs, prunes, apricots, peaches, grapefruit juice, tomato juice, and orange juice. If you are going to have surgery, tell your prescriber or health care professional that you are taking torsemide.

What side effects may I notice from taking torsemide?

Side effects that you should report to your prescriber or health care professional as soon as possible:
- blood in urine
- dry mouth
- increased thirst
- irregular heartbeat, chest pain, weak pulse
- lower back or side pain
- mood changes
- muscle pain or cramps
- nausea, vomiting
- pain or difficulty passing urine
- ringing in the ears, loss of hearing
- skin rash, itching
- unusual tiredness or weakness

Side effects that usually do not require medical attention (report to your prescriber or health care professional if they continue or are bothersome):
- diarrhea or constipation
- dizziness or lightheadedness
- headache
- passing large amounts of urine
- stomach pain or upset, indigestion

Where can I keep my medicine?

Keep out of the reach of children in a container that small children cannot open. Store at room temperature between 15 and 30 degrees C (59 and 86 degrees F). Throw away any unused medicine after the expiration date.

Tramadol tablets

ULTRAM®;
50 mg; Tablet
Janssen Ortho, LLC

TRAMADOL;
50 mg; Tablet
Watson
Pharmaceuticals Inc

What are tramadol tablets ?

TRAMADOL (Ultram®) is an analgesic that can relieve moderate to moderately severe pain following surgery such as cesarean section, hysterectomy, hip replacement or other bone surgery, and dental surgery. This drug also helps relieve chronic pain associated with cancer, nerve pain, or low-back pain. Generic tramadol tablets are available.

What should my health care professional know before I take tramadol?

They need to know if you have any of these conditions:
- an alcohol or drug abuse problem
- breathing difficulty
- head injury or brain tumor
- kidney disease
- liver disease
- seizures (convulsions) or seizure disorder (epilepsy)
- stomach or intestinal problems
- an unusual or allergic reaction to tramadol, codeine, other pain medicines, foods, dyes, or preservatives
- pregnant or trying to get pregnant
- breast-feeding

How should I take this medicine?

Take tramadol tablets by mouth. Follow the directions on the prescription label. Swallow the tablets with a drink of water. If tramadol upsets your stomach, take it with food or milk. Do not take more than 100 mg of tramadol at one time or more than 400 mg of tramadol per day. Older patients (more than 75 years of age) should not take more than 300 mg of tramadol per day. Higher doses may cause severe side effects, do not take more medication than your prescriber has instructed. Contact your pediatrician or health care professional regarding the use of this medicine in children. Special care may be needed.

What if I miss a dose?

If you miss a dose, take it as soon as you can. If it is almost time for your next dose, take only that dose. Do not take double or extra doses.

What may interact with tramadol?

- alcohol
- antihistamines (commonly found in allergy or cold products)
- bupropion
- cocaine
- digoxin
- droperidol
- drugs to regulate heart rhythm such as amiodarone, propafenone, quinidine
- furazolidone
- imatinib
- isoniazid, INH
- linezolid
- medicines called MAO inhibitors-phenelzine (Nardil®), tranylcypromine (Parnate®), isocarboxazid (Marplan®), selegiline (Eldepryl®)
- medicines for anxiety, depression, or sleeping problems
- medicines for nausea or vomiting
- medicines for Parkinson's disease such as entacapone, pramipexole, ropinirole or tolcapone
- medicines for mental problems like schizophrenia
- muscle relaxants
- naloxone
- other medicines for pain such as codeine, morphine, nalbuphine, pentazocine, or propoxyphene
- procarbazine
- rifampin
- ritonavir
- seizure medicines
- stimulants such as amphetamine or dextroamphetamine
- St. John's wort
- warfarin

Tell your prescriber or health care professional about all other medicines you are taking, including non-prescription medicines. Also tell your prescriber or health care professional if you are a frequent user of drinks with caffeine or alcohol, if you smoke, or if you use illegal drugs. These may affect the way your medicine works. Check with your health care professional before stopping or starting any of your medicines.

What should I watch for while taking tramadol?

Tell your prescriber or health care professional if your pain does not go away. Visit your prescriber or health care professional for regular checks on your progress if you are taking tramadol regularly. Do not drive, use machinery, or do anything that needs mental alertness until you know how tramadol affects you. Be careful taking other medicines which may also make you tired. This effect may be worse when taking these medicines with tramadol. Alcohol can increase possible drowsiness, dizziness, confusion and affect your breathing. Avoid alcohol while taking tramadol. Your mouth may get dry. Chewing sugarless gum, sucking hard candy and drinking plenty of water will help. If you are going to have surgery, tell your prescriber or health care professional that you are taking tramadol.

What side effects may I notice from taking tramadol?

Side effects that you should report to your prescriber or health care professional as soon as possible:
Rare or uncommon:
- changes in vision
- difficulty breathing, shortness of breath
- fast or irregular heartbeat
- hallucinations (seeing and hearing things that are not really there)
- passing urine more frequently than usual, or not passing urine as often as usual
- redness, blistering, peeling or loosening of the skin, including inside the mouth
- skin rash, itching
- seizures (convulsions)

More common:
- anxiety, agitation
- nausea
- vomiting

Side effects that usually do not require medical attention (report to your prescriber or health care professional if they continue or are bothersome):
- constipation or diarrhea
- difficulty sleeping
- dizziness, drowsiness
- dry mouth
- false sense of well being, feeling of unreality, mood changes
- headache
- indigestion
- itching

Where can I keep my medicine?

Keep out of reach of children in a container that small children cannot open. Store at room temperature between 15 and 30 degrees C (59 and 86 degrees F). Throw away any unused medicine after the expiration date.

Trandolapril tablets

MAVIK®;
2 mg; Tablet
Abbott
Pharmaceutical
Product Division

MAVIK®;
1 mg; Tablet
Abbott
Pharmaceutical
Product Division

What are trandolapril tablets?

TRANDOLAPRIL (Mavik®) is an antihypertensive (blood pressure lowering agent) known as an ACE inhibitor. Trandolapril controls high blood pressure (hypertension) by relaxing blood vessels; it is not a cure. Generic trandolapril tablets are not yet available.

What should my health care professional know before I take trandolapril?

They need to know if you have any of these conditions:
- autoimmune disease (such as lupus), or suppressed immune function
- previous swelling of the tongue, face, or lips with difficulty breathing, difficulty swallowing, hoarseness, or tightening of the throat (angioedema)
- bone marrow disease
- dehydrated
- diarrhea or vomiting
- diabetes
- heart or blood vessel disease
- liver disease
- low blood pressure
- kidney disease
- stroke
- if you are on a special diet, such as a low-salt diet
- an unusual or allergic reaction to trandolapril, other ACE inhibitors, foods, dyes, or preservatives
- pregnant or trying to get pregnant
- breast-feeding

How should I take this medicine?

Take trandolapril tablets by mouth. Follow the directions on the prescription label. Swallow the tablets with a drink of water. Take your doses at regular intervals. Do not take your medicine more often than directed. Do not stop taking trandolapril except on your prescriber's advice. Contact your pediatrician or health care professional regarding the use of this medicine in children. Special care may be needed.

What if I miss a dose?

If you miss a dose, take it as soon as you can. If it is almost time for your next dose, take only that dose. Do not take double or extra doses. If you take only one dose a day and forget to take it that day, do not take a double dose the next day.

What may interact with trandolapril?

- anti-inflammatory drugs (NSAIDs, such as ibuprofen)
- hawthorn
- heparin
- lithium
- medicines for high blood pressure
- potassium salts or salt substitutes
- water pills

Tell your prescriber or health care professional about all other medicines you are taking, including non-prescription medicines, nutritional supplements, or herbal products. Also tell your prescriber or health care professional if you are a frequent user of drinks with caffeine or alcohol, if you smoke, or if you use illegal drugs. These may affect the way your medicine works. Check with your health care professional before stopping or starting any of your medicines.

What should I watch for while taking trandolapril?

Visit your prescriber or health care professional for regular checks on your progress. Check your blood pressure regularly while you are taking trandolapril. Ask your prescriber or health care professional what your blood pressure should be and when you should contact him or her. Call your prescriber or health care professional if you notice an uneven or fast heart beat. Do not treat yourself for a fever or sore throat; check with your prescriber or health care professional as these may be the result of a trandolapril side effect. Check with your prescriber or health care professional if you get an attack of severe diarrhea, nausea and vomiting, or if you sweat a lot. The loss of body fluid can make it dangerous to take trandolapril. You may get dizzy. Do not drive, use machinery, or do anything that needs mental alertness until you know how trandolapril affects you. To avoid dizzy or fainting spells, do not stand or sit up quickly, especially if you are an older person. Alcohol can make you more dizzy. Avoid alcoholic drinks. If you are going to have surgery, tell your prescriber or health care professional that you are using trandolapril. Avoid salt substitutes or other foods or substances high in potassium salts. Do not treat yourself for coughs, colds, or pain while you are using trandolapril without asking your prescriber or health care professional for advice.

What side effects may I notice from taking trandolapril?

Side effects that you should report to your prescriber or health care professional as soon as possible:
- decreased amount of urine passed
- difficulty breathing, or difficulty swallowing
- dizziness, lightheadedness or fainting spells
- palpitations or chest pain
- fever or chills
- numbness or tingling in your fingers or toes
- skin rash, itching
- swelling of your face, lips, or tongue

Side effects that usually do not require medical attention (report to your prescriber or health care professional if they continue or are bothersome):

- cough
- diarrhea
- headache
- tiredness

Where can I keep my medicine?

Keep out of the reach of children in a container that small children cannot open. Store at room temperature between 15 and 30 degrees C (59 and 86 degrees F). Keep container tightly closed. Throw away any unused medicine after the expiration date.

Trandolapril; Verapamil sustained-release tablets

TARKA®;
1 mg/240 mg;
Tablet, Extended Release
Abbott Pharmaceutical Product Division

TARKA®;
2 mg/180 mg;
Tablet, Extended Release
Abbott Pharmaceutical Product Division

What are trandolapril; verapamil sustained-release tablets?

TRANDOLAPRIL; VERAPAMIL (Tarka®) is a combination of two drugs used to lower blood pressure. They lower, but do not cure high blood pressure. Generic trandolapril; verapamil tablets are not yet available.

What should my health care professional know before I take trandolapril; verapamil?

They need to know if you have any of these conditions:

- autoimmune disease (such as lupus), or suppressed immune function
- bone marrow disease
- collagen-vascular disease (such as scleroderma)
- constipation problems (bowel impaction)
- difficulty swallowing (or narrowing of the esophagus)
- heart or blood vessel disease
- heart rhythm disturbances such as sick sinus syndrome, ventricular arrhythmias, Wolff-Parkinson-White syndrome, or Lown-Ganong-Levine syndrome
- if you are on a special diet, such as a low-salt diet
- liver or kidney disease
- neuromuscular disease such as muscular dystrophy
- previous swelling of the tongue, face, or lips with difficulty breathing, difficulty swallowing, hoarseness, or tightening of the throat (angioedema)
- slow or irregular heartbeat
- stomach problems (obstruction)
- an unusual or allergic reaction to trandolapril, verapamil, other medicines, foods, dyes, or preservatives
- pregnant or trying to get pregnant
- breast-feeding

How should I take this medicine?

Take trandolapril; verapamil tablets by mouth after a meal. Follow the directions on the prescription label. Swallow the tablets whole with a drink of water, do not break, crush or chew. Do not drink grapefruit juice or alcohol with this medicine. Take trandolapril; verapamil regularly. Do not take your medicine more often than directed. Do not stop taking except on your prescriber's advice. Contact your pediatrician or health care professional regarding the use of this medicine in children. Special care may be needed. Elderly patients over 65 years old may have a stronger reaction to this medicine and need smaller doses.

What if I miss a dose?

If you miss a dose, take it as soon as you can. If it is almost time for your next dose, take only that dose. Do not take double or extra doses.

What may interact with trandolapril; verapamil?

Do not take trandolapril; verapamil with any of the following:

- alfuzosin
- astemizole
- cisapride
- disopyramide
- dofetilide
- grapefruit juice
- pimozide
- salt substitutes that contain potassium
- terfenadine

Trandolapril; verapamil may also interact with the following medications:

- alcohol
- alosetron
- aspirin
- azathioprine
- anti-inflammatory drugs (NSAIDs, such as ibuprofen)
- barbiturates such as phenobarbital
- bosentan
- caffeine
- certain antibiotics (clarithromycin, erythromycin, telithromycin, trimethoprim, troleandomycin)
- certain medicines used to treat cancer
- certain medicines to treat migraine (ergotamine, dihydroergotamine, methysergide)
- cevimeline
- cilostazol
- cimetidine
- clonidine
- cyclosporine
- drospirenone; ethinyl estradiol
- fentanyl

- galantamine
- hymenoptera venom
- heparin
- herbal or dietary supplements such as ginger, gingko biloba, ginseng, hawthorn, ma huang (ephedra), melatonin, St. John's wort, went yeast
- lithium
- local anesthetics or general anesthetics
- medicines for anxiety or difficulty sleeping (examples: alprazolam, buspirone, midazolam, triazolam)
- medicines for anxiety, depression or mental problems (imipramine, fluoxetine, fluvoxamine, nefazodone, ziprasidone)
- medicines for diabetes
- medicines for fungal infections (examples: fluconazole, itraconazole, ketoconazole, voriconazole)
- medicines for heart-rhythm problems (amiodarone, digoxin, flecainide, procainamide, quinidine)
- medicines for high cholesterol (atorvastatin, cerivastatin, colesevelam, lovastatin, simvastatin)
- medicines for high blood pressure or heart problems
- medicines for HIV infection or AIDS
- medicines for prostate problems
- medicines for seizures (carbamazepine, clonazepam, ethosuximide, oxcarbazepine, phenobarbital, phenytoin, primidone, zonisamide)
- methadone
- methylprednisolone
- potassium salts (examples: potassium chloride, potassium gluconate)
- rifabutin
- rifampin
- rifapentine
- sildenafil
- sirolimus
- sulfinpyrazone
- tacrolimus
- theophylline or aminophylline
- water pills (diuretics, especially amiloride, triamterene or spironolactone)
- yohimbine
- zafirlukast
- zileuton

Tell your prescriber or health care professional about all other medicines you are taking, including non-prescription medicines, nutritional supplements, or herbal products. Also tell your prescriber or health care professional if you are a frequent user of drinks with caffeine or alcohol, if you smoke, or if you use illegal drugs. These may affect the way your medicine works. Check with your health care professional before stopping or starting any of your medicines.

What should I watch for while taking trandolapril; verapamil?

Check your blood pressure and pulse rate regularly; this is important while you are taking trandolapril-verapamil. Ask your prescriber or health care professional what your blood pressure and pulse rate should be and when you should contact him or her. You may feel dizzy or lightheaded. Do not drive, use machinery, or do anything that needs mental alertness until you know how trandolapril; verapamil affects you. To reduce the risk of dizzy or fainting spells, do not sit or stand up quickly, especially if you are an older patient. Avoid alcoholic drinks; they can make you more dizzy, increase flushing and rapid heartbeats. Do not suddenly stop taking trandolapril-verapamil. Ask your prescriber or health care professional how you can gradually reduce the dose. If you are going to have surgery, tell your prescriber or health care professional that you are taking trandolapril-verapamil. Check with your prescriber or health care professional if you get an attack of severe diarrhea, nausea and vomiting, or if you sweat a lot. The loss of body fluid can make it dangerous to take trandolapril-verapamil. Avoid salt substitutes or other foods or substances high in potassium salts. Do not treat yourself for coughs, colds, or pain while you are taking trandolapril-verapamil without asking your prescriber for advice. This medicine infrequently can cause dental problems for some patients. Clean and floss your teeth carefully and regularly. Check with your dentist if your gums get swollen or inflamed and have the dentist clean your teeth regularly.

What side effects may I notice from taking trandolapril; verapamil?

Side effects that you should report to your prescriber or health care professional as soon as possible:
- decreased amount of urine passed
- difficulty breathing, or swallowing
- dizziness, lightheadedness, confusion, or fainting spells
- persistent dry cough
- persistent muscle pain
- sore throat with fever
- skin rash, itching
- swelling of your legs or ankles
- swelling of your face, lips, or tongue
- tingling, burning or numbness in the fingers and toes
- uneven or fast heartbeat, chest pain, palpitations

Side effects that usually do not require medical attention (report to your prescriber or health care professional if they continue or are bothersome):
- change in taste sensation
- diarrhea or constipation
- drowsiness
- flushed or reddened skin
- headache
- increased sensitivity to sunlight
- nausea
- overgrowth of the gums
- sexual dysfunction
- weakness or tiredness

Where can I keep my medicine?

Keep out of the reach of children in a container that small children cannot open. Store at room temperature between 15 and 25 degrees C (59 and 77 degrees F). Protect from moisture and light. Keep container tightly closed. Throw away any unused medicine after the expiration date.

This drug requires an FDA medication guide. See page xxxvii.

Tranylcypromine tablets

PARNATE®;
10 mg; Tablet
SmithKline Beecham
Pharmaceuticals Div
SmithKline Beecham Co

What are tranylcypromine tablets?

TRANYLCYPROMINE (Parnate®) belongs to a class of drugs called monoamine oxidase inhibitors (MAOIs). Tranylcypromine increases the level of certain chemicals in the brain that help fight depression and other mood problems, including certain anxiety disorders. Tranylcypromine can interact with certain foods and other medicines to cause unpleasant side effects. You must know what foods and medicines to avoid (see below). Generic tranylcypromine tablets are available.

What should my health care professional know before I take tranylcypromine?

They need to know if you have any of these conditions:
- frequently drink alcohol-containing beverages
- asthma or bronchitis
- attempted suicide
- bipolar disorder or mania
- diabetes
- headaches or migraine
- heart or blood vessel disease, or irregular heart beats
- high blood pressure
- kidney disease
- liver disease
- over-active thyroid
- Parkinson's disease
- pheochromocytoma
- recent head trauma
- seizures or convulsions
- schizophrenia or psychosis
- stroke or other cerebrovascular disease
- an unusual or allergic reaction to tranylcypromine, other medicines, foods, dyes, or preservatives
- pregnant or trying to get pregnant
- breast-feeding

How should I take this medicine?

Take tranylcypromine tablets by mouth. Follow the directions on the prescription label. Swallow the tablets with a drink of water. Take your doses at regular intervals. Do not take your medicine more often than directed. Do not stop taking the tablets except on your prescriber's advice. Contact your pediatrician or health care professional regarding the use of this medicine in children. Special care may be needed. Elderly patients over age 65 years may have a stronger reaction to this medicine and should use this medicine with caution.

What if I miss a dose?

If you miss a dose, take it as soon as you can. If it is less than two hours to your next dose, take only that dose and skip the missed dose. Do not take double or extra doses.

What may interact with tranylcypromine?

- alcohol
- barbiturates such as phenobarbital
- bupropion
- buspirone
- caffeine
- carbamazepine
- certain medicines for blood pressure (especially beta-blockers, methyldopa, reserpine, guanadrel, and guanethidine)
- cocaine
- dextromethorphan
- diet pills or stimulants, like amphetamines or ephedra
- disulfiram
- furazolidone
- ginseng
- guarana
- kava kava
- levodopa
- linezolid
- local anesthetics
- medicines for allergies, colds, flu symptoms, sinus congestion and breathing difficulties
- medicines for diabetes
- medicines for migraine headaches
- medicines for movement abnormalities as in Parkinson's disease (examples: entacapone, levodopa, selegiline, tolcapone)
- muscle relaxants
- other medicines for mental depression, anxiety, or mood or mental problems
- meperidine
- procarbazine
- SAM-e
- seizure (convulsion) or epilepsy medicine
- St. John's wort
- tramadol
- tryptophan
- tyramine—see below for foods that contain tyramine
- valerian
- water pills (diuretics)
- yohimbine

Tell your prescriber or health care professional about all other medicines you are taking, including non-prescription medicines, nutritional supplements, or herbal products. Also tell your prescriber or health care professional if you are a frequent user of drinks with caffeine or alcohol, if you smoke, or if you use illegal drugs. These may affect the way your medicine works. Check with your health care professional before stopping or starting any of your medicines.

What should I watch for while taking tranylcypromine?

Visit your prescriber or health care professional for regular checks on your progress. It can take up to 4 weeks to see the full effects of tranylcypromine. Do not suddenly stop taking your medicine; this may make your condition worse or give you withdrawal symptoms. Ask your prescriber or health care professional for advice about gradually reducing your dosage. Even after you stop taking tranylcypromine the effects can last for at least two weeks. Continue to take all precautions and avoid all food and medicines that interact with tranylcypromine. Tranylcypromine can interact with certain foods that contain tyramine to produce severe headaches, a rise in blood pressure, or irregular heart beat. Foods that contain significant amounts of tyramine include aged cheeses; meats and fish (especially aged, smoked, pickled, or processed such as bologna, pepperoni, salami, summer sausage); beer and ale; alcohol-free beer; wine (especially red); sherry; hard liquor; liqueurs; avocados; bananas; figs; raisins; soy sauce; miso soup; yeast/protein extracts; bean curd; fava or broad bean pods; or any over-ripe fruit. Ask your prescriber or health care professional, pharmacist, or nutritionist for a complete listing of tyramine-containing foods. Also, avoid drinks containing caffeine, such as tea, coffee, chocolate, or cola. Call your prescriber or health care professional as soon as you can if you get frequent headaches or have palpitations. You may get drowsy, dizzy or have blurred vision. Do not drive, use machinery, or do anything that needs mental alertness until you know how tranylcypromine affects you. Do not stand or sit up quickly, especially if you are an older patient. This reduces the risk of dizzy or fainting spells. Alcohol may increase dizziness or drowsiness; avoid alcoholic drinks. Tranylcypromine can make your mouth dry. Chewing sugarless gum, sucking hard candy and drinking plenty of water will help. Do not treat yourself for coughs, colds, flu or allergies without asking your prescriber or health care professional for advice. Do not take any medications for weight loss without advice either. Some ingredients in these products may increase possible side effects. If you are diabetic there is a possibility that tranylcypromine may affect your blood sugar. Ask your prescriber or health care professional for advice if there is any change in your blood or urine sugar tests. Notify your health care professional if you are

scheduled to have any surgery, procedure or medical testing (including myelography). You should usually stop taking tranylcypromine at least 10 days before elective surgery; tell your prescriber or health care professional that you have been taking tranylcypromine.

What side effects may I notice from taking tranylcypromine?

Side effects that you should report to your prescriber or health care professional as soon as possible:

- agitation
- chest pain
- confusion
- difficulty breathing
- difficulty passing urine
- enlarged pupils, sensitivity of the eyes to light
- fever, clammy skin, increased sweating
- headache
- lightheadedness or fainting spells
- muscle or neck stiffness or spasm
- sexual dysfunction
- slow, fast, or irregular heartbeat (palpitations)
- yellowing of the skin or eyes

Side effects that usually do not require medical attention (report to your prescriber or health care professional if they continue or are bothersome):

- blurred vision
- constipation
- difficulty sleeping
- drowsiness or dizziness
- dry mouth
- loss of appetite
- muscle aches or pains, trembling
- nausea, vomiting
- swelling of the feet or legs
- unusual tiredness or weakness

Where can I keep my medicine?

Keep out of the reach of children in a container that small children cannot open. Store at room temperature between 15 and 30 degrees C (59 and 86 degrees F). Protect from light. Keep container tightly closed. Throw away any unused medicine after the expiration date.

Trazodone tablets

DESYREL®;
50 mg; Tablet
Bristol Myers Squibb
Co

DESYREL®;
100 mg; Tablet
Bristol Myers Squibb
Co

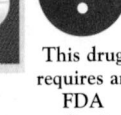
This drug requires an FDA medication guide. See page xxxvii.

What are trazodone tablets?

TRAZODONE (Desyrel®) is an antidepressant, a medicine that helps to lift mental depression. It can help patients whose depression has not responded to other medications, or who have experienced limiting side effects with other antidepressants. Trazodone may also be used to treat other conditions such as problems sleeping, anxiety, and panic attacks. Generic trazodone tablets are available.

What should my health care professional know before I take trazodone?

They need to know if you have any of these conditions:

- attempted or thinking about suicide
- bipolar disorder
- heart disease, or previous heart attack
- irregular heart beat
- kidney disease
- liver disease

- mania
- an unusual or allergic reaction to trazodone, other medicines, foods, dyes or preservatives
- pregnant or trying to get pregnant
- breast-feeding

How should I take this medicine?

Take trazodone tablets by mouth. Follow the directions on the prescription label. Swallow the tablets with a drink of water. Take trazodone shortly after a meal or a light snack. Take your doses at regular intervals. Do not take your medicine more often than directed. Do not stop taking the tablets except on your prescriber's advice. Contact your pediatrician or health care professional regarding the use of this medicine in children. Special care may be needed.

What if I miss a dose?

If you miss a dose, take it as soon as you can. If it is less than four hours to your next dose, take only that dose and skip the missed dose. Do not take double or extra doses.

What may interact with trazodone?

- herbal medicines that contain kava kava, St. John's wort, or valerian
- linezolid
- medicines for high blood pressure
- medicines for seizures
- other medicines for depression

Because trazodone can cause drowsiness, other medicines that also cause drowsiness may increase this effect of trazodone. Some medicines that cause drowsiness are:

- alcohol-containing medicines
- barbiturates such as phenobarbital
- certain antidepressants or tranquilizers
- certain medications used for Parkinson's disease, such as entacapone or tolcapone
- muscle relaxants
- certain antihistamines used in cold medicines

Tell your prescriber or health care professional about all other medicines you are taking, including non-prescription medicines, nutritional supplements, or herbal products. Also tell your prescriber or health care professional if you are a frequent user of drinks with caffeine or alcohol, if you smoke, or if you use illegal drugs. These may affect the way your medicine works. Check with your health care professional before stopping or starting any of your medicines.

What should I watch for while taking trazodone?

Visit your prescriber or health care professional for regular checks on your progress. You may have to take trazodone for two weeks or more before you feel better. If you have been taking trazodone for some time, do not suddenly stop taking it. Your prescriber or health care professional may want you to gradually reduce the dose; ask for advice. You may get drowsy, dizzy or have blurred vision. Do not drive, use machinery, or do anything that needs mental alertness until you know how trazodone affects you. Do not stand or sit up quickly, especially if you are an older patient. This reduces the risk of dizzy or fainting spells. Alcohol may increase dizziness or drowsiness; avoid alcoholic drinks. Trazodone can make your mouth dry. Chewing sugarless gum, sucking hard candy and drinking plenty of water will help. Do not treat yourself for coughs, colds, or allergies without asking your prescriber or health care professional for advice. Some ingredients may increase possible side effects. If you are going to have surgery, tell your prescriber or health care professional that you are taking trazodone.

What side effects may I notice from taking trazodone?

Side effects that you should report to your prescriber or health care professional as soon as possible:
- fainting spells
- fast or irregular heartbeat (palpitations)
- painful erections or other sexual dysfunction
- skin rash
- trembling

Side effects that usually do not require medical attention (report to your prescriber or health care professional if they continue or are bothersome):
- blurred vision
- constipation
- drowsiness, dizziness
- dry mouth
- headache
- muscle aches or pains
- nausea, vomiting
- unusual tiredness or weakness

Where can I keep my medicine?

Keep out of the reach of children in a container that small children cannot open. Store at room temperature, approximately 25 degrees C (77 degrees F). Avoid temperatures above 40 degrees C (104 degrees F). Protect from light. Keep container tightly closed. Throw away any unused medicine after the expiration date.

Tretinoin capsules

VESANOID®;
10 mg; Capsule
Hoffmann La Roche Inc

What are tretinoin capsules?

TRETINOIN (Vesanoid®) is a naturally occurring form of vitamin A. Tretinoin capsules are used to certain cancers, such as acute promyelocytic leukemia or other disorders. Generic tretinoin capsules are not yet available.

What should my health care professional know before I take tretinoin?

They need to know if you have any of these conditions:
- high cholesterol
- liver disease
- an unusual or allergic reaction to tretinoin, vitamin A, parabens, other medicines, foods, dyes, or preservatives
- pregnant or trying to get pregnant
- breast-feeding

How should I take this medicine?

Take tretinoin capsules by mouth. Follow the directions on the prescription label. Swallow the capsules whole with a drink of water. Take with meals. Take your doses at regular intervals; try to take doses at the same time each day. Do not take your medicine more often than directed. Do not stop taking except on your prescriber's advice. Contact your pediatrician or health care professional regarding the use of this medicine in children. Special care may be needed.

What if I miss a dose?

If you miss a dose, take it as soon as you can. If it is almost time for your next dose, take only that dose. Do not take double or extra doses.

What may interact with tretinoin?

- ketoconazole
- medicines that increase your sensitivity to sunlight such as tetracycline or sulfa drugs
- orlistat
- vitamin A supplements
- voriconazole

Tell your prescriber or other health care professional about all other medicines you are taking including nonprescription medicines, nutritional supplements, or herbal products. Also, tell your prescriber or health care professional if you are a frequent user of drinks with caffeine or alcohol, if you smoke or if you use illegal drugs. These may affect the way your medicine works. Check before stopping or starting any of your medications.

What should I watch for while taking tretinoin?

Visit your prescriber or health care professional for regular checks on your progress. You will need to have regular blood checks. Call your prescriber or health care professional for advice if you get a fever, chills or cough. Do not treat yourself. Do not take any vitamin A supplements while receiving tretinoin. Tretinoin is also a form of vitamin A and too much vitamin A can cause many side effects. If you are capable of becoming pregnant, you should have a pregnancy test within one week before you start tretinoin therapy, if possible, and monthly while you are taking tretinoin confirming you are not pregnant. Tretinoin may harm your unborn baby. You should contact your prescriber immediately if you believe or suspect you are pregnant while you are taking tretinoin and until one month after you stop taking tretinoin. You must use effective birth control continuously while taking tretinoin and until one month after you stop taking tretinoin. It is recommended that you use 2 reliable forms of birth control together.

What side effects may I notice from taking tretinoin?

Side effects that you should report to your prescriber or health care professional as soon as possible:
- signs of infection—fever or chills, cough, sore throat, pain or difficulty passing urine
- signs of bleeding—bruising, pinpoint red spots on the skin, black, tarry stools, blood in the urine
- changes in blood pressure
- chest pain
- chills
- difficulty breathing or shortness of breath
- severe headaches
- seizures
- weight gain

Side effects that usually do not require medical attention (report to your prescriber or health care professional if they continue or are bothersome):
- agitation or anxiety
- changes in sight
- changes in skin color
- confusion
- constipation or diarrhea
- decrease in reflexes
- depression
- difficulty sleeping
- dizziness, drowsiness
- dry skin
- earache, fullness in the ear
- flushing
- hair loss
- hallucinations (seeing things that are not really there)
- headache
- heartburn
- increased sweating

- loss of appetite
- muscle aches or pains
- nausea, vomiting
- shivering
- stomach pain
- tingling, numbness, or pain in the hands or feet

- tiredness or weakness
- uncontrollable shaking

Where can I keep my medicine?

Keep out of the reach of children. Store at 15 to 30 degrees C (59 to 86 degrees F) and protect from light.

Triamcinolone tablets

ARISTOCORT®; 4 mg; Tablet Fujisawa Healthcare Inc

ARISTOCORT®; 1 mg; Tablet Fujisawa Healthcare Inc

What are triamcinolone tablets?

TRIAMCINOLONE (Aristocort®, Kenacort®) is a corticosteroid. It helps to reduce swelling, redness, itching, and allergic reactions. Triamcinolone is similar to natural steroid hormone produced by the adrenal gland. Triamcinolone treats severe allergies, skin problems, asthma, arthritis, and many other conditions. Generic triamcinolone tablets are available.

What should my health care professional know before I take triamcinolone?

They need to know if you have any of these conditions:
- blood clotting disorder
- diabetes
- high blood pressure
- infection, including chickenpox, herpes, measles, or tuberculosis
- liver disease
- myasthenia gravis
- osteoporosis
- previous heart attack
- psychosis
- seizures (convulsions)
- stomach or intestinal disease
- under-active thyroid
- an unusual or allergic reaction to triamcinolone, corticosteroids, other medicines, foods, dyes, or preservatives
- pregnant or trying to get pregnant
- breast-feeding

How should I take this medicine?

Take triamcinolone tablets by mouth. Follow the directions on the prescription label. Swallow the tablets with a drink of water. Take with milk or food to avoid stomach upset. If you are only taking triamcinolone once a day, take it in the morning, which is the time your body normally secretes cortisol. Take your doses at regular intervals. Do not take your medicine more often than directed. Do not stop taking triamcinolone except on your prescriber's advice. Contact your pediatrician or health care professional regarding the use of this medicine in children. Special care may be needed.

What if I miss a dose?

If you miss a dose, take it as soon as you can. If it is almost time for your next dose, consult your prescriber or health care professional. You may need to miss a dose

or take a double dose, depending on your condition and treatment. Do not take double or extra doses without advice.

What may interact with triamcinolone?

- anti-inflammatory drugs (NSAIDs, such as ibuprofen)
- aspirin
- barbiturate medicines for inducing sleep or treating seizures (convulsions)
- bosentan
- carbamazepine
- female hormones, including contraceptive or birth control pills
- heart medicine
- medicines for diabetes
- medicines that improve muscle strength or tone for conditions like myasthenia gravis
- phenytoin
- rifampin
- toxoids and vaccines
- water pills

Tell your prescriber or health care professional about all other medicines you are taking, including non-prescription medicines, nutritional supplements, or herbal products. Also tell your prescriber or health care professional if you are a frequent user of drinks with caffeine or alcohol, if you smoke, or if you use illegal drugs. These may affect the way your medicine works. Check with your health care professional before stopping or starting any of your medicines.

What should I watch for while taking triamcinolone?

Visit your prescriber or health care professional for regular checks on your progress. If you are taking corticosteroids for a long time, carry an identification card with your name, the type and dose of corticosteroid, and your prescriber's name and address. Do not suddenly stop taking triamcinolone. You may need to gradually reduce the dose, so that your body can adjust. Follow the advice of your prescriber or health care professional. If you take corticosteroids for a long time, avoid contact with people who have an infection. You may be at an increased risk from infection while taking triamcinolone. Tell your prescriber or health care professional if you are exposed to anyone with measles or chickenpox, or if you develop sores or blisters that do not heal properly. People who are taking certain dosages of triamcinolone may need to avoid immunization with certain vaccines or may need to have changes in their vaccination schedules to ensure adequate protection from certain diseases. Make sure to tell your prescriber or health care professional that you are taking triamcinolone before receiving any vaccine. If you are diabetic, triamcinolone can affect your blood sugar. Check with your prescriber or health care professional if you need help adjusting the dose of your diabetic medicine. If you take triamcinolone tablets every day, you may need to watch your diet. Your body can also lose potassium while you take this medicine. Ask your prescriber or health care professional about your diet, especially about your salt intake. If you are going to have surgery tell your prescriber or health care professional that you are taking triamcinolone, or have taken it within the last 12 months. Alcohol can increase the risk of getting serious side effects while you are taking triamcinolone. Avoid alcoholic drinks. Elderly patients have an increased risk of side effects from triamcinolone. Triamcinolone can interfere with certain lab tests and can cause false skin test results.

What side effects may I notice from taking triamcinolone?

Side effects that you should report to your prescriber or health care professional as soon as possible:

- bloody or black, tarry stools
- confusion, excitement, restlessness, a false sense of well-being
- eye pain, decreased or blurred vision, or bulging eyes
- fever, sore throat, sneezing, cough, or other signs of infection
- frequent passing of urine

- hallucinations (seeing and hearing things that are not really there)
- increased thirst
- irregular heartbeat
- menstrual problems
- mental depression, mood swings, mistaken feelings of self-importance, mistaken feelings of being mistreated
- muscle cramps or muscle weakness
- nausea, vomiting
- pain in hips, back, ribs, arms, shoulders, or legs
- rounding out of face
- skin problems, acne
- stomach pain
- swelling of feet or lower legs
- unusual bruising or red pinpoint spots on the skin
- unusual tiredness or weakness
- weight gain or weight loss
- wounds that will not heal

Side effects that usually do not require medical attention (report to your prescriber or health care professional if they continue or are bothersome):

- diarrhea or constipation
- change in taste
- headache
- increased appetite or loss of appetite
- increased sweating
- nervousness, restlessness, or difficulty sleeping
- unusual increased growth of hair on the face or body
- upset stomach

Where can I keep my medicine?

Keep out of the reach of children in a container that small children cannot open. Store at room temperature between 15 and 30 degrees C (59 and 86 degrees F). Keep container tightly closed. Throw away any unused medicine after the expiration date.

Triamterene capsules

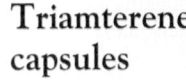

| DYRENIUM®; 50 mg; Capsule Wellspring Pharmaceutical Corp | | DYRENIUM®; 100 mg; Capsule Wellspring Pharmaceutical Corp | |

What are triamterene capsules?

TRIAMTERENE (Dyrenium®) is a diuretic(water or fluid pill). Diuretics increase the amount of urine passed, which causes the body to lose water and salt. Triamterene is used to treat water retention and swelling caused by conditions such as heart, kidney, and liver disease. Triamterene can be combined with hydrochlorothiazide to treat high blood pressure. Triamterene does not cause your body to lose potassium the way that many diuretics do. Generic triamterene capsules are not yet available.

What should my health care professional know before I take triamterene?

They need to know if you have any of these conditions:

- diabetes
- gout
- hearing problems

- high blood levels of potassium
- kidney disease or kidney stones
- liver disease
- low blood levels of sodium
- small amount of urine, or difficulty passing urine
- an unusual or allergic reaction to triamterene, other diuretics, medicines, foods, dyes, or preservatives
- pregnant or trying to get pregnant
- breast-feeding

How should I take this medicine?

Take triamterene capsules by mouth. Follow the directions on the prescription label. Swallow the capsules with a drink of water. If triamterene upsets your stomach, take it with food or milk. Take your doses at regular intervals. Do not take your medicine more often than directed. Contact your pediatrician or health care professional regarding the use of this medicine in children. Special care may be needed.

What if I miss a dose?

If you miss a dose, take it as soon as you can. If it is almost time for your next dose, take only that dose. Do not take double or extra doses.

What may interact with triamterene?

- amantadine
- anti-inflammatory drugs (NSAIDs, such as ibuprofen)
- cyclosporine
- dofetilide
- heparin
- lithium
- medicines for diabetes that are taken by mouth
- medicines for high blood pressure
- potassium salts
- water pills

Tell your prescriber or health care professional about all other medicines you are taking, including non-prescription medicines, nutritional supplements, or herbal products. Also tell your prescriber or health care professional if you are a frequent user of drinks with caffeine or alcohol, if you smoke, or if you use illegal drugs. These may affect the way your medicine works. Check with your health care professional before stopping or starting any of your medicines.

What should I watch for while taking triamterene?

Visit your prescriber or health care professional for regular checks on your progress. Check your blood pressure regularly. Ask your prescriber or health care professional what your blood pressure should be, and when you should contact him or her. You must not get dehydrated, ask your prescriber or health care professional how much fluid you need to drink a day. Watch your diet while you are taking triamterene. Ask your prescriber or health care professional about both potassium and sodium intake. Too much potassium can be very harmful. Elderly patients, the severely ill, diabetics, or patients with kidney problems are more likely to suffer from the effects of too much potassium. Avoid salt-substitutes, unless your prescriber or health care professional tells you otherwise. You may need to avoid foods that are high in potassium, such as bananas, coconuts, dates, figs, prunes, apricots, peaches, grapefruit juice, tomato juice, and orange juice. Check with your prescriber or health care professional if you get severe nausea, vomiting or diarrhea. You must not get dehydrated,

ask your prescriber or health care professional how much fluid you need to drink a day. Triamterene will increase the amount of urine you pass. Do not stop taking triamterene except on your prescriber's advice. If you are diabetic, triamterene may increase your blood sugar levels. Check with your prescriber or health care professional before you change the dose of your diabetic medicine. Triamterene may make your skin more sensitive to sun or ultraviolet light. Keep out of the sun, or wear protective clothing and use a sunscreen. Do not use sun lamps or sun tanning beds or booths. If you are going to have surgery, tell your prescriber or health care professional that you are taking triamterene.

What side effects may I notice from taking triamterene?

Side effects that you should report to your prescriber or health care professional as soon as possible:
- black, tarry stools
- blood in urine
- bright red tongue, burning feeling in tongue, dry mouth, cracked corners of mouth
- confusion, nervousness
- cough, hoarseness
- fast or irregular heartbeat, palpitations, chest pain
- fever, chills
- lower back or side pain
- muscle pain or cramps
- numbness or tingling in hands, feet, or lips
- pain or difficulty passing urine, reduced amount of urine passed
- skin rash, itching
- unusual bleeding or bruising, pinpoint red spots on the skin
- unusual tiredness or weakness
- yellowing of the eyes or skin

Side effects that usually do not require medical attention (report to your prescriber or health care professional if they continue or are bothersome):
- diarrhea
- dizziness
- headache
- increased sensitivity to the sun
- nausea, vomiting

Where can I keep my medicine?

Keep out of the reach of children in a container that small children cannot open. Store at room temperature between 15 and 30 degrees C (59 and 86 degrees F). Protect from light. Throw away any unused medicine after the expiration date.

Triazolam tablets

HALCION®;
0.25 mg; Tablet
Pharmacia and
Upjohn Div Pfizer

HALCION®;
0.125 mg; Tablet
Pharmacia and
Upjohn Div Pfizer

What are triazolam tablets?

TRIAZOLAM (Halcion®) is a benzodiazepine. Benzodiazepines belong to a group of medicines that slow down the central nervous system. Triazolam helps to treat insomnia (difficulty sleeping at night). Federal law prohibits the transfer of triazolam to any person other than the patient for whom it was prescribed. Do not share this medicine with anyone else. Generic triazolam tablets are available.

What should my health care professional know before I take triazolam?

They need to know if you have any of these conditions:
- an alcohol or drug abuse problem
- bipolar disorder, depression, psychosis or other mental health conditions
- kidney disease
- liver disease
- lung disease, such as chronic obstructive pulmonary disease (COPD), sleep apnea or other breathing difficulties
- myasthenia gravis
- Parkinson's disease
- porphyria
- seizures or a history of seizures
- snoring
- suicidal thoughts
- an unusual or allergic reaction to triazolam, other benzodiazepines, foods, dyes, or preservatives
- pregnant or trying to get pregnant
- breast-feeding

How should I take this medicine?

Take triazolam tablets by mouth. Triazolam is only for use at bedtime. Follow the directions on the prescription label. Swallow the tablets with a drink of water. Do not take your medicine more often than directed. Do not stop taking except on your prescriber's advice. Contact your pediatrician or health care professional regarding the use of this medicine in children. Special care may be needed.

What if I miss a dose?

If you miss a dose, take it as soon as you can. It can take up to 2 hours for drowsiness to occur; never repeat the dose before 2 hours have passed. Do not take double or extra doses.

What may interact with triazolam?

Do not take triazolam with any of the following:
- alcohol
- grapefruit juice
- ketoconazole
- itraconazole
- some medicines for HIV infection or AIDS

Triazolam may also interact with the following medications:
- bosentan
- caffeine
- cimetidine
- disulfiram
- female hormones, including contraceptive or birth control pills
- herbal or dietary supplements such as kava kava, melatonin, dehydroepiandrosterone, DHEA, St. John's Wort or valerian
- imatinib, STI-571
- isoniazid
- medicines for anxiety or sleeping problems, such as alprazolam, diazepam or lorazepam
- medicines for depression, mental problems or psychiatric disturbances
- medicines for fungal infections (fluconazole, voriconazole)
- mifepristone, RU-486
- modafinil
- prescription pain medicines
- probenecid
- ranitidine
- rifampin, rifapentine, or rifabutin
- some antibiotics (clarithromycin, erythromycin, troleandomycin)
- some medicines for colds, hay fever or other allergies
- some medicines for high blood pressure or heart problems (amiodarone, diltiazem, nicardipine, verapamil)
- some medicines for seizures (carbamazepine, oxcarbazepine, phenobarbital, phenytoin, primidone)
- theophylline
- zafirlukast
- zileuton

Tell your prescriber or health care professional about all other medicines you are taking, including non-prescription medicines, nutritional supplements, or herbal products. Also tell your prescriber or health care professional if you are a frequent user of drinks with caffeine or alcohol, if you smoke, or if you use illegal drugs. These may affect the way your medicine works. Check with your health care professional before stopping or starting any of your medicines.

What should I watch for while taking triazolam?

Visit your prescriber or health care professional for regular checks on your progress. Triazolam is for short-term periods of use. If sleep medicine is taken every night for a long time it may no longer help you to sleep. Your body can become dependent on triazolam, ask your prescriber or health care professional if you still need to take it. However, if you have been taking triazolam regularly for some time, do not suddenly stop taking it. You must gradually reduce the dose or you may get severe side effects. Ask your prescriber or health care professional for advice. You may get drowsy or dizzy. Do not drive, use machinery, or do anything that needs mental alertness until you know how triazolam affects you. To reduce the risk of dizzy and fainting spells, do not stand or sit up quickly, especially if you are an older patient. Alcohol may increase dizziness and drowsiness. Avoid alcoholic drinks. Do not treat yourself for coughs, colds or allergies without asking your prescriber or health care professional for advice. Some ingredients can increase possible side effects. If you are going to have surgery, tell your prescriber or health care professional that you are taking triazolam.

What side effects may I notice from taking triazolam?

Side effects that you should report to your prescriber or health care professional as soon as possible:

- confusion
- depression
- lightheadedness or fainting spells

- mood changes, excitability or aggressive behavior
- movement difficulty, staggering or jerky movements
- muscle cramps
- tremors
- weakness or tiredness

Side effects that usually do not require medical attention (report to your prescriber or health care professional if they continue or are bothersome):

- dizziness, drowsiness, clumsiness, or unsteadiness; a "hangover" effect
- headache
- increased dreaming
- loss of memory
- nausea, vomiting

Where can I keep my medicine?

Keep out of the reach of children in a container that small children cannot open. Store at room temperature between 15 and 30 degrees C (59 and 86 degrees F). Protect from light. Keep container tightly closed. Throw away any unused medicine after the expiration date.

Trifluoperazine tablets

TRIFLUOPERAZINE;
5 mg; Tablet
Sandoz
Pharmaceuticals

TRIFLUOPERAZINE;
2 mg; Tablet
Mylan
Pharmaceuticals Inc

What are trifluoperazine tablets?

TRIFLUOPERAZINE helps to treat disordered thoughts and some other emotional, nervous, and mental problems. Generic trifluoperazine tablets are available.

What should my health care professional know before I take trifluoperazine?

They need to know if you have any of these conditions:
- blood disorders or disease
- difficulty passing urine
- glaucoma
- head injury or coma
- heart or liver disease
- low blood level of calcium
- Parkinson's disease
- prostate trouble
- Reye's syndrome
- seizures (convulsions)
- stomach problems or peptic ulcer
- an unusual or allergic reaction to trifluoperazine, other medicines foods, dyes, or preservatives
- pregnant or trying to get pregnant
- breast-feeding

How should I take this medicine?

Take trifluoperazine tablets by mouth. Follow the directions on the prescription label. Swallow the tablets with a drink of water. Take trifluoperazine with food or milk if it upsets your stomach. Take your doses at regular intervals. Do not take your medicine more often than directed. Contact your pediatrician or health care

professional regarding the use of this medicine in children. Special care may be needed. Elderly patients over age 65 years may have a stronger reaction to this medicine and need smaller doses.

What if I miss a dose?

If you miss a dose, take it as soon as you can. If it is almost time for your next dose, take only that dose. Try to take your doses at the same time each day. Do not take double or extra doses.

What may interact with trifluoperazine?

- alcohol
- antacids
- some antibiotics
- antidiarrheal medications
- atropine
- bromocriptine
- cimetidine
- cisapride
- dextroamphetamine or amphetamine
- dronabinol or marijuana
- haloperidol or droperidol
- levodopa
- lithium
- medicines for an over-active thyroid gland
- medicines for colds and flu
- medicines for hay fever and other allergies
- medicines for mental depression
- medicines for movement abnormalities as in Parkinson's disease
- medicines to prevent or treat malaria
- medications for treating seizures (convulsions)

- medicines for pain or for use as muscle relaxants, including tramadol
- medicines to treat urine or bladder incontinence
- metoclopramide
- pimozide
- probucol
- some medications for high blood pressure or heart problems
- some weight loss medications

Tell your prescriber or health care professional about all other medicines you are taking, including non-prescription medicines, nutritional supplements, or herbal products. Also tell your prescriber or health care professional if you are a frequent user of drinks with caffeine or alcohol, if you smoke, or if you use illegal drugs. These may affect the way your medicine works. Check with your health care professional before stopping or starting any of your medicines.

What should I watch for while taking trifluoperazine?

Visit your prescriber or health care professional for regular checks on your progress. Do not stop taking trifluoperazine suddenly; this can cause nausea, vomiting, and dizziness. Ask your prescriber or health care professional for advice if you are to stop taking this medicine. You may get drowsy, dizzy, or have blurred vision. Do not drive, use machinery, or do anything that needs mental alertness until you know how trifluoperazine affects you. Do not stand or sit up quickly, especially if you are an older patient. This reduces the risk of dizzy or fainting spells. Alcohol can increase possible dizziness or drowsiness. Avoid alcoholic drinks. Trifluoperazine can reduce the response of your body to heat or cold. Try not to get overheated. Avoid temperature extremes, such as saunas, hot tubs, or very hot or cold baths or showers. Dress warmly in cold weather. Trifluoperazine can make your skin more sensitive to sun or ultraviolet light. Keep out of the sun, or wear protective clothing outdoors and use a sunscreen (at least SPF 15). Do not use sun lamps or sun tanning beds or booths. Wear sunglasses to protect your eyes. Trifluoperazine may make your mouth dry, chewing sugarless gum or sucking hard candy and drinking plenty of water will help. Do not treat yourself for coughs, colds, sore throat, indigestion, diarrhea, or allergies. Ask your prescriber or health care professional for advice. If you are going to have surgery or will need a procedure that uses contrast agents, tell your prescriber or health care professional that you are taking this medicine.

What side effects may I notice from taking trifluoperazine?

Side effects that you should report to your prescriber or health care professional as soon as possible:
- blurred vision
- breast enlargement in men or women
- breast milk in women who are not breast-feeding
- chest pain, fast or irregular heartbeat
- confusion, restlessness
- dark yellow or brown urine
- difficulty breathing or swallowing
- dizziness or fainting spells
- drooling, shaking, movement difficulty (shuffling walk) or rigidity
- fever, chills, sore throat
- hot, dry skin, unable to sweat
- involuntary or uncontrollable movements of the eyes, mouth, head, arms, and legs
- menstrual changes
- puffing cheeks, smacking lips, or worm-like movements of the tongue
- seizures (convulsions)
- slurred speech
- stomach area pain
- sweating
- unusual weakness or tiredness
- unusual bleeding or bruising
- yellowing of skin or eyes

Side effects that usually do not require medical attention (report to your prescriber or health care professional if they continue or are bothersome):
- constipation
- difficulty passing urine
- difficulty sleeping, agitation or restlessness
- drowsiness
- dry mouth
- headache
- increased sensitivity to the sun or ultraviolet light
- sexual difficulties (impotence in men; increased sexual desire in women)
- skin rash, or itching
- stuffy nose
- weight gain

Where can I keep my medicine?

Keep out of the reach of children in a container that small children cannot open. Store at room temperature between 15 and 30 degrees C (59 and 86 degrees F). Throw away any unused medicine after the expiration date.

Trihexyphenidyl tablets or extended-release capsules

ARTANE®;
5 mg; Tablet
Lederle
Pharmaceutical Div
American Cyanamid
Co

TRIHEXYPHENIDYL;
5 mg; Tablet
Watson
Pharmaceuticals Inc

What are trihexyphenidyl tablets or extended-release capsules?

TRIHEXYPHENIDYL (Artane®) can help to improve the stiffness and movement problems associated with Parkinson's disease. Trihexyphenidyl can also help to prevent or control movement-related side effects of other medicines. Generic trihexyphenidyl tablets are available, but generic sustained-release capsules are not available.

What should my health care professional know before I take trihexyphenidyl?

They need to know if you have any of these conditions:
- closed-angle glaucoma
- difficulty passing urine
- heart disease
- high blood pressure
- kidney disease
- prostate trouble
- stomach obstruction
- an unusual or allergic reaction to trihexyphenidyl, other medicines, foods, dyes, or preservatives
- pregnant or trying to get pregnant
- breast-feeding

How should I take this medicine?

Take trihexyphenidyl tablets or capsules by mouth. Follow the directions on the prescription label. Swallow the tablets with a drink of water. If you are taking the extended-release capsules, swallow them whole, do not crush or chew. Take 30 to 60 minutes before meals, unless your prescriber or health care professional tells you otherwise. You can take trihexyphenidyl with food if it upsets your stomach. Take your doses at regular intervals. Do not take your medicine more often than directed. It may take several days to see the full effect of trihexyphenidyl; do not stop taking except on your prescriber's advice. This medicine is not for use in children.

What if I miss a dose?

If you miss a dose, take it as soon as you can. If it is almost time for your next dose, take only that dose. Do not take double or extra doses. If you are taking the extended-release capsules, leave at least 6 to 8 hours between doses.

What may interact with trihexyphenidyl?

- alcohol
- amantadine
- levodopa
- medicines for diarrhea
- medicines for hay fever and other allergies
- medicines for mental depression
- medicines for mental problems and psychotic disturbances
- medicines for movement abnormalities as in Parkinson's disease, or for gastrointestinal problems
- medicines that help relieve anxiety or sleeping problems (such as diazepam or temazepam)

Tell your prescriber or health care professional about all other medicines you are taking, including nonprescription medicines, nutritional supplements, or herbal products. Also tell your prescriber or health care professional if you are a frequent user of drinks with caffeine or alcohol, if you smoke, or if you use illegal drugs. These may affect the way your medicine works. Check with your health care professional before stopping or starting any of your medicines.

What should I watch for while taking trihexyphenidyl?

Visit your prescriber or health care professional for regular checks on your progress. Do not stop taking this medicine abruptly. Your prescriber or health care professional may want to gradually reduce the dose so that you do not get side effects or make your condition worse. Your prescriber or health care professional may want you to have an eye exam from time to time. You may get dizzy or have blurred vision. Do not drive, use machinery, or do anything that requires mental alertness until you know how trihexyphenidyl affects you. To reduce the risk of dizzy or fainting spells, do not sit or stand up quickly, especially if you are an older patient. Alcohol can make you more drowsy, avoid alcoholic drinks. Your mouth may get dry. Chewing sugarless gum or sucking hard candy, and drinking plenty of water, will help. Trihexyphenidyl may cause dry eyes and blurred vision. If you wear contact lenses, you may feel some discomfort. Lubricating drops may help. See your ophthalmologist if the problem does not go away or is severe. Stay out of bright light and wear sunglasses if trihexyphenidyl makes your eyes more sensitive to light. Trihexyphenidyl may increase your chance of a heat stroke (symptoms may include: stomach upset or cramps, fever, heat intolerance). Avoid hot weather and drink plenty of fluids. Report stomach cramps or pain, fever, dizziness, faintness or general inability to handle hot weather to your prescriber immediately.

What side effects may I notice from taking trihexyphenidyl?

Side effects that you should report to your prescriber or health care professional as soon as possible:

- blurred vision
- confusion, hallucinations (seeing or hearing things that are not really there)
- excess sweating or unable to tolerate hot weather
- fast, or irregular heartbeat (palpitations)
- loss of memory
- pain or difficulty passing urine
- skin rash
- slurred speech
- vomiting
- weakness or tiredness

Side effects that usually do not require medical attention (report to your prescriber or health care professional if they continue or are bothersome):

- agitation, nervousness
- constipation
- dizziness, drowsiness
- dry mouth
- headache
- nausea

Where can I keep my medicine?

Keep out of the reach of children in a container that small children cannot open. Store at room temperature between 15 and 30 degrees C (59 and 86 degrees F). Throw away any unused medicine after the expiration date.

Trimethobenzamide capsules

TIGAN®; 250 mg; Capsule Monarch Pharmaceuticals Inc	
TIGAN®; 300 mg; Capsule Monarch Pharmaceuticals Inc	

What are trimethobenzamide capsules?

TRIMETHOBENZAMIDE (Tigan®, Trimazide®) helps to control nausea and vomiting. Generic trimethobenzamide capsules are available.

What should my health care professional know before I take trimethobenzamide?

They need to know if you have any of these conditions:
- dehydration
- recent viral illness
- stomach or intestinal problems
- an unusual or allergic reaction to trimethobenzamide, other medicines, foods, dyes, or preservatives
- pregnant or trying to get pregnant
- breast-feeding
- any other conditions or illnesses you might have

How should I take this medicine?

Take trimethobenzamide capsules by mouth. Follow the directions on the prescription label. Swallow the capsules with a drink of water. Take your doses at regular intervals. Do not take your medicine more often than directed. Contact your pediatrician or health care professional regarding the use of this medicine in children. Special care may be needed. Capsules are typically not recommended for young children and are not used in infants.

What if I miss a dose?

If you miss a dose, use it as soon as you can. If it is almost time for your next dose, use only that dose. Do not use double or extra doses.

What may interact with trimethobenzamide?

- alcohol
- atropine, belladonna alkaloids, hyoscyamine, scopolamine
- medicines for sleep or anxiety
- medicines for pain
- phenobarbital or other barbiturates

Tell your prescriber or health care professional about all other medicines you are taking, including non-prescription medicines, nutritional supplements, or herbal products. Also tell your prescriber or health care professional if you are a frequent user of drinks with caffeine or alcohol, if you smoke, or if you use illegal drugs. These may affect the way your medicine works. Check with your health care professional before stopping or starting any of your medicines.

What should I watch for while taking trimethobenzamide?

If your condition worsens after taking trimethobenzamide, contact your health care professional immediately. Trimethobenzamide may cause blurred vision, dizziness, and drowsiness. Driving or operating machinery, or performing other tasks that require mental alertness requires caution when taking this drug. You should not participate in these activities until you determine how trimethobenzamide affects you. Do not drink alcohol while taking trimethobenzamide. Alcohol can increase side effects.

What side effects may I notice from taking trimethobenzamide?

Side effects that you should report to your prescriber or health care professional as soon as possible:
- difficulty breathing, wheezing, shortness of breath
- tightness in the chest
- sore throat or fever
- shakiness or tremors
- seizures
- severe or continuing vomiting
- skin rash
- swelling of the face, tongue, throat, hands and feet
- yellowing of the eyes or skin
- unusual tiredness

Side effects that usually do not require medical attention (report to your prescriber or health care professional if they continue or are bothersome):

- blurred vision
- diarrhea
- dizziness
- drowsiness
- headache
- muscle cramps

Where can I keep my medicine?

Keep out of the reach of children. Store at room temperature between 15 and 30 degrees C (59 and 86 degrees F). Keep in a well-closed container. Throw away any unused portion after the expiration date.

Trimethoprim tablets

PROLOPRIM®;
100 mg; Tablet
Monarch
Pharmaceuticals Inc

TRIMETHOPRIM;
100 mg; Tablet
Watson
Pharmaceuticals Inc

What are trimethoprim tablets?

TRIMETHOPRIM (Proloprim®, Trimpex®) is an antibiotic used to treat bladder and urinary tract infections. It also can be used to treat or prevent *Pneumocystis carinii* pneumonia. Generic trimethoprim tablets are available.

What should my health care professional know before I take trimethoprim?

They need to know if you have any of these conditions:
- anemia, or other blood disorders
- high blood levels of potassium
- kidney disease
- liver disease
- an unusual or allergic reaction to trimethoprim, other medicines, foods, dyes, or preservatives
- pregnant or trying to get pregnant
- breast-feeding

How should I take this medicine?

Take trimethoprim tablets by mouth. Follow the directions on the prescription label. Trimethoprim works best if you take it on an empty stomach. However, if trimethoprim upsets your stomach, you may take it with food or milk. Do not take your medicine more often than directed. Finish the full course of medicine prescribed by your doctor or health care professional, even if you feel better. Take your doses at regular intervals and at the same time each day.

What if I miss a dose?

If you miss a dose, take it as soon as you can. If it is almost time for your next dose, take only that dose. Do not take double doses. You must leave a suitable interval between doses. If you are taking one dose a day and have to take a missed dose, make sure there is at least 10 to 12 hours between doses. If you are taking two doses a day and have to take a missed dose, make sure there is at least 5 to 6 hours between doses.

What may interact with trimethoprim?

- amiloride
- dapsone
- digoxin
- divalproex
- dofetilide
- methotrexate
- phenytoin
- potassium salts (potassium chloride, potassium phosphate)
- procainamide
- pyrimethamine
- rifampin
- some medicines used to treat blood pressure and/or heart failure (ACE inhibitors such as benazepril, enalapril, lisinopril, moexipril, quinapril, ramipril, and others)
- spironolactone
- tolbutamide
- triamterene
- trimetrexate
- valproic acid
- warfarin

Tell your prescriber or health care professional about all other medicines you are taking, including nonprescription medicines, nutritional supplements, or herbal products. Also tell your prescriber or health care professional if you are a frequent user of drinks with caffeine or alcohol, if you smoke, or if you use illegal drugs. These may affect the way your medicine works. Check with your health care professional before stopping or starting any of your medicines.

What should I watch for while taking trimethoprim?

Tell your prescriber or health care professional if your symptoms do not improve in 3 or 4 days. If you are taking this medicine for a long time, you must visit your prescriber or health care professional for regular checks on your progress.

What side effects may I notice from taking trimethoprim?

Side effects that you should report to your prescriber or health care professional as soon as possible:
- fast or irregular heartbeat, palpitations, chest pain
- fever or chills, sore throat
- bluish fingernails or lips
- difficulty breathing
- joint aches or pains
- muscle aches or pains
- redness, blistering, peeling or loosening of the skin, including inside the mouth
- skin rash, hives, or itching
- unusual bleeding or bruising

- unusual weakness or tiredness
- vomiting

Side effects that usually do not require medical attention (report to your doctor if they continue or are bothersome):

- changes in taste
- diarrhea
- headache
- increased sensitivity to sun and ultraviolet light
- nausea

- skin rash, itching
- stomach pain
- sore mouth

Where can I keep my medicine?

Keep out of the reach of children in a container that small children cannot open. Store at room temperature between 15 and 25 degrees C (59 and 77 degrees F). Protect from light and moisture. Keep container tightly closed. Throw away any unused medicine after the expiration date.

Trimetrexate injection

What is trimetrexate injection?

TRIMETREXATE (Neutrexin®) is an antiprotozoal agent. Trimetrexate treats *Pneumocystis carinii* pneumonia (PCP) in patients who cannot take or have not responded well to more conventional treatments. This infection commonly affects patients whose immune systems are not working properly, such as HIV-infected (AIDS) patients. Another medicine called leucovorin must be used at the same time as trimetrexate to help prevent serious side effects. Generic trimetrexate injections are not yet available.

What should my health care professional know before I take trimetrexate?

They need to know if you have any of these conditions:
- blood disorders
- dental disease
- liver disease
- low blood calcium
- low blood sodium
- recent radiation therapy
- an unusual or allergic reaction to trimetrexate, leucovorin, other medicines, foods, dyes, or preservatives
- pregnant or trying to get pregnant
- breast-feeding

How should I take this medicine?

Trimetrexate is for infusion into a vein.
Trimetrexate is given with another medicine, leucovorin, which prevents some of the serious side effects of trimetrexate. If you are also taking leucovorin, take exactly as directed for the complete length of time prescribed, even if you feel better. It is very important that you complete the full course of treatment and continue to use leucovorin for 3 days after the last dose of trimetrexate. Do not stop taking except on your prescriber's advice.

What if I miss a dose?

If you miss a dose, use it as soon as you can. If it is almost time for your next dose, use only that dose. Do not use double or extra doses.

What may interact with trimetrexate?

- acetaminophen
- bosentan
- cimetidine
- erythromycin
- medicines for fungal infections

Tell your prescriber or health care professional about all other medicines you are taking, including non-prescription medicines, nutritional supplements, or herbal products. Also tell your prescriber or health care professional if you are a frequent user of drinks with caffeine or alcohol, if you smoke, or if you use illegal drugs. These may affect the way your medicine works. Check with your health care professional before stopping or starting any of your medicines.

What should I watch for while taking trimetrexate?

Tell your prescriber or health care professional if your symptoms do not improve. If you get a fever or sore throat, do not treat yourself. Call your prescriber or health care professional for advice.

What side effects may I notice from taking trimetrexate?

Side effects that you should report to your prescriber or health care professional as soon as possible:
- decreased blood pressure leading to dizziness or lightheadedness
- difficulty breathing or shortness of breath
- excessive sweating
- low blood counts—trimetrexate may decrease the number of white blood cells and platelets in your blood. You may be at increased risk for infections and bleeding (see below)
- signs of infection—fever or chills, cough, sore throat, pain or difficulty passing urine
- signs of decreased platelets or bleeding - bruising, pinpoint red spots on the skin, black, tarry stools, blood in the urine

- skin rash
- sores in mouth or throat

Side effects that usually do not require medical attention (report to your prescriber or health care professional if they continue or are bothersome):

- chills
- diarrhea
- nausea, vomiting

Where can I keep my medicine?

This medicine is given in a hospital or clinic setting. You will not store this medicine at home.

This drug requires an FDA medication guide. See page xxxvii.

Trimipramine capsules

SURMONTIL®;
50 mg; Capsule
Odyssey
Pharmaceuticals Inc

SURMONTIL®;
25 mg; Capsule
Odyssey
Pharmaceuticals Inc

What are trimipramine capsules?

TRIMIPRAMINE (Surmontil®) is an antidepressant. Trimipramine can treat your depression by lifting your mood, especially if it is associated with sleep disturbances. Improvement of sleep patterns and anxiety can be the first benefits of treatment. Your prescriber or health care professional may prescribe trimipramine for other conditions, such as relief from nerve pain. Generic trimipramine capsules are not available.

What should my health care professional know before I take trimipramine?

They need to know if you have any of these conditions:
- frequently drink alcohol-containing beverages
- asthma, difficulty breathing
- blood disorders or disease
- diabetes
- difficulty passing urine, prostate trouble
- glaucoma
- heart disease or heart attack
- irregular heart rate
- liver disease
- manic depression
- overactive thyroid
- Parkinson's disease
- schizophrenia
- seizures (convulsions)
- stomach disease
- taking other medicines for depression
- an unusual reaction to trimipramine, other medicines, foods, dyes, or preservatives
- pregnant or trying to get pregnant
- breast-feeding

How should I take this medicine?

Take trimipramine by mouth. Follow the directions on the prescription label. Swallow the capsules with a drink of water. You can take the capsules with or without food. Take your doses at regular intervals. Do not take your medicine more often than directed. Do not stop taking except on your prescriber's advice. Elderly patients over 65 years old and adolescents may have a stronger reaction to this medicine and need smaller doses. Contact your pediatrician or health care professional regarding the use of this medicine in children. Special care may be needed.

What if I miss a dose?

If you miss a dose normally taken only at bedtime, it may be better to miss that dose to avoid daytime drowsiness. Ask your health care professional for advice. If you take more than one dose per day and miss a dose, take it as soon as you can. However, if it is almost time for your next dose, take only that dose. Do not take double or extra doses.

What may interact with trimipramine?

Trimipramine can interact with many other medicines. Some interactions can be very important. Make sure your prescriber or health care professional knows about all other medicines you are taking. Many important interactions are listed below:

Do not take trimipramine with any of the following medications:

- astemizole (Hismanal®)
- cisapride (Propulsid®)
- probucol
- terfenadine (Seldane®)
- thioridazine (Mellaril®)
- medicines called MAO inhibitors-phenelzine (Nardil®), tranylcypromine (Parnate®), isocarboxazid (Marplan®), selegiline (Eldepryl®)
- other medicines for mental depression (may be duplicate therapies or cause additive side effects)

Trimipramine may also interact with any of the following medications:

- alcohol
- antacids
- aprepitant
- atropine and related drugs like hyoscyamine, scopolamine, tolterodine and others
- barbiturate medicines for inducing sleep or treating seizures (convulsions), such as phenobarbital
- blood thinners, such as warfarin
- bromocriptine
- bupropion
- cimetidine
- clonidine
- cocaine
- delavirdine
- diphenoxylate
- disulfiram
- donepezil

- drugs for treating HIV infection
- female hormones, including contraceptive or birth control pills and estrogen
- galantamine
- herbs and dietary supplements like ephedra (Ma huang), kava kava, SAM-e, St. John's wort, valerian, or others
- imatinib, STI-571
- kaolin; pectin
- labetalol
- levodopa and other medicines for movement problems like Parkinson's disease
- lithium
- medicines for anxiety or sleeping problems
- medicines for hay fever or allergies (antihistamines)
- medicines for colds, flu and breathing difficulties, like pseudoephedrine
- medicines for fungus infections (examples: fluconazole, voriconazole)
- medicines for thyroid disease (examples: levothyroxine, methimazole, potassium iodide, sodium iodide, propylthiouracil)
- medicines for weight loss or appetite control
- medicines used to regulate abnormal heartbeat or to treat other heart conditions (examples: amiodarone, bepridil, disopyramide, dofetilide, encainide, flecainide, ibutilide, mibefradil, procainamide, propafenone, quinidine, and others)
- modafinil
- muscle relaxants, like cyclobenzaprine
- naphazoline
- other medicines for mental or mood problems and psychotic disturbances
- oxymetazoline
- phenylephrine
- prescription pain medications like morphine, codeine, tramadol and others
- procarbazine
- seizure (convulsion) or epilepsy medicine such as carbamazepine or phenytoin
- stimulants like dexmethylphenidate or methylphenidate
- some antibiotics (examples: erythromycin, gatifloxacin, levofloxacin, linezolid, moxifloxacin, sotalol, sparfloxacin)
- tacrine
- xylometazoline

Tell your prescriber or health care professional about all other medicines you are taking, including non-prescription medicines, nutritional supplements, or herbal products. Also tell your prescriber or health care professional if you are a frequent user of drinks with caffeine or alcohol, if you smoke, or if you use illegal drugs. These may affect the way your medicine works. Check with your health care professional before stopping or starting any of your medicines.

What should I watch for while taking trimipramine?

Visit your prescriber or health care professional for regular checks on your progress. It can take several days or weeks before you feel the full effect of trimipramine. If you have been taking trimipramine regularly for some time, do not suddenly stop taking it. You must gradually reduce the dose or you may get severe side effects. Ask your prescriber or health care professional for advice. Even after you stop taking trimipramine it can still affect your body for several days. You may get drowsy or dizzy. Do not drive, use machinery, or do anything that needs mental alertness until you know how trimipramine affects you. Do not stand or sit up quickly, especially if you are an older patient. This reduces the risk of dizzy or fainting spells. Alcohol may increase dizziness and drowsiness. Avoid alcoholic drinks. Do not treat yourself for coughs, colds or allergies without asking your prescriber or health care professional for advice. Some ingredients can increase possible side effects. Your mouth may get dry. Chewing sugarless gum or sucking hard candy, and drinking plenty of water will help. Trimipramine may cause dry eyes and blurred vision. If you wear contact lenses you may feel some discomfort. Lubricating drops may help. See your ophthalmologist if the problem does not go away or is severe. Trimipramine may make your skin more sensitive to the sun. Keep out of the sun, or wear protective clothing outdoors and use a sunscreen. Do not use sun lamps or sun tanning beds or booths. Trimipramine can affect blood glucose (sugar) levels. If you are a diabetic, check your blood sugar more often than usual, especially during the first few weeks of treatment. Call your prescriber or health care professional for advice if you notice a change in the results of blood or urine glucose tests. If you are going to have surgery or will need an x-ray procedure that uses contrast agents, tell your prescriber or health care professional that you are taking this medicine.

What side effects may I notice from taking trimipramine?

Side effects that you should report to your prescriber or health care professional as soon as possible:
- abnormal production of milk in females
- blood pressure changes
- blurred vision or eye pain
- breast enlargement in both males and females
- unusual bruising
- confusion, hallucinations (seeing or hearing things that are not really there)
- difficulty breathing
- excess energy
- fainting spells
- fever with increased sweating
- irregular or fast, pounding heartbeat, palpitations
- muscle stiffness, or spasms
- pain or difficulty passing urine, loss of bladder control
- seizures (convulsions)
- sexual difficulties (decreased sexual ability or desire, difficulty ejaculating)
- stomach pain
- swelling of the testicles
- tingling, pain, or numbness in the feet or hands

- unusual weakness or tiredness
- yellowing of the eyes or skin

Side effects that usually do not require medical attention (report to your prescriber or health care professional if they continue or are bothersome):

- anxiety
- constipation, or diarrhea
- drowsiness or dizziness
- dry mouth
- increased sensitivity of the skin to sun or ultraviolet light
- loss of appetite

- nausea, vomiting
- ringing in ears
- skin rash or itching
- unpleasant taste in mouth
- weight gain or loss

Where can I keep my medicine?

Keep out of the reach of children in a container that small children cannot open. Store at room temperature between 15 and 30 degrees C (59 and 86 degrees). Throw away any unused medicine after the expiration date.

Trospium tablets

SANCTURA™;
20 mg; Tablet
Esprit Pharma Inc.

What are trospium tablets?

TROSPIUM (Sanctura™) tablets help to control an overactive bladder, a chronic condition that can be improved with medication. Trospium may reduce the frequency of bathroom visits and may help to control wetting accidents. Generic trospium tablets are not yet available.

What should my health care professional know before I take trospium?

They need to know if you have any of these conditions:
- difficulty passing urine
- glaucoma
- intestinal obstruction
- kidney disease
- liver disease
- stomach problems like pyloric stenosis or reflux, or other problems with proper emptying of the contents of the stomach
- an unusual or allergic reaction to trospium, other medicines, foods, dyes, or preservatives
- pregnant or trying to get pregnant
- breast-feeding

How should I take this medicine?

Take trospium tablets by mouth. Swallow the tablets with a drink of water. Trospium should be taken on an empty stomach, at least one hour before eating. Follow the directions on the prescription label. Take your doses at regular intervals. Do not take your medicine more often than directed. Do not stop taking except on your doctor's advice. Contact your pediatrician or health care professional regarding the use of this medicine in children. Special care may be needed.

What if I miss a dose?

If it is almost time for your next dose, take only that dose on the regular schedule. Do not take double or extra doses.

What may interact with trospium?

- adefovir
- alcohol-containing beverages

- amantadine
- amiloride
- atropine
- caffeine
- cimetidine
- cisapride
- cyclobenzaprine
- donepezil
- entecavir
- galantamine
- hyoscyamine
- itraconazole
- ketoconazole
- lamivudine, 3TC
- megestrol
- memantine
- metformin
- metoclopramide
- midodrine
- morphine
- orphenadrine
- oxybutynin
- quinine
- ranitidine
- rivastigmine
- scopolamine
- some antibiotics such as erythromycin, trimethoprim, and vancomycin
- some medicines for colds, hay fever, or allergies
- some medicines to control the heart rhythm such as digoxin, disopyramide, dofetilide, procainamide, and quinidine
- some medicines for mental depression or psychotic disorders
- tacrine
- tegaserod
- tolterodine
- topiramate
- triamterene
- water pills (diuretics)

Tell your prescriber or health care professional about all other medicines you are taking, including non-pre-

scription medicines, nutritional supplements, or herbal products. Also tell your prescriber or health care professional if you are a frequent user of drinks with caffeine or alcohol, if you smoke, or if you use illegal drugs. These may affect the way your medicine works. Check with your health care professional before stopping or starting any of your medicines.

What should I watch for while taking trospium?

Your health care professional may also recommend techniques that may help improve control of your bladder and sphincter muscles. Such techniques will help train you to need the bathroom less frequently. You may need to limit your intake of tea, coffee, caffeinated sodas, and alcohol. These drinks may aggravate your symptoms. Keeping healthy bowel habits may lessen bladder symptoms. If you currently smoke, quitting smoking may help reduce irritation to the bladder muscle. You may get dizzy or have blurred vision. Do not drive, use machinery, or do anything that requires mental alertness until you know how trospium affects you. Your mouth may get dry. Chewing sugarless gum or sucking hard candy, and drinking plenty of water, will help. Trospium rarely causes dry eyes and blurred vision. If you wear contact lenses, you may feel some discomfort. Lubricating drops may help. See your ophthalmologist if the problem does not go away or is severe.

What side effects may I notice from taking trospium?

Serious side effects are not common. Side effects that you should report to your prescriber or health care professional as soon as possible:

- any signs of an allergic reaction, like itching or hives
- blurred vision or difficulty focusing vision
- confusion
- difficulty passing urine
- severe dizziness

Side effects that usually do not require medical attention (report to your prescriber or health care professional if they continue or are bothersome):

- constipation
- dry eyes
- dry mouth
- headache
- indigestion or stomach upset
- mild dizziness or drowsiness
- nausea

Where can I keep my medicine?

Keep out of the reach of children in a container that small children cannot open. Store at room temperature between 15 and 30 degrees C (59 and 86 degrees F). Throw away any unused medicine after the expiration date.

Ursodeoxycholic Acid, Ursodiol capsules or tablets

URSO 250™;
250 mg; Tablet
Axcan Scandipharm
Inc

URSODIOL;
300 mg; Capsule
Amide
Pharmaceutical Inc

What are ursodiol capsules or tablets?

URSODIOL (Actigall®, URSO®) is a bile acid. The drug helps dissolve gallstones in those who cannot have gallbladder surgery or who do not need the surgery. Ursodiol may be used with a procedural device that fragments the gallstone into smaller pieces; the procedure, called lithotripsy, allows the drug to dissolve the stones more quickly. Ursodiol is also useful for certain liver diseases of adults, children and infants; the drug reduces itching and other symptoms. Generic ursodiol capsules are available.

What should my health care professional know before I take ursodiol?

They need to know if you have any of these conditions:
- pancreatitis (an inflammation of the pancreas)
- an unusual or allergic reaction to ursodiol, bile acids, other medicines, foods, dyes, or preservatives
- pregnant or trying to get pregnant
- breast-feeding

How should I take this medicine?

Take ursodiol capsules or tablets by mouth. Follow the directions on the prescription label. Take the capsules with food or milk to improve absorption and limit stomach or intestinal side effects. Take your doses at regular intervals. Do not take your medicine more often than directed. Contact your pediatrician or health care professional regarding the use of this medicine in children. Special care may be needed. Usually, a pharmacist must prepare this medicine into a suspension for administration to children.

What if I miss a dose?

If you miss a dose, take it as soon as you can. If it is almost time for your next dose, take only that dose. Do not take double or extra doses.

What may interact with ursodiol?

- activated charcoal
- antacids
- cholestyramine
- clofibrate, fenofibrate, or gemfibrozil
- ciprofloxacin
- colesevelam
- colestipol
- dextrothyroxine
- female hormones, including estrogens or birth control pills

Tell your prescriber or health care professional about all other medicines you are taking, including non-prescription medicines, nutritional supplements, or herbal products. Also tell your prescriber or health care professional if you are a frequent user of drinks with caffeine or alcohol, if you smoke, or if you use illegal drugs. These may affect the way your medicine works. Check with your health care professional before stopping or starting any of your medicines.

What should I watch for while taking ursodiol?

Visit your prescriber or health care professional for regular checks on your progress. It may take months of therapy to get the right response. Your prescriber or health care professional will schedule tests to see if your gallstones are dissolving or if your liver problem is improving. Report continued or worsened nausea, vomiting, or abdominal pain to your prescriber. Continue to take your medicine even if you feel better, unless directed otherwise by your prescriber or health care professional. Do not stop taking except on your prescriber's advice. Antacids may interfere with the absorption of ursodiol. Take ursodiol at least 1 hour before or 2 hours after an antacid dose.

What side effects may I notice from taking ursodiol?

Side effects that you should report to your prescriber or health care professional as soon as possible:
- any signs of an allergic reaction (rare): difficulty breathing, hives, skin rash or unusual itching
- severe stomach area pain, especially toward your right side

Side effects that usually do not require medical attention (report to your prescriber or health care professional if they continue or are bothersome):
Less common:
- cough or sore throat
- diarrhea
- hair loss or thinning
- headache
- joint or muscle aches

More common:
- constipation
- gas
- indigestion
- nausea

Where can I keep my medicine?

Keep out of the reach of children in a container that small children cannot open. Store at room temperature below 30 degrees C (86 degrees F). Keep in a well-closed container. Throw away any unused medicine after the expiration date.

Valacyclovir caplets

VALTREX®;
500 mg; Tablet
Glaxo Wellcome Division

What are valacyclovir caplets?

VALACYCLOVIR (Valtrex®) is an antiviral agent. Valacyclovir treats herpes zoster infection (shingles) or genital herpes infection. Valacyclovir is not a cure; it will help the sores heal faster and relieve the pain or discomfort. Valacyclovir can also be used to help prevent a genital herpes infection from coming back. Valacyclovir might help prevent genital herpes from being passed on to a partner who does not have genital herpes if it is used with "safer sex" practices. Generic valacyclovir caplets are not yet available.

What should my health care professional know before I take valacyclovir?

They need to know if you have any of these conditions:
- acquired immunodeficiency syndrome (AIDS)
- any other condition that may weaken the immune system
- dehydration
- kidney disease
- an unusual or allergic reaction to valacyclovir, acyclovir, ganciclovir, valganciclovir, other medicines, foods, dyes, or preservatives
- pregnant or trying to get pregnant
- breast-feeding

How should I take this medicine?

Take valacyclovir caplets by mouth. Follow the directions on the prescription label. Swallow whole with a full glass of water. You can take valacyclovir with or without food. Take your doses at regular intervals. Do not take your medicine more often than directed. Finish the full course prescribed by your prescriber or health care professional even if you think your condition is better. Do not stop taking except on your prescriber's advice. Contact your pediatrician or health care professional regarding the use of this medicine in children. Special care may be needed.

What if I miss a dose?

If you miss a dose, take it as soon as you can. If it is almost time for your next dose, take only that dose. Do not take double or extra doses.

What may interact with valacyclovir?

- cimetidine
- fosphenytoin
- phenytoin
- probenecid

Tell your prescriber or health care professional about all other medicines you are taking, including non-prescription medicines, nutritional supplements, or herbal products. Also tell your prescriber or health care professional if you are a frequent user of drinks with caffeine or alcohol, if you smoke, or if you use illegal drugs. These may affect the way your medicine works. Check with your health care professional before stopping or starting any of your medicines.

What should I watch for while taking valacyclovir?

Tell your prescriber or health care professional if your symptoms do not improve after 1 week. Valacyclovir works best when taken early in the course of an infection, preferably within the first 72 hours. Begin treatment as soon as possible after the first signs of infection (such as tingling, itching, or pain in the affected area). Valacyclovir may be helpful in preventing the spread of infection to others. Valacyclovir will only help prevent the spread of genital herpes if you use 'safer sex' practices. Safer sex practices include not having sexual contact with your partner when you have any symptom or outbreak of genital herpes and using a condom made of latex or polyurethane whenever you have sexual contact.

What side effects may I notice from taking valacyclovir?

Side effects that you should report to your prescriber or health care professional as soon as possible:
- changes in your menstrual cycle
- hives
- reduced amount of urine passed
- skin rash
- stomach pain
- unusual weakness or tiredness

Side effects that usually do not require medical attention (report to your prescriber or health care professional if they continue or are bothersome):
- bone pain
- dizziness
- headache
- nausea, vomiting

Where can I keep my medicine?

Keep out of the reach of children in a container that small children cannot open. Store at room temperature between 15 and 25 degrees C (59 and 77 degrees F). Protect from light and moisture. Throw away any unused medicine after the expiration date.

V

Valdecoxib tablets

This drug is no longer on the market

BEXTRA®;
10 mg; Tablet
GD Searle LLC a
Subsidiary of
Pharmacia Company
Pfizer

BEXTRA®;
20 mg; Tablet
GD Searle LLC a
Subsidiary of
Pharmacia Company
Pfizer

What are valdecoxib tablets?

VALDECOXIB (Bextra®) is a drug used to reduce inflammation and ease mild to moderate pain for such conditions as arthritis or painful menstrual cycles. Generic valdecoxib tablets are not available.
NOTE: This drug is discontinued in the United States. Patients taking Valdecoxib should contact their prescriber regarding discontinuation and alternative therapies. If you have questions about Bextra®, you may call 1-866-6-BEXTRA or 1-866-623-9872.

What should my health care professional know before I take valdecoxib?

They need to know if you have any of these conditions:

- anemia
- asthma, especially aspirin sensitive asthma
- cigarette smoker
- dehydrated
- drink more than 3 alcohol-containing beverages a day
- heart or circulation problems such as heart failure or leg edema (fluid retention)
- high blood pressure
- kidney disease
- liver disease
- recent surgery, especially coronary artery bypass graft surgery (CABG)
- stomach bleeding or ulcers
- taking blood thinners
- taking hormones such as prednisone (steroids)
- an unusual or allergic reaction to valdecoxib, aspirin, other salicylates, other NSAIDs, sulfonamides, other drugs, foods, dyes or preservatives
- pregnant or trying to get pregnant
- breast-feeding

How should I take this medicine?

Take valdecoxib tablets by mouth. Follow the directions on the prescription label. Swallow tablets whole with a full glass of water; take tablets in an upright or sitting position. Taking a sip of water first, before taking the tablets, may help you swallow them. If possible, take bedtime doses at least 10 minutes before lying down. If valdecoxib upsets your stomach, take it with food or milk. Take your doses at regular intervals. Do not take your medicine more often than directed. Contact your pediatrician or health care professional regarding the use of this medicine in children. Special care may be needed.

What if I miss a dose?

If you miss a dose, take it as soon as you can. If it is almost time for your next dose, take only that dose. Do not take double or extra doses.

What may interact with valdecoxib?

- alcohol
- alendronate
- cyclosporine
- cidofovir
- drospirenone; ethinyl estradiol (Yasmin®)
- entecavir
- fluconazole
- herbal products that contain feverfew, garlic, ginger, or ginkgo biloba
- ketoconazole (products taken by mouth only)
- lithium
- medicines for high blood pressure
- methotrexate
- other anti-inflammatory drugs (such as ibuprofen or prednisone)
- pemetrexed
- warfarin
- water pills (diuretics)

Tell your prescriber or health care professional about all other medicines you are taking, including non-prescription medicines, nutritional supplements, or herbal products. Also tell your prescriber or health care professional if you are a frequent user of drinks with caffeine or alcohol, if you smoke, or if you use illegal drugs. These may affect the way your medicine works. Check with your health care professional before stopping or starting any of your medicines.

What should I watch for while taking valdecoxib?

Let your prescriber or health care professional know if your pain continues; do not take with other pain-killers without advice. If you get flu-like symptoms (fever, chills, muscle aches and pains), call your prescriber or health care professional; do not treat yourself. To reduce unpleasant effects on your stomach, take valdecoxib with a full glass of water. Do not smoke cigarettes or drink alcohol; these increase irritation to your stomach and can make it more susceptible to damage from valdecoxib. If you notice black, tarry stools or experience severe stomach pain and/or vomit blood or what looks like coffee grounds, notify your health care prescriber immediately. Avoid taking other prescription or over-the-counter non steroidal anti-inflammatory drugs (NSAIDs), such as ibuprofen (Advil®), naproxen (Aleve®), or ketoprofen (Orudis® KT), while taking valdecoxib. Side effects including stomach upset, heartburn, nausea, vomiting or serious side effects such as ulcers are more likely if valdecoxib is given with other NSAIDs. Many non-prescription products contain NSAIDs; closely read labels before taking any medicines with valdecoxib. Valdecoxib cannot take the place of aspirin for the prevention of heart attack or stroke. If you are currently taking aspirin for this purpose, you should not discontinue taking aspirin without checking with your prescriber or health care professional. It is especially important not to use valdecoxib during the last 3 months of pregnancy unless specifically directed to do so by your health care provider. Valdecoxib may cause problems in the unborn child or complications during delivery.

What side effects may I notice from taking valdecoxib?

Side effects that you should report to your prescriber or health care professional as soon as possible:
- chest pain or pressure
- signs of bleeding from the stomach—black tarry stools, blood in the urine, unusual tiredness or weakness, vomiting blood or vomit that looks like coffee grounds
- signs of an allergic reaction—difficulty breathing, pain while breathing, or wheezing, skin rash, redness, mouth sores, blistering or peeling skin, hives, or itching, swelling of eyelids, throat, lips
- decrease in the amount of urine passed

- difficulty swallowing, severe heartburn or burning, pain in throat
- inability or problems seeing, speaking, or standing
- pain or swelling in an arm or leg
- stomach tenderness, pain, bleeding, or cramps
- swelling of feet or ankles
- unexplained weight gain or edema
- yellowing of eyes or skin

Side effects that usually do not require medical attention (report to your prescriber or health care professional if they continue or are bothersome):
- diarrhea
- dizziness
- gas
- headache
- heartburn
- minor upset stomach
- nausea or vomiting

Where can I keep my medicine?

Keep out of the reach of children in a container that small children cannot open. Store at room temperature between 15 and 30 degrees C (59 and 86 degrees F). Protect from moisture. Keep container tightly closed. Throw away any unused medicine after the expiration date.

Valproic Acid, Divalproex Sodium capsules

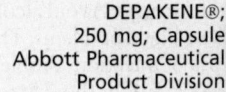

DEPAKENE®;
250 mg; Capsule
Abbott Pharmaceutical
Product Division

What are valproic acid capsules?

VALPROIC ACID capsules (Depakene®) can help with seizure (convulsion) control in certain types of epilepsy. This drug also is used for other conditions, such as treatment of bipolar disorder, mania, migraines, and behavioral problems associated with Alzheimer's disease or dementia. Generic valproic acid capsules are available.

What should my health care professional know before I take valproic acid?

They need to know if you have any of these conditions:
- blood disease
- brain damage or disease
- kidney disease
- liver disease
- low blood proteins
- urea cycle disorder (UCD)
- an unusual or allergic reaction to valproic acid, other medicines, foods, dyes, or preservatives
- pregnant or trying to get pregnant
- breast-feeding

How should I take this medicine?

Take valproic acid capsules by mouth. Follow the directions on the prescription label. Swallow the capsules whole with a drink of water. If valproic acid upsets your stomach, take it with food or milk; do not take with carbonated drinks. Take your doses at regular intervals.

Do not take your medicine more often than directed. Contact your pediatrician or health care professional regarding the use of this medicine in children. Special care may be needed.

What if I miss a dose?

If you take only one dose each day, take the missed dose as soon as you remember. If you do not remember until the next day, skip the missed dose and go on with your regular schedule. Do not take double or extra doses. If you take more than one dose a day and miss a dose, take it if you remember within 6 hours. Space the other doses for that day at regular intervals, do not take two doses at once.

What may interact with valproic acid?

- agents that dissolve blood clots
- alcohol
- antacids
- anti-inflammatory drugs (NSAIDs, such as ibuprofen)
- aspirin
- barbiturate medicines for inducing sleep or treating seizures (convulsions)
- blood thinners
- isoniazid
- medicines for mental depression
- medicines for mental problems and psychotic disturbances
- other seizure (convulsion) or epilepsy medicines

Tell your prescriber or health care professional about all other medicines you are taking, including non-prescription medicines, nutritional supplements, or herbal products. Also tell your prescriber or health care professional if you are a frequent user of drinks with caffeine or alcohol, if you smoke, or if you use illegal drugs. These may affect the way your medicine works. Check with your healthcare professional before stopping or starting any medicines while taking valproic acid.

What should I watch for while taking valproic acid?

Visit your prescriber or health care professional for a regular check on your progress. If you are taking valproic acid to treat epilepsy (seizures), do not stop taking valproic acid suddenly. This increases the risk of seizures. Wear a Medic Alert bracelet or necklace. Carry an identification card with information about your condition, medications, and prescriber or health care professional. Do not change brands or dosage forms of valproic acid without discussing the change with your prescriber or healthcare professional. You may get drowsy, dizzy, or have blurred vision. Do not drive, use machinery, or do anything that needs mental alertness until you know how valproic acid affects you. To reduce dizzy or fainting spells, do not sit or stand up quickly, especially if you are an older patient. Alcohol can increase drowsiness and dizziness. Avoid alcoholic drinks. Valproic acid can cause blood problems. This can mean slow healing and a risk of infection. Problems can arise if you need dental work, and in the day to day care of your teeth. Try to avoid damage to your teeth and gums when you brush or floss your teeth. If you are going to have surgery, tell your prescriber or health care professional that you are taking valproic acid.

What side effects may I notice from taking valproic acid?

Side effects that you should report to your prescriber or health care professional as soon as possible:

- agitation, restlessness, irritability, or other changes in mood
- blurred or double vision or uncontrollable eye movements
- changes in the frequency or severity of seizures
- double vision, or involuntary eye movements
- redness, blistering, peeling or loosening of the skin, including inside the mouth
- skin rash or itching
- stomach pain or cramps
- trembling of hands or arms
- unusual bleeding or bruising or pinpoint red spots on the skin
- unusual swelling of the arms or legs
- unusual tiredness or weakness
- yellowing of skin or eyes

Side effects that usually do not require medical attention (report to your prescriber or health care professional if they continue or are bothersome):

- breast enlargement, unusual production of breast milk
- changes in menstrual periods
- clumsiness or unsteadiness
- diarrhea or constipation
- difficulty speaking
- dizziness or drowsiness
- headache
- increased sensitivity to sun or ultraviolet light
- irregular menstrual cycle
- loss of bladder control
- loss of hair or unusual growth of hair
- loss or increase in appetite
- nausea or vomiting
- skin rash, itching
- weight gain or loss

Where can I keep my medicine?

Keep out of reach of children in a container that small children cannot open. Store at room temperature between 15 and 25 degrees C (59 and 77 degrees F). Keep container tightly closed. Throw away any unused medicine after the expiration date.

Valproic Acid, Divalproex Sodium delayed or extended-release tablets or sprinkle capsules

DEPAKOTE®;
500 mg; Tablet,
Delayed Release
Abbott
Pharmaceutical
Product Division

DEPAKOTE®;
125 mg; Capsule,
Extended Release
Abbott
Pharmaceutical
Product Division

What are divalproex sodium delayed or extended-release tablets or sprinkle capsules?

DIVALPROEX SODIUM (Depakote®, Depakote® ER) can help with seizure (convulsion) control in certain types of epilepsy. This drug is used for other conditions, such as the treatment of bipolar disorder, mania, the prevention of migraines, and control of behavioral problems associated with dementia. Generic dival-proex delayed- or extended-release tablets or capsules are not yet available.

What should my health care professional know before I take divalproex sodium?

They need to know if you have any of these conditions:
- blood disease
- brain damage or disease

- kidney disease
- liver disease
- low blood proteins
- urea cycle disorder (UCD)
- an unusual or allergic reaction to divalproex sodium, other medicines, foods, dyes, or preservatives
- pregnant or trying to get pregnant
- breast-feeding

How should I take this medicine?

Tablets: Take divalproex sodium delayed-release tablets or extended-release tablets by mouth. Follow the directions on the prescription label. Swallow the tablets whole with a drink of water; do not crush or chew. If divalproex sodium upsets your stomach, take it with food or milk; do not take with carbonated drinks. Take your doses at regular intervals. Do not take your medicine more often than directed.

Sprinkle capsules: The capsules can be swallowed whole following the directions for the tablets, or the capsules may be opened carefully and the contents sprinkled on about one teaspoonful of applesauce or pudding. This mixture must be swallowed immediately; do not chew or store for later use. Follow the directions on the prescription label. Take your doses at regular intervals. Do not take your medicine more often than directed. Contact your pediatrician or health care professional regarding the use of this medicine in children. Special care may be needed.

What if I miss a dose?

If you take only one dose each day, take the missed dose as soon as you remember. If you do not remember until the next day, skip the missed dose and go on with your regular schedule. Do not take double or extra doses. If you take more than one dose a day and miss a dose, take it if you remember within 6 hours. Space the other doses for that day at regular intervals, do not take two doses at once.

What may interact with divalproex sodium?

- agents that dissolve blood clots
- alcohol
- antacids
- anti-inflammatory drugs (NSAIDs, such as ibuprofen)
- aspirin
- barbiturate medicines for inducing sleep or treating seizures (convulsions)
- blood thinners
- isoniazid
- medicines for mental depression
- medicines for mental problems and psychotic disturbances
- other seizure (convulsion) or epilepsy medicines

Tell your prescriber or health care professional about all other medicines you are taking, including non-prescription medicines, nutritional supplements, or herbal products. Also tell your prescriber or health care professional if you are a frequent user of drinks with caffeine or alcohol, if you smoke, or if you use illegal drugs. These may affect the way your medicine works. Check

with your health care professional before stopping or starting any of your medicines.

What should I watch for while taking divalproex sodium?

Visit your prescriber or health care professional for a regular check on your progress. If you are taking divalproex to treat epilepsy (seizures), do not stop taking valproic acid suddenly. This increases the risk of seizures. Wear a Medic Alert bracelet or necklace. Carry an identification card with information about your condition, medications, and prescriber or health care professional. Do not change brands or dosage forms of divalproex without discussing the change with your prescriber or healthcare professional. You may get drowsy, dizzy, or have blurred vision. Do not drive, use machinery, or do anything that needs mental alertness until you know how divalproex sodium affects you. To reduce dizzy or fainting spells, do not sit or stand up quickly, especially if you are an older patient. Alcohol can increase drowsiness and dizziness. Avoid alcoholic drinks. Divalproex sodium can cause blood problems. This can mean slow healing and a risk of infection. Problems can arise if you need dental work, and in the day to day care of your teeth. Try to avoid damage to your teeth and gums when you brush or floss your teeth. If you are going to have surgery, tell your prescriber or health care professional that you are taking divalproex sodium.

What side effects may I notice from taking divalproex sodium?

Side effects that you should report to your prescriber or health care professional as soon as possible:

- agitation, restlessness, irritability, or other changes in mood
- blurred or double vision or uncontrollable eye movements
- changes in the frequency or severity of seizures
- double vision, or involuntary eye movements
- redness, blistering, peeling or loosening of the skin, including inside the mouth
- skin rash or itching
- stomach pain or cramps
- trembling of hands or arms
- unusual bleeding or bruising or pinpoint red spots on the skin
- unusual swelling of the arms or legs
- unusual tiredness or weakness
- yellowing of skin or eyes

Side effects that usually do not require medical attention (report to your prescriber or health care professional if they continue or are bothersome):

- breast enlargement, unusual production of breast milk
- changes in menstrual periods
- clumsiness or unsteadiness
- diarrhea or constipation
- difficulty speaking
- dizziness or drowsiness
- headache
- increased sensitivity to sun or ultraviolet light

- irregular menstrual cycle
- loss of bladder control
- loss of hair or unusual growth of hair
- loss or increase in appetite
- nausea or vomiting
- skin rash, itching
- weight gain or loss

Where can I keep my medicine?

Keep out of reach of children in a container that small children cannot open. Store at room temperature between 15 and 25 degrees C (59 and 77 degrees F). Keep container tightly closed. Throw away any unused medicine after the expiration date.

Valsartan tablets

DIOVAN®;
80 mg; Tablet
Novartis
Pharmaceuticals

DIOVAN®;
160 mg; Tablet
Novartis
Pharmaceuticals

What are valsartan tablets?

VALSARTAN (Diovan®) helps lower blood pressure to normal levels. It controls high blood pressure, but it is not a cure. High blood pressure can damage your kidneys, and may lead to a stroke or heart failure. Valsartan helps prevent these things from happening. Generic valsartan is not yet available.

What should my health care professional know before I take valsartan?

They need to know if you have any of these conditions:
- heart failure
- kidney disease, specifically renal artery stenosis
- liver disease
- electrolyte imbalance (e.g. low or high levels of potassium in the blood)
- if you are on a special diet, such as a low-salt diet (e.g. using potassium substitutes)
- an unusual or allergic reaction to valsartan, other medicines, foods, dyes, or preservatives
- pregnant or trying to get pregnant
- breast-feeding

How should I take this medicine?

Take valsartan tablets by mouth. Follow the directions on the prescription label. Swallow the tablets with a drink of water. Valsartan can be taken with or without food. Take your doses at regular intervals. Do not take your medicine more often than directed.

What if I miss a dose?

If you miss a dose, take it as soon as you can. If it is almost time for your next dose, take only that dose. Do not take double or extra doses.

What may interact with valsartan?

- blood pressure medications
- hawthorn
- lithium
- potassium salts or potassium supplements
- water pills (especially potassium-sparing diuretics such as triamterene or amiloride)

Tell your prescriber or health care professional about all other medicines you are taking, including nonprescription medicines, nutritional supplements, or herbal products. Also tell your prescriber or health care professional if you are a frequent user of drinks with caffeine or alcohol, if you smoke, or if you use illegal drugs. These may affect the way your medicine works. Check with your health care professional before stopping or starting any of your medicines.

What should I watch for while taking valsartan?

Check your blood pressure regularly while you are taking valsartan. Ask your prescriber or health care professional what your blood pressure should be and when you should contact him or her. When you check your blood pressure, write down the measurements to show your prescriber or health care professional. If you are taking this medicine for a long time you must visit your prescriber or health care professional for regular checks on your progress. Make sure you schedule appointments on a regular basis. You may experience dizziness. Do not drive, use machinery, or do anything that requires mental alertness until you know how valsartan affects you. To avoid dizziness, do not stand or sit up quickly. Avoid salt substitutes unless you are told otherwise by your prescriber or health care professional. If you are going to have surgery tell your prescriber or health care professional that you are taking valsartan.

What side effects may I notice from taking valsartan?

Side effects that you should report to your prescriber or health care professional as soon as possible:
Rare or uncommon:
- difficulty breathing or swallowing, hoarseness, or tightening of the throat
- swelling of your face, lips, tongue, hands, or feet
- unusual rash

Other:
- decreased amount of urine passed
- confusion, dizziness, lightheadedness or fainting spells
- fast or uneven heart beat, palpitations, or chest pain
- decreased sexual function

Side effects that usually do not require medical attention (report to your prescriber or health care professional if they continue or are bothersome):

- cough
- diarrhea
- fatigue or tiredness
- headache
- nausea or stomach pain

Vardenafil tablets

LEVITRA®;
10 mg; Tablet
Schering Corp

What are vardenafil tablets?

VARDENAFIL (Levitra®) is used to treat erection problems in men. Generic vardenafil tablets are not available.

What should my health care professional know before I take vardenafil?

They need to know if you have any of these conditions:

- anatomical deformity of the penis, Peyronie's disease, or ever had an erection that lasted more than 4 hours
- bleeding disorder
- cancer
- diabetes
- frequent heartburn or gastroesophageal reflux disease (GERD)
- heart disease, angina, high or low blood pressure, a history of heart attack, or other heart problems
- high cholesterol
- HIV infection
- kidney disease
- liver disease
- sickle cell disease
- stroke
- stomach or intestinal ulcers
- eye or vision problems
- an unusual reaction to vardenafil, medicines, foods, dyes, or preservatives
- pregnant or trying to get pregnant
- breast-feeding

How should I take this medicine?

Take vardenafil tablets by mouth with or without food. Follow the directions on the prescription label. The dose is usually taken about 1 hour before sexual activity. Swallow the tablets with a drink of water. Do not take double or extra doses. Contact your pediatrician or health care professional regarding the use of this medicine in children. Special care may be needed. At this time, this medicine is not for use in children.

What if I miss a dose?

This does not apply. However, do not take double or extra doses.

Where can I keep my medicine?

Keep out of the reach of children and in a container that small children cannot open. Store your medicine at room temperature between 15 and 30 degrees C (59 and 86 degrees F). Keep your medicine container tightly closed and protect it from light. Throw away any unused medicine after the expiration date.

What may interact with vardenafil?

Do not take vardenafil if you are taking the following medications:

- nitroglycerin-type drugs for the heart or chest pain such as amyl nitrite, isosorbide dinitrate, isosorbide mononitrate, nitroglycerin, even if these are only taken occasionally. This includes some recreational drugs called 'poppers' which also contain amyl nitrate and butyl nitrate.

Vardenafil may also interact with the following medications:

- alpha blockers such as alfuzosin (Uroxatral®), doxazosin (Cardura®), prazosin (Minipress®), tamsulosin (Flomax®), or terazosin (Hytrin®), used to treat high blood pressure or an enlarged prostate.
- arsenic trioxide
- bosentan
- certain antibiotics such as clarithromycin, erythromycin, sparfloxacin, troleandomycin
- certain medicines used for seizures such as carbamazepine, phenytoin, and phenobarbital
- certain medicines for the treatment of HIV infection or AIDS
- certain medicines to control the heart rhythm (e.g., amiodarone, disopyramide, dofetilide, flecainide, ibutilide, quinidine, procainamide, propafenone, sotalol)
- chloroquine
- cisapride
- diltiazem
- grapefruit juice
- medicines for fungal infections (fluconazole, itraconazole, ketoconazole, voriconazole)
- methadone
- nicardipine
- pentamidine
- pimozide
- rifabutin, rifampin, or rifapentine
- some medicines for treating depression or mood problems (amoxapine, maprotiline, fluoxetine, fluvoxamine, nefazodone, pimozide, phenothiazines, tricyclic antidepressants)
- verapamil

Tell your prescriber or health care professional about all other medicines you are taking, including non-prescription medicines, nutritional supplements, or herbal

products. Also tell your prescriber or health care professional if you are a frequent user of drinks with caffeine or alcohol, if you smoke, or if you use illegal drugs. These may affect the way your medicine works. Check with your health care professional before stopping or starting any of your medicines.

What should I watch for while taking vardenafil?

Contact your physician immediately if the erection lasts longer than 4 hours or if it becomes painful. This may be a sign of priapism and must be treated immediately to prevent permanent damage. If you experience symptoms of nausea, dizziness, chest pain or arm pain upon initiation of sexual activity after vardenafil use, you should refrain from further activity and should discuss the episode with your prescriber or health care professional as soon as possible. If you notice any changes in your vision while taking this drug, notify your prescriber or health care professional as soon as possible. Do not change the dose of your medication. Please call your prescriber or health care professional to determine if your dose needs to be reevaluated. Using vardenafil does not protect you or your partner against HIV infection (the virus that causes AIDS) or other sexually transmitted diseases.

What side effects may I notice from taking vardenafil?

Side effects that you should report to your prescriber or health care professional as soon as possible.

- back pain
- changes in vision
- chest pain or palpitations
- difficulty breathing, shortness of breath
- dizziness
- eyelid swelling
- muscle aches
- prolonged erection (lasting longer than 4 hours)
- skin rash, itching

Side effects that usually do not require medical attention (report to your prescriber or health care professional if they continue or are bothersome):

- flushing
- headache
- indigestion
- nausea
- stuffy nose

Where can I keep my medicine?

Keep out of the reach of children in a container that small children cannot open. Store at room temperature between 15 and 30 degrees C (59 and 86 degrees F). Throw away any unused medicine after the expiration date.

Venlafaxine tablets and extended-release capsules

EFFEXOR®;
50 mg; Tablet
Wyeth Div Wyeth
Pharmaceuticals Inc

EFFEXOR® XR;
150 mg; Capsule,
Extended Release
Wyeth Div Wyeth
Pharmaceuticals Inc

This drug requires an FDA medication guide. See page xxxvii.

What are venlafaxine tablets and extended-release capsules?

VENLAFAXINE (Effexor®, Effexor® XR) is an antidepressant, a medicine that helps to lift mental depression. Venlafaxine can help patients whose depression has not responded to other medications. Venlafaxine is also effective for the treatment of anxiety or other nervous conditions. Occasionally it is prescribed for other purposes. Generic venlafaxine tablets and extended-release capsules are not yet available.

What should my health care professional know before I take venlafaxine?

They need to know if you have any of these conditions:

- anorexia or weight loss
- attempted suicide
- high blood pressure or heart problems
- kidney disease
- liver disease
- mania or bipolar disorder
- seizures (convulsions)
- suicidal thoughts or a previous suicide attempt
- an unusual or allergic reaction to venlafaxine, other medicines, foods, dyes, or preservatives

- pregnant or trying to get pregnant
- breast-feeding

How should I take this medicine?

Take venlafaxine tablets and capsules by mouth. Follow the directions on the prescription label. Swallow the tablets with a drink of water. Take venlafaxine tablets and capsules with food.

Tablets: Take your doses at regular intervals.

Extended-release capsules: Do not cut, crush, chew, or divide the capsule. Try to take your extended-release capsule at the same time each day, in the morning or evening.

Do not take your medicine more often than directed. Do not stop taking the tablets except on your prescriber's advice. Contact your pediatrician or health care professional regarding the use of this medicine in children. Special care may be needed.

What if I miss a dose?

If you miss a dose, take it as soon as you can. If it is less than two hours to your next dose, take only that dose and skip the missed dose. Do not take double or extra doses.

What may interact with venlafaxine?

- alcohol
- amphetamine
- certain migraine headache medicines (almotriptan, eletriptan, frovatriptan, naratriptan, rizatriptan, sumatriptan, zolmitriptan)
- cimetidine
- dextroamphetamine
- furazolidone
- linezolid
- lithium
- medicines for heart rhythm or blood pressure
- medications for weight control or appetite
- medicines called MAO inhibitors-phenelzine (Nardil®), tranylcypromine (Parnate®), isocarboxazid (Marplan®)
- other medicines for mental depression, mania, psychosis, or anxiety
- procarbazine
- selegiline
- St. John's wort, Hypericum perforatum

Tell your prescriber or health care professional about all other medicines you are taking, including non-prescription medicines. Also tell your prescriber or health care professional if you are a frequent user of drinks with caffeine or alcohol, if you smoke, or if you use illegal drugs. These may affect the way your medicine works. Check with your health care professional before stopping or starting any of your medicines.

What should I watch for while taking venlafaxine?

Visit your prescriber or health care professional for regular checks on your progress. You may have to take venlafaxine for 4 weeks before you feel better. If you have been taking venlafaxine for some time, do not suddenly stop taking it. You must gradually reduce the dose to avoid side effects. Ask your prescriber or health care professional for advice. Patients and their families should watch out for worsening depression or thoughts of suicide. Also watch out for sudden or severe changes in feelings such as feeling anxious, agitated, panicky, irritable, hostile, aggressive, impulsive, severely restless, overly excited and hyperactive, or not being able to sleep. If this happens, especially at the beginning of antidepressant treatment or after a change in dose, call your health care professional. Venlafaxine can cause an increase in blood pressure. Check with your prescriber or health care professional; you may be able to measure your own blood pressure and pulse. Find out what your blood pressure and heart rate should be and when you should contact him or her. You may get drowsy, dizzy or have blurred vision. Do not drive, use machinery, or do anything that needs mental alertness until you know how venlafaxine affects you. Do not stand or sit up quickly, especially if you are an older patient. This reduces the risk of dizzy or fainting spells. Alcohol may increase dizziness or drowsiness; avoid alcoholic drinks. Venlafaxine can make your mouth dry. Chewing sugarless gum, sucking hard candy and drinking plenty of water will help. Do not treat yourself for coughs, colds, or allergies without asking your prescriber or health care professional for advice. Some ingredients may increase possible side effects. If you are going to have surgery, tell your prescriber or health care professional that you are taking venlafaxine.

What side effects may I notice from taking venlafaxine?

Side effects that you should report to your prescriber or health care professional as soon as possible:
Rare or uncommon:
- abnormal body movements, for example, of your tongue or upper body
- difficulty breathing
- fainting spells
- problems passing urine (increase or decrease in frequency)
- mania (over-active behavior)
- rapid heartbeat, or palpitations
- seizures (convulsions)

More common:
- agitation, anxiety, or restlessness, especially in the first week of treatment or when doses are changed
- changes in vision (blurred vision)
- sexual difficulties (abnormal ejaculation or orgasm, difficult or painful erections, impotence)
- vomiting

Side effects that usually do not require medical attention (report to your prescriber or health care professional if they continue or are bothersome):
- anxiety
- dry mouth
- constipation
- dizziness, drowsiness
- increased sweating
- loss of appetite, loss of weight
- nausea
- tremor
- weakness or tiredness

Where can I keep my medicine?

Keep out of the reach of children in a container that small children cannot open. Store at a controlled temperature between 20 degrees and 25 degrees C (68 degrees and 77 degrees F), in a dry place. Throw away any unused medicine after the expiration date.

Verapamil sustained-release tablets or capsules

CALAN® SR;
120 mg; Tablet,
Extended Release
GD Searle LLC a
Subsidiary of
Pharmacia Company
Pfizer

CALAN® SR;
240 mg; Tablet,
Extended Release
GD Searle LLC a
Subsidiary of
Pharmacia Company
Pfizer

What are verapamil sustained-release tablets or capsules?

VERAPAMIL (Calan® SR, Covera-HS®, Isoptin® SR, Verelan®, Verelan®-PM) is a calcium-channel blocker. It affects the amount of calcium found in your heart and muscle cells. This results in relaxation of blood vessels, which can reduce the amount of work the heart has to do. Sustained-release verapamil helps reduce high blood pressure (hypertension). It is not a cure. Generic verapamil sustained-release tablets are available. It is not a good idea to change the brand of your sustained-release product. Your body may respond differently. If you do switch between products you will need careful supervision from your prescriber or health care professional.

What should my health care professional know before I take verapamil?

They need to know if you have any of these conditions:
- constipation problems
- difficulty swallowing (or narrowing of the esophagus)
- heart or blood vessel disease
- heart rhythm disturbances such as sick sinus syndrome, ventricular arrhythmias, Wolff-Parkinson-White syndrome, or Lown-Ganong-Levine syndrome
- liver or kidney disease
- neuromuscular disease such as muscular dystrophy
- slow or irregular heartbeat
- stomach problems (obstruction)
- an unusual or allergic reaction to verapamil, other medicines, foods, dyes, or preservatives
- pregnant or trying to get pregnant
- breast-feeding

How should I take this medicine?

Take verapamil sustained-release tablets or capsules by mouth. Follow the directions on the prescription label. Swallow the tablets or capsules with a drink of water. Do not take with grapefruit juice. Sustained-release tablets (except Covera-HS® tablets) can be broken in half, but do not crush or chew the tablets. If you are taking Verelan® extended-release capsules, the capsule may be opened and the medicine poured into a small amount of applesauce. Stir well and swallow without chewing. Take this medicine with food to reduce stomach upset. Take your doses at regular intervals. Covera-HS tablets and Verelan® PM capsules are designed to be taken at bedtime only, do not take at other times of the day. Do not take your medicine more often then directed. Do not stop taking except on your prescriber's advice. Contact your pediatrician or health care professional regarding the use of this medicine in children. Special care may be needed. Elderly patients over 65 years old may have a stronger reaction to this medicine and need smaller doses.

What if I miss a dose?

If you miss a dose, take it as soon as you can. Covera-HS® tablets should only be taken once in 24 hours at bedtime; call your prescriber or health care professional for advice if you forget a dose. For other tablets or capsules, if it is almost time for your next dose (less than 8 hours) take only that dose. Do not take double or extra doses.

What may interact with verapamil?

Do not take verapamil with any of the following:
- astemizole
- cisapride
- disopyramide
- dofetilide
- grapefruit juice
- pimozide
- terfenadine

Verapamil may also interact with the following medications:
- alcohol
- alfuzosin
- alosetron
- anti-inflammatory drugs (NSAIDs, such as ibuprofen)
- barbiturates such as phenobarbital
- bosentan
- caffeine
- certain antibiotics (clarithromycin, erythromycin, telithromycin, troleandomycin)
- certain medicines used to treat cancer
- certain medicines to treat migraine (ergotamine, dihydroergotamine, methysergide)
- cevimeline
- cilostazol
- cimetidine
- clonidine
- cyclosporine
- fentanyl
- galantamine
- herbal or dietary supplements such as ginger, gingko biloba, ginseng, hawthorn, ma huang (ephedra), melatonin, St. John's wort, went yeast
- lithium
- local anesthetics or general anesthetics
- medicines for anxiety or difficulty sleeping (examples: alprazolam, buspirone, midazolam, triazolam)
- medicines for depression or mental problems (examples: imipramine, fluoxetine, fluvoxamine, nefazodone, ziprasidone)

- medicines for fungal infections (fluconazole, itraconazole, ketoconazole, voriconazole)
- medicines for heart-rhythm problems (amiodarone, digoxin, flecainide, procainamide, quinidine)
- medicines for high cholesterol (atorvastatin, cerivastatin, colesevelam, lovastatin, simvastatin)
- medicines for high blood pressure or heart problems
- medicines for HIV infection or AIDS
- medicines for prostate problems
- medicines for seizures (carbamazepine, clonazepam, ethosuximide, oxcarbazepine, phenobarbital, phenytoin, primidone, zonisamide)
- methadone
- methylprednisolone
- rifampin, rifabutin or rifapentine
- sildenafil
- sirolimus
- sulfinpyrazone
- tacrolimus
- theophylline or aminophylline
- water pills (diuretics)
- yohimbine
- zafirlukast
- zileuton

Tell your prescriber or health care professional about all other medicines you are taking, including nonprescription medicines. Also tell your prescriber or health care professional if you are a frequent user of drinks with caffeine or alcohol, if you smoke, or if you use illegal drugs. These may affect the way your medicine works. Check with your health care professional before stopping or starting any of your medicines.

What should I watch for while taking verapamil?

Check your blood pressure and pulse rate regularly; this is important while you are taking verapamil. Ask your prescriber or health care professional what your blood pressure and pulse rate should be and when you should contact him or her. If you are taking the Covera-HS® brand of verapamil, you must take the tablets exactly as prescribed. These tablets are designed to release your medicine at a special time, so that you get the most beneficial effect when you get up in the morning. Do not take the tablets at other times unless your prescriber or health care professional tells you to. You may feel dizzy or lightheaded. Do not drive, use machinery, or do anything that needs mental alertness until you know how verapamil affects you. To reduce the risk of dizzy or fainting spells, do not sit or stand up quickly, especially if you are an older patient. Alcohol can make you more dizzy or increase flushing and rapid heartbeats. Avoid alcoholic drinks. Do not suddenly stop taking verapamil. Ask your prescriber or health care professional how to gradually reduce the dose. If you are going to have surgery, tell your prescriber or health care professional that you are taking verapamil.

What side effects may I notice from taking verapamil?

Side effects that you should report to your prescriber or health care professional as soon as possible:
More common:
- dizziness
- slow heartbeat (less than 50 beats per minute)
- lightheadedness
- swelling of the legs or ankles

Rare or uncommon:
- difficulty breathing
- fast heartbeat, palpitations, irregular heartbeat, chest pain, or
- fainting
- skin rash

Side effects that usually do not require medical attention (report to your prescriber or health care professional if they continue or are bothersome):
- constipation
- facial flushing
- headache
- nausea, vomiting
- sexual dysfunction
- weakness or tiredness

Where can I keep my medicine?

Keep out of the reach of children in a container that small children cannot open. Store at room temperature between 15 and 25 degrees C (59 and 77 degrees F). Protect from light and moisture. Keep container tightly closed.

V

Verapamil tablets

CALAN®;
120 mg; Tablet
GD Searle LLC a
Subsidiary of
Pharmacia Company
Pfizer

CALAN®;
40 mg; Tablet
GD Searle LLC a
Subsidiary of
Pharmacia Company
Pfizer

What are verapamil tablets?

VERAPAMIL (Calan®, Isoptin®) is a calcium-channel blocker. By relaxing blood vessels, it can improve blood flow to the heart. Verapamil reduces attacks of chest pain (angina); lowers blood pressure (treats hypertension); and controls heart rate in certain conditions. Generic verapamil tablets are available.

What should my health care professional know before I take verapamil?

They need to know if you have any of these conditions:
- constipation problems
- heart or blood vessel disease
- heart rhythm disturbances such as sick sinus syndrome, ventricular arrhythmias, Wolff-Parkinson-White syndrome, or Lown-Ganong-Levine syndrome
- liver or kidney disease
- neuromuscular disease such as muscular dystrophy
- slow or irregular heartbeat
- an unusual or allergic reaction to verapamil, other medicines, foods, dyes, or preservatives
- pregnant or trying to get pregnant
- breast-feeding

How should I take this medicine?

Take verapamil tablets by mouth. Follow the directions on the prescription label. Swallow the tablets with a drink of water. Do not take with grapefruit juice. If verapamil upsets your stomach, you can take it with food or milk. Take your doses at regular intervals. Do not take your medicine more often then directed. Do not stop taking except on your prescriber's advice. Contact your pediatrician or health care professional regarding the use of this medicine in children. Special care may be needed. Elderly patients over 65 years old may have a stronger reaction to this medicine and need smaller doses.

What if I miss a dose?

If you miss a dose, take it as soon as you can. If it is almost time for your next dose, take only that dose. Do not take double or extra doses.

What may interact with verapamil?

Do not take verapamil with any of the following:
- astemizole
- cisapride
- disopyramide
- dofetilide
- grapefruit juice
- pimozide
- terfenadine

Verapamil may also interact with the following medications:
- alcohol
- alfuzosin
- alosetron
- anti-inflammatory drugs (NSAIDs, such as ibuprofen)
- barbiturates such as phenobarbital
- bosentan
- caffeine
- certain antibiotics (clarithromycin, erythromycin, telithromycin, troleandomycin)
- certain medicines used to treat cancer
- certain medicines to treat migraine (ergotamine, dihydroergotamine, methysergide)
- cevimeline
- cilostazol
- cimetidine
- clonidine
- cyclosporine
- fentanyl
- galantamine
- herbal or dietary supplements such as ginger, gingko biloba, ginseng, hawthorn, ma huang (ephedra), melatonin, St. John's wort, went yeast
- lithium
- local anesthetics or general anesthetics
- medicines for anxiety or difficulty sleeping (examples: alprazolam, buspirone, midazolam, triazolam)
- medicines for depression or mental problems (examples: imipramine, fluoxetine, fluvoxamine, nefazodone, ziprasidone)
- medicines for fungal infections (fluconazole, itraconazole, ketoconazole, voriconazole)
- medicines for heart-rhythm problems (amiodarone, digoxin, flecainide, procainamide, quinidine)
- medicines for high cholesterol (atorvastatin, cerivastatin, colesevelam, lovastatin, simvastatin)
- medicines for high blood pressure or heart problems
- medicines for HIV infection or AIDS
- medicines for prostate problems
- medicines for seizures (carbamazepine, clonazepam, ethosuximide, oxcarbazepine, phenobarbital, phenytoin, primidone, zonisamide)
- methadone
- methylprednisolone
- rifampin, rifabutin or rifapentine
- sildenafil
- sirolimus
- sulfinpyrazone
- tacrolimus
- theophylline or aminophylline
- water pills (diuretics)
- yohimbine
- zafirlukast
- zileuton

V

Tell your prescriber or health care professional about all other medicines you are taking, including non-prescription medicines. Also tell your prescriber or health care professional if you are a frequent user of drinks with caffeine or alcohol, if you smoke, or if you use illegal drugs. These may affect the way your medicine works. Check with your health care professional before stopping or starting any of your medicines.

What should I watch for while taking verapamil?

Check your blood pressure and pulse rate regularly; this is important while you are taking verapamil. Ask your prescriber or health care professional what your blood pressure and pulse rate should be and when you should contact him or her. You may feel dizzy or lightheaded. Do not drive, use machinery, or do anything that needs mental alertness until you know how verapamil affects you. To reduce the risk of dizzy or fainting spells, do not sit or stand up quickly, especially if you are an older patient. Alcohol can make you more dizzy or increase flushing and rapid heartbeats. Avoid alcoholic drinks. Do not suddenly stop taking verapamil. Ask your prescriber or health care professional how to gradually reduce the dose. If you are going to have surgery, tell your prescriber or health care professional that you are taking verapamil.

What side effects may I notice from taking verapamil?

Side effects that you should report to your prescriber or health care professional as soon as possible:

More common:
- dizziness
- slow heartbeat (less than 50 beats per minute)
- lightheadedness
- swelling of the legs or ankles

Rare or uncommon:
- difficulty breathing
- fast heartbeat, palpitations, irregular heartbeat, chest pain, or
- fainting
- skin rash

Side effects that usually do not require medical attention (report to your prescriber or health care professional if they continue or are bothersome):
- constipation
- facial flushing
- headache
- nausea, vomiting
- sexual dysfunction
- weakness or tiredness

Where can I keep my medicine?

Keep out of the reach of children in a container that small children cannot open. Store at room temperature between 15 and 30 degrees C (59 and 86 degrees F). Protect from light. Keep container tightly closed.

Voriconazole tablets

VFEND®;
200 mg; Tablet
Roerig Division of Pfizer

What are voriconazole tablets?

VORICONAZOLE (VFEND®) is an antifungal type of antibiotic. It treats serious fungal infections found throughout the body. These infections include aspergillosis, which is often found in the lung, and other types of mold or yeast infections. Generic voriconazole tablets are not yet available.

What should my health care professional know before I take voriconazole?

They need to know if you have any of these conditions:
- eye disease
- kidney disease
- liver disease
- other chronic illness
- an unusual or allergic reaction to voriconazole, or other azole medicines, other foods, dyes or preservatives
- pregnant or trying to get pregnant
- breast-feeding

How should I take this medicine?

Take voriconazole tablets by mouth. Follow the directions on the prescription label. You should take the tablets 1 hour before or 1 hour after a meal. Do not drink grapefruit juice while taking voriconazole. Take your doses at regular intervals. Do not take your medicine more often than directed. Finish the full course of tablets prescribed by your prescriber or health care professional even if you feel better. Do not stop taking except on your prescriber's advice. Contact your pediatrician or health care professional regarding the use of this medicine in children. Special care may be needed.

What if I miss a dose?

If it is almost time for your next dose, take only that dose. Do not take double or extra doses.

What may interact with voriconazole?

Voriconazole has the potential to interact with many other drugs. Some of the possible interactions are listed:

- alosetron
- amiodarone
- amphotericin B
- astemizole
- barbiturates, like phenobarbital
- bromocriptine

- calcium channel blockers like amlodipine, diltiazem or verapamil
- cevimeline
- cilostazol
- cisapride
- cocaine
- cyclosporine
- dapsone
- dextromethorphan
- disopyramide
- dofetilide
- donepezil
- ergotamine or dihydroergotamine
- ethanol
- galantamine
- grapefruit juice
- halofantrine
- isoniazid, INH
- levomethadyl
- medicines for depression, anxiety, psychosis or other mood problems
- medicines for diabetes
- medicines for HIV infection
- medicines for insomnia (sleep problems)
- medicines for seizures like carbamazepine, clonazepam, ethosuximide, phenobarbital, phenytoin, valproic acid and others
- medicines for treating high cholesterol, like atorvastatin, fluvastatin, lovastatin or simvastatin
- methadone
- mifepristone, RU-486
- modafinil
- nystatin
- omeprazole
- prescription pain medications or muscle relaxants
- quinidine
- quinine
- rifampin
- sibutramine
- sildenafil
- sirolimus
- some medicines for treating cancers
- St. John's wort
- tacrolimus
- tamoxifen
- terfenadine
- warfarin
- went yeast (Cholestin™)

Tell your prescriber or health care professional about all other medicines you are taking, including non-prescription medicines, nutritional supplements, or herbal products. Also tell your prescriber or health care professional if you are a frequent user of drinks with caffeine or alcohol, if you smoke, or if you use illegal drugs. These may affect the way your medicine works. Check with your health care professional before stopping or starting any of your medicines.

What should I watch for while taking voriconazole?

Tell your prescriber or health care professional if your symptoms do not improve in a few weeks. Some fungal infections need many weeks or months of treatment to cure. Keep taking your medicine regularly for as long as your prescriber or health care professional tells you to. You may need to visit your prescriber or health care professional for regular blood, kidney and liver function tests. Do not drive at night or perform other hazardous tasks at night while taking voriconazole. Changes in your vision, such as blurring or sensitivity to light may occur. Do not drive at all or operate machinery if you notice any change in your vision. Do not drink grapefruit juice while receiving voriconazole therapy. Grapefruit juice may lead to higher levels of voriconazole in your blood. Drinking alcohol can increase possible damage to your liver. Do not drink alcoholic beverages while you take this medicine. Avoid strong, direct sunlight during treatment with voriconazole. Your skin or eyes may be more sensitive to sunlight. Voriconazole should not be taken during pregnancy. If you are pregnant or think you may be pregnant, tell you prescriber or health care professional immediately. Women who may become pregnant should use effective birth control while receiving voriconazole treatment.

What side effects may I notice from taking voriconazole?

Side effects that you should report to your prescriber or health care professional as soon as possible:
- dark yellow or brown urine
- difficulty breathing
- severe problems with your eyesight or eye pain
- redness, blistering, peeling or loosening of the skin, including inside the mouth
- skin rash, itching
- stomach pain
- unusual bruising or bleeding
- yellowing of the eyes or skin

Side effects that usually do not require medical attention (report to your prescriber or health care professional if they continue or are bothersome):
- blurred vision
- flashing lights or bright spots in your field of vision
- headache
- hotness or flushing of the skin
- loss of appetite
- nausea, vomiting

Where can I keep my medicine?

Keep out of the reach of children in a container that small children cannot open. Store at room temperature below 30 degrees C (86 degrees F). Keep container tightly closed. Throw away any unused medicine after the expiration date.

Warfarin tablets

COUMADIN®;
5 mg; Tablet
Bristol Myers Squibb
Pharma Co

COUMADIN®;
7.5 mg; Tablet
Bristol Myers Squibb
Pharma Co

What are warfarin tablets?

WARFARIN (Coumadin®) is an anticoagulant. Warfarin helps to treat or prevent clots in the veins, arteries, lungs, or heart. Warfarin stops clots from forming or getting bigger, and lets the body naturally dissolve the clots. Sometimes warfarin is called a blood thinner because you may bleed more easily while taking it; however, warfarin does not actually thin the blood. Generic warfarin tablets are available.

What should my health care professional know before I take warfarin?

They need to know if you have any of these conditions:
- If you frequently drink alcohol-containing beverage
- blood disease, bleeding disorders, hemorrhage, hemophilia or aneurysm
- bowel disease, diverticulitis, or ulcers
- diabetes
- heart valve infection
- high blood pressure
- kidney disease
- liver disease
- protein or vitamin deficiency
- psychosis
- recent surgery
- thyroid problems
- an unusual or allergic reaction to warfarin, other medicines, foods, dyes, or preservatives
- pregnant or trying to get pregnant
- breast-feeding

How should I take this medicine?

Take warfarin tablets by mouth. Follow the directions on the prescription label. Warfarin is usually taken once a day. Swallow the tablets with a drink of water. Take your dose at the same time each day. Record your daily dose on a calendar when you take it. Do not take warfarin more often than directed. Contact your pediatrician or health care professional regarding the use of this medicine in children. Special care may be needed.

What if I miss a dose?

Try not to miss doses. If you do miss a dose, take it as soon as you can that same day. If it is almost time for your next dose, take only that dose. Do not double doses, and do not take two doses in one day unless your prescriber or health care professional tells you to; this can increase the risk of bleeding. If you miss a dose, record the date of the missed dose and tell your prescriber or health care professional at your next visit. If you miss doses for two or more days, call your doctor for instructions.

What may interact with warfarin?

Warfarin interacts with many other medicines; some are listed below:
- agents that dissolve blood clots
- agents that lower cholesterol
- alcohol
- allopurinol
- amiodarone
- antibiotics or medicines for treating bacterial, fungal or viral infections
- anti-inflammatory drugs, NSAIDs, such as ibuprofen
- aprepitant
- aspirin
- acetaminophen
- azathioprine
- barbiturate medicines for inducing sleep or treating seizures
- bosentan
- cimetidine
- cyclosporine
- disulfiram
- female hormones, including contraceptive or birth control pills
- fish oil (omega-3 fatty acids) supplements
- herbal products such as danshen, garlic, ginkgo, ginseng, green tea, or kava kava
- influenza virus vaccine
- male hormones
- medicines for some types of cancer
- certain medicines for heart rhythm problems
- certain medicines for high blood pressure
- quinidine, quinine
- seizure or epilepsy medicine such as carbamazepine, phenytoin, and valproic acid
- testolactone
- thyroid medicine
- tolterodine
- vitamin K (including vitamin, mineral, and food supplements that contain vitamin K)

Tell your prescriber or health care professional about all other medicines that you are taking, including non-prescription medicines, nutritional supplements, or herbal products. Also tell your prescriber or health care professional if you are a frequent user of drinks with caffeine or alcohol, if you smoke, or if you use illegal drugs. These may affect the way your medicine works. Check with your health care professional before stopping or starting any of your medicines.

What should I watch for while taking warfarin?

Visit your prescriber or health care professional for regular checks on your progress. You will need to have your blood checked regularly to make sure you are getting the right dose of warfarin. The blood test that is used to monitor warfarin therapy is called the protime

W

(PT) or INR. Your prescriber or health care professional will check your PT or INR and decide whether or not your dose of warfarin needs to be changed. When you first start warfarin, these tests are done frequently. Once the correct dose is determined and you take your medication properly, these tests can be done less often. While you are taking warfarin, carry an identification card with your name, the name and dose of medicine(s) being used, and the name and phone number of your prescriber or health care professional or person to contact in an emergency. You should discuss your diet with your prescriber or health care professional. Many foods contain high amounts of vitamin K, which can interfere with the effect of warfarin. Your prescriber or health care professional may want you to limit your intake of foods that contain vitamin K. Foods that have moderate to high amounts of vitamin K include brussel sprouts, kale, green tea, asparagus, avocado, broccoli, cabbage, cauliflower, collard greens, liver, soybean oil, soybeans, certain beans, mustard greens, peas (black-eyed peas, split peas, chick peas), turnip greens, parsley, green onions, spinach, and lettuce. Warfarin can cause birth defects or bleeding in an unborn child. Women of childbearing age should use effective contraception while receiving warfarin therapy. If a woman becomes pregnant while taking warfarin, she should discuss the potential risks and her options with her health care professional. Do not change brands of warfarin without talking to your prescriber or health care professional. Also, always check the color of your medicine when you get a new prescription. If you notice a change in the color of your warfarin tablet, check with your pharmacist or health care professional to make sure you received the correct medicine. Alcohol can affect the way warfarin works. Ask your prescriber or health care professional how much, if any, alcohol you may consume. Do not take any over-the-counter medicines without first talking to your prescriber or health care professional. Do not take any aspirin or aspirin-containing products, ibuprofen (Motrin®, Advil®, or Nuprin®) naproxen (Aleve®), ketoprofen (Orudis-KT®) or other medicines known as nonsteroidal anti-inflammatory agents without talking to your prescriber or health care professional first. Be careful to avoid sports and activities that might cause injury while you are using warfarin. Severe falls or injuries can cause unseen bleeding. Be careful when using sharp tools or knives.

Consider using an electric razor. Take special care brushing or flossing your teeth. Report any injuries, bruising, or red spots on the skin to your prescriber or health care professional. If you have an illness that causes vomiting, diarrhea, or fever for more than a few days, contact your doctor. Also check with your doctor if you are unable to eat for several days. These problems can change the effect of warfarin. Even after you stop taking warfarin, it takes several days before your body recovers its normal ability to clot blood. Ask your prescriber or health care professional how long you need to be cautious. If you are going to have surgery or dental work, tell your prescriber or health care professional that you have been taking warfarin.

What side effects might I notice from taking warfarin?

Side effects that you should report to your prescriber or health care professional as soon as possible:

- signs and symptoms of bleeding such as bloody or black, tarry stools, red or dark-brown urine, spitting up blood or brown material that looks like coffee grounds, red spots on the skin, unusual bruising or bleeding from the eye, gums, or nose
- back or stomach pain
- chest pain; fast or irregular heartbeat (palpitations)
- difficulty breathing or talking, wheezing
- fever or chills
- heavy menstrual bleeding or vaginal bleeding
- nausea, vomiting
- painful, blue, or purple toes
- prolonged bleeding from cuts
- skin rash, itching or skin damage
- unusual swelling or sudden weight gain
- unusual tiredness or weakness
- yellowing of skin or eyes

Side effects that usually do not require medical attention (report to your prescriber or health care professional if they continue or are bothersome):

- diarrhea
- loss of appetite
- unusual hair loss

Where can I keep my medicine?

Keep out of the reach of children in a container that small children cannot open. Store at room temperature between 15 and 30 degrees C (59 and 86 degrees F). Protect from light. Throw away any unused medicine after the expiration date.

W

Zafirlukast tablets

ACCOLATE®;
20 mg; Tablet
AstraZeneca Pharmaceuticals
LP

What is zafirlukast?

ZAFIRLUKAST (Accolate®) helps to reduce asthma symptoms (coughing, wheezing, shortness of breath, or chest tightness) and control your asthma. It does not provide instant relief and cannot be used to treat a sudden asthma attack. It works only when used on a regular basis to help reduce inflammation and prevent asthma attacks. Zafirlukast is effective in adults and older children. Generic zafirlukast tablets are not yet available.

What should my health care professional know before I take zafirlukast?

They need to know if you have any of these conditions:
- an acute asthma attack
- are on corticosteroid therapy, like prednisone or inhalers
- liver disease, like hepatitis
- an unusual or allergic reaction to zafirlukast, other medicines, foods, dyes, or preservatives
- pregnant or trying to get pregnant
- breast-feeding

How should I take this medicine?

Take zafirlukast by mouth (i.e., swallowed) on an empty stomach. This means you should take this medicine at least 1 hour before or 2 hours after a meal. Follow the directions on the prescription label. You should take zafirlukast every day, even when you are not having asthma symptoms. Do not take your medicine more often than directed. Contact your pediatrician or health care professional regarding the use of this medicine in children under the age of 5 years old. Special care may be needed.

What if I miss a dose?

If you miss a dose, use it as soon as you can. If it is almost time for the next dose, skip the previous dose. Do not use double or extra doses.

What may interact with zafirlukast?

- alprazolam
- aspirin
- astemizole
- carbamazepine
- cilostazol
- cisapride
- clarithromycin
- cyclosporine
- diazepam
- diltiazem
- dofetilide
- erythromycin
- phenytoin
- sildenafil
- some medicines for lowering cholesterol (examples: lovastatin, simvastatin)
- some medicines for lowering heart rate or blood pressure (examples: diltiazem, felodipine, nifedipine, quinidine, verapamil)
- terfenadine
- theophylline
- tolbutamide
- voriconazole
- warfarin

Tell your prescriber or health care professional about all other medicines that you are taking, including non-prescription medicines. Also tell your prescriber or health care professional if you are a frequent user of drinks with caffeine or alcohol, if you smoke, or if you use illegal drugs. These may affect the way your medicine works. Check with your health care professional before stopping or starting any of your medicines.

What should I watch for while taking zafirlukast?

Zafirlukast is only used to help prevent asthma attacks; it is not used as a "quick-relief" medicine to treat an asthma attack. Therefore, you should always have your "quick-relief" medicine with you to treat an asthma attack. Talk with your prescriber about what you should do if you have an acute asthma attack. Tell your prescriber or health care professional if your symptoms do not improve or if your asthma gets worse while you are using zafirlukast. If you find that your medicines become less effective in treating your asthma, you should contact your health care professional as soon as possible. Do not to stop taking or decrease the use of your other asthma treatments, including steroids, when starting zafirlukast unless otherwise directed by their health care prescriber. Follow your prescriber's directions exactly. Zafirlukast works best if you use it regularly even when you do not have asthma symptoms. Do not stop using your medication without your prescriber's advice. If you are going to have surgery, tell your health care professional that you take zafirlukast.

What side effects may I notice from taking zafirlukast?

Side effects that you should report to your prescriber or health care professional as soon as possible:
- wheezing or continued coughing

Rare or uncommon—signs of allergic reactions:
- skin rash and itching (hives)
- swelling of face, lips, or eyelids
- difficulty breathing

Z

Rare—signs of liver problems:
- brown or dark urine
- fatigue
- loss of appetite
- nausea and vomiting
- severe itching
- yellowing of the eyes or skin

Side effects that usually do not require medical attention (report to your prescriber or health care professional if they continue or are bothersome):

- cough, sore throat
- headache
- indigestion or mild stomachache
- runny or stuffy nose

Where can I keep my medicine?

Keep out of the reach of young children. Store at room temperature; do not freeze. Protect from light and moisture. Throw away any unused medicine after the expiration date.

Zalcitabine, ddC tablets

HIVID®;
0.375 mg; Tablet
Hoffmann La Roche
Inc

HIVID®;
0.75 mg; Tablet
Hoffmann La Roche
Inc

What are zalcitabine tablets?

ZALCITABINE, ddC (Hivid®) is an antiviral drug called a nucleoside reverse transcriptase inhibitor or NRTI. Zalcitabine is used to treat human immunodeficiency virus (HIV) infection. Zalcitabine may reduce the amount of HIV in the blood and increase the number of CD4 cells (T-cells) in the blood. Zalcitabine is used in combination with other drugs to treat the HIV virus. Zalcitabine will not cure or prevent HIV infection or AIDS. You may still develop other infections or conditions associated with HIV. Generic zalcitabine tablets are not yet available.

What should my health care professional know before I take zalcitabine?

They need to know if you have any of these conditions:
- if you frequently drink alcohol-containing beverages
- high cholesterol
- kidney disease
- liver disease
- pancreatitis
- tingling or numbness in the hands or feet
- an unusual or allergic reaction to zalcitabine, other medicines, foods, dyes, or preservatives
- pregnant or trying to get pregnant
- breast-feeding

How should I take this medicine?

Take zalcitabine tablets by mouth. Follow the directions on the prescription label. Swallow tablets with a drink of water. Take zalcitabine on an empty stomach, 1 hour before or 2 hours after food. Take your doses at regular intervals. Do not take your medicine more often than directed. To help to make sure that your anti-HIV therapy works as well as possible, be very careful to take all of your medicine exactly as prescribed. Do not stop taking except on your prescriber's advice. Contact your pediatrician or health care professional regarding the use of this medicine in children. Special care may be needed.

What if I miss a dose?

If you miss a dose, take it as soon as you can. If it is almost time for your next dose, take only that dose. Do not take double or extra doses.

What may interact with zalcitabine?

- alcohol
- amphotericin
- certain antibiotics (usually given in the hospital)
- didanosine, ddI
- foscarnet
- lamivudine, 3TC
- stavudine, d4T
- ribavirin

Tell your prescriber or health care professional about all other medicines you are taking, including nonprescription medicines, nutritional supplements, or herbal products. Also tell your prescriber or health care professional if you are a frequent user of drinks with caffeine or alcohol, if you smoke, or if you use illegal drugs. These may affect the way your medicine works. Check with your health care professional before stopping or starting any of your medicines.

What should I watch for while taking zalcitabine?

Visit your prescriber or health care professional for regular checks on your progress. Discuss any new symptoms with your prescriber or health care professional. Alcohol can increase the risk of developing severe side effects when taken with zalcitabine. Avoid alcoholic drinks while you are taking zalcitabine. Do not treat yourself for nausea, vomiting, or stomach pain. Call your prescriber or health care professional for advice. Tell your prescriber or health care professional if you get tingling, pain or numbness in your hands or feet. Zalcitabine will not cure HIV and you can still get other illnesses or complications associated with your disease. Taking zalcitabine does not reduce the risk of passing HIV infection to others through sexual or blood contact. It is best to avoid sexual contact so that you do not spread the disease to others. For any sexual contact, use a condom. Be careful about cuts, abrasions and other possible sources of blood contact. Never share a needle or syringe with anyone.

What side effects may I notice from taking zalcitabine?

Side effects that you should report to your prescriber or health care professional as soon as possible:
- back pain
- changes in body appearance (such as weight gain or loss around the waist and/or face)
- fever or chills, sore throat
- nausea, vomiting
- stomach pain
- tingling, pain or numbness in the hands or feet
- unusual bleeding or bruising
- unusual tiredness or weakness

Side effects that usually do not require medical attention (report to your prescriber or health care professional if they continue or are bothersome):
- muscle and joint pain
- skin rash, itching
- sore or ulcerated mouth

Where can I keep my medicine?

Keep out of the reach of children in a container that small children cannot open. Store at room temperature between 15 and 30 degrees C (59 and 86 degrees F). Keep container tightly closed. Throw away any unused medicine after the expiration date.

Zaleplon capsules

SONATA®; 5 mg; Capsule Wyeth Laboratories Div Wyeth Ayerst Pharmaceuticals Inc	SONATA®; 10 mg; Capsule Wyeth Laboratories Div Wyeth Ayerst Pharmaceuticals Inc

What are zaleplon capsules?

ZALEPLON (Sonata®) is a sedative-type drug that helps to treat difficulty falling asleep (insomnia). If your main sleep problem is waking up after falling asleep, then zaleplon will not be helpful for you. Zaleplon helps people with problems falling asleep and should not be taken for long periods, except on your prescriber's advice. Do not share your medicine with anyone else. Generic zaleplon capsules are not yet available.

What should my health care professional know before I take zaleplon?

They need to know if you have any of these conditions:
- an alcohol or drug abuse problem
- attempted suicide
- breathing difficulty, such as chronic obstructive pulmonary disease (COPD), untreated asthma, or sleep apnea
- liver disease
- mental depression
- an unusual or allergic reaction to zaleplon, other medicines, foods, dyes, or preservatives
- pregnant or trying to get pregnant
- breast-feeding

How should I take this medicine?

Take zaleplon capsules by mouth. Follow the directions on the prescription label. Swallow the capsules with a drink of water. It is better to take zaleplon on an empty stomach (without food). Take zaleplon immediately before going to bed or after you have gone to bed and are having trouble falling asleep. Do not take your medicine more often than directed. Contact your pediatrician or health care professional regarding the use of this medicine in children. Special care may be needed. Elderly patients over age 65 years or seriously ill patients may have a stronger reaction to this medicine and need smaller doses.

What if I miss a dose?

This does not apply. Zaleplon should only be taken immediately before getting into bed or after getting in bed and having trouble falling asleep. Do not take double or extra doses.

What may interact with zaleplon?

- alcohol and alcoholic beverages
- barbiturate medicines for inducing sleep or treating seizures (convulsions)
- carbamazepine
- cimetidine
- kava kava
- melatonin
- muscle relaxants
- phenytoin
- rifampin
- valerian
- certain medications for allergies, such as azatadine, clemastine, diphenhydramine
- certain medications for depression, anxiety, or other emotional or psychiatric problems.
- certain medications for pain
- certain medications for sleep

Tell your prescriber or health care professional about all other medicines you are taking, including non-prescription medicines, nutritional supplements, or herbal products. Also tell your prescriber or health care professional if you are a frequent user of drinks with caffeine or alcohol, if you smoke, or if you use illegal drugs. These may affect the way your medicine works. Check with your health care professional before stopping or starting any of your medicines.

What should I watch for while taking zaleplon?

Visit your prescriber or health care professional for regular checks on your progress. If sleep medicine is taken every night for a long time it may no longer help you to sleep. In most cases zaleplon should only be taken for a few days and for not longer than 1 or 2 weeks.

Z

Consult your prescriber or health care professional if you still have difficulty in sleeping. Be sure to take only the amount of zaleplon prescribed by your health care provider. If you feel you need a higher dose, contact your health care provider to discuss your options. If you have been taking zaleplon regularly and suddenly stop taking it, you may get unpleasant withdrawal symptoms. Your prescriber or health care professional may want to gradually reduce the dose. Do not stop taking except on your prescriber's advice. After you stop taking zaleplon you may get rebound insomnia. This means that for a few nights you may have trouble sleeping, but this usually goes away after 1 or 2 nights. After taking zaleplon you may get a residual hangover effect that leaves you drowsy or dizzy the next day. Do not drive, use machinery, or do anything that needs mental alertness until you know how zaleplon affects you. To reduce dizzy or fainting spells, do not sit or stand up quickly, especially if you are an older patient. Alcohol can increase the drowsy or dizzy effects. Avoid alcoholic drinks. If you are going to have surgery, tell your prescriber or health care professional that you are taking zaleplon.

What side effects may I notice from taking zaleplon?

Side effects that you should report to your prescriber or health care professional as soon as possible:

- confusion
- difficulty breathing
- hallucinations (seeing, hearing, or feeling things that are not really there)
- hostility, restlessness, excitability
- lightheadedness or fainting spells
- mental depression or worsening of depression
- slurred speech
- unusual weakness
- staggering, tremors
- suicidal thoughts
- vision problems

Side effects that usually do not require medical attention (report to your prescriber or health care professional if they continue or are bothersome):

- difficulty with coordination
- dizziness, drowsiness 'hangover' effect
- nightmares
- stomach upset
- diarrhea
- loss of memory

Where can I keep my medicine?

Keep out of the reach of children in a container that small children cannot open. Store at room temperature between 20 and 25 degrees C (68 and 77 degrees F). Throw away any unused medicine after the expiration date.

Zidovudine, ZDV capsules

RETROVIR®;
100 mg; Capsule
Glaxo Wellcome Division

What are zidovudine capsules?

ZIDOVUDINE, ZDV (AZT or Retrovir®) is an antiviral drug called a nucleoside reverse transcriptase inhibitor or NRTI. Zidovudine is used to treat human immunodeficiency virus (HIV) infection. Zidovudine may reduce the amount of HIV in the blood and increase the number of CD4 cells (T-cells) in the blood. Zidovudine is usually used in combination with other drugs to treat the HIV virus. Zidovudine will not cure or prevent HIV infection or AIDS. You may still develop other infections or conditions associated with HIV. Generic zidovudine capsules are available.

What should my health care professional know before I take zidovudine?

They need to know if you have any of these conditions:

- If you frequently drink alcohol-containing beverages
- anemia
- dental disease
- kidney disease
- liver disease
- recent chemotherapy or radiation therapy
- an unusual or allergic reaction to zidovudine, other medicines, foods, dyes, or preservatives
- pregnant or trying to get pregnant
- breast-feeding

How should I take this medicine?

Take zidovudine capsules by mouth. Follow the directions on the prescription label. Swallow capsules with plenty of water, especially at bedtime to prevent throat irritation. If zidovudine upsets your stomach, you can take it with food. Take your doses at regular intervals. Do not take your medicine more often than directed. To help to make sure that your anti-HIV therapy works as well as possible, be very careful to take all of your medicine exactly as prescribed. Do not stop taking except on your prescriber's advice. Contact your pediatrician or health care professional regarding the use of this medicine in children. Special care may be needed.

What if I miss a dose?

If you miss a dose, take it as soon as you can. If it is almost time for your next dose, take only that dose. Do not take double or extra doses.

What may interact with zidovudine?

- antiviral agents (such as acyclovir, cidofovir, foscarnet, ganciclovir, valganciclovir)
- atovaquone
- certain antibiotics (such as clarithromycin)
- dapsone

- doxorubicin
- fluconazole
- flucytosine
- interferon alfa or beta
- methadone
- phenytoin
- probenecid
- pyrimethamine
- ribavirin
- rifampin
- stavudine, d4T
- sulfamethoxazole; trimethoprim, SMX-TMP (co-trimoxazole, Bactrim®)
- valproic acid

Tell your prescriber or health care professional about all other medicines you are taking, including nonprescription medicines, nutritional supplements, or herbal products. Also tell your prescriber or health care professional if you are a frequent user of drinks with caffeine or alcohol, if you smoke, or if you use illegal drugs. These may affect the way your medicine works. Check with your health care professional before stopping or starting any of your medicines.

What should I watch for while taking zidovudine?

Visit your prescriber or health care professional for regular checks on your progress. Discuss any new symptoms with your prescriber or health care professional. Tell your prescriber or health care professional if you get tingling, pain or numbness in your hands or feet. Zidovudine can cause blood problems. This can mean slow healing and a risk of infection. Try to avoid cutting or injuring yourself. Problems can arise if you need dental work, and in the day to day care of your teeth. Try to avoid damage to your teeth and gums when you brush or floss your teeth. Tell your dentist you are taking zidovudine. Zidovudine will not cure HIV and you can still get other illnesses or complications associated with your disease. Taking zidovudine does not reduce the risk of passing HIV infection to others through sexual or blood contact. It is best to avoid sexual contact so that you do not spread the disease to others. For any sexual contact, use a condom. Be careful about cuts, abrasions and other possible sources of blood contact. Never share a needle or syringe with anyone.

What side effects may I notice from taking zidovudine?

Side effects that you should report to your prescriber or health care professional as soon as possible:
- changes in body appearance (weight gain around waist and/or face)
- fever or chills, sore throat
- muscle pain or weakness
- joint pain
- pain or difficulty swallowing
- seizures or convulsions
- signs of low platelet counts such as unusual bleeding or bruising
- signs of low red blood cell counts such as increased tiredness or weakness
- skin rash, itching, or rash with symptoms such as fever, blisters, eye irritation, edema, redness, peeling or loosening of the skin, including inside the mouth
- sores or ulcers in the mouth or throat
- swelling of the eyelids, face, hands, or feet
- unusual tiredness or weakness
- tingling, pain, burning, or numbness in the hands or feet

Side effects that usually do not require medical attention (report to your prescriber or health care professional if they continue or are bothersome):
- constipation
- difficulty sleeping
- discolored nails and skin
- dizziness
- drowsiness
- headache
- loss of appetite
- nausea, vomiting
- stomach pain

Where can I keep my medicine?

Keep out of the reach of children in a container that small children cannot open. Store at room temperature between 15 and 25 degrees C (59 and 77 degrees F). Protect from light and moisture. Throw away any unused medicine after the expiration date.

Zileuton tablets

ZYFLO®;
600 mg; Tablet
Abbott Pharmaceutical
Product Division

What are zileuton tablets?

Zileuton (Zyflo®) is used to treat asthma. It helps to reduce recurring symptoms of asthma, but it is not for rapid relief of asthma attacks. Generic zileuton tablets are not available. NOTE: This drug will be discontinued in the US. Zyflo® should be available until December 2003. Talk to your healthcare provider as soon as possible to switch to a different medication to help control your asthma.

What should my health care professional know before I take zileuton?

They need to know if you have any of these conditions:
- liver disease
- fever or infection

- an unusual or allergic reaction to zileuton, other medicines, foods, dyes, or preservatives
- pregnant or trying to get pregnant
- breast-feeding

How should I take this medicine?

Take zileuton tablets by mouth. Follow the directions on the prescription label. Take your doses at regular intervals. Zileuton may be taken with meals and at bedtime. Do not take your medicine more often than directed. Contact your pediatrician or health care professional regarding the use of this medicine in children. Special care may be needed.

What if I miss a dose?

If you miss a dose, take it as soon as you can. If it is almost time for your next dose, take only that dose. Do not take double or extra doses.

What may interact with zileuton?

- alosetron
- astemizole
- bosentan
- caffeine
- carbamazepine
- certain drugs for anxiety, insomnia, or difficulty sleeping (such as alprazolam, diazepam, midazolam, or triazolam)
- certain drugs used to lower cholesterol (atorvastatin, cerivastatin, lovastatin, simvastatin)
- certain drugs used for HIV infection or AIDS (such as indinavir, ritonavir, or saquinavir)
- certain heart or high blood pressure medicines (such as bepridil, diltiazem, felodipine, lidocaine, nicardipine, nifedipine, nimodipine, nisoldipine, propranolol, quinidine, or verapamil)
- cisapride
- clarithromycin or erythromycin
- cyclosporine
- donepezil
- ergot alkaloids (such as dihydroergotamine, ergotamine, methysergide or methylergonovine)
- guarana
- imatinib, STI-571
- pimozide
- sirolimus
- steroid drugs (such as prednisone, hydrocortisone, dexamethasone)
- tacrolimus
- terfenadine
- theophylline or aminophylline
- voriconazole
- warfarin
- went yeast
- zonisamide

Tell your prescriber or health care professional about all other medicines you are taking, including non-prescription medicines, nutritional supplements, or herbal products. Also tell your prescriber or health care professional if you are a frequent user of drinks with caffeine or alcohol, if you smoke, or if you use illegal drugs. These may affect the way your medicine works. Check with your health care professional before stopping or starting any of your medicines.

What should I watch for while taking zileuton?

It is important that you go on taking your medicine even when you do not have any symptoms. Tell your prescriber or health care professional if your symptoms do not start to improve after several days. Only stop taking zileuton on your prescriber's advice. Visit your prescriber or health care professional for regular checks on your progress. Liver tests will need to be done on a regular basis while taking zileuton.

What side effects may I notice from taking zileuton?

Side effects that you should report to your prescriber or health care professional as soon as possible:

- chest pain
- difficulty breathing, wheezing
- flu-like symptoms (chills, fatigue, fever, muscle aches)
- nausea
- pruritus
- skin rash or itching
- unusual weakness or tiredness
- yellowing of the skin

Call your prescriber or health care professional immediately if you get any of these side effects. Side effects that usually do not require medical attention (report to your prescriber or health care professional if they continue or are bothersome):

- back pain
- dizziness
- drowsiness
- dyspepsia
- headache
- insomnia
- numbness or tingling in the hands or feet
- stomach pain
- weakness

Where can I keep my medicine?

Keep out of the reach of children in a container that small children cannot open. Store at room temperature between 20 and 25 degrees C (68 and 77 degrees F). Throw away any unused medicine after the expiration date.

Ziprasidone capsules

GEODON®;
60 mg; Capsule
Roerig Division of Pfizer

What are ziprasidone capsules?

ZIPRASIDONE (Geodon®) treats the symptoms of schizophrenia. Such symptoms may include hearing or seeing things that others do not, suspiciousness of others, mistaken beliefs, or withdrawal from normal activities, family and friends. This drug may also help treat some other emotional problems, such as bipolar disorder (also known as manic depression). Generic ziprasidone capsules are not yet available.

What should my health care professional know before I take ziprasidone?

They need to know if you have any of these conditions:
- frequently drink alcohol or alcohol-containing beverages
- diabetes or high blood sugar
- difficulty swallowing
- history of breast cancer
- heart disease, including heart failure
- history of head injury
- previous heart attack or stroke
- irregular heartbeat
- liver disease
- low blood pressure
- low potassium level in the blood
- Parkinson's disease
- seizures (convulsions)
- tardive dyskinesia (uncontrollable movement disorder)
- thoughts of suicide
- an unusual or allergic reaction to ziprasidone, other medicines, foods, dyes, or preservatives
- pregnant or trying to get pregnant
- breast-feeding

How should I take this medicine?

Take ziprasidone capsules by mouth with food. Follow the directions on the prescription label. Swallow the capsules with a drink of water and take each dose with food. Take your doses at regular intervals, usually at the same times each day. Do not take your medicine more often than directed. Do not stop taking except on your prescriber's advice. Contact your pediatrician or health care professional regarding the use of this medicine in children. Special care may be needed.

What if I miss a dose?

If you miss a dose, take it as soon as you can. If it is almost time for your next dose, take only that dose. Do not take double or extra doses.

What may interact with ziprasidone?

Do not take ziprasidone with any of the following medications:

- certain antibiotics (clarithromycin, erythromycin, gatifloxacin, grepafloxacin, levofloxacin, moxifloxacin, sparfloxacin, telithromycin, troleandomycin)
- certain antidepressants (check with your health care professional)
- arsenic trioxide
- astemizole
- bepridil
- chlorpromazine
- cisapride
- daunorubicin
- diltiazem
- dolasetron
- doxorubicin
- droperidol
- halofantrine
- haloperidol
- halothane
- levomethadyl
- mesoridazine
- octreotide
- pentamidine
- pimozide
- probucol
- risperidone
- some medicines for treating heart-rhythm problems (examples: amiodarone, dofetilide, flecainide, procainamide, quinidine, sotalol)
- tacrolimus
- terfenadine
- thioridazine
- verapamil

Ziprasidone may also interact with the following medications:

- alcohol
- bromocriptine
- cabergoline
- carbamazepine
- cimetidine
- cocaine
- danazol
- dronabinol
- medicines for anxiety, depression or difficulty sleeping
- medicines for diabetes
- medicines for fungal infections (fluconazole, itraconazole, ketoconazole, voriconazole)
- medicines for Parkinson's disease
- other medicines for treating thought disorders such as schizophrenia
- phenobarbital
- phenytoin
- prescription medicines for muscle relaxation or pain
- primidone
- quinine

- rifabutin
- rifampin
- some medications for high blood pressure
- some medicines for HIV infection
- some medicines for infertility
- some medicines for the hormonal treatment of cancer
- stimulants (amphetamine, dextroamphetamine)
- troglitazone
- water pills (diuretics)

Tell your prescriber or health care professional about all other medicines you are taking, including non-prescription medicines. Also tell your prescriber or health care professional if you are a frequent user of drinks with caffeine or alcohol, if you smoke, or if you use illegal drugs. These may affect the way your medicine works. Check with your health care professional before stopping or starting any of your medicines.

What should I watch for while taking ziprasidone?

Visit your prescriber or health care professional for regular checks on your progress. It may be several weeks before you see the full effects of ziprasidone. Do not suddenly stop taking ziprasidone. Your doctor may want you to gradually reduce the dose. Only stop taking ziprasidone on your prescriber's advice. You may get dizzy or drowsy. Do not drive, use machinery, or do anything that needs mental alertness until you know how ziprasidone affects you. Alcohol can increase dizziness and drowsiness. Avoid alcoholic drinks. Do not stand or sit up quickly, especially if you are an older patient. This reduces the risk of dizzy or fainting spells. If you notice an increased thirst or hunger, different from your normal hunger or thirst, or if you find that you must frequently use the restroom (excessive urination), you should contact your health care provider as soon as possible. You may need to have your blood sugar monitored. Ziprasidone may cause your skin to become more sensitive to the sun or ultraviolet light. If this reaction occurs, it can cause a severe sunburn and damage the skin. Keep out of the sun, or wear protective clothing outdoors and use a sunscreen (at least SPF 15). Do not use sun lamps or sun tanning beds or booths. Wear sunglasses to protect your eyes. Ziprasidone can change the response of your body to heat or cold. Try not to get overheated. Avoid temperature extremes, such as saunas, hot tubs, or very hot or cold baths or showers. Dress warmly in cold weather. If you experience dry mouth while taking ziprasidone, make sure to drink plenty of water. It may also be helpful to suck on sugarless hard candy or crushed ice. If your dry mouth is severe, ask your doctor about a saliva substitute. If you are going to have surgery tell your prescriber or health care professional that you are taking ziprasidone.

What side effects may I notice from taking ziprasidone?

Side effects that you should report to your prescriber or health care professional as soon as possible:
Because the following side effects could mean you are having a heart rhythm problem, contact your prescriber immediately for:
- chest pain
- fast or irregular heartbeat or palpitations
- difficulty breathing
- fainting or falling spells

Other side effects to report to your prescriber as soon as possible for:
- change in emotion or behavior such as feeling depressed, angry, or anxious
- difficulty swallowing
- fever
- inability to control muscle movements in the face, hands, arms, or legs
- increased thirst or hunger
- increased need to pass urine
- loss of balance or difficulty walking
- menstrual changes
- prolonged erection
- seizures
- skin rash or hives
- stiff muscles or jaw
- tremor
- uncontrollable movements or spasms of the face, tongue or mouth
- weakness or loss of strength

Side effects that usually do not require medical attention (report to your prescriber or health care professional if they continue or are bothersome):
Less common or rare:
- breast enlargement (men or women)
- breast milk in women who are not breast-feeding
- changes in sexual desire or ability
- diarrhea
- dry mouth
- increased sensitivity to the sun
- intolerance to heat or cold
- restlessness or need to keep moving
- stuffy or runny nose
More common:
- constipation
- mild dizziness; especially on standing from a sitting or lying position
- drowsiness
- headache
- nausea or vomiting
- upset stomach

Where can I keep my medicine?

Keep out of the reach of children in a container that small children cannot open. Store at room temperature between 15 degrees and 30 degrees C (59 degrees and 86 degrees F). Throw away any unused medicine after the expiration date.

Zolmitriptan tablets and disintegrating tablets

ZOMIG;
5 mg; Tablet
AstraZeneca
Pharmaceuticals LP

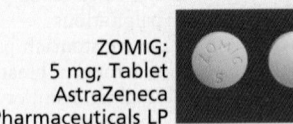

ZOMIG;
2.5 mg; Tablet,
Orally
Disintegrating
AstraZeneca
Pharmaceuticals LP

What are zolmitriptan tablets and disintegrating tablets?

ZOLMITRIPTAN (Zomig®, Zomig-ZMT®) helps to relieve a migraine attack that starts with or without aura (a peculiar feeling or visual disturbance that warns you of an attack). Generic zolmitriptan tablets and disintegrating tablets are not yet available.

What should my health care professional know before I take zolmitriptan tablets?

They need to know if you have any of these conditions:
- abdominal pain
- bowel disease, colitis or bloody diarrhea
- diabetes
- headaches that are different from your usual migraine
- heart or blood vessel disease, angina (chest pain), or previous heart attack
- family history of heart disease
- high blood pressure
- high cholesterol
- history of stroke, transient ischemic attacks (TIAs or "mini-strokes"), or intracranial bleeding
- fast or irregular heartbeat
- postmenopausal or surgical removal of uterus and ovaries
- kidney disease
- liver disease
- overweight
- poor circulation
- Raynaud's disease
- seizure disorder
- tobacco smoker
- an unusual or allergic reaction to zolmitriptan, other medicines, foods, dyes, or preservatives
- pregnant or trying to get pregnant
- breast-feeding

How should I take this medicine?

Take zolmitriptan tablets by mouth. Follow the directions on the prescription label. Zolmitriptan is taken at the first symptoms of a migraine attack; it is not for everyday use.
Tablets: Swallow the tablets with a drink of water.
Disintegrating tablets: Leave the zolmitriptan disintegrating tablet in the foil package until you are ready to take it. Do not push the tablet through the blister pack. Peel open the blister pack with dry hands and place the tablet on your tongue. The tablet will dissolve rapidly and be swallowed in your saliva. It is not necessary to drink any water to take this medicine.
If your migraine headache returns after one dose, you can take another dose as directed. You must allow at least 2 hours between doses, and do not take more

than 10 mg total in any 24 hour period. If there is no improvement at all after the first dose, do not take a second dose without talking to your prescriber or health care professional. Do not take your medicine more often than directed. Contact your pediatrician or health care professional regarding the use of this medicine in children. Special care may be needed.

What if I miss a dose?

This does not apply, zolmitriptan is not for regular use.

What may interact with zolmitriptan?

Do not take zolmitriptan with any of the following medicines:

- amphetamine or cocaine
- dihydroergotamine, ergotamine, ergoloid mesylates, methysergide, or ergot-type medication—do not take within 24 hours of taking zolmitriptan.
- almotriptan, eletriptan, naratriptan, rizatriptan, sumatriptan—do not take within 24 hours of taking zolmitriptan.
- medicines for weight loss such as dexfenfluramine, dextroamphetamine, fenfluramine, or sibutramine
- monoamine oxidase inhibitors (MAOIs) such as phenelzine (Nardil®), tranylcypromine (Parnate®), isocarboxazid (Marplan®), and selegiline (Carbex®, Eldepryl®)—do not take zolmitriptan within 2 weeks of stopping MAOI therapy.

Check with your doctor or pharmacist if you take any of these medications:

- birth control pills
- cimetidine
- cough syrup or other products containing dextromethorphan
- feverfew
- lithium
- medicines for mental depression, anxiety or mood problems such as buspirone, citalopram, fluoxetine, fluvoxamine, mirtazapine, nefazodone, paroxetine, sertraline, trazodone, tricyclic antidepressants, or venlafaxine
- meperidine
- propranolol
- St. John's wort
- tryptophan

Tell your physician or health care provider: about all other medicines you are taking, including non-prescription medicines; if you are a frequent user of drinks with caffeine or alcohol; if you smoke; or if you use illegal drugs. These may affect the way your medicine works. Check with your health care professional before stopping or starting any of your medicines.

Z

What should I watch for while taking zolmitriptan?

Only take zolmitriptan tablets for a migraine headache. Take it if you get warning symptoms or at the start of a migraine attack. Zolmitriptan is not for regular use to prevent migraine attacks. Do not take migraine products that contain ergotamine while you are taking zolmitriptan; this combination can affect your heart. You may get drowsy, dizzy. Do not drive, use machinery, or do anything that needs mental alertness until you know how zolmitriptan affects you. To reduce dizzy or fainting spells, do not sit or stand up quickly, especially if you are an older patient. Alcohol can increase drowsiness, dizziness and flushing. Avoid alcoholic drinks. Smoking cigarettes may increase the risk of heart-related side effects from using zolmitriptan.

What side effects may I notice from taking zolmitriptan?

Rare or uncommon:
- chest or throat pain, tightness
- dizziness or faintness
- fast or irregular heart beat

- feeling of chest heaviness or pressure
- increased blood pressure
- palpitations
- severe stomach pain and cramping, bloody diarrhea
- shortness of breath, wheezing, or difficulty breathing
- tingling, pain, or numbness in the face, hands or feet
- unusual reaction or swelling of the skin, eyelids, face, or lips

Side effects that usually do not require medical attention (report to your prescriber or health care professional if they continue or are bothersome):
- drowsiness
- dry mouth
- feeling warm, flushing, sweating or redness of the face
- muscle pain or cramps
- nausea, vomiting, stomach upset, or difficulty swallowing
- tiredness or weakness

Where can I keep my medicine?

Keep out of the reach of children in a container that small children cannot open. Store at room temperature between 20 and 25 degrees C (68 and 77 degrees F). Protect from light and moisture. Throw away any unused medicine after the expiration date.

Zolpidem tablets

AMBIEN®;
10 mg; Tablet
Sanofi-Synthelabo
Inc

AMBIEN®;
5 mg; Tablet
Sanofi-Synthelabo
Inc

What are zolpidem tablets?

ZOLPIDEM (Ambien®) is a sedative-type drug that helps to relieve insomnia (sleeplessness). Trouble falling asleep, waking up too early in the morning, or waking up too often during the night are symptoms of insomnia. Zolpidem helps treat these problems with sleep, and is usually used for no longer than a few days to a few weeks. Sleep medicines should not be taken for long periods of time, except on your prescriber's advice. Do not share your medicine with anyone else. Generic zolpidem tablets are not yet available.

What should my health care professional know before I take zolpidem?

They need to know if you have any of these conditions:
- frequently drink alcohol
- depression
- history of a drug abuse problem
- liver disease
- lung or respiratory disease (breathing difficulties, like emphysema or sleep apnea)
- an unusual or allergic reaction to zolpidem, other medicines, foods, dyes, or preservatives
- pregnant or trying to get pregnant
- breast-feeding

How should I take this medicine?

Take zolpidem tablets by mouth. Follow the directions on the prescription label. Swallow the tablets with a drink of water. It is better to take zolpidem on an empty stomach (without food) and only when you are ready for bed. Do not take your medicine more often than directed. Do not share your medicine with anyone else. Contact your pediatrician or health care professional regarding the use of this medicine in children. Special care may be needed. Elderly patients over age 65 years may have a stronger reaction to this medicine and need smaller doses.

What if I miss a dose?

This does not apply. Zolpidem should only be taken immediately before going to sleep. Do not take double or extra doses.

What may interact with zolpidem?

- bupropion
- caffeine
- flumazenil
- certain antidepressants, like citalopram, fluoxetine, fluvoxamine, paroxetine, sertraline, or venlafaxine
- medications for fungal infections, like ketoconazole, fluconazole, or itraconazole
- some medicines used to treat HIV infection or AIDS, like ritonavir
- St. John's wort

Certain medications may cause additive drowsiness or decrease alertness with zolpidem:

- alcohol
- allergy, cough, or cold medications (antihistamines)
- kava kava
- melatonin
- medicines for anxiety
- medicines for pain
- medicines for treating mental problems
- melatonin
- other sedatives given for sleep
- some medicines for Parkinson' s disease or other movement disorders
- valerian

Tell your prescriber or health care professional about all other medicines you are taking, including non-prescription medicines, nutritional supplements, or herbal products. Also tell your prescriber or health care professional if you are a frequent user of drinks with caffeine or alcohol, if you smoke, or if you use illegal drugs. These may affect the way your medicine works. Check with your health care professional before stopping or starting any of your medicines.

What should I watch for while taking zolpidem?

Visit your prescriber or health care professional for regular checks on your progress. In most cases zolpidem should only be taken for a few days and for not longer than 1 or 2 weeks. Keep a regular sleep schedule by going to bed at about the same time nightly. Avoid caffeine-containing drinks in the evening hours, as caffeine can cause trouble with falling asleep. Consult your prescriber or health care professional if you still have difficulty in sleeping. Sleep medicines sometimes cause a type of memory loss, in which the person may not remember what has happened in the several hours after taking the medication. This type of memory loss is usually not a problem since zolpidem is taken right before bedtime. Be sure to talk to your doctor if you think you are having memory problems while on this medication. If you have been taking zolpidem for several weeks and suddenly stop taking it, you may get unpleasant withdrawal symptoms. Your prescriber or health care professional may want to gradually reduce the dose. Do not stop taking zolpidem on your own. Always follow your prescriber's advice. After you stop taking your zolpidem prescription, you may notice some trouble with falling asleep. This is sometimes called "rebound insomnia." Do not get discouraged, because this problem usually goes away on its own after 1 or 2 nights. You may get drowsy or dizzy. Do not drive, use machinery, or do anything that needs mental alertness until you know how zolpidem affects you. To reduce dizzy or fainting spells, do not sit or stand up quickly, especially if you are an older patient. Alcohol can increase possible unpleasant effects. Do not drink alcoholic drinks while taking medications to help you sleep. If you are going to have surgery, tell your prescriber or health care professional that you are taking zolpidem.

What side effects may I notice from taking zolpidem?

Side effects that you should report to your prescriber or health care professional as soon as possible:
- confusion
- depressed mood
- hallucinations (seeing, hearing, or feeling things that are not really there)
- lightheadedness, fainting spells or falls
- slurred speech or difficulty with coordination
- vision changes
- restlessness, excitability, or feelings of agitation

Side effects that usually do not require medical attention (report to your prescriber or health care professional if they continue or are bothersome):
- diarrhea
- dizziness, or daytime drowsiness, sometimes called a "hangover" effect
- headache
- strange dreams
- slight stomach upset

Where can I keep my medicine?

Keep out of the reach of children in a container that small children cannot open. Store at controlled room temperature, 20 to 25 degrees C (68 to 77 degrees F). Throw away any unused medicine after the expiration date.

Z

Zonisamide
capsules

ZONEGRAN®;
25 mg; Capsule
Eisai Inc

ZONEGRAN®;
100 mg; Capsule
Eisai Inc

What are zonisamide capsules?

ZONISAMIDE (Zonegran®) is used to help control partial seizures (convulsions) in adults with epilepsy. Zonisamide is usually prescribed with other medications that also help to control the convulsions. Generic zonisamide capsules are available.

What should my health care professional know before I take zonisamide?

They need to know if you have any of these conditions:
- dehydrated
- kidney disease, including history of kidney stones
- liver disease
- an unusual or allergic reaction to zonisamide, sulfa drugs, other medicines, foods, dyes, or preservatives
- pregnant or trying to get pregnant
- breast-feeding

How should I take this medicine?

Take zonisamide capsules by mouth. Follow the directions on the prescription label. Swallow the capsules whole with a drink of water. Do not bite into or break open the capsule. Zonisamide may be taken with or without food. Take your doses at regular intervals. Do not take your medicine more often than directed. Contact your pediatrician or health care professional regarding the use of this medication in children. Special care may be needed.

What if I miss a dose?

If you miss a dose, take it as soon as you can. If it is almost time for your next dose, take only that dose. Do not take double or extra doses.

What may interact with zonisamide?

- acetazolamide
- atropine
- barbiturates such as butalbital, phenobarbital, secobarbital, and others
- bosentan
- certain drugs used to treat HIV infection or AIDS (such as indinavir, ritonavir, or saquinavir)
- certain heart or high blood pressure medicines such as diltiazem, nicardipine, nifedipine, and verapamil
- carbamazepine
- certain antibiotics such as clarithromycin, erythromycin, telithromycin, or troleandomycin
- dexamethasone
- dronabinol, THC
- drugs used to treat fungal infections such as fluconazole, itraconazole, ketoconazole or voriconazole
- fluoxetine
- fluvoxamine
- grapefruit juice
- imatinib, STI-571
- hyoscyamine
- methazolamide

- nefazodone
- phenytoin
- rifampin, rifabutin, or rifapentine
- scopolamine
- St. John's wort
- sulfinpyrazone
- zafirlukast
- zileuton

Tell your prescriber or health care professional about all other medicines you are taking, including non-prescription medicines, nutritional supplements, or herbal products. Also tell your prescriber or health care professional if you are a frequent user of drinks with caffeine or alcohol, if you smoke, or if you use illegal drugs. These may affect the way your medicine works. Check with your health care professional before stopping or starting any of your medicines.

What should I watch for while taking zonisamide?

Visit your prescriber or health care professional for a regular check on your progress. Wear a Medic Alert bracelet or necklace. Carry an identification card with information about your condition, medications, and prescriber or health care professional. It is important to take zonisamide exactly as instructed by your health care professional. When first starting zonisamide treatment, you prescriber may have to adjust your dosage. It may take weeks or months before your dose is stable. You should contact your prescriber or health care professional if your seizures get worse or if you have any new types of seizures. Do not stop taking zonisamide or any of your seizure medicines unless instructed by your prescriber or health care professional. Stopping your medicine suddenly can increase your seizures or their severity. Drink 6 to 8 glasses of water a day. This may help to prevent kidney stones. You may get drowsy or dizzy or have coordination problems. Do not drive, use machinery, or do anything that needs mental alertness until you know how zonisamide affects you. To reduce dizzy spells, do not sit or stand up quickly, especially if you are an older patient. Alcohol can increase drowsiness and dizziness. Avoid alcoholic drinks or medicines containing alcohol. If you are going to have surgery, tell your prescriber or health care professional that you are taking zonisamide.

What side effects may I notice from taking zonisamide?

Side effects that you should report to your prescriber or health care professional immediately:
- changes in seizure type or frequency
- decreased sweating or a rise in body temperature, especially in patients under 17 years old
- depression
- difficulty breathing or tightening of the throat

- fever, sore throat, sores in your mouth, or bruising easily (signs of a blood problem)
- seeing or hearing things or people that are not really there (hallucinations)
- redness, blistering, peeling or loosening of the skin, including inside the mouth
- skin rash or itching
- severe drowsiness, difficulty concentrating, or coordination problems
- speech or language problems
- sudden back pain, abdominal pain, pain when urinating, bloody or dark urine (signs of kidney stones)
- swelling of lips or tongue
- unusual thoughts
- vomiting

Side effects that usually do not require medical attention (report to your prescriber or health care professional if they continue or are bothersome):

- agitation
- anorexia (loss of appetite)
- dizziness
- drowsiness
- headache
- irritability
- nausea

These side effects can occur at any time, but most often occur in the first 4 weeks.

Where can I keep my medicine?

Keep out of reach of children in a container that small children cannot open. Store at room temperature between 15 and 30 degrees C (59 and 86 degrees F). Keep in a dry place protected from light. Throw away any unused medicine after the expiration date.

Z

Disease and Disorder Index

Bold text indicates disease or disorder.

Index of Generic and Brand-Name Drugs

Bold text are trade names and regular text are generic drug names